Clinical Essays on The Heart

Volume I

Clinical Essays on The Heart

Volume I

Edited by

J. Willis Hurst, M.D.

Candler Professor of Medicine (Cardiology)
Chairman, Department of Medicine
Emory University School of Medicine

Chief of Medicine, Emory University Hospital

Chief of Medicine, Grady Memorial Hospital

Head, Medical Section
Emory University Clinic
Atlanta, Georgia

McGraw-Hill Book Company

New York St. Louis San Francisco Auckland Bogotá Guatemala Hamburg
Johannesburg Lisbon London Madrid Mexico Montreal New Delhi
Panama Paris San Juan São Paulo Singapore Sydney Tokyo Toronto

This book was set in Times Roman by Jay's Publishers Services, Inc.; the editors were Robert P. McGraw and Donna McIvor; the production supervisor was Jeanne Skahan.
Halliday Lithograph Corporation was printer and binder.

Library of Congress Cataloging in Publication Data
Main Entry under title:

Clinical essays on the heart.

   Bibliography: p.
   1. Cardiovascular system—Diseases—Addresses, essays, lectures.   I. Hurst, J. Willis (John Willis), date.
RC667.C55   1983   616.1'2   83–734
ISBN 0–07–031494–2 (v. 1)

NOTICE

Medicine is an ever-changing science. As new research and clinical experience broaden our knowledge, changes in treatment and drug therapy are required. The editors and the publisher of this work have made every effort to ensure that the drug dosage schedules herein are accurate and in accord with the standards accepted at the time of publication. Readers are advised, however, to check the product information sheet included in the package of each drug they plan to administer to be certain that changes have not been made in the recommended dose or in the contraindications for administration. This recommendation is of particular importance in regard to new or infrequently used drugs.

To N.W.H. with love

J.W.H.

Contents

List of Contributors

Michael G. Baird, M.D.
Associate Professor of Medicine (Cardiology), Department of Medicine, University of Ottawa, Cardiac Unit, Ottawa, Ontario, Canada

Donald S. Beanlands, M.D.
Professor of Medicine (Cardiology), Chief of Division of Cardiology, Department of Medicine, University of Ottawa, Ottawa, Ontario, Canada

I. Belenkie, M.D.
Associate Professor of Medicine, University of Calgary, Director, Noninvasive Laboratory, Foothills Hospital, Calgary, Alberta, Canada

Walter Bleifeld, M.D.
Professor, Department of Cardiology, University Hospital Eppendorf, Hamburg, West Germany

I. Sylvia Crawley, M.D.
Associate Professor of Medicine (Cardiology), Emory University School of Medicine, Chief, Cardiology Division, Atlanta Veterans Administration Medical Center, Atlanta, Georgia

Ross A. Davies, M.D.
Assistant Professor of Medicine (Cardiology), Department of Medicine, University of Ottawa, Cardiac Unit, Ottawa, Ontario, Canada

James E. Doherty, M.D.
Professor of Medicine, Professor of Pharmacology, University of Arkansas for Medical Sciences; Director of Cardiovascular Research, Little Rock Veterans Administration Medical Center, Little Rock, Arkansas

Kenneth J. Dooley, M.D.
Associate Professor of Pediatrics, Emory University School of Medicine, Atlanta, Georgia

Gordon A. Ewy, M.D.
Professor of Medicine, Chief, Section of Cardiology, University of Arizona, College of Medicine; Director of Diagnostic Cardiology, Arizona Health Sciences Center, Tucson, Arizona

Azhar M. A. Faruqui, M.D.
Associate Professor and Physician, National Institute of Cardiovascular Diseases, Karachi, Pakistan

Paul E. Fenster, M.D.
Assistant Professor of Internal Medicine, University of Arizona Health Sciences Center; Director of Coronary Care Unit, University Hospital, Tucson, Arizona

Charles Fisch, M.D.
Distinguished Professor of Medicine, Director, Cardiovascular Division Indiana University School of Medicine; Director, Krannert Institute of Cardiology, Indianapolis, Indiana

Robert A. Guyton, M.D.
Assistant Professor of Surgery, Department of Surgery; Director, Cardiothoracic Research Laboratory, Carlyle Fraser Heart Center, Crawford W. Long Memorial Hospital, Emory University School of Medicine, Atlanta, Georgia

James J. Heger, M.D.
Associate Professor of Medicine, Indiana University School of Medicine; Research Associate, Krannert Institute of Cardiology, Indianapolis, Indiana

Eberhard Henze, M.D.
Assistant Professor of Radiological Sciences, Laboratory of Nuclear Medicine, School of Medicine, University of California at Los Angeles, Los Angeles, California

Lyall A. J. Higginson, M.D.
Assistant Professor of Medicine (Cardiology), Department of Medicine, University of Ottawa, Cardiac Unit, Ottawa, Ontario, Canada

Michael Jones, M.D.
Staff Surgeon, Cardiac Surgery, National Heart, Lung and Blood Institute, Bethesda, Maryland

Robert M. Kolodner, M.D.
Assistant Professor of Psychiatry, Emory University School of Medicine, Staff Psychiatrist, Atlanta Veterans Administration Medical Center, Atlanta, Georgia

Hans-Joachim Krebber, M.D.
Department of Cardiovascular Surgery, University Hospital Eppendorf, Hamburg, West Germany

Karl-Heinz Kuck, M.D.
Department of Cardiology, University Hospital Eppendorf, Hamburg, West Germany

Byron D. McLees, M.D.
Chief of Pulmonary Medicine, Bowman-Gray School of Medicine, Winston-Salem, North Carolina

Frank I. Marcus, M.D.
Distinguished Professor of Internal Medicine (Cardiology), University of Arizona Health Sciences Center, Tucson, Arizona

Robert C. Marshall, M.D.
Assistant Professor of Medicine, Department of Medicine, Division of Cardiology, University of California at Los Angeles, Los Angeles, California

Detlef G. Mathey, M.D.
Professor, Department of Cardiology, University Hospital Eppendorf, Hamburg, West Germany

Richard E. Michalik, M.D.
Fellow in Surgery (Thoracic), Emory University School of Medicine, Atlanta, Georgia

Harry G. Mond, M.D.
Specialist Physician to Pacemaker Clinic, Department of Cardiology, The Royal Melbourne Hospital, Victoria, Australia

Richard Montz, M.D.
Professor, Department of Nuclear Medicine, University Hospital Eppendorf, Hamburg, West Germany

Spyridon D. Moulopoulos, M.D.
Chairman, Department of Therapeutics, University of Athens Medical School; Rector, The National University, Athens, Greece

Nicholas M. Papadopoulos, Ph.D.
Clinical Biochemist, Clinical Chemistry and Pathology, National Institutes of Health Branch, Bethesda, Maryland

George Rodewald, M.D.
Professor, Department of Cardiovascular Surgery, University Hospital Eppendorf, Hamburg, West Germany

Heinrich R. Schelbert, M.D.
Professor of Radiological Sciences, Laboratory of Nuclear Medicine, School of Medicine, University of California at Los Angeles, Los Angeles, California

Jochen Schofer, M.D.
Department of Cardiology, University Hospital Eppendorf, Hamburg, West Germany

Hans R. Schön, M.D.
Technical University School of Medicine, Division of Cardiology, Munich, Germany: Formerly Fellow, Division of Nuclear Medicine, UCLA

E. R. Smith, M.D.
Professor of Physiology and Medicine, Head, Cardiology Division, University of Calgary; Chief of Cardiology and Director, Cardiovascular Laboratories, Foothills Hospital, Calgary, Alberta, Canada

Volkmar Tilsner, M.D.
Professor, Department for Blood Coagulation Disorders, University Hospital Eppendorf, Hamburg, West Germany

W. Dean Wilcox, M.D.
Assistant Professor of Pediatrics (Pediatric Cardiology), Emory University School of Medicine, Atlanta, Georgia

William L. Williams, M.D.
Assistant Professor of Medicine (Cardiology), Department of Medicine, University of Ottawa, Cardiac Unit, Ottawa, Ontario, Canada

Preface

The Change of the Name

The new name of this series about *The Heart* is *Clinical Essays on the Heart*. The former title, *Update: The Heart,* has been changed for a number of reasons. Some readers believed that the *Updates* simply provided more recent information about the material covered in the last edition of *The Heart*. The new series will maintain that role, as well as accomplish much more, its purpose being to:

- Continue to update the information presented in *The Heart,* which is published every four years. For example, a new procedure, such as nuclear magnetic resonance, may become available after *The Heart* is published; it would be presented to the readership as quickly as possible in the *Essays*.

- Present more detailed information on a subject that is discussed in the last edition of *The Heart*. An old subject such as atrial fibrillation, for example, should be reviewed every few years. The discussion might be one page in *The Heart* but an in-depth discussion of the subject might use thirty pages in an edition of the series.

- Present interesting subjects in the field of cardiology that are seldom discussed.

- Present more illustrations and more complete bibliographies than are possible in the textbook. Space allocations do not permit an author to use an unlimited number of illustrations or listings in a bibliography in a textbook such as *The Heart*. Rather, he or she is forced to bear the pain of omitting a favorite figure or reference in order to keep the book at a manageable size. The new series offers much more freedom.

- Consequently, each edition of the series will be well illustrated and the bibliographies for each article quite complete.

- Permit me, as Editor, to present material not necessarily suited to a textbook or a journal. Accordingly, the series may contain articles on: medical history, controversial subjects not dealt with in a textbook, and many other categories of manuscripts.

Most of the volumes in this series will not have a theme. Volume II, however, does have a central subject, "The Treatment of Atherosclerotic Coronary Heart Disease (Drugs, Coronary Bypass Surgery, and Coronary Angioplasty)."

I would like to thank my colleagues, worldwide, for their warm reception of the *Update* series upon its appearance. It is my hope that *Clinical Essays on the Heart* will enjoy the same enthusiastic response that the *Updates* received.

J. Willis Hurst, M.D.

Four editions of the *Essays* will appear between editions of *The Heart*.

April 1983	*Essays I*
November 1983	*Essays II*
April 1984	*Essays III*
November 1984	*Essays IV*

Pacemaker Faultfinding

HARRY G. MOND, M.D.

The success of an implanted cardiac pacemaker is dependent on the establishment of a harmonious relationship between the artificial pacemaker and the human receiver. Failure of a pacemaker system may result from an electronic or mechanical defect within the pacemaker, a physiologic problem, or from a poor relationship between the normal function of both. In this article, the methods of pacemaker testing and a logical system for investigating patients with suspected pacemaker malfunction will be outlined. Only the ventricular-inhibited pacing system will be discussed.

THE NORMAL VENTRICULAR PACEMAKER ELECTROCARDIOGRAM

The pacemaker QRS (depolarization) consists of a stimulus artifact and the subsequent ventricular response (Fig. 1). The stimulus artifact represents the energy delivered by the pulse generator and is seen as a perpendicular voltage deflection from the ECG baseline. As the energy is dissipated through the myocardium, the stimulus artifact returns to the baseline as a decay curve. It is during this period that actual ventricular depolarization occurs, and thus the QRS is a summation of true depolarization and the decay curve. As seen in Fig. 1, the decay curve can on occasion be as large or larger than the actual QRS. Thus in order to establish true ventricular depolarization, it is important to recognize ventricular repolarization, i.e., the T wave, and a number of ECG leads may be required before satisfactory tracings are obtained.

The major pacing system used today is the ventricular-inhibited (demand or synchronous) system. Here the lead lies at the apex of the right ventricular chamber (endocardial) or is placed on the outer surface of either ventricle (epicardial).

Characteristic ECG patterns are recognized when

*From the Department of Cardiology, The Royal Melbourne Hospital, Victoria, Australia.

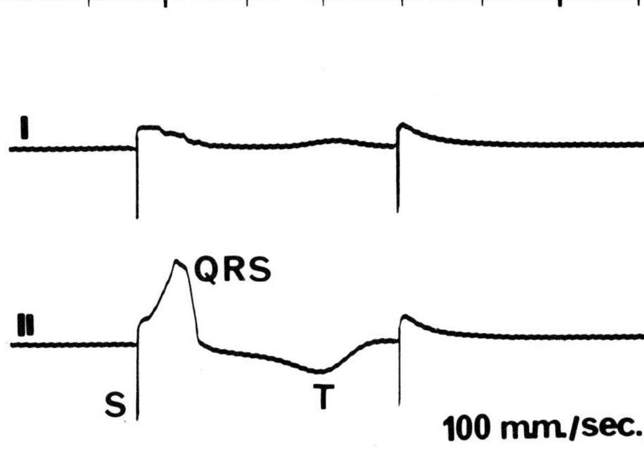

FIGURE 1 Unipolar endocardial lead in right ventricle. The pacemaker ECG consists of a stimulus artifact (S), depolarization (QRS), and repolarization (T). In lead I, first complex, the stimulus artifact is followed by a small QRS and T wave. The second complex is composed of a stimulus artifact and no QRS or T wave, i.e., a failed-paced beat. Note that the stimulus artifact deforms the baseline, and this could be misinterpreted as a QRS. However, there is no T wave. In lead II, the QRS and T wave are prominent, and despite the deformity of the baseline in the second complex, there is no doubt about failed pacing. This illustrates the value of taking more than one lead in interpreting the ECG in patients with pacemakers. The predominant R wave in lead II suggests that the lead has become dislodged and the electrode is in the right ventricular outflow tract.

pacing is established from various parts of the heart. Unipolar endocardial pacing from the apex of the right ventricle results in a left bundle branch block configuration, and the frontal plane vector is to the extreme left (Fig. 2). However, if the electrode is in the right ventricular outflow tract, then the bundle branch block is the same, but the front plane vector is now normal or to the right (Fig. 3). Epicardial left ventricular pacing has a right bundle branch block configuration with an axis depending on the position of the electrode on the left ventricular surface.

With ventricular-inhibited systems, pacing will continue at a regular interval unless inhibited by a premature spontaneous ventricular depolarization (own QRS), such as a ventricular extrasystole or a return to sinus rhythm faster than the pacemaker rate (Fig. 4). Sensing of the spontaneous rhythm occurs via the lead that transmits the electrical information to the sensing circuit of the pulse generator. The other type of pacing is fixed-rate, or asynchronous. Here pacing occurs irrespective of the underlying cardiac rhythm (Fig. 5).

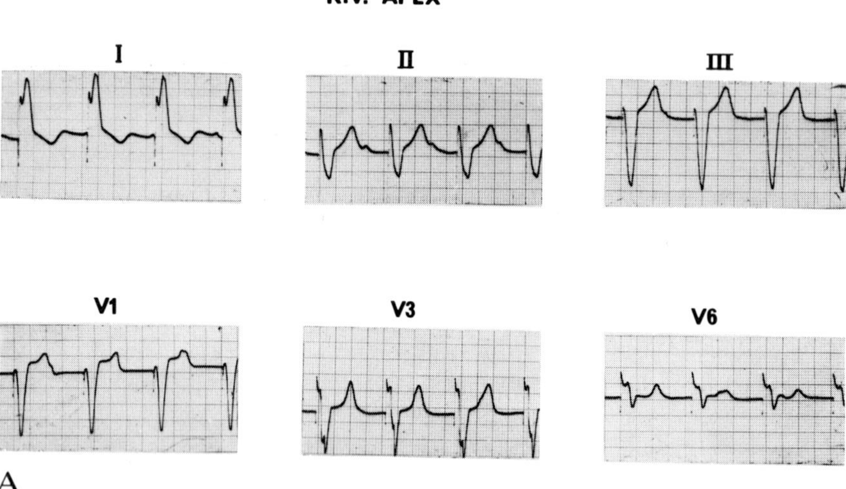

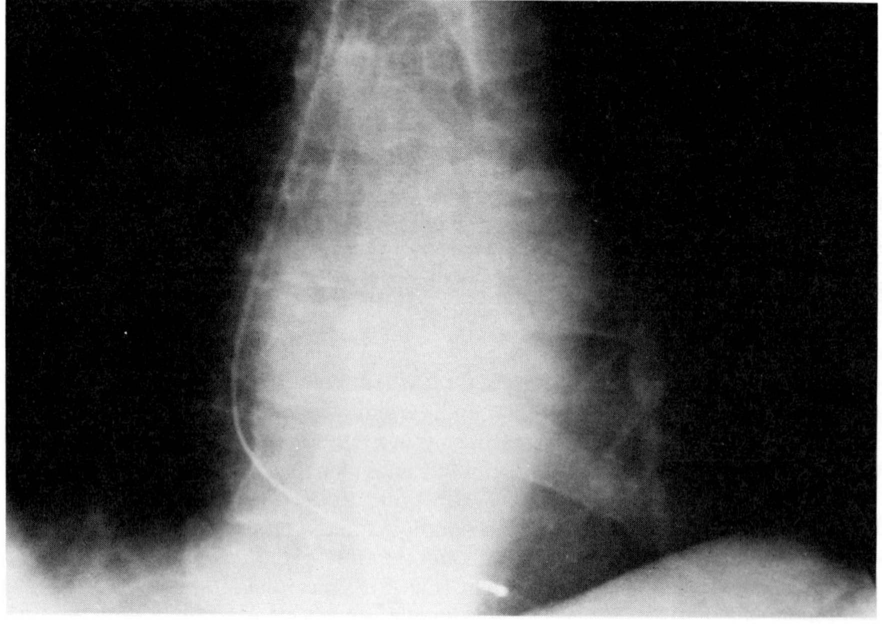

FIGURE 2 (*A*) Typical ECG appearance of a right ventricular endocardial lead with electrode at apex of right ventricle. There is left bundle branch block with a frontal plane axis markedly to the left. (*B*) Chest radiograph to show position of electrode at apex of right ventricle.

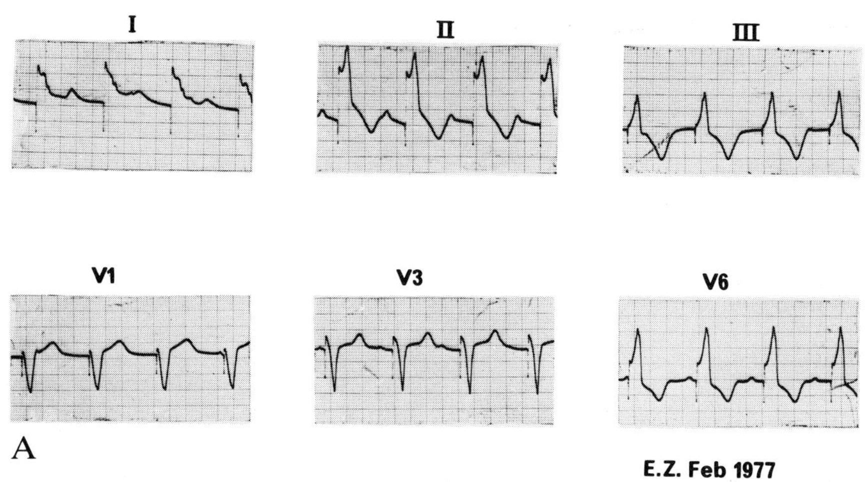

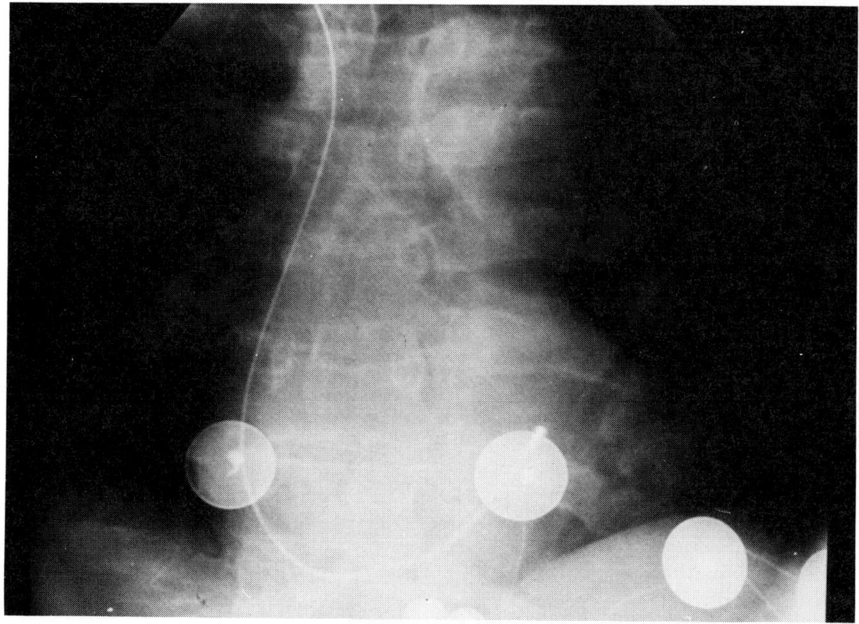

FIGURE 3 (*A*) ECG appearance of endocardial electrode within the right ventricular outflow tract. There is left bundle branch block and a normal frontal plane axis. (*B*) Chest radiograph to show dislodgement toward the right ventricular outflow tract. Monitoring leads lie on the chest.

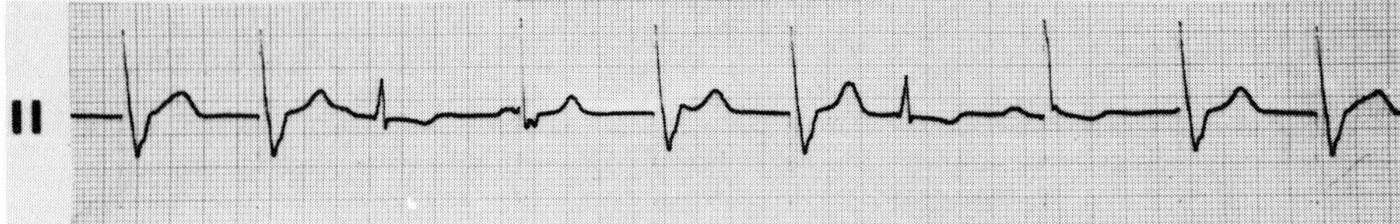

FIGURE 4 ECG, lead II. Ventricular-inhibited pacing with normal sensing. Complexes 1, 2, 5, 6, 9, and 10 are normal-paced beats. Complexes 3 and 7 are spontaneous ventricular complexes that successfully inhibit the pacemaker. Complexes 4 and 8 are fusion beats.

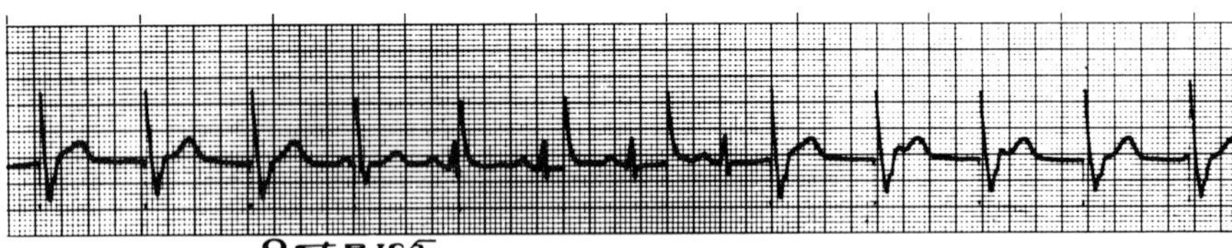

FIGURE 5 ECG, lead II. Asynchronous pacing. The first three and the last five complexes are normal-paced beats. In the middle of the tracing the stimulus artifacts continue at a regular repetition rate irrespective of the sinus beats. Stimulus artifacts that occur within the refractory period of the sinus QRS complexes obviously do not pace the heart. A similar appearance may occur when the sensing mechanism fails (undersensing) or a magnet is placed above the implanted pulse generator.

METHODS USED IN THE EVALUATION OF PACEMAKER FUNCTION

Routine Pacemaker Assessment

Routine pacemaker assessment involves an ECG together with electronic pulse-generator testing. Baseline levels are established and then patients are tested usually at 6 monthly intervals. Oscilloscopic display of the stimulus artifact together with fluoroscopic and radiographic chest examinations should also be carried out shortly after implant to provide baseline data.

ELECTROCARDIOGRAPH

A baseline 12-lead ECG during pacing is necessary postoperatively. At follow-up visits a rhythm strip to confirm pacing is performed. With ventricular-inhibited pacing systems, pacing may be inhibited by the patient's spontaneous rhythm. In this situation testing is performed by positioning a special magnet on the skin over the pulse generator. This activates a reed switch that dislocates the demand function and establishes asynchronous pacing. The stimulus artifact will now occur in competition with the spontaneous rhythm, and pacing will be evident where a QRS and T wave follow the stimulus artifact (Fig. 5).

ELECTRONIC PULSE-GENERATOR TESTING

The two parameters tested are the pulse repetition rate (interval between stimulus artifacts, which is measured in milliseconds or expressed in pulses per minute) and the pulse duration (width or time duration of the stimulus artifact). Both these parameters can now be measured using a variety of inexpensive testing devices. Testing is performed in the synchronous mode and then repeated in the asynchronous mode using a magnet applied over the pulse generator. The results are compared with previous recordings, and usually a fall of 6 to 8 beats per minute of pulse repetition rate and an increase in pulse duration represents impending power-source depletion. However, it must be stressed that each manufacturer has characteristic end-of-life pulse-generator indicators, and these should be known to the physician.

Methods Used in Pacemaker Faultfinding

Initial investigations include routine testing and a clinical examination. Usually, sufficient information is obtained from these simple investigations to diagnose the general cause of malfunction. Further investigations may be necessary. These include the following:

CLINICAL FINDINGS, INCLUDING HISTORY AND EXAMINATION

An unwell patient is examined clinically. Symptomatic patients, with normal routine testing, can often have their symptoms traced to a nonpacemaker cause, such as vertebrobasilar insufficiency. However, should the patient history indicate a return of original symptoms, such as Stokes-Adams attacks, then the possibility of an intermittent-failed pacemaker system should be entertained.

OSCILLOSCOPIC EXAMINATION

Although still widely used, oscilloscopic examination of the stimulus artifact as a routine procedure in pacemaker clinics diminished with the introduction of simpler methods of measuring pulse duration and repetition rate. Despite this, oscilloscopic examination continues to be a very important tool in the investigation of pacemaker malfunction, especially with pulse-generator electronic faults and lead fracture.[1] Consequently, all personnel responsible for a pacemaker clinic must have a working knowledge of oscilloscopic testing and analysis. It is advisable that all patients undergo such testing soon after implant to obtain baseline documentation of the stimulus artifact so that comparison studies can be made at a later date if indicated (Fig. 6).

ECG MONITORING

In cases of suspected intermittent pacemaker system malfunction, prolonged ECG monitoring may be very valuable. Such systems include 24-h ambulatory monitoring, ECG telemetry, direct bedside monitoring, and telephone transmission of the ECG.

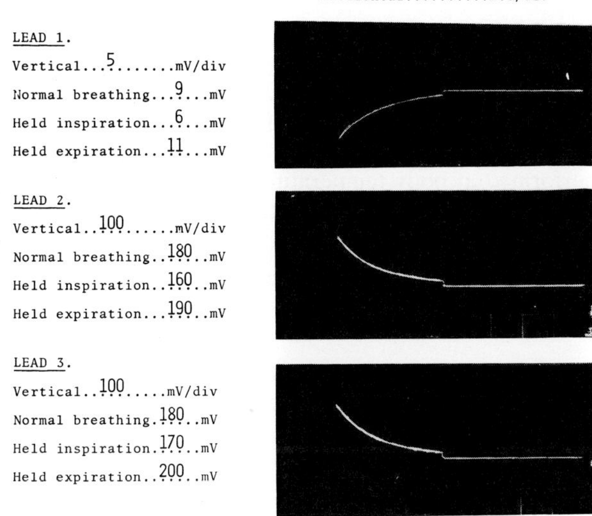

FIGURE 6 Oscilloscopic appearance of the stimulus artifact in leads I, II, and III. The vertical axis is the pulse amplitude and is measured in millivolts. There is a slight fall in voltage on inspiration and a rise on expiration. The horizontal time base is the pulse duration and is, in this case, about 1.75 m/s.

CHEST RADIOGRAPH AND FLUOROSCOPY

These are particularly important noninvasive tools used in the evaluation of suspected pacemaker malfunction. Originally, x-rays were used to judge the depletion of zinc-mercury batteries. Today, however, the chest radiograph and fluoroscopy are essential in determining lead position and possible lead fracture.

PROVOCATIVE MOVEMENTS

Specific movements likely to reproduce symptoms should be performed with ECG monitoring. These include rapid arm movements for skeletal muscle inhibition or unusual postures to demonstrate lead fracture. An intermittent lead fracture or poor connection between setscrew and lead pin can also be demonstrated by abruptly moving the pulse generator beneath the skin. Concomitant fluoroscopy or oscilloscopic analysis are also valuable during provocative movements.

CHEST-WALL STIMULATION

Electric stimuli too weak to affect the heart will inhibit an implanted ventricular-inhibited pulse generator, thus testing its sensing function (Fig. 7). These electric signals can be applied to the chest wall by an external pulse generator.[2,3] As demonstrated in Fig. 7, the technique of inhibiting a pulse generator will allow the physician to examine the patient's underlying, or intrinsic, cardiac rhythm. The technique is also useful in differentiating a pulse generator from a myocardial cause for lack of sensing (undersensing). Successful inhibition of the pulse generator by this technique will exclude a pulse-generator component failure.

SURGICAL EXPLORATION WITH PACING SYSTEM ANALYSIS AND FLUOROSCOPY

On occasion, surgical intervention is necessary as a means of investigating suspected pacemaker malfunction. Many cases of pacemaker malfunction determined by other means will also require surgical intervention. Whether a cause has been established or not, the procedures performed during surgical intervention remain essentially the same. Pulse generator and lead system are mobilized and inspected; both are tested using the pacing system analyzer. The lead system can be observed by fluoroscopy, and where necessary, tension is applied to the lead to demonstrate fractured ends. Any site where nonabsorbable suture material is tied around the lead should be very carefully inspected. Blood inside the lead insulator suggests an insulation break and a possible site for current leakage.

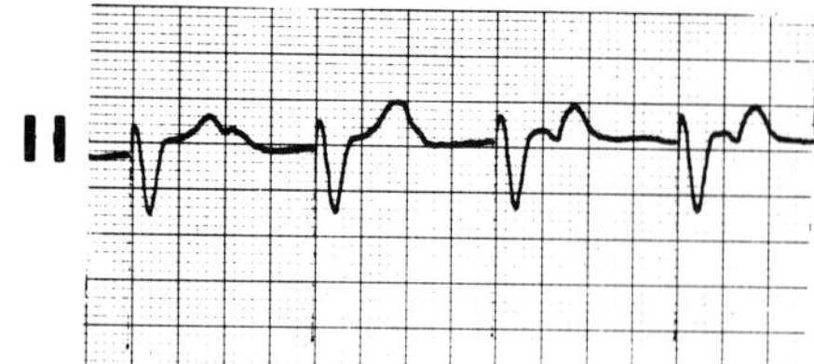

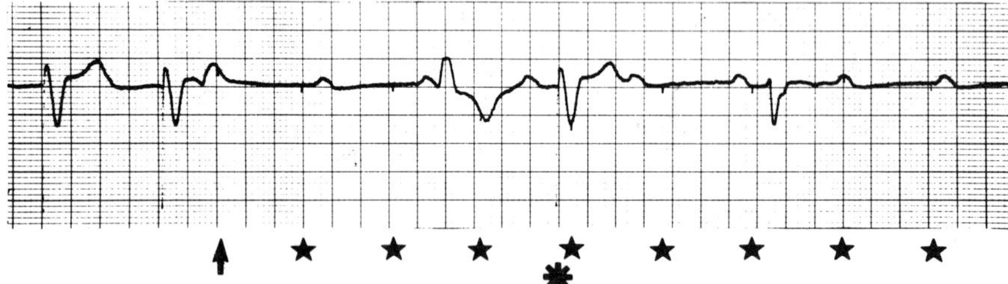

FIGURE 7 Inhibition of an implanted pulse generator by an external pulse generator with the electrodes placed over the anterior chest wall. In the top tracing, normal pacing is recorded prior to turning on the external pulse generator. In the bottom tracing, the external pulse generator is turned on (arrow) and the attenuated stimulus artifact (stars) represents the impulses from the external power source. The implanted pacemaker system assumes that the impulses are coming from the heart and is thus inhibited, revealing the underlying rhythm (complete heart block). However, one paced beat is seen during external inhibition (*). This occurs because a spontaneous QRS complex also inhibits the pulse generator and the next impulse from the external pulse generator occurs in the refractory period of the implanted pulse generator and is not sensed. A normal-paced beat occurs after the appropriate recycling time.

INTRACARDIAC ELECTROGRAPHY

The unipolar intracardiac electrogram is a simple means of recording electric potentials from the heart. Using a battery-operated ECG machine, the V lead is attached to the exposed lead pin of the implanted lead and a recording is taken. With a bipolar lead system, a bipolar recording can be obtained using lead I of the ECG. When the electrode makes contact with the right ventricular endocardium, "a current of injury" pattern characterized by ST elevation and T wave inversion occurs. In contrast, coronary sinus recordings have no such pattern. This current of injury disappears with time, leaving T wave inversion. In about 60 percent of cases, the unipolar ventricular electrogram is biphasic, with the R wave at least 10 percent of the S wave amplitude. In 30 percent of cases, the R wave is less than 10 percent of the S wave (Fig. 8). In the remaining 10 percent there is a dominant R wave without a discrete S wave.[4]

As well as being useful for lead placement, such electrograms are valuable for correct diagnosis of right ventricular perforation. Recordings are performed as the electrode is withdrawn from the epicardial surface.[5]

TESTING OF AN EXPLANTED PULSE GENERATOR

Prior to testing, the explanted pulse generator should be thoroughly washed in a detergent solution and then soaked in 10 percent formaldehyde. This procedure prevents transmission of any infective agent, such as hepatitis B virus.[6] Pulse-generator testing must be performed at body temperature using a water bath or an incubator. The characteristics examined should be compared with the initial test performed and those specified by the manufacturers. These tests are divided into three major categories.

Pulse-generator output This is tested at 37° under a 510-Ω load. Testing is performed with and without the magnet.

Oscilloscope Output pulse voltage shape and pulse duration. The leading- and trailing-edge voltages and pulse duration are recorded.

Rate Counter Pulse repetition rate.

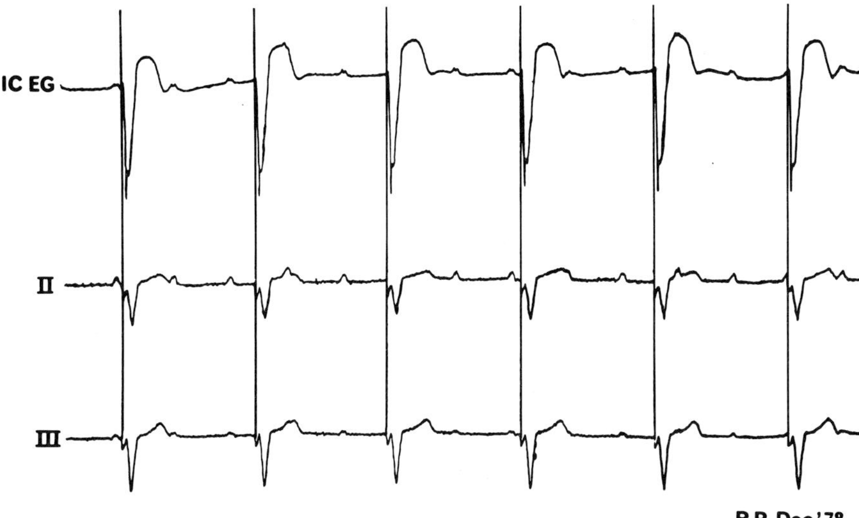

FIGURE 8 Unipolar endocardial electrogram (ICEG) and standard leads II and III of a normal pacing rhythm. The electrogram shows a deep S wave and a current of injury pattern.

Demand function This is performed using a simulated QRS complex having the characteristics of approximately 25 Hz and 4-mV amplitude. Tests include R wave sensitivity, refractory period, and interference frequency.

Missing-pulse detection If a pulse generator passes the preceding tests but there is doubt about performance over a long period, the unit should be tested specifically to identify intermittent failure of operation.[6]

CAUSES OF PACEMAKER MALFUNCTION

In devising a practical classification of pacemaker malfunction, the ECG appearances of pacing, both in the synchronous and asynchronous (magnet or test) modes, are used.

Three principles must be fulfilled to establish normal pacing:

1 A normal stimulus artifact is produced regularly at the preset rate in the asynchronous mode.

2 The stimulus artifact is followed by ventricular depolarization (QRS) and repolarization (T).

3 The pacemaker senses normally.

Using these principles, a flow diagram has been constructed (Fig. 9). The first part investigates the stimulus artifact, and thus the magnet must be applied. The second part investigates the QRS and T wave, and magnet application is not essential. The third part investigates demand function, and the magnet is not used. Within each section of the flow diagram there are a number of end points. One is "normal," indicating that the pacemaker malfunction under investigation is not within this section, since the basic ECG principle being examined has been fulfilled. The other end points represent a pacemaker malfunction group as identified by an ECG abnormality, and specific causes of each malfunction are tabulated (Tables 1 through 6). The tables are subdivided into true malfunctions and pseudomalfunctions. Pseudomalfunctions usually result from misinterpretation or faulty documentation of test data or from a poor understanding of the pacemaker system. Such errors may therefore be human or mechanical.

A second flow diagram (Fig. 10) investigates situations that are not strictly pacemaker malfunction but rather physical or psychologic side effects of pacing (Table 7). This flow diagram also classifies those problems unrelated to the pacemaker system and those where no diagnosis is made but the patient is symptomatic.

Stimulus Artifact

The first principle of normal function stated: "A normal stimulus artifact is produced regularly at the present rate in the asynchronous mode." Figure 9

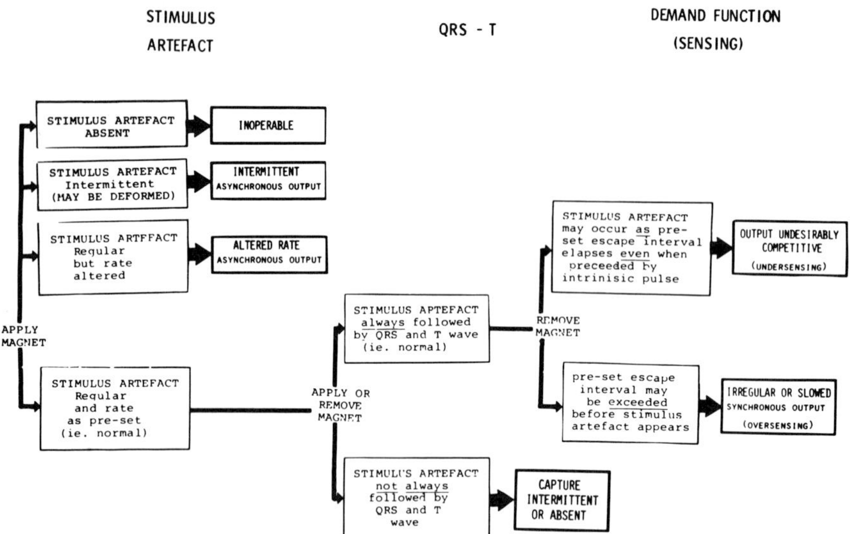

FIGURE 9 Flow diagram to demonstrate steps in faultfinding procedure. The stimulus artifact in the asynchronous mode is inspected, and three abnormalities are recognized: absent, intermittent, or altered rate. The QRS and T wave are then inspected to determine capture. Demand function is investigated in the synchronous mode, and two major abnormalities are recognized: undersensing and oversensing.

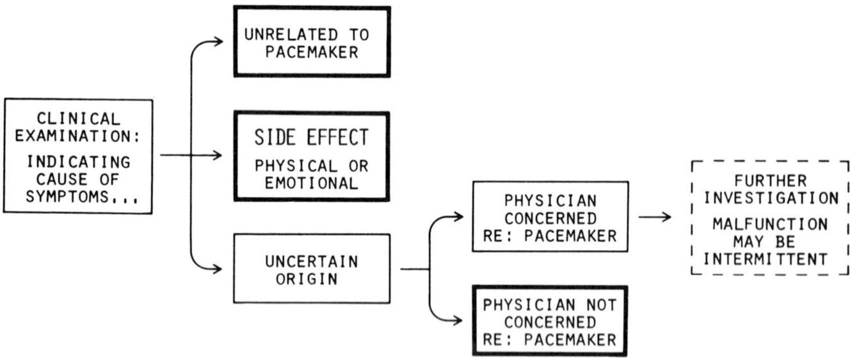

FIGURE 10 The clinical examination suggests that the patient's symptoms are unrelated to the pacemaker system, are due to side effects of the pacing system, or are of uncertain origin. The last group may need further investigation.

investigates the stimulus artifact in the asynchronous mode and identifies three abnormalities.

1 Stimulus artifact absent (inoperable pacemaker system).

2 Stimulus artifact intermittent (may be deformed).

3 Stimulus artifact present but at an altered rate.

STIMULUS ARTIFACT ABSENT—INOPERABLE PACEMAKER SYSTEM (Table 1)

There is no detectable stimulus artifact and thus no pulse-generator output in the asynchronous mode.

There are four major true malfunctions: power-source failure, random component failure in the output circuit, a break at some point in the pacemaker-patient electric circuit, and a pacemaker-patient electric short circuit. Clarification of the actual malfunction may be difficult by routine noninvasive testing because the stimulus artifact is absent. Chest radiography and fluoroscopy are usually diagnostic for electrode-lead system fractures with complete discontinuity (Fig. 11). The treatment of all true malfunctions requires surgical intervention. Pseudomalfunctions are extremely important because surgical intervention is not indicated.

TABLE 1
Stimulus artifact absent—inoperable pacemaker system

True malfunction

1 Power-source failure:
  Battery components depleted
    Expected
    Accelerated, e.g., large electrode surface area, loss
      of insulation
  Battery components not depleted, e.g., internal short
    circuit
2 Output circuit failure
3 Pacemaker-patient electrical circuit incomplete, e.g.,
  lead fracture
4 Pacemaker-patient electrical short circuit, e.g., within a
  bipolar lead, within pulse generator

Pseudomalfunction

5 Misinterpretation, ECG:
  Pulse artifact overlooked
6 Testing-equipment problem:
  Equipment battery failure, faulty or misuse

STIMULUS ARTIFACT INTERMITTENT (MAY BE DEFORMED) (Table 2)

Here, intermittently in the asynchronous mode, the stimulus artifact is not recorded on the ECG or detected with electronic testing equipment. The causes of an intermittent stimulus artifact are similar to the absent stimulus artifact, but they are reversible. The most important cause is an intermittent break in the pacemaker-patient electric circuit. A typical example is the all-or-nothing effect of a fractured lead conductor

TABLE 2
Stimulus artifact intermittent (may be deformed)

True malfunction
1 Power-source failure, battery components not depleted 2 Timing of output circuit, intermittent component failure 3 Pacemaker-patient electrical circuit imcomplete,   intermittent 4 Pacemaker-patient electrical short circuit, intermittent

Pseudomalfunction
(As in Table 1, problem intermittent)

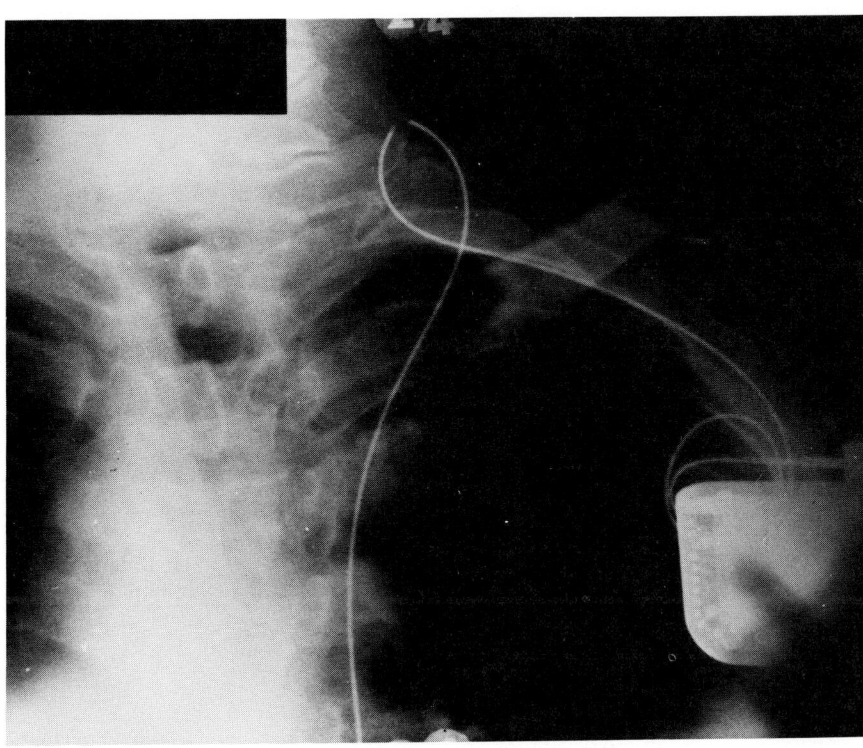

FIGURE 11 Chest radiograph to show fractured lead conductor at point of entry into left external jugular vein. This is a stress point where the lead turns on itself.

in which the fractured ends intermittently make contact. This is seen in Fig. 12, where the patient in whom a pacemaker had been implanted 3 years previously had a typical Stokes-Adams attack earlier that day. No abnormality was noted on testing and fluoroscopy, but hand pressure over the pulse generator resulted in failure of pacing and reversion to complete heart block.

At surgery, a lead-conductor fracture was noted near the connector.

However, this situation may not always give an all-or-nothing effect. On occasion, a deformed or attenuated stimulus artifact is present (Fig. 13). This "small" stimulus artifact is usually subthreshold and represents a reduced current reaching the heart. The

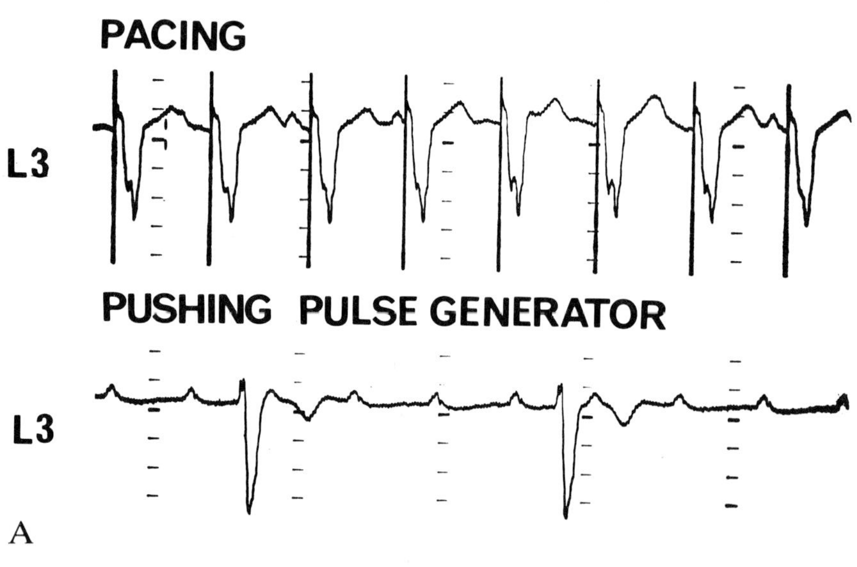

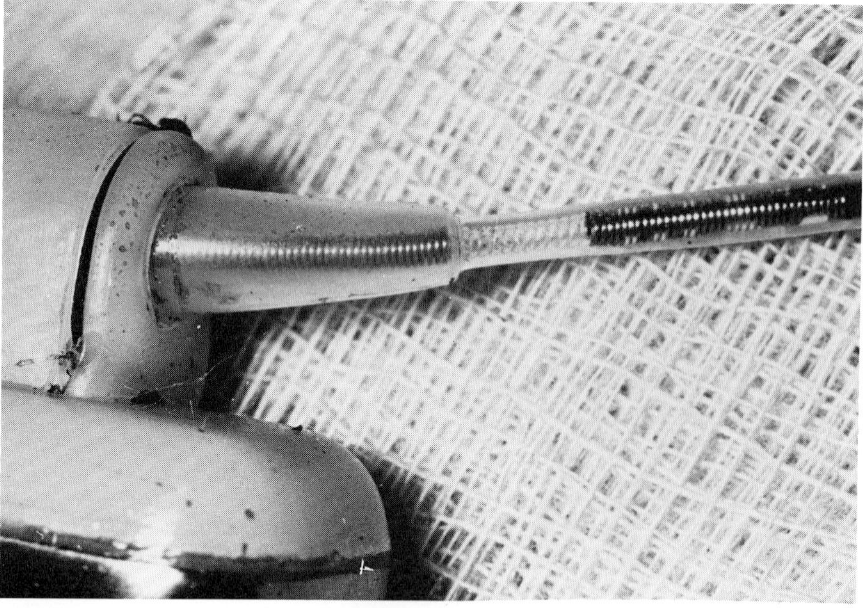

FIGURE 12 (A) ECG, lead III. Normal pacing. Hand pressure on implanted pulse generator resulted in an inoperable system and complete heart block. (B) At operation a conductor fracture was found at point where lead entered the connector. To demonstrate the fractured ends, the insulator has been stretched. When first visualized, the fractured ends were in contact.

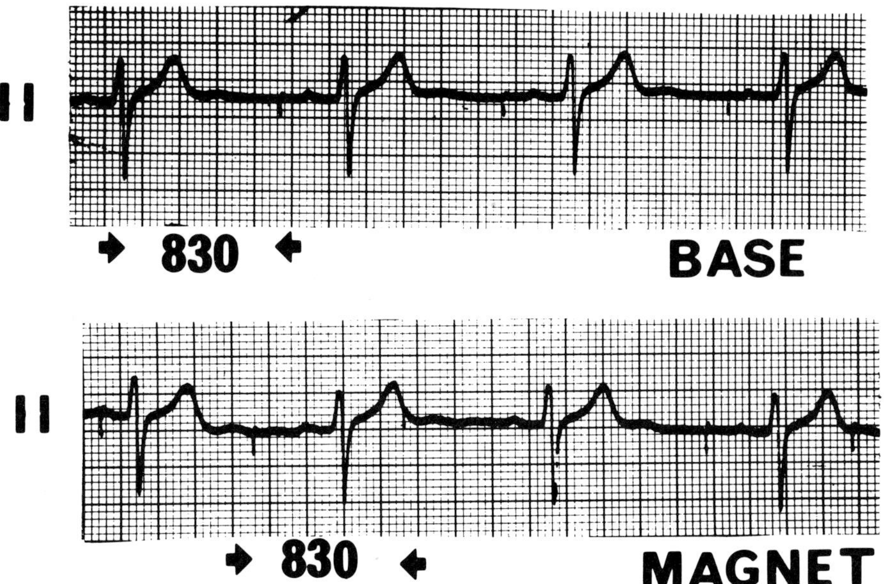

FIGURE 13 ECG, lead II. Conductor with contact through fluid bridge (ruptured insulator). On the first line the stimulus artifact is attenuated and subthreshold, but sensing is retained. The stimulus artifact occurs 830 m/s after the sinus QRS. Line two is similar except that the stimulus artifacts occur asynchronously (magnet).

cause may be a fractured conductor that makes contact but results in a high lead impedance. Such a high lead impedance may be due to tissue fluid bridging the fractured conductor gap and thus may occur with a ruptured insulator as well. An attenuated stimulus artifact may also occur when battery components are almost depleted or when there is a patient-pacemaker electric short circuit.

The group with an intermittent or deformed stimulus artifact is presented separately from the group with an absent stimulus artifact because the diagnosis of malfunction may not be obvious. An intermittent problem may be very difficult to observe and thus detect. Occasionally, prolonged ambulatory monitoring is necessary. Treatment, however, is usually surgical intervention and follows the same principle as the first group.

STIMULUS ARTIFACT IS PRESENT BUT AT AN ALTERED RATE (Table 3)

True malfunctions are peculiar to the pulse generator. Minor rate changes within 6 months of implantation are common and usually represent maturation changes in the power source or timing circuit. In contrast, marked rate changes suggest impending power-source failure. Inadvertent or phantom reprogramming of programmable pulse generators may occur in the manufacturer's facilities or during shipment to the implanting center. Thus these pulse generators must be tested prior to implantation. *Runaway pulse generator* usually

TABLE 3
Stimulus artifact at altered rate

True malfunction

1 Power-source failure (see Table 1)
2 Timing circuit:
    Component maturation: rate drift first year after
     implantation
    Inadvertent reprogramming of programmable pulse
     generator
    Random component failure
     Runaway pulse generator
     Slow

Pseudomalfunction

3 Misinterpretation:
    Lack of understanding of rate change with
     Temperature change: room to body at implant
     Power-source depletion
     Activation of reed switch (magnet or test rate)
4 Faulty recording:
    Asynchronous and synchronous testing confused
    ECG recorder
     Speed variable
     Sticking paper delivery, intermittent
5 Testing-equipment problem
    Equipment faulty

refs to an increasing pacing rate beyond 150 beats per minute with sufficient output to capture the heart.[7] Improved pacemaker technology has significantly decreased the probability of runaway in modern pulse generators.

The QRS and T Wave

The second principle of normal function stated: "The stimulus artifact is followed by ventricular depolarization (QRS) and repolarization (T)." The importance of recognizing the T wave has been illustrated in Fig. 1. Thus pacemaker malfunction can be recognized when the following occurs:

THE STIMULUS ARTIFACT IN THE ASYNCHRONOUS OR SYNCHRONOUS MODE DEMONSTRATES INTERMITTENT OR ABSENT CAPTURE (Table 4):

This malfunction is unrelated to demand function, and thus sensing may be retained (Fig. 14). The problem of a lead incorrectly placed at implant should be overcome by good surgical technique. New lead designs, such as the incorporation of tines behind the electrode, have markedly reduced lead displacement.[8] The major cause of a pulse-generator voltage output below pacing threshold is power-source depletion (see Table 1). An increased pacing threshold above conventional pulse-generator output (5 V) may occur early or appear some years after implantation and is usually due to fibrosis around the electrode. A special group is those patients in whom acute elevation in pacing threshold occurs following myocardial infarction. Severe metabolic disturbances, such as changes in acid-base balance and myxedema, as well as drugs, may elevate the pacing threshold. Pacing may also be intermittent or absent in situations of high resistance in the electrode-lead system. This may result from a small stimulating electrode or partial lead fracture.

Demand Function

The third principle of normal function stated: "The pacemaker senses normally." The two major abnormalities of sensing function are *undersensing* (output undesirably competitive) or *oversensing* (synchronous output is slowed or irregular). These malfunctions are correctable by magnet conversion to the asynchronous mode.

PULSE-GENERATOR OUTPUT IS UNDESIRABLY COMPETITIVE (Table 5 and Figure 5)

Failure to sense the QRS may result from a fault in the pulse generator or electrode-lead system or from the size and type of potentials produced by the myocardium. Pulse-generator faults include impending power-source failure, reed switch lodged in the asynchronous or test mode after removal of the magnet, and random component failure within the sensing circuit. Electrode-lead system problems resulting in undersensing include loss of insulation and improper electrode-lead position. A high resistance in the electrode-lead system, such as

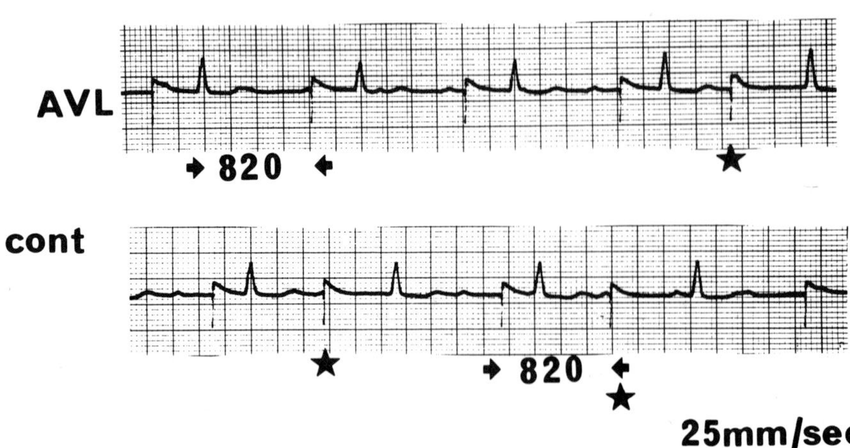

FIGURE 14 ECG, AVL. High threshold with failure of pacing. No QRS or T wave follows the stimulus artifact. However, there is retained sensing. The stimulus artifact occurs 820 m/s after the spontaneous QRS. However, if a spontaneous QRS occurs 300 m/s or less after a stimulus artifact, then the spontaneous QRS is not sensed and another stimulus artifact occurs 820 m/s later (★).

TABLE 4
Capture intermittent or absent (sensing may be retained)

True malfunction

1 Improper electrode-lead position:
    Incorrectly placed at implant, e.g., coronary sinus displacement:
        Dislodgement
        Perforation
        Retraction of electrode from endocardium
2 Pulse-generator voltage output to heart below pacing threshold:
    Power-source failure (see Table 1)
    Current leakage, loss of insulation
    Voltage too low at implant (variable-voltage pulse generator)
    Output circuit, random component failure
3 Increased pacing threshold:
    Exit block:
        Early, 4 to 6 weeks
        Late, fibrosis
    Myocardial infarction
    Severe metabolic imbalance
    Drug overdose, e.g., antiarrhythmics, antidepressants
4 High resistance in electrode-lead system
    Lead design
    Electrode-lead system partial fracture

Pseudomalfunction

5 Misinterpretation, ECG:
    Pulse artifact occurs during refractory period of previous spontaneous beat as a result of competition
        Asynchronous pulse generator
        Magnet applied
    Lack of understanding of "vario" pulse-generator function (threshold testing)

TABLE 5
Output undesirably competitive (undersensing)

True malfunction

1 Pulse generator:
    Power-source failure (see Table 1)
    Reed switch lodged in asynchronous mode after magnet removed
    Asynchronous pulse generator
    Sensing circuit, random component failure
    Reprogramming of sensitivity in programmable pulse generator
    Previous spontaneous beat in refractory period
2 Electrode-lead system:
    Loss of insulation (see Table 1)
    Improper electrode-lead position or high resistance (see Table 4)
3 Myocardium (size of QRS):
    Broad QRS (poor slew rate)
    Reduced size of QRS:
        Idiopathic, especially bipolar leads
        Myocardial infarction or fibrosis
        Severe metabolic imbalance or drugs

Pseudomalfunction

4 Misinterpretation, ECG:
    Fusion beats
    Ventricular-triggered pacing
    Low-voltage marker spike
5 Faulty recording
    Magnet applied during test of synchronous mode
    Asynchronous testing labeled as synchronous mode

small-surface-area electrode, can also lead to failure of sensing. The size of the QRS potential produced by the myocardium is particularly important. Most patients who require permanent pacing are elderly and have generalized degenerative or atherosclerotic heart disease. The underlying disease process may result in a poorly generated QRS, especially with bipolar lead systems. Signals appropriate at the time of implant may become inappropriate postoperatively.

Sinus rhythm with right bundle branch block or late left ventricular ectopics may not be sensed by the pulse generator if depolarization is delayed in reaching the electrode in the right ventricle.[9] In these cases, the *slew rate,* or rate of voltage change in the electrogram, is important for accurate sensing by the pulse generator. As discussed earlier, chest-wall stimulation is useful in differentiating a pulse generator from a myocardial cause for undersensing.

The major causes of pseudomalfunction are misin-

terpretation of normal ECG patterns, such as fusion beats or ventricular-triggered pacing. It is surprisingly simple to confuse test data. Inadvertent application of the magnet during testing of the synchronous mode or incorrectly labeling the asynchronous testing as that during the synchronous mode are common problems.

PULSE-GENERATOR OUTPUT IN THE SYNCHRONOUS MODE IS SLOWED OR IRREGULAR (Table 6)

Slowing of the pulse-generator output in the synchronous mode only implies oversensing. Intermittent oversensing produces an irregular output (Fig. 15), whereas persistent oversensing may appear as a decreased rate or total inhibition of synchronous output. Oversensing may occur from four sources: cardiac, pacemaker, skeletal, and extracorporeal.

P wave sensing may occur if an epicardial ventricular lead is implanted near the left atrium or ventricular pacing has been established using the coronary sinus. T wave sensing, although apparently obvious from the ECG, is almost impossible to differentiate from

TABLE 6
Synchronous output slowed or irregular (oversensing)

True malfunction

1 Cardiac source: P wave, T wave, or concealed ectopics
2 Pacemaker source:
    After potentials
    Partial lead fracture
    Inactive lead
    Current leakage, pulse generator
    False signals, loose connections, insulation break,
      short circuits
3 Skeletal source:
    Muscle beneath implanted pulse generator
    Diaphragm
4 Extracorporeal source:
    Electromagnetic
    Radio frequency

Pseudomalfunction

5 Misinterpretation, ECG:
    Pulse-generator inhibition owing to test magnet place-
      ment or removal
    Hysteresis interpreted as oversensing
    VVT interpreted as VVI
6 Faulty recording:
    Monitoring equipment undersensitive and does not de-
      tect weaker signals, e.g., transtelephonic recording
    ECG recorder:
      Speed variable or sticking paper delivery

pacemaker afterpotentials, although in some cases the combined effect of both may lead to pulse-generator inhibition.[10] T wave sensing is rare today because the pulse-generator refractory period is set beyond the period of the T wave. Concealed ventricular ectopics can inhibit a pulse generator and are usually abolished with an antiarrhythmic agent such as lidocaine.

The pacemaker system may be the source of inappropriate sensing. Afterpotentials may result from the pulse generator delivering to the heart nonsymmetrical biphasic wave forms. Afterpotential inhibition can also occur with intermittent lead fracture, where momentary interruption of the fractured ends may result in sudden changes in lead resistance. This increases the potential at the electrode site, allowing the afterpotential to be sensed. Oversensing owing to spurious electric potentials may occur when an inactive lead makes contact with the active lead in the cavity of a ventricle. It may also occur if a lead pin of an inactive permanent lead is not insulated and left in contact with skeletal muscle.

Myopotentials produced by contracting skeletal muscle represent a common cause of oversensing, but despite an apparent high incidence of this problem,

significant clinical symptoms are unusual (Fig. 15).

Extracorporeal pulse-generator interference resulting in oversensing is a vast topic which, although it has generated a great deal of interest and publicity, is nevertheless only very occasionally a significant clinical problem today. Exteriorized early model demand pulse generators were very sensitive to electromagnetic and radio-frequency interference. However, once implanted, the pacemaker system became shielded from most of these interferences. Later, such improvements as electronic barriers, metal encapsulation of the pulse generator, and reversion to the asynchronous mode in the presence of recognized interference further shielded and protected the patient. A number of common potential problems appear unfounded. Microwave oven irradiation represents high-frequency interference that is easily rejected by modern pacemaker systems. Airport security magnetometers do not affect conventional implanted pulse generators. However, potential interference may still occur with electrosurgical diathermy and arc welding.

Normal Function of Pacemaker System (Fig. 10)

Investigation of apparent pacemaker system malfunction frequently reveals no abnormality either with the implanted hardware or with the patient's physical response. On occasion, the problem may be a side effect of the pacemaker system, whereas in other patients, the origin of the symptoms remains uncertain and routine investigations are unrewarding. If, however, the physician remains concerned, and especially if the symptoms are recurrent or persistent, then further investigation, such as long-term monitoring, becomes essential.

PACEMAKER SYSTEM PRODUCES SIDE EFFECTS (Table 7)

Pacemaker side effects can be divided into physical or psychologic. The problems of pulse-generator erosion and infection have diminished significantly in recent years. Pre-erosion can be diagnosed when an area of reddening develops usually on a corner of a pulse-generator site. Although bacterial endocarditis on an endocardial lead is rare, sustained bacteremia or septicemia may occur in 1 to 3 percent of patients, and the usual organism is a staphylococcus.[11] It is more common with temporary leads and in patients with infected intravenous lines.

Pain at the pulse-generator site is uncommon following normal healing from the surgical incision and

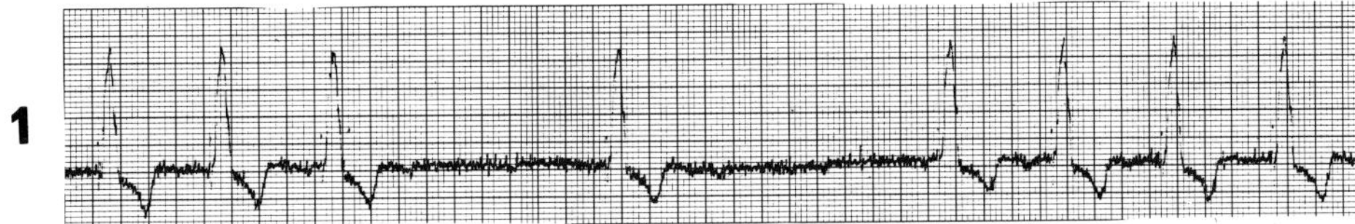

1

FIGURE 15 ECG, lead I. Muscle inhibition of pulse-generator output. Skeletal myopotentials (somatic tremor on baseline) are sensed, and consequently, there are long periods of pulse-generator inhibition.

TABLE 7
Pacemaker causes side effects (functioning normally)

Physical side effects

1 Placement of pacemaker system causing:
    Erosion or pre-erosion
    Infection:
      Local
      Septicemia or endocarditis
    Failure to heal
    Pain:
      Local
      Remote, anginal or pericardial
    Venous thrombosis or stenosis
    Pulmonary emboli or lead migration into pulmonary artery
    Pacemaker-twiddler's syndrome (lead dislodgement may occur)
    Allergy to components
    Pericardial tamponade owing to lead perforation
    Surgical myocardial infarction
    Knotting of endocardial leads
    Carcinoma of breast
2 Pacing causing undesirable stimulation:
    Skeletal muscle stimulation:
      Local, indifferent electrode unipolar system or loss of insulation (see Table 1)
      Diaphragmatic, direct or via phrenic nerve
    Paroxysmal cough
    Ventricular fibrillation, asynchronous pacing
3 Defibrillation or electrosurgery causing
    Pacemaker malfunction
    Cardiac burning or infarction at electrode site
4 Pysiotherapy shortwave treatment with local heat production
5 Pulse-generator characteristics:
    Inappropriate programming
    "Pacemaker syndrome"

Psychological side effects

6 Frequent self-detection of ectopic beats or hysteresis distressing patient
7 Enforced reliance on pacing system by patient causing a psychologic disturbance
8 Attempted suicide using pacemaker system

usually denotes infection, pre-erosion, or pressure on surrounding structures. Angina may on occasion be exacerbated on initiating pacing. This may be due to an inappropriate pacing rate, and thus in patients with preexisting angina, rate-programmable pulse generators should be considered. Pericardial pain may result from endocardial-lead perforation or following epicardial-lead placement. Pericardial tamponade resulting from endocardial-lead perforation is a life-threatening complication that can be minimized by not having the stiffening stylet at the tip of the lead as the electrode is being positioned at the right ventricular apex.

Clinical evidence of recurrent pulmonary emboli secondary to thrombosis around a permanent lead is surprisingly rare, even if the thrombotic material is infected. Symptomatic local venous thrombosis induced by pacemaker leads is also very uncommon.

The pacemaker-twiddler's syndrome is a psychologic disturbance with significant physical overtones.[12] Repeated turning of the implanted pulse generator under the skin may result in lead retraction from the endocardium. Carcinoma of the breast in a pectoral pulse-generator pocket is rare and may be coincidental. Skeletal muscle may be stimulated locally by the indifferent plate of a unipolar system or from a loss of lead insulation. Direct diaphragmatic pulsation following endocardial-lead placement is an infrequent troublesome complication that is usually transient. Indirect diaphragmatic pacing may result from phrenic nerve stimulation by an epicardial electrode.

In the presence of ischemic heart disease, ventricular fibrillation may occur with asynchronous pacing when the impulse falls in the vulnerable period. This is more common with bipolar or unipolar anodal pacing. DC electro-cardioversion may result in permanent or temporary damage to the implanted pulse generator. Myocardial burning may occur with dc electro-cardioversion or surgical diathermy and is due to the electric discharge transmitted along the lead. Physiotherapy shortwave treatment may result in local heat production, thus damaging the pulse generator or surrounding tissues.

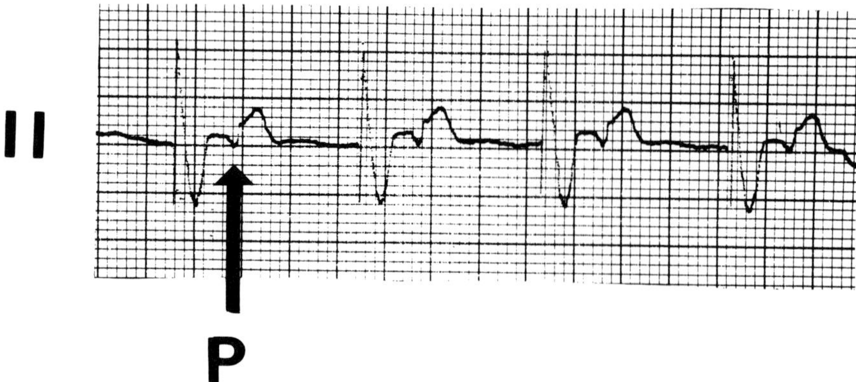

FIGURE 16 ECG, lead II. "Pacemaker syndrome" (see text). Following each paced QRS there is an inverted P wave, suggesting retrograde conduction.

The "pacemaker syndrome" is a physiologic disturbance caused by a normal ventricular-inhibited pacemaker system inserted in a patient with intact ventriculoatrial conduction. A retrograde P wave follows each ventricular complex (Fig. 16). In patients dependent on an atrial contraction prior to ventricular systole for an adequate cardiac output, this retrograde atrial contraction may have a negative effect on cardiac output. There is resultant vertigo, lightheadedness, syncope, and hypotension.[13] In these patients, a sequential pacemaker system is indicated.

Psychologic side effects following pacemaker system implantation can be minimized through careful explanation of the procedure to the patient and relatives beforehand. In the elderly age group, depression may not be uncommon. The patient may fear that the inevitable battery failure will introduce a further crisis in his or her life or that he or she is being run by an artificial device. Attempts at suicide by endeavoring to damage the pacemaker system have recently been reported.[14]

CONCLUSION

All implanted pacemaker systems will eventually fail with power-source depletion. On occasion, systems will prematurely develop a defect. To determine rapidly and correctly the cause, the physician must not only be conversant with the range of malfunctions that may arise, but also be able to distinguish pseudomalfunctions from true malfunctions. It is hoped that by using the principles and tables described that the physician new to the field of pacing will be able to determine logically the cause of a pacemaker system malfunction.

REFERENCES

1 Smith, D., McDonald, R., and Sloman, G.: Implanted Cardiac Pacemakers. Experience with Electronic Testing, *Cardiovasc. Res.,* 5:236, 1971.

2 Varenne, A., and Barold, S. S.: Therapeutic Usefulness of Chest Wall Stimulation in Patients with Demand Pacemakers, *J. Electrocardiol.,* 8:91, 1975.

3 Castellanos, A., Bloom, M. G., Sung, R. J., Rozanski, J. J., and Myerburg, R. J.: Mode of Operation Induced by Rapid External Wall Stimulation in Patients with Normally Functioning QRS Inhibited VVI Pacemakers, *PACE,* 2:2, 1979.

4 Furman, S., Hurzeler, P., and DeCaprio, V.: The Ventricular Endocardial Electrogram and Pacemaker Sensing, *J. Thorac. Cardiovasc. Surg.,* 73:258, 1977.

5 Mond, H. G., Stuckey, J. G., and Sloman, G.: The Diagnosis of Right Ventricular Perforation by an Endocardial Pacemaker Electrode, *PACE,* 1:62, 1978.

6 Mond, H., Tartaglia, S., Cole, A., and Sloman, G.: The Refurbished Pulse Generator, *PACE,* 3:311, 1980.

7 Runaway Protection of CPI Implantable Pacemakers. CPI Tech. Issues. Number 11. Cardiac Pacemakers Incorporated. St. Paul, Minnesota.

8 Mond, H., and Sloman, G.: The Small Tined Pacemaker Lead—Absence of Dislodgement, *PACE,* 3:171, 1980.

9 Vera, Z., Mason, D. T., Awan, N. A., Hilliard, G., and Massumi, R. A.: Lack of Sensing by Demand Pacemakers Due to Intraventricular Conduction Defects, *Circulation,* 51:185, 1975.

10 Gould, L., Reddy, C. V. R., Singh, B. K., and Zen, B.: Inappropriate Slowing of the Pacemaker Rate with Programmable Demand Pacemaker, *PACE,* 2:370, 1979.

11 Morgan, G., Ginks, W., Siddons, H., and Leatham, A.: Septicemia in Patients with an Endocardial Pacemaker, *Am. J. Cardio.,* 44:221, 1979.

12 Bayliss, C. E., Beanlands, D. S., and Baird, R. J.: The Pacemaker-Twiddler's Syndrome: A New Complication of Implantable Transvenous Pacemakers, *Can. Med. Assoc. J.,* 99:371, 1968.

13 Miller, M., Fox, S., Jenkins, R., Schwartz, J., and Toonder, R. G.: Pacemaker Syndrome: A Non-Invasive Means to Its Diagnosis and Treatment, *PACE,* 4:503, 1981.

14 Simon, A. B., Kleinman, P., and Janz, N.: Suicide Attempt by Pacemaker System Abuse: A Case Report with Comments on the Psychological Adaptation of Pacemaker Patients, *PACE,* 3:224, 1980.

Advances in
Echocardiographic Diagnosis[*]

I. BELENKIE, M.D., and E. R. SMITH, M.D.

Those, who are engaged in studying the heart and its defects by means of special instruments, are fully conscious of the burden which awaits the student or practitioner who has yet to bring himself abreast of the times in this field of knowledge.

SIR THOMAS LEWIS, 1911[1]
Clinical Disorders of the Heartbeat: A Handbook for Practitioners and Students

Both M-mode and two-dimensional echocardiography are firmly established as valuable noninvasive methods of cardiac diagnosis. The two techniques should not be considered exclusive, but rather as complementary methods in the thorough assessment of the patient with known or suspected heart disease. The M-mode approach is limited by the relatively small portion of the total cardiac structure that can be visualized, by the lack of lateral resolution, and by the inability to adequately determine the spatial orientation of imaged structures. The resolution in the axial plane is excellent, however, and the high repetition rate (1,000 pulses per second) provides a crisp image that allows accurate measurement of the distances between interfaces. By contrast, the two-dimensional approach allows imaging of most of the cardiac structure and provides excellent spatial orientation. Although resolution (in the axial plane) remains high, the slower sampling rate (30 frames per second) limits the ability to identify interfaces, particularly when viewed in stop frame. A combination of the two approaches provides an imaging technique that is capable of providing detailed information concerning both the structure and function of the heart. In most instances, therefore, M-mode recordings should be obtained at the same time as two-dimensional echocardiographic studies. The use of a cursor superimposed on the two-dimensional image directs the M-mode beam, thereby ensuring accurate definition of the structures being studied.

In this overview, it is our intention to describe some of the recent advances in the utilization of echocardiography. We have not attempted to deal with every application of the technique, nor are the discussions of individual applications necessarily comprehensive.

TECHNICAL CONSIDERATIONS

Technical advances in two-dimensional echocardiography have been considerable over the past few years.

Basically, two types of instruments are available: one has a mechanically operated transducer(s), and the other uses a phased array of transducers. Mechanical sector scanners either have a single, rapidly oscillating transducer or three or four rotating elements. At the present time, most mechanical scanners do not provide simultaneous M-mode and two-dimensional images, a feature that is clearly desirable. The phased-array instruments use a large number of transducer elements with the direction of the wave front altered by the firing sequence of the individual elements. M-mode and two-dimensional images can be obtained simultaneously with this equipment. Since each approach has both advantages and limitations, equipment should be purchased to meet the specific needs of the laboratory. If portability is important, or if the pediatric case load is significant, the choice may well be different than if patients are mainly adult and examinations are performed in the laboratory.

In understanding the application of two-dimensional echocardiography, the resolution capability of currently available equipment is a major consideration. Optimal resolution is obtained with the highest transducer frequency and minimum gain settings.[1a] Axial resolution (in the plane of the beam) is very satisfactory (approximately 2 mm) and is independent of distance from the transducer. Lateral resolution (the plane perpendicular to the beam) is much less satisfactory, varying from 2 to 4 mm in the near field but increasing progressively at greater distances from the transducer. A recent study found the lateral resolution capability to be only 17 mm at a distance of 20 cm from the transducer.[2] There is little difference between the resolution capabilities of the mechanical and phased-array instruments currently available. However, it is technically more difficult to use transducers having frequencies greater than 3.5 MHz with phased-array equipment, although prototypes are being tested at the time of this writing.

TWO-DIMENSIONAL ECHOCARDIOGRAPHIC ANATOMY

Most of the cardiac anatomy can be assessed from two standard transducer positions, one at the left sternal border and the other at the apex. The long-axis parasternal view is shown in Fig. 1. It is a particularly useful view to assess interventricular septal and posterior wall motion, as well as to visualize the mitral and aortic valves, the proximal ascending aorta, and the left

*From the Department of Medicine, University of Calgary and the Foothills Provincial Hospital Calgary, Alberta, Canada.

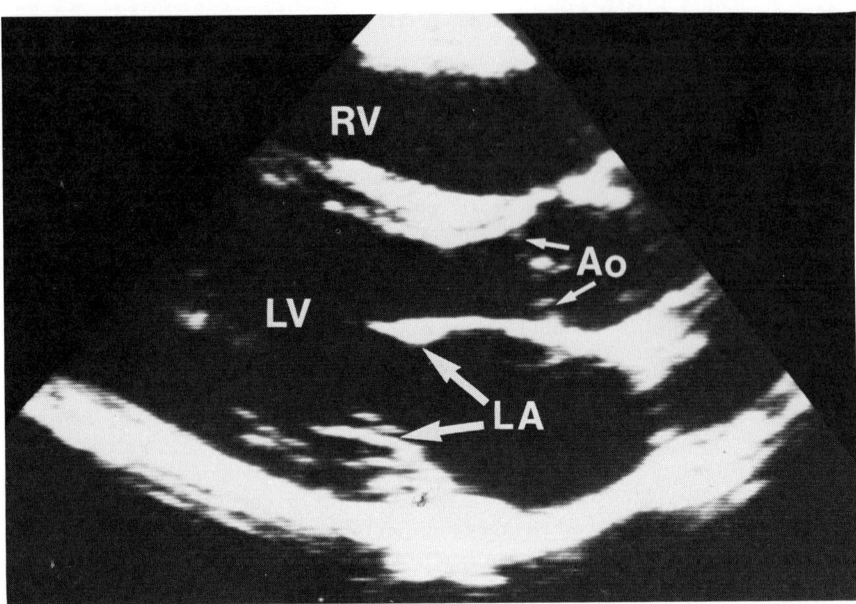

FIGURE 1 A left parasternal long-axis view from a normal person. Small arrows point to the right (anterior) and noncoronary (posterior) cusps of the aortic valve. Large arrows point to the anterior and posterior leaflets of the mitral valve.

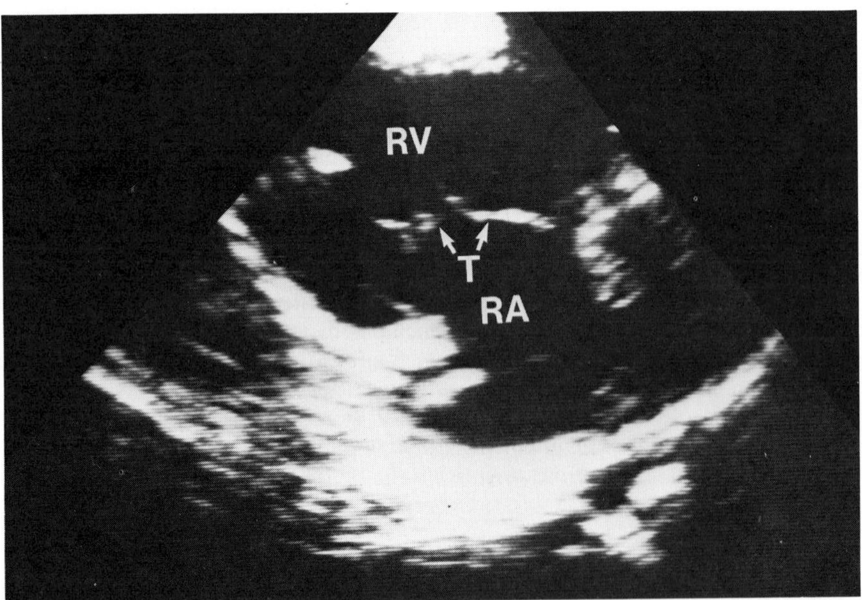

FIGURE 2 A left parasternal view of the right atrium (RA) and right ventricle (RV). T = tricuspid valve.

atrium. Utilizing the cursor on the two-dimensional image, M-mode recordings can be easily obtained from these structures. It is usually not possible to image the apex from the parasternal location, but often this can be accomplished by moving the transducer toward the apex. The right ventricle and right atrium can be imaged in their long axis from the left parasternal position by pointing the transducer toward the patient's right hip (Fig. 2). By rotating the transducer 90°, one can examine short-axis views from the base of the heart

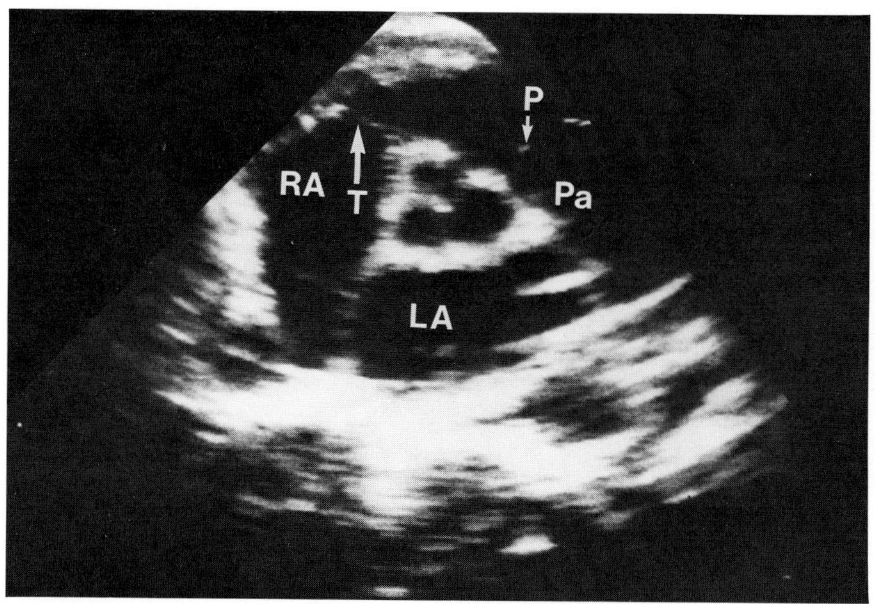

FIGURE 3 A left parasternal short-axis view taken at the level of the aortic valve. At this level, the aortic, pulmonic (P), and tricuspid (T) valves can be seen. When, as shown here, all three of the aortic cusps are seen, the appearance resembles the Mercedes-Benz emblem— the "mercedes sign." Pa = pulmonary artery; LA = left atrium; RA = right atrium.

and great vessels to the apex. With the transducer angled cephalad, the aortic, pulmonary, and tricuspid valves can be seen, as well as the aorta, left and right atria, interatrial septum, and, on occasion, the left main coronary artery (Fig. 3). The transducer can then be directed caudad to obtain a series of short-axis views of the left and right ventricles (Fig. 4). The mitral valve apparatus is also easily examined from this position.

The other commonly utilized position is at the cardiac apex with the transducer directed toward the right shoulder (Fig. 5). From this position it is possible to view all four cardiac chambers and the two atrioventricular valves; by directing the transducer slightly anteriorly, the aortic valve may also be imaged. Rotation of the transducer through 90° provides the apical two-chamber view. The apex, true posterior and anterior free walls of the left ventricle, the left atrium, and the mitral and aortic valves can be visualized in this plane (Fig. 6). One can move the transducer to a large number of locations between the two standard positions to acquire additional information. Several other transducer locations are occasionally very useful: the subcostal view may be helpful in patients with chronic obstructive pulmonary disease and is extremely useful to image the interatrial and interventricular septa (Fig. 7) as well as the inferior vena cava. The right parasternal view allows visualization of the interatrial septum, and the suprasternal view is of help in assessing the great vessels. It should be stressed that proper utilization of any of these views requires that the echocardiog-

rapher be completely familiar with planar cardiac anatomy and with the characteristics of cardiac pathology.

LEFT VENTRICULAR VOLUME MEASUREMENTS

A major goal of echocardiographers over the past decade has been to determine left ventricular volumes and ejection fractions with results comparable with those obtained by contrast angiography. Left ventricular dimensions obtained by M-mode echocardiography can be used to provide reasonably accurate estimates of volumes in people with normal hearts (Fig. 8). However, this method is unreliable in the presence of either enlarged hearts or when segmental wall-motion abnormalities exist. These concerns do not exist with two-dimensional echocardiography, which allows the operator to obtain multiple tomographic images in several planes. However, there are significant limitations to using two-dimensional echocardiography to obtain such quantitative information. First, it is not possible to acquire technically satisfactory studies in as many as 25 percent of patients, particularly in the older age groups. Second, endocardial recognition lateral to the plane of the transducer is often difficult or impossible. This is particularly troublesome in apical views, where the entire length of the endocardial surface may

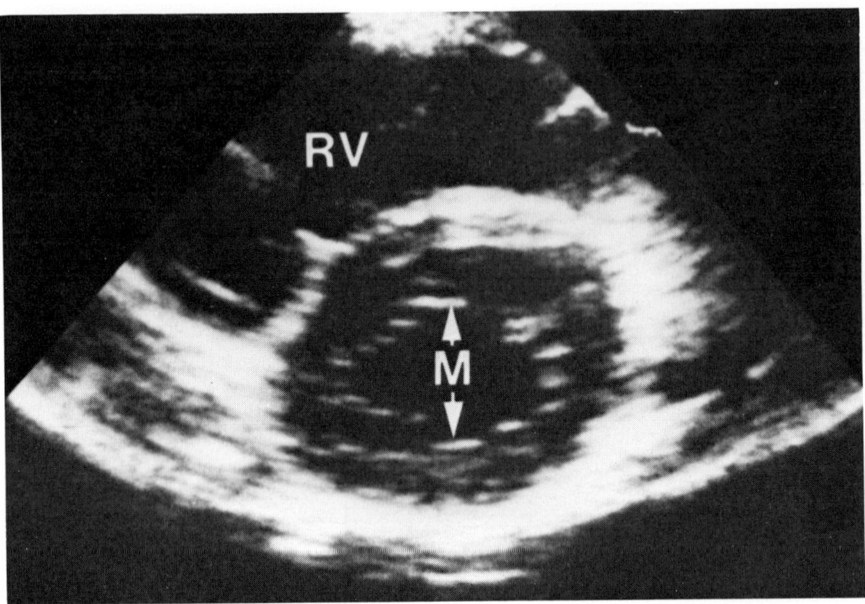

A

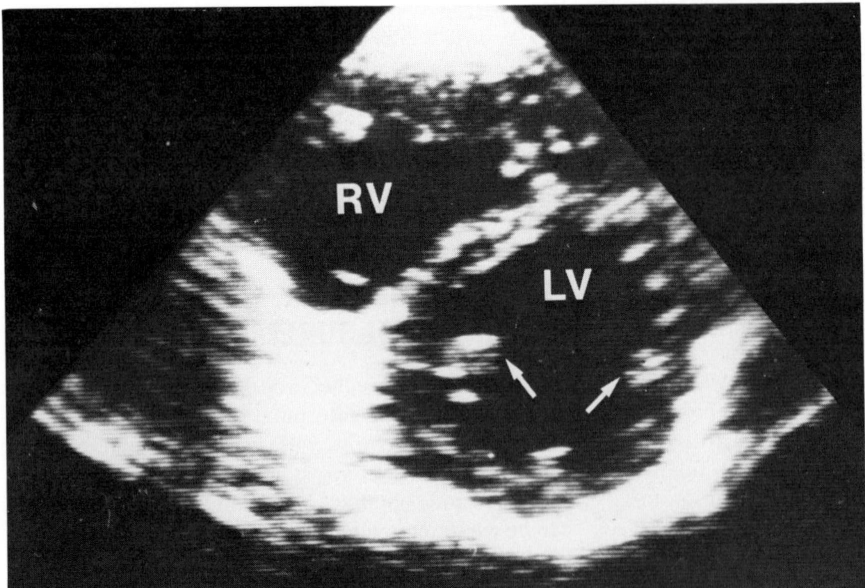

B

FIGURE 4 Left parasternal short-axis views at the level of the mitral (M) leaflets (*A*) and papillary muscles (*B*). The arrows point to the papillary muscles. RV = right ventricle; LV = left ventricle.

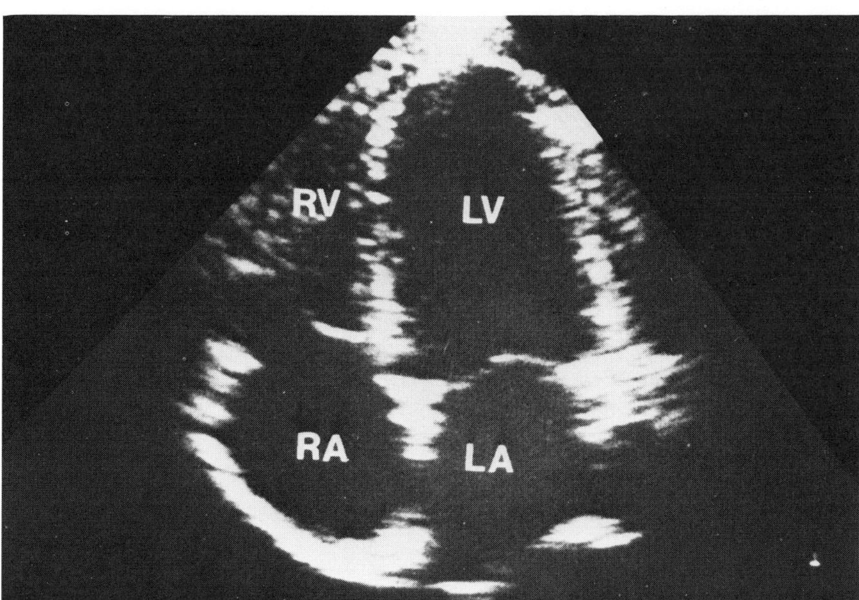

FIGURE 5 An apical four-chamber view from a normal person. The mitral and tricuspid valves can be seen between the ventricles and atria. Note that the attachment of the tricuspid valve to the septum is normally closer to the apex than that of the mitral valve. RV = right ventricle; LV = left ventricle; RA = right atrium; LA = left atrium.

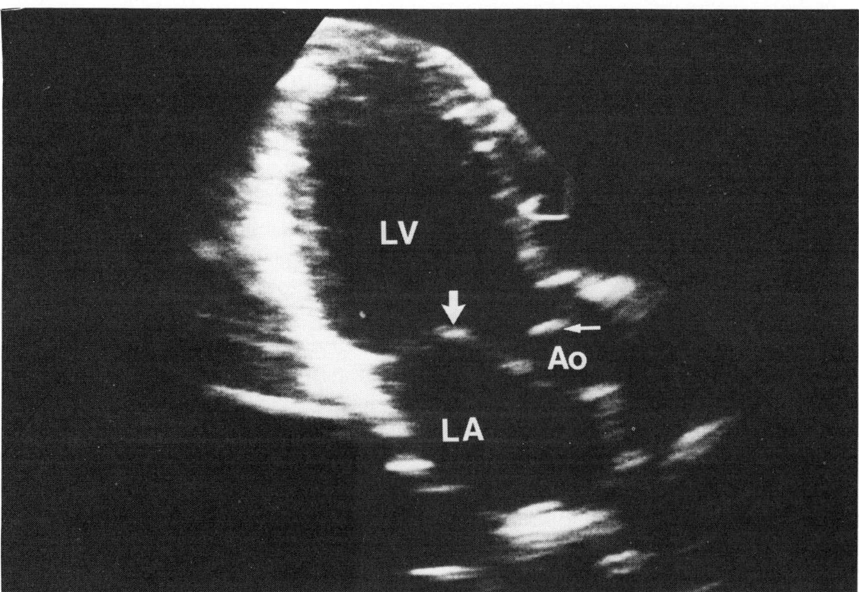

FIGURE 6 An apical two-chamber view of the left ventricle (LV), left atrium (LA), and the mitral valve (arrow).

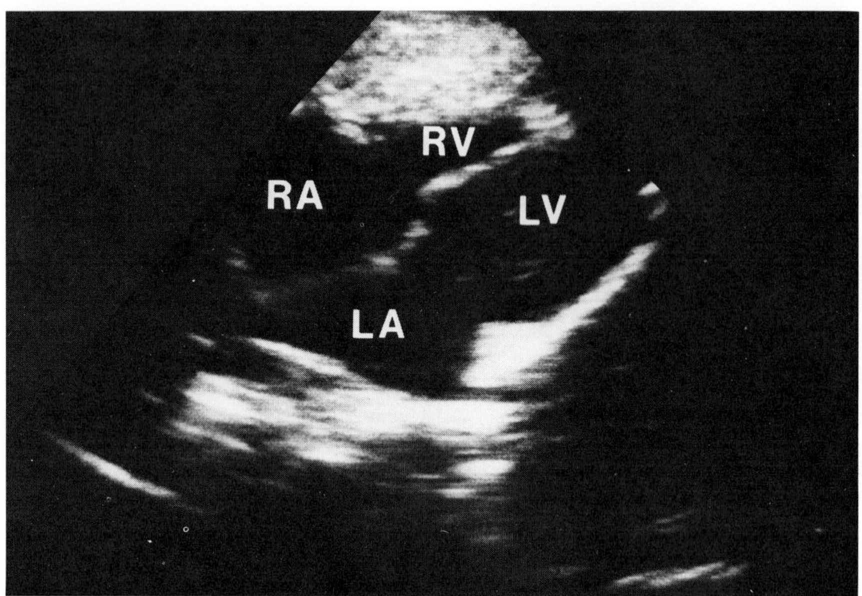

FIGURE 7 A subcostal four-chamber view from a normal person. The atrial and ventricular septa are almost perpendicular to the ultrasound beam, particularly in the region of the endocardial cushion.

be inadequately visualized. Finally, the poor lateral resolution of current instruments can contribute to significant errors in measurements even if the endocardium is visible. It is important to note that endocardium may be well recognized when the study is viewed in real time, since the eye integrates the images over several frames. However, when viewed in stop frame for the purpose of obtaining measurements, the endocardial detail may be considerably more difficult to appreciate. Despite these limitations, left ventricular volumes and ejection fractions obtained with two-dimensional echocardiography correlate reasonably well with those obtained by both contrast and nuclear angiographic techniques.[3–6] Commercially available microprocessor based light-pen systems facilitate these measurements and calculations. A simplified technique to determine ejection fraction using two-dimensional echocardiography has recently been reported, although to date this has not been confirmed in other laboratories.[7]

Although M-mode echocardiography is not a technique that should be used to estimate left ventricular volumes, it does provide an important reproducible method for assessing left ventricular function in patients without regional wall-motion abnormalities. Care must be taken to direct the beam across the left ventricle at or just below the level of the tips of the mitral valve (Fig. 8). Fractional shortening of the diastolic dimension and circumferential fiber-shortening velocity can both be derived from this record and have been found to be helpful in detecting and quantitating left ventricular dysfunction. Since there is significant beat-to-beat variability in left ventricular diameters, data from several consecutive beats should be averaged.[8] Another useful measurement in both normal-sized and enlarged left ventricles is the mitral E point–interventricular septal separation; an increase in this measurement has been noted to have a reasonably close inverse correlation with ejection fraction.[9,10]

M-mode echocardiography can be used in a variety of other ways to describe systolic and diastolic function of the left ventricle. One such method involves digitizing the left ventricular septal and posterior wall interfaces and plotting dimensional change against time.[11] From these data it is possible to calculate peak rates of dimension change. Simultaneous measurement of left ventricular pressure allows construction of pressure-dimension loops and calculation of ventricular efficiency. Other examples of the utility of this technique include the demonstration that peak circumferential fiber-shortening velocity may occasionally be more useful than fractional shortening or mean circumferential fiber-shortening velocity in detecting left ventricular dysfunction[12] and that the decrease in the peak rate of diastolic increase in left ventricular dimension can be extremely helpful in assessing the severity of mitral stenosis[13] or detecting prosthetic mitral valve dysfunction.

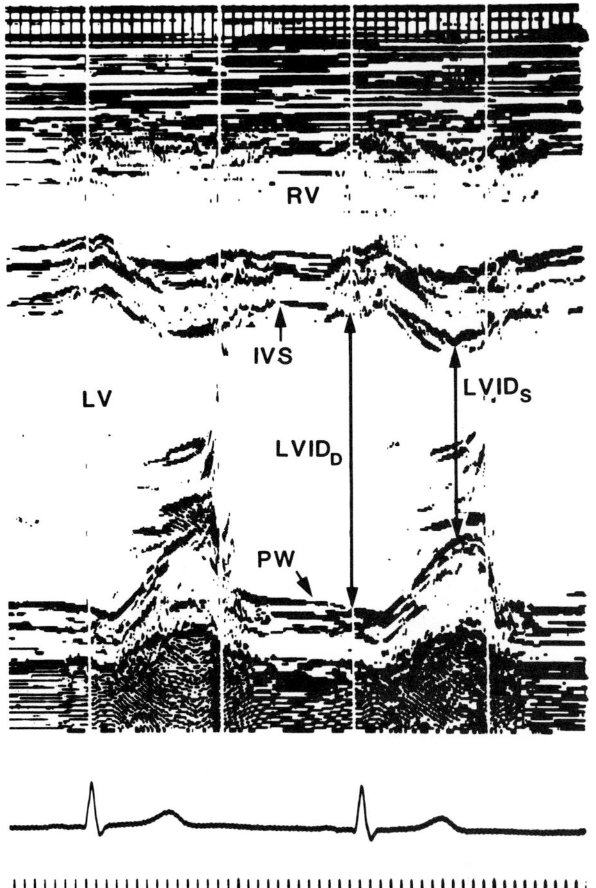

FIGURE 8 An M-mode tracing taken at the level of the tip of the mitral valve. RV = right ventricle; IVS = interventricular septum; LV = left ventricle; LVID$_D$ and LVID$_S$ = left ventricular internal diameters at end-diastole and end-systole, respectively; PW = posterior wall.

ACQUIRED HEART DISEASE
Coronary Artery Disease
DETECTION OF MYOCARDIAL DAMAGE

Because of the "ice-pick" view, M-mode echocardiography is of limited value in assessing the effects of coronary artery disease on the left ventricle. Since virtually all the left ventricle can be imaged by two-dimensional echocardiography, this technique can be used to great advantage in these patients. In addition, by obtaining simultaneous M-mode data from selected areas, wall thickness can be assessed throughout the cardiac cycle. Infarcted segments of myocardium may appear as thin, echo-dense areas that do not thicken during systole; myocardium that has normal diastolic thickness but fails to thicken appropriately during

systole may represent areas with reversible ischemia.[14] This may prove an important consideration when one attempts to assess patients for coronary bypass grafting procedures.

The accuracy in detecting regional wall-motion abnormalities by two-dimensional echocardiography compares well with that of contrast angiography[7,15] (Fig. 9). Whereas it is possible to detect abnormal wall motion in most instances, the size of an abnormally moving segment may be underestimated because the imaging plane does not always traverse the largest diameter of the involved region. The technique has also been shown to provide an accurate means to detect[16] and localize[17–19] acute myocardial infarction. Indeed, the demonstration of normal wall motion several hours after the onset of chest pain is strong evidence against there being acute transmural damage.[16,20] However, subendocardial infarction cannot be excluded by the finding of normal wall motion. Two-dimensional echocardiography may also prove useful in estimating the size of a myocardial infarction. However, as long as wall motion is the parameter being assessed, considerable error must be expected.[18] This simply reflects the fact that hypokinesis might occur secondary to reversible ischemia or subendocardial infarction or because of proximity to an infarcted segment. Despite these potential problems, two-dimensional echocardiographic estimates of the amount of muscle damage have been reported to correlate well with hemodynamically determined subsets,[16,21] serum creatine kinase levels, and the frequency of complications.[19,22] Early after an acute myocardial infarction, a wall-motion index may predict hemodynamic deterioration before other indicators of a poor prognosis are clinically evident.[16,22] The detection of infarct expansion during the evolution of acute infarction suggests a poor prognosis,[23] as well as predicting subsequent left ventricular dilatation and chronically diminished functional capacity.[24] An echocardiographic index of residual functioning myocardium in the presence of a myocardial aneurysm has correlated well with clinical status and prognosis and may prove helpful in the selection of patients for aneurysmectomy.[25]

Regional wall-motion abnormalities may also be seen in areas of the left ventricle other than those suggested by the infarction pattern on the electrocardiogram. This usually suggests multivessel coronary artery stenosis, which, when detected during acute myocardial infarction, is associated with a higher incidence of complications and mortality.[16]

Regional wall-motion abnormalities of the right ventricle have also been detected echocardiographically in patients with right ventricular infarction.[26] However, the accuracy of the technique in this situation has not yet been established. Certainly, in this clinical setting and in the presence of marked elevation of

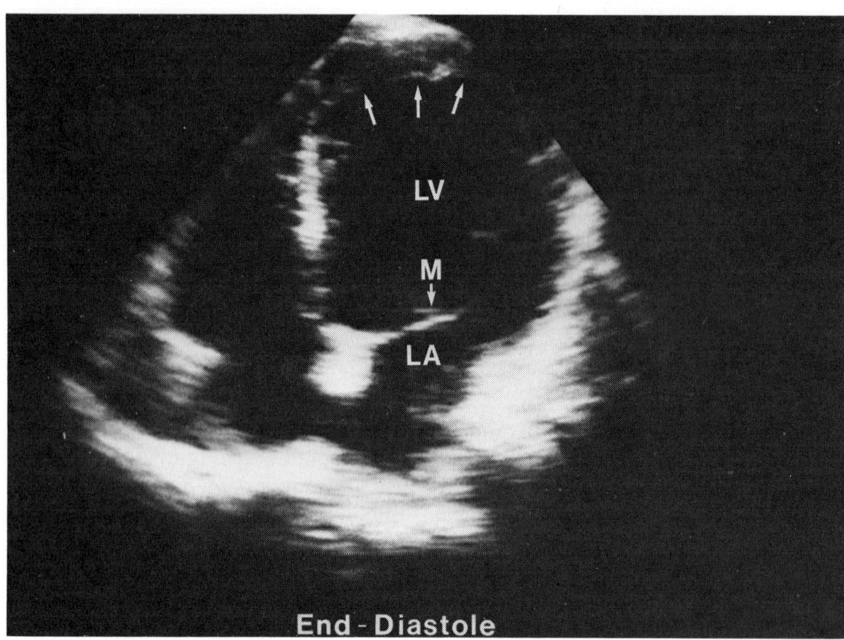

A

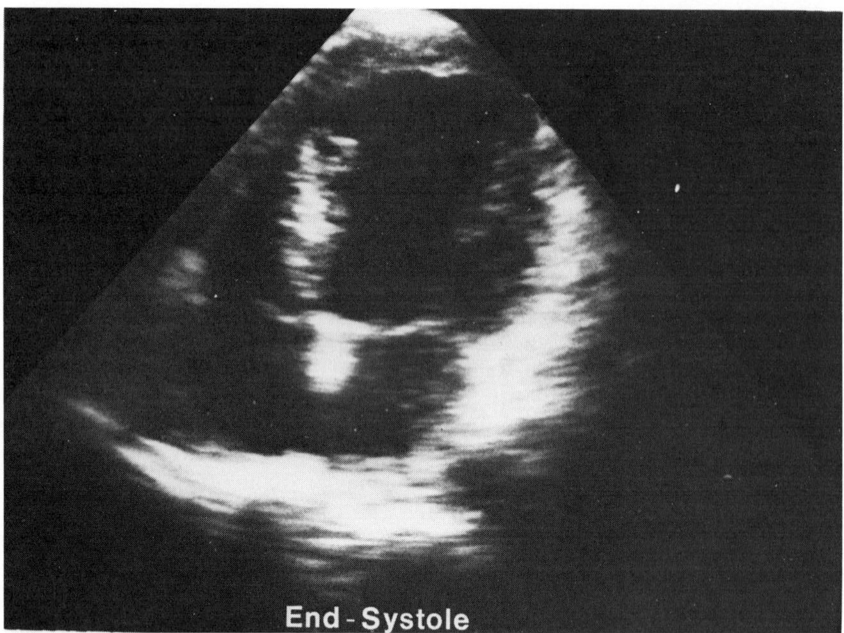

B

FIGURE 9 Apical four-chamber views from a patient with an apical aneurysm and a mural thrombus (arrows). (*A*) At end-diastole. (*B*) At end-systole. There is little change at end-systole at the apex, which is largely akinetic, except for the most apical portion, which is dyskinetic. LV = left ventricle; LA = left atrium; M = mitral valve.

right-sided pressures, echocardiography can be useful in distinguishing right ventricular infarction from pericardial tamponade.

DIAGNOSIS OF CORONARY ARTERY DISEASE

Exercise echocardiography has recently been evaluated as a method for detecting significant coronary artery disease in patients with exertional symptoms. M-mode features in the affected segment reported to be indicators of significant coronary artery stenosis include decreases in systolic wall thickening, velocity of wall thinning, and fractional shortening.[27] The detection of new regional wall-motion abnormalities during exercise by two-dimensional echocardiography is a specific but relatively insensitive method of detecting coronary artery disease.[28–30] A decrease in ejection fraction at peak exercise may prove to be a more sensitive method of detecting significant coronary artery stenosis and, at least theoretically, could be superior to rest and exercise gated radionuclide angiography.[31] The relatively long sampling period required during radioisotope studies may preclude the detection of a decrease in ejection fraction occurring only at peak exercise. Two-dimensional echocardiography allows assessment of each beat, thereby avoiding the loss of sensitivity associated with the averaging of data obtained over many cardiac cycles. Although initial reports have been encouraging, it must be remembered that this procedure has many technical difficulties. These include the problem of obtaining satisfactory images during exercise and the previously mentioned problems with obtaining accurate ventricular volumes owing to poor lateral definition of the endocardium and the error associated with poor lateral resolution.

Some interest has developed in the potential use of echocardiography to image directly coronary arteries. To date, this has been limited to detecting stenosis in left main coronary artery disease.[32–34] Success in detecting these lesions is highly skill dependent, and currently, two-dimensional echocardiography is not widely utilized in this application. Coronary artery fistulas have occasionally been detected echocardiographically.[35]

COMPLICATIONS OF ACUTE MYOCARDIAL INFARCTION

Recent data suggest that two-dimensional echocardiography is useful in detecting and localizing ventricular septal rupture following acute myocardial infarction, and by utilizing a wall-motion index, it provides a means to predict survival.[36–38] This may prove to be the technique of choice to distinguish ventricular septal

defect from papillary muscle rupture.[38] The latter can be identified by the resultant disordered motion of the involved leaflet,[38,39] and on occasion, the detached portion of the papillary muscle may also be visualized. Papillary muscle dysfunction usually does not result in distinctive echocardiographic abnormalities, but on occasion, there may be prolapse of a mitral leaflet or increased echo density of the involved muscle.[40]

Until recently, there has been no method to detect reliably left ventricular mural thrombus. Two-dimensional echocardiography has now been shown to be a sensitive and specific means to demonstrate left ventricular clot following myocardial infarction[41–43] (Figs. 9 and 10). The apical four-chamber view is usually best for this purpose, although care must be taken to avoid artifact when using this transducer position. The vast majority of demonstrable thrombi are found in an akinetic or dyskinetic apex, the data suggesting that patients with akinesis or dyskinesis in this region have an approximately 50 percent risk of developing a mural thrombus early after an acute myocardial infarction. The natural history of these thrombi has not been established. Some resolve while under therapy with anticoagulants or spontaneously; recurrence may or may not develop after medication is discontinued.[41] The risk of embolization is small; currently, a means to predict patients most likely to suffer this complication has not been established. The question of whether or not to use anticoagulants when a left ventricular thrombus is detected echocardiographically remains to be resolved.

The differentiation of true aneurysms from pseudoaneurysms of the left ventricle is important because of the potential for spontaneous rupture of the latter. This has been shown to be possible with two-dimensional echocardiography, but the predictive accuracy is still uncertain.[44–46]

Valvular Heart Disease

M-mode and two-dimensional echocardiography have proved to be valuable in detecting and assessing the severity of a variety of forms of valvular heart disease. This ability, plus the additional capability to measure chamber dimensions and wall thickness, as well as to assess left ventricular function, has made it possible to opt for operation in many patients based on clinical and noninvasive data without resorting to preoperative cardiac catheterization.[47]

STENOSIS OF THE ATRIOVENTRICULAR VALVES

The diagnosis of mitral stenosis is usually possible from M-mode echocardiography by detecting thickened leaf-

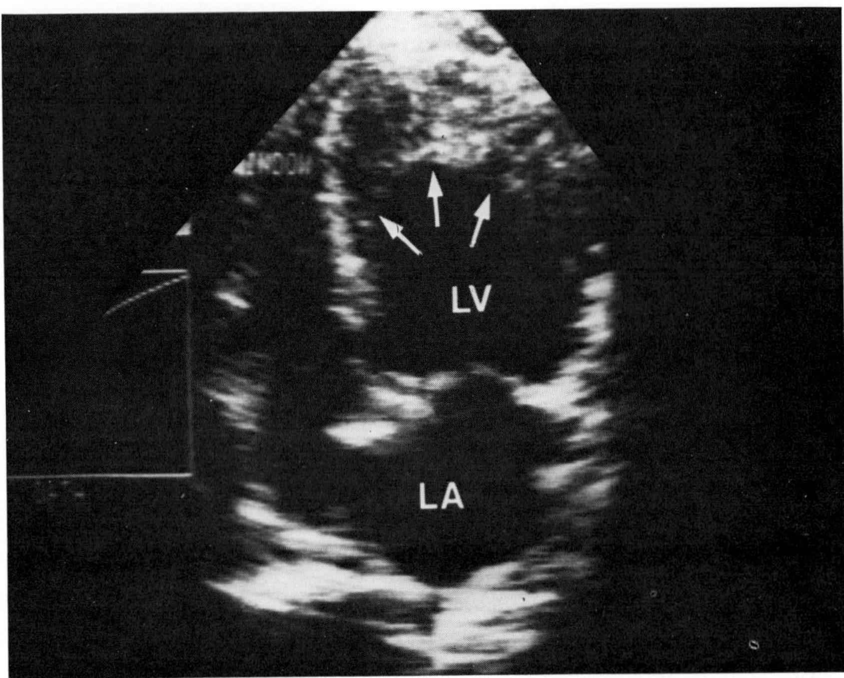

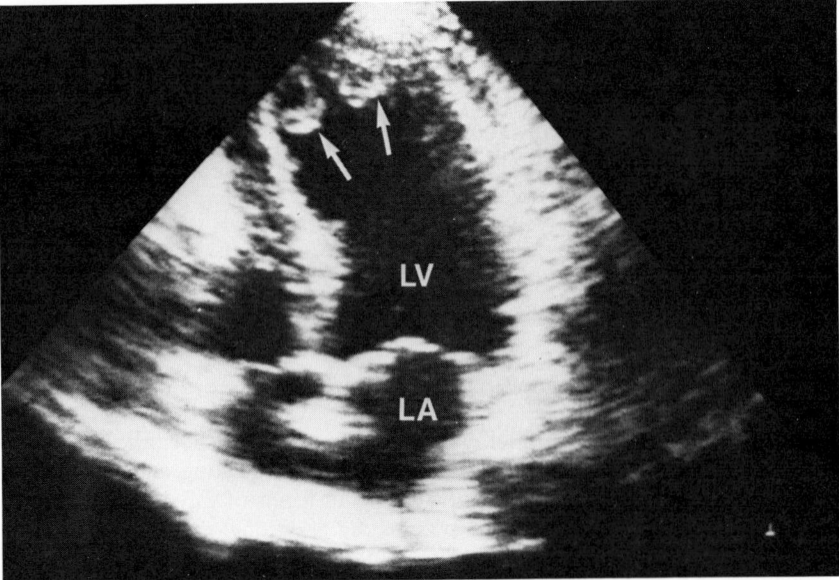

FIGURE 10 (*A*) Apical four-chamber views showing clots in the apices of the left ventricles (arrows). The view in (*B*) was taken in a patient after he had an embolus to his leg following an acute myocardial infarction. LA = left atrium; LV = left ventricle.

lets, a reduced E-F slope, and an anterior movement of the posterior leaflet during diastole. However, since the mitral E-F slope can be decreased in a number of other conditions and the posterior leaflet can move posteriorly during diastole in mild stenosis, the occasional echocardiogram may prove difficult to interpret. This should occur only rarely if one correlates all the echocardiographic and clinical features in each case. The assessment of the severity of mitral stenosis from M-mode echocardiograms has proved more difficult than initially reported. Measurement of the E-F slope of the anterior leaflet is now recognized to be unreliable,[13,48,49] although mild stenosis may be distinguished from severe disease by estimates of the left ventricular diastolic filling rate.[13] Two-dimensional echocardiography offers a more direct means to assess severity of mitral stenosis. Measurements of the mitral valve orifice area during diastole correlate well with hemodynamically derived estimates and those measured directly during surgery[48,49] (Fig. 11). For reliability, however, it is important to ensure that the area measurement is made at the level of the mitral orifice

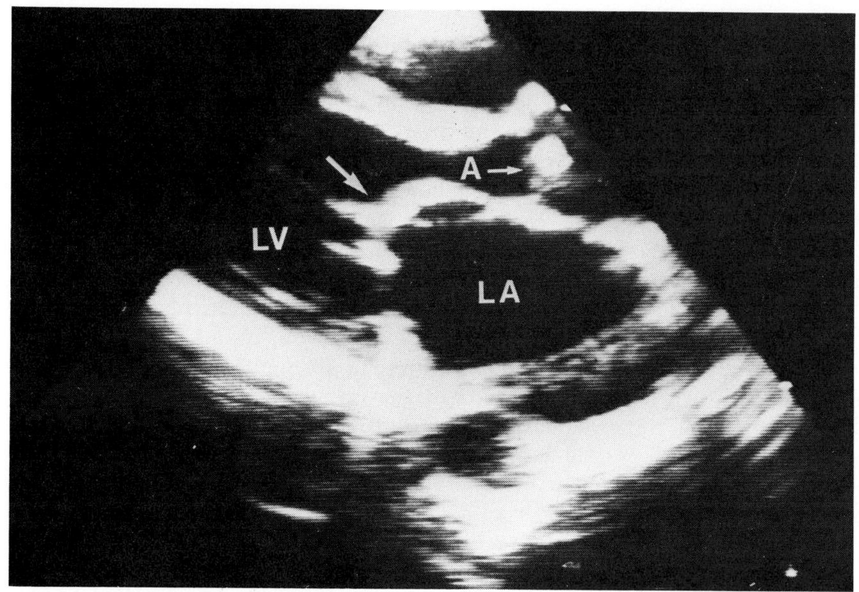

A

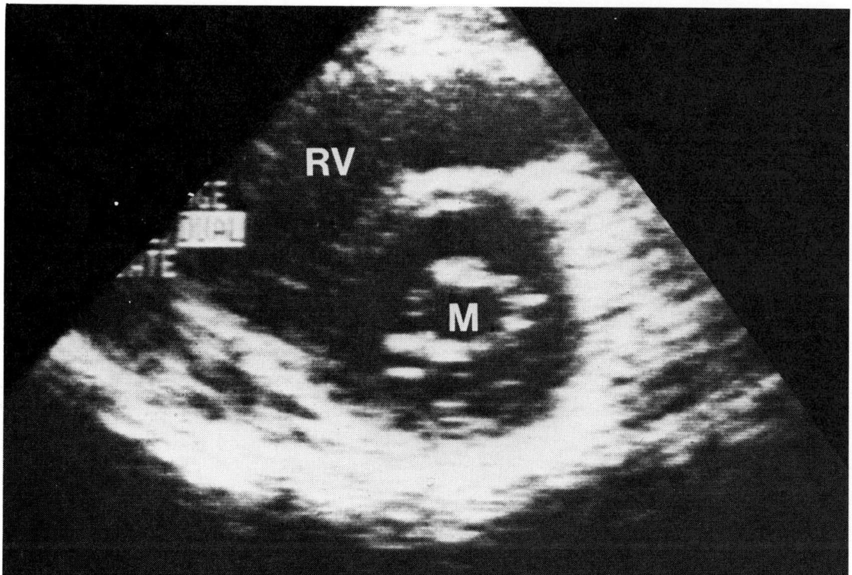

B

FIGURE 11 (*A*) Left parasternal long-axis and (*B*) short-axis views from patients with mild mitral stenosis. In (*A*) note the thickened anterior leaflet (large arrow), which bows upward because of its restricted motion away from the posterior leaflet. The left atrium (LA) is mildly enlarged and the aortic valve (A) is thickened. In (*B*) the mildly narrowed mitral orifice (M) is seen. LV = left ventricle; LA = left atrium; RV = right ventricle.

rather than more proximally in the mitral funnel and that the proper gain settings are utilized.

In tricuspid stenosis, abnormal motion and thickening of the tricuspid leaflets similar to that found in mitral stenosis may be seen. In such patients, small but important pressure gradients across the valve may be appreciated only by careful hemodynamic study.

REGURGITATION AT THE ATRIOVENTRICULAR VALVES

The etiology of mitral regurgitation can usually be determined by echocardiography.[50,51] Measurement of left atrial and left ventricular chamber sizes[52] as well as other indices of left ventricular function, may be helpful in assessing the severity of the lesion. However, a sensitive and reliable index of left ventricular dysfunction in this condition has not yet been validated.

Controversy continues regarding the echocardiographic features of mitral valve prolapse, largely owing to the lack of a reliable diagnostic gold standard.[53,54] Accordingly, there remains some question as to the best echocardiographic criteria. Mid or late systolic prolapse of at least 3 mm posterior to the CD line of the mitral valve is a frequently used M-mode criterion.

Pansystolic hammocking is also a generally accepted criterion, at least if care is taken to avoid excessive inferior angulation of the transducer. Other findings may include thickening of the leaflets and dense echoes posterior to the anterior leaflet, which, on occasion, may suggest the presence of either a vegetation or left atrial myxoma[55] (Fig. 12). Left atrial and left ventricular enlargement as well as excessive septal motion suggesting left ventricular volume overload can all be helpful in assessing the hemodynamic importance of the lesion. False positive diagnoses can be minimized with careful attention to the transducer position and angulation, although even with good technique it is not possible to demonstrate prolapse in some patients with the click-murmur syndrome.

Using two-dimensional echocardiography, one or both mitral leaflets may be seen to bulge to the atrial side of the mitral ring during ventricular systole (Fig. 12). Although the apical four-chamber view has been suggested[53] to be the best one to detect prolapse, the other standard views should also be carefully assessed. Tricuspid valve prolapse has been reported to occur in 20 to 50 percent of cases of mitral valve prolapse, and aortic cusp prolapse may be seen in as many as 15 to 20 percent of such patients[53] (some of whom will also have aortic regurgitation).

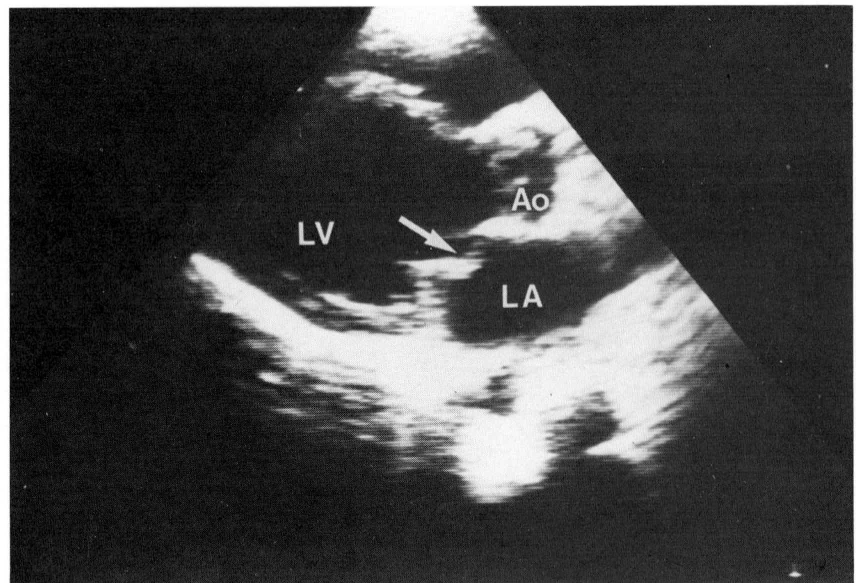

A

FIGURE 12 (*A*) Left parasternal long-axis view showing prolapse of the anterior leaflet of the mitral valve (arrow). (*B,* opposite) An apical two-chamber view showing prolapse of the posterior leaflet of the mitral valve (arrow). (*C,* opposite) An apical four-chamber view from a patient with prolapse of the anterior leaflet of the mitral valve (arrow). (*D,* p. 32) An M-mode tracing from a patient with mitral valve prolapse. Multiple echoes (arrows) posterior to the anterior mitral valve leaflet (AM) resemble those seen in left atrial myxoma. LV = left ventricle; LA = left atrium; Ao = aorta.

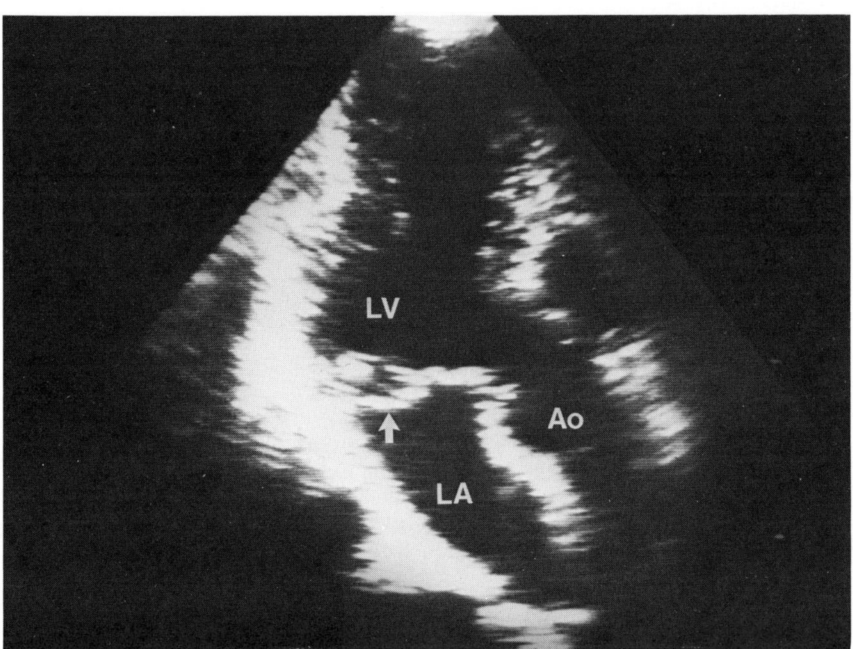

B

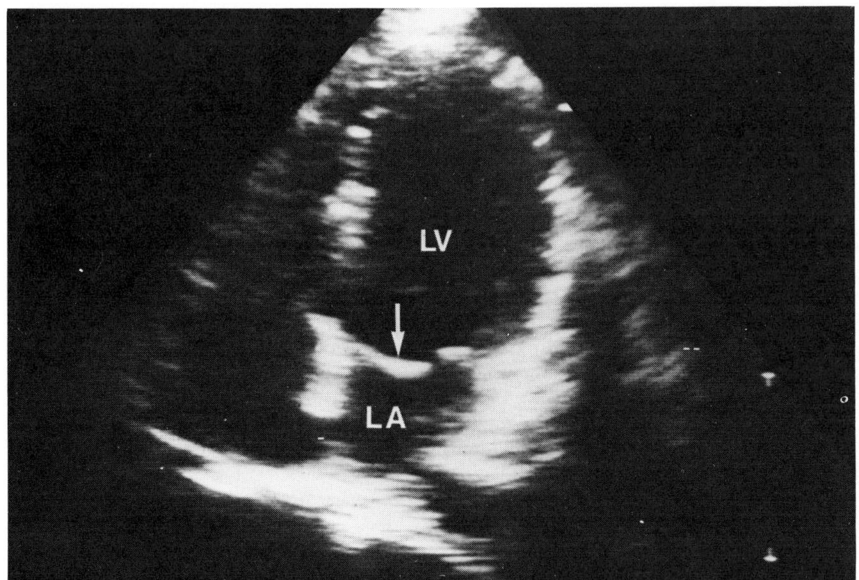

C

In some cases it may be difficult or impossible to distinguish severe mitral valve prolapse from a flail mitral leaflet, the latter often resulting from ruptured chordae tendineae or infective endocarditis. A flail leaflet is suggested on an M-mode examination by the presence of chaotic diastolic motion and systolic flutter-ing of a leaflet. On two-dimensional studies, abnormal echoes may be imaged in the left atrium with a lack of systolic coaptation of the leaflets.[56,57] This latter finding, however, is not necessarily diagnostic of ruptured chordae tendineae (see Fig. 16). It is important to note that patients with mitral valve prolapse who develop

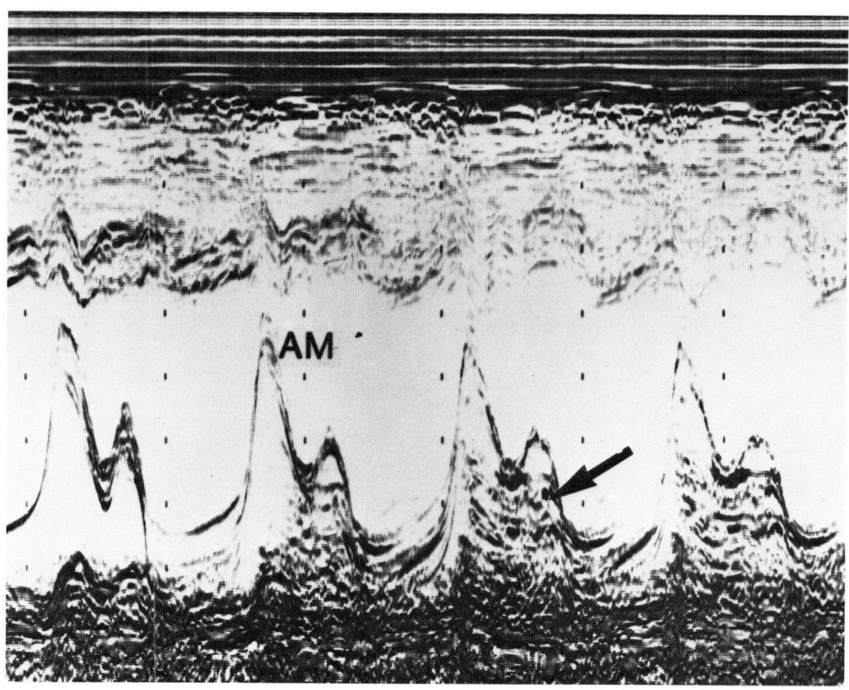

D

significant mitral regurgitation will frequently be found at surgery to have ruptured chordae to the posterior leaflet.[51] If infective endocarditis is present, a vegetation is often visualized.

Rheumatic mitral regurgitation can usually be distinguished from other causes of regurgitation by the frequent presence of thickened leaflets and concomitant commissural fusion typical of some degree of stenosis.

Echocardiography is a very sensitive method for detecting calcification in the mitral valve apparatus.[58] Mitral annular calcification is frequently seen in older subjects; in patients with aortic valve disease, hypertrophic cardiomyopathy, and chronic renal failure; and in some young individuals with no other apparent cardiac abnormality. Although hemodynamically important mitral regurgitation can result from annular calcification, the importance of minor degrees of involvement is not known.

BICUSPID AORTIC VALVE

Bicuspid aortic valve is the most common congenital cardiac defect, being a cause of stenosis as well as regurgitation. The M-mode criterion of an eccentric diastolic closure point of the valve cusps is probably not as reliable a diagnostic feature as previously believed.[59] However, it is frequently possible to determine the number of leaflets present by two-dimensional echocar-

diography, providing the image is of high quality (Fig. 13) and the valve is not significantly distorted by fibrosis or calcification.

AORTIC REGURGITATION

Since the presence of aortic regurgitation is generally apparent on clinical examination, the echocardiographic features of diastolic flutter of the mitral leaflets and the interventricular septum,[60] as well as of the volume-overloaded left ventricle, are usually of little importance in diagnosis of the lesion. However, the underlying etiology of the process can often be inferred echocardiographically.[61] A rheumatic etiology is suggested if mitral stenosis is also present. A bicuspid aortic valve, bacterial endocarditis, aortic aneurysm with or without dissection,[61–64] and prolapsed aortic cusps can all be detected by two-dimensional echocardiography. It is occasionally possible to detect aortic valve echoes in the left ventricular outflow tract, suggesting either a flail or prolapsed aortic cusp or a vegetation secondary to endocarditis (see Figs. 13 and 15).

Echocardiographic measurements of left ventricular dimensions and systolic function have been assessed as a possible means to select the optimal time for operative intervention in patients with chronic aortic regurgitation. Despite limitations in extrapolating volume calculations from a single diameter[65] and the variability

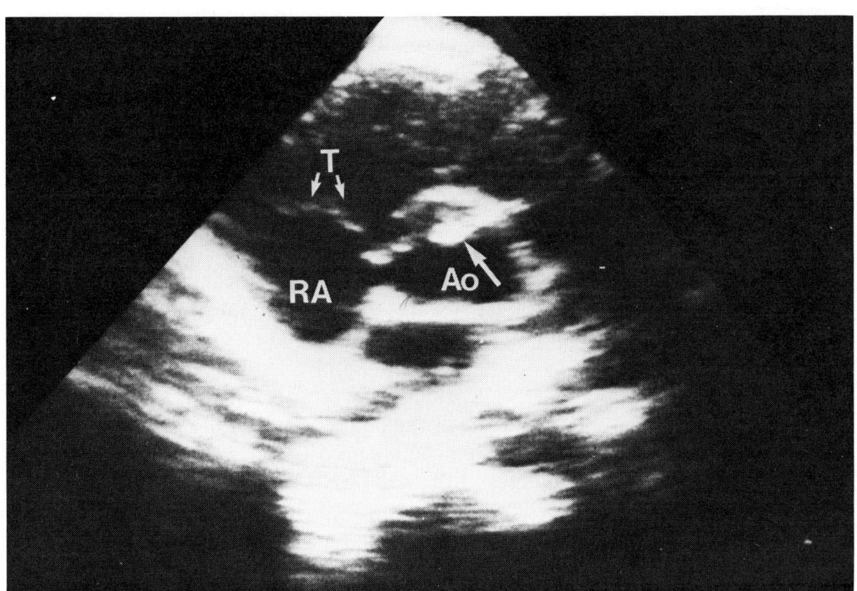

A

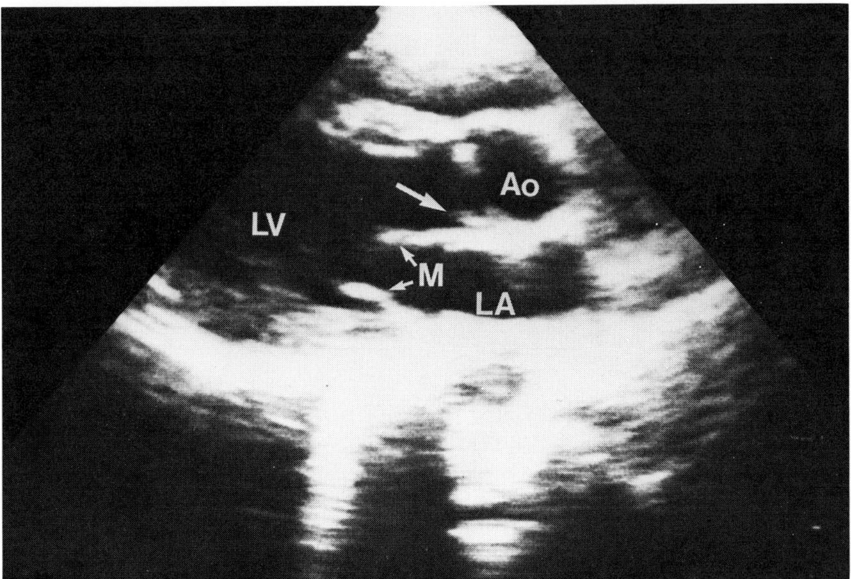

B

FIGURE 13 (*A*) Left parasternal short-axis view at the level of the aortic valve from a patient with a bicuspid aortic valve and aortic regurgitation. The large arrow points to the eccentric location of the valve closure line. The small arrows indicate two leaflets of the tricuspid valve (T). (*B*) Left parasternal long-axis view in the same patient. The posterior cusp (large arrow) prolapses into the left ventricular outflow tract and presumably is the reason for the aortic regurgitation. Ao = aorta; LA = left atrium; RA = right atrium; LV = left ventricle; M = mitral.

in these measurements over a period of time,[66] serial determinations of end-systolic diameter,[67–69] wall stress,[68] and end-diastolic radius/wall thickness ratio[70] all promise to be helpful in this situation. Exercise echocardiography may also prove useful, with a sub-normal rise in peak circumferential fiber-shortening velocity during exercise suggesting the presence of significant left ventricular dysfunction.[12] In acute aortic regurgitation, premature mitral valve closure detected by M-mode echocardiography suggests a very high left ventricular end-diastolic pressure secondary to a large regurgitant volume into a relatively normal sized cavity. Animal studies in our laboratory have documented that the left ventricular size increases only slowly after the onset of acute aortic regurgitation.[71] Patients with this finding almost always require urgent valve replacement despite the apparent initial beneficial response to medical therapy experienced by some of them.

AORTIC STENOSIS

M-mode echocardiography is useful in the detection of aortic valve disease, as indicated by thickened or calcified cusps with or without decreased cusp excursion. In adults with a significant gradient across the valve, thickening and calcification are almost always present (Fig. 14); in children, the aortic leaflets may appear essentially normal, since the beam may traverse a valve plane more proximal than the stenotic orifice. In neither children nor adults does the M-mode assessment of the aortic valve provide reliable data concerning the severity of stenosis. Two-dimensional echocardiography facilitates the measurement of leaflet separation at the valve orifice and therefore may prove more reliable in assessing the severity of obstruction. In addition, the actual aortic valve area can be measured

in a minority of patients. In one study,[72] separation of the aortic cusps of less than 8 mm at the orifice was highly predictive of severe stenosis; greater than 12 mm separation was highly predictive of mild stenosis. Measurements between 8 and 12 mm, which were present in approximately 50 percent of cases, were of little help. Analysis of cusp motion in the short-axis view may also be useful: the greater the degree of restricted motion, the greater the likelihood of more severe stenosis. In children, the peak left ventricular systolic pressure can be estimated echocardiographically by obtaining the left ventricular radius/systolic wall thickness ratio. The simultaneous measurement of systolic blood pressure by the cuff technique allows calculation of the peak systolic gradient.[73] In adults, the relationship between the left ventricular radius/wall thickness ratio and left ventricular systolic pressure is not as close as that in children. However, this technique is usually reliable in identifying those patients with severe aortic stenosis.[74,75]

Infective Endocarditis

Both M-mode and two-dimensional echocardiography are very useful in detecting vegetations and complications of infective endocarditis.[76–79] Two-dimensional

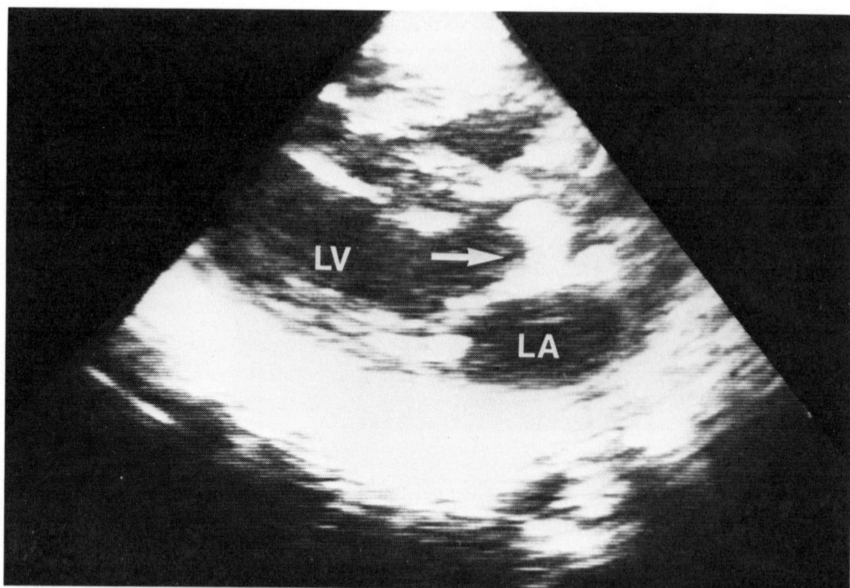

FIGURE 14 (*A*) Left parasternal long-axis view from a patient with considerable thickening and calcification of the aortic valve (arrow). The left ventricular posterior wall and the interventricular septum are hypertrophied. (*B,* opposite) A short-axis view at the level of the aortic valve from another patient with severe aortic stenosis. There is dense calcification of the valve (arrow) with no clearly identifiable leaflet structure. LV = left ventricle; LA = left atrium.

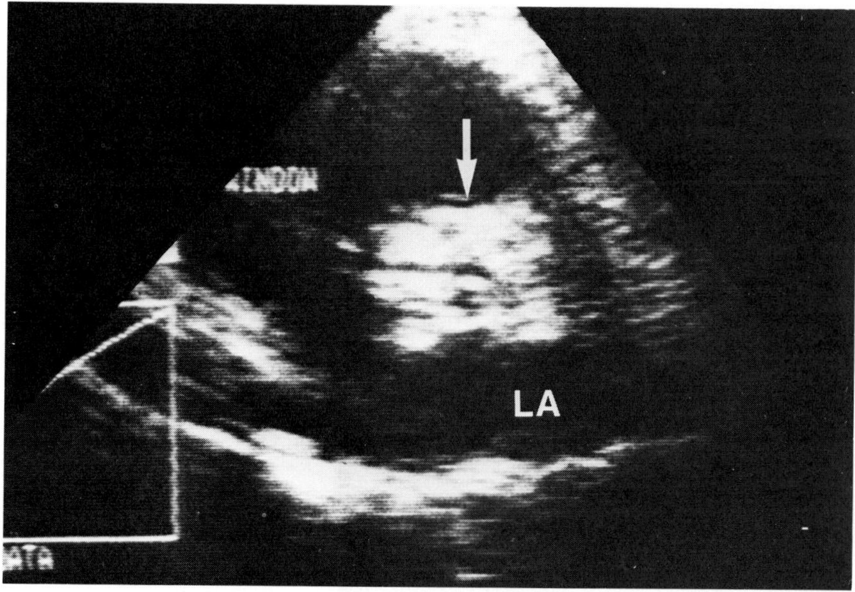

B

echocardiography is preferable to the M-mode technique, vegetations being detected in approximately 50 to 75 percent of documented cases (Fig. 15). Obviously, small vegetations are difficult to detect with certainty when present on prosthetic valves or natural valves with excessive fibrosis or calcification. Occasionally, other abnormalities, such as mitral valve prolapse or a left atrial myxoma, can be confused with a mitral valve vegetation (Fig. 12). Vegetations are generally visualized as masses of variable shape and size, usually with a movement pattern that is independent of the valve motion. In addition, there may also be evidence of complications of endocarditis, such as a flail leaflet owing to a ruptured chorda tendinea or damage to the leaflet itself (Fig. 16). If the initial echocardiographic examination for vegetations is negative in a patient suspected of having endocarditis, subsequent studies may occasionally detect vegetations despite appropriate antibiotic therapy. Patients in whom vegetations are detected have a greater incidence of complications, although there is little correlation between size or shape of the vegetation and subsequent course. For unclear reasons, right-sided vegetations are often larger than those on the left (Fig. 15). Serial studies in patients with vegetations reveal that they may become larger, smaller, or disappear; the latter may be seen following a clinically obvious embolic event (Fig. 15). However, size often changes very little with time, although echo density may increase. Importantly, it does not appear possible to determine accurately if a vegetation is new or old, nor can a change in size over time be considered proof of effective or ineffective antibiotic treatment. Although clinical evidence of

heart failure remains the major criterion for surgical intervention, echocardiographic demonstration of disruption of a mitral leaflet or premature closure of the mitral valve in aortic valve endocarditis correlates well with the need for valvular surgery. Serial observations of left ventricular chamber size and function in some patients may also prove useful in assessing the hemodynamic importance of the lesion. An uncommon complication of infective endocarditis is mitral ring abscess, a condition that has been detected echocardiographically.[80]

Prosthetic Valves

The large variety of prosthetic heart valves currently in use and the several ways that each can malfunction make it necessary for the echocardiographer to be familiar with both the normal and abnormal echocardiographic features of each type of valve. It has been possible to detect abnormalities or prosthetic valves with the use of echocardiography and phonocardiography in approximately 70 percent of documented patients.[81] However, these techniques are generally used to confirm what is clinically suspected, with auscultation continuing to be a sensitive means to detect prosthetic malfunction.[82]

With the ball-in-cage type of prosthesis, delayed or incomplete opening may be due to ball variance, clots, or fibrous ingrowth impeding movement. This is usually easily detected echocardiographically,[83] although a simultaneously recorded phonocardiogram is extremely helpful for timing events. Similarly, a clotted disk valve

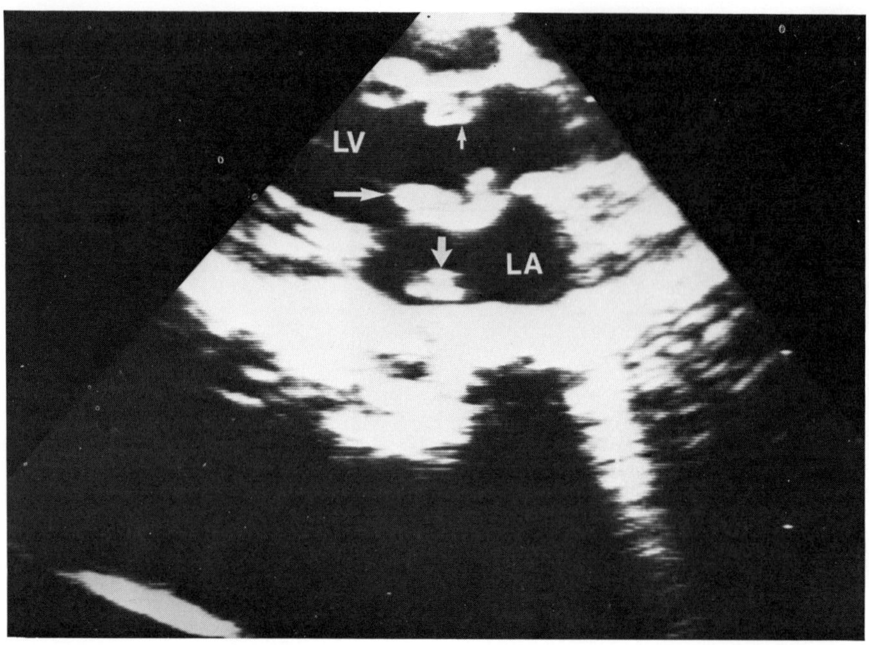

A

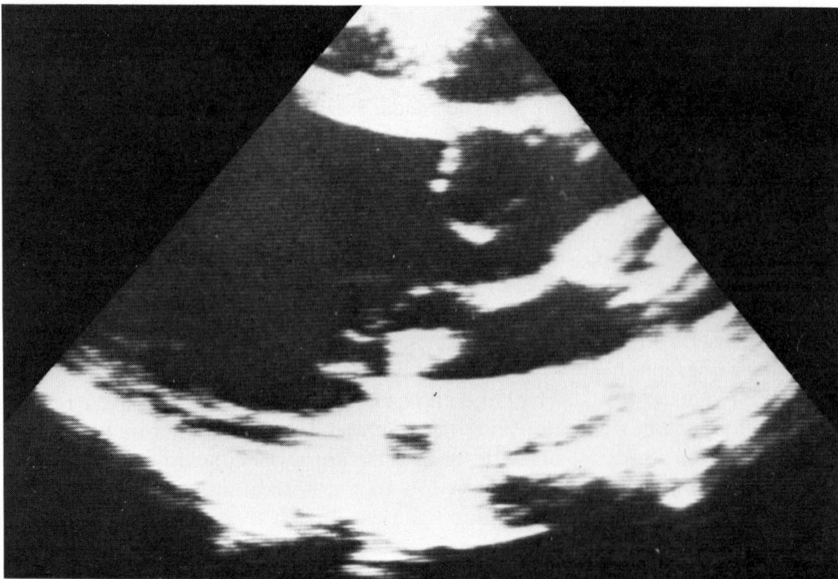

B

FIGURE 15 (*A*) Left parasternal long-axis view from a patient with bacterial endocarditis showing vegetations on the right coronary cusp of the aortic valve (arrow pointing up), the base of the anterior leaflet of the mitral valve (horizontal arrow), and in the left atrium (arrow pointing down). (*B*) A similar view taken after the patient had a cerebral vascular accident. The aortic vegetation could still be found (not shown here), but the one attached to the base of the anterior mitral leaflet could not be seen. It presumably embolized to the cerebral vessel. (*C*, opposite) An off-axis apical four-chamber view from a patient with extensive burns who had a subclavian catheter in place before this study and had a clinical picture suggestive of pulmonary embolism. A large vegetation is present on the tricuspid valve (arrow). LV = left ventricle; LA = left atrium; RV = right ventricle; RA = right atrium.

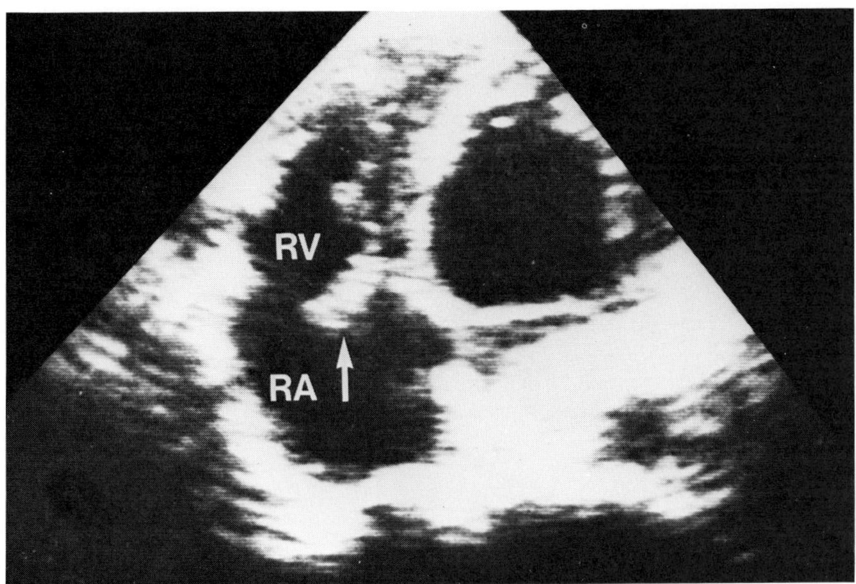

C *(Figure 15)*

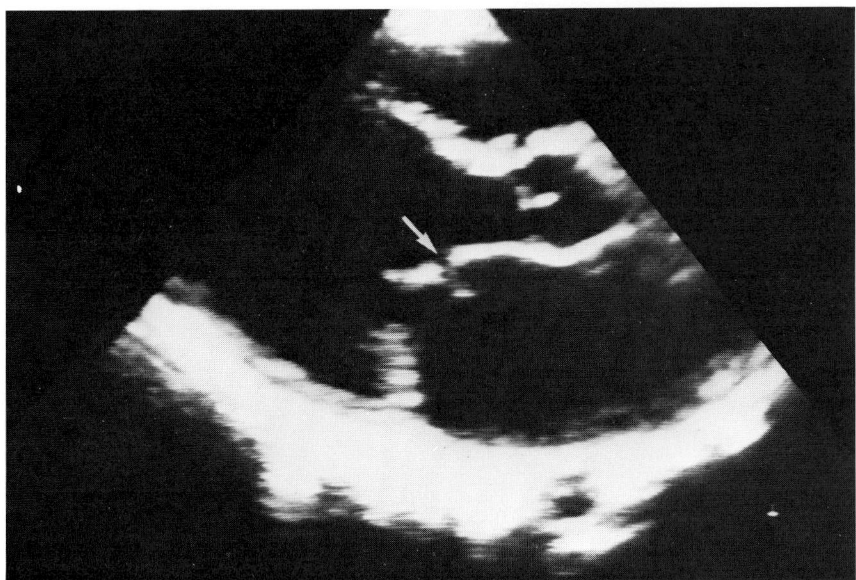

A

FIGURE 16 Left parasternal long-axis views in diastole (*A*) and systole (*B*, p. 38) from a patient with bacterial endocarditis and a perforated anterior leaflet of the mitral valve (upper arrow). The defect in the echo of the anterior mitral leaflet was seen throughout the cardiac cycle in real time. Despite the suggestion of ruptured chordae tendineae of the posterior leaflet in (*B*) (lower arrow), they were intact at surgery. (*C*, p. 38) An off-axis apical four-chamber view from the same patient showing the severe degree of prolapse of the posterior mitral leaflet into the left atrium (LA) (arrow). LV = left ventricle.

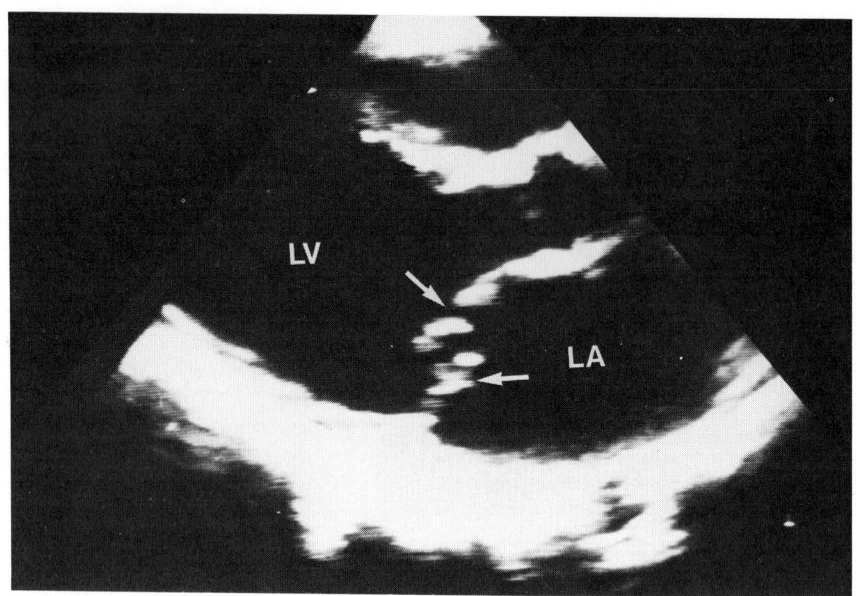

B

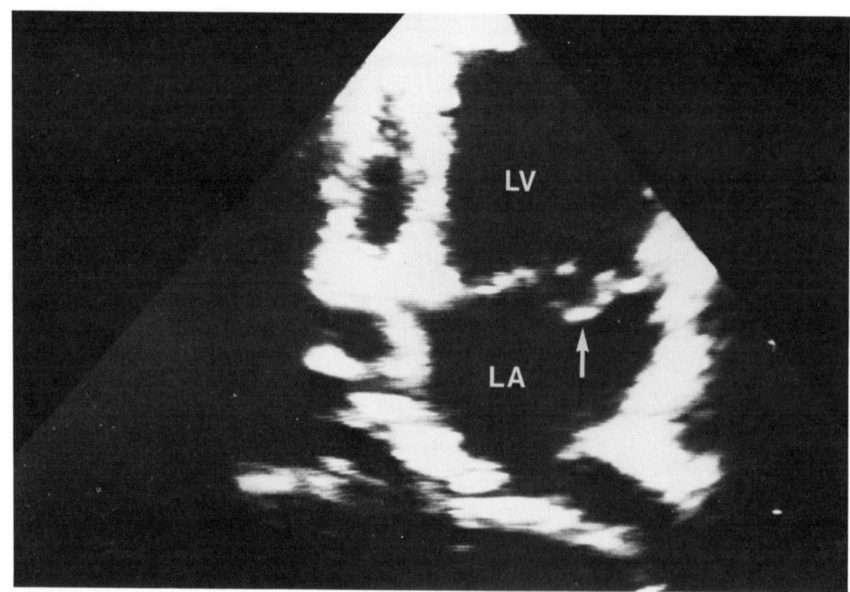

C

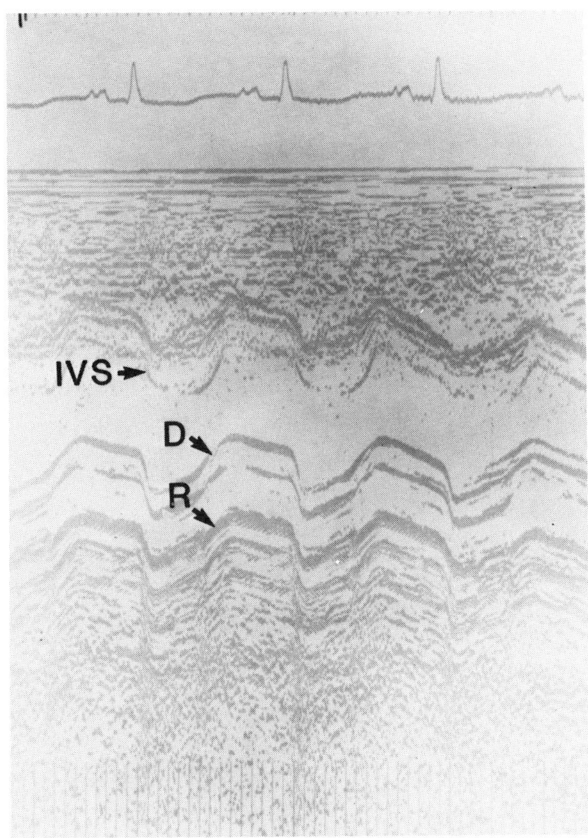

A

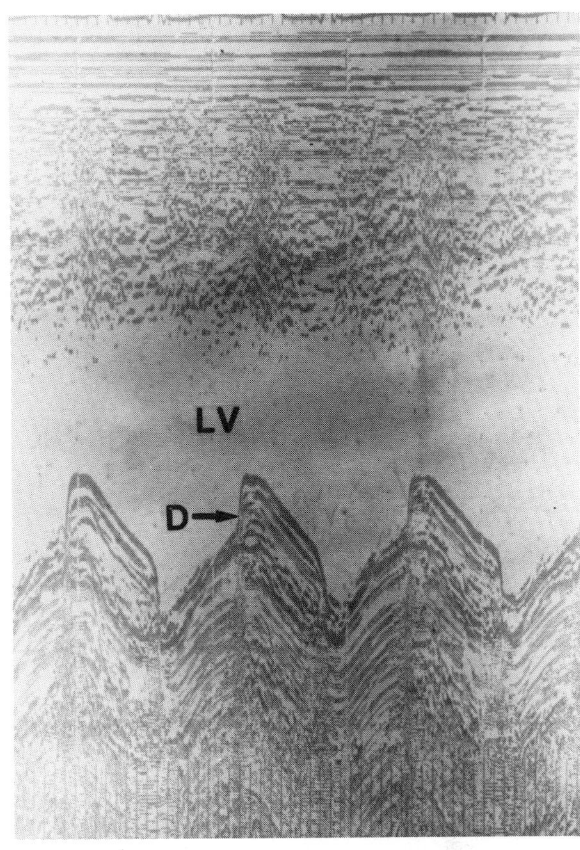

B

FIGURE 17 (*A*) An M-mode tracing from a patient with a clotted Bjork-Shiley mitral prosthetic valve. Note the slow opening motion of the disk (D). (*B*) A postoperative trace from the same patient in whom the valve was replaced. Note the rapid opening motion of the disk. R = prosthetic ring; IVS = interventricular septum; LV = left ventricle.

may be detected by diminished motion of the disk on the M-mode recording (Fig. 17) and by the presence of dense echoes at the orifice on the two-dimensional study. Ring dehiscence can be detected by abnormal mobility of the valve ring compared with that of the surrounding tissues. Vegetations on a prosthetic valve are generally difficult to detect echocardiographically because of the dense echoes produced by the prosthesis itself. Thickened, calcified, and stenotic leaflets of bioprosthetic valves are generally well visualized echocardiographically, the normal leaflet thickness being less than 3 mm. Characteristic features of a torn mitral bioprosthetic leaflet are similar to those of a flail natural one; systolic fluttering is usually evident and valvular echoes are imaged in the left atrium during systole.[84,85]

It is also necessary to be prepared for previously unreported findings associated with complications of prosthetic valves. An example is shown in Fig. 18, which is an M-mode tracing from a patient with a Wada-Cutter prosthesis in the mitral position. No disk motion is evident, but unusual echoes are visible in the left atrium. These obviously were produced from the disk which was found to be free in that chamber at autopsy. Another example is presented in Fig. 19, where the disk of a Beall mitral prosthesis was seen to frequently move abnormally during systole, causing incomplete closure and massive mitral regurgitation.

Cardiomyopathy

HYPERTROPHIC CARDIOMYOPATHY

Hypertrophic cardiomyopathy is associated with a number of M-mode echocardiographic markers, including systolic anterior motion of the mitral valve, disproportionate septal thickness, systolic preclosure of the aortic valve, anterior position of the mitral valve, decreased systolic thickening, and hypokinesis of the septum and small left ventricular cavity with excessive movement of the posterior wall (Fig. 20). None of these markers is found in more than about 85 percent of cases,[86] nor are any of these signs specific for hypertrophy cardiomyopathy. Two-dimensional echocar-

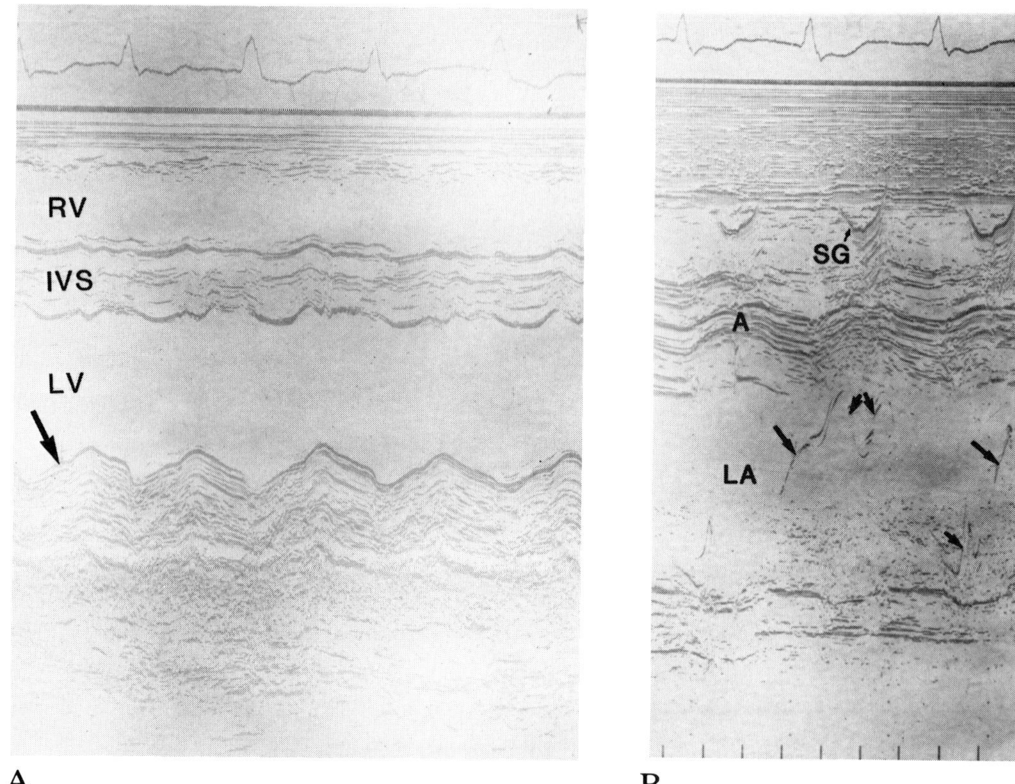

FIGURE 18 M-mode tracings taken at the level of the mitral ring (*A*) and the aortic valve (*B*) from a patient with a Wada-Cutter mitral prosthesis. In (*A*) the mitral ring motion (arrow) is seen, but no disk motion can be appreciated. In (*B*) echoes (arrows) in the left atrium (LA) are from the disk that had broken off the prosthesis and was free in that chamber at necropsy. RV = right ventricle; IVS = interventricular septum; LV = left ventricle; SG = Swan-Ganz flow-directed catheter; A = aortic valve.

diographic has shown that there is considerable variability in the distribution of left ventricular hypertrophy in individual patients.[87] A characteristic stippled appearance of the echoes from the hypertrophied muscle is also frequently apparent (Fig. 21).

Systolic anterior motion (SAM) of the mitral valve is generally considered to be the cause of, or at least contribute to, outflow-tract obstruction in this disorder. SAM is usually not apparent in the absence of an outflow gradient, and if it is marked and prolonged, a resting gradient is almost always present[88,89] (Fig. 20). Effective symptomatic treatment is frequently accompanied by abolition of or a decrease in SAM, although there is not a particularly close correlation between the presence of this sign and symptoms in general. It should also be noted that SAM has been noted in normal subjects,[90] as well as in a variety of pathologic conditions, including fixed subaortic stenosis, pulmonary hypertension, concentric left ventricular hypertrophy, hyperkinetic states, cardiac amyloidosis,[91] mitral valve prolapse, and pericardial effusion, and it is particularly frequent in d-transposition of the great vessels.[89] De-

spite this long list of associations, the prevalence in the general population is very low, so its detection is suggestive of hypertrophic cardiomyopathy.[89]

Asymmetrical septal hypertrophy, although initially considered to be pathognomonic of hypertrophic cardiomyopathy, has proven to be a relatively nonspecific finding, having been reported in a wide variety of conditions as well as in normal subjects.[86,91,92] If the criterion is changed to a septal/posterior wall thickness ratio of 1.6 rather than 1.3, the specificity increases but the sensitivity decreases.[93] Certainly, the two-dimensional echocardiographic appearance of the distribution of the hypertrophy in some patients provides an explanation for the absence of asymmetrical septal hypertrophy on M-mode examination.[87,94] Hypertrophy is confined to the anterior septum in approximately 10 percent of patients and to both the anterior and posterior portions in 20 percent, whereas in 50 percent of patients both septum and free wall are involved. However, in approximately 20 percent of patients the anterior basal septum is normal or only-minimally thickened, thereby explaining the occasional

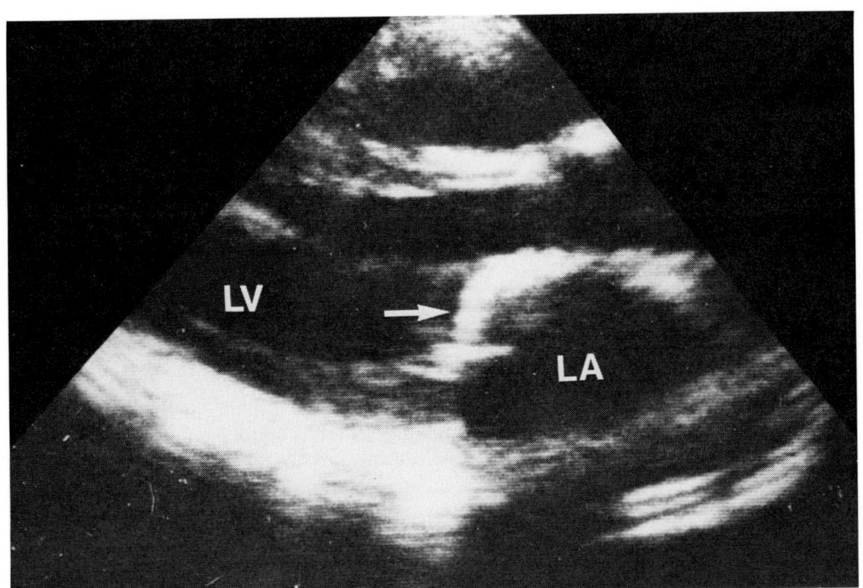

A

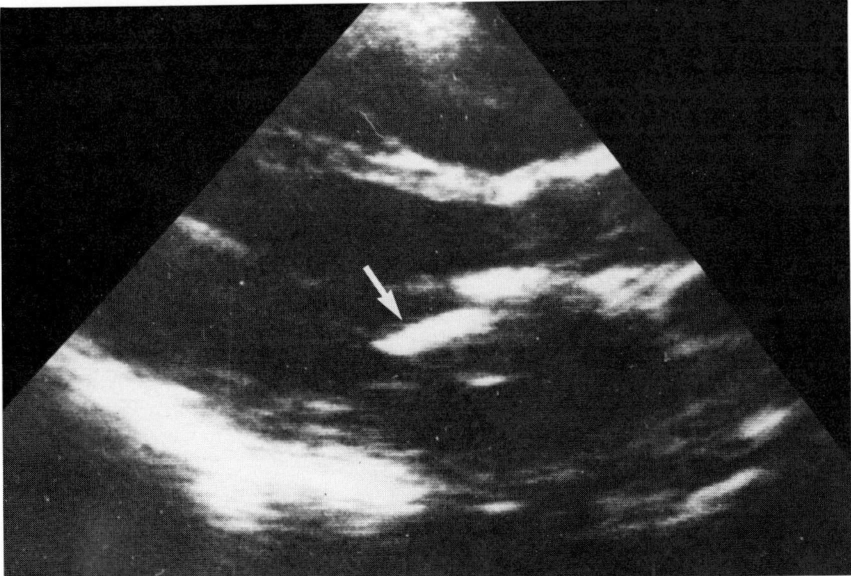

B

FIGURE 19 Left parasternal long-axis views from a patient with a malfunctiong Beall mitral prosthesis. In (*A*) the disk (arrow) is normally oriented in midsystole. In (*B*) the disk is at an abnormal angle in early systole, the posterior part not moving toward the left atrium (LA). The patient had an intermittent murmur consistent with mitral regurgitation and was in severe heart failure. LV = left ventricle.

finding of a normal septal/free wall thickness ratio on an M-mode echocardiogram. Conversely, if the septum is sharply angulated anteriorly from the anterior aortic root in normal subjects, a false impression of discrepant septal hypertrophy may be apparent on an M-mode tracing. Although most false negative and false positive diagnoses can be avoided by use of the two-dimensional technique, the broad spectrum of this disease makes it important that the echocardiographic findings always be carefully correlated with the clinical presentation.

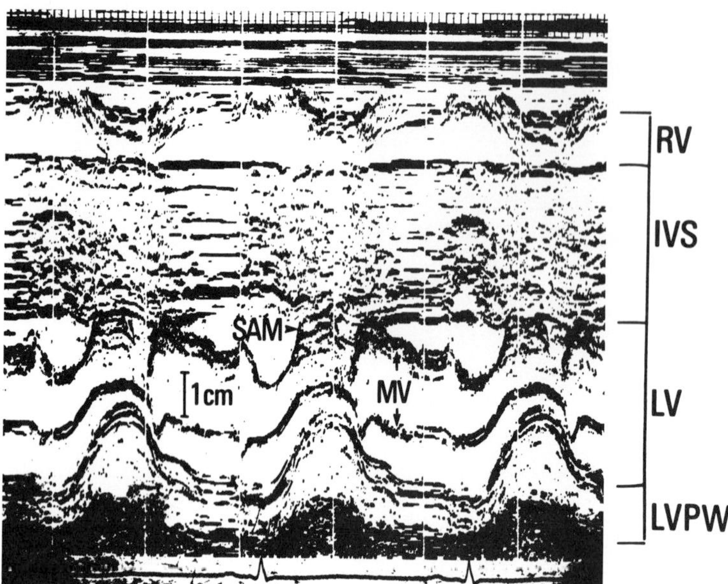

FIGURE 20 An M-mode recording from a patient with hypertrophic obstructive cardiomyopathy. There is systolic anterior motion of the mitral valve (SAM), a reduced mitral E-F slope, an almost akinetic and very thick interventricular septum (IVS) with virtually no systolic thickening, no hypertrophy of the left ventricular posterior wall (LVPW), and a relatively small left ventricle (LV). RV = right ventricle.

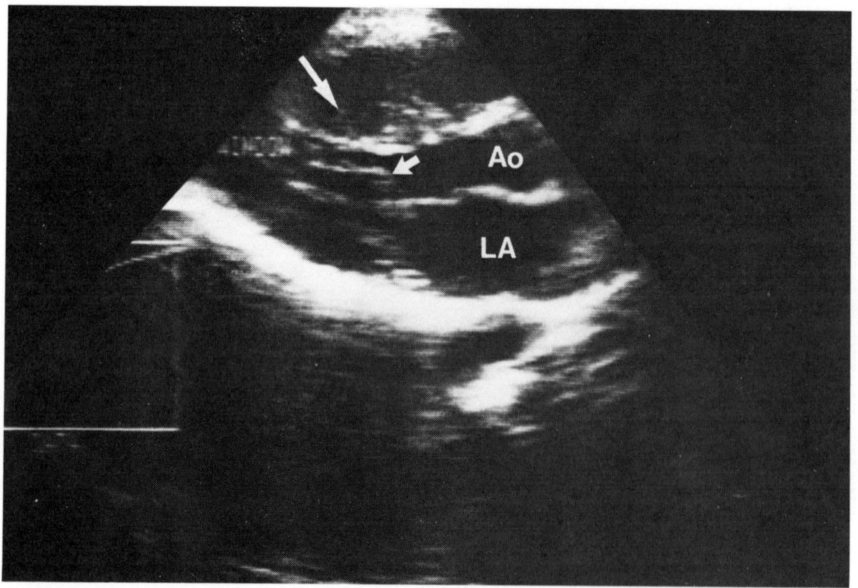

A

FIGURE 21 (*A*) A left parasternal long-axis view from a patient with hypertrophic obstructive cardiomyopathy. The interventricular septum (large arrow) is considerably hypertrophied, and systolic anterior motion of the chordae tendineae of the anterior mitral leaflet is seen (small arrow). (*B* and *C*, opposite) Apical four-chamber views from two patients with the same disease. The interventricular septa (arrows) are very thick, and there is increased echo-density as well. LA = left atrium; Ao = aorta; LV = left ventricle.

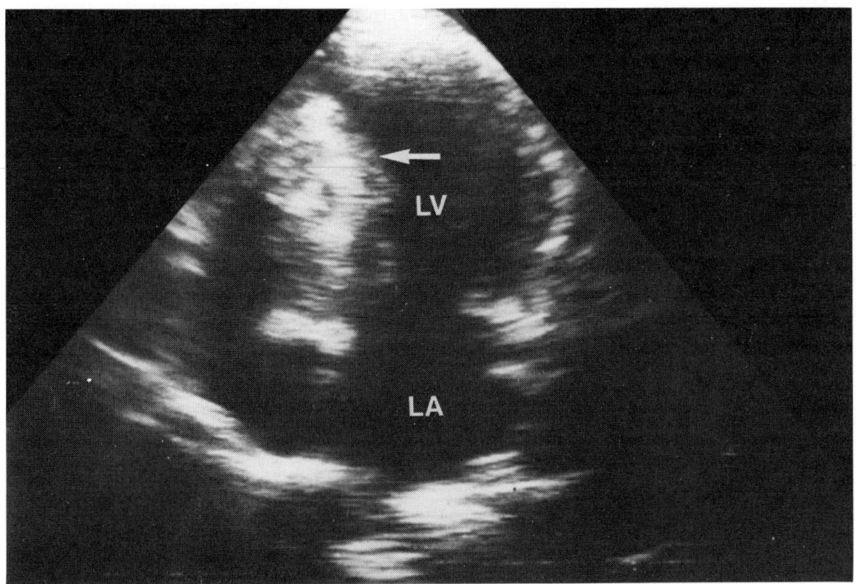

B

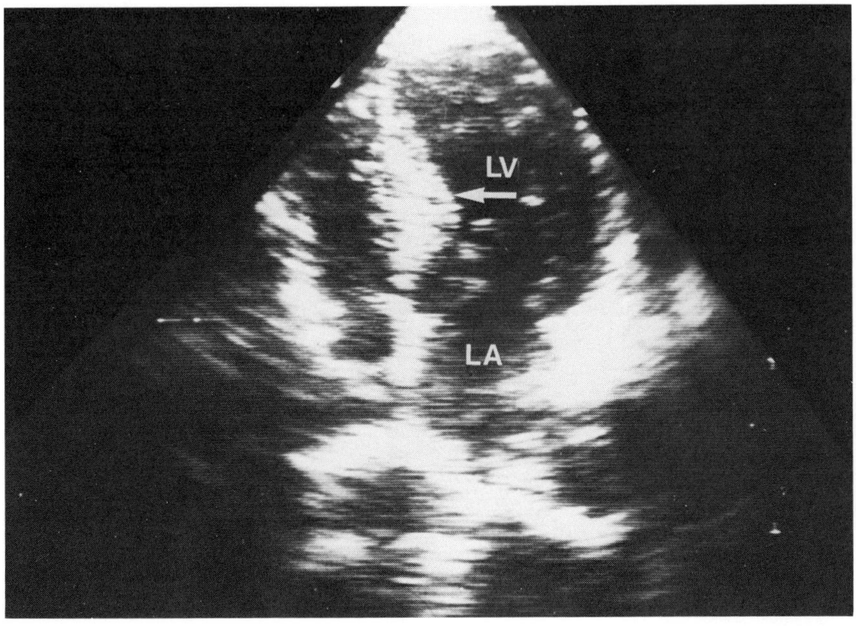

C

CONGESTIVE CARDIOMYOPATHY

Echocardiography is very helpful in the detection of congestive cardiomyopathy. This diagnosis is suggested by the presence on M-mode examination of enlarged left ventricular systolic and diastolic dimensions with reduced wall-thickening indices. Other indicators of decreased systolic function, such as increased mitral E-point–septal separation, decreased excursion of the posterior aortic wall, and enlargement of other cardiac chambers, are usually present. Although the M-mode examination provides suggestive evidence for this diagnosis, two-dimensional studies are clearly desirable. In this way, the entire left ventricle can be assessed, and the chance of missing a segmental wall-motion abnormality secondary to ischemic heart disease is considerably reduced.

RESTRICTIVE CARDIOMYOPATHY

The sensitivity of echocardiography in detecting various forms of restrictive cardiomyopathy has not been determined, with most of the reports to date dealing with amyloid heart disease. The characteristic M-mode findings in amyloidosis are those of a normal or small left ventricular cavity, increased wall thickness with decreased systolic thickening, and increased left atrial size. A small pericardial effusion is usually present. Two-dimensional echocardiographic findings may also include the detection of thickened papillary muscles, right ventricular free wall, valves, and the interatrial septum[91] (Fig. 22). There is frequently a sparkling appearance of the myocardium, the septum being more frequently involved than the posterior wall. An extremely important clue to the diagnosis of cardiac amyloid is an inverse relationship between electrocardiographic voltage and echocardiographic measures of wall thickness.[95] The differentiation between amyloid and constrictive pericarditis can be facilitated by echocardiography, since increased wall thickness is not an expected finding in the latter condition. In hemochromatosis, left ventricular wall thickness and cavity size may be increased, but the findings are not specific.[96]

Pericardial Disease
PERICARDIAL EFFUSION

Echocardiography remains the most useful technique for the detection of pericardial effusion. M-mode echocardiography is usually all that is required to detect fluid and to provide a rough estimate of the size of an effusion. However, on occasion, two-dimensional

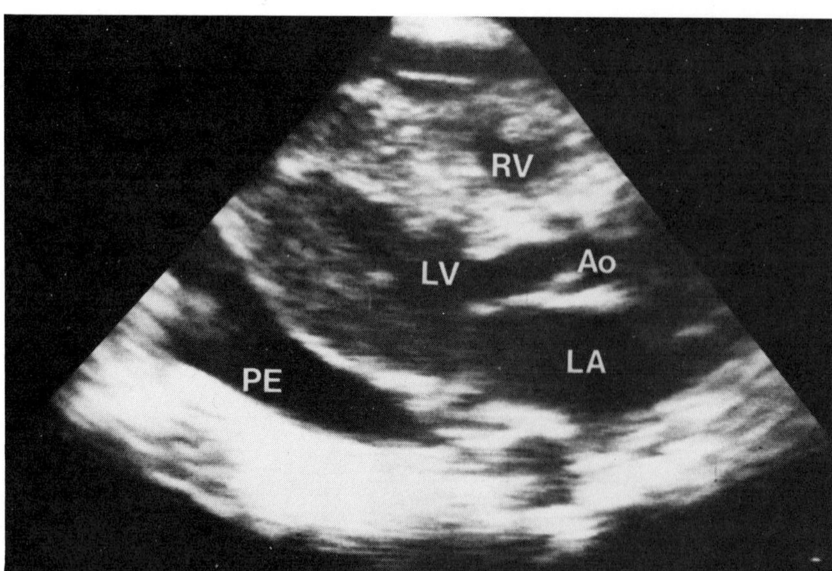

A

FIGURE 22 (*A*) A left parasternal long-axis view from a patient with cardiac amyloidosis showing the thick-walled left and right ventricles, a small left ventricular cavity, and a pericardial effusion (PE). (*B*, opposite) A four-chamber view from the same patient. The septum and right ventricular wall appear particularly echo-dense. RV = right ventricle; LV = left ventricle; RA = right atrium; LA = left atrium; PE = pericardial effusion; Ao = aorta.

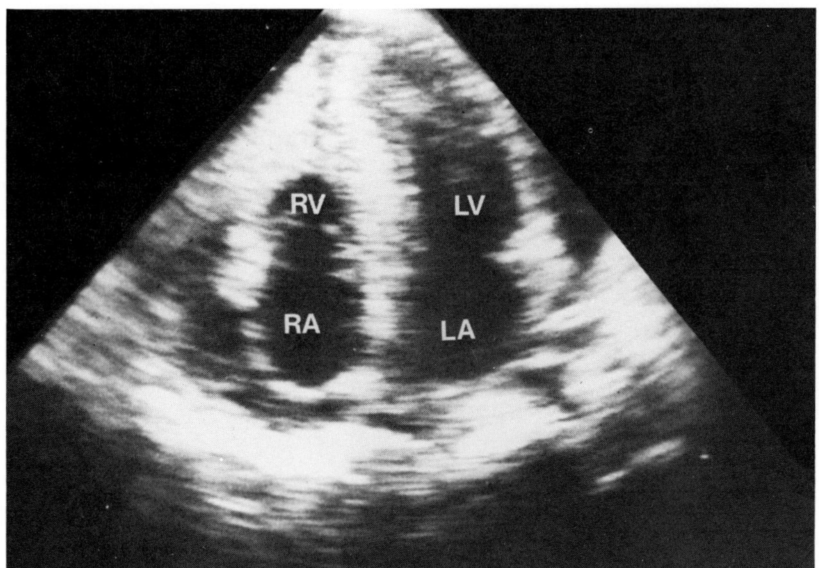

B   (*Figure 22*)

echocardiography is required to avoid confusing pericardial effusion with a number of other conditions, including mitral annular calcification, enlarged left atrium, tumor, fibrosis, medial angulation of the transducer, pleural effusion, and unrecognized imaging of the descending aorta. In addition, a loculated effusion will occasionally be missed if only the M-mode technique is employed. The distribution of fluid around the heart is relatively uniform in moderate-sized effusions, although small effusions tend to collect posteriorly near the atrioventricular groove or more apically. In large effusions, disproportionately greater amounts of fluid tend to be found posteriorly and toward the apex[97] (Fig. 23).

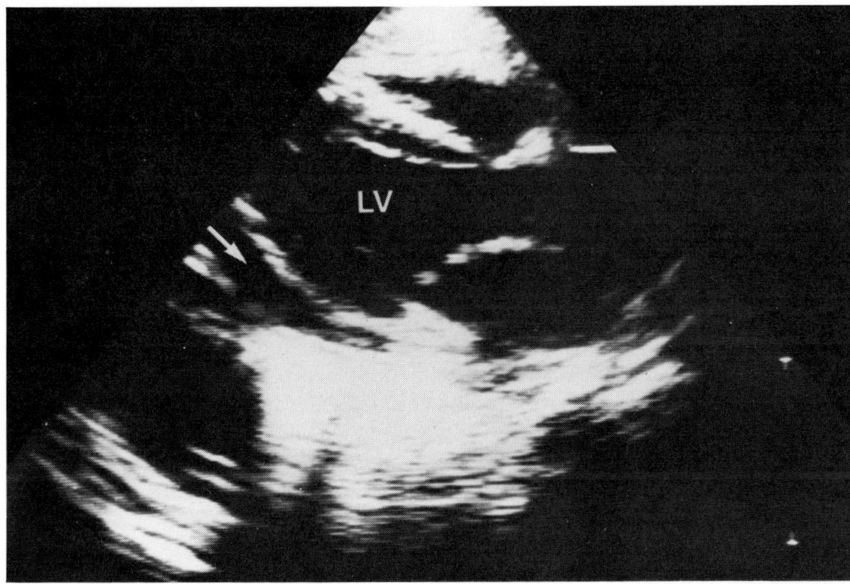

A

FIGURE 23 (*A*) A left parasternal long-axis view from a patient with a small posterior pericardial effusion (arrow). (*B*, opposite) An apical four-chamber view from a patient with a very large malignant pericardial effusion (PE). LV = left ventricle; RV = right ventricle.

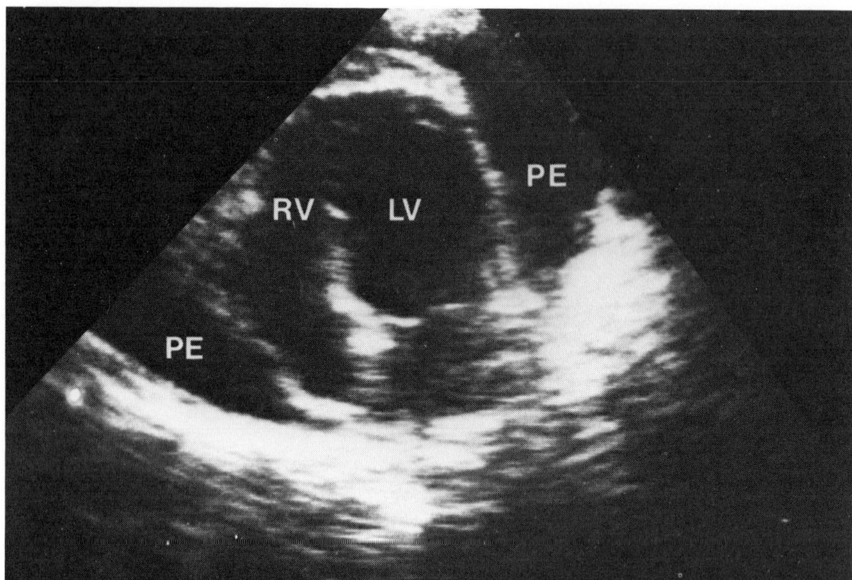

B

Cardiac tamponade remains a clinical diagnosis, although there are a number of echocardiographic features that may be helpful in suggesting the presence of a hemodynamically important effusion.[98] Marked swinging of the heart, with or without some rotation, exaggerated anterior right ventricular wall motion, and a decreased early diastolic closing velocity of the mitral valve have all been noted. An inspiratory increase in the right ventricular diameter and decrease in the left ventricular diameter are suggestive of tamponade, although these also may be present in some patients with obstructive pulmonary disease with a paradoxical pulse.[98] All these findings tend to decrease or disappear after pericardiocentesis. Pseudoprolapse of the mitral valve, found in some patients with large pericardial effusions, is thought to be due to a posterior swing of the entire heart during ventricular systole.

Pericardial metastases may be recognized by two-dimensional echocardiography as irregular, mobile, cauliflower-like masses protruding into the pericardial space.[99] Pericardial adhesions can also occasionally be identified.

CONSTRICTIVE PERICARDITIS

Although findings are not specific, echocardiography may be helpful in suggesting pericardial thickening with hemodynamically important constriction. A variety of M-mode features have been noted in fibrous, calcific, effusive-constrictive, and fibroplastic pericardial disease.[100,101] Parallel motion of visceral and parietal pericardial echoes with or without an intervening echo-free space suggests fibrosis, adhesions, or calcification.

A posterior echo-free space with an apparent thick band of echoes from the visceral pericardium suggests effusive-constrictive pericarditis, whereas numerous random echoes in the pericardium may represent coagulated pericardial exudate of fibroplastic pericarditis. A number of other abnormalities have been noted in some patients with constrictive pericarditis. These include abnormal septal motion and the absence of continued left ventricular enlargement during the latter part of diastole. The presence of normal wall thickness and systolic muscle thickening is helpful in distinguishing constrictive pericarditis from restrictive cardiomyopathy; increased wall thickness and decreased systolic wall thickening are common features in the latter condition.

CONGENITAL HEART DISEASE

Echocardiography is now firmly established as a reliable diagnostic method in patients with known or suspected congenital heart disease. The technique is harmless and can be performed on ill neonates without sedation. Although M-mode echocardiography has proved useful in the diagnosis of even complex anomalies, the two-dimensional technique with superior capability for spatial orientation of structures has greatly improved the accuracy of anatomic definition. The utilization of contrast studies[102] and, more recently, Doppler ultrasound usually allows the examiner to determine the physiologic significance of the anatomic abnormalities. It must be stressed, however, that proper utilization of the technique requires that the examiner be totally familiar with the spectrum of possible defects. Given this, careful echocardiographic examination usually results in accurate diagnostic information, thereby obviating the need for cardiac catheterization in some and allowing the invasive procedure to be more focused in others.

The utility of two-dimensional echocardiography in congenital heart disease is enhanced by the use of two views not routinely used in acquired disease, namely, the subcostal[103] and the suprasternal approaches.[104] From the subcostal four-chamber view both the ventricular and atrial septa lie perpendicular to the ultrasound beam, their definition thereby being enhanced (see Fig. 7). The suprasternal view allows detailed assessment of the proximal great vessels and is particularly useful in patients suspected of having coarctation of the aorta.

Left-to-Right-Shunts

ATRIAL SEPTAL DEFECT

M-mode echocardiography has proved to be a sensitive tool in detecting atrial septal defects. The finding of an enlarged right ventricle with paradoxic interventricular septal movement (Fig. 24) is not specific, however, and is observed in a variety of conditions that cause volume

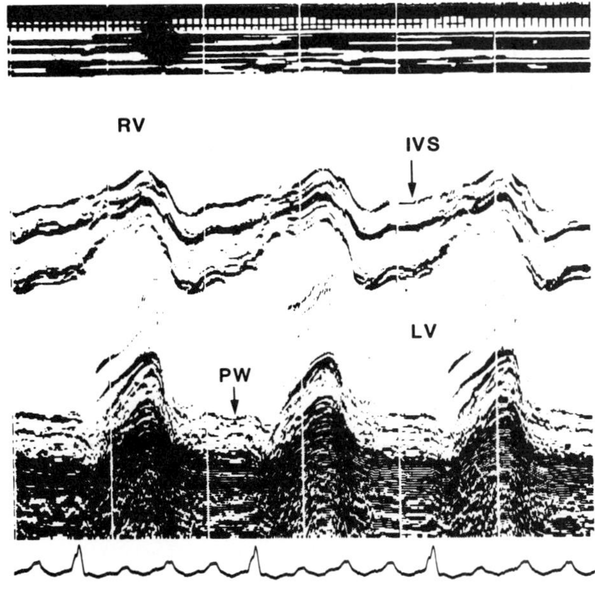

FIGURE 24 An M-mode tracing from a patient with a secundum atrial septal defect and a large left-to-right shunt. IVS = interventricular septum; RV = right ventricle; LV = left ventricle; PW = left ventricular posterior wall.

(or extreme pressure) overload on the right ventricle.[105,106] Indeed, data from our laboratory[107] and others[108,109] suggest that the abnormal septal movement is the result of a reversal in the normal transseptal diastolic pressure gradient such that the right ventricular pressure transiently exceeds that in the left ventricle. This results in a leftward shift in the septum, so that at the onset of systole it may be bulging into the left ventricular cavity. Credence is given to this by two-dimensional echocardiographic findings[110] (Fig. 25). In the left parasternal short-axis view, the normal curvature of the ventricular septum is flattened at end-diastole but reassumes its normal shape at end-systole. This abnormal shape of the septum at end-diastole not only explains movement toward the transducer during systole but also accounts in part for the increase in right ventricular diastolic dimension.

Early reports of direct visualization of atrial septal defects by two-dimensional echocardiography utilized the apical four-chamber view. This approach is not reliable, however, because of echo dropout. The subcostal transducer position has proved far superior.[111] Secundum defects can be distinguished from primum and sinus venosus locations. In patients with primum defects, an associated cleft in the anterior mitral leaflet can be directly imaged in the parasternal short-axis view.[112] The injection of saline or other contrast media into a peripheral vein has also proved useful in the detection of atrial septal defect. Apical four-chamber views allow visualization of contrast medium traversing the atrial septum into the left atrium in those with increased pulmonary vascular resistance.[113] Even in those with uncomplicated atrial septal defects, some microbubbles usually cross the septum and are visible in the left atrium,[114] a phenomenon that can be accentuated by imaging during a Valsalva maneuver.[113] Finally, even in those patients without bidirectional shunting, the presence of a defect in the atrial septum can often be inferred by detecting a negative contrast effect in the right atrium; the contrast medium near the septal defect is cleared by blood free of the contrast medium entering from the left atrium.[115]

VENTRICULAR SEPTAL DEFECT

Occasionally, a large ventricular septal defect can be visualized with M-mode echocardiography by the absence of septal echoes on scans from the aortic root to the left ventricle.[116] In the presence of a ventricular septal defect without pulmonary arterial hypertension, the magnitude of the shunt can be estimated by determining the ratio of left atrial dimension to aortic root size.[117] The use of two-dimensional echocardiography, particularly with the subcostal views, allows direct visualization of the defect in the majority of

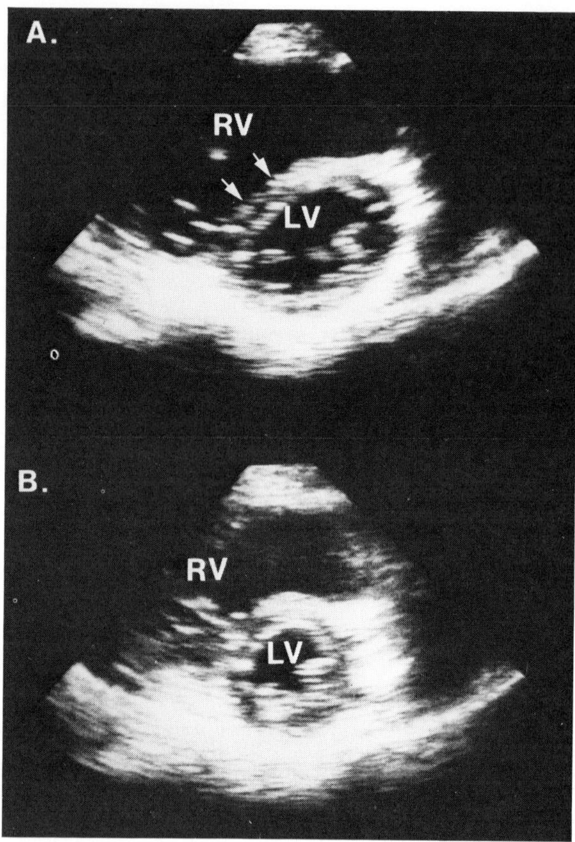

FIGURE 25 Left parasternal short-axis views from a patient with an atrial septal defect. (*A*) A diastolic frame showing the flattened curvature of the septum (arrows). (*B*) A systolic frame that shows the normal circular shape of the left ventricle (LV). The right ventricle (RV) is enlarged.

cases.[118] False positive diagnoses are minimized by utilizing multiple views[119] and also by the detection of broadened septal echoes at the margin of the defect, the so-called T sign. Injection into peripheral veins is also useful, since negative contrast (in the right ventricle) can be readily appreciated in the uncomplicated cases, and in those with raised pulmonary vascular resistance, some contrast medium will cross the defect and be imaged in the left ventricle.[118]

PATENT DUCTUS ARTERIOSUS

As with ventricular septal defect, there are no M-mode findings characteristic of a patent ductus arteriosus; an indication of the shunt size can be obtained from measurements of the left atrial and left ventricular size.[117] The two-dimensional technique, utilizing the parasternal short-axis view, does allow direct visualization of the ductus[120] and provides additional information concerning the shape and size of the defect.

ENDOCARDIAL CUSHION DEFECTS

The most consistent M-mode echocardiographic abnormality noted in patients with endocardial cushion defect is the apparent movement of the anterior leaflet of the mitral valve across the ventricular septum,[121] a feature that is noted in both the partial and complete forms. Two-dimensional imaging from the cardiac apex or the subcostal position, however, allows visualization of the ostium primum atrial septal defect, as well as the attachment of the atrioventricular valve to the crest of the septum, and characterization of the common anterior valve leaflet.[122] In addition, the left parasternal short-axis view allows direct visualization of the associated cleft anterior mitral leaflet.[112,122]

Right-to-Left Shunts

Except for the Eisenmenger reaction occurring in those abnormalities discussed earlier, right-to-left shunting generally reflects complex congenital heart disease. Echocardiography by the experienced observer will allow accurate definition of the anatomy in most instances; the simultaneous use of contrast medium and/or Doppler echocardiography is frequently sufficient to determine the physiologic importance of each aspect of the lesion.

Arriving at a detailed anatomic and physiologic diagnosis is facilitated if a systematic approach is used to determine ventricular situs, as well as great artery relations to each other, to the ventricles, to atrioventricular valves, and to the ventricular septum. The venous atrium can be correctly identified by following the course of the inferior vena cava with the transducer in the subcostal position. Identification of the arterial atrium is facilitated by observing pulmonary vein entry either from the apical or subcostal four-chamber views. Ventricular situs is suggested by a number of echocardiographic features. The morphologic right ventricle is characterized by a tricuspid valve, chordal insertion in the septum, the presence of a moderator band, a conus separating the tricuspid valve from the semilunar valve, and a triangular-shaped cavity with an irregular endocardial surface. A morphologic left ventricle is characterized by a bicuspid (mitral) valve, two discrete papillary muscles, and a smooth endocardium in a circular or oval cavity. By far the most useful sign is the identification of the atrioventricular valves. Although other features may be helpful, the most reliable aid in identification of the tricuspid valve is its more distal attachment to the interventricular septum compared with that of the mitral valve. This is best appreciated from an apical four-chamber view (see Fig. 5). The parasternal short-axis is best for determining the relationship of the great arteries. Normally, the aorta is visualized as a circular structure with the right ventricular outflow tract and pulmonary artery positioned anteriorly and wrapping around in a clockwise direction (see Fig. 3). In transposition of the great arteries, the two vessels run parallel with the aorta anterior to the pulmonary artery. Once the great vessels have been identified, then it is possible to determine from which chamber each arises. Determination of mitral-semilunar valve continuity and the relationship of each great artery to the ventricular septum completes the exercise.

CONDITIONS WITH AORTIC OVERRIDE

Tetralogy of Fallot, truncus arteriosus, and pulmonary atresia–ventricular septal defect all are associated with an enlarged aorta that overrides the crest of the ventricular septum, thereby resulting in a septal defect (Fig. 26). With care in technique, these anatomic features can be detected by M-mode echocardiography, although the left parasternal long-axis two-dimensional view is most reliable.[123,124] This view will also document the normal mitral-aortic valve continuity present in these anomalies. Visualization of the pulmonary valve and a hypoplastic right ventricular outflow tract distinguishes tetralogy of Fallot from both truncus and pulmonary atresia–ventricular septal defect. In patients with pulmonary atresia–ventricular septal defect, a recent report indicates that it is possible to reliably image and measure the size of the right pulmonary

artery utilizing the suprasternal transducer position.[125] This is important in planning operative therapy; if the right pulmonary artery is large, then a one-staged correction can be carried out without the need for a palliative shunt to stimulate arterial growth.

TRANSPOSITION OF THE GREAT ARTERIES

In transposition, two great arteries leave the heart, although these run parallel rather than exhibiting the normal clockwise rotation of the right ventricular outflow tract. There is normal ventricular situs and mitral-semilunar valve (pulmonary) and ventricular septum–great artery continuity. In the parasternal short-axis view obtained through the great vessels,[126] two circular structures are imaged, with the aorta being anterior to the pulmonary artery (Fig. 27). Identification of the vessels is aided by angulating the transducer superiorly and detecting the posterior angulation of the pulmonary artery and its subsequent bifurcation. Other views are required to fully determine the extent of associated anomalies.

DOUBLE-OUTLET RIGHT VENTRICLE

In this uncommon condition, the ventricular situs is normal, but no great vessel can be identified to leave the left ventricle. In the parasternal long-axis view, no

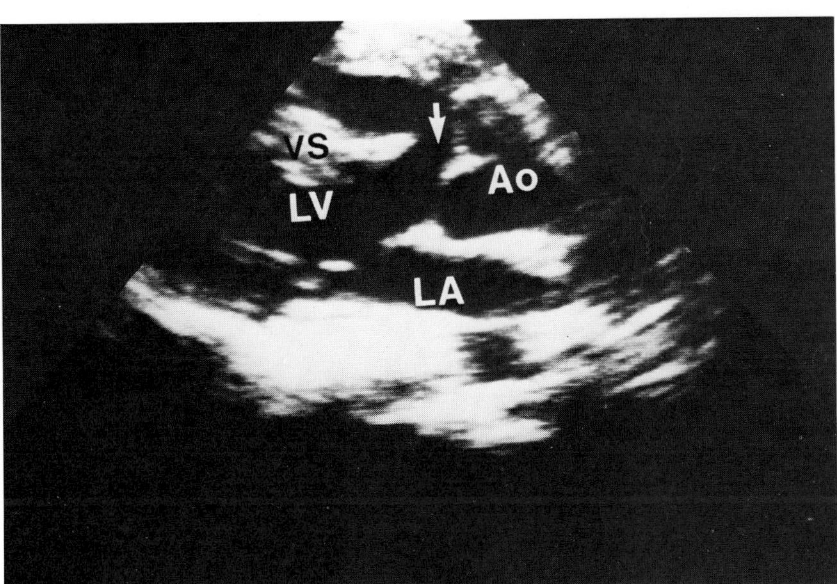

FIGURE 26 A left parasternal long-axis view from a patient with tetralogy of Fallot. Note the large aortic root (Ao) overriding the interventricular septum (VS) with a large ventricular septal defect (arrow). The pulmonary outflow tract is very small. LV = left ventricle; LA = left atrium.

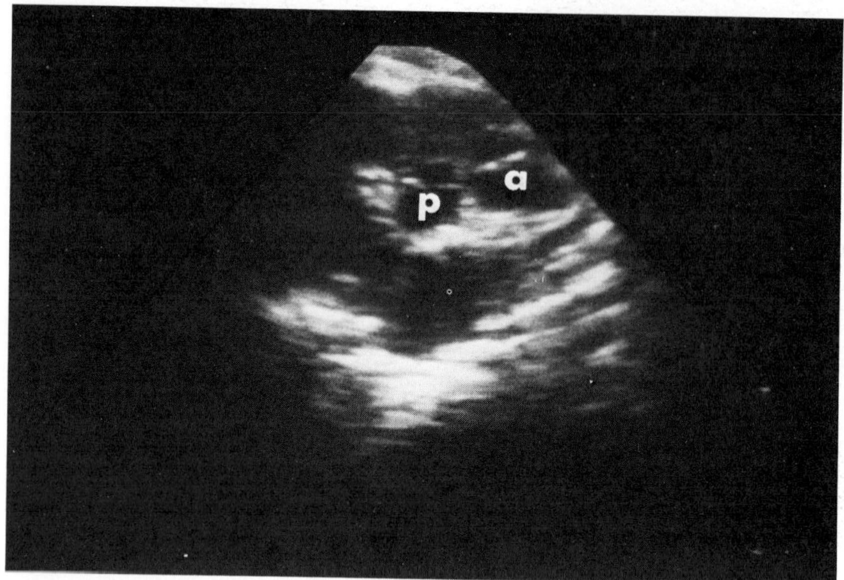

FIGURE 27 A left parasternal short-axis view at the level of the great vessels from a patient with transposition of the great arteries. The aorta (a) is anterior and to the left of the pulmonary artery (p).

continuity is detected between the anterior mitral leaflet and either semilunar valve; this is identified as an area of echo-dense conal tissue at the hinge point of the anterior mitral leaflet.[127] In the parasternal short-axis views, it is possible to recognize that both great arteries arise anteriorly to the ventricular septum and lie side by side in an anterior position.[126] A ventricular septal defect of variable position is present and can usually be visualized from the subcostal transducer position.

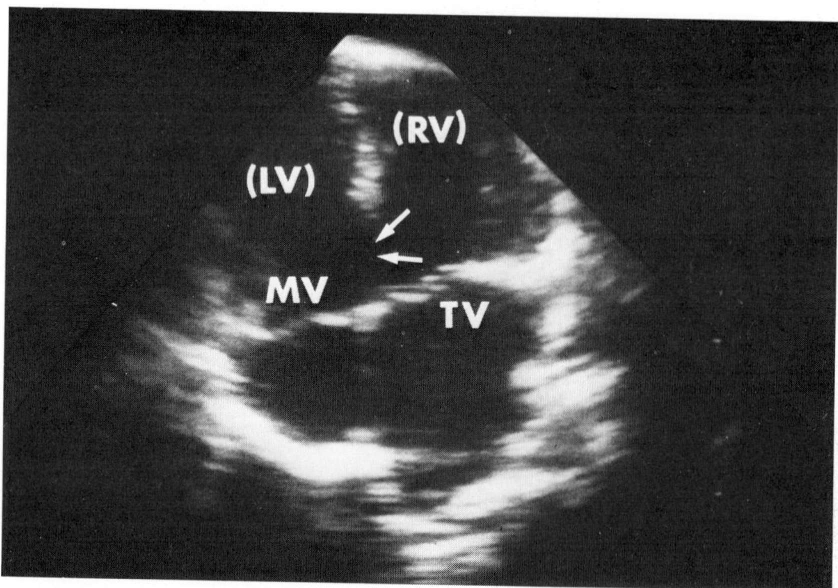

FIGURE 28 An apical four-chamber view from an adult with corrected transposition of the great arteries. The tricuspid valve (TV) is on the left and the mitral valve (MV) is on the right. A large ventricular septal defect (arrows) is also well visualized. RV = anatomic right ventricle; LV = anatomic left ventricle.

CORRECTED TRANSPOSITION OF THE GREAT ARTERIES

In this condition there is atrioventricular and ventriculoarterial discordance.[128] Thus a morphologic right ventricle lies to the left and posterior to the morphologic left ventricle and attaches to an anteriorly positioned aorta. Utilizing the apical four-chamber view, the left-sided and posterior ventricle has a tricuspid atrioventricular valve best identified by its more distal attachment to the ventricular septum[128,129] (Fig. 28). From the parasternal short-axis view at the level of the great vessels the aorta is identified occupying a position anterior and to the left of the pulmonary artery. Other anomalies, such as a ventricular septal defect, are commonly observed.

TOTAL ANOMALOUS PULMONARY VENOUS DRAINAGE

The clinical spectrum of this disorder is great, varying from right ventricular volume overload to severely ill neonates with cyanosis and pulmonary edema. The M-mode features of this disorder are not specific, but the ability to directly image pulmonary veins entering the left atrium, from either the apical or subcostal four-chamber views by two-dimensional echocardiography, proves very useful in excluding this diagnosis.[130]

EBSTEIN'S ANOMALY OF THE TRICUSPID VALVE

Although not strictly a complex congenital malformation, patients with Ebstein's anomaly present the differential diagnosis of cyanotic heart disease. The M-mode features of this disorder, which include a large right-sided cavity, a large excursion to the tricuspid valve, and delayed tricuspid valve closure,[131] are useful but are neither totally sensitive nor specific. The two-dimensional apical four-chamber view (Fig. 29) allows direct imaging of the displaced tricuspid valve structure.[132] The injection of contrast medium into the peripheral vein allows detection of the associated tricuspid regurgitation[133] and, if present, right-to-left shunting across a patent foramen ovale.

Two-dimensional echocardiographic features of single ventricle, straddling tricuspid valve, tricuspid atresia, and hypoplastic left heart syndrome have all been characterized.[124]

Ventricular Inflow and Outflow Abnormalities

Pulmonary valvular stenosis is suggested on M-mode examination by a large *a* wave on the pulmonary valve. However, this is both insensitive and nonspecific, the *a*

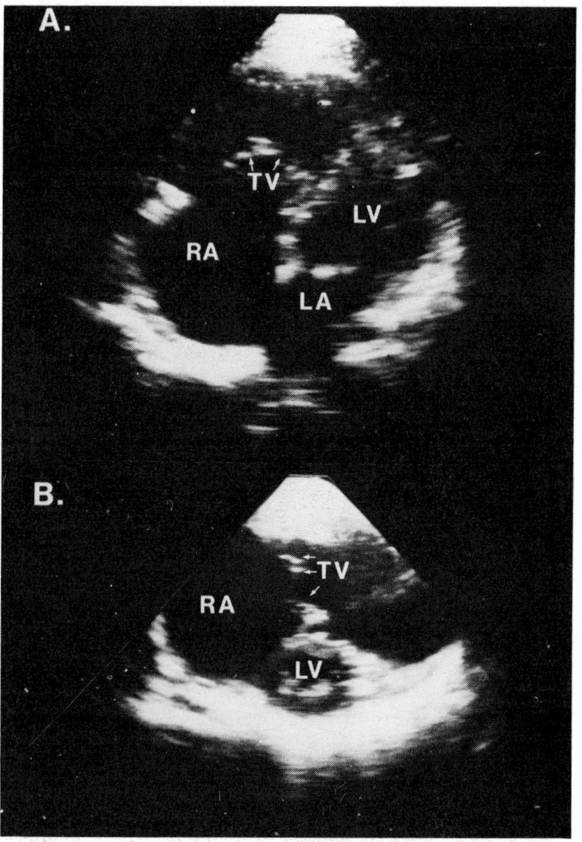

FIGURE 29 Two-dimensional echocardiograms from a patient with Ebstein's anomaly of the tricuspid valve (TV). (*A*) An apical four-chamber view that shows the apically displaced tricuspid leaflet(s) with a large "atrialized" chamber superiorly (RA). (*B*) A left parasternal short-axis view demonstrating a small left ventricle (LV), a large right side of the heart (RA), and anteriorly displaced tricuspid valve.

wave occasionally exceeding 10 mm in normal individuals. With two-dimensional echocardiography, doming of the valve cusps is best visualized in the parasternal short-axis as the right ventricular outflow tract curves around the aorta.[134]

Cor triatriatum and congenital mitral stenosis are uncommon abnormalities that can be recognized by echocardiography. Again the two-dimensional technique offers the more accurate mode of diagnosis.

Abnormalities of the left ventricular outflow tract are also well delineated by echocardiography. Hypertrophic cardiomyopathy and biscuspid aortic valve have been described previously. Subvalvular stenosis can result from a fibromuscular ridge or a discrete membrane. Both can be imaged from the left parasternal long-axis transducer position. Supravalvular aortic stenosis can be readily detected on a long-axis view of the ascending aorta.[135]

Coarctation of the aorta is a common problem that

52

is also detectable by echocardiography. The M-mode examination may only suggest an associated bicuspid aortic valve or left ventricular hypertrophy secondary to the pressure overload. Using the two-dimensional echocardiographic suprasternal approach, the arch and descending aorta can be imaged and the area of coarctation identified.[136]

REFERENCES

1 Lewis, T.: "Clinical Disorders of the Heartbeat: A Handbook for Practitioners and Students," Shaw & Son, London, 1911, p. iii.

1A Latson, L. A., Cheatham, J. P., and Gutgesell, H. P.: Resolution and Accuracy in Two Dimensional Echocardiography, *Am. J. Cardiol.*, 48:106, 1981.

2 Jacobs, L. E., Hall, J. D., Gubernick, I., Meister, S. G., and Barrett, M. J.: Axial versus Lateral Resolution: Inherent Errors in Two-Dimensional Echocardiography Imaging, *Am. J. Cardiol.*, 49:1020, 1982. (Abstract.)

3 Schiller, N. B., Acquatella, H., Ports, T. A., Drew, D., Georke, J., Ringertz, H., Silverman, N. H., Bundage, B., Botvinick, E. H., Boswell, R., Carlsson, E., and Parmley, W. W.: Left Ventricular Volume from Paired Biplane Two-Dimensional Echocardiography, *Circulation*, 60:547, 1979.

4 Starling, M. R., Crawford, M. H., Sorensen, S. G., Levi, B., Richards, K. L., and O'Rourke, R. A.: Comparative Accuracy of Apical Biplane Cross-Sectional Echocardiography and Gated Equilibrium Radionuclide Angiography for Estimating Left Ventricular Size and Performance, *Circulation*, 63:1075, 1981.

5 Silverman, N. H., Ports, T. A., Snider, A. R., Schiller, N. B., Carlsson, E., and Heilbron, D. C.: Determination of Left Ventricular Volume in Children: Echocardiographic and Angiographic Comparisons, *Circulation*, 62:548, 1980.

6 Folland, E. D., Parisi, A. F., Moynihan, P. F., Jones, D. R., Feldman, C. L., and Tow, D. E.: Assessment of Left Ventricular Ejection Fraction and Volumes by Real Time, Two-Dimensional Echocardiography, *Circulation*, 60:760.1979.

7 Quinones, M. A., Waggoner, A. D., Reduto, L. A., Nelson, J. G., Young, J. B., Winters, W. L., Jr., Ribeiro, L. G., and Miller, R. R.: A New, Simplified and Accurate Method for Determining Ejection Fraction with Two-Dimensional Echocardiography, *Circulation*, 64:744, 1981.

8 Belenkie, I.: Beat-to-Beat Variability of Echocardiographic Measurements of Left Ventricular End Diastolic Diameter and Performance, *J. Clin. Ultrasound*, 7:263, 1979.

9 Child, J. S., Krivokapich, J., and Perloff, J. K.: Effect of Left Ventricular Size on Mitral E Point to Ventricular Septal Separation in Assessment of Cardiac Performance, *Am. Heart J.*, 101:797, 1981.

10 Massie, B. M., Schiller, N. B., Ratshin, R. A., and Parmley, W. W.: Mitral-Septal Separation: New Echocardiographic Index of Left Ventricular Function, *Am. J. Cardiol.*, 39:1008, 1977.

11 Upton, M. T., and Gibson, D. G.: The Study of Left Ventricular Function from Digitized Echocardiograms, *Prog. Cardiovasc. Dis.*, 20:359, 1978.

12 Paulsen, W., Boughner, D. R., Persaud, J., and DeVries, L.: Aortic Regurgitation. Detection of Left Ventricular Dysfunction by Exercise Echocardiography, *Br. Heart J.*, 46:380, 1981.

13 Hall, R., Austin, A., and Hunter, S.: M-Mode Echogram as a Means of Distinguishing between Mild and Severe Mitral Stenosis, *Br. Heart J.*, 46:486, 1981.

14 Dumesnil, J. G., Gagné, S., Rouleau, J., and Dagenais, G. R.: The Use of Nitroglycerine in 2-D Echocardiographic Studies of Regional Ventricular Function, *Am. J. Cardiol.*, 49:1020, 1982. (Abstract.)

15 Kisslo, J. A., Robertson, D., Gilbert, B. W., von Ramm, O., and Behar, V. S.: A Comparison of Real Time, Two-Dimensional Echocardiography and Cineangiography in Detecting Left Ventricular Asynergy, *Circulation*, 55:134, 1977.

16 Gibson, R. S., Bishop, H. L., Stamm, R. B., Crampton, R. S., Beller, G. A., and Martin, R. P.: Value of Early Two-Dimensional Echocardiography in Patients with Acute Myocardial Infarction, *Am. J. Cardiol.*, 49:1110, 1982.

17 Heger, J. J., Weyman, A. E., Wann, L. S., Dillon, J. C., and Feigenbaum, H.: Cross-Sectional Echocardiography in Acute Myocardial Infarction: Detection and Localization of Regional Left Ventricular Asynergy, *Circulation*, 60:531, 1979.

18 Weiss, J. L., Bulkley, B. H., Hutchins, G. M., and Mason, S. J.: Two-Dimensional Echocardiographic Recognition of Myocardial Injury in Man: Comparison with Postmortem Studies, *Circulation*, 63:401, 1981.

19 Visser, C. A., Lie, K. I., Kan, G., Meltzer, R., and Durrer, D.: Detection and Quantification of Acute Myocardial Infarction by Two-Dimensional Echocardiography, *Am. J. Cardiol.*, 47:1020, 1981.

20 Horowitz, R. S., Morganroth, J., Parrotto, C., Chen, C. C., Soffer, J., and Pauletto, F. J.: Immediate Diagnosis of Acute Myocardial Infarction by Two-Dimensional Echocardiography, *Circulation*, 65:323, 1982.

21 Heger, J. J., Weyman, A. E., Wann, L. S., Rogers, E. W., Dillon, J. C., and Feigenbaum, H.: Cross-Sectional Echocardiographic Analysis of the Extent of Left Ventricular Asynergy in Acute Myocardial Infarction, *Circulation*, 61:1113, 1980.

22 Horowitz, R. S., and Morganroth, J.: Immediate Detection of Early High-Risk Patients with Acute Myocardial Infarction Using Two-Dimensional Echocardiographic Evaluation of Left Ventricular Regional Wall Motion Abnormalities, *Am. Heart J.*, 103:814, 1982.

23 Eaton, L. W., Weiss, J. L., Bulkley, B. H., Garrison, J. B., and Weisfeldt, M. L.: Regional Cardiac Dilatation after Acute Myocardial Infarction, *N. Engl. J. Med.,* 300:57, 1979.

24 Erlebacher, J. A., Weiss, J. L., Eaton, L. W., Kallman, C., Weisfeldt, M. L., and Bulkley, B. H.: Late Effects of Acute Infarct Dilatation on Heart Size: A Two-Dimensional Echocardiographic Study, *Am. J. Cardiol.,* 49:1120, 1982.

25 Barrett, M. J., Charuzi, Y., and Corday, E.: Ventricular Aneurysm: Cross-Sectional Echocardiographic Approach, *Am. J. Cardiol.,* 46:1133, 1980.

26 D'Arcy, B., and Nanda, N. C.: Two-Dimensional Echocardiographic Features of Right Ventricular Infarction, *Circulation,* 65:167, 1982.

27 Mason, S. J., Weiss, J. L., Weisfeldt, M. L., Garrison, J. B., and Fortuin, N. J.: Exercise Echocardiography: Detection of Wall Motion Abnormalities during Ischemia, *Circulation,* 59:50, 1979.

28 Wann, L. S., Faris, J. V., Childress, R. H., Dillon, J. C., Weyman, A. E., and Feigenbaum, H.: Exercise Cross-Sectional Echocardiography in Ischemic Heart Disease, *Circulation,* 60:1300, 1979.

29 Morganroth, J., Chen, C. C., David, D., Sawin, H. S., Naito, M., Parrotto, C., and Meixell, L.: Exercise Cross-Sectional Echocardiographic Diagnosis of Coronary Artery Disease, *Am. J. Cardiol.,* 47:20., 1981.

30 Maurer, G., and Nanda, N. C.: Two-Dimensional Echocardiographic Evaluation of Exercise-Induced Left and Right Ventricular Asynergy: Correlation with Thallium Scanning, *Am. J. Cardiol.,* 48:720, 1981.

31 Crawford, M. H., Amon, K. W., Vance, W. S., Sorensen, S. G., and Rabinowitz, A. C.: Advantage of Two-Dimensional Echo over Radionuclide Angiography for Detecting Acute Changes in LV Performance during Exercise, *Circulation* 64 (suppl. 2):IV–13, 1981. (Abstract.)

32 Morganroth, J., Chen, C. C., David, C., Naito, M., and Mardelli, T. J.: Echocardiographic Detection of Coronary Artery Disease, *Am. J. Cardiol.,* 46:1178, 1980.

33 Friedman, M. J., Sahn, D. J., Goldman, S., Eisner, D. R., Gittinger, N. C., Lederman, F. L., Puckette, C. M., and Tiemann, J. J.: High Predictive Accuracy for Detection of Left Main Coronary Artery Disease by Antilog Signal Processing of Two-Dimensional Echocardiographic Images, *Am. Heart J.,* 103:194, 1982.

34 Rink, L. D., Feigenbaum, H., Godley, R. W., Weyman, A. E., Dillon, J. C., Phillips, J. F., and Marshall, J. E.: Echocardiographic Detection of Left Main Coronary Artery Obstruction, *Circulation,* 65:719, 1982.

35 Yoshikawa, J., Katao, H., Yanagihara, K., Takagi, Y., Okumachi, F., Yoshida, K., Tomita, T., Fukaya, T., and Baba, K.: Noninvasive Visualization of the Dilated Main Coronary Arteries in Coronary Artery Fistulas by Cross-Sectional Echocardiography, *Circulation,* 65:600, 1982.

36 Bishop, H. L., Gibson, R. S., Stamm, R. B., Beller, G. A., and Martin, R. P.: Role of Two-Dimensional Echocardiography in the Evaluation of Patients with Ventricular

37 Farcot, J. C., Boisante, L., Rigaud, M., Bardet, J., and Bourdarias, J. P.: Two Dimensional Echocardiographic Visualization of Ventricular Septal Rupture after Acute Anterior Myocardial Infarction, *Am. J. Cardiol.,* 45:370, 1980.

38 Mintz, G. S., Victor, M. F., Kotler, M. N., Parry, W. R., and Segal, B. L.: Two-Dimensional Echocardiographic Identification of Surgically Correctable Complications of Acute Myocardial Infarction, *Circulation,* 64:91, 1981.

39 Parisi, A. F., Moynihan, P. F., Folland, E. D., Strauss, W. E., Sharma, G. V. R. K., and Sasahara, A. A.: Echocardiography in Acute and Remote Myocardial Infarction, *Am. J. Cardiol.,* 46:1205, 1980.

40 Ogawa, S., Hubbard, F. E., Mardelli, T. J., and Dreifus, L. S.: Cross-Sectional Echocardiographic Spectrum of Papillary Muscle Dysfunction, *Am. Heart J.,* 97:312, 1979.

41 Asinger, R. W., Mikell, F. L., Elsperger, J., and Hodges, M.: Incidence of Left-Ventricular Thrombosis after Acute Transmural Myocardial Infarction, *N. Engl. J. Med.,* 305:297, 1981.

42 Asinger, R. W., Mikell, F. L., Sharma, B., and Hodges, M.: Observations on Detecting Left Ventricular Thrombus with Two Dimensional Echocardiography: Emphasis on Avoidance of False Positive Diagnoses, *Am. J. Cardiol.,* 47:145, 1981.

43 DeMaria, A. N., Bommer, W., Neumann, A., Grehl, T., Weinart, L., DeNardo, S., Amsterdam, E. A., and Mason, D. T.: Left Ventricular Thrombi Identified by Cross-Sectional Echocardiography, *Ann. Intern. Med.* 90:14, 1979.

44 Katz, R. J., Simpson, A., DiBianco, R., Fletcher, R. D., Bates, H. R., and Sauerbrunn, B. J. L.: Noninvasive Diagnosis of Left Ventricular Pseudoaneurysm, *Am. J. Cardiol.,* 44:372, 1979.

45 Levy, R., Rozanski, A., Charuzi, Y., Childs, W., Waxman, A., Corday, E., and Berman, D. S.: Complementary Roles of Two-Dimensional Echocardiography and Radionuclide Ventriculography in Ventricular Pseudoaneurysm Diagnosis, *Am. Heart J.,* 102:1066, 1981.

46 Gatewood, R. P., Jr., and Nanda, N. C.: Differentiation of Left Ventricular Pseudoaneurysm from True Aneurysm with Two Dimensional Echocardiography, *Am. J. Cardiol.,* 46:869, 1980.

47 St. John Sutton, M. G., St. John Sutton, M., Oldershaw, P., Sacchetti, R., Paneth, M., Lennox, S. C., Gibson, R. V., and Gibson, D. G.: Valve Replacement without Preoperative Cardiac Catheterization, *N. Engl. J. Med.,* 305:1233, 1981.

48 Nichol, P. M., Gilbert, B. W., and Kisslo, J. A.: Two-Dimensional Echocardiographic Assessment of Mitral Stenosis, *Circulation,* 55:120, 1977.

49 Martin, R. P., Rakowski, H., Kleiman, J. H., Beaver, W., London, E., and Popp, R. L.: Reliability and Reproducibility of Two-Dimensional Echocardiographic Mea-

surement of the Stenotic Mitral Valve Orifice Area, *Am. J. Cardiol.,* 43:560, 1979.

50 Mintz, G. S., Kotler, M. N., Segal, B. L., and Parry, W. R.: Two Dimensional Echocardiographic Evaluation of Patients with Mitral Insufficiency, *Am. J. Cardiol.,* 44:670, 1979.

51 Guy, F. C., MacDonald, R. P. R., Fraser, D. B., and Smith, E. R.: Mitral Valve Prolapse as a Cause of Hemodynamically Important Mitral Regurgitation, *Can. J. Surg.,* 23:166, 1980.

52 Gehl, L. G., Mintz, G. S., Kotler, M. N., and Segal, B. L.: Left Atrial Volume Overload in Mitral Regurgitation: A Two-Dimensional Echocardiographic Study, *Am. J. Cardiol.,* 49:33, 1982.

53 Morganroth, J., Jones, R. H., Chen, C. C., and Naito, M.: Two Dimensional Echocardiography in Mitral, Aortic, and Tricuspid Valve Prolapse, *Am. J. Cardiol.,* 46:1164, 1980.

54 Smith, E. R., Fraser, D. B., Purdy, J. W., and Anderson, R. N.: Angiographic Diagnosis of Mitral Valve Prolapse: Correlation with Echocardiography, *Am. J. Cardiol.,* 40:165, 1977.

55 Liedtke, A. J., Babb, J. D., and DeJoseph, R. L.: Mitral Valve Echoes in Patients with Mitral Valve Prolapse Syndrome, *Am. Heart J.,* 97:286, 1979.

56 Child, J. S., Skorton, D. J., Taylor, R. D., Krivokapich, J., Abbasi, A. S., Wong, M., and Shah, P. D.: M Mode and Cross-Sectional Echocardiographic Features of Flail Posterior Mitral Leaflets, *Am. J. Cardiol.,* 44:1383, 1979.

57 Mintz, G. S., Kotler, M. N., Parry, W. R., and Segal, B. L.: Statistical Comparison of M Mode and Two Dimensional Echocardiographic Diagnosis of Flail Mitral Leaflets, *Am. J. Cardiol.,* 45:253, 1980.

58 D'Cruz, I., Panetta, F., Cohen, H., and Glick, G.: Submitral Calcification or Sclerosis in Elderly Patients: M Mode and Two Dimensional Echocardiography in "Mitral Anulus Calcification," *Am. J. Cardiol.,* 44:31, 1979.

59 Kececioglu-Draelos, Z., and Goldberg, S. J.: Role of M Mode Echocardiography in Congenital Aortic Stenosis, *Am. J. Cardiol.,* 47:1267, 1981.

60 Skorton, D. J., Child, J. S., and Perloff, J. K.: Accuracy of the Echocardiographic Diagnosis of Aortic Regurgitation, *Am. J. Med.,* 69:377, 1980.

61 Imaizumi, T., Orita, Y., Koiwaya, Y., Hirata, T., and Nakamura, M.: Utility of Two-Dimensional Echocardiography in the Differential Diagnosis of the Etiology of Aortic Regurgitation, *Am. Heart J.,* 103, 887, 1982.

62 DeMaria, A. N., Bommer, W., Neumann, A., Weinert, L., Bogren, H., and Mason, D. T.: Identification and Localization of Aneurysms of the Ascending Aorta by Cross-Sectional Echocardiography, *Circulation, 59:755, 1979.*

63 Victor, M. F., Mintz, G. S., Kotler, M. N., Wilson, A. R., and Segal, B. L.: Two Dimensional Echocardiographic Diagnosis of Aortic Dissection, *Am. J. Cardiol.,* 48:1155, 1981.

64 Smuckler, A. L., Nomeir, A., Watts, L. E., and Hackshaw, B. T.: Echocardiographic Diagnosis of Aortic Root Dissection by M-Mode and Two-Dimensional Techniques, *Am. Heart J.* 103:897, 1982.

65 Abdulla, A. M., Frank, M. J., Canedo, M. I., and Stafadouros, M. A.: Limitations of Echocardiography in the Assessment of Left Ventricular Size and Function in Aortic Regurgitation, *Circulation,* 61:148, 1980.

66 McDonald, I. G., and Jelinek, V. M.: Serial M-Mode Echocardiography in Severe Chronic Aortic Regurgitation, *Circulation,* 62:1291, 1980.

67 Henry, W. L., Bonow, R. O., Rosing, D. R., and Epstein, S. E.: Observations on the Optimum Time for Operative Intervention for Aortic Regurgitation. II. Serial Echocardiographic Evaluation of Asymptomatic Patients, *Circulation,* 61:484, 1980.

68 Kumpuris, A. G., Quinones, M. A., Waggoner, A. D., Kanon, D. J., Nelson, J. G., and Miller, R.: Importance of Preoperative Hypertrophy, Wall Stress and End-Systolic Dimension as Echocardiographic Predictors of Normalization of Left Ventricular Dilatation after Valve Replacement in Chronic Aortic Insufficiency, *Am. J. Cardiol.,* 49:1091, 1982.

69 Henry, W. L., Bonow, R. O., Borer, J. S., Ware, J. H., Kent, K. M., Redwood, D. R., McIntosh, C. L., Morrow, A. G., and Epstein, S. E.: Observations on the Optimal Time for Operative Intervention for Aortic Regurgitation. I. Evaluation of the Results of Aortic Valve Replacement in Symptomatic Patients, *Circulation,* 61:471, 1980.

70 Gaasch, W. H., Andrias, C. W., and Levine, H. J.: Chronic Aortic Regurgitation: The Effect of Aortic Valve Replacement on Left Ventricular Volume, Mass and Function, *Circulation,* 58:825, 1978.

71 Belenkie, I., and Rademaker, A.: Acute and Chronic Changes after Aortic Valve Damage in the Intact Dog, *Am. J. Physiol.,* 241:H95, 1981.

72 Godley, R. W., Green, D., Dillon, J. C., Rogers, E. W., Feigenbaum, H., and Weyman, A. E.: Reliability of Two-Dimensional Echocardiography in Assessing the Severity of Valvular Aortic Stenosis, *Chest,* 79:657,1981.

73 Gewitz, M. H., Werner, J. C., Kleinman, C. S., Hellenbrand, W. E., and Talner, N. S.: Role of Echocardiography in Aortic Stenosis: Pre- and Postoperative Studies, *Am. J. Cardiol.,* 43:67, 1979.

74 Gaasch, W. H.: Left Ventricular Radius to Wall Thickness Ratio, *Am. J. Cardiol.,* 43:1189, 1979.

75 Reichek, N., and Devereux, R. B.: Reliable Estimation of Peak Left Ventricular Systolic Pressure by M-Mode Echographic-Determined End-Diastolic Relative Wall Thickness: Identification of Severe Valvular Aortic Stenosis in Adult Patients, *Am. Heart J.,* 103:202, 1982.

76 Wann, L. S., Hallam, C. C., Dillon, J. C., Weyman, A. E., and Feigenbaum, H.: Comparison of M-Mode and Cross-Sectional Echocardiography in Infective Endocarditis, *Circulation,* 60:728, 1979.

77 Melvin, E. T., Berger, M., Lutzker, L. G., Goldberg, E., and Mildvan, D.: Noninvasive Methods for Detection of Valve Vegetations in Infective Endocarditis, *Am. J. Cardiol.,* 47:271, 1981.

78 Martin, R. P., Meltzer, R. S., Chia, B. L., Stinson, E. B., Rakowski, H., and Popp, R. L.: Clinical Utility of Two Dimensional Echocardiography in Infective Endocarditis, *Am. J. Cardiol.,* 46:379, 1980.

79 Stewart, J. A., Silimperi, D., Harris, P., Wise, N. K., Fraker, T. D., and Kisslo, J. A.: Echocardiographic Documentation of Vegetative Lesions in Infective Endocarditis: Clinical Implications, *Circulation,* 61:374, 1980.

80 Nakamura, K., Suzuki, S., Satomi, G., Hayashi, H., and Hirosawa, K.: Detection of Mitral Ring Abscess by Two-Dimensional Echocardiography, *Circulation,* 65:816, 1982.

81 Cunha, C. L. P., Giuliani, E. R., Callahan, J. A., and Pluth, J. R.: Echophonocardiographic Findings in Patients with Prosthetic Heart Valve Malfunction, *Mayo Clin. Proc.,* 55:231, 1980.

82 Mintz, G. S., Carlson, E. B., and Kotler, M. N.: Comparison of Noninvasive Techniques in Evaluation of the Nontissue Cardiac Valve Prosthesis, *Am. J. Cardiol.,* 49:39, 1982.

83 Belenkie, I., Carr, M., Schlant, R. C., Nutter, D. O., and Symbas, P. N.: Malfunction of a Cutter-Smeloff Mitral Ball Valve Prosthesis. Diagnosis by Phonocardiography and Echocardiography, *Am. Heart J.,* 86:399, 1973.

84 Alam, M., Madrazo, A. C., Macgilligan, D. J., and Goldstein, S.: M Mode and Two Dimensional Echocardiographic Features of Porcine Valve Dysfunction, *Am. J. Cardiol.,* 43:502, 1979.

85 Schapira, J. N., Martin, R. P., Fowles, R. E., Rakowski, H., Stinson, E. B., French, J. W., Shumway, N. E., and Popp, R. L.: Two Dimensional Echocardiographic Assessment of Patients with Bioprosthetic Valves, *Am. J. Cardiol.,* 43:510, 1979.

86 Doi, Y. L., McKenna, W. J., Gehrke, J., Oakley, C. M., and Goodwin, J. F.: M Mode Echocardiography in Hypertrophic Cardiomyopathy: Diagnostic Criteria and Prediction of Obstruction, *Am. J. Cardiol.,* 45:6, 1980.

87 Maron, B. J., Gottdiener, J. S., and Epstein, S. E.: Patterns and Significance of Distribution of Left Ventricular Hypertrophy in Hypertrophic Cardiomyopathy, *Am. J. Cardiol.,* 48:418, 1981.

88 Gilbert, B. W., Pollick, C., Adelman, A. G., and Wigle, E. D.: Hypertrophic Cardiomyopathy: Subclassification by M Mode Echocardiography, *Am. J. Cardiol.,* 45:861, 1980.

89 Maron, B. J., and Epstein, S. E.: Hypertrophic Cardiomyopathy, *Am. J. Cardiol.,* 45:141, 1980.

90 Gardin, J. M., Talano, J. V., Stephanides, L., Fizzano, J., and Lesch, M.: Systolic Anterior Motion in the Absence of Asymmetric Septal Hypertrophy, *Circulation,* 63:181, 1981.

91 Siqueira-Filho, A. G., Cunha, C. L. P., Tajik, A. J., Seward, J. B., Schattenberg, T. T., and Giuliani, E. R.: M-Mode and Two-Dimensional Echocardiographic Features in Cardiac Amyloidosis, *Circulation,* 63:188, 1981.

92 Kansal, S., Roitman, D., and Sheffield, L. T.: Interventricular Septal Thickness and Left Ventricular Hypertrophy, *Circulation,* 60:1058, 1979.

93 Smith, E. R., Heffernan, L. P., Sangalang, V. E., Vaughan, L. M., and Flemingtom, C. S.: Voluntary Muscle Involvement in Hypertrophic Cardiomyopathy: A Study of Eleven Patients, *Ann. Intern. Med.,* 85:566, 1976.

94 Maron, B. J., Gottdiener, J. S., Bonow, R. O., and Epstein, S. E.: Hypertrophic Cardiomyopathy with Unusual Locations of Left Ventricular Cardiomyopathy with Unusual Locations of Left Ventricular Hypertrophy Undetectable by M-Mode Echocardiography, *Circulation,* 63:409, 1981.

95 Carroll, J. D., Gaasch, W. H., and McAdam, K. P. W. J.: Amyloid Cardiomyopathy: Characterization by a Distinctive Voltage/Mass Relation, *Am. J. Cardiol.,* 49:9, 1982.

96 Borer, J. S., Henry, W. L., and Epstein, S. E.: Echocardiographic Observations in Patients with Systemic Infiltrative Disease Involving the Heart, *Am. J. Cardiol.,* 39:184, 1977.

97 Martin, R. P., Rakowski, H., French, J., and Popp, R. L.: Localization of Pericardial Effusion with Wide Angle Phased Array Echocardiography, *Am. J. Cardiol.,* 42:904, 1978.

98 Settle, H. P., Adolph, R. J., Fowler, N. O., Engel, P., Agruss, N. S., and Levenson, N. I.: Echocardiographic Study of Cardiac Tamponade, *Circulation,* 56:951, 1977.

99 Chandraratna, P. A. N., and Aronow, W. S.: Detection of Pericardial Metastases by Cross-Sectional Echocardiography, *Circulation,* 63:197, 1981.

100 Horowitz, M. S., Rossen, R., and Harrison, D. C.: Echocardiographic Diagnosis of Pericardial Disease, *Am. Heart J.,* 97:420, 1979.

101 Schnittger, I., Bowden, R. E., Abrams, J., and Popp, R. L.: Echocardiography: Pericardial Thickening and Constrictive Pericarditis, *Am. J. Cardiol.,* 42:388, 1978.

102 Seward, J. B., Tajik, A. J., Spangler, J. G., and Ritter, D. G.: Echocardiographic Contrast Studies, *Mayo Clin. Proc.,* 50:163, 1975.

103 Lange, L. W., Sahn, D. J., Allen, H. D., and Goldberg, S. J.: Subxiphoid Cross-Sectional Echocardiography in Infants and Children with Congenital Heart Disease, *Circulation,* 59:513, 1979.

104 Allen, H. D., Goldberg, S. J., Sahn, D. J., Ovitt, T. W., and Goldberg, B. B.: Suprasternal Notch Echocardiography: Assessment of its Clinical Utility in Pediatric Cardiology, *Circulation,* 55:605, 1977.

105 Meyer, R. A., Schwartz, D. C., Benzing, G., and

Kaplan, S: Ventricular Septum in Right Ventricular Volume Overload: An Echocardiographic Study, *Am. J. Cardiol.,* 30:349, 1972.

106 Hagan, A. D., Francis, G. S., Sahn, D. J., Karliner, J. S., Friedman, W. F., and O'Rourke, R. A.: Ultrasound Evaluation of Systolic Anterior Septal Motion in Patients with and without Right Ventricular Volume Overload, *Circulation,* 50:248, 1974.

107 Kingma, I., MacDonald, R., Groves, G. Tyberg, J., and Smith, E: Paradoxic Interventricular Septal Motion: Effects of Diastolic Transseptal Pressure Gradient on Septal Position, Shape and Movement, *Clin. Invest. Med.,* in press. (Abstract.)

108 Tanaka, H., Tei, C., Nakao, S., Tahara, M., Sakurai, S., Kashima, T., and Kanehisa, T: Diastolic Bulging of the Interventricular Septum toward the Left Ventricle, *Circulation,* 62:558, 1980.

109 Brinker, J. A., Weiss, J. L., Lappé, D. L., Rabson, J. L., Summer, W. R., Permutt, S., and Weisfeldt, M. L.: Leftward Septal Displacement during Right Ventricular Loading in Man, *Circulation,* 61:626, 1980.

110 Weyman, A. E., Wann, S., Feigenbaum, H., and Dillon, J. C.: Mechanism of Abnormal Septal Motion in Patients with Right Ventricular Volume Overload, *Circulation,* 54:179, 1976.

111 Bierman, F. Z., and Williams, R. G.: Subxiphoid Two-Dimensional Imaging of the Interatrial Septum in Infants and Neonates with Congenital Heart Disease, *Circulation,* 60:80, 1979.

112 Beppu, S., Nimura, Y., Sakakibara, H., Nagata, S., Park, Y., Baba, K., Naito, Y., Ohta, M., Kamiya, T., Koyanagi, H., and Fujita, T.: Mitral Cleft in Ostium Primum Atrial Septal Defect Assessed by Cross-Sectional Echocardiography, *Circulation,* 62:1099, 1980.

113 Kronik, G., Slany, J., and Moesslacher, H.: Contrast M-Mode Echocardiography in Diagnosis of Atrial Septal Defect in Acyanotic Patients, *Circulation,* 59:372, 1979.

114 Fraker, T. D., Harris, P. J., Behar, V. S., and Kisslo, J. A.: Detection and Exclusion of Interatrial Shunts by Two-Dimensional Echocardiography and Peripheral Venous Injection, *Circulation,* 59:379,1979.

115 Weyman, A. E., Wann, L. S., Caldwell, R. L., Hurwitz, R. A., Dillon, J. C., and Feigenbaum, H.: Negative Contrast Echocardiography: A New Method for Detecting Left-to-Right Shunts, *Circulation,* 59:498, 1979.

116 King, D. L., Steeg, C. N., and Ellis, K.: Visualization of Ventricular Septal Defects by Cardiac Ultrasonography, *Circulation,* 48:1215, 1973.

117 Bloom, K. R., Rodrigues, L., and Swan, E. M.: Echocardiographic Evaluation of Left-to-Right Shunt in Ventricular Septal Defect and Persistent Ductus Arteriosus, *Br. Heart J.,* 39:260, 1977.

118 Funabashi, T., Yoshida, H., Nakaya, S., Maeda, T., and Taniguchi, N.: Echocardiographic Visualization of Ventricular Septal Defect in Infants and Assessment of Hemodynamic Status Using a Contrast Technique, *Circulation,* 64:1025,1981.

119 Canale, J. M., Sahn, D. J., Allen, H. D., Goldberg, S. J., Valdes-Cruz, L. M., and Ovitt, T. W.: Factors Affecting Real-Time Cross-Sectional Echocardiographic Imaging of Perimembranous Ventricular Septal Defects, *Circulation,* 63:689, 1981.

120 Sahn, D. J., and Allen, H. D.: Real-Time Cross-Sectional Echocardiographic Imaging and Measurement of the Patent Ductus Arteriosus in Infants and Children, *Circulation,* 58:343, 1978.

121 Williams, R. G., and Rudd, M.: Echocardiographic Features of Endocardial Cushion Defects, *Circulation,* 49:418, 1974.

122 Hagler, D. J., Tajik, A. J., Seward, J. B., Mair, D. D., and Ritter, D. G.: Real-Time Wide-Angle Sector Echocardiography: Atrioventricular Canal Defects, *Circulation,* 59:140, 1979.

123 Hagler, D. J., Tajik, A. J., Seward, J. B., Mair, D. D., and Ritter, D. G.: Wide-Angle Two-Dimensional Echocardiographic Profiles of Conotruncal Abnormalities, *Mayo Clin. Proc.,* 55:73, 1980.

124 Kotler, M. N., Mintz, G. S., Parry, W. R., and Segal, B. L.: Two Dimensional Echocardiography in Congenital Heart Disease, *Am. J. Cardiol.,* 46:1237, 1980.

125 Huhta, J. C., Piehler, J. M., Tajik, A. J., Hagler, D. J., Mair, D. D., Julsrud, P. R., And Seward, J. B.: Two Dimensional Echocardiographic Detection and Measurement of the Right Pulmonary Artery in Pulmonary Atresia-Ventricular Septal Defect: Angiographic and Surgical Correlation, *Am. J. Cardiol.,* 49:1235, 1982.

126 Henry, W. L., Maron, B. J., and Griffith, J. M.: Cross-Sectional Echocardiography in the Diagnosis of Congenital Heart Disease, *Circulation,* 56:267, 1977.

127 DiSessa, T. G., Hagan, A. D., Pope, C., Samtoy, L., and Friedman, W. F.: Two Dimensional Echocardiographic Characteristics of Double Outlet Right Ventricle, *Am. J. Cardiol.,* 44:1146, 1979.

128 Hagler, D. J., Tajik, A. J., Seward, J. B., Edwards, W. D., Mair, D. D., and Ritter, D. G.: Atrioventricular and Ventriculoarterial Discordance (Corrected Transposition of the Great Arteries), *Mayo Clin. Proc.,* 56:591, 1981.

129 Foale, R., Stefanini, L., Rickards, A., and Sommerville, J.: Left and Right Ventricular Morphology in Complex Congenital Heart Disease Defined by Two Dimensional Echocardiography, *Am. J. Cardiol.,* 49:93, 1982.

130 Sahn, D. J., Allen, H. D., Lange, L. W., and Goldberg, S. J.: Cross-Sectional Echocardiographic Diagnosis of the Sites of Total Anomalous Pulmonary Venous Drainage, *Circulation,* 60:1317, 1979.

131 Lundstrom, N.-R.: Echocardiography in the Diagnosis of Ebstein's Anomaly of the Tricuspid Valve, *Circulation,* 47:597, 1973.

132 Ports, T. A., Silverman, N. H., and Schiller, N. B.: Two-

Dimensional Echocardiographic Assessment of Ebstein's Anomaly, *Circulation,* 58:336, 1978.

133 Meltzer, R. S., Van Hoogenhuyze, D., Serruys, P. W., Haalebos, M. M. P., Hugenholtz, P. G., and Roelandt, J.: Diagnosis of Tricuspid Regurgitation by Contrast Echocardiography, *Circulation,* 63:1093, 1981.

134 Heger, J. J., and Weyman, A. E.: A Review of M-Mode and Cross-Sectional Echocardiographic Findings of the Pulmonary Valve, *J. Clin. Ultrasound,* 7:98, 1979.

135 Weyman, A. E., Caldwell, R. L., Hurwitz, R. A., Girod, D. A., Dillon, J. C., Feigenbaum, H., and Green, D.: Cross-Sectional Echocardiographic Characterization of Aortic Obstruction. 1. Supravalvular Aortic Stenosis and Aortic Hypoplasia, *Circulation,* 57:491, 1978.

136 Snider, A. R., and Silverman, N. H.: Suprasternal Notch Echocardiography: A Two-Dimensional Technique for Evaluating Congenital Heart Disease, *Circulation,* 63:165, 1981.

Prediction of Outcome following Acute Myocardial Infarction Using Noninvasive Techniques[*]

LYALL A. J. HIGGINSON, M.D., WILLIAM L. WILLIAMS, M.D., MICHAEL G. BAIRD, M.D., ROSS A. DAVIES, M.D., and DONALD S. BEANLANDS, M.D.

Any man's death diminishes me because I am involved in mankind; And therefore, never send to know for whom the bell tolls; It tolls for thee.

JOHN DONNE, 1572–1631[1]

Coronary artery disease claims more lives and inflicts more prolonged disability than any other single disease in North America. It has been estimated that a North American male has a 20 percent chance of suffering myocardial infarction or sudden death before the age of 65.[2] Six percent of patients who survive the first 24 hours of acute myocardial infarction will die in the ensuing month and about 8 percent in the subsequent 5 months.[3] After 6 months, the rate of cardiac death falls to approximately 4 percent per year, which is similar to the death rate for patients with chronic ischemic disease. However, a threefold to fourfold excess risk of death persists for 10 years after infarction compared with a similar population with no history of coronary heart disease.

Despite extensive investigation it is difficult to predict which postinfarction patient will develop recurrent infarction, angina, or sudden death. Dr. S. Levine, in 1929, wrote, "There are few diseases in which the prognosis in any individual case is more difficult to predict than in coronary thrombosis." Several studies have attempted to stratify patients in the early postinfarct period into high- or low-risk groups. There are several reasons why accurate prediction of survival and mortality would be valuable. Although unproven, perhaps our management will be improved by knowledge of prognosis, with more aggressive intervention in high-risk subsets. Risk stratification may also identify a group at low risk, the members of which have little chance of dying in the subsequent 6 to 12 months. These people may warrant early discharge, rapid rehabilitation, and few medications. Stratification of risk is also important in designing therapeutic trials, and it can be argued that low-risk patients have little to gain from a therapeutic intervention, are just as susceptible as high-risk subsets to the adverse effects of a therapeutic trial, and increase the numbers required to evaluate an intervention.[4] We intend to review the factors influencing prognosis after myocardial infarction using preinfarction characteristics, clinical profiles during hospitalization, routine laboratory measurements, predischarge ambulatory electrocardiographic monitoring, exercise testing, and nuclear imaging. Furthermore, we will report our experience with 226 consecutive patients discharged from the University of Ottawa Cardiac Unit following hospitalization for acute myocardial infarction. The descriptive characteristics of this population are outlined in Table 1.

TABLE 1
Descriptive characteristics of the University of Ottawa study population

Eligible patients*	233
Enrolled patients†	226
Treadmill tested	205/226 (91%)
Ambulatory ECG monitoring	214/226 (95%)
Timing of tests	12 days postinfarction (6–33 days)
Mean age	56 years
Follow-up	1 year in all patients
1-Year mortality	16/226 (7%)

*Patients were not eligible if they were over 69 years of age or demonstrated persistent postinfarction angina, hypotension, or severe heart failure. Patients transferred from other hospitals and those with severe physical or psychiatric handicap were also excluded.

†Seven of the 233 eligible patients refused to be enrolled.

PREINFARCTION CHARACTERISTICS
Age

The age of the patient significantly influences risk following myocardial infarction (Table 2). This risk is not linear but increases exponentially after age 55.[5] Several postinfarction studies have pointed to increasing age as an important determinant of future prognosis. Norris et al. demonstrated that age above 70 years at the time of infarction is associated with an increased mortality 3 and 6 years later.[6] Moss et al. in an unrestricted age population, found that age is one of the most important factors in identifying patients with increased mortality.[7] In our study, we excluded patients

*From the Division of Cardiology, Department of Medicine, University of Ottawa, Cardiac Unit, Ottawa, Ontario, Canada.

59

TABLE 2
Reported factors adversely affecting prognosis following myocardial infarction

Preinfarction characteristics
Age > 55
History of myocardial infarction angina
Female gender
History of hypertension
History of hypercholesterolemia
History of diabetes

Physical examination
Killip class

Electrocardiogram
Anterior location of the infarct
Q waves in multiple leads
Persistent ST depression
Intraventricular conduction defects
Prolonged QT
Left ventricular hypertrophy
Atrial fibrillation

Chest x-ray
Cardiomegaly

Laboratory data
Markedly elevated cardiac enzymes
Elevated BUN

Hemodynamic data
C.I. < 2 L/(m^2)(min), LVEDP > 20 mm Hg

over the age of 69 and found that the age factor exerts a negligible influence on outcome 1 year following infarction.

Sex

Women appear to have the same prognosis following myocardial infarction as do their male counterparts. A few studies have indicated a worse short-term prognosis for women than for men, but most investigators have found no significant differences between the sexes.[8,9] Women have a lower incidence of coronary heart disease than men. However, once infarction has occurred, women no longer have the same protection against subsequent mortality and morbidity.

Previous History of Infarction or Angina

A prior history of myocardial infarction has an important bearing on prognosis following the index infarction. Patients with prior infarction have less myocardial reserve, which is reflected in the higher hospital mortality and greater long-term morbidity and mortality. Norris and Peel found that a previous myocardial infarct was associated with a significantly increased posthospital mortality.[6,8] Vedin et al. reported a 1-year mortality for first infarctions of 8 percent versus a 22 percent mortality following reinfarction.[10] Henning et al. reported that late mortality was doubled in patients with prior infarction.[11] A prior history of angina pectoris also has a detrimental effect on prognosis following infarction. Moss et al. in a 3-year follow-up, and Norris et al., in a 6-year follow-up, found that prior history of angina pectoris had a significant effect on postinfarction mortality.[6,7]

Prior Risk Factors

Opinions vary as to whether a prior history of hypertension influences prognosis after infarction. In the New York Health Insurance study, the 3-year postinfarction mortality was 28 percent for those with initial blood pressures greater than 160/95 mm Hg compared with 9 percent for those with normal blood pressure recordings.[5] Moss et al. also demonstrated an important relationship between prior history of hypertension and posthospital mortality.[7] This has not been corroborated by other studies, and our experience is that a prior history of hypertension does not significantly influence postinfarction mortality. Diabetes mellitus and hypercholesterolemia present before an index infarction do not increase mortality during the hospital phase or following discharge. The importance of a history of cigarette smoking prior to infarction is controversial, but most authors agree that post infarction mortality is not influenced by the patient's prior smoking habits.

CLINICAL DATA OBTAINED DURING HOSPITALIZATION
Left Ventricular Function

Left ventricular function is the most important determinant of short- and long-term survival following acute myocardial infarction. Killip and Kimball divided patients into four different classes based on the severity of clinical left ventricular failure at the time of admission. They found that hospital mortality correlated with the degree of failure.[12] Norris et al. observed that the simple demonstration of cardiomegaly on chest x-ray is associated with an increased mortality 3 years after discharge.[13] Patients free of heart failure have a 1-year mortality of 5 percent or less, those with pulmonary rales have an annual mortality of 10 to 30 percent, and 50 percent of patients with pulmonary edema are dead within a year.[14]

Invasive monitoring of cardiac output and left ventricular filling pressure has been used to assess more accurately hemodynamics in the infarct period. Patients with elevated left ventricular filling pressures (LVFP > 20 mm Hg) and reduced cardiac output [< 2 L/(m^2)(min)] have a particularly guarded short- and long-term prognosis.[11] Left ventricular dysfunction assessed by physical examination or hemodynamic monitoring is usually a sequela of extensive left ventricular damage. It is not surprising, therefore, that enzymatic measurements of infarct size correlate with short- and long-term prognosis.

Electrocardiographic Infarct Location

The electrocardiogram can be used to classify infarcts as transmural or nontransmural and, if the infarct is transmural, can further be divided into anterior or inferior involvement. Although controversy still exists, it appears that transmural infarction characterized by pathologic Q waves on the electrocardiogram has the same short- and long-term prognostic significance as subendocardial infarction.[15–18] Clinical heart failure and enzyme peaks are lower in subendocardial infarction, but hospital and 1-year mortality are similar. This similarity in outcome may be a reflection of comparable coronary anatomy or of an inability of the electrocardiogram to precisely distinguish subendocardial from transmural involvement.[18] Several authors have suggested that anterior transmural infarction denotes a worse prognosis in follow-up than inferior transmural infarction.[15,18–20] In one study the 3-year survival rate was 85 percent for anterior infarction and 92 percent for infarction in other locations.[19]

Anterior wall infarctions may be associated with increased mortality because they have more left ventricular necrosis and hence more left ventricular dysfunction than comparably sized infarcts involving the inferior wall and portions of the right ventricle. The major determinant, however, is the extent of infarction rather than its location.

Conduction Disturbances

Bundle branch block occurs at some time during hospitalization in 13 percent of patients with acute myocardial infarction.[20] The inhospital mortality of uncomplicated myocardial infarction is usually 10 to 15 percent but rises to 28 percent or higher if complicated by bundle branch block.[20] This poor prognosis is a result of the extent of myocardial damage, causing pulmonary edema or cardiogenic shock, rather than a result of the conduction disturbance itself. The hospital survivors of myocardial infarction complicated by bundle branch block have an increased risk during the subsequent year.[20–22] Hindman et al. reported a 28 percent mortality in the first-year follow-up of 309 patients discharged from hospital after infarction complicated by bundle branch block. One year after discharge, mortality was highest in patients with left or alternating bundle branch block (33 percent) compared with patients with any one of right bundle branch block, right bundle branch block plus left anterior fascicular block, or right bundle branch block plus left posterior fascicular block (23 percent). This, compared with 15 percent in patients with normal intraventricular conduction, again suggests the importance of extensive myocardial damage in determining long-term prognosis.

Coronary Care Unit (CCU) Arrhythmias

Supraventricular arrhythmias occurring in the early phase of acute myocardial infarction are often associated with signs of congestive heart failure and, therefore, a greater overall early mortality. Luria et al. found that atrial arrhythmias in the CCU were associated with a significant increase in 2-year mortality.[23] Bigger et al. could not substantiate the prognostic usefulness of these atrial arrhythmias. They felt that atrial arrhythmias were not of value as independent variables in predicting prognosis.[24] Our experience also indicates that atrial arrhythmias in the CCU are not useful predictors for future cardiac events. Ventricular arrhythmias recorded in the early phase of myocardial infarction are generally felt to be unreliable predictors of future prognosis. Survivors of inhospital ventricular fibrillation, providing that it is primary ventricular fibrillation and not secondary to congestive heart failure, have the same long-term prognosis as those not suffering cardiac arrest.

Postinfarction 12-Lead Electrocardiogram

The electrocardiogram following infarction may give us valuable information that is independent of the other clinical characteristics mentioned earlier. The Coronary Drug Project looked at several ECG findings and followed patients for 3 years.[25] ST-segment depression on the resting electrocardiogram was found to be the single most powerful predictor of subsequent death.

We have found that ST-segment depression on the resting ECG prior to discharge denotes a fourfold risk of death in the ensuing year compared with patients without this ECG abnormality. Patients with inferior infarction and concomitant anterior ST-segment depression may be at particular risk for future cardiac events. We have demonstrated that 95 percent of patients with an acute inferior infarct plus ST-segment depression in one or more leads from V_1 to V_4 have concomitant LAD disease,[26] as well as obstruction to the artery supplying the inferior wall. These patients have larger infarcts assessed enzymatically, greater depression of left ventricular ejection fraction, and more extensive coronary artery disease compared with patients having inferior infarction without anterior ST-segment depression.[26,27]

The size, location, and extent of Q waves are also an aid in predicting future outcome. Other changes reported to be of value by the Coronary Drug Project included tall R waves in lead II, deep inverted T waves in lead V_5, and frequent VPBs.[25] Prolongation of the QT segment has been associated with ventricular irritability and an increased incidence of sudden death. Schwartz reported that a prolonged QT segment on the resting predischarge electrocardiogram doubles the incidence of sudden death following infarction.[28]

Multivariate Analysis

In any individual patient, multiple factors influence clinical outcome both during the hospitalization and in the subsequent follow-up period. Very few of these factors are independent, and their interaction is exceedingly complex. Henning et al. looked at 158 variables in 221 patients over 26 months and found only three independent markers that identified late deaths, namely, (1) a history of previous infarction, (2) increased heart size on x-ray, and (3) an elevated left ventricular filling pressure more than 20 mm Hg at the time of infarction. No other independent variables were helpful in predicting late outcome.[11]

Risk Index

Reliance on a few single variables has frustrated attempts to assess prognosis. Consequently, several statistical techniques have been employed to identify variable interactions as they may pertain to risk stratification. The development of a risk index is one technique in which attempts are made to assign weighted significance to historical data, clinical findings, and routine laboratory measurements. The value placed on each variable is arbitrary and dependent on the clinical impression of its relative importance. An index is then developed for grading the severity of infarction and is

used in predicting prognosis. Peel developed an index based on age, sex, prior history of infarction, heart failure, shock, and certain ECG abnormalities. Summation of this score was used to stratify four patient groups.[8] High scores were able to predict patients at increased risk, but the technique proved less valuable in correctly predicting death in patients with lower scores. Other studies have since shown this prognostic system to be imprecise.[29]

Prognostic Stratification

Prognostic stratification is another technique in which selected individual variables are used in bivariate or trivariate combination (two or three variables together) to separate patients into low- and high-risk groups. Using this technique, Bigger et al. followed 100 post-infarction patients for 6 months. They suggested that of the variables they examined, the most predictive of mortality included a peak creatine kinase (CK) level of more than 585 IU, a blood urea nitrogen level of 20 mg/dl or more, and left ventricular failure in the coronary care unit. Fifty percent of patients with these three variables had died within 6 months.[24]

Discriminant Analysis

A large number of variables are involved in any clinical problem, and because of this, the physician attaches a subjective weight to each component of clinical information according to its importance. The weighted sum of these clinical variables may then indicate the severity of the disease and perhaps the prognosis of the patient. Discriminant analysis is a formal statistical method that is analogous to the subjective method of the physician. Once the predictive variables have been chosen, they $(X_1,\ldots,X_M)$ are weighted by $(a_1,\ldots,a_M)$ and expressed mathematically as $a_1X_1 + \cdots + a_2X_2 + a_MX_M$. This linear function, a weighted sum, is termed the *discriminant function*. The resulting number obtained from any particular patient is the *discriminant score* for that patient. This score can be converted into a probability of survival for that patient. Several studies using a multivariate stepwise discriminant function are detailed in Table 3.

Luria et al. followed 143 patients for 2 years and found that the discriminant function components included admission systolic blood pressure, highest blood urea nitrogen level in the CCU, atrial arrhythmias in the CCU, prior history of angina or infarction, and more than one VPB per hour on an 8-h Holter monitor recording performed prior to discharge. This provided an overall predictive efficiency of 83 percent,[23] but only 11 of 27 deaths (41 percent) could be predicted.

TABLE 3
Factors influencing long-term prognosis using multivariate regression analysis

	Luria et al.[23]	Vedin et al.[10]	Geltman et al.[16]	Henning et al.[11]	Univ. of Ottawa
Number of patients	143	292 (1st MI)	173 (1st MI)	175	226
Age (upper limits)	No limit	67	65	79	69
Follow-up (months)	24	24	22	6	12
Predictors of mortality	Syst. BP BUN S.V. arrhythmias Prior Hx. CAD VPB/h (Holter)	Dyspnea Serum SGOT CHF Cardiomegaly Atrial fibrillation	Infarct size Peak CK CHF Age Gender	Syst. BP < 100 mm Hg Chronic lung disease Anterior MI Hx. of CHF	ST depression at rest Hx. of MI Highest Killip class Serum CK Angina after MI
Predictive efficiency*(%)	83	†	92	92	80
Correctly predicted deaths (%)	41	†	40	24	63

*Predictive efficiency = correct classification/population size.

†Not easily obtainable from the published data. Sixty percent of mortality was concentrated in the highest-risk subset.

Vedin et al. followed 292 men with first infarctions for 2 years and believed the five most important variables were (1) dyspnea with the infarction, (2) serum SGOT, (3) congestive heart failure, (4) cardiomegaly on chest x-ray, and (5) atrial fibrillation recorded during the admission.[10] The total group was divided into 10 groups with increasing risk profiles. Thirty deaths were noted in a 2 year follow-up, and 18 (60 percent) were in the highest-risk subset.

Geltman et al., using a multivariate maximum-likelihood estimation analysis on 173 patients with first myocardial infarction, found that the two most significant variables associated with late mortality were infarct size measured by CK enzyme curves and the presence of congestive heart failure during hospitalization. Peak CK level, age, and gender were also related to mortality. Although the analysis indicated that these five variables were significantly related to survival, the best predictive power correctly identified only 40 percent of the deaths.[16]

Henning et al., using a linear discriminant analysis with 158 variables collected from history, physical examination, and noninvasive assessment, were able to identify correctly 73 percent of early deaths (8 to 30 days) and 97 percent of survivors. The analysis proved less valuable in predicting mortality beyond 30 days. Four variables were selected to predict mortality between 30 days and 6 months. They were (1) systolic blood pressure less than 100 mm Hg, (2) chronic obstructive lung disease, (3) anterior location of infarction, and (4) history of congestive heart failure during hospitalization. Using these variables, mortality in the group predicted to die between 30 days and 6 months was 63 percent (5 of 8) compared with the 7.2 percent mortality for the group predicted to survive beyond 6 months (16 of 223). This analysis, therefore, correctly identified only 5 of 21 deaths (24 percent) beyond 30 days.[11]

At the University of Ottawa Cardiac Unit we have used a stepwise discriminant analysis to follow 226 consecutive patients for at least 1 year following acute infarction. The five most important clinical variables in this discriminant analysis were (1) ST-segment depression on the predischarge ECG greater than 1 mm, (2) history of previous infarction, (3) highest Killip class, (4) serum CK level, and (5) persistent postinfarctional angina. Maximum ST-segment elevation on the resting electrocardiogram prior to discharge and female sex also contributed somewhat to the discriminant analysis. In the first year, 16 of the 226 patients died (7 percent). The overall accuracy using discriminant analysis was 80 percent, and 10 of the deaths were correctly predicted (62.5 percent).

The studies to date all indicate the importance of extensive myocardial damage and left ventricular dysfunction as major determinants of outcome after my-ocardial infarction. Furthermore, admission variables have a very good short-term prognostic value but are of less value in predicting late outcome. This is not surprising in view of the importance of distribution, extent, and progression of underlying coronary artery disease, which exerts a dominant influence on mortality during long-term follow-up. The difficulty in predicting long-term prognosis using the information obtained from history, bedside examination, and laboratory measurements is apparent. Consequently, this problem has been approached with sophisticated noninvasive testing early after infarction. Exercise testing, ECG ambulatory monitoring prior to discharge, and various nuclear investigations have been examined in anticipation that the prediction of long-term prognosis may be improved.

PREDICTIVE IMPLICATIONS OF EXERCISE TESTING
Historical Background

Our appreciation of exercise testing is the result of an enduring relationship that has successfully adapted to changing circumstances. Beyond confirming our suspicions of ischemic heart disease, exercise testing may provoke arrhythmias or may be used to assess adequacy of therapy. However, its apparent ability to reduce the vagaries of the future in the patient with ischemic heart disease by predicting cardiac events has provoked much recent activity.

The predictive capacity of stress testing is well established in large numbers of patients with chronic coronary disease.[30,31] In a study of 2,700 subjects, Ellestad and Wan[30] performed a maximal treadmill test with a positive response defined as ST-segment depression of 1.5 mm or more. The results were correlated with progression of angina, myocardial infarction, or death. ST-segment depression predicted an incidence of some new coronary event of 9.5 percent per year compared with 1.2 percent in the negative respondents. As single events, death and myocardial infarction, but not progression of angina, were associated with a positive test. Other studies have demonstrated that exercise testing may predict coronary anatomy. Marked ST depression, especially at low work loads, correlates with high-grade left main or severe triple vessel disease.[32–36] Dagenais and associates[37] assessed the prognosis of 220 medically treated patients with a strongly positive treadmill test defined as at least 2 mm of ST-segment depression. The 5-year survival related directly to exercise duration. All patients who achieved stage IV of the Bruce protocol survived, 86 percent lived who stopped during stage III, but only 52 percent survived 5 years when they terminated their exercise during stage I.

In chronic ischemic disease, Bruce and colleagues[38] have emphasized three exercise variables that help predict outcome, the most important being maximal systolic blood pressure less than 130 mm Hg. The other two are exercise duration and exertionally induced ventricular dysrhythmia. Furthermore, a low maximal heart rate during exercise predicts a worse outcome. Low exercise tolerance and poor blood pressure response reflect left ventricular dysfunction, the major determinant of a poor prognosis.[39] This experience with stress testing in patients with chronic coronary disease holds out the tantalizing prospect of being able to identify the high-risk individual. These results have been extended to patients convalescing from acute myocardial infarction in an attempt to identify those likely to sustain another cardiac event.

For many patients, a myocardial infarction is the introduction to an uncertain future clouded by the threat of early, sudden death.[40] The evident prognostic utility of exercise testing has provoked a search for the postinfarction patient who carries a disproportionately high risk for a recurrent cardiac event.

Stress testing has a number of attractive features when performed before discharge. It offers an objective assessment of exercise tolerance that can be adapted to an activity prescription during convalescence. Important clues concerning a patient's attitude may be reflected by the motivation displayed during the test. Testing may reveal information relating to residual myocardial ischemia, left ventricular dysfunction, and electrical irritability as reflected by angina, poor endurance, or exertional dysrhythmia. Since these factors influence prognosis following myocardial infarction, early exercise testing may help to identify the high-risk survivor following infarction. Furthermore, it has been postulated that the type of coronary event may be predicted by the ischemia or arrhythmia provoked by the stress test. These provocative questions have generated considerable recent interest and will be reviewed in the next aspect of this report.

SAFETY OF EXERCISE TESTING EARLY AFTER MYOCARDIAL INFARCTION

Granath and associates, in Sweden, demonstrated the safety of low-level treadmill tests on 100 patients 3 weeks following myocardial infarction.[41] Follow-up was restricted to 3 months, during which 5 patients died. Although little correlation with the variables of the treadmill test was attempted, the safety of low-level exercise testing soon after myocardial infarction was well established. The initial report on 46 men from the Stanford Cardiac Rehabilitation Center[42] is in agree-

ment with others[43] in concluding that exercise testing soon after myocardial infarction can safely provide objective information concerning the capacity for physical exercise. This initial experience has been corroborated by many subsequent reports attesting to the feasibility and safety of submaximal exercise testing within 2 weeks of a myocardial infarction.[44-50]

A WORD OF CAUTION

As a prelude to assessing the literature concerning the ability of exercise testing to predict future cardiac events, we offer a note of caution. The influence of several important variables must be borne in mind. A precise description of the study population, uniform criteria for events, adequate sample size, and meticulous follow-up are essential components of a competent study. The selection process may bias the study group by including patients with differing rates of previous myocardial infarction or functional class differences. Post-myocardial infarction exercise studies have reported first-year mortality from 2.2 to 10 percent, reflecting an important difference in the composition of the study population (Table 4). Comparison of reports is confounded by differing exercise protocols and lead-monitoring systems. The intercurrent use of such drugs as digitalis, betablockers, and antiarrhythmic agents are not uniform and may influence exercise measurements. The definition of cardiac events, especially unstable angina, and the manner in which they are grouped together for correlation with exercise variables may influence the conclusions drawn. Differences in definition are a likely explanation for the great variation in subsequent unstable angina from 2.8 to 21.0 percent during a 1 year follow-up period.[45,47] If bypass grafting is considered one of a constellation of "cardiac events," then it should not be surprising that "cardiac events" are associated with a positive treadmill test. Assessment of the decision responses of many cardiologists would indicate that a positive treadmill test is a potent predictor of subsequent bypass surgery. Cardiac mortality, reinfarction, and unstable angina are the cardiac events most investigators are trying to predict with early exercise testing.

The metabolic milieu of the recently infarcted heart is constantly changing, so timing of the exercise test may be prognostically important. Most studies have performed tests within 2 to 3 weeks of the index event to determine exercise capability just prior to discharge. With a view to optimizing timing, DeBusk, Sami, and coworkers performed serial treadmill tests at 3, 5, 7, 9, and 11 weeks as well as at 6, 9, and 12 months following infarction.[44] In their experience, most important recurrent events occurred within 1 month of infarction, making the 3-week test most strategically situated as a potential predictor.

TABLE 4
Comparison of treadmill characteristics and coronary event rates in studies using predischarge treadmill testing to assess prognosis

Investigator	Number of patients	Exercise limit	Percentage TMT* positive	Angina during TMT	Percentage lost to CABG	1-year mortality	Percentage Re-MI	Percentage unstable angina
Sami et al.[44]	200	Symptom limited	21.2	—	11.1	2.7	4.9	—
Théroux et al.[45]	210	Submax. 70% MPHR	31.0	10.0	6.2	9.5	6.2	2.8
Koppes et al.[46]	90	Submax. 50% MPHR	3.0	10.0	—	2.2	—	—
Starling et al.[47]	130	Submax. 70% MPHR	32.3	26.9	—	7.7	9.0	21.0
Weld et al.[48]	236	Submax. to 4 METS	22.0	21.0	—	8.5	4.0	—
Smith et al.[49]	62	Submax. 60% MPHR	32.0	—	—	10.0	4.8	—
Davidson et al.[50]	195	Symptom limited	21.8	15.4	9.7	2.6	—	—
University of Ottawa	205	Submax. 85% MPHR	46.3	22.9	11.7	5.9	6.8	3.4

*Abbreviations: TMT = treadmill test; CABG = 5 coronary artery bypass grafting; Re-MI = recurrent myocardial infarction; MPHR = maximum predicted heart rate.

Prognostic Value of ST-Segment Deviation

ST-SEGMENT DEPRESSION

The prognostic value of exercise induced ST depression during convalescence from a myocardial infarction is supported by three reports[44,45,49] as detailed in Table 5. Théroux et al.[45] and Sami et al.[44] used a Naughton type of treadmill protocol, attaining a target work load of approximately 3 METS. In the study of Théroux et al., the 1-year mortality rate was 2.1 percent (3 of 146) in patients without ST-segment changes during exercise, compared with 27 percent (17 of 64) in patients with a positive test ($p < .001$). This predictive power of ST-segment depression has not been supported by subsequent studies.[46–48] The initial report of Sami et al., from Stanford, held that 40 percent (4 of 10) of patients with ST-segment depression of 2 mm or more had a cardiac arrest or died. No deaths were reported among the 8 patients who had ST-segment depression of 1 to 1.9 mm, suggesting that high-grade ST-segment depression is required to predict outcome. However, no such relationship between the magnitude of ST deviation and cardiac events was noted by Théroux et al.

Weld et al.[48] reported a weaker association of ST depression and posthospital cardiac mortality. As an independent variable, ST depression was associated with 1-year mortality in 11.9 percent of patients compared with 7.1 percent when not present ($p > .05$). The poor correlation of ST depression with cardiac mortality is supported by the study of Starling and associates,[47] as detailed in Table 5. In these reports, the ST segment was not any more successful in predicting other events, namely, progression of angina or recurrent infarction. Hence a detailed review of the literature underscores the inconsistency of ST-segment depression as a predictor of subsequent cardiac events.

ST-segment depression is correlated with exercise-induced angina in some reports[48] but not in others. While angina during a predischarge exercise test is of little prognostic value for mortality, it can predict subsequent stable angina during follow-up.[45–49,51]

SIGNIFICANCE OF EXERCISE-INDUCED ST DEPRESSION: UNIVERSITY OF OTTAWA CARDIAC UNIT EXPERIENCE

At the University of Ottawa Cardiac Unit, we treadmill-tested 205 consecutive patients 12 (6 to 33) days following acute myocardial infarction (see Table 1). This represented 91 percent of all enrolled patients. Complicated infarcts transferred from other hospitals were excluded in an attempt to assemble a study population that was generalizable to a primary care hospital serving as initial contact to infarct patients.

Efforts were made to stop cardiac medications prior to the test, but this was not feasible in all patients. Drugs such as digoxin, beta blockers, and antiarrhythmic agents may confound some treadmill results, but their use represents the pharmacologic realities of treating cardiac patients.

We used a standard Bruce protocol starting at a workload of 4 METS. Electrocardiographgic leads V_1, V_5, and a V_F were monitored continuously, and 12-lead electrocardiograms were recorded at rest and every 3 minutes during exercise and recovery. Stress testing was stopped because of symptoms in 80 percent of patients, ST-segment abnormalities in 5 percent, and attainment of 85 percent of maximum predicted heart rate in 15 percent.

Horizontal ST depression of at least 1 mm below the resting base line was required for a positive test. Follow-up is complete for all entrants. Cardiac events were classified as sudden death (24 h from onset), recurrent myocardial infarction, and unstable angina. Coronary artery bypass grafting was considered a

TABLE 5
Relation of exercise-induced ST-segment depression ($\geq$1 mm) to cardiac mortality following myocardial infarction

Investigator	TMT response		Cardiac mortality		Odds ratio	*p* Value
Sami et al.[44]	−	67	0	0	−	<.01
	+	18	4	18.2%		
Théroux et al.[45]	−	146	3	2.1%	12.93	<.001
	+	64	17	27.0%		
Weld et al.[48]	−	183	14	7.1%	1.76	>.05
	+	52	7	11.9%		
Starling et al.[47]	−	88	6	6.4%	1.40	>.05
	+	42	4	8.7%		
Smith et al.[49]	−	42	1	2.4%	8.40	<.025
	+	20	4	20.0%		
University of Ottawa	−	109	9	8.3%	0.40	>.05
	+	94	3	3.2%		

unique event resulting from conscious decision and occurred in 12 percent of our patients. This became an end point that disqualified the patients from further prognostic analysis.

During the year following myocardial infarction, cardiac mortality was 5.9 percent (see Table 4). This is intermediate between the 2.2 and 10 percent reported in the literature.[46,49] Recurrent infarction occurred in 6.8 percent and unstable angina in 3.4 percent. At least one of these major cardiac events occurred in 16.1 percent of our patients.

An ischemic ST-segment response was noted in 46.3 percent of patients exercised. This is a higher yield than other groups have reported (see Table 4) and may reflect the generally higher workloads used in our study. In addition, all 12 ECG leads were analyzed for ischemic changes, a factor known to improve efficiency.[52] Definite or probable angina was provoked in 23 percent of our patients, and the average exercise load that provoked pain was 5.3 METS.

The relationship of ST-segment depression to cardiac events observed at the University of Ottawa is detailed in Table 6. There is absolutely no correlation between ST-segment depression and cardiac death, recurrent infarction, or unstable angina in the first year following the treadmill test. Patients with a negative test had a mortality rate of 8.3 percent, compared with 3.2 percent for those with a positive test.

DISCREPANCIES BETWEEN STUDIES

The marked discrepancy between studies is difficult to explain on the basis of available information. Inclusion of a number of patients with more severe left ventricular dysfunction may prevent these patients from attaining adequate exercise to provoke ST depression. Once left ventricular failure supervenes in ischemic heart disease, outcome may depend more on the state of the left ventricle than on residual ischemia. However, similar rates of positive treadmill tests and of first-year mortality[45,48] in studies with differing conclusions regarding the value of ST depression militate against this (see Table 4).

Théroux et al. found ST-segment depression useful in predicting future events and asserted that a precise level of exercise must be chosen to best discriminate between high- and low-risk patients. They used 70 percent of predicted maximal heart rate or 5 METS.[45] However, other studies using low exercise loads[46] judged ST depression to be a poor predictor. When we analyzed the patients who had 1-mm ST depression at low workloads of 5 METS, the yield of positive tests fell from 46.3 to 21.7 percent and the predictive power of the ST segment was not enhanced. There appears to be no optimal level of exercise at the present time that ensures detection of the high-risk patient.

Perhaps a multiple-lead monitoring system enhances the sensitivity of the test at the expense of a reduced specificity. If our analysis of the ST segment is reduced from 11 leads to 1, lead V_5, the incidence of positive tests falls to 17.7 percent, a figure compatible with other reports. Unfortunately, this maneuver did not influence the predictive value of ST-segment depression. The poor predictive value of ST-segment depression in our study is consistent with that of other reports.[46–48] This should not be surprising when one considers the all-pervasive influence of left ventricular dysfunction on prognosis.

SIGNIFICANCE OF ST-SEGMENT ELEVATION

Persistent ST-segment elevation at rest and during exercise is common following myocardial infarction. Exercise-induced ST-segment elevation several weeks following infarction is commonly associated with a left ventricular aneurysm.[53] Concomitant ST depression in other leads predicts multivessel coronary disease. The prognostic significance of ST elevation provoked by predischarge exercise testing has been explored only recently. The Seattle group suggests that ST elevation in this setting identifies a small group of patients who are at a considerably higher risk for cardiac death in the first 6 months after infarction.[54]

We analyzed the clinical and prognostic significance of ST elevation in our patient population exercised within 2 weeks of myocardial infarction. Resting ST

TABLE 6
Exercise-induced ST-segment depression as a predictor of unstable angina, recurrent infarction, and death 1 year following acute myocardial infarction, University of Ottawa experience

	No event		Unstable angina		Re-MI		Death		
ST response	Number	Percentage	Number	Percentage	Number	Percentage	Number	Percentage	Total
ST↓ <1.0 mm	88	80.7	3	2.8	9	8.3	9	8.3	109
ST↓ 1–1.9 mm	43	87.8	3	6.1	3	6.1	0	0	49
ST↓ ≥ 2	39	86.7	1	2.2	2	4.4	3	6.7	45
Total	170	83.7	7	3.5	14	6.9	12	5.9	203

Note: Two patients with left bundle branch block were not analyzed for ST deviation.

elevation was noted in one-third of all patients. Among those with an anterior infarction, the serum creatine kinase concentration was significantly higher in those with ST elevation on the resting ECG. This reflects a tendency for larger anterior wall infarcts to be associated with persistent ST elevation. While additional ST elevation with exercise is common, it does not add to the strength of this correlation. Compared with patients without ST-segment elevation, there were no differences detected in the incidence of subsequent myocardial infarction or unstable angina. When analyzed for cardiac mortality at 1 year, twice as many patients with resting ST elevation had died (9 versus 4.4 percent, $p > .05$). This relationship is not strengthened by exercise-induced ST elevation.

In our experience, persistent ST elevation is associated with large infarcts and is commonly exaggerated by exercise but adds little to the prognostic usefulness of its resting counterpart. It remains a relatively insensitive marker of subsequent coronary events.

Stress Testing for Ventricular Dysfunction

The common denominator for poor survival following acute infarction is the cumulative amount of myocardial damage. The requirement that postinfarction patients be able to perform a submaximal treadmill test introduces a selection bias in favor of a healthier study population. In our experience, the group of patients disqualified from participating in exercise tests soon after myocardial infarction owing to cardiovascular disability sustains considerably more cardiac complications. While 30 percent of patients not medically qualified to exercise died, only 5.9 percent succumbed who performed early stress tests.

In the study of Weld et al.,[48] exercise tolerance of less than 6 min was associated with clinical variables indicating ventricular dysfunction, such as digitalis therapy, pulmonary rales, S_3 gallop, or pulmonary vascular congestion on x-ray. In their study, exercise variables were ranked by logistic regression analysis for strength of association with cardiac mortality. The following were selected: (1) exercise duration, (2) ventricular ectopic activity (VEA), and (3) ST-segment depression. This indicates the importance of exercise endurance when analyzing treadmill variables.

In our study, the 1-year mortality rate was 14 percent in patients exercising 3 min or less, compared with 7 percent in those exercising 3 to 6 min. No deaths occurred in those exercising longer than 6 min (Fig. 1). The relative risk of dying is 3.4 times greater in patients failing to complete stage I of the Bruce protocol. We agree with Weld's statement that left ventricular function that permits modest performance in an exercise

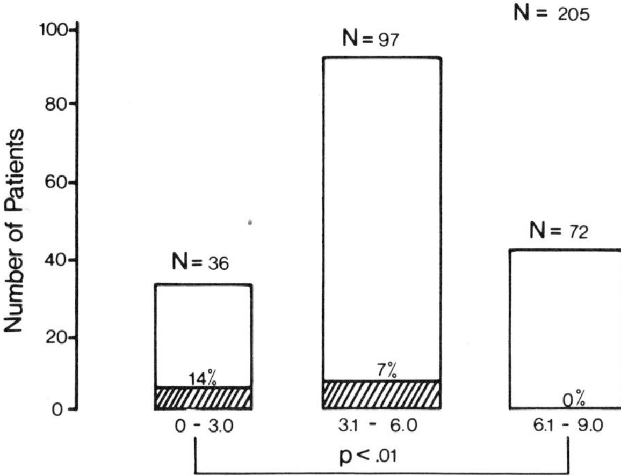

FIGURE 1 The total population and 1-year mortality are grouped by stage of exercise. Total height of each bar represents the number of patients (N) reaching each stage. The hatched portion of each bar represents the number of cardiac deaths in 1 year. The percentage represents the proportion of patients in each stage who died.

protocol implies a favorable outcome even in the presence of rather profound ST depression, arrhythmias, or clinical left ventricular failure.[48] This observation agrees with the relationship between poor endurance and poor outcome established in the setting of chronic ischemic heart disease.[38]

Stress Testing for Ventricular Ectopic Activity

Exercise-induced ventricular ectopic activity during the convalescent phase has been correlated with an increased risk of cardiac death or reinfarction.[41,44,55] This is particularly true when ventricular ectopic activity (VEA) is associated with poor exercise endurance and ventricular dysfunction.[48]

In our study, VEA was analyzed by 24-h ambulatory monitoring as well as by exercise testing prior to discharge (Table 7). Complex VEA consisting of multiform ectopics and pairs and runs of three or more was detected more readily by ambulatory monitoring than by treadmill testing (37 versus 11 percent). Complex VEA provoked by exercise testing was three times more predictive of recurrent myocardial infarction (17.4 percent) than was simple VEA (6 percent) (Table 8). However, complex VEA was not helpful in predicting subsequent cardiac death.

SUMMARY OF THE STATUS OF PREDISCHARGE EXERCISE TESTING

It has been reported by some authors that exercise-induced ST depression occurs in postinfarct patients

TABLE 7
Distribution of the highest grade of VEA in simple and complex categories

	Simple VEA		Complex VEA	
	Lown 0	Lown 1,2	Lown 3,4A,4B,5	Total
Ambulatory monitoring group	33 (15%)	102 (48%)	79 (37%)	214 (100%)
Treadmill group	114 (56%)	68 (33%)	23 (11%)	205 (100%)

who have a higher risk of dying in the near future. These observations have not been confirmed by other investigators. The discrepancies may be explained in part by differing populations and methodologies. Cardiac events such as unstable angina and recurrent myocardial infarction continue to evade prediction by the convalescent exercise test. If exercise variables are joined with other clinical and historical features, the predictive power is increased so that we may be able to detect a few patients who deserve more detailed observation and investigation. It is our feeling that other observations made during the predischarge treadmill test are as useful as, if not more useful than, the isolated ST-segment response.

AMBULATORY ELECTROCARDIOGRAPHIC MONITORING

Ambulatory electrocardiograms recorded during the late hospital phase or during the first 3 months after acute myocardial infarction record three variables that have potential value for predicting prognosis in the ensuing years: supraventricular ectopy, ST-segment changes, and ventricular ectopy.

Supraventricular Ectopy

Atrial arrhythmias may influence the prognosis of patients with chronic and acute coronary artery disease. In an actuarial study of life insurance applicants with coronary artery disease, those with paroxysmal or chronic atrial fibrillation had a higher mortality than expected.[56] Atrial fibrillation during an acute myocardial infarction is associated with an increased mortality rate,[57] and mortality is higher if it occurs with anterior wall compared with inferior wall infarcts. Although atrial dysrhythmias are common in the late hospital phase of acute infarction and during the subsequent 3 months,[58,59] they are not of prognostic importance. In the Coronary Drug Project study, 12-lead electrocardiograms were recorded on 2,035 male survivors of myocardial infarction a minimum of 3 months after their infarct. The mortality among the 110 men with supraventricular beats was not excessive. Even when the subjects with ventricular ectopy were excluded, the mortality rate of 19.4 percent was not significantly higher than the 12.4 percent mortality rate in those without supraventricular beats.[59]

ST-Segment Changes

The prognostic value of ST-segment changes recorded during ambulatory monitoring is not known. Their diagnostic importance is still being determined, and this must be settled before any predictive usefulness can be studied. When these changes occur with symptoms of chest pain or dyspnea, they may confirm the true ischemic nature of a patient's symptoms,[60] but when they occur without symptoms, their significance is uncertain. Silent ST-segment depression is reported to occur more frequently in patients with known coronary artery disease.[61]

TABLE 8
Predictive value of simple and complex VEA on predischarge treadmill testing and 24-h ambulatory monitoring for coronary events in the first year after infarction

	Treadmill testing			24-h ambulatory monitoring		
	n	Simple VEA	Complex VEA	n	Simple VEA	Complex VEA
Myocardial infarction	15	6.0%*	17.4%*	14	5.9%	7.6%
Unstable angina	12	6.6%	0.0%	14	6.7%	6.3%
Death	12	6.0%	4.3%	15	3.7%†	12.7%†

*$p < .05$
†$p < .02$

Ventricular Ectopy

The only ambulatory ECG monitoring variable that has been related to prognosis following an acute infarction is ventricular ectopic activity (VEA). Although any ventricular ectopy increases risk after an infarct, the risk is higher in those with frequent and complex forms. Complex ventricular ectopy usually includes ventricular bigeminy, ventricular couplets or pairs, multiform beats, runs of three or more beats in a row, and R-on-T beats. The latter are especially difficult to recognize on commercially available scanning systems. The criteria for frequent ventricular ectopy vary.

Much of the success of intensive and coronary care units in reducing the inhospital mortality of acute infarction is a result of the prophylactic suppression of VEA likely to progress to ventricular tachycardia or fibrillation. Schulze et al. clarified the relationship between ventricular ectopy, infarct size, and death.[62] In this study, 81 patients had nuclear angiograms and 24-h ambulatory electrocardiograms 2 weeks after their infarction and before hospital discharge. In the subsequent follow-up period of 2 to 16 months (mean 7 months), 8 patients died suddenly; all 8 were in the subgroup of 26 patients with an ejection fraction of less than 40 percent and complex ventricular arrhythmias. There were no deaths in the 19 patients with a low ejection fraction but no complex VEA or in the 36 patients with an ejection fraction greater than 40 percent. Patients with a recent infarct but without complex ventricular ectopics are more likely to have single-vessel rather than multivessel coronary disease and usually have less severe left ventricular dysfunction.[63] Despite this relationship between VEA and left ventricular dysfunction, VEA is considered by some to have an independent effect on the risk of sudden death.[64,65]

Review of published reports on the value of ambulatory monitoring for detecting VEA and the subsequent prediction of future coronary events in survivors of the hospital phase of an acute infarct reveals the marked diversity in methodology and usefulness of the technique. Table 9 lists some of the differences in methodology that must be considered in evaluating and comparing these reports.

TYPE OF RECORDING INSTRUMENT

Ventricular ectopy is often unrecognized by the patient, so continuous ECG recorders rather than patient-initiated recorders have been used almost exclusively. A few early reports used one-channel recorders. Two-channel recorders, usually recording a V_5 and a V_1-like lead, are more popular and allow accurate recognition of ventricular ectopics with different morphology. There is also less chance for loss of information owing to lead displacement.

TABLE 9
Ambulatory monitoring after infarction: differences in methodology

Type of recording instrument
Accuracy of arrhythmia analysis
Method of grading ventricular ectopic activity
Duration of the monitoring period
Timing of the monitoring period
Activity of the subject at the time of ambulatory monitoring
Spontaneous variability of VEA frequency
Control of antiarrhythmic medications
Patient population
Duration of follow-up
Definition of study end points

ACCURACY OF ARRHYTHMIA ANALYSIS

Some authors[66] have very accurately recorded the number and type of VEA by hand counting and classification or by using custom-designed arrhythmia analysis computers.[67] Such techniques have very high sensitivity and specificity for detecting arrhythmias but are extremely time-consuming and impractical in the clinical situation. Time constraints and the use of commercially available scanning systems with less sophisticated arrhythmia detection computers make routine classification of these arrhythmias less than perfect. Prognosis is related to both the frequency and the complexity of the VEA, and these scanning systems detect most subjects fulfilling either or both of these criteria.

METHOD OF GRADING VENTRICULAR ECTOPIC ACTIVITY

Ventricular ectopy is classified by frequency and/or by complexity. Risk increases directly with both.[67] There is no widely accepted definition of *frequent*, but generally, this refers to more than 10 ventricular ectopics per hour; neither is there uniformity in the definition of *complex,* or *complicated,* VEA.[62]

The Lown grading system[68] is popular and defines different levels of simple and complex ventricular ectopy (Table 10). The original system was not designed for ambulatory monitoring analysis, and although it has been modified for this purpose, it still has shortcomings. The basic premise of the method is that the higher the VEA grade, the greater is the risk. This has recently been challenged.[67] Bigger was unable to demonstrate a difference in risk between Lown grades 5, 4A, and 4B in postinfarction patients without incorporating VEA frequency as well. The Lown system does not account for the additional risk imparted to complex VEA by the presence of frequent ventricular ectopics. It is also mutually exclusive in its classification. Different complex forms of VEA may be

TABLE 10
The Lown classification of ventricular ectopic activity

Grade 0	No VEA
Grade 1	Less than 30 ventricular ectopics per hour
Grade 2	30 or more ventricular ectopics per hour
Grade 3	Multiform ventricular ectopics
Grade 4A	Ventricular couplets
Grade 4B	Three or more ventricular ectopics in a row
Grade 5	R-on-T ventricular ectopics

detected on an individual monitoring tape, but the patient is assigned to the highest grade in the hierarchy without recognition of the other complex forms.

DURATION OF THE MONITORING PERIOD

Prognostic importance has been attached to VEA detected on recordings of different lengths. Recording times have varied from less than 1 min in the Coronary Drug Project, where only 11.5 percent of the patients showed ventricular ectopics, to 24 h, where 94 percent of 216 Holter tapes contained at least one ventricular ectopic.[69] The relationship between the duration of the monitoring period and VEA complexity and frequency was examined in detail by Winkle et al.,[66] and a number of important observations were made. First, recordings of longer than 24 h detect many more patients with complex ventricular ectopic activity of all types. In this particular study, most patients who were going to develop a particular type of complex VEA had done so by 72 h. The study involved 57 ambulatory patients on whom three consecutive 24-h ambulatory ECG recordings were made prior to discharge following infarction. By 72 h 21 percent had demonstrated ventricular tachycardia, 32 percent had ventricular bigeminy, 32 percent had couplets, 53 percent had shown the R-on-T phenomenon, and 65 percent had demonstrated multiform ectopics. In all, 79 percent of the 57 patients had demonstrated at least one type of complex ventricular ectopic during the 72 h. Although 86 percent of patients who were to manifest any complex VEA at 72 h had done so by 24 h, this was not so for all specific types. Only 42 percent of those who were to show ventricular tachycardia had done so by 24 h. Second, there is a direct relationship between frequency of VEA and complexity, and this holds for each type of complex VEA. In this study, virtually all patients with more than 100 ventricular ectopics in 24 h had complex forms as well. This also has been demonstrated by other studies.[67]

The predictive value of VEA may vary with the duration of the monitoring period. Winkle et al.[66] reported that subjects who have complex VEA detected by short-duration monitoring are those who have these arrhythmias during much of the time. They also pointed out that most studies showing a predictive

value for ventricular ectopy after infarction are of less than 12 h in duration, whereas in studies utilizing 24 h of monitoring, only one of four at the time of this writing showed such a relationship.

It appears that with increasing length of the monitoring period, more and more ventricular ectopic activity, both simple and complex, is seen, and one suspects that when it is recorded in such a manner, it tends to lose its specificity and predictive value.

TIME OF THE MONITORING PERIOD

The ambulatory ECG has been recorded while the patient is still in the hospital, early after discharge,[70] or as long as 3 months later.[71,72] Since mortality drops quickly during the first 6 months after infarction,[24] the predictive value of VEA may differ depending on when it is recorded. The optimal timing of ambulatory monitoring in this situation has not been established.

ACTIVITY OF THE SUBJECT AT THE TIME OF AMBULATORY MONITORING

The prognostic value of ventricular premature beats recorded by ambulatory monitoring may differ depending on whether the recording was obtained while the patient was resting inhospital or at home, where there is more likely to be physical and social stress with its resulting increase in sympathetic tone. Recordings of less than 24 h in duration are likely to show more ventricular ectopic activity per hour during the day than during the night.

SPONTANEOUS VARIABILITY OF VEA FREQUENCY

This is an important consideration in antiarrhythmic drug studies, where day-to-day variation in VEA frequency may mimic drug effects. Its effect in the postinfarction period is uncertain. It is probably minimal, since the variability is rarely so much as to cause complex ventricular ectopics to disappear or to effect a great reduction in VEA frequency.[73]

CONTROL OF ANTIARRHYTHMIC MEDICATIONS

Studies do not usually control for antiarrhythmic medications, which would be expected to decrease VEA frequency and complexity. In only one report[70] were there no patients taking antiarrhythmic medications.

PATIENT POPULATION

Most investigations have excluded some patients from their study population. Patient refusal, technical problems with ambulatory monitoring instrumentation,[62,74,75] the exclusive use of males,[59,71] exclusion of patients with complicated infarcts,[73] and exclusion of people over the age of 65 or 70[65,73,75] all affect the applicability of these studies to a general population.

DURATION OF FOLLOW-UP

Ventricular ectopy has been correlated with death as early as 7 months after infarction[62] and as long as 5 years after the index event.[71]

DEFINITION OF STUDY END POINTS

Most reports relate the frequency or complexity of ventricular ectopy to the risk of cardiac death. This usually implies sudden death, but nonsudden death has also been used.[65] Other end points include all-cause mortality,[71] recurrent infarction, and postinfarction angina.[75]

The Predictive Value of Ventricular Ectopic Activity

The majority of reports show a direct relationship between frequency and/or complexity of ventricular ectopic activity and future coronary events; some do not.

STUDIES SHOWING NO CORRELATION BETWEEN VEA AND FUTURE CARDIAC EVENTS

DeBusk et al.[73] were unable to demonstrate any prognostic value in ventricular ectopy recorded by 12 h of monitoring for recurrent coronary events (sudden death, recurrent infarction, or cardiac arrest) over a 2-year follow-up period. Patients with evidence of left ventricular dysfunction were excluded, which explains the low incidence of events, 11 of 90 (12.2 percent), in this study. Other studies[62] have demonstrated a lack of predictive power of VEA in the absence of left ventricular dysfunction. Manger Cats et al.[70] did not exclude patients with complicated infarcts but did exclude those taking antiarrhythmic medications. There were 21 coronary events (sudden death, fatal recurrent infarctions, and nonfatal recurrent infarc-

tions) in their 200 subjects followed over 12 months; 16 of these occurred in the first 6 months. Although more events occurred in patients with a higher Lown grade of VEA (grades 3, 4A, 4B) than in lower grades, the difference was not significant. In another study,[24] patients with one or more ventricular ectopics per hour had a higher death rate than those with a lower frequency.

STUDIES SHOWING A CORRELATION BETWEEN FREQUENT OR COMPLEX VEA AND FUTURE CARDIAC EVENTS

The Coronary Drug Project research group[59] demonstrated an increased mortality associated with ventricular premature beats double that of those without on a 12-lead electrocardiogram recorded at least 3 months after infarction. VEA was predictive of excess mortality independent of other risk factors known to increase mortality in these men. In this study, the risk of VEA persisted for 3 years without decline.

Increased risk of death is related to both frequency and complexity of the VEA. Within each Lown grade of complexity, Bigger and Weld demonstrated that ventricular ectopic frequency exerts a significant influence on mortality.[67] For example, in patients who had VEA Lown grades 4A, 4B, and 5, persons with 10 or more ectopics had a higher mortality than persons in the same grade who had less than 10 ventricular ectopics per hour. In this study, the best predictors of death were VEA frequency, ventricular couplets, and ventricular tachycardia.

Some studies have indicated that ventricular ectopy is an independent predictor of outcome,[59,64,65] but it may be more useful in describing high-risk subsets of patients when used with other risk factors in a multivariate fashion. Complex VEA, when found in patients with anterior wall infarcts and left ventricular dysfunction, for example, has a higher mortality than in those with complex VEA alone. Such a subgroup made up 15 percent of 940 patients in Moss's study and carried a survival rate of 85 percent in 6 months and 70 percent for 3 years.[65] The 5-year mortality in survivors of acute myocardial infarction in the HIP study[71] was 18.5 percent in those with any VEA, and it rose to 35 percent in those who had congestive heart failure or ST-segment depression on their resting electrocardiogram. It climbed to 52 percent in those who had both congestive heart failure and ST-segment depression as well as VEA. A corollary of these observations is that patients without complex or frequent ventricular ectopics and other factors considered to increase risk have a very good prognosis.[65,72,76] It would appear that those patients with a low risk can be spared the expense and adverse effects of pharmacotherapy or other procedures.

Ambulatory Monitoring: University of Ottawa Cardiac Unit Experience

Ambulatory electrocardiograms were obtained in 214 of the 226 patients enrolled in the University of Ottawa study (see Table 1). They were recorded on portable two-channel recorders monitoring a V_1-like lead and a modified bipolar V_5 lead. The mean recording time was 22 h. The ECG tapes were reviewed with a rapid playback system at 60 times real time and analyzed by an experienced nurse with extensive knowledge in arrhythmia analysis. The highest Lown grade (grade 0 to grade 5) of VEA recorded during any hour of the ambulatory ECG determined whether a patient was considered to have simple (Lown grade 0, 1, 2) VEA or complex (Lown grade 3, 4A, 4B, 5) VEA. Frequency of VEA was not taken into account during this study. For the majority of patients, the highest grade of ventricular ectopic activity achieved was grade 0, 1, or 2 (see Table 7).

Subsequent coronary events occurring in the first year following the index infarction were then correlated with the highest grade of ventricular ectopic activity recorded. The predictive value of complex or simple ventricular ectopy was defined as the percentage of patients with one or the other types of ventricular ectopy having a coronary event (recurrent infarction, angina, or death). We were unable to demonstrate a significant difference between the prognostic value of simple and complex ventricular ectopy for recurrent infarction or angina. However, complex ventricular ectopy was three times more predictive of death than simple ventricular ectopy, 12.7 versus 3.7 percent (see Table 8).

The predictive value of complex ventricular ectopy recorded during ambulatory monitoring for any of the three coronary events was 23 percent (Table 11). Perhaps of more importance, 77 percent of the patients with complex ventricular ectopy did not have a coronary event in the first year after their infarction.

The study confirmed that the predictive value of complex ventricular ectopy for cardiac death is greater than that of simple ventricular ectopy in certain circumstances, and yet, even in the best instance, it is still only 12.7 percent. That is, of 100 patients with complex ventricular ectopy, 12.7 or fewer will die from a cardiac cause in the first year after the index infarction (see Table 8). We are led to conclude that, by itself, complex ventricular ectopy recorded by ambulatory monitoring in our patient population is of limited clinical prognostic value.

SUMMARY

It is difficult to reconcile the many differences between studies to arrive at a concensus concerning the predictive value of VEA recorded by ambulatory monitoring following acute infarction. It appears that they do have predictive value. Studies to the contrary might have demonstrated this if a larger study population[70] had been used or they had allowed fewer exclusions.[73] The predictive value increases with increasing VEA frequency and complexity. When used in conjunction with other variables known to suggest a poor prognosis, such as left ventricular dysfunction, congestive heart failure, prior infarction, low ejection fraction, or anterior wall infarction, VEA frequency can be used to detect subgroups of patients with mortality rates approaching 50 to 80 percent in the first year after infarction.

THE SIGNIFICANCE OF VENTRICULAR TACHYCARDIA EARLY AFTER ACUTE MYOCARDIAL INFARCTION

A *run of ventricular tachycardia* (VT) is usually defined as three or more ventricular ectopics in a row with a rate of 100 per minute or greater. When so defined, it occurs in 1 to 21 percent of patients who have ambulatory monitoring prior to hospital discharge following an acute myocardial infarction. In serial recordings of 289 patients, ventricular tachycardia occurred in 3.4 percent 2 weeks after infarction, 11.1 percent at 1 month, and it stabilized at about 7 percent between 2 months and 1 year.[77] Over 30 percent of those patients who had eight 10-h recordings in the first year had at least one run at some time. Three consecutive 24-h monitoring periods recorded the arrhythmia in 21 percent of patients just prior to hospital discharge.[66]

Ventricular tachycardia in the postinfarct period does not differ in characteristics from that recorded at other times. Most (30 to 50 percent) runs are of three beats in duration and self-limiting; they are rarely associated with palpitations.[78,79] The relationship between ventricular tachycardia and subsequent mortality is not yet clear, although it appears to increase risk. Ruberman et al.[80] and Kotler et al.[81] demonstrated that runs of ventricular tachycardia are associated with

TABLE 11
The predictive value of VEA recorded on predischarge 24-h ambulatory monitoring (AM) or treadmill testing (TM) for any coronary event in the first year after an acute myocardial infarction

	Simple VEA		Complex VEA	
	AM	TM	AM	TM
n	135	182	79	23
Coronary event	13%	16%	23%	17%
No coronary event	87%	84%	77%	83%

an increased risk of sudden death; Schulze et al.[62] and Kleiger et al.[77] did also, but only in patients with severe left ventricular dysfunction. Kleiger et al. concluded that "the presence of ventricular runs...seemed to be a marker of severe cardiac disease rather than an independent factor for increased incidence of sudden death." Bigger et al.,[79] however, demonstrated an overall 1-year mortality rate of 38 percent in the 50 patients with ventricular tachycardia in his study of 430 patients who survived the CCU phase of acute myocardial infarction. Death was not necessarily sudden. Only 11.6 percent of the group without ventricular tachycardia died—the difference was highly significant. The 36-month cumulative mortality rate was 54 percent in those with ventricular tachycardia compared with 19.4 percent in the group without. When analyzed in relation to other predictors of subsequent death, this arrhythmia was more powerful than 15 other variables commonly associated with increased risk, and moreover, it was independently associated with 1-year mortality. Patients who had VT were five times as likely to die within 1 year as were those who did not. Neither the number of episodes, the length of the episodes, nor the maximum rate of the arrhythmia correlated with risk of death.

By the end of a 4-year follow-up period, Anderson et al.[78] was able to demonstrate a twofold increase in the risk of dying for postinfarction patients with the arrhythmia. Eleven of 66 patients (16.6 percent) with ventricular tachycardia and 11 of 132 (8.3 percent) without it died. This difference was not statistically significant. Those patients who died tended to have more severe heart disease as manifested by a higher Peel index, history of previous myocardial infarction, and a higher NYHA class of heart failure.

Ventricular tachycardia, then, like complex ventricular ectopy, is associated with an increased risk of death in the years subsequent to a myocardial infarction. Whether it is an independent risk factor for death is not yet clarified, but it appears that it occurs more commonly in patients with severe left ventricular dysfunction.

VENTRICULAR ECTOPY DURING AMBULATORY MONITORING VERSUS TREADMILL TESTING

In the postinfarction patient, ambulatory monitoring documents more ventricular ectopy, both simple and complex, than treadmill testing, whether the tests are performed prior to hospital discharge or months later. DeBusk et al.[73] observed that the prevalence of treadmill-induced VEA was 42 percent 3 weeks after an infarction and 52 percent at 11 weeks or later, whereas 77 percent of patients had ventricular ectopy at 3 weeks

on 10-h of ambulatory monitoring, and this remained the same at 11 weeks or more. In addition, the overall prevalence of complex VEA during monitoring was significantly higher than during treadmill testing, 42 versus 27 percent. In 100 coronary artery disease patients, 81 of whom had a previous infarct, ventricular ectopics were present in 56 during maximal treadmill or bicycle stress testing and in 88 during 24-h monitoring.[82] The difference in prevalence of complex ventricular ectopy in the two techniques was even more marked. Ventricular tachycardia was seen in 7 patients during exercise and in 16 during monitoring; exercise provoked ventricular couplets in 13 and multiform ventricular ectopics in 5, whereas ambulatory monitoring detected similar arrhythmias in 24 and 55 patients, respectively. For maximum efficiency in detection of ventricular ectopics, both tests should be performed. There are patients who will demonstrate ectopy on one test and not on the other.

The greater ability of ambulatory monitoring to detect simple or complex ventricular ectopics does not translate into greater predictive power. In our study,[75] complex ventricular ectopy on ambulatory monitoring was an independent predictor of death but not of recurrent infarction. However, complex VEA during treadmill testing was predictive of recurrent myocardial infarction but not of death (see Table 8). Ventricular ectopics recorded by either technique are of no predictive value in a population free of clinically significant left ventricular dysfunction.[73]

NUCLEAR CARDIAC IMAGING

A large post-myocardial infarction angiographic study found that ejection fraction, the number of diseased vessels, and the occurrence of heart failure in the coronary care unit were the most important predictors of survival.[83] Since nuclear cardiac imaging comprises several noninvasive methods of evaluating both ventricular function and myocardial perfusion, it is not surprising that these techniques have some prognostic value following myocardial infarction.

There are three radionuclide techniques that are in widespread clinical use. Infarct-avid imaging agents, commonly technetium-99m stannous pyrophosphate, allow detection of recent myocardial necrosis. Myocardial perfusion imaging, usually performed with thallium-201, is used to assess regional myocardial blood flow and may be performed at rest or with exercise. Radionuclide ventriculography, generally using technetium-99m, allows assessment of right and left ventricular volume, regional wall motion, and ejection fraction. It may also be performed at rest or during exercise. None of these techniques provides the same detailed anatomic resolution as coronary angiography.

However, they may provide more functional information, particularly when coupled with exercise. These tests are noninvasive with essentially no morbidity and are suitable for evaluation of patients following myocardial infarction.

Infarct-Avid Imaging with Technetium-99m Stannous Pyrophosphate

The intensity of Tc-99m pyrophosphate uptake does not relate closely to the extent of infarction. However, the area of uptake correlates with infarct size.[84–86] This correlation is better with anterior infarctions because of the geometric difficulty in imaging the inferoposterior surface of the heart by conventional techniques. Tomographic techniques may extend this application. The complication rate after acute myocardial infarction relates to both the area and pattern of pyrophosphate uptake. Holman et al.[87] performed Tc-99m pyrophosphate scintigraphy in 100 consecutive patients admitted to the coronary care unit with suspected acute myocardial infarction and followed the patients for 6 months. The area of Tc-99m pyrophosphate uptake correlated with the inhospital complication rate. Massive uptake (8 patients) and intense focal uptake (12 patients) was associated with a higher complication rate than focal uptake (37 patients), diffuse uptake (22 patients), or normal scintigrams (21 patients). The inhospital complication rate associated with massive uptake was extremely high, at 88 percent, and the complication rate (death, recurrent infarction, or unstable angina) following hospital discharge was high with both massive uptake (50 percent) and intense focal uptake (42 percent). A specific pattern of uptake, the so-called doughnut pattern, found with large anterior infarctions is associated with a poor prognosis.[86–90] this doughnut pattern may be due to uptake in the partially perfused border zone of the infarct but not in the necrotic center of the infarct, or it may reflect left ventricular dilatation. With uncomplicated acute myocardial infarction, the Tc-99m pyrophosphate scintigram becomes negative in 1 to 2 weeks. However, up to 50 percent of patients have persistent positive scans, often with diffuse uptake. This predicts a worse outcome with a higher incidence of persistent angina, recurrent infarction, heart failure, arrhythmias, and death within 1 to 2 years.[91–94] Poliner et al. suggested that persistent uptake is caused by continuing cell damage and necrosis.[95]

It has been assumed that a positive Tc-99m pyrophosphate scintigram in unstable angina is a false positive result. However, histologic studies have shown that there may be unrecognized multifocal necrosis.[96] In addition, a positive scan in unstable angina identifies a group of patients with a higher risk of sudden death or nonfatal infarction following hospital discharge,[87,97,98] possibly because they have more extensive coronary artery disease than patients with unstable angina and normal scans.

Although Tc-99m pyrophosphate scintigraphy has some prognostic value with acute myocardial infarction, its role is primarily diagnostic. For example, it is capable of detecting necrosis in clinical situations where conventional methods are limited, such as left bundle branch block and perioperative infarction. The area of Tc-99m pyrophosphate uptake reflects infarct size. However, unlike exercise thallium-201 scintigraphy or exercise radionuclide ventriculography, it provides no insight into the extent of ischemic but noninfarcted myocardium, which is so important in predicting future cardiac events.

Resting Thallium-201 Myocardial Perfusion Imaging

Viable myocardium incorporates thallium-201 roughly in proportion to regional blood flow. Unfortunately, image quality, namely, myocardial to background separation, in the resting thallium-201 scintigram is poor compared with that of exercise scintigraphy. Imaging is performed immediately following injection and is usually repeated 2 to 4 h later without further radionuclide administration (delayed or redistribution imaging). A perfusion defect unchanged on delayed imaging is often considered to represent scar, whereas one that is smaller on delayed imaging is considered to represent transient ischemia. It is now appreciated that interpretation is not so simple, since failure of redistribution does not always imply irreversible necrosis and may be delayed or absent in the presence of severe coronary artery stenosis without infarction.[99]

Resting thallium-201 imaging immediately following myocardial infarction is sensitive for detecting infarction. However, this sensitivity depends on the size of infarction and the time interval following infarction.[100] The size of the initial perfusion defect decreases with time, which may represent peri-infarction ischemia.[100,101] Although there is a correlation between infarct size estimated from the in vivo thallium-201 defect size and actual infarct size at autopsy,[102] the role of thallium-201 for determining infarct size in human beings is limited. The size of the initial thallium defect includes old as well as recent infarction and cannot differentiate between acute infarction and associated peri-infarctional ischemia.

Resting thallium-201 myocardial perfusion imaging is primarily a diagnostic method, although it has some prognostic ability following acute myocardial infarction. The resting scintigram summates the area of acute infarction, peri-infarction ischemia, and previous infarction. Silverman et al.[103] found that the extent of the thallium-201 scintigraphic defect within hours of acute myocardial infarction was predictive of subsequent mortality and was more predictive than the best combination of clinical parameters, including a history of previous infarction. In this study, resting thallium-201 scintigraphy was performed in 42 consecutive patients with Killip class I or II heart failure a mean of 8 ± 4 h after the onset of acute myocardial infarction. They found that a high thallium defect score corresponding to a 40 percent reduction in perfusion in two views identified a subgroup of 13 patients with higher inhospital mortality (46 percent versus overall 17 percent) and mortality at 6 months (62 percent versus overall 24 percent). When the size of an infarct was assessed by thallium imaging and compared with left ventricular performance assessed by radionuclide ventriculography, a defect size less than 25 percent was associated with a near normal global ejection fraction, whereas a defect size greater than 25 percent was associated with a depressed ejection fraction.[104]

Resting Radionuclide Ventriculography

The importance of left ventricular function in determining prognosis has been established by contrast ventriculography in patients with ischemic heart disease[105] and following acute myocardial infarction.[83] That similar observations have been made with radionuclide ventriculography is hardly surprising given the close correlation of the two methods. The ability of radionuclide ventriculography to predict outcome after myocardial infarction reflects in part its ability to summate the cumulative effect of both new and old infarctions on left ventricular performance. A depressed left ventricular ejection fraction predicts what would be expected, namely, death, heart failure, and ventricular arrhythmias.

Battler et al.[106] performed radionuclide angiography in 102 patients 1 to 4 days after admission with acute myocardial infarction. Mortality at 30 days was not influenced by the admission ejection fraction. However, mortality at 1 year was greater among patients with a reduced ejection fraction (< 0.52) on admission. Marmor et al.[107] performed radionuclide ventriculography 48 to 96 h after onset of infarction in 50 patients with nontransmural infarction and followed them for 9 months. Although global left ventricular ejection fraction was higher in survivors, the only independent noninvasive variable that predicted survival was a higher wall-motion score by their grading method.

Radionuclide ventriculography is predictive of survival among patients suffering an out-of-hospital cardiac arrest. Ptacin et al.[108] assessed 36 such patients

within 24 h of hospital admission. Not surprisingly, there was a high incidence of severe left ventricular dysfunction, with 18 patients having an ejection fraction less than 30 percent. There was a significantly higher mortality at 1 month among patients with ejection fractions less than 30 percent (56 percent mortality) compared with patients with ejection fractions over 30 percent (22 percent mortality). In addition, there was no short-term mortality among 7 patients with normal regional wall motion compared with 14 deaths among 29 patients with abnormal regional wall motion.

Exercise Thallium-201 Myocardial Perfusion Imaging

The use of exercise thallium-201 scintigraphy following myocardial infarction is relatively recent, and its value has not yet been clearly defined. The majority of studies assessing its value have looked at its ability to detect multivessel disease[109–113] rather than prognosis.[114]

In patients without prior myocardial infarction, exercise thallium imaging is relatively sensitive in detecting the presence of coronary artery disease. However, it is less useful in predicting the extent and distribution of disease.[112,115] This may be explained because the interpretation of thallium-201 scintigrams involves comparison of the relative uptake of thallium-201 in different walls of the left ventricle, assuming uptake in one wall is normal. This may be less accurate in the presence of a previous scar, since it is difficult to compare normal versus ischemic versus infarcted myocardium.

Over half of asymptomatic patients following myocardial infarction have multivessel disease. The number of diseased vessels is predictive of survival.[83] Thus if exercise thallium-201 scintigraphy can identify multivessel disease in this setting, it may have prognostic value. From data currently available, it appears that the ability of thallium-201 scintigraphy to detect multivessel diseases is limited,[109,113] being more reliable following inferior than anterior infarction.[112,113]

Gibson et al.[109] performed submaximal exercise thallium-201 scintigraphy and coronary angiography in 42 patients prior to hospital discharge following infarction. Multiple thallium-201 defects were more predictive of multivessel disease than other parameters, including ischemic ST-segment depression. Ischemic ST-segment depression with exercise identified only 45 percent of patients with multivessel disease, whereas multiple thallium-201 defects with exercise identified 88 percent. When submaximal exercise thallium-201 imaging 2 weeks after infarction was compared with symptom-limited studies at 3 months, there was no additional information provided by the late postinfarction study, although a higher heart rate and workload was achieved.[110] Exercise studies at 2 weeks correctly identified 24 of 36 patients (67 percent) with multivessel disease and hence falsely predicted single-vessel disease in 12 patients (33 percent). At 2 weeks all 24 patients with single-vessel disease were correctly identified. However, 2 had multiple thallium defects at 3 months, suggesting multivessel disease. In a separate publication, the same group analyzed the significance of increased pulmonary uptake of thallium-201 during exercise 2 weeks after infarction compared with exercise radionuclide ventriculography and coronary angiography.[116] Those with increased pulmonary uptake had a more frequent history of previous infarction, a higher Norris coronary prognostic index, more frequent exercise-induced ST-segment depression, more anterior perfusion defects, a lower resting ejection fraction, and more asynergic wall-motion segments.

Rigo et al.[112] performed exercise thallium-201 scintigraphy and coronary angiography in 101 patients with prior infarction. Of the 35 patients with a single previous anterior infarction, exercise thallium-201 scintigraphy only identified 3 of the 16 patients with multivessel disease. Forty-three patients had single inferior or lateral infarctions, of whom 34 patients had multivessel disease. Exercise thallium imaging was predictive of multivessel disease in 25 of 34 patients (74 percent) and left anterior descending involvement in 20 of 29 patients (69 percent) compared with one false positive prediction among the 9 patients with single-vessel disease.

At the University of Ottawa Cardiac Unit we studied 40 patients following first inferior infarction by symptom-limited exercise thallium-201 scintigraphy and coronary angiography.[117] Ischemic ST-segment depression with exercise and an additional anteroseptal perfusion defect were equally sensitive (60 versus 60 percent) and specific (80 versus 70 percent) in detecting multivessel disease. The predictive accuracy of a positive stress test or imaging study for multivessel disease was good at 83 and 75 percent, respectively. However, the predictive accuracy of a negative stress test or imaging study for single-vessel disease was low at 55 and 48 percent, respectively. This relates partly to the high prevalence of multivessel disease after inferior infarction (62.5 percent in our study).

Brown et al.[114] examined the prognostic value of exercise thallium-201 scintigraphy compared with angiographic left ventricular function and the number of diseased coronary arteries in 138 medically treated patients over a 3.7-year follow-up. For patients without a previous myocardial infarction, they found that the number of transient perfusion defects was the only predictor of subsequent cardiac events. The number of stenosed coronary arteries was only predictive when

thallium-201 data were not included. Among patients with a previous myocardial infarction, resting angiographic ejection fraction was the only predictor of a subsequent cardiac event when all the data were considered together, and when the angiographic data were excluded, the number of persistent thallium defects and thallium lung activity became predictive.

Exercise Radionuclide Ventriculography

Unlike exercise thallium-201 scintigraphy studies that have attempted to identify multivessel disease rather than predict outcome, there have been several studies assessing the prognostic capability of exercise radionuclide ventriculography.[118–121] The resting ejection fraction determined by radionuclide techniques has been shown to be a powerful predictor of subsequent mortality. An abnormal radionuclide response to exercise (defined as a failure to increase ejection fraction, a drop in ejection fraction, or development of a new wall-motion abnormality) has the capability of detecting residual ischemia in the distribution of stenosed noninfarct vessels.

Borer et al.[118] performed supine multigated radionuclide cineangiography prior to hospital discharge and 6 to 14 months later in 45 patients to determine the natural history of left ventricular function after infarction and its relation to survival. Resting left ventricular ejection fraction was low (39 ± 5 percent) at the early study and did not change significantly with submaximal exercise (37 ± 5 percent). A low resting ejection fraction at the early study correlated with complex ventricular ectopy on 24-h electrocardiographic recording and with death at 1 year. Exercise ejection fraction at the predischarge study did not predict mortality at 1 year. Resting ejection fraction at the late study (42 ± 4 percent) was not significantly different from that at the early study, except for a subgroup of 17 patients whose predischarge ejection fraction was greater than 40 percent and who showed a small but significant rise in resting ejection fraction at the late study, perhaps indicating they had greater cardiac reserve. Similar results were found by Morris et al.[120] Upright bicycle multigated radionuclide angiography was performed in 102 patients 3 and 8 weeks after infarction, and the patients were followed for 1 year. Resting ejection fraction 3 weeks after infarction was most predictive of death at 1 year, mortality being 7, 12, and 35 percent for ejection fraction above 50 and 30 to 49 percent and under 30 percent, respectively. The change in ejection fraction with exercise did not predict mortality, but it did predict total cardiac events, including death, recurrent nonfatal infarction, and rehospitalization for unstable angina or coronary bypass surgery. The additional study 8 weeks after infarction added no further information, especially since 5 patients died between the 3- and 8-week studies.

Corbett et al.[119] performed submaximal supine multigated radionuclide ventriculography in 61 patients, a mean of 19 days after infarction and followed the patients a mean of 9.6 months. Failure to increase left ventricular ejection fraction by 5 percent, an increase of end-systolic volume by 5 percent, or failure to increase the ratio of systolic blood pressure to end-systolic volume by 35 percent were three scintigraphic variables they found to be more predictive of future cardiac events than clinical or exercise electrocardiographic parameters. A normal response by these three radionuclide criteria accurately predicted a cardiac event–free follow-up period.

Nicod et al.[121] compared the prognostic value of coronary angiography and exercise radionuclide ventriculography in 44 patients after infarction over a 6-month follow-up period. They found that the two tests were equally predictive of subsequent cardiac complications among patients with multivessel disease, but with single-vessel disease, an abnormal exercise ejection fraction response (failure to increase by 5 percent or more) provided more prognostic information than coronary angiography.

Although not applied specifically to postinfarction patients, the ability of exercise radionuclide cineangiography to identify prognostic critical coronary stenosis has been established, and presumably this would also apply to postinfarction patients. Among 250 patients with at least 50 percent coronary artery narrowing in one vessel, Phillips et al.[122] found that a rise of left ventricular ejection fraction with exercise excluded left main or three-vessel disease, whereas a drop of 10 percent or more was highly suggestive of left main or three-vessel disease.

SUMMARY

Of the nuclear imaging techniques, resting radionuclide ventriculography best predicts fatal cardiac events. Nonfatal cardiac events, such as recurrent infarction or unstable angina, which depend on the extent of coronary artery disease may be best predicted by exercise radionuclide ventriculography. Although infarct-avid imaging with Tc-99m pyrophosphate and resting thallium-201 myocardial perfusion imaging have some predictive value, they are primarily diagnostic tests. The value of exercise thallium-201 scintigraphy following myocardial infarction has yet to be clearly defined. Its ability to detect multivessel disease is limited particularly following anterior infarction.

REFERENCES

1 Donne, J.: Devotions Upon Emergent Occasions, in "Oxford Dictionary of Quotations," 2d ed., Oxford University Press, London, England, 1953. p. 186.

2 Stamler, J.: The Primary Prevention of Coronary Heart Disease. The Myocardium, in "Failure and Infarction," H. P. Publishing Co., Inc., New York, 1974, p. 219.

3 Weinblatt, E., Shapiro, S., Frank, C. W. et al.: Prognosis of Men after First Myocardial Infarction: Mortality and First Recurrence in Relation to Selected Parameters, *Am. J. Public Health,* 58:1329, 1968.

4 Bigger, J. T., Jr.: New Directions and New Uses for Risk Stratification in the Posthospital Phase of Acute Myocardial Infarction, *Am. J. Med.,* 67:1, 1979.

5 Shapiro, S., Weinblatt, E., and Frank, C.: The HIP Study of Incidence and Prognosis of Coronary Heart Disease: Work Tables and Figures, in "The Health Insurance Plan of Greater New York," New York, 1970.

6 Norris, R. M., Caughey, D. E., Mercer, C. J., Deeming, L. W., and Scott, P. J.: Coronary Prognostic Index for Predicting Survival after Recovery from Acute Myocardial Infarction, *Lancet,* 2:485, 1970.

7 Moss, A., DeCamilla, J., Engstrom, F., Hoffman, W., Odoroff, C., and Davis, H.: The Posthospital Phase of Myocardial Infarction, *Circulation,* 49:460, 1974.

8 Peel, A. A. F., Semple, T., Wang, I., Lancaster, W. M., and Dall, J. L. G.: A Coronary Prognostic Index for Grading the Severity of Infarction, *Br. Heart J.,* 24:745, 1962.

9 Weinblatt, E., Shapiro, S., and Frank, C.: Prognosis of Women with Newly Diagnosed Coronary Heart Disease— A Comparison with Course of Disease among Men, *Am. J. Public Health,* 63:577, 1973.

10 Vedin, A., Wilhelmsen, L., Wedel, H., et al.: Prediction of Cardiovascular Deaths and Non-Fatal Reinfarctions after Myocardial Infarction, *Acta Med. Scand.,* 201:309, 1977.

11 Henning, H., Gilpin, E. A., Covell, J. W., Swan, E. A., O'Rourke, R. A., and Ross, J., Jr.: Prognosis after Acute Myocardial Infarction: A Multivariate Analysis of Mortality and Survival, *Circulation,* 59:1124, 1979.

12 Killip, T., and Kimball, J. T.: Treatment of Myocardial Infarction in a Coronary Care Unit. A Two Year Experience with 250 Patients, *Am. J. Cardiol.,* 20:457, 1967.

13 Norris, R., Caughey, D., Mercer, C., and Scott, P.: Prognosis after Myocardial Infarction—Six-Year Follow-Up, *Br. Heart J.,* 36:786, 1974.

14 Humphries, J.: Survivors of Recent Myocardial Infarction: Prognosis and Management, *Prim. Cardiol.,* 4(9):28, 1978.

15 Sobel, B. E., Bresnahan, G. F., Shell, W., and Yoder, R.: Estimation of Infarct Size in Man and Its Relation to Prognosis, *Circulation,* 46:640, 1972.

16 Geltman, E. M., Ehsani, A. A., Campbell, M. K.,

Schechtman, K., Roberts, R., and Sobel, B. E.: The Influence of Location and Extent of Myocardial Infarction on Long-Term Ventricular Dysrhythmia and Mortality, *Circulation,* 60:805, 1979.

17 Thanavaro, S., Krone, R. J., Kleiger, R. E., et al.: In-hospital Prognosis of Patients with First Nontransmural and Transmural Infarctions, *Circulation,* 61:29, 1980.

18 Madias, J. E., and Gorlin, R.: The Myth of Acute "Mild" Myocardial Infarction, *Ann. Intern. Med.,* 86(3):347, 1977.

19 Moss, A. J.: Factors Influencing Prognosis after Myocardial Infarction, *Curr. Prob. Cardiol.,* 4:5, 1979.

20 Hindman, M. C., Wagner, G. S., JaRo, M., et al.: The Clinical Significance of Bundle Branch Block Complicating Acute Myocardial Infarction, *Circulation,* 58:679, 1978.

21 Mullins, C., and Atkins, J.: Prognosis and Management of Ventricular Conduction Blocks in Acute Myocardial Infarction, *Mod. Concepts Cardiovasc. Dis.,* 45:129, 1976.

22 Waugh, R., Wagner, G., Haney, T., Rosati, R., and Morris, J.: Immediate and Remote Prognostic Significance of a Fascicular Block during Acute Myocardial Infarction, *Circulation,* 47:765, 1973.

23 Luria, M. H., Knoke, J. D., Margolis, R. M., Hendricks, F. H., and Kuplic, J. B.: Acute Myocardial Infarction: Prognosis after Recovery, *Ann. Intern. Med.,* 85:561, 1976.

24 Bigger, J. T., Heller, C. A., Wenger, T. L., and Weld, F. M.: Risk Stratification after Acute Myocardial Infarction, *Am. J. Cardiol.,* 42:202, 1978.

25 Coronary Drug Project Research Group: The Prognostic Importance of the Electrocardiogram after Myocardial Infarction: Experience in the Coronary Drug Project, *Ann. Intern. Med.,* 77:677, 1972.

26 Salcedo, J. R., Baird, M. G., Chambers, R. J., and Beanlands, D. S.: Significance of Reciprocal S-T Segment Depression in Anterior Precordial Leads in Acute Inferior Myocardial Infarction: Concomitant Left Anterior Descending Coronary Artery Disease? *Am. J. Cardiol.,* 48:1003, 1981.

27 Shah, R. K., Pichler, M., Berman, D. S., et al.: Noninvasive Identification of a High Risk Subset of Patients with Acute Inferior Myocardial Infarction, *Am. J. Cardiol.,* 46:915, 1980.

28 Schwartz, P., and Wolf, S.: QT Interval Prolongation as Predictor of Sudden Death in Patients with Myocardial Infarction, *Circulation,* 57:1074, 1978.

29 Norris, R. M., Brandt, P. W. T., Caughey, D. E., Lee, A. J., and Scott, P. J.: A New Coronary Prognostic Index, *Lancet,* 1:274, 1969.

30 Ellestad, M. H., and Wan, M. K. C.: Predictive Implications of Stress Testing. Follow-Up of 2700 Subjects after Maximum Treadmill Stress Testing, *Circulation,* 51:363, 1975.

31 Ellestad, M. H., Cook, B. M., and Greenberg, P. S.: Stress Testing: Clinical Applications and Predictive Capacity, *Prog. Cardiovasc. Dis.,* 21:431, 1979.

32 Goldman, S., Tselos, S., and Cohn, K.: Marked Depth of ST-Segment Depression during Treadmill Exercise Testing. Indicator of Severe Coronary Disease, *Chest,* 69:729, 1976.

33 Goldschlager, N., Selzer, A., and Cohn, K.: Treadmill Stress Tests as Indicators of Presence of Severity of Coronary Artery Disease, *Ann. Intern. Med.,* 85:277, 1976.

34 Cohn, K., Kamm, B., Fetiah, N., Brand, R., and Goldschlager, N.: Use of Treadmill Score to Quantify Ischemic Response and Predict Extent of Coronary Disease, *Circulation,* 59:286, 1979.

35 Weiner, D. A., McCabe, C. H., and Ryan, T. J.: Identification of Patients with Left Main and Three-Vessel Coronary Disease with Clinical and Exercise Test Variables, *Am. J. Cardiol.,* 46:21, 1980.

36 Podrid, J. P., Graboys, T. B., and Lown, B.: Prognosis of Medically Treated Patients with Coronary-Artery Disease with Profound ST-Segment Depression during Exercise Testing, *N. Engl. J. Med.,* 305:1111, 1981.

37 Dagenais, G. R., Rouleau, J. R., Christen, A., and Fabia, J.: Survival of Patients with a Strongly Positive Exercise Electrocardiogram, *Circulation,* 65:452, 1982.

38 Bruce, R. A., DeRouen, T., Peterson, B. R., Irving, J. B., Chinn, N., Blake, B., and Hofer, V.: Non-Invasive Predictors of Sudden Cardiac Death in Men with Coronary Heart Disease. Predictive Value of Maximal Stress Testing, *Am. J. Cardiol.,* 39:833, 1977.

39 Hammermeister, K. E., DeRouen, T. A., and Dodge, H. T.: Variables Predictive of Survival in Patients with Coronary Disease. Selection by Univariate and Multivariate Analysis from the Clinical, Electrocardiographic, Exercise, Arteriographic, and Quantitative Angiographic Evaluations, *Circulation,* 59:421, 1979.

40 Moss, A. J., DeCamilla, J., and Davis, H.: Cardiac Death in the First Six Months after Myocardial Infarction: The Potential for Coronary Reduction in the Early Post-Hospital Period, *Am. J. Cardiol.,* 39:816, 1977.

41 Ericsson, M., Granath, A., Ohlsen, E., Sodermark, T., and Volpe, U.: Arrhythmias and Symptoms during Treadmill Testing Three Weeks after Myocardial Infarction in 100 Patients, *Br. Heart J.,* 35:787, 1973.

42 Markowicz, W., Houston, N., and DeBusk, R. F.: Exercise Testing Soon after Myocardial Infarction, *Circulation,* 56:26, 1977.

43 Styperek, J., Ibsen, H., Cajoller, E., and Petersen, A.: Exercise ECG in Patients with Acute Myocardial Infarction before Discharge from the CCU, *Am. J. Cardiol.,* 35:172, 1975. (Abstract.)

44 Sami, M., Kramer, H., and DeBusk, R. F.: The Prognostic Significance of Serial Exercise Testing after Myocardial Infarction, *Circulation,* 60:1238, 1979.

45 Théroux, P., Waters, D. D., Halphen, P., Debaisieux, J. C., and Mizgala, H. F.: Prognostic Value of Exercise Testing Soon after Myocardial Infarction, *N. Engl. J. Med.,* 301:341, 1979.

46 Koppes, G. M., Kruyer, W., Beckman, C. H., and Jones, F. G.: Response to Exercise Early after Uncomplicated Myocardial Infarction in Patients Receiving No Medication: Long Term Follow-Up, *Am. J. Cardiol.,* 46:764, 1980.

47 Starling, M. R., Crawford, M. H., Kennedy, G. T., and O'Rourke, R. A.: Exercise Testing Early after Myocardial Infarction: Predictive Value for Subsequent Unstable Angina and Death, *Am. J. Cardiol.,* 46:909, 1980.

48 Weld, F. M., King-Lee, C., Bigger, T. J., and Romitzky, L. M.: Risk Stratification with Low Level of Exercise Testing Two Weeks after Acute Myocardial Infarction, *Circulation,* 64:306, 1981.

49 Smith, J. W., Dennis, C. A., Gassman, A., et al.: Exercise Testing Three Weeks after Myocardial Infarction, *Chest,* 75:12, 1979.

50 Davidson, D. M., and DeBusk, R. F.: Prognostic Value of a Single Exercise Test 3 Weeks after Uncomplicated Myocardial Infarction, *Circulation,* 61:236, 1980.

51 Waters, D. D., Théroux, P., Halphen, E., et al.: Clinical Predictors of Angina Following Myocardial Infarction, *Am. J. Med.,* 66:991, 1979.

52 Chaitman, B. R., Bourassa, M. G., Wagnairt, P., et al.: Improved Efficiency of Treadmill Exercise Testing Using a Multiple Lead ECG System and Basic Hemodynamic Exercise Response, *Circulation,* 57:71, 1978.

53 Weiner, D. A., McCabe, C., Klein, M. D., and Ryan, T. J.: ST-Segment Changes Post-Infarction: Predictive Value for Multivessel Coronary Disease and Left Ventricular Aneurysm, *Circulation,* 58:887, 1978.

54 Hossack, K. F., Sivarajan, E. S., Almes, M. J., Belanger, L. G., Green, B., and Bruce, R. A.: Prognostic Value of ST Evaluation during Low Level Treadmill Testing Early after Myocardial Infarction, *Am. J. Cardiol.,* 49:932, 1982. (Abstract.)

55 Granath, A., Sodermark, T., Winge, T., Volpe, U., and Zetterquist, S.: Early Work Load Tests for Evaluation of Long-Term Prognosis of Acute Myocardial Infarction, *Br. Heart J.,* 39:758, 1977.

56 Gajewski, J., and Singer, R. B.: Mortality in an Insured Population with Atrial Fibrillation, *J.A.M.A.,* 245:1540, 1981.

57 Cristal, N., Szwarcberg, J., and Guern, M.: Supraventricular Arrhythmias in Acute Myocardial Infarction. Prognostic Importance of Clinical Setting: Mechanism of Prediction, *Ann. Intern. Med.,* 82:35, 1975.

58 Lindsay, J., Jr., and Gorfinkel, H. J.: Arrhythmias in the Post CCU Phase of Myocardial Infarction. Their Correlation with the Acute Illness, *Chest* 72:571, 1977.

59 Coronary Drug Project Research Group: Prognostic Importance of Premature Beats following Myocardial Infarction, *J.A.M.A.,* 223:1116, 1973.

60 Kennedy, H. L.: "Ambulatory Electrocardiography," 1st ed., Lea & Febiger, Philadelphia, 1981, p. 224.

61 Allen, R. D., Gettes, L. S., Phalan, C., and Avington, M. D.: Painless ST-Segment Depression in Patients with Angina Pectoris, *Chest,* 69:467, 1976.

62 Schulze, R. A., Strauss, H. W., and Pitt, B.: Sudden Death in the Year following Myocardial Infarction. Relation to Ventricular Premature Contractions in the Late Hospital Phase and Left Ventricular Ejection Fraction, *Am. J. Med.,* 62:192, 1977.

63 Taylor, G. J., Humphries, J. O., Mellits, E. D., et al.: Predictors of Clinical Course, Coronary Anatomy and Left Ventricular Function after Recovery from Acute Myocardial Infarction, *Circulation,* 62:960, 1980.

64 Davis, H. T., DeCamilla, J., Bayer, L. W., and Moss, A. J.: Survivorship Patterns in the Posthospital Phase of Myocardial Infarction, *Circulation,* 60:1252, 1979.

65 Moss, A. J., Davis, H. T., DeCamilla, J., and Bayer, L. W.: Ventricular Ectopic Beats and Their Relation to Sudden and Nonsudden Cardiac Death after Myocardial Infarction, *Circulation,* 60:998, 1979.

66 Winkle, R. A., Peters, F., and Hall, R.: Characterization of Ventricular Tachyarrhythmias on Ambulatory ECG Recordings in Post-Myocardial Infarction Patients: Arrhythmia Detection and Duration of Recording, Relationship between Arrhythmia Frequency and Complexity, and Day-to-Day Reproducibility, *Am. Heart J.,* 102:162, 1981.

67 Bigger, J. T., and Weld, F. M.: Analysis of Prognostic Significance of Ventricular Arrhythmias after Myocardial Infarction. Shortcomings of Lown Grading System, *Br. Heart J.,* 45:717, 1981.

68 Lown, B., and Wolf, M.: Approaches to Sudden Death from Coronary Heart Disease, *Circulation,* 44:130, 1971.

69 Thanavaro, S., Kleiger, R. E., Hieb, R. B., Krone, R. J., DeMello, V. R., and Oliver, G. C.: Effect of Electrocardiographic Recording Duration on Ventricular Dysrhythmia Detection after Myocardial Infarction, *Circulation,* 62:262, 1980.

70 Manger Cats, V., Lie, K. I., Van Capelle, F. J. L., and Durrer, D.: Limitations of 24 Hour Ambulatory Electrocardiographic Recording in Predicting Coronary Events after Acute Myocardial Infarction, *Am. J. Cardiol.,* 44:1257, 1979.

71 Ruberman, W., Weinblatt, E., Goldberg, J. D., Frank, C. W., Chaudhary, B. S., and Shapiro, S.: Ventricular Premature Complexes and Sudden Death after Myocardial Infarction, *Circulation,* 64:297, 1981.

72 Ivanova, L. A., Mazur, N. A., Smirnova, T. M., Sumarokov, A. B., Nazarenko, V. A., and Svet, E. A.: Electrocardiographic Exercise Testing and Ambulatory Monitoring to Identify Patients with Ischemic Heart Disease at High Risk of Sudden Death, *Am. J. Cardiol.,* 45:1132, 1980.

73 DeBusk, R. F., Davidson, D. M., Houston, N., and Fitzgerald, J.: Serial Ambulatory Electrocardiography and Treadmill Exercise Testing after Uncomplicated Myocardial Infarction, *Am. J. Cardiol.,* 45:547, 1980.

74 Luria, M. H., Knoke, J. D., Wachs, J. S., and Luria, M. A.: Survival after Recovery from Acute Myocardial Infarction. Two and Five Year Prognostic Indices, *Am. J. Med.,* 67:7, 1979.

75 Baird, M. G., Williams, W. L., Nair, R., Allan, K., Higginson, L. A., and Beanlands, D. S.: The Limited Prognostic Value of Ventricular Ectopy Recorded Early after Myocardial Infarction, *Circulation,* 64 (suppl. 4):306, 1981.

76 Taylor, G. J., Humphries, J. O., Pitt, B., Griffith, L. S. C., and Achuff, S. C.: Complex Ventricular Arrhythmias after Myocardial Infarction during Convalescence and Follow-Up: A Harbinger of Multi-Vessel Coronary Disease, Left Ventricular Dysfunction and Sudden Death, *Johns Hopkins Med. J.,* 149:1, 1981.

77 Kleiger, R. E., Miller, J. P., Thanavaro, S., Province, M. A., Martin, T. F., and Oliver, G. C.: Relationship between Clinical Features of Acute Myocardial Infarction and Ventricular Runs 2 Weeks to 1 Year after Infarction, *Circulation,* 63:64, 1981.

78 Anderson, K. P., DeCamilla, J., and Moss, A. J.: Clinical Significance of Ventricular Tachycardia (3 Beats or Longer) Detected during Ambulatory Monitoring after Myocardial Infarction, *Circulation,* 57:890, 1978.

79 Bigger, J. T., Weld, F. M., and Rolnitzky, L. M.: Prevalence, Characteristics and Significance of Ventricular Tachycardia (Three or More Complexes) Detected with Ambulatory Electrocardiographic Recording in the Late Hospital Phase of Acute Myocardial Infarction, *Am. J. Cardiol.,* 48:815, 1981.

80 Ruberman, W., Weinblatt, E., Goldberg, J. D., Frank, C. W., and Shapiro, S.: Ventricular Premature Beats and Mortality after Myocardial Infarction, *N. Engl. J. Med.,* 297:750, 1977.

81 Kotler, M. N., Tabatznik, B., Mower, M. M., and Tominga, S.: Prognostic Significance of Ventricular Ectopic Beats with Respect to Sudden Death in the Late Postinfarction Period, *Circulation,* 47:959, 1973.

82 Ryan, M., Lown, B., and Horn, H.: Comparison of Ventricular Ectopic Activity during 24-Hour Monitoring and Exercise Testing in Patients with Coronary Heart Disease, *N. Engl. J. Med.,* 292:224, 1975.

83 Sanz, G., Castaner, A., Magrina, J., et al.: Determinants of Prognosis in Survivors of Myocardial Infarction: A Prospective Clinical Angiographic Study, *N. Engl. J. Med.,* 306:1065, 1982.

84 Botvinick, E., Shamos, D., Lappain, H., Tyberg, J. V., Townsend, R., and Parmley, W. W.: Non-Invasive Quantification of Myocardial Infarction with Technetium-99m Pyrophosphate, *Circulation,* 52:909, 1975.

85 Stokley, E. M., Buja, L. M., Lewis, S. E., et al.: Measurement of Acute Myocardial Infarcts in Dogs with ^{99m}Tc-Stannous Pyrophosphate Scintigrams, *J. Nucl. Med.,* 17:1, 1975.

86 Henning, H., Schelbert, H. R., Righetti, A., Ashburn, W. L., and O'Rourke, R. A.: Dual Myocardial Imaging with Technetium-99m Pyrophosphate and Thallium-201 for Detecting, Localizing and Sizing Acute Myocardial Infarction, *Am. J. Cardiol.,* 40:147, 1977.

87 Holman, B. L., Chisholm, R. J., and Braunwald, E.: The Prognostic Implications of Acute Myocardial Infarct Scintigraphy with 99m-Tc Pyrophosphate, *Circulation,* 57:320, 1978.

88 Ahmad, M., Logan, K. W., and Martin, R. H.: Doughnut Pattern of Technetium-99m Pyrophosphate Myocardial Uptake in Patients with Acute Myocardial Infarction. A Sign of Poor Long-Term Prognosis, *Am. J. Cardiol.,* 44:13, 1973.

89 Rude, R. E., Parkey, R. W., Bonte, F. J., et al.: Clinical Implications of the Technetium-99m Stannous Pyrophosphate Myocardial Scintigraphic "Doughnut" Pattern in Patients with Acute Myocardial Infarcts, *Circulation,* 59:721, 1979.

90 Aldor, E., Heeger, H., Kahn, P., and Kainz, W.: Long-Term Follow-Up Scintigraphy with 99m-Tc Pyrophosphate after Myocardial Infarction, *Z. Kardiol.,* 68:461, 1979.

91 Olson, H. G., Lyons, K. P., Aronow, W. S., Brown, W. T., and Greenfield, R. S.: Follow-Up Technetium-99m Stannous Pyrophosphate Myocardial Scintigrams after Acute Myocardial Infarction, *Circulation,* 56:181, 1977.

92 Olson, H. G., Lyons, K. P., Aronow, W. S., Kuperus, J., Orlando, J., and Hughes, D.: Prognostic Value of a Persistently Positive Technetium-99m Stannous Pyrophosphate Myocardial Scintigram after myocardial Infarction, *Am. J. Cardiol.,* 43:889, 1979.

93 Malin, F. R., Rollo, F. D., and Gertz, E. W.: Sequential Myocardial Scintigraphy with Technetium-99m Stannous Pyrophosphate following Myocardial Infarction, *J. Nucl. Med.,* 19:1111, 1978.

94 Nicod, P., Lewis, S. E., Buja, L. M., et al.: Increased Incidence of "Persistently Positive" Technetium Pyrophosphate Myocardial Scintigrams following Myocardial Infarction in Diabetics, *Am. J. Cardiol,* 49:1016, 1982. (Abstract.)

95 Poliner, L. R., Buja, L. M., Parkey, R. W., Bonte, F. J., and Willerson, J. T.: Clinicopathologic Findings in 52 Patients Studied by Technetium-99m Stannous Pyrophosphate Myocardial Scintigraphy, *Circulation,* 59:257, 1979.

96 Platt, M. R., Parkey, R. W., Willerson, J. T., Bonte, F. J., Shapiro, W., and Sugg, W. L.: Technetium Stannous Pyrophosphate Myocardial Scintigrams in the Recognition of Myocardial Infarction in Patients Undergoing Coronary Artery Revascularization, *Ann. Thorac. Surg.,* 21:311, 1976.

97 Jaffe, A. S., Klein, M. S., Patel, B. R., Siegel, B. A., and

Roberts, R.: Abnormal Technetium-99m Pyrophosphate Images in Unstable Angina: Ischemia versus Infarction, *Am. J. Cardiol.,* 44:1035, 1979.

98 Olson, H. G., Lyons, K. P., Aronow, W. S., Stinson, P. J., Kuperus, J., and Waters, H. J.: The High Risk Angina Patient. Identification by Clinical Features, Hospital Course, Electrocardiography and Technetium-99m Pyrophosphate Scintigraphy, *Circulation,* 64:674, 1981.

99 Berger, B. C., Watson, D. D., Burwell, L. R., et al.: Redistribution of Thallium at Rest in Patients with Stable and Unstable Angina and the Effect of Coronary Artery Bypass Surgery, *Circulation,* 60:1114, 1979.

100 Wackers, F. J. Th., Sokole, E. B., Swanson, G., et al.: Value and Limitations of Thallium-201 Scintigraphy in the Acute Phase of Myocardial Infarction, *N. Engl. J. Med.,* 295:1, 1976.

101 Smitherman, T. C., Osborne, R. C., Jr., Narahara, K. A.: Serial Myocardial Scintigraphy after a Single Dose of Thallium-201 in Men after Acute Myocardial Infarction, *Am. J. Cardiol.,* 42:177, 1978.

102 Wackers, F. J. Th., Becker, A. E., Samson, G., et al.: Location and Size of Acute Transmural Myocardial Infarction Estimated from Thallium-201 Scintigrams, *Circulation,* 56:72, 1977.

103 Silverman, K. J., Becker, L. C., Bueldey, B. H., et al.: Value of Early Thallium-201 Scintigraphy for Predicting Mortality in Patients with Acute Myocardial Infarction, *Circulation,* 61:996, 1980.

104 Shiraishi, T., Kobayaski, A., Hasegewa, T., et al.: A Study of the Quantification of 201-T1 Myocardial Scintigrams of Prior Myocardial Infarctions and Their Influence on Left Ventricular Function, *Radioisotopes,* 29:479, 1980.

105 Mock, M. B., Ringqvist, I., Fisher, L., et al.: The Survival of Nonoperated Patients with Ischemic Heart Disease: The CASS Experience, *Am. J. Cardiol.,* 49:1007, 1982. (Abstract.)

106 Battler, A., Slutsky, R., Karliner, J., Froelicher, V., Ashburn, W., and Ross, J., Jr.: Left Ventricular Ejection Fraction and First Third Ejection Fraction Early after Acute Myocardial Infarction: Value for Predicting Mortality and Morbidity, *Am. J. Cardiol.,* 45:197, 1980.

107 Marmor, A., Geltman, E. M., Schechtman, K., Biello, D., and Roberts, R.: Segmental Wall Motion Impairment, an Indicator of Long-Term Prognosis after Non-Transmural as well as Transmural Infarction, *Am. J. Cardiol.,* 49:1019, 1982. (Abstract.)

108 Ptacin, M. J., Tresch, D. D., Soin, J. S., and Brooks, H. L.: Evaluation of Postresuscitation Left Ventricular Global and Segmental Function by Radionuclide Ventriculography in Sudden Coronary Death Survivors of Prehospital Cardiac Arrest: Correlation to Short Term Prognosis, *Am. Heart J.,* 103:54, 1982.

109 Gibson, R. S., Taylor, G. J., Watson, D. D., et al.: Predicting the Extent and Location of Coronary Artery Disease during the Early Post-Infarction Period by Quantitative Thallium-201 Scintigraphy, *Am. J. Cardiol.,* 47:1010, 1981.

110 Gibson, R. S., Watson, D. D., and Beller, G. A.: Comparison of Submaximal Exercise T1-201 Stress Testing at 2 Weeks and Symptom-Limited Maximum Testing at 3 Months Post Myocardial Infarction, *J. Nucl. Med.,* 23:62, 1982. (Abstract.)

111 Turner, J. D., Schwartz, K. M., Logic, J. R., et al.: Detection of Residual Jeopardized Myocardium 3 Weeks after Myocardial Infarction by Exercise Testing with Thallium-201 Myocardial Scintigraphy, *Circulation,* 61:729, 1980.

112 Rigo, P., Bailey, I. K., Griffith, L. S. C., Pitt, P., Wagner, H. N., and Becker, L. C.: Stress Thallium-201 Myocardial Scintigraphy for the Detection of Individual Coronary Artery Lesions in Patients with and without Previous Myocardial Infarction, *Am. J. Cardiol.,* 48:209, 1981.

113 Madsen, E., Juban, J., Froelicher, V., and Ashburn, W. L.: Value of Radionuclide Technique in Assessment of Ischemia in Patients with Previous Myocardial Infarction, *Am. J. Cardiol.,* 49:1016, 1982. (Abstract.)

114 Brown, K. A., Boucher, C. A., Okada, R. D., Newell, J., Strauss, H. W.: The Prognostic Value of Serial Exercise Thallium-201 Imaging in Patients Presenting for Evaluation of Chest Pain: Comparison to Contrast Angiography, Exercise Electrocardiography and Clinical Data, *Am. J. Cardiol.,* 49:967, 1982. (Abstract.)

115 Rigo, P., Bailey, I. K., Griffith, L. S. C., et al.: Value and Limitations of Segmental Analysis of Stress Thallium Myocardial Imaging for Localization of Coronary Artery Disease, *Circulation,* 61:973, 1980.

116 Gibson, R. S., Watson, D. D., Carbello, B. A., Holt, N. D., and Beller, G. A.: Clinical Implications of Increased Lung Uptake of Thallium-201 during Exercise Scintigraphy 2 Weeks after Myocardial Infarction, *Am. J. Cardiol.,* 49:1586, 1982.

117 Davies, R. A., Beanlands, D. S., and Deimel, J.: Exercise Thallium-201 Myocardial Imaging after Inferior Infarction to Detect Multi-Vessel Coronary Artery Disease: Accepted for Presentation at the Canadian Cardiovascular Society, Calgary, October, 1982. (Abstract.)

118 Borer, J. S., Dosing, D. R., Miller, R. H., et al.: Natural History of Left Ventricular Function during 1 Year after Acute Myocardial Infarction, Comparison with Clinical, Electrocardiographic and Biochemical Determinations, *Am. J. Cardiol.,* 46:1, 1980.

119 Corbett, J. R., Dehmer, G. J., Lewis, S. E., et al.: The Prognostic Value of Submaximal Exercise Testing with Radionuclide Ventriculography before Hospital Discharge in Patients with Recent Myocardial Infarction, *Circulation,* 64:535, 1981.

120 Morris, K. G., Califf, R. M., Sebastian, T., et al.: Significance of Serial Rest and Exercise Radionuclide

Angiography after Acute Myocardial Infarction, *Am. J. Cardiol.*, 49:901, 1982. (Abstract.)

121 Nicod, P., Corbett, J. R., Firth, B. G., et al.: Prognostic Assessment after Myocardial Infarction: Comparison between Coronary Angiography and Submaximal Exercise Testing with Radionuclide Ventriculography, *Am. J. Cardiol.*, 49:991, 1982. (Abstract.)

122 Phillips, P., Borer, J. S., Jacobstein, J., et al.: Prognostically Critical Coronary Stenoses: Identification by Radionuclide Cineangiography, *Am. J. Cardiol.*, 49:991, 1982. (Abstract.)

Research performed at the University of Ottawa Cardiac Unit in this field was supported in part by Ontario Heart Foundation Grant No. T5-15. We would like to acknowledge the research assistance of Mrs. Kathy Allan, R.N., and Rama Nair, Ph.D. We also appreciate the secretarial assistance and support of Miss Heather Cross, Ms. Margaret Bruce, Mrs. Elaine Halliday, and Mrs. Cheryl Nurse.

Reliability of the LD–1/LD–2 Ratio in the Diagnosis of Perioperative Myocardial Infarction in Cardiac Surgical Patients[*]

RICHARD E. MICHALIK, M.D., NICHOLAS M. PAPADOPOULOS, PH.D., BYRON D. MCLEES, M.D., and MICHAEL JONES, M.D.

An accurate estimate of myocardial damage in cardiac surgical patients would be an important index of the adequacy of intraoperative myocardial protection.[1] Reliable early detection of perioperative infarction would aid in the management of the immediate postoperative course. To this end, the electrocardiogram (ECG),[2-3] the vectorcardiogram,[4] radionuclide myocardial perfusion imaging,[5-7] and quantitation of the serum enzymes lactate dehydrogenase (LD), creatine kinase (CK),[8,9] and their respective isoenzymes[10-12] have been studied as diagnostic tools. Shortcomings in sensitivity or specificity have been found with each method. Usually preoperative and serial postoperative determinations over 3 or more days are required. The radionuclide studies are difficult to perform in critically ill patients in the first hours or day following operation, require special equipment, and may often require a repeat study to delineate ischemia from infarction. Combinations of these tests may improve diagnostic accuracy, but with added cost. These considerations emphasize the need for a single, reliable test to detect significant perioperative myocardial infarction.

The LD isoenzyme-1 (LD-1) is relatively cardiac specific. Determinations of LD isoenzymes and estimations of the ratio of LD-1 to LD-2 isoenzyme fractions have been established as useful biochemical indexes of myocardial infarction (MI) in nonsurgical patients.[13] A change in the LD-1/LD-2 ratio from a value less than 1.0 to one greater than 1.0, the so-called reversal or flip, occurs after myocardial infarction. Galen and others,[13] however, consider the ratio of LD-1 to LD-2 to have limited value in the diagnosis of myocardial infarction in cardiac surgical patients in view of the contamination of serum LD-1 (myocardial fraction) by hemolysis. The improved technique of Papadopoulos[14,15] offers enhanced electrophoretic resolution, permitting accurate quantitation of these isoenzymes. The electrophoretic test has been applied successfully in patients undergoing either revascularization or valve replacement[17] and is further validated in the present investigation.

Our study was undertaken to examine the usefulness of the reversal or flip of the LD-1/LD-2 ratio as an indicator of myocardial infarction in patients undergoing a variety of cardiac surgical procedures.

[*]From the Surgery Branch, National Heart, Lung and Blood Institute, and the Departments of Clinical Pathology and Critical Care Medicine, National Institutes of Health, Bethesda, Maryland.

MATERIALS AND METHODS

Forty patients were chosen for study: 9 underwent revascularization procedure, 9 valve replacement, 9 ventricular myotomy and myectomy (LV M and M) for obstructive asymmetric septal hypertrophy (ASH), and 10 for anatomic correction of congenital cardiac anomalies. Three additional patients underwent combined revascularization and valve replacement. Ages ranged from 5 to 71 years; there were 30 men and 10 women. Each operation employed cardiopulmonary bypass with moderate systemic hypothermia (25 to 30°C) and aortic cross-clamping. Hypothermic (30°C) coronary perfusion, cold crystalloid cardioplegia, and topical hypothermia were all used in this study either alone or in combination.

The data base was comprised of the assessments of the postoperative clinical course, serial electrocardiograms, and serial determinations of serum LD and CK enzymes and isoenzymes. Clinical assessments were based on the postoperative hemodynamic data and the need for pharmacologic support and/or intraaortic balloon counterpulsation. Twelve-lead ECGs were obtained from each patient 48 h prior to operation, 24 h after the completion of cardiopulmonary bypass, and on the mornings of postoperative days 2, 3, 5, and 7. In patients not undergoing ventriculotomies, the appearance of new Q waves was equated with the occurrence of infarction. The persistence of injury currents for more than 48 h postoperatively or the appearance of new bundle branch blocks was considered suggestive of myocardial injury. The ECGs of those patients undergoing left ventricular myotomy and myectomy were reviewed for evidence of injury other than might be expected resulting from the myocardial incisions per se, i.e., left bundle branch block. A single cardiologist reviewed all ECGs without adjunctive clinical information except for patient age and operative procedure.

Serum samples were obtained preoperatively and at 0, 4, and 24 h, as well as 2, 3, 5, and 7 days postoperatively. The 0 time was taken as 30 min following separation from cardiopulmonary bypass. Serum samples with visible hemolysis were discarded. Samples from the first 10 patients were separated into two portions, one analyzed the same day it was obtained and one stored at −72°C routinely and analyzed within 3 months.

85

Measurement of the total LD and CK activities was made spectrophotometrically using the SMAC analyzer.* Determination of CK isoenzymes was performed by an electrophoretic fluorometric procedure using agarose gel plates.† The relative percentages of CK isoenzymes were determined by densitometric scanning and the absolute values were calculated.

Determinations of LD isoenzymes were performed by a quantitative 0.5% agarose gel electrophoretic technique,[14,15] which has recently been improved[16] and evaluated in patients undergoing cardiac operations.[17] The main features of this technique are (1) electrophoretic separation of LD isoenzymes on agarose gel–covered microscope slides, (2) colorimetric development of the isoenzymatic activity by a tetrazolium reduction procedure, and (3) quantitation of the isoenzyme zones by densitometric scanning.

RESULTS

Validation of Assay Technique

In order to exclude hemolysis in determining the reversal of the LD-1/LD-2 ratio, the improved method of Papadopoulos was used to quantitate the LD isoenzymes in normal serum, erythrocyte lysates, and myocardial extracts. The results in Table 1 show the relative percentages of LD-1 and LD-2 in normal serum to be approximately 30 and 40 percent, respectively, yielding an LD-1/LD-2 ratio of 0.75 in normal serum. By this technique, however, the LD isoenzyme ratio in erythrocyte lysates is also less than unity (0.95). Consequently, hemolysis alone, while increasing total LD, cannot result in an LD-1/LD-2 ratio greater than unity by our method. This observation is further substantiated by the test results shown in Fig. 1. Addition of aliquots from erythrocyte lysate to a normal human serum sample caused an increase in LD-1 that approached but did not exceed the LD-2 value. However, a reversal of the LD-1/LD-2 ratio can occur following myocardial injury owing to the release of the myocardial LD with its preponderance of LD-1, as demonstrated in extracts of biopsy specimens and fresh samples obtained at postmortem examination.

Additional evidence that a reversal of the ratio does not occur with hemolysis is the fact that even those patients who received 10 or more units of blood in transfusion did not exhibit a flip as a consequence of either or both of these events.

Clinical Studies

The combined analysis of the clinical, ECG, and enzymatic courses of the 40 patients, grouped by operative procedures, are summarized in Table 2. The ECGs could be evaluated for the occurrence of the perioperative infarction in 24 patients undergoing revascularization procedures, valve replacements, or repairs of congenital anomalies via atriotomies (groups I to VI). In these 24 patients, the electrocardiographic findings are designated + for infarction, − for no infarction, and −/+ for those patients in whom the ECG was highly suggestive of but not diagnostic of myocardial infarction. In the remaining 16 patients, the ECG could not be interpreted reliably for the appearance of new myocardial infarction, and the ECG results are designated as 0.

All 40 patients had at least 30 IU CK-MB activity in two or more consecutive samples during the postoperative period, and thus the CK-MB level was of little use in the determination of clinically significant myocardial infarction.

In 19 of the 24 patients (groups I to VI) in whom the ECGs could be interpreted for the presence or absence of myocardial infarction, there was full agreement between the clinical course, ECG, and the behavior of the LD-1/LD-2 ratio. Six patients (numbers 1 through 6) who underwent revascularization, 7 patients (numbers 10 through 16) who had valve replacements, and 3 patients (numbers 22 through 24) who had congenital anomalies repaired via atriotomies had no evidence of ischemic infarction by any of the techniques. Two

TABLE 1

Relative percentage distribution of lactate dehydrogenase isoenzyme fractions*

	n	1	2	3	4	5
Normal serum	100	29.9 ± 0.4	40.4 ± 0.34	20.3 ± 0.4	5.7 ± 0.2	3.6 ± 0.2
Erythrocyte hemolysates	12	37.9 ± 1.2	40.1 ± 0.9	19.3 ± 2.0	1.5 ± 0.5	1.0 ± 0
Myocardial extracts	4	56	35	6	2	1

*Results expressed as mean ± standard deviation.

*Technicon Corp., Tarrytown, N.Y. 10591.

†Croning, Medfield, Mass. 02052.

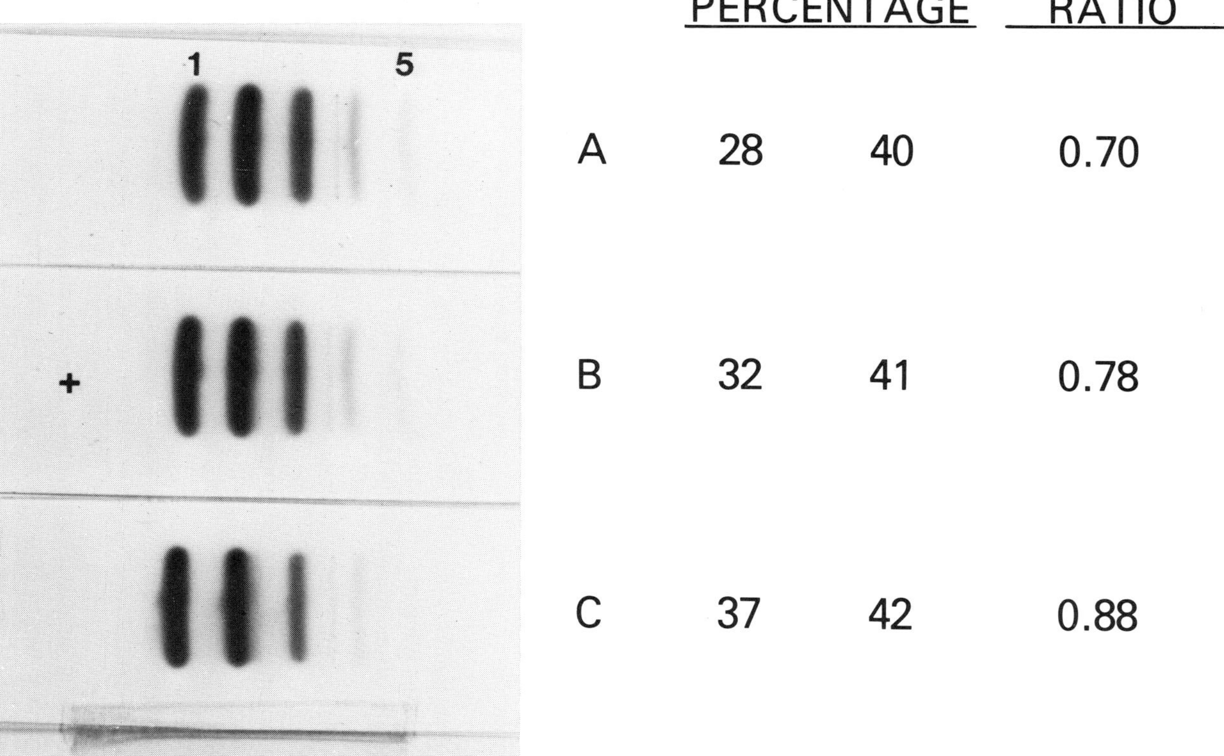

	LD-1	LD-2	LD-1/LD-2
	PERCENTAGE		RATIO
A	28	40	0.70
B	32	41	0.78
C	37	42	0.88

FIGURE 1 Lactate dehydrogenase isoenzymes of a normal human serum (*A*), of mixtures of the same serum with an erythrocyte lysate in a 1:4 ratio (*B*), and in a 1:1 ratio (*C*). The values of the isoenzymes were obtained by densitometric scanning and their ratios estimated.

88

TABLE 2
Display of the clinical, ECG and enzymatic course of 40 patients

Groups	Patient number	Clinical course	ECG	LD-1/LD-2 ratio > 1.0
I. Myocardial revascularization	1–6	– – –	– – –	– – –
	7	– – –	– – –	+ + +
	8	– – –	+ + +	+ + +
	9	+ + +	+/–	+ + +
II. Valve replacement	10–16	– – –	– – –	– – –
	17	– – –	– – –	+ + +
	18	+/–	+/–	+/–
III. Combined valve replacement and revascularization	19–20	+ + +	+ + +	+ + +
	21	+ + +	+/–	– – –
IV. Congenital repair without ventriculotomy	22–24	– – –	– – –	– – –
V. Left ventriculomyotomy and myectomy	25–29	– – –	0	– – –
	30–32	+/–	0	– – –
	33	– – –	0	+ + +
VI. Congenital repair with ventriculotomy	34	– – –	0	– – –
	35–36	– – –	0	+ + +
	37–38	+ + +	0	– – –
	39–40	+ + +	0	+ + +

patients (numbers 19 and 20), both elderly, who underwent combined aortic valve replacements and revascularization procedures experienced infarctions by all three study modes. The remaining patient (number 18) had marked transient ECG changes of injury after refractory ventricular arrhythmias progressed to cardiac arrest. Within hours after resuscitation, this patient's LD-1/LD-2 ratio rose to 1.0 and then returned to normal within 48 h.

Five of the 24 patients showed conflicts of interpretations of the three study modes with respect to occurrence of infarction. One revascularization patient (number 8) had an unremarkable operative procedure and postoperative clinical course, but clearly had a myocardial infarction, evidenced by significant new Q waves and a clearcut pattern of LD%1/LD-2 reversal. One revascularization patient (number 7) and one aortic valve replacement patient (number 17) had benign postoperative courses with no significant ECG changes, but they both had LD isoenzyme evidence of infarction. Another myocardial revascularization patient (number 9) required inotropic agent support during the first 24 h following operation, had a flipped LD-1/LD-2 ratio, but exhibited no new ECG findings of infarction compared with his preoperative tracing. Another patient (number 21), age 70, underwent mitral and aortic valve replacements with revascularization. He required mechanical ventilation and pressor support for the duration of the study and intraaortic balloon counterpulsation for the first 3 postoperative days. He expired in renal failure and sepsis some 60 days following operation. There was no flip of the LD ratio and only anterior ST-T wave abnormalities on ECG. At autopsy, he was found to have a large midseptal infarction of indeterminate age.

The results in the remaining 16 patients (groups V and VI), in whom the ECG was not useful, are described below. In the NIH experience, the postoperative ECGs of patients with obstructive hypertrophic cardiomyopathy are variable. Owing to severe septal and left ventricular hypertrophy, patients may have changes consistent with lateral or inferior myocardial infarction preoperatively. Following the septal incisions and resection, new left bundle branch block may occur in more than 60 percent of patients after left ventricular myotomy and myectomy[18] and obscure the changes of myocardial infarction. The 7 patients who had right ventriculotomies for repair of congenital cardiac anomalies had multiple ECG abnormalities preoperatively, including intraventricular conduction delay and right bundle branch block; so that the postoperative ECG was of limited diagnostic value. The clinical course remains the only standard for comparison in this group, but adjunctive LD and CK data are presented. Group V contains nine patients (numbers 25 through 33) who underwent left ventricular myotomy and myectomy for asymmetric septal hypertrophy with left ventricular outflow obstruction. One patient (number 30) also underwent triple saphenous vein coronary artery bypass grafting. Each had documented relief of obstruction. Three patients (numbers 30 through 32) who exhibited congestive failure preoperatively required mild inotropic support during the first 24 h following operation. Electrocardiograms of the three patients provided no evidence of new myocardial injury. None of the three exhibited enzymatic evidence of significant myocardial injury by LD-1/LD-2 ratio. One of the remaining 6 myotomy and myectomy patients (number 33), an otherwise healthy 32-year-old male, had an uncomplicated course and no ECG changes (including no new left bundle branch block), but had a flip of magnitude and duration consistent with the perioperative injury pattern. The 5 patients in this group who had no ECG or enzymatic evidence of infarction experienced unremarkable postoperative courses.

Group VI contains the 7 patients (numbers 34 through 40) who had right ventriculotomies as part of procedures for correction of congenital anomalies and also have no corroborative ECG data. The results in these patients are difficult to categorize. Three patients clearly had benign postoperative courses. One (number 34) was a 55-year-old male with a ventricular septal defect (VSD) who underwent closure of the VSD through a right ventriculotomy and exhibited no flip of the L-1/L-2 ratio. The other two (numbers 35 and 36) were children, one of whom underwent VSD closure while the other received a right ventricular-to-pulmonary artery conduit for correction of type IV truncus anteriosus. Both these patients exhibited flipped LD-1/LD-2 ratios so as to indicate myocardial infarction. The remaining 4 patients in group VI had complex congenital anomalies. All were cyanotic and polycythemic, all required inotropic agent support postoperatively, and 2 did not survive. Of the 4, one survivor and one nonsurvivor flipped the LD ratio, while one survivor and one nonsurvivor evidenced no flip.

DISCUSSION

Intraoperative infarction in the patient receiving inadequate myocardial protection may range from focal myocardial ischemia to transmural infarction. The operative procedure itself may result in direct injury to the myocardium through manipulation, incision, suture lines, and so forth. Each procedure is accompanied by some skeletal muscle injury, and a degree of hemolysis is associated with cardiopulmonary bypass and transfusion. The subsequent changes in serum enzymes (LD and CK) and their isoenzymes reflect these factors. Changes in these enzymes, as well as the ECG and radionuclide myocardial perfusion imaging studies, have been evaluated as indicators of myocardial infarction. Recently, studies have suggested that the reversal, or flip, of the LD-1/LD-2 ratio is a reliable indicator of myocardial infarction in nonsurgical patients.[13] The findings of our study indicate that a clearcut flip may be indicative of perioperative myocardial infarction.

The LD isoenzyme proportions in normal human serum, as established at our institution, indicate the ratio of LD-1/LD-2 to be 0.75 (see Table 1). No other organ is known to approach the myocardium in its preponderance of LD-1, whereas the amount of LD-1 in erythrocytes is always slightly less than that of LD-2. Consequently, hemolysis associated with mechanical factors such as cardiopulmonary bypass or cardiac valvular prostheses cannot cause the amount of LD-1 in serum to exceed that of LD-2. Should the ratio exceed 1.0, a source relatively rich in LD-1 must be sought. It has been suggested that the hemolysis may facilitate the flip by bringing the ratio closer to 1. While this is conceptually possible, as the hemolysis is increased, the relative proportions of LD-1 and LD-2 would remain unchanged, and absolute excess of LD-2 would increase with increased hemolysis.

The diagnosis of myocardial infarction by LD isoenzymes in this study required the demonstration of the reversal of the LD-1/LD-2 ratio in 3 or more consecutive samples, thus ruling out chance errors in technique or sample handling. The serum collected at 24 h was always one of the 3 or more samples exhibiting the flip, suggesting that patients could be screened for infarction by obtaining a single blood sample. This simplicity contrasts with that of nuclear imaging techniques and methods requiring serial sampling.

All 40 patients had at least 30 IU CK-MB activity in 2 or more consecutive samples at some point during the postoperative myocardial infarction. If CK-MB appears in nearly all patients after cardiac operations, then numerical thresholds must be established for the diagnosis of infarction.[19] Such thresholds probably would vary according to surgical procedure, surgeon, and the mode of myocardial protection.

The results in the 33 patients (Table 2) not undergoing ventriculotomy indicate that the LD-1/LD-2 ratio is the best single index of clinically significant myocardial infarction. This group includes patients undergoing revascularization, valve replacement, left ventricular myotomy and myectomy, and repair of congenital anomalies without a ventriculotomy. No patient in this group with electrocardiographic evidence of myocardial infarction failed to show a flipped ratio. Of those 24 in whom the ECG might be useful, 4 patients (numbers 7, 8, 9, and 17) showed ratio changes characteristic of infarction without clinical or electrocardiographic evidence to support the diagnosis. A single patient had an uncomplicated course but unmistakable ECG and enzyme changes indicative of infarction. Given the limitations of the ECG and the clinical course assessments, we feel that the reversal of the isoenzyme ratio in these 5 patients (numbers 7, 8, 9, 17, and 33) reflects the occurrence of significant myocardial infarction. This is supported by the autopsy findings of myocardial infarction in 1 patient.

Several trends support the accuracy of the flip. Preoperative total LD values ranged up to 300 U/liter with the exception of 1 patient known to have anemia secondary to mechanical valve hemolysis. The total LD value in those patients not demonstrating a flip rose no higher than 600 U/liter, while patients experiencing reversal of the ratio had higher LD values. Occasional isolated samples showing evaluations in total LD that did not fit the expected time course for LD postoperatively were usually associated with secondary procedures such as cardioversion. These appeared at various times throughout the study period, were far in excess of the values derived from neighboring samples, and were accompanied in no instance by the return of CK-MB. The patients involved all had benign clinical courses with no evidence of myocardial infarction.

The small number of patients in the ventriculotomy group (group VI), the complexity of the intracardiac procedures, and the variable postoperative courses observed permit only general conclusions. The reversal of the LD-1/LD-2 ratio in some patients indicated myocardial infarction beyond that expected from the operation alone. For this reason, this ratio can be used to identify such patients for additional study, particularly with radionuclide myocardial imaging, and may show that variations in operative technique are responsible for the infarction. Further studies also may provide explanations in those cases where a seemingly good technical procedure yields less than the expected clinical results.

In conclusion, the reversal, or flip, of the LD-1/LD-2 ratio was an accurate indicator of the occurrence of myocardial infarction in patients undergoing myocardial revascularization, valve replacements, left ventricular myotomy and myectomy, and repair of congenital cardiac malformation via atriotomies. Mechanical hemolysis associated with cardiopulmonary bypass did not result in a serum LD-1/LD-2 ratio greater than 1.0, as determined by the method of Papadopoulos. All patients with LD isoenzyme reversal exhibited this finding in the sample collected 24 h after cardiopulmonary bypass, suggesting that patients may be accurately screened for significant perioperative ischemic infarction using a single LD isoenzyme determination drawn 1 full day after operation. Serial determinations, 4, 12, 24, and 48 h after operation, may allow estimation of the extent of myocardial infarction, particularly when total LD and CK are considered.

CONCLUSIONS

Serial determinations of lactate dehydrogenase (LD), creatine kinase (CK), and their isoenzymes were performed in serum samples of 40 patients undergoing a variety of cardiac operations. The electrocardiograms and evaluations of the clinical courses were used as determinants of the occurrence of perioperative myocardial injury. These patients were divided into four categories: myocardial revascularization, valve replacement, left ventriculomyotomy and myectomy, and repair of intracardiac congenital defects. LD isoenzymes were determined by an improved electrophoretic method minimizing the effect of hemolysis. The ratio of LD isoenzyme-1 to LD isoenzyme-2 was found to be the best indicator of significant myocardial infarction, whereas ventricular incisions per se did not produce the reversal pattern. The consistent early appearance of CK isoenzyme MB in all patients limited its usefulness in diagnosing perioperative myocardial infarction. However, the LD-1/LD-2 ratio in a single serum sample obtained 24 h following operation did predict accurately the occurrence of perioperative myocardial infarction.

REFERENCES

1 Spencer, F. C.: The Significance of Myocardial Preservation and Subclinical Myocardial Infarction Following Coronary Bypass, *Ann. Thorac. Surg.*, 26:197, 1978.

2 Warren, S. G., Wagner, G. S., Bethea, C. F., Row, C. R., Oldham, H. N., and Kong, Y: Diagnostic and Prognostic Significance of Electrocardiographic and CPK Isoenzyme Changes Following Coronary Bypass Surgery, *Am. Heart J.*, 93:189, 1977.

3 Shirey, E. K., Proudfit, W. L., and Sones, F. M.: Serum Enzyme and Electrocardiographic Changes after Coronary Artery Surgery, *Chest,* 57:122, 1970.

4 Fennel, W. H., Chua, K. G., Cohen, L., Morgan, J., Karunaratne, H. B., Resnekov, L., Al-Sadir, J., Lin, C. Y., Lamberti, J. L., and Anagnostopoulos, C. E.: Detection, Prediction and Significance of Perioperative Myocardial Infarction Following Aortocoronary Bypass, *J. Thorac. Cardiovasc. Surg.*, 78:244, 1979.

5 Righetti, M. A., Crawford, M. H., O'Rourke, R. A., Hardarson, T., Schelbert, H., Daily, P. O., DuLuca, M., Ashburn, W., and Ross, J.: Detection of Perioperative Myocardial Damage after Coronary Artery Bypass Graft Surgery, *Circulation,* 55:173, 1977.

6 Hung, J., Kelly, D. T., McLaughlin, A. F., Uren, R. E., and Baird, D. K.: Preoperative and Postoperative Technetium-99m Pyrophosphate Myocardial Scintigraphy in the Assessment of Operative Infarction in Coronary Artery Surgery, *J. Thorac. Cardiovasc. Surg.,* 78:68, 1979.

7 Roberts, A. J., Combes, J. R., Jacobstein, J. G., Alonso, D. R., Post, M. R., Subramanian, V. A., Abel, R. M., Brachfeld, N., Kline, S. A., and Gay, W. A.: Perioperative Myocardial Infarction Associated with Coronary Artery Bypass Graft Surgery: Improved Sensitivity in the Diagnosis within 6 Hours after Operation with Tcglucoheptonate Myocardial Imaging and Myocardial Specific Isoenzymes, *Ann. Thorac. Surg.,* 27:42, 1978.

8 DePonti, C., Pioselli, D., and DeVita, C.: Serum Enzyme Changes Following Coronary Bypass Surgery, *Am. Heart J.,* 90:535, 1975.

9 Alderman, E. L., Matlof, H. J., Shumway, N. E., and Harrison, D. C.: Evaluation of Enzyme Testing for the Detection of Myocardial Infarction Following Direct Coronary Surgery, *Circulation,* 48:135, 1973.

10 Krafft, J., Fink, R., and Rosalki, S. B.: Serum Enzymes and Isoenzymes after Surgery, *Ann. Clin. Biochem.,* 14:294, 1977.

11 Codd, J. E., Kaiser, G. C., Wiens, R. D., Barner, H. M., and Willman, V. L.: Myocardial Injury and Bypass Grafting, *J. Thorac. Cardiovasc. Surg.,* 70:489, 1975.

12 Dixon, S. H., Limbird, L. E., Roe, C. R., Wagner, G. S., Oldham, H. N., and Sabiston, D. C.: Recognition of Postoperative Acute Myocardial Infarction, *Circulation,* 48 (suppl. 3):137, 1973.

13 Galen, R. S.: The Enzyme Diagnosis of Myocardial Infarction, *Hum. Pathol.,* 6:141, 1975.

14 Papadopoulos, N. M., and Kintzios, J.: Quantitative Electrophoretic Determination of Lactate Dehydrogenase Isoenzymes, *Am. J. Clin. Pathol.,* 47:96, 1967.

15 Papadopoulos, N. M.: Clinical Applications of Lactate Dehydrogenase Isoenzymes, *Ann. Clin. Lab. Sci.,* 7:506, 1977.

16 Papadopoulos, N. M., and Hufnagel, C.: Detection of Complications in Cardiac Operations by Lactate Dehydrogenase Isoenzymes, *Clin. Chem.,* 25:1087, 1979.

17 Papadopoulos, N. M., and Hufnagel, C.: Evaluation of Lactate Dehydrogenase Isoenzyme Patterns in Serum of Patients Undergoing Cardiac Surgery, *J. Thorac. Cardiovasc. Surg.,* 76:173, 1978.

18 Morrow, A. G., Reitz, B. A., Epstein, S. E., Henry, W. L., Conkle, D. M., Itscoitz, S. B., and Redwood, D. R.: Operative Treatment in Hypertrophic Subaortic Stenosis: Techniques, and the Results of Pre- and Postoperative Assessment in 83 Patients, *Circulation,* 52:88, 1975.

19 Delva, E., Maille, J. G., Solymoss, B. C., Chabot, M., Grondin, C. M., and Bourassa, M. G.: Evaluation of Myocardial Damage during Coronary Artery Grafting with Serial Determinations of Serum CPK MB Isoenzyme, *J. Thorac. Cardiovasc. Surg.,* 75:467, 1978.

Radionuclide Imaging in Patients with Chronic Chest Pain[*]

EBERHARD HENZE, M.D., ROBERT C. MARSHALL, M.D., and HEINRICH R. SCHELBERT, M.D.

Traditional rest-exercise electrocardiographic evaluation of patients with chronic chest pain provides important diagnostic information about the presence of coronary artery disease. However, the temporal disappearance of Q waves after myocardial infarction and the nonspecific ST-T wave changes produced by ventricular hypertrophy, conduction disturbances, drugs, and metabolic abnormalities limit the diagnostic accuracy of the electrocardiogram in many patients. In addition, no information is obtained about the functional consequences of coronary artery obstruction with respect to myocardial perfusion, metabolism, and contraction.

Because of the limitations of electrocardiography, radionuclide imaging techniques have been applied to patients with chronic chest pain in an attempt to improve the noninvasive diagnosis of coronary artery disease. In contrast to the electrocardiogram, radionuclide techniques provide additional, unique physiologic information about the functional consequences of coronary artery obstruction. Based on their documented clinical utility, rest and exercise evaluation of myocardial perfusion with thallium-201 and myocardial function with technetium-99m have become routine procedures in the work-up of patients with chronic chest pain. However, specific limitations of these approaches have been observed, and these are primarily related to the tracers, imaging equipment, and image analysis currently employed.

This article will review the nuclear medicine techniques employed in the evaluation of patients with chronic chest pain. Attention will be focused on the diagnostic and functional information provided, possible future developments, and the potential limitations of these techniques so that a guide for their proper use can be developed.

RADIONUCLIDE EVALUATION OF MYOCARDIAL PERFUSION

The major ionic perfusion indicator currently employed, thallium-201 (^{201}Tl), is a potassium analogue with a low-energy photon emission that can be imaged with standard gamma cameras. Thallium-201 has a physical half-life of 72 h. Given the standard dose of 1.5

*From the Department of Medicine, Division of Cardiology, and Laboratory of Nuclear Medicine, School of Medicine, University of California at Los Angeles.

to 2.0 mCi, there is a whole-body radiation dose of 350 to 400 mrad (approximately equal to one abdominal x-ray).[1]

Physiologic Distribution and Imaging Procedure

Following isotope introduction, ^{201}Tl initially accumulates in the myocardium in direct proportion to regional blood flow.[2] The flow-dependent distribution of ^{201}Tl reflects its high affinity for the myocardium, as manifested by a single-pass extraction fraction of 80 to 90 percent.[2-4] Metabolic factors that affect intracellular cation flux and extreme conditions of high or low flow may alter the relative distribution of ^{201}Tl in the myocardium.[2] Although the physiologic kinetics of ^{201}Tl have been assumed to be analogous to those of potassium, recent evidence suggests that there are differences in transmembranous uptake, cellular distribution, and efflux.[5] These differences do not appear to affect the clinical use of ^{201}Tl as a blood flow indicator.

Immediately following the flow-related accumulation of ^{201}Tl in the myocardium, equilibration of intracellular and total-body ^{201}Tl pools begin.[6,7] The direction and rate of exchange across the sarcolemma is primarily determined by the intracellular-to-extracellular concentration gradient. In cells with normal blood flow and a high intracellular tracer concentration, there is a net efflux of ^{201}Tl out of the cell as ^{201}Tl moves down its concentration gradient. In cells with low flow and a low intracellular tracer concentration, efflux of ^{201}Tl occurs at a much slower rate or there than can be continued influx of ^{201}Tl. Over time, equilibration of intracellular and extracellular ^{201}Tl pools leads to the disappearance of flow-induced regional differences in myocardial tracer concentration—a phenomenon known as *redistribution*. Following redistribution, the final regional concentration of thallium reflects myocardial mass instead of blood flow.

Although patients with coronary artery disease frequently have reduced regional perfusion at rest,[8-10] these differences may be subtle, and ^{201}Tl perfusion imaging is usually performed after maximal symptom-limited exercise in order to exaggerate regional differences in coronary reserve. In patients whose exercise capacity is limited, dipyridamole administration can be substituted for stress provocation.[11,12] Because redistribution begins immediately, imaging in the anterior and 30 to 40° and 70° left anterior oblique views should be completed within 30 min after introduction of ^{201}Tl.

To evaluate the presence of redistribution, delayed views are obtained approximately 3 to 4 h after exercise.

Image interpretation is usually performed qualitatively on both the analogue images (allowing evaluation of the quality of the data) and on computer-enhanced images (allowing improvement of the target-to-background ratio). By comparing stress and delayed scintigrams, different patterns of ^{201}Tl uptake and redistribution can be discerned consistent with normal, ischemic, and infarcted myocardium. In normal hearts, ^{201}Tl tracer activity is distributed homogeneously throughout the left ventricular wall with a central zone of decreased radioactivity corresponding to the left ventricular cavity. The stress and redistribution images are identical in appearance. In hearts made transiently ischemic with exercise, a perfusion defect is observed on the exercise study that completely or partially disappears on delayed views owing to tracer redistribution[7,13] (see also Fig. 1). In hearts with a previous infarction, an unchanged, persistent perfusion defect is observed in both the exercise and delayed images.

Clinical Application in Patients with Chronic Chest Pain

Evaluation of patients with chronic chest pain with rest-exercise ^{201}Tl scintigraphy provides clinically important information in two general areas. The first and more extensively evaluated is the noninvasive diagnosis of coronary artery disease. The second is the assessment of the functional significance of known disease.

From 1976 to 1979, the sensitivity and specificity of rest-exercise ^{201}Tl perfusion imaging in the diagnosis of coronary artery disease was evaluated in a total of 1,817 patients.[14] The sensitivity (true positives divided by all patients with coronary artery disease) ranged from 67 to 100 percent and averaged 82 percent. The specificity (true negatives divided by all patients without coronary artery disease) ranged from 50 to 100 percent and averaged 91 percent. The considerable scatter in the reported sensitivity and specificity probably reflects variations in the disease prevalence and criteria used in image interpretation. The specificity of ^{201}Tl perfusion

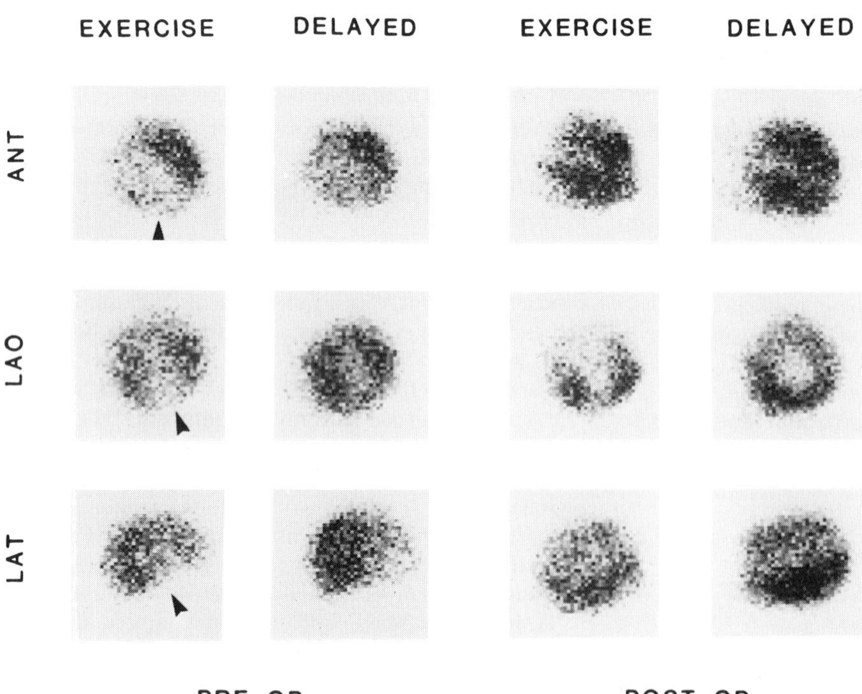

FIGURE 1 Two sets of ^{201}Tl perfusion images obtained before (preoperative) and after (postoperative) double bypass graft surgery in a patient with right and circumflex coronary artery lesions. The preoperative study demonstrates an inferior perfusion defect (arrow) after exercise with complete redistribution on the delayed images. The postoperative study was performed 4 months after surgery for persistent atypical chest pain and demonstrates almost uniform distribution of ^{201}Tl throughout the left ventricular myocardium on both the postexercise and the delayed images, thus indicating successful bypass grafting and patency.

imaging appears to be reduced in women compared with men, possibly owing to breast attenuation of the low-energy ^{201}Tl radiation[15] (Fig. 2). In addition, sensitivity of ^{201}Tl scintigraphy is decreased in patients who receive inadequate exercise or who take beta blocking drugs.[15,16] When compared with the diagnostic accuracy of the rest-exercise electrocardiogram, Tl-201 perfusion scintigraphy is significantly more sensitive (72 versus 60 percent, $p < .001$) and specific (91 versus 81 percent, $p < .05$).[14] These results, acquired in many different laboratories, demonstrate that application of rest-exercise ^{201}Tl myocardial perfusion imaging to patients with chest pain has improved the noninvasive diagnosis of coronary artery disease.[17-22]

Compared with the diagnostic application of ^{201}Tl scintigraphy, use of myocardial perfusion imaging to evaluate the functional significance of coronary artery

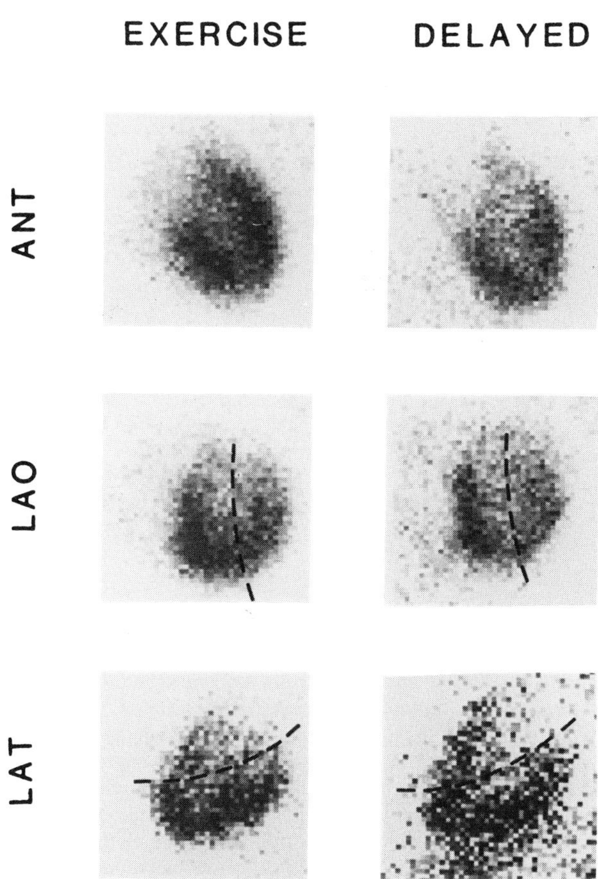

FIGURE 2 Thallium-201 rest-exercise perfusion images in a female patient with normal coronary arteries and no evidence of previous myocardial infarction. The "defects" in the posterolateral and high anterior walls in LAO and LAT views, respectively, are caused by breast attenuation and illustrate one of the limitations of this technique. The breast silhouette is marked by the dashed lines.

obstruction is more difficult. For example, in attempting to assess the significance of a specific coronary lesion, the inaccuracies of coronary arteriography and documented interobserver variability in assessing the degree of obstruction,[23-25] the arbitrary approach to defining a given obstruction as significant, and the effect of collaterals are all variables that must be considered.[26,27] Further, since ^{201}Tl scintigraphy provides information that is not routinely available with other techniques, there is no "gold standard" to assess the accuracy of the physiologic information obtained with ^{201}Tl scintigraphy.

Accepting these limitations, several groups of investigators have attempted to define the accuracy with which ^{201}Tl perfusion imaging detects individual coronary artery obstructions. In general, severe coronary artery obstruction present as single-vessel disease was detected with reasonable sensitivity, while lesser degrees of obstruction in the presence of multivessel disease were not identified.[28,29] Since the presence of a defect was highly specific for coronary artery obstruction, these data indicate that abnormal regional radiotracer activity indicates significant coronary artery obstruction, while normal regional ^{201}Tl concentration does not exclude the presence of a critical coronary artery stenosis.

Rest-exercise ^{201}Tl perfusion imaging also has been used to assess coronary bypass graft patency or the success of percutaneous transluminal angioplasty.[30-32] In patients with complete revascularization and 100 percent graft patency, normal ^{201}Tl scintigrams are routinely obtained (Fig. 1). However, in patients with incomplete revascularization or graft occlusion, normal exercise ^{201}Tl images are obtained in up to 35 percent of instances. These data are similar to those reported for the detection of individual coronary artery obstructions and indicate that a postoperative exercise perfusion defect is highly specific for incomplete revascularization or graft occlusion while a normal exercise ^{201}Tl scintigram does not exclude unrelieved coronary artery obstruction.

Recently there has been increasing interest in using the redistribution kinetics of ^{201}Tl to distinguish between regional wall-motion disturbances owing to "ischemia" from those owing to infarction. Regions with dysynergy and redistribution of ^{201}Tl into a stress-induced defect are felt to be "ischemic," while dysfunctional regions with persistent defects on delayed images are interpreted as having sustained a myocardial infarction. Several groups of investigators have reported that this approach accurately predicts reversible regional dysfunction, as judged by intervention ventriculography or response to coronary artery bypass grafting.[33-35] However, in another study, two-thirds of persistent resting defects were observed to disappear after successful bypass grafting.[36] Difficulties related to quantification of dynamic changes in regional background might account for these discrepancies.[37] Further evaluation of this potentially important clinical application of ^{201}Tl myocardial perfusion imaging will be necessary to reconcile these conflicting results.

Current Limitations and Future Directions

Despite the documented diagnostic accuracy of rest-exercise ^{201}Tl scintigraphy, individual patients are encouraged with either false positive or false negative images. There are several technical limitations inherent in current ^{201}Tl perfusion imaging that might account for these apparent inaccuracies. First, image interpretation is qualitative with documented significant interobserver variability.[38] The specific interpretation of a given ^{201}Tl image is, therefore, somewhat dependent on the individual interpreting the study. Several groups of investigators have developed a variety of methods of quantitative image analysis using interpolative background subtraction with regional quantitation of ^{201}Tl uptake, redistribution, and washout characteristics.[7,13,39,40] Although widespread evaluation or standardization of these approaches has not been accomplished, it is hoped that quantitative image analysis might overcome problems associated with subjective image interpretation. The second technical limitation results from the two-dimensional display and analysis of a three-dimensional structure. Because of the superimposition of different myocardial regions, independent analysis of specific myocardial segments is limited. To overcome this problem, three-dimensional tomographic reconstruction of ^{201}Tl myocardial perfusion images is currently being evaluated using either specifically designed collimators (longitudinal tomography)[41-43] or rotating camera systems (transaxial tomography).[44,45] Although the initial experience with longitudinal tomography has been disappointing,[46] different collimator designs and transaxial tomography have yet to be adequately evaluated and might provide better results. Finally, there is significant tissue attenuation of the low-energy radiation of [201]Tl. Although new flow tracers with higher radiation energies are currently being evaluated,[47] tissue attenuation of single-photon-emitting radionuclides remains an unsolved problem at the present time.

In contrast, tomographic evaluation of positron-emitting radionuclides overcomes many of the problems inherent in single-photon planar or tomographic imaging.[48] Upon annihilation, positrons emit two high-energy photons 180° apart. Using electronic coincidence detection, only radiation occurring between two opposing detectors is recorded. In combination with three-dimensional reconstruction techniques, regional tissue tracer concentrations can be detected quantitatively, spatial resolution is depth-independent, and exact correction for photon attenuation is possible. Using ^{13}N ammonia as a flow tracer, it has been shown[12,49] that a coronary artery obstruction of 47 percent or greater can be detected and that patients with coronary artery disease can be identified with a sensitivity of 100 percent (see also Fig. 3). Widespread application of positron computed tomography is currently limited because of the necessity of an on-side cyclotron to produce the short-lived radioisotopes.

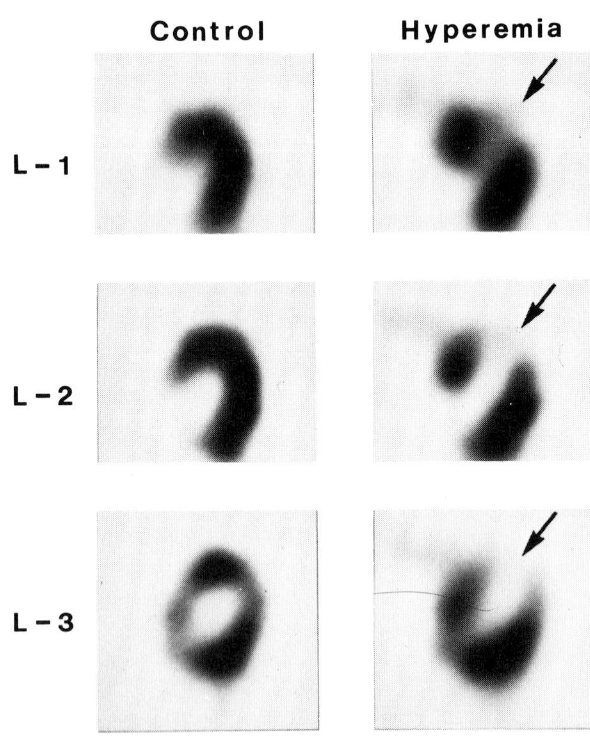

FIGURE 3 Control and hyperemic cross-sectional positron computed tomographic images of the myocardial ^{13}N ammonia distribution in a 67-year-old woman with 100 percent stenosis of the proximal left anterior descending coronary artery. Level 1 (L-1) is recorded through the high anterior and lateral wall, level 2 (L-2) through the mid-left ventricle, and level 3 (L-3) through the middle to lower left ventricle. The control images reveal uniform ^{13}N activity throughout the left ventricular myocardium, suggesting adequate collateral flow to the anterior wall at rest. However, in the hyperemic images, ^{13}N activity was greatly reduced in the anterior wall. Nitrogen-13 activity increased from rest to hyperemia by 32 percent in the lateral wall and by 40 percent in the interventricular septum, but only by 13 percent in the anterior wall. The appearance of a defect in the hyperemic images therefore does not indicate a decrease in flow from the control state to hyperemia but an attenuated response to pharmacologic coronary vasodilation.

With the development of small, dedicated medical cyclotrons and continued demonstration of the clinical utility of this approach, widespread dissemination of positron computed tomography might occur in the near future.

RADIONUCLIDE EVALUATION OF VENTRICULAR PERFORMANCE

Radionuclide evaluation of ventricular function is accomplished using technetium-99m (^{99}Tc). The physical half-life of ^{99m}Tc is 6 h. The standard dose is 20 to 25 mCi, resulting in whole radiation dose similar to that received with ^{201}Tl (200 to 300 mrad).[1,50]

Imaging Techniques

Two procedures are currently in use: first-pass radionuclide angiocardiography and multiple-gated equilibrium cardiac blood pool imaging. First-pass radionuclide angiocardiography is performed immediately after the peripheral venous introduction of a bolus of ^{99m}Tc.[51–55] Real-time count rate data are recorded as the isotope traverses the central circulation. A count-based ejection fraction is calculated from a high-time-resolution count versus a time (or relative ventricular volume) curve constructed from a region of interest placed over the left or right ventricle. Regional wall motion can be evaluated either from images of end-diastole and end-systole or from a computer-reconstructed cine-type display of the entire cardiac cycle.

Multiple-gated equilibrium cardiac blood pool imaging is performed 5 to 10 min following equilibration of autologous red blood cells labeled in vivo or in vitro with ^{99m}Tc.[56,57] Using the R wave of the ECG as a signal of the onset of systole, high-time-resolution images of the entire central circulation are acquired repetitively into computer memory throughout each cardiac cycle.[58–61] A summed cardiac cycle is formed from data acquired over several hundred heart beats and can be viewed as an endless-loop movie for qualitative analysis of regional wall motion. Similar to first-pass radionuclide angiocardiography, a count-based ejection fraction can be determined from a count versus time curve generated from a region of interest placed over the left or right ventricle (Fig. 4).

Both techniques have been shown to accurately measure left ventricular ejection fraction, to accurately evaluate regional ventricular function, and to have suitable interobserver and interstudy variability for the sequential analysis of ventricular function.[51–55,58–67]

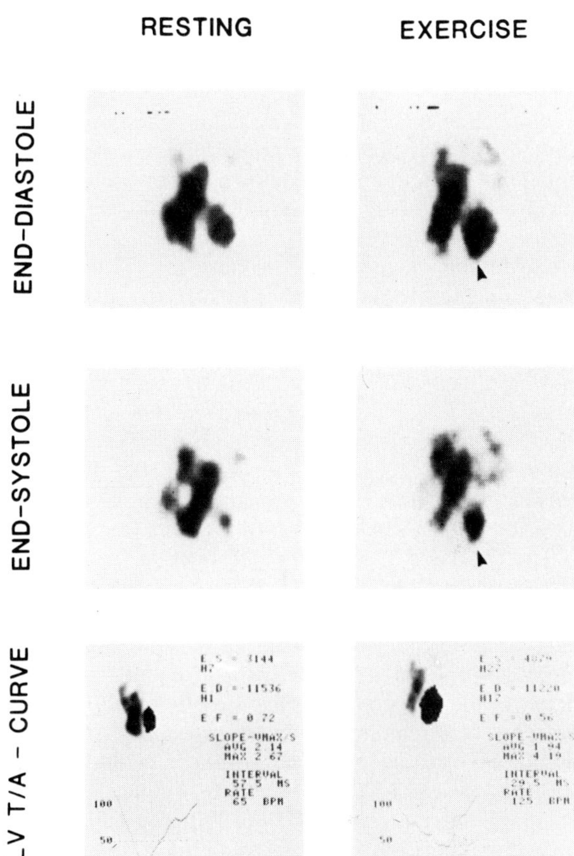

FIGURE 4 End-diastolic and end-systolic frames of a cardiac cycle obtained from a gated equilibrium blood pool study. The lower panel shows the computer display of the results after data processing. A variable region of interest was placed over the left ventricle, resulting in the time-activity curve. End-diastolic (E.D.) and end-systolic (E.S.) counts are used to determine the left ventricular ejection fraction (E.F.). In this patient, the global left ventricular ejection fraction fell from 72 to 65 percent, the left ventricular end-diastolic and end-systolic volumes increased, and an apical akinesis developed (arrow) in response to exercise, indicative of coronary artery disease probably in the LAD distribution. This finding was subsequently confirmed by coronary arteriography.

However, each approach has specific attributes when compared with the other. An advantage of the multiple-gated technique is the ability to perform sequential studies with a single radionuclide injection. In addition to allowing for assessment of regional wall motion in several views, serial evaluation of a variety of physiologic and pharmacologic interventions is possible. The major advantages of first-pass radionuclide angiocardiography are (1) shorter imaging time, (2) more accurate evaluation of right ventricular function, and (3) more accurate evaluation of cardiac shunts and chamber-to-chamber transit times.

Clinical Application in Patients with Chronic Chest Pain

Radionuclide analysis of ventricular function can be used to diagnose coronary artery disease, assess the functional consequences of known disease, and evaluate the effects of therapeutic interventions on cardiac performance. Application of radionuclide ventriculography to the diagnosis of coronary artery disease is based on the evaluation of both regional and global ventricular function at rest and during exercise. In most studies, abnormal ventricular reserve reflecting the presence of coronary artery disease has been defined as less than a 5 to 7 percent exercise-related increase in the absolute ejection fraction value.[61,62,68,69] Averaging the results of 427 patients reported in the literature between 1978 and 1980, coronary artery disease was detected with a sensitivity of 87 percent (range 73 to 100 percent) and a specificity of 93 percent (range 67 to 100 percent).[14] In those studies comparing exercise ventricular performance with electrocardiographic data, radionuclide ventriculography was significantly more sensitive ($p < 0.001$) with an equivalent specificity. In the absence of cardiac surgery or trauma, the presence of a regional wall-motion disturbance at rest or during exercise predicted coronary artery disease with a specificity of 100 percent but a reduced sensitivity of 73 percent (range 47 to 100 percent). As with myocardial perfusion imaging, radionuclide analysis of rest and exercise ventricular performance provides less accurate diagnostic information in women compared with men and in patients who obtain inadequate exercise or who take beta blocking drugs.[73,74]

More recently, several reports have questioned the specificity of using the single criterion of an absolute increase in exercise ejection fraction of 5 to 7 percent to separate normal and abnormal ventricular reserve.[70–72] In a group of 60 catheterization-documented normal subjects, 13 percent of men and 28 percent of women actually demonstrated a decline in exercise left ventricular ejection fraction. In addition to coronary artery disease, resting left ventricular ejection fraction, peak workload, age, sex, body surface area, and the exercise-related change in end-diastolic volume were found to be univariate predictors of the change in ejection fraction during exercise.[72] Based on these findings, a multivariate approach was developed to differentiate normal and abnormal ventricular reserve, and this resulted in improved specificity.

In patients with chronic chest pain, assessment of the functional significance of known disease has received scant investigative attention. In one study, abnormalities in right ventricular function during exercise were demonstrated in a substantial number of patients with coronary artery disease.[75] Abnormal right ventricular exercise reserve appeared to be dependent primarily on concomitant left ventricular dysfunction, although the effect of proximal right coronary artery obstruction is, at present, unclear.[76] In a more recent study, the effect of the location of left anterior obstruction on exercise ventricular reserve was evaluated: More severe exercise left ventricular dysfunction was observed in patients with proximal compared with distal left anterior stenosis, suggesting that the loss of exercise ventricular reserve is related to the amount of myocardium made ischemic with exercise.[77]

In contrast to the functional assessment of known disease in patients with chronic chest pain, numerous investigations have evaluated the effect of many of the commonly used therapeutic modalities on rest-exercise regional and global left ventricular performance. Although the effect on resting left ventricular function is variable, nitrates, propanolol, and coronary artery bypass grafting have all been shown to improve exercise ventricular reserve in many patients with coronary artery disease.[73,78–81] In the future, decisions between these therapeutic modalities in individual patients might be based, in part, on their respective abilities to improve exercise ventricular function documented by radionuclide studies.

Current Limitations and Future Directions

The 100 percent specificity of regional left ventricular dysfunction in the diagnosis of coronary artery disease emphasizes the clinical importance of accurate regional wall-motion analysis. However, the inaccuracies inherent in evaluating regional ventricular function documented for contrast angiography[82] also apply to radionuclide ventriculography. Recently, Fourier analysis has been applied to multiple-gated equilibrium cardiac blood pool imaging, allowing the description of both the amplitude and temporal sequence of regional contraction.[83,84] This approach is particularly attractive because it is quantitative and nonsubjective and provides temporal data unavailable with other techniques. Another potential approach to improving regional wall-motion analysis is through the tomographic reconstruction of multiple-gated equilibrium cardiac blood pool images. Although only preliminary data are available, improved visualization of septal, diaphragmatic, and basal segmental contraction compared with planar imaging was reported.[85]

Recently, equilibrium gated cardiac blood pool images have been used to measure left ventricular volumes using a count-based non-geometry-dependent approach. Although initial studies ignored the variable effect of tissue attenuation,[86,87] a recent investigation has proposed a means of addressing this issue.[88] Since absolute end-diastolic and end-systolic pressures are important functional parameters reflecting overall ventricular performance, widespread application of this technique might improve the diagnostic and functional information obtained with radionuclide ventriculography.

Owing to the prognostic and therapeutic implications of compromised left ventricular performance, evaluation of the functional relationship of coronary artery obstruction to regional and global ventricular reserve during exercise could become an important area of clinical research. In a recent report, a general trend was noted between the extent of coronary artery disease and the degree of exercise left ventricular dysfunction.[70] Since the ability of stress electrocardiography to predict short- and long-term prognosis has recently been questioned,[90] a potentially important clinical application of exercise radionuclide ventriculography could be the demonstration of a poorer prognosis in patients with markedly reduced ventricular reserve during exercise compared with patients with reasonably preserved exercise ventricular function and similar degrees of coronary artery obstruction. Additional important pathophysiologic information might be obtained by evaluating the relationship between exercise ventricular reserve and the severity of coronary artery obstruction, the presence of collaterals, and the existence of prior myocardial infarction. Such prognostic and pathophysiologic information might provide important insights into the timing and implementation of medical or surgical interventions.

Rationale for Use in Patients with Chronic Chest Pain

Application of radionuclide perfusion imaging and ventriculography to patients with chronic chest pain involves two fundamental questions. First, in what patient subgroups should these procedures be performed? Second, should radionuclide perfusion imaging or radionuclide ventriculography be the procedure of choice?

For the detection of coronary artery disease, we do not recommend performing either radionuclide procedure as the first diagnostic maneuver in patients with an interpretable electrocardiogram because of the increased expense and small but significant radiation exposure. In patients with a nondiagnostic rest-exercise ECG stress test, considerations based on Bayes' theorems delineate those specific patient subsets in whom clinically useful information is obtained.[89] As shown in Fig. 5, exercise radionuclide perfusion imaging and ventriculography provide important diagnostic information in patients with a pretest disease prevalence of 30 to 70 percent (e.g., middle-aged males with atypical chest pain, multiple major risk factors for

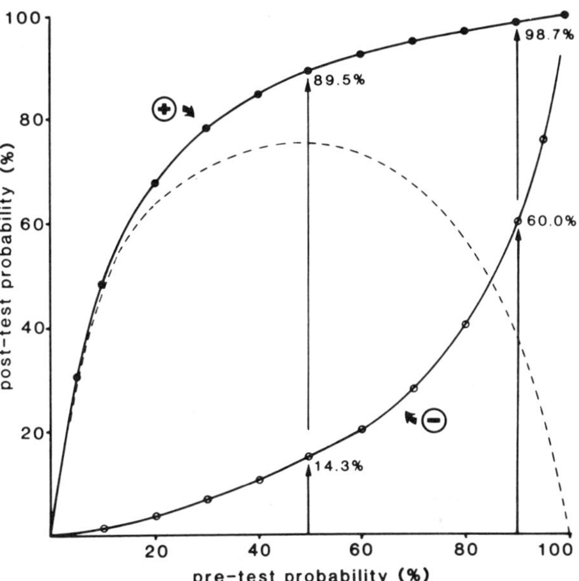

FIGURE 5 Evaluation of the posttest probability of coronary artery disease after rest-exercise thallium-201 perfusion imaging or rest-exercise radionuclide angiography using Bayes' theorem. The curves plotted for a positive test result (solid circles) or for a negative test result (open circles) are based on an 85 percent sensitivity and a 90 percent specificity for the detection of coronary artery disease. In order to determine the posttest probability in a given patient, the pretest probability is estimated from the patient's age, clinical symptoms, ECG, and risk factors. As shown by two examples, a patient with high pretest probability, i.e., typical angina and positive ECG treadmill test, has a pretest probability of approximately 90 percent. As the posttest results indicate, neither of the radionuclide imaging procedures will significantly alter this probability. However, in a patient with a pretest probability of about 50 percent, i.e., atypical chest pain and equivocal ECG treadmill test, the posttest probability will increase to 89.5 percent if the test is abnormal and will decrease to approximately 14 percent in the presence of a negative study. The predictive accuracy of both tests is thus best in a range of 30 to 70 percent, as indicated by the dashed line.

coronary artery disease, or an asymptomatic positive ECG stress test).

The choice between radionuclide perfusion imaging and ventriculography should be guided by the specific expertise and experience of the laboratory performing the test. If equal expertise is present and the sole reason for performing the test is diagnostic, then rest-exercise ^{201}Tl perfusion scintigraphy is the recommended procedure based on its somewhat higher specificity and equivalent sensitivity compared with rest-exercise radionuclide ventriculography demonstrated in 315 patients in whom both tests were performed.[14] However, if additional functional information is desired, no overall guidelines can be set. For example, in patients with symptoms of left ventricular dysfunction, a history of congestive heart failure, or a previous myocardial infarction, the extra information obtained through analysis of left and right ventricular function recommends radionuclide ventriculography as the procedure of choice.

SUMMARY

In summary, the noninvasive diagnostic accuracy of detecting coronary artery disease has been improved through the application of radionuclide evaluation of myocardial perfusion and ventricular function at rest and during exercise. This improvement is more apparent in men than in women. Functional information about the consequences of coronary artery obstruction can be obtained with these radionuclide techniques that is otherwise not routinely available.

REFERENCES

1 Brown, M. L.: Myocardial Scan, in J. W. Keyes, Jr. (ed.), "Manual of Nuclear Medicine Procedures," CRC Press, West Palm Beach, Fl., 1978, p. 31.

2 Strauss, H. W., Harrison, K., Langan, J. K., Lebowitz, E., and Pitt, B.: Thallium-201 for Myocardial Imaging; Relation of Thallium-201 to Regional Myocardial Perfusion, *Circulation,* 51:641, 1975.

3 Grunwald, A. M., Watson, D. D., Hoezgrefe, H. H., Irving, J. F., and Beller, G. A.: Myocardial Thallium-201 Kinetics in Normal and Ischemic Myocardium, *Circulation,* 64:610, 1981.

4 DiCola, V. C., Downing, S. E., Donabedian, R. K., and Zaret, B. L.: Pathophysiological Correlates of Thallium-201 Myocardial Uptake in Experimental Infarction, *Cardiovasc. Res.,* 11:141, 1977.

5 Okada, R. D., Marshall, L. J., Daggett, W. M., et al.: Thallium-201 Kinetics in Nonischemic Canine Myocardium, *Circulation,* 65:70, 1982.

6 Pohost, G. M., Alpert, N. M., Ingall, J. S., and Strauss, H. W.: Thallium Redistribution: Mechanism and Clinical Utility, *Semin. Nucl. Med.,* 10:70, 1980.

7 Pohost, G. M., Zir, L. M., Moore, R. H., McKusick, K. A., Guiney, T. E., and Beller, G. A.: Differentiation of Transiently Ischemic from Infarcted Myocardium by Serial Imaging after a Single Dose of Thallium-201, *Circulation,* 55:294, 1977.

8 Klocke, F. J., Bunnell, I. L., Green, D. G., Wittenberg, S. M., and Visco, J. P.: Average Coronary Flow per Unit Weight of the Left Ventricle with and without Coronary Artery Disease, *Circulation,* 50:547, 1974.

9 Cannon, P. J., Schmidt, D. H., Weiss, M. B., et al.: The Relationship between Regional Myocardial Perfusion at Rest and Arteriographic Lesions in Patients with Coronary Atherosclerosis, *J. Clin. Invest.,* 56:1442, 1977.

10 Mymin, D., and Shanma, G. P.: Total and Effective Coronary Blood Flow in Coronary and Noncoronary Disease, *J. Clin. Invest.,* 53:363, 1974.

11 Albro, P. C., Gould, K. L., Westcott, R. J., Hamilton, G. W., Ritchie, J. L., and Williams, D. L.: Noninvasive Assessment of Coronary Stenoses by Myocardial Imaging during Pharmacologic Coronary Vasodilatation: III. Clinical Trial, *Am. J. Cardiol.,* 42:751, 1978.

12 Schelbert, H. R., Wisenberg, G., Phelps, M. E., et al.: Noninvasive Assessment of Coronary Stenoses by Myocardial Imaging during Pharmacologic Coronary Vasodilatation: VI. Detection of Coronary Artery Disease in Man with Intravenous N-13 Ammonia and Positron Computed Tomography, *Am. J. Cardiol.,* 49:1197, 1982.

13 Beller, G. A., Watson, D. D., and Pohost, G. M.: Kinetics of Thallium Distribution and Redistribution: Clinical Applications in Sequential Myocardial Imaging, in H. W. Strauss and B. Pitt (eds.), "Cardiovascular Nuclear Medicine," 2d ed., St. Louis, C. V. Mosby, 1979, p. 225.

14 Okada, R. D., Boucher, C. A., Strauss, H. W., and Pohost, G. M.: Exercise Radionuclide Imaging Approaches to Coronary Artery Disease, *Am. J. Cardiol.,* 46:1188, 1980.

15 Botvinick, E. H., Dunn, R. F., Hattner, R. S., and Massie, B. M.: A Consideration of Factors Affecting the Diagnostic Accuracy of Thallium-201 Myocardial Perfusion Scintigraphy in Detecting Coronary Artery Disease, *Semin. Nucl. Med.,* 10:157, 1980.

16 Osbakken, M. D., Boucher, C. A., Okada, R. D., Strauss, H. W., and Pohost, G. M.: The Effect of Propranolol on the Diagnostic Accuracy of Exercise Thallium-201 and Gated Blood Pool Scans for Detecting Coronary Artery Disease, *Circulation,* 62 (suppl. 3): 230, 1980.

17 Bailey, I. K., Griffith, L. S. C., Rouleau, J., Strauss, H. W., and Pitt, B.: Thallium-201 Myocardial Perfusion Imaging at Rest and during Exercise: Comparative Sensitivity to Electrocardiography in Coronary Artery Disease, *Circulation,* 55:79, 1977.

18 Ritchie, J. L., Trobaugh, G. B., Hamilton, G. W., et al.: Myocardial Imaging with Thallium-201 at Rest and during Exercise: Comparison with Coronary Arteriography and Resting and Stress Electrocardiography, *Circulation,* 56:66, 1977.

19 Ritchie, J. L., Zaret, B. L., Strauss, H. W., et al.: Myocardial Imaging with Thallium-201: A Multicenter Study in Patients with Angina Pectoris or Acute Myocardial Infarction, *Am. J. Cardiol.,* 42:345, 1978.

20 McCarthy, D. M., Blood, D. K., Sciacca, R. R., and Cannon, P. J.: Single dose Myocardial Perfusion Imaging with Thallium-201: Application in Patients with Nondiagnostic Electrocardiographic Stress Tests, *Am. J. Cardiol.,* 43:899, 1979.

21 Botvinick, E. H., Taradash, M. R., Shames, D. M., and

Parmley, W. W.: Thallium-201 Myocardial Perfusion Scintigraphy for the Clinical Clarification of Normal, Abnormal and Equivocal Electrocardiographic Stress Tests, *Am. J. Cardiol.*, 41:43, 1978.

22 Caralis, D. G., Bailey, I., Kennedy, H. L., and Pitt, B.: Thallium-201 Myocardial Imaging in Evaluation of Asymptomatic Individuals with Ischaemic ST Segment Depression on Exercise Electrocardiogram, *Br. Heart J.*, 42:562, 1979.

23 Zir, L. M., Miller, S. W., Dinsmore, R. E., Gilbert, J. P., and Hawthorne, J. W.: Interobserver Variability in Coronary Angiography, *Circulation*, 53:627, 1976.

24 Gray, C. R., Hoffman, H. A., Hammond, W. S., Miller, K. I., and Oceasohn, R. Q.: Correlation of Arteriographic and Pathologic Findings in the Coronary Arteries in Man, *Circulation*, 26:494, 1962.

25 Hutchins, G. M., Bulkley, B. H., Ridolfi, R. L., Griffith, L. S. C., Ohr, F. T. L., and Piaso, M. A.: Correlation of Coronary Arteriograms and Left Ventriculograms with Postmortem Studies, *Circulation*, 56:32, 1977.

26 Rigo, P., Becker, L. C., Griffith, L. S. C., et al.: Influence of Coronary Collateral Vessels on the Results of Thallium-201 Myocardial Stress Imaging, *Am. J. Cardiol.*, 44:452, 1979.

27 Berger, B. C., Watson, D. D., Taylor, G. J., Burwell, L. R., Martin, R. P., and Beller, G. A.: Effect of Coronary Collateral Circulation on Regional Myocardial Perfusion Assessed with Quantitative Thallium-201 Scintigraphy, *Am. J. Cardiol.*, 46:365, 1980.

28 Rigo, P., Bailey, I. K., Griffith, L. S. C., Pitt, B., Wagner, H. N., and Becker, L. C.: Stress Thallium-201 Myocardial Scintigraphy for the Detection of Individual Coronary Artery Lesions in Patients with and without Previous Myocardial Infarction, *Am. J. Cardiol.*, 48:209, 1981.

29 Massie, B. M., Botvinick, E. H., and Brundage, B. H.: Correlation of Thallium-201 Scintigrams with Coronary Anatomy: Factors Affecting Region by Region Sensitivity, *Am. J. Cardiol.*, 44:616, 1979.

30 Hirzel, H. O., Neusch, K., Gruentzig, A. R., and Luetlof, U. M.: Short- and Long-Term Results in Myocardial Perfusion after Percutaneous Transluminal Angioplasty Assessed by Thallium-201 Exercise Scintigraphy, *Circulation*, 63:1001, 1981.

31 Ritchie, J. L., Nakahara, K. A., Trobaugh, G. B., Williams, O. L., and Hamilton, G. W.: Thallium-201 Myocardial Imaging in Assessment of Results of Aortocoronary Bypass Surgery, *Circulation*, 56:830, 1977.

32 Iskandrian, A. S., Haaz, W., Segal, B. L., and Kane, S. A.: Exercise Thallium-201 Scintigraphy in Evaluating Aortocoronary Bypass Surgery, *Chest*, 80:11, 1981.

33 Bodenheimer, M. M., Banka, V. S., Fooshee, C., Herman, G. A., and Helfant, R. H.: Relationship Between Regional Myocardial Perfusion and the Presence, Severity and Reversibility of Asynergy in Patients with Coronary Heart Disease, *Circulation*, 58:789, 1978.

34 Massie, B. M., Botnivick, E. H., Brundage, B. H., Greenberg, B., Shames, D., and Gelbert, H.: Relationship of Regional Myocardial Perfusion to Segmental Wall Motion, *Circulation*, 58:1154, 1978.

35 Rozanski, A., Berman, D. S., Gray, R., et al.: Use of Thallium-201 Scintigraphy in the Preoperative Differentiation of Reversible and Nonreversible Myocardial Asynergy, *Circulation*, 64:936, 1981.

36 Berger, B. C., Watson, D. D., Bunwell, L. R., et al.: Redistribution of Thallium at Rest in Patients with Stable and Unstable Angina and the Effect of Coronary Artery Bypass Surgery, *Circulation*, 60:1114, 1979.

37 Steingart, R. M., Bontempo, R., Scheuer, J., and Yipintsoi, J.: Gamma Camera Quantification of Thallium-201 Redistribution at Rest in a Dog Model, *Circulation*, 65:542, 1982.

38 Trobaugh, G. B., Wackers, F. J., Sokole, E. B., DeRowen, T. A., Ritchie, J. L., and Hamilton, G. W.: Thallium-201 Myocardial Imaging: An Interinstitutional Study of Observer Variability, *J. Nucl. Med.*, 19:359, 1978.

39 Burow, R. D.., Pond, M., Schafer, A. W., and Becker, L.: Circumferential Profiles: A New Method for Computer Analysis of Thallium-201 Myocardial Perfusion Images, *J. Nucl. Med.*, 20:771, 1979.

40 Maddahi, J., Garcia, E. V., Berman, D. S., Waxman, A., Swan, H. J. C., and Forrester, J.: Improved Noninvasive Assessment of Coronary Artery Disease by Quantitative Analysis of Regional Stress Myocardial Distribution and Washout of Thallium-201, *Circulation*, 64:1981.

41 Vogel, R. A., Kirch, D. L., LeFree, M. T., Rainwater, J. O., Jensen, D. P., and Steele, P. P.: Thallium-201 Myocardial Perfusion Scintigraphy: Results of Standard and Multi-Pinhole Tomographic Techniques, *Am. J. Cardiol.*, 43:787, 1979.

42 Ritchie, J. L., Williams, D. L., Caldwell, J. H., et al.: Seven-Pinhole Emission Tomography with Thallium-201 in Patients with Prior Myocardial Infarction, *J. Nucl. Med.*, 22:107, 1981.

43 Ratib, O., Henze, E., Hoffman, E., Phelps, M. E., and Schelbert, H. R.: Performance of the Rotating Slant Hole Collimator in Detection of Myocardial Perfusion Abnormalities, *J. Nucl. Med.*, 23:34, 1982.

44 Keyes, J. W.: Emission Computed Tomography of the Myocardium, in H. W. Strauss and B. Pitt (eds.), "Cardiovascular Nuclear Medicine," 2d ed., C. V. Mosby, St. Louis, 1979, pp. 46–56.

45 Holman, B. L., Hill, T. C., Wynne, J., Lovette, R. D., Zimmerman, R. E., and Smith, E. M.: Single-Photon Transaxial Emission Computed Tomography of the Heart in Normal Subjects and in Patients with Infarction, *J. Nucl. Med.*, 20:736, 1979.

46 Vogel, R., Alderson, P., Berman, D., et al.: A Multicenter Comparison of Standard and Seven-Pinhole Tomographic Scintigraphy, *Circulation*, 62 (suppl. 2): 9, 1980. (Abstract.)

47 Deutsch, E., Libson, K., Vanderheyden, J. L., Nosco, O. L., Sodd, V. J., and Nishiyama, H.: Chemistry and Preparation of the Potential Myocardial Imaging Agent [^{99m}Tc(dmpe)$_2$ Cl$_2$] and Tc-99 DMPE, *J. Nucl. Med.*, 23:9, 1982. (Abstract.)

48 Schelbert, H. R., Henze, E., and Phelps, M. E.: Emission Tomography of the Heart, *Semin. Nuc. Med.*, 10:355, 1980.

49 Gould, K. L., Schelbert, H. R., Phelps, M. E., and Hoffman, E. J.: Noninvasive Assessment of Coronary Stenoses by Myocardial Perfusion Imaging during Pharmacologic Coronary Vasodilatation: V. Detection of 47 Per Cent Diameter Coronary Stenosis with Intravenous Nitrogen-13 Ammonia and Emission-Computed Tomography in Intact Dogs, *Am. J. Cardiol.*, 43:200, 1979.

50 Syed, I. B., Flowers, N., Granlick, D., and Samols, E.: Radiation Exposure in Nuclear Cardiovascular Studies, *Health Phys.*, 42:159, 1982.

51 Schelbert, H. R., Verba, J. W., Johnson, A. D., et al.: Nontraumatic Determination of Left Ventricular Ejection Fraction by Radionuclide Angiocardiography, *Circulation*, 51:902, 1975.

52 Berger, H. J., Matthay, R. A., Pytlik, L. M., Gottschalk, A., and Zaret, B. L.: First-Pass Radionuclide Assessment of Right and Left Ventricular Performance in Patients with Cardiac and Pulmonary Disease, *Semin. Nucl. Med.*, 9:275, 1979.

53 Marshall, R. C., Berger, H. J., Costin, J. C., et al.: Assessment of Cardiac Performance with Quantitative Radionuclide Angiocardiography: Sequential Left Ventricular Ejection Fraction, Normalized Left Ventricular Ejection Rate, and Regional Wall Motion, *Circulation*, 56:820, 1977.

54 Berger, H. J., Gottschalk, A., and Zaret, B. L.: Radionuclide Assessment of Left and Right Ventricular Performance, *Radiol. Clin. North Am.*, 18:441, 1980.

55 Rerych, S. K., Scholz, P. M., Newman, G. E., Sabiston, D. C., and Jones, R. H.: Cardiac Function at Rest and during Exercise in Normals and in Patients with Coronary Heart Disease: Evaluation by Radionuclide Angiocardiography, *Ann. Surg.*, 187:449, 1978.

56 Pavel, D. G., Zimmer, A. M., and Patterson, V. N.: In Vivo Labeling of Red Blood Cells with ^{99m}Tc: A New Approach to Blood Pool Visualization, *J. Nucl. Med.*, 18:305, 1977.

57 Smith, T. D., and Richards, P.: A Simple Kit for the Preparation of ^{99m}Tc-Labeled Red Blood Cells, *J. Nucl. Med.*, 17:126, 1976.

58 Burow, R. D., Strauss, H. W., Singleton, R., et al.: Analysis of Left Ventricular Function from Multiple Gated Acquisition Cardiac Blood Pool Imaging: Comparison to Contrast Angiography, *Circulation*, 56:1024, 1977.

59 Green, M. V., Ostrow, H. G., Douglas, M. A., et al.: High Temporal Resolution ECG-Gated Scintigraphic Angiocardiography, *J. Nucl. Med.*, 16:95, 1975.

60 Bacharach, S. L., Green, M. V., Borer, J. S., Douglas, M. A., Ostrow, H. G., and Johnston, G. S.: A Real-Time System for Multi-Image Gated Cardiac Studies, *J. Nucl. Med.*, 18:79, 1977.

61 Borer, J. S., Bacharach, S. L., Green, M. V., Kent, K. M., Epstein, S. E., and Johnston, G. S.: Real-Time Radionuclide Cineangiography in the Noninvasive Evaluation of Global and Regional Left Ventricular Function at Rest and during Exercise in Patients with Coronary-Artery Disease, *N. Engl. J. Med.*, 296:839, 1977.

62 Jengo, J. A., Oren, V., Conant, R., et al.: Effects of Maximal Exercise Stress on Left Ventricular Function in Patients with Coronary Artery Disease Using First Pass Radionuclide Angiocardiography: A Rapid, Noninvasive Technique for Determining Ejection Fraction and Segmental Wall Motion, *Circulation*, 59:60, 1979.

63 Ashburn, W. L., Schelbert, H. R., and Verba, J. W.: Left Ventricular Ejection Fraction: A Review of Several Radionuclide Angiographic Approaches Using the Scintillation Camera, *Prog. Cardiovasc. Dis.*, 20:267, 1978.

64 Wackers, F. J., Berger, H. J., Johnstone, D. E., et al.: Multiple Gated Cardiac Blood Pool Imaging for Left Ventricular Ejection Fraction: Validation of the Technique and Assessment of Variability, *Am. J. Cardiol.*, 43:1159, 1979.

65 Sorenson, S. G., Hamilton, G. W., Williams, D. L., and Ritchie, J. L.: R-Wave Synchronized Blood Pool Imaging. A Comparison of Accuracy and Reproducibility of Fixed and Computer-Automated Varying Region of Interest for Determining the Left Ventricular Ejection Fraction, *Radiology*, 131:473, 1979.

66 Marshall, R. C., Berger, H. J., Reduto, L. A., Gottschalk, A., and Zaret, B. L.: Variability in Sequential Measures of Left Ventricular Performance Assessed with Radionuclide Angiocardiography, *Am. J. Cardiol.*, 41:531, 1978.

67 Okada, R. D., Kirshenbaum, H. D., Kushner, F. G., et al.: Observer Variance in the Qualitative Evaluation of Left Ventricular Wall Motion and Quantitation of Left Ventricular Ejection Fraction Using Rest and Exercise Multigated Blood Pool Imaging, *Circulation*, 61:137, 1980.

68 Caldwell, J. H., Hamilton, G. W., Sorenson, S. G., Ritchie, J. L., Williams, D. L., and Kennedy, J. W.: The Detection of Coronary Artery Disease with Radionuclide Techniques: A Comparison of Rest-Exercise Thallium Imaging and Ejection Fraction Response, *Circulation*, 61:610, 1980.

69 Berger, H. J., Reduto, L. A., Johnstone, D. E., et al.: Global and Regional Left Ventricular Response to Exercise in Coronary Artery Disease: Assessment by Quantitative Radionuclide Angiocardiography, *Am. J. Med.* 66:13, 1979.

70 Jones, R. H., McEwan, P., Newman, G. E., et al.: Accuracy of Diagnosis of Coronary Artery Disease by Radionuclide Measurement of Left Ventricular Function during Rest and Exercise, *Circulation*, 64:586, 1981.

71 Port, S., Cobb, F. R., Coleman, R. E., and Jones, R. H.:

Effect of Age on the Response of the Left Ventricular Ejection Fraction to Exercise, *N. Engl. J. Med.*, 303:1133, 1980.

72 Gibbons, R. H., Lee, J. L., Cobb, F. R., and Jones, R. H.: Ejection Fraction Response to Exercise in Patients with Chest Pain and Normal Coronary Arteriograms, *Circulation*, 64:752, 1981.

73 Marshall, R. C., Wisenberg, G., Schelbert, H. R., and Henze, E.: Effect of Oral Propranolol on Rest, Exercise and Postexercise Left Ventricular Performance in Normal Subjects and Patients with Coronary Artery Disease, *Circulation*, 63:572, 1981.

74 Berger, H. J., and Zaret, B. L.: Nuclear Cardiology, *N. Engl. J. Med.*,305:799, 1981.

75 Berger, H. J., Johnstone, D. E., Sands, J. M., Gottschalk, A., and Zaret, B. L.: Response of the Right Ventricular Ejection Fraction to Upright Bicycle Exercise in Coronary Artery Disease, *Circulation*, 60:1292, 1979.

76 Johnson, L. L., McCarthy, P. M., Sciacca, R. R., and Cannon, P. J.: Right Ventricular Ejection Fraction during Exercise in Patients with Coronary Artery Disease, *Circulation*, 60:1284, 1979.

77 Loeng, K., and Jones, R. H.: Influence of the Location of Left Anterior Descending Coronary Artery Obstruction on Left Ventricular Function during Exercise, *Circulation*, 65:109, 1982.

78 Ritchie, J. L., Sorenson, S. G., Kennedy, J. W., and Hamilton, G. W.: Radionuclide Angiography: Noninvasive Assessment of Hemodynamic Changes after Administration of Nitroglycerin, *Am. J. Cardiol.*, 43:278, 1979.

79 Borer, J. S., Bacharach, S. L., Green, M. V., Kent, K. M., Johnston, G. S., and Epstein, S. E.: Effect of Nitroglycerin on Exercise-Induced Abnormalities of Left Ventricular Regional Function and Ejection Fraction in Coronary Artery Disease: Assessment by Radionuclide Cineangiography in Symptomatic and Asymptomatic Patients, *Circulation*, 57:314, 1978.

80 Kent, K. M., Borer, J. S., Green, M. V., et al.: Effects of Coronary Artery Bypass on Global and Regional Left Ventricular Function During Exercise, *N. Engl. J. Med.*, 298:1434, 1978.

81 Marshall, R. C., Berger, H. J., Reduto, L. A., Cohen, L. S., Gottschalk, A., and Zaret, B. L.: Assessment of Cardiac Performance with Quantitative Radionuclide Angiocardiography: Effects of Oral Propranolol on Global and Regional Left Ventricular Function in Coronary Artery Disease, *Circulation*, 58:808, 1978.

82 Chaitman, B. R., DeMots, H., Bristow, J. D., Roach, J., and Rahemtoola, S. H.: Objective and Subjective Analysis of Left Ventricular Cineangiograms, *Circulation*, 52:420, 1975.

83 Links, J. M., Douglas, K. H., and Wagner, H. N., Jr.: Patterns of Ventricular Emptying by Fourier Analysis of Gated Blood Pool Studies, *J. Nucl. Med.*, 21:978, 1980.

84 Ratib, O., Henze, E., Schon, H., and Schelbert, H. R.: Phase Analysis of Radionuclide Ventriculograms for the Detection of Coronary Artery Disease, *Am. Heart J.*, 104:1, 1982.

85 Maublant, J., Bailey, P., Mestas, D., et al.: Gated Single Photon Emission Computerized Tomography (SPECT) of the Cardiac Cavities, *J. Nucl. Med.*, 23 (suppl.):25, 1982. (Abstract.)

86 Slutsky, R., Karliner, J., Ricci, D., et al.: Ventricular Volumes by Gated Equilibrium Radionuclide Angiography: A New Method, *Circulation*, 60:556, 1980.

87 Dehmer, G. J., Lewis, S. E., Hillis, L. D., et al.: Nongeometric Determination of Left Ventricular Volumes from Equilibrium Blood Pool Scans, *Am. J. Cardiol.*, 45:293, 1980.

88 Links, J. M., Becker, L. C., Shindledecker, J. G., et al.: Measurement of Absolute Left Ventricular Volumes from Gated Blood Pool Studies, *Circulation*, 65:82, 1982.

89 Hamilton, G. W., Trobaugh, G. B., Ritchie, J. L., Gould, K. L., DeRowen, T. A., and Williams, D. L.: Myocardial Imaging with [201]Thallium: An Analysis of Clinical Usefulness Based on Bayes' Theorem, *Semin. Nucl. Med.*, 8:358, 1978.

90 Podrid, P. H., Graboys, T. B., and Lown, B.: Prognosis of Medically Treated Patients with Coronary Artery Disease with Profound ST-Segment Depression during Exercise Testing, *N. Engl. J. Med.*, 305:1111, 1981.

Radionuclide Evaluation of Patients with Acute Myocardial Infarction[*]

HANS R. SCHÖN, M.D., ROBERT C. MARSHALL, M.D., and HEINRICH R. SCHELBERT, M.D.

Patients admitted to the hospital for evaluation of a possible myocardial infarction frequently pose a diagnostic dilemma if there are equivocal electrocardiographic and serum enzyme changes in addition to an atypical chest pain history. In contrast, patients with a large infarction do not present a diagnostic problem but pose a therapeutic challenge because impaired ventricular performance results in clinically apparent hemodynamic compromise. Patients with an initial small infarction but postinfarct extention, intractible ventricular arrhythmia, or sudden death pose both a diagnostic and therapeutic challenge because proper identification and therapeutic manipulation might alter the unfavorable clinical result.

Because nuclear medicine techniques provide the capability of assessing the functional consequences of acute myocardial infarction with respect to perfusion, contraction, and metabolism, radionuclide evaluation of patients with acute myocardial infarction can provide potentially important information related to the diagnosis and management of each of these three infarct patient subgroups. This article will review the application of radionuclide techniques to acute infarct patients with attention focused on diagnosis, assessing potential therapeutic manipulations, and defining short- and long-term prognosis.

RADIONUCLIDE DIAGNOSIS OF ACUTE MYOCARDIAL INFARCTION

Radionuclide diagnosis of acute myocardial infarction has been achieved through the evaluation of resting myocardial perfusion with thallium-201 (^{201}Tl) and by using infarct-avid agents such as technetium-99m stannous pyrophosphate (^{99m}Tc-PYP).[1] Although radionuclide assessment of regional and global ventricular function could provide potentially important diagnostic information, this possibility has not been systematically evaluated and will not be reviewed here.

Infarct-Avid Imaging

Although a number of different infarct-avid agents are available, the current imaging agent of choice is technetium-99m stannous pyrophosphate (^{99m}Tc-PYP). Other radiotracers with infarct-avid properties, such as technetium-99m–labeled tetracycline and glucoheptonate, have not proven clinically useful.[2] Recently, myosin-specific antibody labeled with iodine-131 or indium-111 has been shown to concentrate in regional infarction in the dog.[3,4] Clinical evaluation of this new radiopharmaceutical has not been undertaken.

PYROPHOSPHATE IMAGING TECHNIQUE AND DISTRIBUTION PHYSIOLOGY

Infarct-avid imaging is performed 2 h following the peripheral venous introduction of 15 to 20 mCi of ^{99m}Tc-PYP.[5,6] Imaging is routinely performed in the anterior, 35° left anterior blight, and left lateral positions. For maximum sensitivity, pyrophosphate imaging should be performed 36 to 72 h after the onset of chest pain: images acquired before 36 h and after 7 days are often normal despite the presence of documented infarction. Image interpretation is based on both the site and intensity of radiotracer accumulation.[7] The site is generally categorized as either focal or diffuse (Fig. 1). Since ^{99m}Tc-PYP is a bone-imaging agent, the intensity of radiotracer accumulation is judged by comparison with skeletal activity. Images with diffuse cardiac tracer accumulation equal in intensity to adjacent bone activity or slightly less intense focal uptake are considered to be consistent with the presence of acute myocardial infarction.

The pathophysiologic factors governing the distribution of ^{99m}Tc-PYP into acutely ischemic myocardium appear to be residual myocardial blood flow and severity of tissue necrosis.[8] In experimental infarction, maximum ^{99m}Tc-PYP uptake is found in peripheral infarct areas with 30 to 40 percent of normal blood flow. Compared with regions of maximal radiotracer accumulations, ^{99m}Tc-PYP accumulation actually decreases in central infarct zones with less relative blood flow. The resulting "doughnut" pattern is also observed in patients with large transmural infarcts,[9] suggesting that residual blood flow is necessary for ^{99m}Tc-PYP to gain access to infarcted myocardium in both clinical and experimental myocardial infarction.

At the cellular level, the biochemical mechanisms determining ^{99m}Tc-PYP uptake are controversial. Since ^{99m}Tc-PYP is a bone-imaging agent and there is excessive accumulation of calcium in the mitochondria of acutely necrotic myocardium, there might be a relation-

[*]From the Divisions of Cardiology and Nuclear Medicine, UCLA School of Medicine, University of California, Los Angeles.

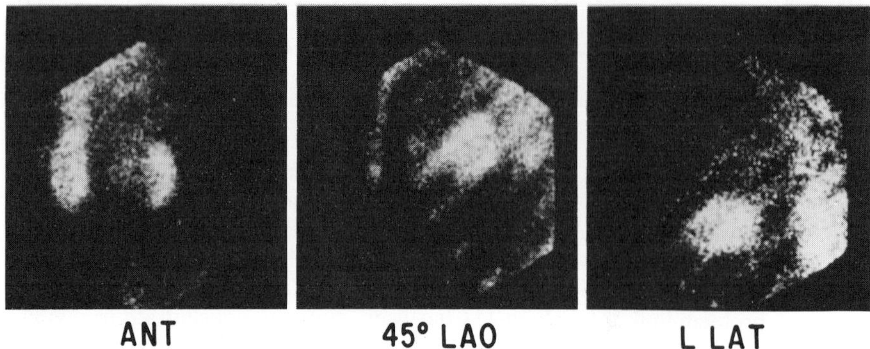

FIGURE 1 ^{99m}Tc-PYP myocardial images obtained in a 61-year-old male with acute myocardial infarction. Note the markedly increased focal uptake of tracer in the region corresponding to the posterior and lateral wall of the left ventricle.

ship between myocardial calcium and ^{99m}Tc-PYP up-date. In support of this hypothesis, a close temporal and spacial correlation between calcium and ^{99m}Tc-PYP accumulation has been observed in regional infarction in the dog.[10,11] However, evidence against a central role for calcium in infarct-avid tracer accumulation in necrotic myocardium is that the major fraction of intracellular ^{99m}Tc-PYP is bound in the cytoplasm, not the mitochondria.[12] This latter observation suggests that radiotracer accumulation might be more closely related to denatured proteins than to calcium uptake. In addition, in a fetal heart model, no significant correlation could be demonstrated between calcium and ^{99m}Tc-PYP accumulation.[13] Therefore, although ^{99m}Tc-PYP uptake appears related to calcium sequestration in experimental regional infarction, a central mechanistic role for calcium has not been established, and the close correlation between ^{99m}Tc-PYP and calcium accumulation might reflect residual blood flow and their mutual delivery to the myocardium.

INFARCT-AVID DIAGNOSIS OF ACUTE MYOCARDIAL INFARCTION

Infarct-avid imaging with ^{99m}Tc-PYP is an extremely sensitive approach for the identification of patients with large transmural infarctions. The overall sensitivity of pyrophosphate imaging in 2,625 patients reported in the literature between 1974 and 1979 was 89 percent, with some series reporting a sensitivity of 100 percent.[1,2,6] However, the results of pyrophosphate imaging are more variable in patients with small transmural or subendocardial infarctions.[14] Depending on the criteria used for image interpretation, focal myocardial tracer accumulation is observed in less than 50 percent of such patients. Although less intense, diffuse tracer activity is frequently observed in patients with non-transmural myocardial infarction; this pattern is also present in patients with stable and unstable angina pectoris.[15,16] Furthermore, positive pyrophosphate scintigrams are not specific for acute myocardial infarction, because patients with left ventricular aneurysm, calcified aortic and/or mitral valves, thoracic or cardiac trauma, recent cardioversion, pericarditis, and neoplastic diseases have been observed with myocardial pyrophosphate accumulation.[17]

The reported inaccuracies of pyrophosphate imaging make it clear that infarct-avid imaging is not generally applicable to the majority of patients suspected of having an acute myocardial infarction. However, clinically useful information can be obtained in specific patient subsets. A potentially important application of pyrophosphate scintigraphy is in patients undergoing cardiac surgery in whom conventional assessment of infarction is unreliable.[18] Similarly, infarct-avid imaging is useful in patients who present to the hospital more than 24 to 48 h after onset of symptoms, at which time the electrocardiogram and serum enzymes can be nondiagnostic. In patients with inferior myocardial infarction, pyrophosphate scintigraphy may allow definition of right ventricular myocardial necrosis.

Myocardial Perfusion Imaging

The physiology of tracer distribution and imaging procedure were reviewed in the preceding article. The details of tracer kinetics and imaging technique are identical in patients with acute myocardial infarction and in patients with chronic chest pain.

PERFUSION IMAGING IN THE DIAGNOSIS OF ACUTE MYOCARDIAL INFARCTION

The sensitivity of resulting ^{201}Tl scintigraphy in the detection of acute myocardial infarction appears to depend on the time that has elapsed since the onset of symptoms.[19] In patients evaluated within the first 24 h after the onset of symptoms, perfusion defects have been noted in 94 percent with a documented infarction. In patients evaluated after 24 h, ^{201}Tl scintigraphy detected only 72 percent of documented infarcts, primarily because of its inability to accurately identify small inferior and nontransmural infarcts. The loss of sensitivity 24 h or more after the onset of symptoms appears to be due to a time-dependent reduction in perfusion defect size.[19–21] These data indicate that myocardial perfusion imaging is a highly sensitive technique for the diagnosis of both transmural and nontransmural infarctions if scintigrams are obtained early after the onset of symptoms (Fig. 2).

Abnormal resting ^{201}Tl images are not specific for acute myocardial infarction. Resting perfusion defects have been observed in patients with severe coronary artery disease and no evidence of acute ischemia or infarction.[22–24] This observation is not surprising in view of earlier reports that demonstrated abnormal regional or global myocardial perfusion using diffusible indicators to quantitate regional and global myocardial blood flow in patients with severe coronary artery disease in the absence of acute ischemia or infarction.[25–27] In addition, thallium-201 perfusion scintigraphy cannot distinguish between remote and acute infarction. Although regional perfusion defects are reasonably specific for regional coronary artery obstruction, perfusion defects have been noted in infiltrative,[28] hypertrophic,[29] and dilated[30] cardiomyopathies. These observations indicate that ^{201}Tl scintigraphy is not specific for acute myocardial infarction and suggests that the diagnosis of acute myocardial infarction should be established with additional enzymatic and electrocardiographic data.

Several investigators have advocated the use of early myocardial perfusion scintigraphy as a screening procedure for triage of patients presenting to the emergency room with chest pain and no prior history of ischemic heart disease.[31,32] However, a significant portion of patients with unstable angina and severe coronary artery disease have normal resting ^{201}Tl images. Since patients with severe coronary artery disease and prolonged resting chest pain warrant intensive monitoring, prospective clinical trials demonstrating the clinical feasibility and cost-effectiveness of this approach will be necessary prior to its widespread clinical application.

RADIONUCLIDE EVALUATION OF THERAPY IN ACUTE MYOCARDIAL INFARCTION

Exclusive of investigative attempts to salvage jeopardized myocardium, the goals of therapeutic intervention in patients with acute myocardial infarction are to maintain hemodynamic compensation and electric stability. In recent years, there has been increasing application of radionuclide ventriculography to directly assess residual myocardial performance prior to the institution of specific therapeutic interventions with potentially important hemodynamic effects. Although only preliminary data are available, some predictions can be made concerning the use of radionuclide ventriculography to provide therapeutically useful information in specific clinical subsets of acute infarction patients.

Several studies have shown that patients with anterior myocardial infarctions exhibit reduced regional and global left ventricular performance, while patients

Rest Thallium - 201 - Image S/P Infarction

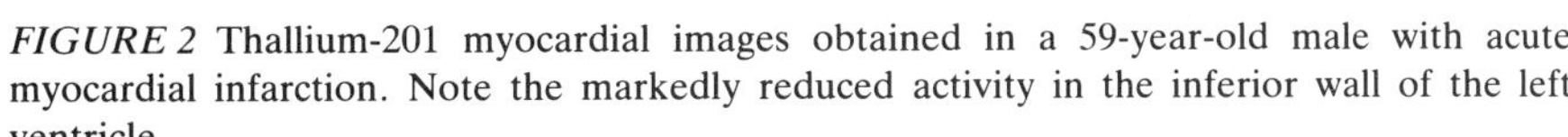

FIGURE 2 Thallium-201 myocardial images obtained in a 59-year-old male with acute myocardial infarction. Note the markedly reduced activity in the inferior wall of the left ventricle.

with inferior myocardial infarction have less left ventricular and more right ventricular dysfunction.[33-36] Therefore, in patients with cardiogenic shock and anterior myocardial infarction, inadequate hemodynamic compensation is almost certainly due to a severe reduction in left ventricular performance. Little additional information will be obtained with radionuclide ventriculography. In contrast, in patients with an inferior myocardial infarction and cardiogenic shock, hemodynamic decompensation can be due either to poor left or right ventricular contraction. Since therapeutic priorities are somewhat different in cardiogenic shock owing to right versus left ventricular failure, radionuclide ventriculography can be used to guide the choice of interventions in these patients.

In a recent study, only a rough correlation between physical or chest x-ray evidence of congestive heart failure and radionuclide-determined ventricular performance was observed.[37] Using a multivariate approach to predict left ventricular ejection fraction from electrocardiographic, physical, and chest x-ray findings, poor predictive accuracy was noted in 55 percent of patients. Occasional patients were observed with chest x-ray or physical evidence of severe congestive heart failure and reasonably well-preserved systolic ventricular performance. The observed near-normal ventricular function in these patients is consistent with a small infarct size, suggesting that medical or surgical therapy designed to reduce myocardial ischemia might

benefit these patients (Fig. 3). More frequently, patients without clinical evidence of congestive heart failure were found to have a severely depressed left ventricular ejection fraction. This finding is consistent with extensive myocardial infarction and might suggest the need for more careful and prolonged clinical evaluation for the development of congestive heart failure and the need for slower ambulation and discharge. In addition, institution of negative inotropic drugs in such patients should be performed cautiously. Since severe ventricular ectopy occurring greater than 48 h after infarction is strongly associated with extensive infarction and reduced left ventricular function,[38-42] patients with a severely depressed left ventricular ejection fraction might also benefit from an aggressive search for malignant ventricular arrhythmias.

Based on current knowledge and the pathophysiologic implications of left ventricular dysfunction, it seems reasonable to use radionuclide ventriculography to guide therapeutic decisions in many patients with acute myocardial infarction. However, clinical studies demonstrating the feasibility of this approach are not currently available. Completion of such studies should document the utility of radionuclide evaluation of ventricular performance and provide more precise therapeutic guidelines for using both clinical and radionuclide information in specific subsets of patients with acute myocardial infarction.

Post-infarct Patient with C.H.F.
LAO View

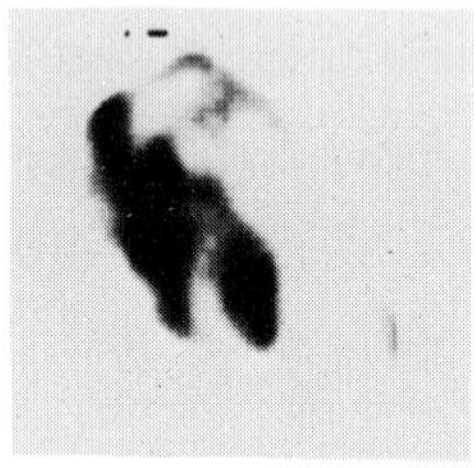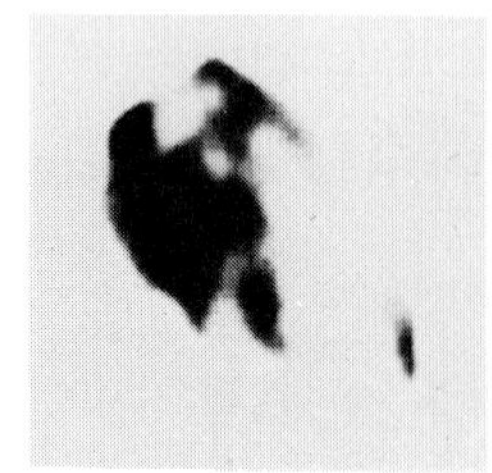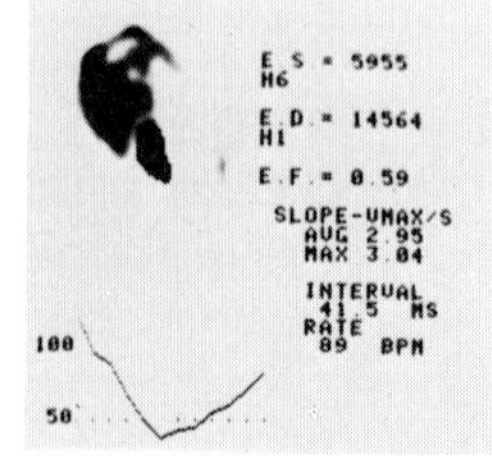

FIGURE 3 Multiple-gated equilibrium cardiac blood pool images in the LAO view from a 73-year-old patient admitted to the hospital 5 days prior to radionuclide ventriculography with pulmonary edema and subendocardial infarction. The patient manifested rales and an intermittent S$_3$ with frequent bouts of chest pain after successful clearing of his pulmonary edema and institution of digitalis, diuretic, and long-acting nitrate therapy. Following radionuclide ventriculography and the demonstration of normal global systolic function, the patient's therapeutic regimen was switched to propranalol and intravenous nitroglycerin. Failure to control chest pain ultimately resulted in coronary arteriography and coronary artery bypass grafting.

RADIONUCLIDE EVALUATION OF PROGNOSIS IN ACUTE MYOCARDIAL INFARCTION

The prognosis for patients with acute myocardial infarction varies from a few hours to well over a decade. In addition to maintaining hemodynamic and electric stability, ideal management of patients with acute myocardial infarction should include identification of individual patients with a poor short- or long-term prognosis. Since it is doubtful that any acute therapeutic intervention would significantly alter the life expectancy of a patient destined to live 10 years or longer, the ability to accurately assess the prognosis of acute infarct patients would allow definition of specific patient subsets that might benefit from the institution of therapeutic manipulations designed to reduce ischemic myocardial damage.

In patients dying of pump failure following an acute myocardial infarction, the underlying left ventricular dysfunction reflects the cumulative extent of irreversible damage from old and recent myocardial necrosis.[43,44] Similarly, in many infarct patients dying without clinical evidence of left ventricular failure, extensive myocardial damage is present on pathologic examination.[45] However, not all patients who die following acute infarction have large infarcts.[46] Several investigators have suggested that the presence of additional viable but ischemic myocardium adversely affects prognosis.[46–48] Therefore, clinical evaluation of patients presenting with an acute myocardial infarction to define the cumulative extent of myocardial infarction and ischemia should provide information about short- and long-term prognosis.

Many studies have attempted to derive prognostic indices using a multitude of clinically defined variables with varying degrees of success.[49–55] The insensitivity of individual clinical parameters and the statistical difficulties related to patient selection and statistical analysis probably account for the variable success of these studies. Because of the unique functional information available with nuclear medicine techniques, improved assessment of life expectancy might be possible through the radionuclide evaluation of patients with acute myocardial infarction. To date, preliminary studies have supported this possibility.[9,39,40,56–60]

Infarct-Avid Imaging

In experimental myocardial infarction evaluated more than 24 h following left anterior descending occlusion, the extent of ^{99m}Tc-PYP accumulation has been shown to correlate with overall infarct size.[52,59,60] Similarly, in human beings, the scintigraphic infarct area provides a good estimate of infarct size in anterior myocardial infarction.[61] Presumably owing to the unfavorable angle of the inferior wall to the detector, the extent of inferior myocardial infarction is not well estimated by pyrophosphate imaging.[3,61] Application of tomographic or three-dimensional volume reconstruction techniques to the estimation of infarct size with pyrophosphate might further improve the accuracy of this approach.[5,7] The reported data indicate that information about prognosis in patients with anterior myocardial infarction can be obtained by quantifying the extent of infarct-avid tracer accumulation. The major limitations of infarct size evaluation with ^{99m}Tc-PYP are the necessity of waiting more than 24 h following onset of symptoms and the potential effect of time from infarction on the extent of pyrophosphate uptake in necrotic myocardium.[31]

Of interest is the observation that two high-risk postinfarct patient subgroups can be identified from routine analysis of ^{99m}Tc-PYP scintigrams. Patients who exhibit a "doughnut" image pattern have a significantly higher mortality than patients who do not have this pattern.[9] Similarly, patients with persistently positive pyrophosphate images several months after infarction have a higher than expected morbidity and mortality.[58] The pathophysiologic basis for the doughnut image pattern is presumably the presence of extensive transmural infarction with a central zone of markedly diminished perfusion, while the underlying mechanism of continued late myocardial infarct-avid tracer accumulation is postulated to be continued myocardial necrosis in the infarct zone.

Prognosis and Myocardial Perfusion Imaging

Unlike ^{99m}Tc-PYP, which detects only acutely necrotic myocardium, regionally reduced ^{201}Tl tissue concentration occurs with both acute and remote infarction and myocardial ischemia. Since it is likely that prognosis in most acute infarct patients is determined by the cumulative amount of ischemic and age-independent infarcted myocardium, ^{201}Tl myocardial perfusion imaging might provide more accurate prognostic information than scintigraphic techniques that evaluate only the extent of acute myocardial necrosis. Previous studies have reported that the size of the ^{201}Tl perfusion defect agrees well with the volume of acutely infarcted myocardium in patients with acute myocardial infarction and with the percentage of the left ventricle with regional contraction abnormalities in patients with remote myocardial infarction.[78–80] Reported evidence supporting the use of myocardial perfusion imaging to evaluate resting myocardial ischemia are the observations that (1) occasional patients who die with pathologic small infarcts have large premorbid ^{201}Tl defects,[46] (2) the demonstration of resting perfusion defects in patients with severe coronary artery disease and no evidence of acute or remote myocardial infarction,[22–24] and (3) transient perfusion abnormalities in patients without acute myocardial infarction following documented coronary arterial spasm.[81] In a study evaluating the prognostic accuracy of thallium scintigraphy compared with conventional clinical parameters, early ^{201}Tl imaging was found to be the most powerful predictor of short-term survival,[56] providing direct evidence for the use of myocardial perfusion imaging to provide prognostic information in patients with acute myocardial infarction. Despite the disadvantage posed by the necessity of maintaining a shelf supply of this expensive cyclotron-produced isotope in order to image patients early after the onset of symptoms, confirmation of these preliminary findings in larger patient studies could provide a basis for the use of ^{201}Tl scintigraphy to identify high-risk patients with acute myocardial infarction in whom a specific therapeutic intervention might alter clinical outcome.

In patients surviving the hospital phase of acute myocardial infarction, the detection of multivessel coronary artery disease has been accomplished with predischarge rest-exercise ^{201}Tl scintigraphy.[62–64] The frequent finding of abnormally increased ^{201}Tl lung uptake also has been observed to indicate decreased resting ventricular function and exercise reserve.[65] Although no information is available directly relating rest-exercise ^{201}Tl imaging to prognosis, presumably, postinfarction patients with extensive coronary disease and poor rest-exercise ventricular function have a poorer life expectancy than patients without these findings.

Prognosis and Radionuclide Ventriculography

Similar to myocardial perfusion imaging, the severity of left ventricular dysfunction demonstrated with radionuclide ventriculography most likely reflects the cumulative amount of infarcted and ischemic myocardium. Therefore, important prognostic information should be available with radionuclide evaluation of ventricular performance in patients with acute myocardial infarction. To date, studies evaluating resting ventricular performance early after infarction and exercise ventricular reserve prior to hospital discharge provide supportive evidence for this potentially important clinical application of radionuclide ventriculography.[39,40,66] In addition, the inability to predict left ventricular ejection fraction from the physical examination or chest x-ray in acute infarct patients[37] suggests that radionuclide evaluation of ventricular performance might provide additional prognostic information not available with the more commonly used clinical parameters.

Clinical trials documenting improved survival following institution of specific therapeutic interventions in prospectively defined high-risk patients are currently unavailable. In part, performing such studies has been limited by the difficulties in identifying individual patients with a poor prognosis from clinical variables alone in the absence of invasive hemodynamic monitoring.[53,54] This problem might be overcome through the continued demonstration of the ability of infarct-avid imaging, myocardial perfusion imaging, and radionuclide ventriculography used alone or in combination to accurately identify patients destined for limited survival. Prospective identification of high-risk patients with acute myocardial infarction would allow institution and evaluation of therapeutic interventions in those patients who might receive the most benefit.

Positron Computed Tomography and Prognosis

Not all patients identified with a poor short- or long-term prognosis are likely to have a favorable response to therapeutic manipulation: Limited therapeutic benefit is predictable in patients with completed extensive infarction and severe left ventricular dysfunction. Although radionuclide evaluation of myocardial necrosis, perfusion, and function will probably result in improved prognostic accuracy in patients with acute myocardial infarction, there has been no documentation that these approaches can differentiate patients with additional potentially reversible myocardial ischemia from patients with completed irreversible infarction.

The development of positron computed tomography has made it possible to noninvasively evaluate in vivo regional biochemical processes, obtaining information analogous to in vitro autoradiography.[82] Use of the positron-emitting radionuclides ^{13}N, ^{15}O, ^{11}C, and ^{18}F allows labeling of a variety of biologically important compounds whose physiologic fate is either identical to or altered in a predictable fashion compared with their naturally occurring analogues. Evaluation of regional myocardial metabolism can be achieved with positron computed tomography and positron-emitting tracers of substrates used by the myocardium for energy metabolism. Current evidence suggest that distinctive patterns of substrate utilization exist in normal, ischemic, and infarcted myocardium.[67] Evaluation of acute infarct patients with PCT and positron-labeled myocardial substrates might, therefore, provide a method of differentiating patients with a poor prognosis owing to the presence of additional jeopardized myocardium from those patients with a poor prognosis owing to extensive infarction.

Palmitate labeled with ^{11}C has received extensive evaluation as a tracer of nonesterified fatty acid metabolism.[83] Under fasting, normoxic conditions, nonesterified fatty acids are the preferred substrate to supply reducing equivalents for oxidative phosphorylation.[67] During myocardial ischemia, oxidation of nonesterified fatty acids is decreased and there is increased conversion of extracted nonesterified fatty acids to tissue neutral and phospholipids. In myocardial infarction, both the extraction and oxidation of nonesterified fatty acids are markedly reduced. These three distinctive patterns of myocardial monosterified fatty acid metabolism have been observed in experimental and myocardial ischemia and clinical myocardial infarction with positron computed tomography and ^{11}C-labeled palmitate.[68,69]

Using [^{18}F]-2-fluoro-2-deoxyglucose (FDG) and [^{13}N]ammonia as tracers of exogenous glucose utilization and perfusion,[72] respectively, a dual tracer approach has been used in our laboratory to identify and differentiate ischemic from infarcted myocardium in human beings. In myocardial ischemia, regional perfusion is decreased while glucose utilization is maintained, as reflected by the development of lactate production.[67,70,71] In myocardial infarction, both perfusion and exogenous glucose utilization are reduced concordantly. Patterns consistent with normal, ischemic, and infarcted myocardial perfusion and glucose utilization have been observed in patients after recent infarction with positron computed tomography, FDG, and [^{13}N]ammonia that correlated with clinical, electrocardiographic, and angiographic evaluation[73–77] (Fig. 4).

These initial studies demonstrating distinctive metabolic patterns in ischemic and infarcted myocardium with positron computed tomography and positron-

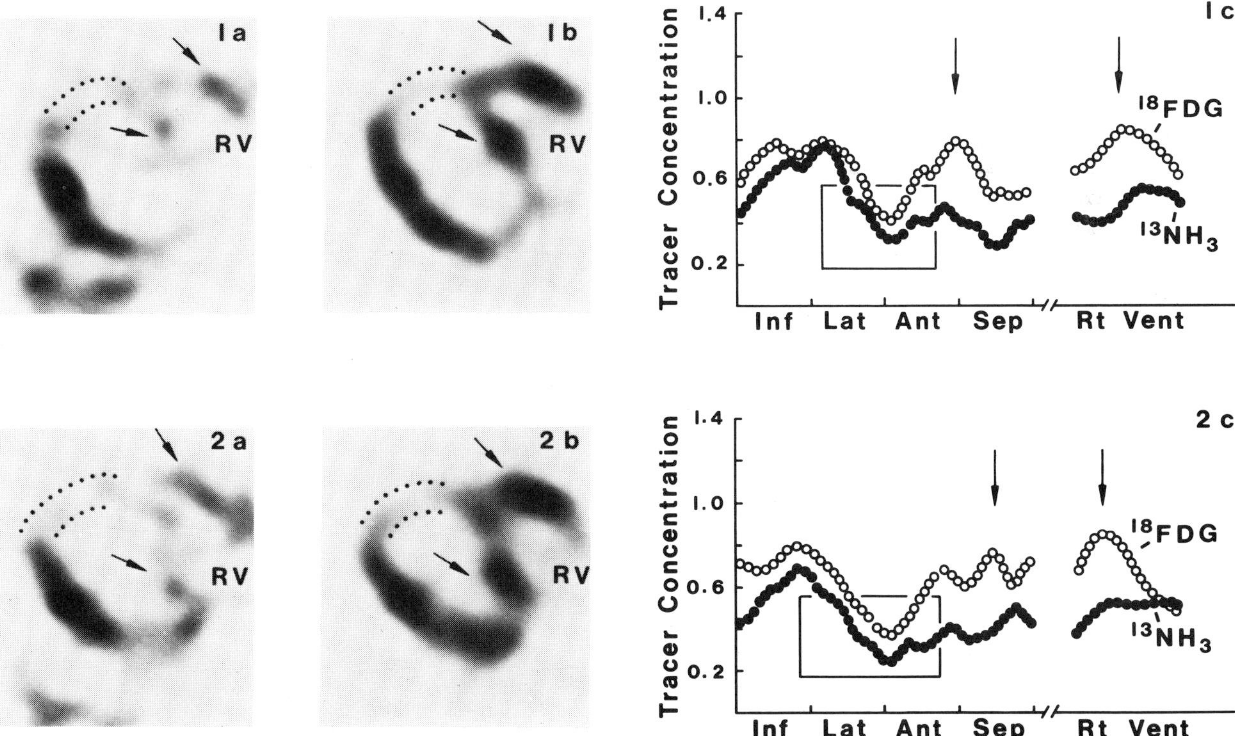

FIGURE 4 Relative regional perfusion (1A,2B) and exogenous glucose utilization (1B,2B) from a patient with refractory postinfarction angina, severe proximal triple-vessel coronary artery disease, and elevated pulmonary arterial and venous pressures at the time of imaging. Both transaxial cross-sectional pairs are through the body of the left ventricle. The corresponding superimposed normalized regional tissue tracer concentrations are shown in the graphs (1C,2C). The anterior wall of the left ventricle is superior, the septum to the right, and the inferior wall at the bottom. Unlike patients without pulmonary hypertension, both left and right ventricles are visualized. However, the left ventricle has both an area of infarct-related depressed perfusion and glucose utilization (which is outlined) and an area of ischemia manifested as a discordant increase in FDG activity relative to [^{13}N]ammonia (arrows). The right ventricle also demonstrates ischemic exogenous glucose utilization. The tracer discordance in the inferior wall was not considered significant.[76]

emitting tracers of free fatty acid and glucose utilization provide a demonstration of the potential for further refining the noninvasive identification of high-risk post-infarct patients into subsets with and without the presence of additional jeopardized myocardium with presumably different responses to therapeutic manipulation.

SUMMARY

Myocardial perfusion imaging early after the onset of symptoms has been shown to be a highly sensitive technique in the diagnosis of acute myocardial infarction. Radionuclide evaluation of left ventricular function can provide potentially important therapeutic information. Although in its infancy, evaluation of prognosis in acute infarct patients with radionuclide techniques has been shown to accurately identify high-risk patients who might benefit from therapeutic interventions designed to reduce ischemic myocardial damage.

REFERENCES

1 Berger, H. J., and Zaret, B. L.: Nuclear Cardiology, *N. Engl. J. Med.*, 305:799, 1981.

2 Holman, B. L.: Infarct Avid Radiopharmaceuticals, in D. S. Berman and D. T. Mason (eds.), "Clinical Nuclear Cardiology," Grune & Stratton, New York, 1981, p. 144.

3 Khaw, B. A., Beller, G. A., and Haber, E.: Experimental Myocardial Infarct Imaging Following Intravenous Administration of Iodine-131 Labeled Antibody (Fab')$_2$ Fragment Specific for Cardiac Myosin, *Circulation*, 57:743, 1978.

4 Khaw, B. A., Fallon, J. T., Strauss, H. W., and Haber, E.: Myocardial Infarct Imaging of Antibodies to Canine Cardiac Myosin with Indium-111-Diethylenetriamine Pentaacetic Acid, *Science*, 209:295, 1980

5 Parkey, R. W., Bonte, F. J., Meyer, S. L., et al.: A New Method for Radionuclide Imaging of Acute Myocardial Infarction in Humans, *Circulation*, 50:540, 1974.

6 Willerson, J. T., Parkey, R. W., Bonte, F. J., Meyer, S. L., Atkins, J. M., and Stokely, E. M.: Technetium Stannous Pyrophosphate Myocardial Scintigrams in Patients with Varying Chest Pain Syndromes, *Circulation*, 51:1049, 1975.

7 Berman, D. S., Amsterdam, E. A., Hines, H. H., et al.: New Approach to Interpretation of Technetium-99m Pyrophosphate Scintigraphy in Detection of Acute Myocardial Infarction: Clinical Assessment of Diagnostic Accuracy. *Am. J. Cardiol.*, 39:341, 1977.

8 Zaret, B. L., DiCola, V. C., Donadedin, R. K., et al.: Dual Radionuclide Study of Myocardial Infarction: Relationship between Myocardial Uptake of Potassium-43, Technetium-99m Stannous Pyrophsptate, Regional Myocardial Blood Flow and Creatine Phosphokinase Depletion, *Circulation*, 53:422, 1976.

9 Ahmad, M., Logan, K. W., and Martin, R. H.: Doughnut Pattern of Technetium-99m Pyrophosphate Myocardial Uptake in Patients with Acute Myocardial Infarction: A Sign of Poor Long-Term Prognosis, *Am. J. Cardiol.*, 44:13, 1977.

10 Buja, L. M., Parkey, R. W., Stokely, E. M., Bonte, F. J., and Willerson, J. T.: Pathophysiology of Technetium-99m Stannous Pyrophosphate and Thallium-201 in Acute Anterior Myocardial Infarction in Dogs, *J. Clin. Invest.*, 57:1508, 1976.

11 Buja, L. M., Tofe, A. J., Kalkarmi, P. V., et al.: Sites and Mechanisms of Localization of Technetium-99m Phosphorus Radiopharmaceuticals in Acute Myocardial Infarction and Other Tissues, *J. Clin. Invest.*, 60:724, 1977.

12 Dewanjee, M. K., and Kahn, P. C.: Mechanisms of Localization of ^{99m}Tc-Labeled Pyrophosphate and Tetracycline in Infarcted Myocardium, *J. Nucl. Med.*, 17:639, 1976.

13 Schelbert, H. R., Ingwall, J. S., Sybers, H. D., and Ashburn, W. L.: Uptake of Myocardial Infarct Agents in Reversibly and Irreversibly Injured Myocardium in Cultured Fetal Mouse Heart, *Circ. Res.*, 39:860, 1976.

14 Massie, B. M., Botnivich, E. H., Werner, J. A., Chaterjee, and Parmley, W. W.: Myocardial Scintigraphy with Technetium-99m Stannous Pyrophosphate, *Am. J. Cardiol.*, 43:186, 1979.

15 Donsky, M. S., Curry, G. C., Parkey, R. W., et al.: Unstable Angina Pectoris: Clinical Angiographic and Myocardial Scintigraphic Observations, *Br. Heart J.*, 38:257, 1976.

16 Prasquier, R., Taradash, M. R., Botnivich, E. H., Shames, D. H., and Parmeley, W. W.: The Specificity of the Diffuse Pattern of Cardiac Uptake in Myocardial Infarct Imaging with Technetium-99m Stannous Pyrophosphate, *Circulation*, 55:61, 1977.

17 Holman, B. L., and Wynne, J.: Infarct Avid (Hot Spot) Myocardial Scintigraphy, *Radiol. Clin. North Am.*, 18:487, 1980.

18 Platt, M. R., Parkey, R. W., Willerson, J. T., Bonte, F. J., Shapiro, W., and Sugg, W. L.: Technetium Stannous Pyrophosphate Myocardial Scintigrams in the Recognition of Myocardial Infarction in Patients Undergoing Coronary Revascularization, *Ann. Thorac. Surg.*, 21:311, 1976.

19 Wackers, F. J., Sokole, E. B., Samson, G., et al.: Value and Limitations of Thallium-201 Scintigraphy in the Acute Phase of Myocardial Infarction, *N. Engl. J. Med.*, 295:1, 1976.

20 Umbach, R. E., Lange, R. C., Lee, J. C., and Zaret, B. L.: Temporal Changes in Sequential Quantitative Thal-

lium-201 Scintigraphy Following Myocardial Infarction in Dogs: Comparison of Four and Twenty-Four Hour Infarct Images, *Yale J. Biol. Med.*, 51:597, 1978.

21 Smitherman, T. C., Osborn, R. C., and Narahara, K. A.: Serial Myocardial Scintigraphy after a Single Dose of Thallium-201 in Men after Acute Myocardial Infarctions, *Am. J. Cardiol.*, 42:177, 1978.

22 Wackers, F. J. T., Lie, K. I., Liem, K. L., et al.: Thallium-201 Scintigraphy in Unstable Angina Pectoris, *Circulation*, 57:738, 1978.

23 Berger, B. C., Watson, D. D., Bunwell, L. R., Crosby, I. K., Wellons, H. A., Teates, C. D., and Beller, G. A.: Redistribution of Thallium at Rest in Patients with Stable and Unstable Angina and the Effect of Coronary Artery Bypass Surgery, *Circulation*, 60:1114, 1979.

24 Gewirtz, H., Beller, G. A., Strauss, H. W., Dinsmore, R. E., Zir, L. M., and McKussick, K. A.: Transient Defects of Resting Thallium Scans in Patients with Coronary Artery Disease, *Circulation*, 59:707, 1979.

25 Klocke, F. J., Bunnel, I. L., Green, D. G., Wittenberg, S. M., and Visco, J. P.: Average Coronary Flow per Unit Weight of the Left Ventricle with and without Coronary Disease, *Circulation*, 50:547, 1974.

26 Cannon, P. J., Schmidt, D. H., Weiss, M. B., Fowler, D. L., Sciacca, R. R., Ellis, K., and Casarella, W. J.: The Relationship between Regional Myocardial Perfusion at Rest and Arteriographic Lesions in Patients with Coronary Atherosclerosis, *J. Clin. Invest.*, 56:1442, 1975.

27 Mymin, D., and Sharma, G. P.: Total and Effective Blood Flow in Coronary and Noncoronary Heart Disease, *J. Clin. Invest.*, 53:363, 1974.

28 Bulkley, B. H., Rouleau, J., Strauss, H. W., et al.: Sarcoid Heart Disease: Diagnosis by Thallium-201 Myocardial Perfusion Imaging, *Am. J. Cardiol.*, 37:125, 1976.

29 Bulkley, B. H., Rouleau, J., Strauss, H. W., et al: Idiopathic Hypertrophnic Subaortic Stenosis: Detection by Thallium-201 Myocardial Perfusion Imaging, *N. Engl. J. Med.*, 293:113, 1975.

30 Bulkley, B. H., Hutchins, G. M., Barby, I., Strauss, H. W., and Pitt, B.: Thallium-201 Imaging and Gated Cardiac Blood Pool Scans in Patients with Ischemic and Congestive Cardiomyopathy: A Clinical and Pathologic Study, *Circulation*, 55:753, 1977.

31 Pitt, B., and Thrall, J. H.: Thallium-201 versus Technetium-99m Pyrophosphate Myocardial Imaging in Detection and Evaluation of Patients with Acute Myocardial Infarction, *Am. J. Cardiol.*, 46:1215, 1980.

32 Wackers, F. J. T., Lie, K. I., Liem, K. L., et al.: Potential Value of Thallium-201 Scintigraphy as a Means of Selecting Patients for the Coronary Care Unit, *Br. Heart J.*, 41:111, 1979.

33 Rigo, P., Murray, M., Strauss, H. W., et al.: Left Ventricular Function in Acute Myocardial Infarction Evaluated by Gated Scintigraphy, *Circulation*, 50:678, 1974.

34 Reduto, L. A., Berger, H. J., Cohen, L. S., Gottschalk, A., and Zaret, B. L.: Sequential Radionuclide Assessment of Left and Right Ventricular Performance after Acute Transmural Infarction, *Ann. Intern. Med.*, 89:441, 1978.

35 Schelbert, H. R., Henning, H., Ashburn, W. L., Verba, J. W., Karliner, J., and O'Rourke, R. A.: Serial Measurements of Left Ventricular Ejection Fraction Early and Late after Myocardial Infarctions, *Am. J. Cardiol.*, 38:407, 1976.

36 Rigo, P., Murray, M., Taylor, D. R., et al.: Right Ventricular Dysfunction Detected by Gated Scintigraphy in Patients with Acute Inferior Myocardial Infarctions, *Circulation*, 52:268, 1975.

37 Sanford, C. F., Corbett, J., Nicod, P., et al.: Value of Radionuclide Ventriculography in the Immediate Characterization of Patients with Acute Myocardial Infarctions, *Am. J. Cardiol.*, 49:632, 1982.

38 Schultz, R. A., Strauss, H. W., and Pitt, B.: Sudden Death in the Year Following Acute Myocardial Infarction: Relation to Ventricular Premature Contractions in the Late Hospital Phase and Left Ventricular Ejection Fraction, *Am. J. Med.*, 62:192, 1977.

39 Shah, P. K., Pichler, M., Berman, D. S., Singh, B. N., and Swan, H. J. C.: Left Ventricular Ejection Fraction and First Third Ejection Fraction Determined by Radionuclide Ventriculography in Early Stages of First Transural Infarction: Relation to Short-Term Prognosis, *Am. J. Cardiol.*, 45:542, 1980.

40 Maddahi, J., Shah, P. K., Berman, D. S., et al.: Assessment of Right Ventricular Ejection Fraction in Early Acute Myocardial Infarction by Multiple Gated Equilibrium Scintigraphy: Hemodynamic Correlates and Prognostic Significance, *Am. J. Cardiol.*, 43:371, 1979.

41 Schulze, R. A., Humphries, J. O., Griffith, L. S. C., Ducci, H., Aschuff, S., Baird, M. G., Mellits, E. D., and Pitt, B.: Left Ventricular and Coronary Angiographic Anatomy: Relationship to Ventricular Irritability in the Late Hospital Phase of Acute Myocardial Infarction, *Circulation*, 55:839, 1977.

42 Taylor, J. G., Humphries, J. O., Mellits, E. D., Pitt, B., Schulze, R. A., Griffith, L. S. C., and Ashuff, S. C.: Predictors of Clinical Course, Coronary Anatomy and Left Ventricular Function after Recovery from Acute Myocardial Infarctions, *Circulation*, 62:960, 1980.

43 Page, D. L., Caulfield, J. B., Kastor, J. A., DeSanctis, R. W., and Sanders, C. A.: Myocardial Changes Associated with Cardiogenic Shock, *N. Engl. J. Med.*, 285:133, 1971.

44 Caulfield, J. B., Leinbach, R., and Gold, H.: The Relationship of Myocardial Infarct Size and Prognosis, *Circulation*, 53 (suppl. 1):1, 1976.

45 Roeske, W. R., Savage, R. M., O'Rourke, R. A., and Bloor, C. M.: Clinicopathologic Correlations in Patients after Myocardial Infarction, *Circulation*, 63:36, 1981.

46 Bulkley, B. H., Silverman, K., Weisfeldt, M. L., Burow, R., Pond, M., and Becker, L. C.: Pathologic Basis of

Thallium-201 Scintigraphic Defects in Patients with Fatal Myocardial Injury, *Circulation,* 60:785, 1979.

47 Schuster, E. H., and Bulkley, B. H.: Ischemia at a Distance after Acute Myocardial Infarction: A Cause of Early Post-Infarction Angina, *Circulation,* 62:509, 1980.

48 Schuster, E. H., and Bulkley, B. H.: Early Post-Infarction Angina: Ischemia at a Distance and Ischemia in the Infarct Zone, *N. Engl. J. Med.,* 305:1101, 1981.

49 Norris, R. M., Caughey, P. E., Mercer, C. J., and Scott, P. J.: Prognosis after Myocardial Infarction: Six-Year Follow-Ups, *Br. Heart J.,* 36:786, 1974.

50 Peel, A. A. F., Semple, T., Wang, I., Lancaster, W. M., and Dall, J. L. G.: A Coronary Prognostic Index for Grading Severity of Myocardial Infarctions, *Br. Heart J.,* 24:745, 1962.

51 Davis, H. J., DeCamilla, J., Bayer, L. W., and Moss, A. J.: Survivorship Patterns after Myocardial Infarction, *Circulation,* 60:1252, 1979.

52 Bigger, J. J., Jr., Heller, C. A., Wenger, T. L., and Weld, F. M.: Risk Stratification after Acute Myocardial Infarction, *Am. J. Cardiol.,* 42:202, 1978.

53 McHugh, J. J., and Swan, H. J. C.: Prognostic Indicators in Acute Myocardial Infarction, *Geriatrics,* 26:72, 1971.

54 Henning, H., Gilpin, E. A., Covell, J. W., Swan, E. A., O'Rourke, R. A., and Ross, J., Jr.: Prognosis after Myocardial Infarction: A Multivariate Analysis of Mortality and Survival, *Circulation,* 59:1124, 1979.

55 Battler, A., Karliner, J. S., Higgins, C. B., Slutsky, R., Gilpin, E. A., Froelicher, V. F., and Ross, J., Jr.: The Initial Chest X-Ray in Acute Myocardial Infarction, Prediction of Early and Late Mortality and Survival, *Circulation,* 61:1004, 1980.

56 Silverman, K. J., Becker, L. C., Bulkley, B. H., Burow, R. D., Mellits, E. D., Kaliman, C. H., and Weisfeldt, M. L.: Value of Early Thallium-201 Scintigraphy for Predicting Mortality in Patients with Acute Myocardial Infarction, *Circulation,* 61:996, 1980.

57 Lewis, M., Buja, L. M., Saffer, S., et al: Experimental Infarct Sizing Using Computer Processing and a Three-Dimensional Model, *Science,* 197:167, 1977.

58 Buja, L. M., Poliner, L. R., Parkey, R. W., et al.: Clinicopathologic Study of Persistently Positive Technetium-99m Stannous Pyrophosphate Myocardial Scintigrams and Myocytolytic Degeneration after Myocardial Infarction, *Circulation,* 56:1016, 1977.

59 Holman, B. L., Chisolm, R. J., and Braunwald, E.: The Prognostic Implications of Acute Myocardial Infarct Scintigraphy with ^{99m}Tc-Pyrophosphate, *Circulation,* 57:320, 1978.

60 Botnivich, E. H., Shames, D., Lappin, H., et al.: Noninvasive Quantification of Myocardial Infarction with Technetium-99m Pyrophosphate, *Circulation,* 52:909, 1975.

61 Henning, H. Schelbert, H., Righetti, A., Ashburn, W. L., and O'Rourke, R. A.: Dual Myocardial Imaging with Technetium-99m Pyrophosphate and Thallium-201 for Detecting, Localizing and Sizing Acute Myocardial Infarction, *Am. J. Cardiol.,* 40:147, 1977.

62 Turner, J. D., Schwartz, K. M., Logic, R. J., et al.: Detection of Residual Jeopardized Myocardium 3 Weeks after Myocardial Infarction by Exercise Testing with Thallium-201 Myocardial Infarction, *Circulation,* 61:729, 1980.

63 Dunn, R. F., Freedman, B., Bailey, I. K., Uren, R., and Kelley, D. T.: Noninvasive Prediction of Multivessel Disease after Myocardial Infarction, *Circulation,* 62:726, 1980.

64 Gibson, R. S., Taylor, G. J., Watson, D. D., et al.: Predicting the Extent and Location of Coronary Artery Disease during the Early Post-Infarction Period by Quantitative Thallium-201 Scintigraphy, *Am. J. Cardiol.,* 47:1010, 1981.

65 Gibson, R. S., Watson, D. D., Carabello, B. A., Holt, N. D., and Beller, G. A.: Clinical Implications of Increased Lung Uptake of Thallium-201 during Exercise Scintigraphy 2 Weeks after Myocardial Infarction, *Am. J. Cardiol.,* 49:1586, 1982.

66 Corbett, J. R., Dehmer, G. J., Lewis, S. E., Woodward, W., Henderson, E., Parkey, R. W., Blomqvist, C. G., and Willerson, J. T.: The Prognostic Value of Submaximal Exercise Testing with Radionuclide Ventriculography before Hospital Discharge in Patients with Recent Myocardial Infarction, *Circulation,* 64:535, 1981.

67 Liedtke, J. A.: Alterations of Carbohydrate and Lipid Metabolism in the Acutely Ischemic Heart, *Prog. Cardiovasc. Dis.,* 23:321, 1981.

68 Ter-Pogossian, M. M., Klein, M. S., Markham, J., Roberts, R., and Sobel, B. E.: Regional Assessment of Myocardial Metabolic Integrity in Vivo by Positron-Emission Tomography with ^{11}C-Palmitate, *Circulation,* 61:242, 1980.

69 Lerch, R. A., Ambos, H. D., Bergman, S. R., Welch, M. J., Ter-Pogossian, M. M., and Sobel, B. E.: Localization of Viable, Ischemic Myocardium by Positron-Emission Tomography with ^{11}C-Palmitate, *Circulation,* 64:689, 1981.

70 Helfant, R. H., Forrester, J. S., Hampton, J. R., et al.: Differential Hemodynamic, Metabolic and Electrocardiographic Effects in Subjects with and without Angina Pectoris during Atrial Pacing, *Circulation,* 42:601, 1970.

71 Marshall, R. C., Nash, W. W., Shine, K. I., Phelps, M. E., and Ricchiuti, N.: Glucose Metabolism during Ischemia Due to Excessive Oxygen Demand or Altered Coronary Flow in the Isolated Arterially Perfused Rabbit Septum, *Circ. Res.,* 49:640, 1981.

72 Phelps, M. E., Huang, S. C., Hoffman, E. J., et al.: Tomographic Measurement of Local Cerebral Glucose

Metabolic Rate in Humans with ^{18}F-2-Fluoro-2-Deoxy-glucose: Validation of Methods, *Ann. Neurol.*, 6:371, 1979.

73 Ratib, O., Phelps, M. E., Huang, S. C., et al.: The Deoxyglucose Method for the Estimation of Local Myocardial Glucose Metabolism without Positron Computed Tomography, *J. Nucl. Med.*, in press.

74 Schelbert, H. R., Phelps, M. E., Huang, S. C., et al.: N-13 Ammonia as an Indicator of Myocardial Blood Flow, *Circulation*, 63:1259, 1981.

75 Marshall, R. C., Schelbert, H. R., Tillisch, J. H., Phelps, M. E., and Henze, E.: Identification of Ischemic Myocardium Using 18-Fluorodeoxyglucose, N-13 Ammonia and Positron Computed Tomography, *J. Nucl. Med. (suppl.)*, 22:39, 1981. (Abstract.)

76 Marshall, R. C., Huang, S. C., Tillisch, J. H., et al.: Development of Regional Criteria to Assess the Significance of Changes in 18-Fluorodeoxyglucose and N-13-Ammonia Activities Evaluated with Positron Computed Tomography, *J. Nucl. Med. (suppl.)*, 23:33, 1982. (Abstract.)

77 Marshall, R. C., Tillisch, J. H., Phelps, M. E., Huang, S. C., Carson, R., Henze, E., and Schelbert, H. R.: Identification and Differentiation of Resting Myocardial Ischemia and Infarction in Man with Positron Computed Tomography, ^{18}F-Labeled Fluorodeoxyglucose and N-13 Ammonia, *Circulation*, submitted for publication.

78 Shuster, E. H., Bulkley, B. H., Jugdutt, B. I., et al.: Assessment of the Extent of Myocardial Infarction by Computer Analysis of Thallium-201 Scintigrams, *Circulation*, 60:11, 1979.

79 Wackers, F. J., Becker, A. E., Samson, G., et al.: Location and Size of Acute Myocardial Infarction Estimated from Thallium-201 Scintigrams: A Clinical Pathologic Study, *Circulation*, 56:72, 1977.

80 Zaret, B. L., Vlay, S. C., Freedman, G. S., et al.: Quantitative Relationships between Potassium-43 Imaging and Left Ventricular Cineangiography following Myocardial Infarction in Man, *Circulation*, 52:1076, 1975.

81 Maseri, A., Parodi, O., Severi, S., et al.: Transient Transmural Reduction of Myocardial Blood Flow Demonstrated by Thallium-201 Scintigraphy, as a Cause of Variant Angina, *Circulation*, 54:280, 1976.

82 Phelps, M. E.: Emission Computed Tomography, *Semin. Nucl. Med.*, 7:337, 1977.

83 Goldstein, R. A., Klein, M. S., Welch, M. J., Sobel, B. E.: External Assessment of Myocardial Metabolism with ^{11}C-Palmitate in Vivo, *J. Nucl. Med.*, 21:342, 1980.

This work was supported in part by Investigate Group Fellowship Award 617IG1 by the Greater Los Angeles Affiliate of the American Heart Association.

Use of Antidysrhythmic Drugs[*]

PAUL E. FENSTER, M.D., and FRANK I. MARCUS, M.D.

> Premature beats or extrasystoles are so common and unimportant except as a source of discomfort in some people and as evidence of digitalis intoxication on occasion in others that little needs to be said about their long follow-up. We have always supposed that premature beats with slight to moderate frequency are normal events in healthy people. It is rather surprising that they are not present in all people all the time, since the myocardium of all heart chambers is so sensitive.
>
> P. D. WHITE AND H. DONOVAN, 1967
> *Hearts—Their Long Follow-Up.*[1]

SUDDEN DEATH DUE TO CARDIAC DYSRHYTHMIA

Antidysrhythmic Therapy and Ventricular Ectopic Depolarizations

Sudden cardiac death due to ventricular fibrillation is the single greatest cause of death from coronary artery disease. The identification of the patient at risk, and appropriate therapy to prevent death due to ventricular dysrhythmias, is the major goal of antidysrhythmic therapy. The risk of sudden cardiac death is related to two major factors: first, the presence of any underlying organic heart disease; and second, the nature and severity of the ventricular dysrhythmia.

In the absence of heart disease, the occurrence of ventricular ectopy does not indicate a worsened prognosis. Hinkle and associates found ventricular ectopic depolarizations (VEDs) on a 6-h ambulatory electrocardiographic recording in 62 percent of 301 asymptomatic, actively employed, middle-aged American males.[1a] During a 2½-year follow-up, there was no increased cardiac mortality in those subjects who did not have major coronary risk factors. Similar findings were reported in the Tecumseh heart study.[2] A number of other studies confirm the common occurrence of ventricular ectopy in apparently healthy adults. Unless symptomatic, such individuals require no treatment for these dysrhythmias.

In contrast, in the setting of ischemic heart disease, VEDs are associated with an increased risk of sudden cardiac death. In the Coronary Drug Project, 271 of 2,035 survivors of an acute myocardial infarction had one or more VEDs on a standard 12-lead electrocardiogram.[3] During a 3-year follow-up, the total mortality, as well as the incidence of sudden death, was twice as frequent in the group with VEDs as for the entire study population. Several recent studies have documented that the presence of certain forms of ventricular ectopy is the single greatest prognostic factor for sudden cardiac death in the postinfarction patient.[4,5] Ventricular ectopy thus identifies a population at risk. In these individuals, the rationale for treatment with antidysrhythmic agents is to attempt to prevent sudden death.

Although VEDs are also a risk factor for sudden death in other forms of heart disease, the association is not as well documented as in coronary artery disease. Ventricular ectopy is common in cardiomyopathies. Hypertrophic cardiomyopathy is associated with a high incidence of sudden death, presumably owing to ventricular tachydysrhythmias. Savage et al. performed ambulatory ECG recordings on 100 patients with hypertrophic cardiomyopathy.[6] High-grade VEDs were found in over 50 percent, including ventricular tachycardia in 19 percent. Two patients with ventricular tachycardia experienced cardiac arrest. Studies such as this suggest that ventricular ectopy, especially if high grade, may identify a subset of patients with hypertrophic cardiomyopathy at high risk for sudden cardiac death.

Ventricular ectopy is also an important prognostic sign in congestive cardiomyopathy. In one study of over 115 patients with idiopathic congestive cardiomyopathy, the overall 5-year survival rate was 65 percent.[7] However, those with complex ventricular ectopy recorded at any time during their illness had a 5-year survival of 54 percent. Of note was the fact that ventricular tachycardia was significantly associated with sudden cardiac death. These studies document that in certain forms of heart disease, the presence of ventricular ectopy identifies a high-risk subgroup.

An important factor in defining this risk is the nature and severity of the dysrhythmia. Recent reports indicate that risk of sudden death is associated with certain complex forms of ventricular ectopy and not with isolated, unifocal VEDs. Ruberman and associates obtained 1-h ambulatory electrocardiographic recordings on 1,739 men within 1 year after a myocardial infarction.[4] Total mortality and sudden cardiac death were compared among the following groups: (1) those with no ventricular ectopy, (2) those with unifocal VEDs, and (3) those with complex VEDs (bigeminal, multifocal, pairs, runs, or early-cycle VEDs). During a follow-up period averaging 2 years, the presence of unifocal VEDs was not associated with an increase in mortality, regardless of the total number of VEDs. The presence of complex VEDs during the monitoring hour was associated with a threefold increase in sudden cardiac death. Among those with

*From the University of Arizona Health Sciences Center, Tucson, Arizona.

complex forms, there was a greater overall frequency of VEDs and in this group of patients, the greater the frequency, the greater the mortality.

Ruberman and associates analyzed the contribution of complex VEDs to the increased mortality and compared this risk to that associated with a number of clinical variables, such as age, duration of heart disease, congestive heart failure, and other factors known to influence prognosis. Controlling for all these variables, the presence of complex VEDs was associated with a threefold increase in risk of sudden death. Complex VEDs constituted the strongest single variable relating to prognosis.

Quite similar findings were reported by Moss and associates in an evaluation of 6-h ambulatory electrocardiographic recordings obtained in 940 survivors of an acute myocardial infarction.[5] Complex VEDs (bigeminal, multiform, repetitive, or R on T) were associated with a significantly increased cardiac death rate. This association was independent of 10 other clinical variables.

In summary, the mere presence of ventricular ectopy is not an indication for treatment in the asymptomatic patient. However, the patient should be evaluated to determine whether heart disease, particularly coronary artery disease, is present and whether complex forms of ventricular ectopy are present. In the high-risk patient, therapy with antidysrhythmic drugs is warranted in an attempt to prevent sudden cardiac death.

Therapeutic Options

Antidysrhythmic *drugs* are the mainstay of therapy. However, prior to the initiation of drug therapy, a vigorous search should be made for noncardiac abnormalities that may contribute to the occurrence of ectopy. These include pulmonary disease, anemia, thyroid disease, infection, electrolyte imbalance, and sympathomimetic drugs. In addition, congestive failure should be optimally treated.

If the dysrhythmia is refractory to drug therapy, there are a few other options. In some patients, episodes of ventricular tachycardia can be prevented by chronic overdrive atrial or ventricular *pacing,* usually at a rate of less than 100 beats per minute.[8–11]

The demonstration that ventricular tachycardia can usually be terminated by programmed premature stimuli led to the use of implanted pacemakers to terminate recurrent ventricular tachycardias.[12–14] The success of this technique may depend on the rate of the tachycardia and on the position of the pacing wire. The method usually involves either use of a magnet held over the pacemaker to produce a fixed rate or use of a permanently implanted radio-frequency receiver that

can be activated to induce burst pacing.[13,14] Both magnetic and radio-frequency pacemakers can be patient-activated. Some pacemakers are designed to sense ventricular tachycardia and/or ventricular flutter. The pacer then produces a sequence of pulses until normal rhythm is restored.[13]

In patients in whom drug therapy is ineffective in controlling malignant ventricular dysrhythmias, a number of surgical procedures may be employed. Coronary artery disease is the most common form of organic heart disease associated with severe ventricular dysrhythmias. However, revascularization by bypass surgery has not been generally successful therapy for ventricular dysrhythmias.[15,16]

An association between ventricular aneurysm and refractory ventricular dysrhythmias is well established. An area of ischemic tissue in the border of the aneurysm provides the electrophysiologic substrate for the reentry pathway producing the ventricular tachycardia. However, resection of the aneurysm has proven an unreliable means of treating refractory dysrhythmias because the origin of the ventricular tachycardia is in the border of the aneurysm, a site not routinely resected during aneurysmectomy. This has led to the use of electrophysiologic mapping techniques to localize the site of the origin of the dysrhythmia and to guide the surgical operation. The dysrhythmia usually originates in the endocardium and frequently within 2 cm of the border of the aneurysm. Endocardial mapping can substantialy improve the success of surgical therapy for dysrhythmia.[17,18]

ANTIDYSRHYTHMIC DRUGS
Conventional Antidysrhythmic Drugs
PROCAINAMIDE

Procainamide is effective in the treatment of both supraventricular and ventricular dysrhythmias. (Table 1). The drug has been in clinical use since 1951.

Clinical electrophysiology Procainamide depresses spontaneous diastolic depolarization and reduces the maximum rate of rise of the action potential in atrial and ventricular muscle, as well as in Purkinje fibers. This is associated with depression of the conduction velocity, an increase of the threshold for excitability, and prolongation of the effective refractory period. These direct effects are opposed by a vagolytic action of the drug. Consequently, therapeutic levels have a variable effect on atrioventricular nodal conduction, although a slight prolongation is usually observed. The drug significantly slows His-Purkinje conduction.[19]

TABLE 1
Procainamide

Pharmacology:
  Bioavailability 75 to 85 percent
  Peak level 1 h after ingestion
  Rapid distribution; volume of distribution 2 liters/kg
  Metabolized in liver to *N*-acetylprocainamide
  Fifty percent excreted unchanged in urine
  Half-life 2.5 to 4.0 h
Dosing:
  Intravenous loading dose 10 mg/kg
  Intravenous infusion rate 2 to 4 mg/min
  Oral maintenance dose 50 to 100 mg/(kg·day)
  Decrease doses in heart failure and renal failure
Uses:
  Ventricular dysrhythmias
  Conversion of atrial fibrillation
  Supraventricular dysrhythmias
  Wolff-Parkinson-White syndrome
Adverse effects:
  Hypotension
  Anorexia, nausea, vomiting
  Malaise, fatigue, insomnia
  Lupus erythematosus-like syndrome

Clinical pharmacology Procainamide is rapidly absorbed from the gastrointestinal tract, and peak plasma levels are reached approximately 1 h after oral ingestion.[20,21] Bioavailability of oral procainamide is approximately 75 to 85 percent.[20,21] Absorption may be delayed and bioavailability may be decreased in the patient with an acute myocardial infarction.[22] When administered intramuscularly, peak plasma levels are reached in about 30 min and absorption is generally complete.[22,23]

Procainamide is approximately 10 to 20 percent bound to plasma protein and is rapidly distributed to the body tissues. The drug is extensively bound to heart, liver, kidney, and lung. The volume of distribution is approximately 2 liters/kg.

Procainamide is both eliminated by the kidneys and metabolized in the liver. Approximately 50 percent of a dose is excreted unchanged in the urine.[24,25] The rate of procainamide elimination varies directly with creatinine clearance. In normal individuals, the half-life of elimination of procainamide is approximately 3 to 4 h. This is markedly prolonged in the patient with renal failure.

Approximately 20 percent of administered procainamide is recovered as the major metabolite, N-acetylprocainamide (NAPA).[25,26] The extent of hepatic metabolism is related to the activity of the hepatic acetyltransferase enzyme system.[27] Individuals may be classified as either slow or fast acetylators. This enzyme activity is genetically determined and is distributed bimodally in the population. NAPA is an active metabolite that is eliminated predominantly by the kidneys. In renal failure, NAPA is retained and the ratio of serum NAPA to procainamide is increased. In patients with renal failure, NAPA may account for much of the antidysrhythmic effect achieved by procainamide administration.[28] Therefore, it is important to obtain both procainamide and NAPA levels in order to properly adjust the dose of procainamide in patients with renal failure.

Dosing considerations The therapeutic effect of procainamide may be rapidly achieved by intravenous administration of a loading dose. The usual loading dose is approximately 10 mg/kg, but dosage must be individualized. Procainamide may be administered by continuous intravenous infusion, at a rate not exceeding 40 mg/min. The electrocardiogram must be monitored continuously to watch for excessive QRS prolongation, and the blood pressure must be closely checked during the intravenous infusion, because hypotension may occur. An alternative method of loading consists of the administration of 100 mg of the drug every 5 min up to a maximum of 1,000 mg.[29] Myocardial depression may occur with excessively rapid loading. After achieving a therapeutic effect, procainamide may be given intravenously as a continuous infusion, usually at a rate of 2 to 4 mg/min.

When administered orally, a therapeutic effect is usually maintained with doses between 50 and 100 mg/(kg·day). A satisfactory therapeutic effect is usually maintained when the total dose is given as four divided doses. Use of a slow-release formulation allows for an 8- to 12-h dosing interval.[30,31]

In the presence of cardiac or renal failure, the clearance of procainamide is decreased, a smaller dose is advisable, and the dosing interval may be prolonged. Patients on hemodialysis may be administered procainamide once every 12 to 24 h. Indexes of efficacy and toxicity should be carefully monitored. Dosing may be guided by measurement of serum concentrations of both procainamide and NAPA.

The usual therapeutic range of procainamide is 4 to 8 μg/ml. Higher levels are required in a significant number of patients. Generally, procainamide concentrations greater than 12 μg/ml are associated with a high incidence of adverse effects.[32] The therapeutic range of NAPA is not well defined. A wide range of effective levels has been reported.[33,34] NAPA appears to be well tolerated over a wide range. The relative contributions of procainamide and NAPA to therapeutic and toxic effects requires further investigation.

Indications for use The efficacy of procainamide against ventricular dysrhythmias is well documented. Procainamide may be useful in abolishing ventricular dysrhythmias in the coronary care unit,[35] particularly in patients with dysrhythmias not well controlled by lidocaine.[36] Procainamide is effective for the chronic suppression of ventricular ectopy. High-dose procainamide has been used successfully in the treatment of recurrent ventricular tachycardia refractory to other agents.[37]

Procainamide is effective for the prevention of supraventricular dysrhythmias.[38,39] It is effective in converting atrial fibrillation to sinus rhythm, particularly when this rhythm disturbance is of short duration.[40] Procainamide may be used to prevent recurrences of atrial fibrillation once sinus rhythm is restored.

Procainamide prolongs the refractory period during both antegrade and retrograde conduction through accessory pathways in most patients. The drug may therefore be effective in slowing the ventricular response to atrial fibrillation in patients with the Wolff-Parkinson-White (WPW) syndrome who have antegrade conduction in the accessory pathway.[41] An exception to this, however, is the patient with an initially short (less than 270 msec) refractory period in the accessory pathway. In these individuals, the refractory period is not consistently prolonged after procainamide.[41a]

Adverse effects Rates of intravenous administration of procainamide greater than 40 mg/min may be associated with hypotension or aggravation of dysrhythmias. Cardiac toxicity may also be manifested by marked prolongation of the QRS or Q-T interval. Prolongation of these intervals by up to 30 percent is not uncommon and should not be considered a sign of toxicity. The development of atrioventricular or intraventricular conduction defects is uncommon.

Procainamide may produce anorexia, nausea, malaise, fatigue, or insomnia. These adverse effects are generally associated with high serum concentrations. Uncommon adverse effects include fever, vomiting, disorientation, hallucinations, or seizures. Agranulocytosis rarely occurs.

The most common adverse effect from chronic administration of procainamide is the occurrence of a syndrome resembling systemic lupus erythematosus.[42,43] Manifestations of this syndrome are seen in approximately 30 percent of patients after long-term administration. This complication occurs after a shorter duration of therapy in slow acetylators.[44] Clinical manifestations of the syndrome include fever, rash, arthritis, arthralgia, myalgia, pleurisy, and pericarditis. The LE cell and antibodies to denatured DNA are usually present. The syndrome is reversible after discontinuation of procainamide. The syndrome has not been reported in patients taking NAPA, and patients who have developed the lupus-like syndrome have been given NAPA without recurrence of this condition.

QUINIDINE

Quinidine is one of the oldest and most widely used antidysrhythmic agents in the prevention and termination of both ventricular and supraventricular dysrhythmias (Table 2).

Clinical electrophysiology Quinidine depresses spontaneous diastolic depolarization and markedly prolongs the effective refractory period in atrial and ventricular muscle, as well as in Purkinje fibers. The drug has antiadrenergic effects and vagolytic actions that have opposing electrophysiologic effects. The vagolytic effect usually produces a slight increase in heart rate and enhances atrioventricular nodal conduction.[45] The effects on ventricular conduction result in a prolongation of the QRS and Q-T intervals in a dose-dependent manner.[45] Quinidine depresses conduction and increases refractoriness in accessory pathways.[41]

Clinical pharmacology Quinidine sulfate contains 82 percent quinidine. This preparation is well absorbed after oral administration.[46] Absorption is enhanced at low gastric pH. Peak levels occur approximately 2 h after ingestion.[46] Bioavailability is approximately 80 percent, owing to first-pass hepatic metabolism. Quinidine gluconate contains 62 percent quinidine and is more slowly absorbed. Peak levels occur 4 to 5 h after dosing.[47] The gluconate is approximately 70 percent bioavailable.

Quinidine is about 80 percent bound to serum albumin. However, changes in protein binding are of little clinical consequence, because the drug is highly

TABLE 2
Quinidine

Pharmacology:
  Bioavailability 70 to 80 percent
  Peak level 2 h (sulfate) or 4 to 5 h (gluconate) after ingestion
  Highly tissue bound; volume of distribution 2 to 4 liters/kg
  Hydroxylated in the liver to inactive products
  Ten to 30 percent unchanged in urine
  Half-life 6 to 8 h
Dosing:
  Oral loading dose 600 to 1,000 mg in 4 to 8 h
  Oral maintenance dose 800 to 1,600 mg/day (sulfate)
  Decrease doses in hepatic dysfunction
Uses:
  Ventricular dysrhythmias
  Conversion of atrial fibrillation
  Supraventricular dysrhythmias
Adverse effects:
  Gastrointestinal irritation
  Cinchonism
  Exacerbation of ventricular dysrhythmias
  Fever, dermatitis, thrombocytopenia

bound to myocardium, liver, kidney, and skeletal muscle. The volume of distribution is 2 to 4 liters/kg.

Quinidine is mostly hydroxylated in the liver to inactive products.[48,49] Metabolism is accelerated by phenytoin and some other anticonvulsant drugs. Approximately 10 to 30 percent of the drug is eliminated unchanged by the kidneys. Renal excretion increases as urine pH decreases. Quinidine clearance is only slightly decreased in renal failure, but the metabolites accumulate. The elimination half-life of quinidine is usually 6 to 8 h, but it ranges from 5 to 12 h.

Quinidine profoundly alters the pharmacokinetics of digoxin and digitoxin. Quinidine decreases the renal and nonrenal clearances of digoxin in a dose-dependent fashion.[50] Quinidine decreases digoxin volume of distribution, probably by displacing the glycoside from tissue binding sites. The quinidine-induced rise in serum digoxin level is associated with an increased risk of digitalis toxicity. Digoxin administration raises serum quinidine levels, although the mechanism is unknown.

Quinidine decreases the total-body clearance of digitoxin without altering volume of distribution.[51] The result is a prolongation of half-life. The clinical significance of the quinidine-digitoxin interaction is unclear.

Dosing considerations Quinidine sulfate is usually given in doses of 0.8 to 1.6 g/day in three or four divided doses. Oral loading with the drug may be accomplished by an initial dose of 600 mg. An alternate method is to administer 200 mg every 2 h for five doses. Rapid loading by the intravenous route is seldom used, because a rapid rate of administration of quinidine may produce vasodilation and myocardial depression, leading to hypotension, dysrhythmias, and death. The ECG should be continuously monitored, and the blood pressure should be checked frequently. Quinidine gluconate may be administered as a maintenance dose of 324 to 972 mg every 8 h.

Quinidine should not be given by the intramuscular route, because this is painful and may produce tissue necrosis, and absorption after intramuscular injection is erratic.[52]

The therapeutic range of quinidine is 2 to 5 μg/ml. Toxicity is common at levels greater than 8 μg/ml.

Quinidine kinetics are little affected by changes in cardiac output or renal function. Inactive metabolites may accumulate and may be measured as quinidine, if a nonspecific assay method is used. Quinidine dosage should be decreased if liver dysfunction is present, although there are few studies that have explored this problem.

Indications for use Quinidine in doses of 200 to 400 mg four times daily is frequently effective in converting atrial fibrillation or flutter to sinus rhythm. The vagolytic effect of quinidine may enhance atrioventricular

conduction as well as slow the fibrillatory rate, thereby enhancing AV nodal conduction, resulting in a more rapid ventricular response. Therefore, it is recommended that verapamil, digitalis, or a beta adrenergic blocking drug be administered prior to quinidine in this situation. After conversion to sinus rhythm, chronic quinidine therapy should be used to prevent recurrences of atrial fibrillation.

Quinidine is frequently effective in treating supraventricular tachycardia due to AV nodal reentry as well as in reducing the frequency of episodes of paroxysmal supraventricular tachycardia. The drug suppresses the atrial or ventricular ectopy that initiates the tachycardia and depresses retrograde fast pathway conduction.

Quinidine is frequently effective in suppressing ventricular ectopic beats and preventing ventricular tachycardia.

Adverse effects More than one-third of patients treated with quinidine have adverse reactions. Gatrointestinal side effects, including anorexia, nausea, vomiting, diarrhea, and abdominal pain, are most common. These effects are due to gastric irritation and may be less severe with quinidine gluconate or polygalacturonate than with the sulfate preparation.

"Therapeutic" concentrations of quinidine may induce serious ventricular dysrhythmias in some individuals, particularly those with bradycardia or those who have a long Q-T interval prior to therapy. "Quinidine syncope" may be due to nonsustained ventricular tachycardia or ventricular fibrillation. In the majority of reported cases, the patients were also taking digitalis, and it is suspected that at least some deaths due to quinidine may have been due to digitalis-induced ventricular fibrillation as a result of the digitalis-quinidine pharmacokinetic interaction. Therapeutic or toxic levels of quinidine may be present when these dysrhythmias occur.

High concentrations of quinidine may produce cinchonism. Mild symptoms consist of tinnitus, blurred vision, headache, or vertigo. In more severe cases, confusion, delirium, and psychosis may occur.

Quinidine may cause fever, urticaria, maculopapular rash, or exfoliative dermatitis. Thrombocytopenia is uncommon, but it may be severe and associated with bleeding. The mechanism is antibody formation against platelet-quinidine complexes. Hepatotoxicity and bone marrow depression are other rare complications of quinidine therapy.

Quinidine has well-known effects on the electrocardiogram, which should be monitored during therapy. The prolongation of the Q-T interval is dose-dependent, but the degree of prolongation shows considerable interindividual variation. The dose should be decreased if either the QRS or Q-T interval increases by more than 50 percent. If an intraventricular conduction defect is present before the quinidine is given, a QRS prolongation of greater than 25 percent should be cause for decreasing the dose of quinidine.

DISOPYRAMIDE

Although the antidysrhythmic effects of disopyramide have been recognized since 1962, the drug has been available for clinical use in the United States only since 1977 (Table 3).

Clinical electrophysiology Disopyramide is a membrane-active agent that decreases automaticity and prolongs both action potential duration and effective refractory period in atrial and ventricular tissue in human beings without depressing AV nodal or His-Purkinje conduction.[53] The observed effects on AV nodal conduction are due to direct depressant action and the anticholinergic properties of this drug. Disopyramide prolongs the QRS and Q-T intervals, especially in the presence of preexisting abnormality of intraventricular conduction.

Clinical pharmacology In normal subjects, orally administered disopyramide is rapidly and completely absorbed.[54,55] The peak plasma level occurs about 2 h after oral ingestion. The bioavailability of the drug ranges from 57 to 87 percent, owing in part to hepatic first-pass metabolism.[54–56]

Disopyramide is bound to serum proteins. Total levels of disopyramide demonstrate nonlinear kinetics. The percent bound decreases as the serum drug concentration rises.[57] Since drug clearance is related to unbound drug, there is a less than proportional increase

TABLE 3
Disopyramide

Pharmacology:
    Bioavailability 57 to 87 percent
    Peak level 2 h after ingestion
    Bound to serum proteins; volume of distribution 1 liter/kg
    Metabolized in the liver
    Fifty-five percent excreted unchanged in urine
    Half-life 7 h
Dosing:
    Oral loading dose 300 mg
    Oral maintenance 300 to 1,200 mg/day
    Decrease doses in heart failure and renal or hepatic insufficiency
Uses:
    Ventricular dysrhythmias
Adverse effects:
    Negative inotropic effect
    Anticholinergic

in total drug level as dose is increased. However, the concentration of free drug changes linearly with dose. The volume of distribution of disopyramide is approximately 1.0 liter/kg.

Disopyramide is cleared both by renal excretion and hepatic metabolism. Approximately 55 percent is excreted unchanged in the urine.[54,57] The major metabolite has weak antidysrhythmic activity.

In healthy subjects, disopyramide elimination half-life ranges from 4 to 10 h with a mean of 7 h. The half-life is prolonged in older patients, and this may be due to decreased renal function.

Dosing considerations The usual therapeutic plasma concentration is 2 to 5 µg/ml. This level is achieved with doses of 300 to 1,200 mg daily, given as three or four divided doses. For rapid attainment of steady-state levels, an oral loading dose of 300 mg may be administered. The loading and maintenance doses should be decreased in the setting of low cardiac output, renal insufficiency, or hepatic insufficiency.

Indications for use Disopyramide has been shown to be as effective as quinidine or procainamide in the treatment of chronic ventricular ectopy.[58,59] The drug may be effective in some cases of ventricular tachycardia refractory to other agents.[60]

Some studies have demonstrated efficacy of disopyramide in the treatment of supraventricular dysrhythmias.[61,62] However, at this time, the role of disopyramide in the management of atrial dysrhythmias is uncertain.

Adverse effects The most common side effects are those due to the anticholinergic action of disopyramide. These include dry mouth and tongue, blurred vision, constipation, and urinary retention. These effects are dose-dependent. Disopyramide is contraindicated in patients with glaucoma. A serious adverse effect is depression of ventricular function.[63] Either rapid intravenous administration or an oral loading dose may precipitate pulmonary edema, particularly in patients with underlying ventricular dysfunction.[64,65]

Disopyramide may exacerbate the sick sinus syndrome, produce widening of the QRS or prolongation of the Q-T interval.

The therapeutic and toxic effects of disopyramide are enhanced in the presence of hyperkalemia. Conversely, the therapeutic effect may be decreased in hypokalemia.

Uncommon adverse effects include skin rash, psychosis, cholestatic jaundice, hypoglycemia, and agranulocytosis. These have all been reversible in reported cases. The safety of disopyramide in pregnancy and lactation has not been established.

LIDOCAINE

Lidocaine was introduced to clinical medicine in the 1940s as a local anesthetic agent (Table 4). It was first reported to be effective in life-threatening dysrhythmias by Southworth et al. in 1950.[66] They described its beneficial effect in treating an episode of ventricular tachycardia and fibrillation that occurred during cardiac catheterization. In the 1950s, it was used primarily by anesthesiologists for the treatment of intraoperative ventricular dysrhythmias. It was not until 1959 that it began to be used for the treatment of dysrhythmias complicating cardiac surgery.[67]

Clinical electrophysiology In therapeutic doses lidocaine has a minimal effect on atrioventricular and intraventricular conduction.[68] However, in patients with intraventricular conduction delay, especially bifascicular or trifascicular block, lidocaine has caused complete AV block distal to the His bundle,[69] but this complication, fortunately, is rare.

Lidocaine has an inconsistent effect on AV node refractoriness.[70,71] In addition, lidocaine causes no alteration of right ventricular refractoriness in clinical doses in human beings.[72] Bigger et al.[73] noted that lidocaine has electrophysiologic properties that resemble diphenylhydantoin or propranolol more closely than procainamide or quinidine.

Clinical pharmacology Orally administered lidocaine does not provide effective therapeutic levels, because lidocaine is metabolized primarily in the liver and is largely inactivated prior to reaching the systemic circulation. It is possible to partially avoid first-pass metabolism through the liver by rectal administration. When given by this route, there is a 70 percent systemic availability.[74]

Seventy percent of lidocaine is bound to plasma proteins. Alpha-1-acid glycoprotein is the major plasma binding protein for lidocaine. The concentration of this glycoprotein increases in patients following an acute myocardial infarction. This may account for the observed rise in total-blood lidocaine concentrations during constant infusion in patients with myocardial infarction. However, since the concentration of the alpha-1-glycoprotein increases, the rise in free drug concentration is less than the increase in total drug level. Therefore, the observed increase in total lidocaine concentration during constant infusion in patients with myocardial infarction may be misleading with regard to toxicologic implications of lidocaine accumulation. Enhanced binding may reduce drug clearance.[75]

Over 90 percent of administered lidocaine is rapidly and extensively converted to metabolites.[76,77] There

TABLE 4
Lidocaine

Pharmacology:
  Seventy percent bound to serum proteins; volume of distribution 1.2 liter/kg
  Extensive hepatic metabolism; active metabolite
  Increased levels and prolonged half-life with prolonged infusion
  Half-life 1.5 h
Dosing:
  Intravenous loading dose 100 to 200 mg
  Intravenous maintenance infusion 2 to 4 mg/min
  Decrease doses in heart failure and hepatic dysfunction, and in presence of propranolol or cimetidine
Uses:
  Acute suppression or prophylaxis against ventricular dysrhythmias
Adverse effects:
  Nausea, drowsiness, confusion, seizure
  Rarely depresses cardiac conduction system

are two active metabolities, monoethylglycinexylidide (MEGX) and glycinexylidide (GX). In guinea pig atria, MEGX had a potency of 80 percent relative to lidocaine, and GX was only 10 percent as potent.[77] The concentration of MEGX may vary from 50 percent of lidocaine concentration to a concentration greater than that of lidocaine.[76] Therefore, MEGX may contribute to the antidysrhythmic activity of lidocaine. It has also been postulated that under certain circumstances, such as congestive heart failure, MEGX and GX may accumulate and contribute to CNS toxicity.[78]

The distribution volume of lidocaine is 1.2 liters/kg. The half-life of elimination is 1.5 h in normal as well as cardiac patients.[79] The elimination half-life of lidocaine may be increased to 2 to 4 h (mean 3.22 h) in patients with uncomplicated myocardial infarction when measured after discontinuation of lidocaine infusion lasting more than 24 h. The mechanism by which a prolonged infusion of lidocaine impairs its own elimination in human beings is not known.[80] Patients with heart failure have a decrease in the volume of distribution and plasma clearance, while patients with liver disease show a marked increase in the volume of distribution, a marked decrease in plasma clearance, and an increase in half-life that averages 4.5 h.[81] Alterations in cardiac dynamics, such as hypotension, shock, or coadministration of such drugs as propranolol or cimetidine, will decrease lidocaine clearance.[82,83]

Dosing considerations Lidocaine is generally used for the treatment or prevention of life-threatening dysrhythmias. Therefore, the object of therapy is to achieve blood levels of lidocaine promptly and maintain these levels. The most common circumstance under which lidocaine is administered is in the first 24 h following an acute myocardial infarction. Several drug regimens have been suggested, all of which require a loading dose to achieve therapeutic levels. In a patient who does not have shock, heart failure, or hepatocellular disease, 100 mg of lidocaine may be given over 2 min. Since the blood level will fall rapidly during the distribution phase, a repeat loading dose of 75 to 100 mg should be given in 10 to 15 min.[84] Alternate schemes for loading with lidocaine are as follows: 50 mg in 1 min given four times, 5 min apart, or 20 mg/min infused for 10 min. In order to maintain plasma concentrations, a continuous infusion of lidocaine, 2 to 4 mg/min, should be administered. In shock, heart failure, or hepatocellular disease, both the loading dose and infusion rate should be reduced by one-half. If ventricular dysrhythmias recur, it is necessary to administer an additional loading dose of 50 mg over 1 min in order to rapidly raise the plasma concentration. At the same time, the infusion rate should also be increased, but by no greater than 5 mg/min. There is no need to gradually decrease the infusion rate when one wishes to discontinue the drug, because abrupt cessation of the infusion will cause the plasma concentration to fall gradually to one-half the original level in 1 to 3 h.

Indications for use The major indication for the use of lidocaine is the prevention of ventricular tachycardia and ventricular fibrillation within the first hours or day following acute myocardial infarction. The study of Lie and colleagues demonstrates that lidocaine, given at a loading dose of 100 mg followed by an infusion of 3 mg/min, is highly effective in preventing primary ventricular fibrillation under these circumstances. None of the 107 treated patients developed primary ventricular fibrillation compared with 11 of 105 controls.[85] Similarly impressive results were reported by Wyman and Hammersmith, who treated 1,165 patients who had an acute myocardial infarction with lidocaine. They reported an incidence of primary ventricular fibrillation in the coronary care unit of only 0.3 percent.[86] A review of lidocaine in acute myocardial infarction showed a greater protective effect in the trials that excluded patients with severe congestive heart failure and shock, as well as in those which excluded patients over the age of 70, who appear to have a lower incidence of primary ventricular fibrillation with acute myocardial infarction.[87]

It has been reported that intramuscular administration of 300 mg of lidocaine reduces the incidence of sudden death in the prehospital phase of infarction.[88] However, another study cast doubt on the efficacy of intramuscular lidocaine in this dosage, because it was not found to be effective in preventing primary ventricular fibrillation.[89]

Lidocaine is used extensively in patients undergoing cardiovascular surgery for treatment of ventricular dysrhythmias. The dosing considerations are similar to those outlined for patients with acute myocardial infarction.

Lidocaine is not effective in the treatment of supraventricular dysrhythmias, except for the treatment of paroxysmal atrial tachycardia associated with digitalis intoxication.[90]

Lidocaine has deservedly earned the reputation of being an extremely safe antidysrhythmic agent. In therapeutic doses, it has minimal negative inotropic effects and can be given safely to patients with congestive heart failure.

Adverse effects There have been rare case reports of severe sinus bradycardia, sinus arrest, or complete heart block following lidocaine administration.[91] In patients with complete heart block due to block below the bundle of His, lidocaine can cause a marked decrease in the ventricular escape rate. Therefore, lidocaine should not be used in patients with complete heart block. The most frequent side effects of lidocaine are confined to the central nervous system and include nausea, drowsiness, speech disturbances, confusion, respiratory depression, and seizures. These side effects are more common in elderly individuals and those with congestive heart failure, particularly those who have a low body weight.

BRETYLIUM TOSYLATE

Bretylium tosylate, a benzyl quaternary ammonium compound, is an adrenergic neural blocking drug that was introduced in the 1950s as an antihypertensive agent (Table 5). Its antihypertensive effect is a result of inhibition of norepinephrine release from postganglionic nerve terminals of the sympathetic nervous system.[92] Bretylium is highly concentrated in the postganglionic nerve terminal of adrenergic nerves and interferes with norepinephrine release. This inhibition of norepinephrine release is preceded by an initial release of catecholamines from adrenergic nerve endings into the general circulation.[92] Leveque first reported that bretylium had antidysrhythmic activity in 1965.[93]

Clinical electrophysiology The cardiac electrophysiologic actions of bretylium are complicated by the dual actions of the drug on the sympathetic nervous system and the ventricular myocardium. Initial bretylium administration results in the release of norepinephrine from sympathetic nerve terminals followed by an inhibition of neuronal catecholamine release.[93] Be-

TABLE 5
Bretylium tosylate

Pharmacology:
  Bioavailability 10 to 30 percent after oral ingestion
  Completely free in plasma
  Volume of distribution 3.4 liters/kg
  Ninety percent excreted unchanged in urine
  Half-life 13.6 h after I.V. administration
Dosing:
  Intravenous loading dose 5 to 10 mg/kg, repeated to a
    maximum of 30 mg/kg
  Intravenous maintenance infusion 1 to 2 mg/min
  Decrease doses in renal failure
Uses:
  Recurrent ventricular tachycardia or fibrillation refractory
    to other antidysrhythmic drugs
Adverse effects:
  Hypotension
  Nausea, vomiting

cause of this dual action, it has been difficult to separate the electrophysiologic effects of the sympathetic nervous system from the direct effects of the drug on the heart. However, this was accomplished by giving bretylium intravenously to conscious dogs with surgically denervated hearts with chronically implanted electrodes over the sinus node, bundle of His, and right bundle branch. In this preparation, there was an increase in the effective refractory period of the atria and ventricles.[94] The drug was found to slow atrioventricular conduction and produced second-degree AV block in this intact dog preparation. However, when bretylium is given intravenously to patients, the functional refractory period of the AV node is decreased. This directional change, which is opposite to that found in the denervated dog, suggests that the indirect action of bretylium resulting from the release of norepinephrine from adrenergic nerve terminals counters the direct effect of the drug. In human beings there is an increase in the effective refractory period of the right atrium but not of the ventricle.[95] Bretylium has been classified as a type III agent because its electrophysiologic effects as studied in ventricular muscle–Purkinje fiber preparations are similar to those of amiodarone. It prolongs the action potential and lengthens refractory period without slowing conduction.[96]

Clinical pharmacology Bretylium has poor systemic availability after oral administration. Only 10 to 30 percent of the drug is absorbed. It has certain pharmacokinetic features that are rather unique. It is virtually 100 percent free (unbound) in plasma. Greater than 90 percent is excreted unchanged in the urine. Therefore, in the presence of decreased renal function,

it is anticipated that the drug will have an increase in half-life and the dosage should be decreased. The volume of distribution is 3.4 liters/kg. The elimination half-life after intravenous administration to normal subjects is 13.6 h, and after oral administration, 6 h. The cause of the difference in elimination half-life after oral and intravenous bretylium is not clear. It may relate to concentration-dependent renal clearance.[97]

Dosing considerations The use of this drug for the treatment of dysrhythmias is limited almost entirely to the parenteral route. The usual dose of bretylium tosylate by the intravenous or intramuscular route is 5 to 10 mg/kg of body weight. For intravenous administration, bretylium tosylate should be diluted and given over 8 to 10 min to avoid nausea and vomiting. For emergency administration, it may be given rapidly by intravenous infusion, and the dose may be repeated at 15 to 30 min intervals, but not to exceed a total of 30 mg/kg. The maintenance dose can be administered by constant intravenous infusion at the rate of 1 to 2 mg/min. This dose should be decreased in patients with impaired renal function.

Indications for use This drug is used primarily to treat life-threatening dysrhythmias in the setting of cardiac arrest, because continued use either intravenously or orally is associated with an unacceptably high incidence of intolerable side effects.

Bretylium is often effective in preventing recurrent ventricular fibrillation or ventricular tachycardia in patients in whom conventional antiarrhythmic drugs fail to maintain sinus rhythm.[98,99] It is not known how the overall effectiveness of bretylium for the treatment of recurrent ventricular tachycardia and fibrillation compares with that of other drugs, since control studies have not been done. However, it is remarkable that the intravenous administration of bretylium tosylate resulted in chemical defibrillation in 5 of 7 patients.[100] Since established ventricular fibrillation in human beings rarely reverts spontaneously, this finding is striking, and similar findings have not been reported with any other antidysrhythmic drug. It should be noted, however, that several studies using experimental animals have failed to document an antifibrillatory effect of bretylium.[101,102]

Adverse effects The major undesirable side effect of bretylium is hypotension due to adrenergic and neuronal blockade. Hypotension of variable severity occurs in most patients and may occur even in the supine position. This adverse effect can be reversed with plasma volume expansion or catecholamine infusion. Nausea and vomiting are common when bretylium is given rapidly by the intravenous route. Carotid pain and swelling have been observed with chronic oral therapy with bretylium, but not during short-term parenteral administration.[103,104]

VERAPAMIL

Verapamil is a calcium channel blocking agent that is exceptionally potent in the treatment and prevention of paroxysmal supraventricular tachycardias (PSVT) (Table 6). The drug also has antianginal and antihypertensive as well as negative inotropic properties.

Clinical electrophysiology Verapamil has a direct depressant effect on fast and slow channel fibers in the AV node. The drug thereby depresses AV nodal conduction and prolongs the effective refractory period directly.[105] This mechanism of action is different from that of beta adrenergic blocking drugs and vagotonic drugs, which affect AV nodal function indirectly via alterations in autonomic traffic. Verapamil does not affect intraatrial or intraventricular conduction,[106] and it has little effect on the R-R, QRS, and Q-T intervals.[107] Early investigations indicated that verapamil also has little effect on anterograde or retrograde conduction or refractoriness in accessory pathways.[108] However, a recent electrophysiologic study[108a] demonstrated that, in some patients with WPW, verapamil may shorten the refractory period of the accessory pathway during both antegrade and retrograde conduction.

Clinical pharmacology Verapamil is almost completely absorbed after oral ingestion. However, bioavailability is only 10 to 20 percent owing to extensive hepatic first pass metabolism.[109] Measurable effects on the AV node are first noted approximately 30 min after oral administration. Peak effect occurs after approximately 5 h.[110] Following intravenous administration, the onset of action occurs within 2 min and the peak effect within 15 min. The duration of effect on the atrioventricular nodes exceeds the duration of the hemodynamic effect, suggesting preferential binding in the nodal tissues.[110]

Verapamil undergoes extensive metabolism, to produce *N*-demethylated and *N*-dealkylated metabolites of uncertain antidysrhythmic potency. The serum levels of metabolites may double that of verapamil. Both the parent drug and the metabolites are renally excreted. The elimination half-life of verapamil varies from 3 to 7 h.

Dosing considerations For the termination of reentrant supraventricular tachycardia, the usual dose is 0.10 to 0.15 mg/kg, administered over 1 to 3 min. The blood pressure must be checked frequently for hypotension, and the electrocardiogram should be con-

TABLE 6
Verapamil

Pharmacology:
  Bioavailability 10 to 20 percent
  Extensive hepatic metabolism
  Half-life 3 to 7 h
Dosing:
  Acute intravenous dose 0.1 to 0.15 mg/kg in 1 to 3 min
  Continuous infusion rate 0.005 mg/(kg·min)
  Oral maintenance dose 240 to 480 mg/day
Uses:
  Termination of reentry supraventricular tachycardia
  Control of ventricular response to atrial fibrillation
Adverse effects:
  Gastrointestinal intolerance
  Headache
  Edema
  Sinus bradycardia, atrioventricular block
  Hypotension
  Negative inotropic effect

tinuously monitored. The dose may be repeated in 30 min. Verapamil may be administered as a continuous intravenous infusion, at a rate of 0.005 mg/(kg · min). Doses should be reduced in patients with acute myocardial infarction.

Verapamil may be administered chronically for the prevention of paroxysmal supraventricular tachycardia. The usual oral dose range is 80 to 120 mg three to four times daily.

Indications for use The potent depressant effect of verapamil on atrioventricular conduction accounts for the drug's remarkable efficacy in terminating paroxysmal supraventricular tachycardia due to reentry. The onset of action is within 2 to 5 min after intravenous administration. The tachycardia is usually abruptly terminated, with restoration of sinus rhythm, but a variety of transitional dysrhythmias may occur. Atrioventricular dissociation with junctional escape rhythm or transient atrial fibrillation have been reported. Verapamil is successful in terminating reentrant supraventricular tachycardia in over 80 percent of cases.[111–113]

Verapamil may be used to slow the ventricular response to atrial fibrillation either acutely or chronically. This is achieved rapidly after an intravenous dose. The inhibitory effect on the AV node decreases gradually over 30 min. Verapamil may also regularize the ventricular response to atrial fibrillation. Conversion of atrial fibrillation or flutter to sinus rhythm is uncommon after verapamil.

In some patients with WPW, verapamil may decrease the refractory period of the accessory pathway, thereby increasing the ventricular response to atrial fibrillation or atrial flutter.[108a] Therefore, the drug should not be given to treat a wide QRS tachycardia in patients suspected of having the Wolff-Parkinson-White syndrome. However, verapamil may be used to treat a supraventricular dysrhythmia when the QRS is narrow, since the pathway is antegrade via the AV node and retrograde by the accessory pathway. Verapamil would terminate the dysrhythmia by its effect on the AV node. Verapamil should not be used to prevent supraventricular tachycardia in patients with WPW who have had episodes of atrial fibrillation.

Verapamil is usually not useful in treating ventricular ectopy. However, efficacy has been documented in some cases of recurrent sustained ventricular tachycardia.[114,115]

Adverse effects Oral verapamil is usually well tolerated. Side effects severe enough to require drug discontinuation occur in less than 1 percent of users.[110] The most common adverse effects include gastrointestinal intolerance, headache, nervousness, vertigo, and edema. Intravenous verapamil may induce bradycardia, AV block, or hypotension. These are uncommon except in patients receiving concomitant beta blockers, in patients with sick sinus syndrome, particularly in elderly patients, and in patients with intrinsic AV conduction system disease. The electrophysiologic effects of verapamil may be rapidly reversed by intravenous isoproterenol. Verapamil is a negative inotropic agent and may exacerbate left ventricular dysfunction. This effect may be reliably overcome by the intravenous infusion of dopamine, 1 to 5 μg/(kg · min), and has been reported to be reversed by the intravenous administration of calcium.

The major contraindications to the use of verapamil are sinus node disease, AV block, hypotension (unless due to rapid reentry supraventricular tachycardia), suspected or definite left ventricular failure, and digitalis toxicity.

PHENYTOIN

Phenytoin has been in clinical use for more than 30 years, but its precise role in the treatment of dysrhythmias is still uncertain (Table 7). Harris and Kokernot reasoned that the discharge of impulses in the area of a myocardial infarction may bear some similarity to epileptogenic spikes in boundary zones of certain cerebral lesions.[116] These investigators demonstrated that the survival of dogs following occlusion of the anterior descending coronary artery was enhanced by phenytoin. Mosey and Tyler demonstrated the effectiveness of phenytoin in abolishing ouabain-induced ventricular tachycardia.[117] The earlier clinical experience with phenytoin was first summarized by Conn.[118]

Other reviews of phenytoin as an antidysrhythmic drug have appeared subsequently.[119–122]

Clinical electrophysiology Phenytoin enhances atrioventricular conduction in the majority of patients and has little or no effect on intraventricular conduction. These effects of phenytoin on atrioventricular and intraventricular conduction differ from those of other antidysrhythmic agents, such as procainamide and propranolol.[123,124] It has been suggested that the enhancement of atrioventricular conduction may be due to an anticholinergic effect, since phenytoin, when given to dogs with chronic cardiac denervation, causes suppression of sinus rate and prolongation of atrioventricular conduction.[125] The effects of phenytoin on the refractory periods of the atria and AV node are inconsistent, but the functional refractory period of the His-Purkinje system is shortened.[124]

Clinical pharmacology Phenytoin has a systemic availability of approximately 85 percent.[126] In normal patients, 93 percent of phenytoin is protein-bound.[127] There is decreased binding of phenytoin in patients with uremia.[127] Albumin is an important plasma protein for binding of phenytoin. When the concentration of albumin is decreased, as in hepatic or renal disease, the percent of drug bound may be decreased. Reduction in the extent of protein binding of phenytoin may result in higher concentrations of the free drug. Therefore, unless free levels of the drug can be measured, patients with renal and hepatic insufficiency should be maintained at total phenytoin plasma concentrations that are generally considered to be below the optimal therapeutic range in order to avoid toxic effects.[128]

Phenytoin is primarily metabolized by the liver, and

TABLE 7
Phenytoin

Pharmacology:
  Bioavailability 85 percent
  Highly bound to plasma protein; displaced by several drugs
  Volume of distribution 0.5 to 0.8 liter/kg
  Metabolized in the liver
  Half-life 8 to 60 h, depending on dose
Dosing:
  Loading dose (oral or intravenous) 1 g
  Oral maintenance dose 300 to 500 mg/day
Uses:
  Ventricular dysrhythmias due to digitalis toxicity
  Ventricular dysrhythmias in the prolonged Q-T syndromes
  Ventricular tachycardia in children
Adverse effects:
  Rash
  Gingival hyperplasia
  Pseudolymphoma
  Megaloblastic anemia

the major metabolites are eliminated by renal excretion.[129] The kinetics of phenytoin disposition are nonlinear. The half-life is dose-dependent and may range from 8 to 6 h. The volume of distribution is 0.5 to 0.8 liter/kg.

Salicylic acid, sulfonamides, phenylbutazone, and hyperbilirubinemia all displace phenytoin from plasma proteins and elevate the free phenytoin level.[130]

Dosing considerations Since phenytoin has a variable but long half-life, a loading dose is generally necessary to reach therapeutic plasma levels within 24 h. The usual loading dose is 1 g given over 24 h either orally or intravenously. Bigger et al.[131] found that phenytoin could be given intravenously in doses of 100 mg every 5 min until the loading dose was achieved. Phenytoin is insoluble in standard intravenous solutions and will precipitate if diluted in an alkaline solution. Therefore, the drug should be given undiluted. After the loading dose, phenytoin should be given on the second and third day at a dose of 500 to 600 mg/day. Thereafter the maintenance dose is 300 to 500 mg/day. For most patients, once-daily administration provides continuously therapeutic plasma concentrations.[132]

Indications for use The major indications for the use of phenytoin are digitalis intoxication, particularly when there is AV block, ventricular dysrhythmias associated with a long Q-T syndrome, and ventricular tachycardia in children with organic heart disease.

Digitalis-induced dysrhythmias in animals are promptly and effectively treated with phenytoin.[117,133–135] Phenytoin is effective in abolishing VEDs or ventricular tachycardia caused by digitalis in human beings and in suppressing VEDs after cardioversion in digitalized patients. It is also effective in converting digitalis-induced atrial tachycardia with block but not necessarily in suppressing digitalis-induced atrioventricular junctional tachycardia.[136]

A most striking case of the efficacy of phenytoin in the treatment of AV block due to massive digitalis overdose was reported by Rumack et al.[137] The patient had complete heart block, and phenytoin restored conduction to a first-degree block. The effect of phenytoin to enhance atrioventricular conduction was well demonstrated by Helfant et al.[138] Quabain produced a prolongation of the P-R interval in patients. This prolongation was promptly reversed to control values following the infusion of phenytoin. The mechanism for this enhanced atrioventricular conduction by phenytoin may be a central effect of the drug rather than a direct effect of phenytoin on the AV node. Gillis et al.[139] demonstrated that phenytoin in doses as low as 2 mg/kg reduced sympathetic activity. This drug also depresses vagal and phrenic nerve activity.

Phenytoin shortens the Q-T interval, abolishes alternans phenomena, and suppresses tachydysrhythmias in patients with the Romano-Ward syndrome.[140] In contrast, quinidine and procainamide have the opposite effect. Phenytoin is suggested for the treatment of malignant ventricular arrhythmias in patients with the long Q-T syndrome.[141]

Although phenytoin has been generally ineffective for the prevention of recurrent ventricular tachycardia in patients with coronary heart disease,[142] it may be extremely effective in preventing recurrent ventricular tachycardia in children with congenital heart disease.[143,144] There was a higher percentage of success in preventing recurrent ventricular dysrhythmias in patients who had severely abnormal hemodynamics as compared with those with moderately abnormal hemodynamics.

Phenytoin did not significantly reduce the mortality in the year following an acute myocardial infarction in two long-term trials.[145,146]

Adverse effects Many of the adverse drug reactions reported in clinical administration of phenytoin have occurred in the context of its use as an anticonvulsant drug rather than as an antidysrhythmic compound. However, there have been case reports of sinus arrest and atrioventricular block.[131,147]

Long-term side effects are infrequent at therapeutic plasma levels. Gingival hyperplasia occurs frequently but does not necessarily require stopping the drug. Rash is the most common side effect, necessitating cessation of therapy in 3 to 5 percent of patients.[148] Other unusual reactions to phenytoin include systemic lupus erythematosus, pseudolymphoma, and a variety of dermatologic disorders, including pigmentation and hirsutism. Megaloblastic anemia associated with low serum folate levels is also encountered.

Investigational Antidysrhythmic Drugs

MEXILETINE

Mexiletine is a new antidysrhythmic agent that is structurally similar to lidocaine (Table 8). Mexiletine is a local anesthetic and an anticonvulsant whose antidysrhythmic action has been recognized since 1972. It is in clinical use in Ireland and Britain but is presently only approved for investigational studies in the United States.

Clinical electrophysiology Mexiletine decreases the spontaneous firing rate of ventricular pacemaker tissue in a manner similar to that of quinidine and procainamide. Mexiletine shortens the action potential duration in Purkinje fibers, an effect similar to that of

TABLE 8
Mexiletine

Pharmacology:
  Bioavailability 80 to 88 percent
  Seventy percent plasma protein bound
  Peak level 2 to 4 h after ingestion
  Rapid and extensive tissue distribution; volume of distribu-
    tion 7 to 8 liters/kg
  Extensively metabolized
  Half-life 10 to 17 h
Dosing:
  Intravenous loading dose 150 to 250 mg in 5 to 10 min
  Intravenous maintenance infusion 20 to 40 mg/h
  Oral maintenance dose 10 to 15 mg/(kg·day)
Uses:
  Ventricular dysrhythmias
Adverse effects:
  Nausea, vomiting
  Tremor, dizziness, blurred vision
  Hypotension, bradycardia, conduction defects

lidocaine. The drug has little effect on sinus node automaticity or sinoatrial conduction. It prolongs the A-V node refractory period and has a variable effect on His-Purkinje refractory period.[149] However, a prolongation of the H-V interval is usually observed after mexiletine in patients with underlying abnormality in the His-Purkinje system.[149]

Clinical pharmacology Mexiletine may be administered orally or intravenously. In healthy volunteers, the drug is well absorbed after oral administration, and peak blood levels are reached within 2 to 4 h.[150,151] The systemic availability of the drug after oral administration is approximately 80 to 88 percent.

In patients with a recent myocardial infarction, the extent of absorption is decreased, and the peak blood level is reached later.[150] These findings are most marked in patients receiving narcotic analgesics, which retard gastric emptying. In these patients, the peak blood levels are not reached until 4 to 6 h after the dose.

Following intravenous injection, mexiletine is rapidly and extensively distributed to body tissues. After distribution, less than 1 percent of the total amount of drug in the body is found in the blood. Blood levels after intravenous injection are best described by a three-compartment model.

The apparent volume of distribution has been estimated at 7 to 8 liters/kg. This large volume is a reflection of the extensive tissue binding of the drug. Mexiletine is approximately 70 percent protein-bound in the blood.[152] However, this is a small fraction of the total amount of the drug in the body, and changes in protein binding would not be expected to have clinical significance.

Mexiletine undergoes extensive metabolism. The major metabolites are parahydroxymexiletine, hydroxymethylmexiletine, and their alcohols.[153] The antidysrhythmic activity of these metabolites is unknown. In normal individuals, less than 10 percent of the drug is excreted unchanged in the urine. However, renal clearance of mexiletine increases as urine pH decreases.[154] Acidification of the urine produces a shorter plasma half-life of the drug and increases the percent excreted as unchanged drug.

Despite the relatively small role of the kidney in mexiletine disposition, subjects with renal failure (creatinine clearance less than 40 ml/min) demonstrate a longer half-life than those with normal renal function.[155] A slight decrease in dosage may therefore be appropriate in patients with renal failure.

Mexiletine has a relatively long plasma half-life, averaging 10 h in normal individuals. The half-life is prolonged to approximately 17 h in patients with acute myocardial infarction.[150,156] The prolongation of half-life occurs with both oral and intravenous administration and so does not reflect slowed absorption. The effect is probably related to decreased hepatic blood flow and reduced rate of drug metabolism.

Dosing considerations Mexiletine may be given rapidly by vein, followed by a constant infusion, to achieve prompt control of ventricular dysrhythmias.

An initial intravenous injection of 150 to 250 mg should be administered over at least 5 to 10 min to avoid hypotension or serious conduction disturbances and to minimize subjective adverse effects. This may then be followed by a maintenance infusion of 20 to 40 mg/h. This regimen must be individualized, because mexiletine has a narrow therapeutic index and there is individual variability in sensitivity and pharmacokinetics, especially in acutely ill patients.

For chronic oral administration, doses of 10 to 15 mg/(kg · day) or 200 to 300 mg three to four times daily will produce a therapeutic steady-state level in the majority of patients.[157] The usual therapeutic range is 0.75 to 2.0 µg/ml of plasma.

Indications for use Mexiletine is effective in suppression of ventricular ectopic depolarizations of diverse etiologies. Efficacy against supraventricular dysrhythmias has not been adequately evaluated.

Mexiletine suppresses ventricular ectopy, including ventricular tachycardia, from a variety of causes, including myocardial infarction, cardiac surgery, and digitalis toxicity.[152] In acute myocardial infarction, intravenous mexiletine has been shown to suppress the frequency of ventricular ectopy, as well as prevent ventricular tachycardia and fibrillation.[158,159] Long-term use of oral mexiletine is effective for suppression of chronic ventricular ectopy.[160,161] Adequate plasma

130

levels are readily maintained with long-term dosing. However, the therapeutic range is relatively narrow, and careful dosage adjustment is necessary.

In comparison with conventional agents, mexiletine has been found more effective than beta blockers and as effective as procainamide.[162] Mexiletine has been effective in patients refractory to other antidysrhythmic agents, although the proportion of refractory patients responding to this drug has varied in different reports.[163–165]

Adverse effects Mexiletine is usually well tolerated during chronic oral dosing. Side effects may occur during loading with the drug or after dose increases. Most common side effects are gastrointestinal, including nausea and vomiting. The gastrointestinal effects may be decreased by giving the drug with or immediately after meals. Central nervous system effects may occur, including a fine tremor of the hands, dizziness, blurred vision, dysarthria, ataxia, drowsiness, and confusion.

At high serum levels, cardiac toxicity may be manifest as hypotension, sinus bradycardia, or atrioventricular and intraventricular conduction defects.

TOCAINIDE

Tocainide is a primary amine analogue of lidocaine, which can be administered intravenously and orally (Table 9). It has been available in the United States only for emergency use in patients with intractable ventricular dysrhythmias.

Clinical electrophysiology Tocainide is electrophysiologically similar to its congener lidocaine. Both drugs depress membrane responsiveness and shorten the effective refractory period and action potential duration while increasing the ratio of effective refractory period to action potential duration in atrial and ventricular tissue. The effects on atrioventricular conduction are minimal. The drug raises the threshold for ventricular fibrillation.

Clinical pharmacology Tocainide, unlike lidocaine, may be administered orally. The compounds differ in that tocainide lacks the two ethyl groups that contribute to the first-pass hepatic degradation of lidocaine when administered orally. Tocainide is rapidly and almost completely absorbed after oral administration, with bioavailability approaching 100 percent.[166] Peak serum levels are reached 60 to 90 min after oral ingestion. Administration of drug 5 min after a meal decreases peak blood levels without significantly decreasing bioavailability. Tocainide is extensively metabolized, but approximately 50 percent of a dose is excreted unchanged in the urine. The elimination half-life of the drug is approximately 12 h.[166,167] Thus the drug may be administered two or three times daily. The pharmacokinetics is linear over a dose range of 10 mg to 1 g. Fifty percent of the drug is bound to plasma protein at clinically effective concentrations.

Dosing considerations When administered orally in 400- to 600-mg doses at 8-h intervals, a therapeutic plasma concentration of greater than 6 μg/ml can be anticipated.[167,168] At an oral dosing interval of 8 h, a mean steady-state plasma concentration of approximately 1.7 μg/ml is obtained for every 100 mg of drug administered.[167] On a similar dosing interval, an average peak plasma concentration of 2.3 μg/ml is obtained for every 100 mg administered, with the peak occurring 1.3 h after the dose is given. Intravenous loading may be achieved by infusing tocainide at a rate of 0.5 to 0.75 mg/(kg · min) for 15 min.

Indications for use Numerous studies report the utility of tocainide treatment for the suppression of chronic stable ventricular ectopy or ventricular tachycardia resulting from acute myocardial ischemia, valvular heart disease, or cardiomyopathies.

Initial studies in patients focused on suppression of chronic ventricular ectopic depolarizations from a variety of causes. In one study,[167] tocainide produced a 91 percent average reduction in the frequency of VEDs, at a plasma tocainide concentration greater than 6 μg/ml, in 11 of 15 subjects. Similar results were achieved by McDevitt et al.,[169] who demonstrated a 63 to 98 percent reduction in VEDs over a 5-h period after a single 400- to 800-mg oral dose.

The antidysrhythmic effect of tocainide has been

TABLE 9
Tocainide

Pharmacology:
  Rapid and nearly complete absorption
  Peak serum level 60 to 90 min after absorption
  Fifty percent eliminated unchanged in urine
  Significant hepatic metabolism
  Half-life 12 h
Dosing:
  Intravenous loading infusion 0.5 to 0.75 mg/(kg·min) for 15 min
  Oral maintenance dose 400 to 600 mg every 8 h
Uses:
  Ventricular dysrhythmias
Adverse effects:
  Nausea, vomiting, abdominal pain
  Impaired memory, alertness, concentration
  Tremor, diplopia, ataxia, vertigo
  Bradycardia, hypotension

compared to that of a placebo in a randomized double-blind trial of 146 patients after acute myocardial infarction.[170] At intervals over a 6-month period, 24-h ECG recordings were obtained. There was a consistent increase in the number of ventricular ectopic depolarizations as the placebo-treated patients increased mobilization. This was not observed in the tocainide-treated groups. Forty-two of the 146 patients developed significant ventricular dysrhythmias requiring withdrawal from the study. Ten of these patients had effective (>3.5 μg/ml) plasma levels of tocainide; 27 were placebo-treated patients. Tocainide produced intolerable side effects in 11 patients.

A similar double-blind placebo-controlled study of 112 patients after acute myocardial infarction was reported by Ryden et al.[171] During the first 24 h, tocainide-treated subjects had significantly fewer VEDs and episodes of ventricular tachycardia compared with placebo-treated patients. There was also a statistically significant reduction in exercise-induced ventricular tachycardia in the tocainide-treated patients at 6 months.

A number of studies have assessed antidysrhythmic efficacy of tocainide in ventricular dysrhythmias refractory to conventional agents. In most of these studies, tocainide reduced or abolished these refractory dysrhythmias in a substantial percentage of patients. Winkle et al.[172] assessed the efficacy of tocainide in 38 patients with refractory ventricular dysrhythmias. Tocainide produced nearly complete elimination of ventricular ectopy and/or prevented recurrent ventricular tachycardia in 61 percent of the patients. The average daily dose of tocainide was 1,600 mg (range 600 to 2,400). The plasma concentration in responders was 8.9 ± 3.1 μg/ml. The response to lidocaine frequently predicted tocainide responsiveness. Lidocaine was effective in 26 patients, and 16 (63 percent) of these responded to tocainide. However, only 2 of 12 in whom lidocaine was ineffective responded to tocainide.

Similarly, Ryan et al.[173] studied 30 patients with ventricular dysrhythmias refractory to quinidine, propranolol, and procainamide. Treatment with tocainide in dosage of 400 to 800 mg every 8 h provided a mean drug level of 10.3 μg/ml. Thirteen patients had an average decrease of 88 percent in the frequency of ventricular ectopy. Overall, 60 percent of patients responded to tocainide therapy. Of particular interest was the observation that 14 of 21 patients with refractory ventricular tachycardia had complete abolition of this dysrhythmia.

Adverse effects Side effects from tocainide have ranged from 10 to 100 percent of subjects in various series. In general, these adverse reactions have not been sufficiently severe to warrant discontinuation of therapy.

Gastrointestinal and central nervous system effects have been most common. The former include nausea, vomiting, abnormal pain, and constipation. Central nervous system symptoms include memory impairment, decreased mental alertness, difficulty in concentrating, paresthesia, aberrations of sensation, and, more rarely, confusion. Tremor, diplopia, ataxia, blurred vision, slurred speech, dizziness, and vertigo have also been reported.

Other unusual reactions include bradycardia and hypotension, lupus erythematosus reaction with pericarditis, and allergic reaction manifested by an erythematous maculopapular rash and eosinophilia. Allergic alveolitis has been reported. Occurrence of adverse reactions has not correlated with plasma tocainide levels.

ENCAINIDE

Encainide is a benzanilide derivative that is an effective and well-tolerated antidysrhythmic drug (Table 10). Chemically, the drug is unlike any conventional antidysrhythmic agent.

Clinical electrophysiology Encainide prolongs intraatrial and intraventricular conduction times and increases atrial, AV nodal, and ventricular refractory periods.[174] The drug produces a dose-dependent prolongation of H-V and QRS intervals.

Clinical pharmacology There is marked interpatient variation in the pharmacokinetics of encainide. In one study of 11 patients, peak plasma concentrations ranged from 2.4 to 135 ng/ml after a single 25-mg dose.[175] The area under the plasma concentration versus time curve varied over a wide range, suggesting marked differences in systemic bioavailability. The elimination half-life averaged 2.7 ± 0.2 h. During steady state, the half-life increased to 3.4 ± 0.3 h. In

TABLE 10
Encainide

Pharmacology:
    Nonlinear kinetics
    Marked interpatient variation in bioavailability
    Active metabolite
Dosing:
    Half-life during chronic dosing 3 to 4 h
    12.5 mg every 6 h, to a maximum of 8 mg/(kg·day)
Uses:
    Ventricular dysrhythmias
Adverse effects:
    Exacerbation of dysrythmia
    Dizziness, ataxia, tremor, headache, visual disturbances
    Gastrointestinal upset

addition, measurement of plasma levels after steady-state dosing indicated nonlinear kinetics. A tripling of the dose caused a 12-fold rise in trough plasma concentration.

It is possible that the metabolite contributes significantly to the antidysrhythmic effect. Roden et al.[175] found higher plasma encainide levels and a longer half-life in one patient who did not respond clinically. This patient was the only subject in whom *O*-demethylated encainide was not detected in the plasma. These findings were supported by Winkle et al.[176] In their study, each of 9 subjects was given a 75-mg intravenous or oral dose of encainide on different days. After oral dosing, the peak plasma level ranged from 36 to 587 ng/ml, reflecting the wide range of bioavailability in the patients (average 42 percent, range 7 to 82 percent). The time to peak concentration ranged from 1.5 to 3.0 h, and the elimination half-life ranged from 2.1 to 6.9 h with a mean of 3.4 h. These investigators noted that the minimal effective plasma concentration was higher after intravenous dosing than after oral dosing, suggesting an active metabolite formed after oral dosing.

Indications for use Encainide effectively suppresses ventricular ectopy. Roden et al.[175] assessed the efficacy of encainide for the treatment of ventricular ectopy in a placebo-controlled crossover study of 11 patients. Encainide was administered orally, starting with 12.5 or 25 mg every 6 h. Efficacy was assessed by a 12-h ECG recording. The dose was increased every 2 days until VEDs were abolished, side effects occurred, or a maximum dose of 8 mg/(kg · day) was reached. In 10 of 11 patients, encainide reduced ectopic frequency by over 99 percent. Ventricular tachycardia was abolished in all 5 patients in whom this dysrhythmia had frequently occurred prior to treatment.

A similarly high degree of efficacy against ventricular ectopy was reported by Winkle et al.[176] In 8 of 9 patients studied, a single dose of encainide reduced ectopic frequency by at least 90 percent compared with a 1-h control period; the duration of effect was at least 1 h. Complex ventricular ectopy was also virtually abolished.

Encainide has also been found effective in some patients with ventricular ectopy refractory to conventional agents. In one report, 38 patients with recurrent ventricular tachycardia were studied.[177] All patients had required previous hospitalization for treatment of ventricular tachycardia, and all had failed therapy with two or more antidysrhythmic drugs. Eleven of the 38 patients failed to respond to encainide. Twenty-one of the 27 responders were treated for more than 1 month. Seven of these had late drug failures after 2 to 15 months of treatment. Thus approximately 50 percent of a group of patients with severe refractory ventricular tachycardia appear to have responded to encainide.

Duff et al.[177a] evaluated the relationship between the electrocardiographic response to encainide and the response during programmed electrical stimulation of the right ventricle. Suppression of ventricular ectopy did not correlate with the response to programmed stimulation. Four patients showed increased ease of inducibility of the repetitive ventricular response at a time when encainide had suppressed spontaneous ventricular dysrhythmias. The clinical implications of these findings are that suppression of ventricular ectopy may not be predictive of a favorable response in preventing recurrent ventricular tachycardia. A corollary is that patients with recurrent ventricular tachycardia who appear to respond favorably to encainide should have this response verified by programmed stimulation. Further study is required to determine whether ease of inducibility by programmed stimulation following encainide administration predicts adverse clinical outcome.

Adverse effects The most serious adverse effect of encainide is exacerbation of dysrhythmia, particularly precipitation of sustained ventricular tachycardia. This may have occurred in 2 of 9 patients studied by Winkle et al.,[176] in 4 of 38 patients studied by Mason and Peters,[177] and in 3 of 20 patients reported by DiBianco et al.[174]

The most common adverse effects from encainide are nonspecific central nervous system phenomena. These include dizziness, ataxia, tremor, headaches, and visual disturbances. Gastrointestinal upset also occurs, although it is less commonly reported. Often the side effects resolve with decreases in dose.

FLECAINIDE

Flecainide is structurally unlike any other antiarrhythmic drug, although part of the molecule resembles procainamide (Table 11).

Clinical electrophysiology The intracardiac conduction time is prolonged within all parts of the heart in a dose-dependent manner.[178] These measurements include the interval from the high right atrium to the atrial spike, the A-H interval and H-V times. On the surface ECG there is a dose-dependent increase in the P-R interval and in the width of the QRS complex. In contrast, there is only an insignificant increase in the refractoriness of the atrium and a slight but significant prolongation of the ventricular effective refractory period.[179] Administration of flecainide can unmask or exacerbate the sick sinus syndrome.

Clinical pharmacology Only preliminary reports have been published regarding the pharmacokinetics of

TABLE 11
Flecainide

Pharmacology:
  Nearly complete absorption
  Plasma protein bound 32 to 47 percent
  Half-life 14 to 20 h
Dosing:
  Intravenous loading dose 1 to 2 mg/kg
  Oral maintenance dose 100 to 200 mg twice daily
Uses:
  Ventricular dysrhythmias
  Wolff-Parkinson-White syndrome with antegrade conduc-
    tion through accessory pathway
Adverse effects
  Atrioventricular and intraventricular conduction defects
  Negative inotropic effect
  Visual disturbances
  Dizziness, nausea, headaches

this drug in human beings.[180] Flecainide is almost completely absorbed as the unchanged drug. Binding to plasma protein ranges from 32 to 47 percent.[181] The plasma half-life in normal subjects has been reported to range between 7 and 22 h, and with a mean of 14 h. However, in patients with ventricular premature beats, the half-life is longer, with a range of 12 to 27 h and a mean of near 20 h.[182,183]

Dosing considerations The intravenous dose is 1 to 2 mg/kg. The oral dose ranges from 100 to 200 mg twice daily. The drug may be given in a twice-daily dosing interval to diminish side effects.

Indications for use Flecainide is highly effective in decreasing and frequently totally eliminating all VEDs. At a dose of 200 mg twice daily, the mean percent suppression is over 90 percent. Complex as well as single VEDs are also suppressed, often totally.[182–184] However, the effectiveness of this drug in preventing recurrent ventricular tachycardia or ventricular fibrillation has not been adequately assessed. A paradoxical increase in the frequency of VEDs has been documented, particularly at low dosages or after the drug has been stopped, during the decline from therapeutic plasma levels.

Flecainide may be useful in patients with Wolff-Parkinson-White syndrome who have antegrade conduction through the bypass tract during dysrhythmias. In 3 patients with WPW, flecainide was found to completely block antegrade conduction in the accessory pathway, and to delay conduction in a fourth.[185]

Adverse effects Since flecainide increases the P-R interval and widens the QRS complex, high-degree antrioventricular block can be anticipated in some patients, particularly those who have intraventricular

conduction defects. Both second-degree Wenckebach block and Mobitz II block have been reported in patients who have had underlying intraventricular conduction defects.[178]

In studies in animals, a negative inotropic effect has been observed. In patients who do not have heart failure, administration of flecainide has not been found to have negative inotropic effects.[182–184] The major side effects include blurred vision and dizziness, which occurs in over 20 percent of patients and appears to be dose-related. Nausea and headaches have been observed in approximately 10 percent of subjects given flecainide.

LORCAINIDE

Lorcainide is a benzene-acetamide hydrochloride derivative (Table 12). It is not closely related structurally to other antidysrhythmic drugs.

Clinical electrophysiology Lorcainide may prolong sinus node recovery time in patients with sinus node disease; therefore, it should be used with caution in these patients.[186] Atrioventricular conduction is minimally prolonged, and the refractory period of the AV node is unchanged.[187] The most consistent electrophysiologic effects are an increase in the H-V interval and widening of the QRS interval. This widening appears to be dose-related, and this phenomenon is most marked in patients who have a conduction delay below the His bundle.[188] In fact, complete block below the bundle of His has been induced by lorcainide in

TABLE 12
Lorcainide

Pharmacology:
  Saturable first-pass effect; bioavailability 80 to 90 percent
    with chronic dosing
  Highly bound to plasma proteins; volume of distribution
    12.8 liters/kg
  Metabolized to the active compound norlorcainide
  Half-life 7 to 8 h
  Norlorcainide half-life 20 h
Dosing:
  Intravenous loading dose 2 mg/kg, at rate of 10 to 20 mg/min
  Oral maintenance dose 100 mg twice daily
  Decrease dose in presence of heart failure, hepatic insuffi-
    ciency, concomitant beta blocker
Uses:
  Ventricular dysrhythmias
  Wolff-Parkinson-White syndrome with atrial fibrillation
Adverse effects:
  Sinus node dysfunction
  Intraventricular conduction defects
  Sleep disturbances
  Dizziness, nausea, vomiting

134

patients with preexisting prolongation of the H-V interval. The hemodynamic effects appear to be minor and of short duration.

Clinical pharmacology The kinetics of the unchanged drug may not be directly relevant to its dynamic effects because of the importance of an active metabolite, the N-dealkylated metabolite, norlorcainide. Levels of this compound are minimal after intravenous drug administration but increase gradually after chronic oral treatment and may exceed those of lorcainide itself.[189] The drug is well absorbed, but at low doses the systemic bioavailability is low because of a marked first-pass effect. This effect appears to be saturable, and the bioavailability is greater at higher doses or after the drug is administered for a few days.[189] Bioavailability may be as low as 40 percent but usually is in the range of 80 to 90 percent.[189] The drug is extensively (80 to 90 percent) bound to plasma proteins and has a large (12.8 liters/kg) volume of distribution.

In patients with VEDs, the half-life of elimination is 7 to 8 h, but it may be greatly prolonged in patients with impaired liver function or decreased hepatic blood flow, such as in congestive heart failure. The half-life of the active metabolite, norlorcainide, is 20 h.[190] As previously noted, the dynamic half-life of the drug may be longer than the measured half-life of the unchanged drug because of the long half-life of norlorcainide. Two-thirds of the drug is eliminated in the urine; almost all of which consists of metabolites.[189]

Dosing considerations Lorcainide may be given intravenously in a dose of 2 mg/kg, at a rate of infusion of 10 mg/min. The rate should not exceed 20 mg/min.

The average oral dose is 100 mg twice daily, but occasionally, up to 400 mg/day may be required. The dose should be decreased in patients with heart failure, hepatic insufficiency, or with concomitant administration of beta adrenergic blocking drugs.

Indications for use Treatment with lorcainide almost completely suppresses VEDs in patients with heart disease.[191] It appears to be effective in preventing recurrent ventricular tachycardia, even in patients who are refractory to conventional antidysrhythmic drugs.[192] The efficacy of lorcainide may not necessarily be adequately assessed by electrophysiologic stimulation. Several investigators have noted that ventricular tachycardia can be induced in most patients with recurrent ventricular tachycardia after a single intravenous dose, although lorcainide appears to be effective in a large percentage of patients.[187,193] One explanation for this possible lack of predictability of lorcainide efficacy using electrophysiologic testing is the absence of norlorcainide with the acute intravenous route of administration.

Lorcainide may be effective in the treatment of patients with Wolff-Parkinson-White syndrome, particularly in those patients with atrial fibrillation who conduct antegrade through the accessory pathway.[187] It is not clear whether lorcainide will prevent atrial fibrillation in these patients or if the drug will be beneficial primarily by its effect on increasing the antegrade refractory period of the accessory bypass tract, thus slowing the ventricular response.

The effect of lorcainide in the treatment or prevention of PSVT has not been adequately evaluated in controlled trials; however, the electrophysiologic effects suggest that it may be more useful for the prevention of recurrent ventricular tachydysrhythmias or in patients with Wolff-Parkinson-White syndrome.[187]

Adverse effects Lorcainide should be used cautiously, if at all, in patients who have the sick sinus syndrome because of its effect in depressing sinus node function. In patients who have an intraventricular conduction defect, it may cause further and marked QRS widening because of its effect in slowing His-Purkinje conduction.[187] It is not known if measurement of the baseline H-V interval will predict whether it can be used safely in these patients. Only minor hemodynamic effects have been identified to date, suggesting that it may be used safely in patients with congestive heart failure. A major side effect is sleep disturbance, which occurs in nearly 20 percent of patients given this drug. Patients complain of difficulty falling asleep, as well as of nightmares and vivid dreams. Sleep disturbance may be prevented, particularly in the first 2 weeks of drug administration, by the use of benzodiazepines.[192] Other side effects include dizziness, nausea, and vomiting.

AMIODARONE

Amiodarone is a benzofuran derivative (Table 13). It was marketed as an antianginal agent in Belgium in 1967 and soon thereafter was introduced in France. Within a few years after its introduction to clinical medicine for the tretment of angina, its antidysrhythmic effects became recognized.

Clinical electrophysiology Amiodarone causes an increase in the effective refractory periods of the right atrium, AV node, and right ventricle.[194] Its action on intraatrial and intraventricular conduction is variable. After chronic oral administration, there is a decrease in AV nodal conduction. In the Wolff-Parkinson-White syndrome, amiodarone increases the refractory period of the accessory pathway in the antegrade direction in the majority of patients and prolongs the refractory period in the retrograde direction in about half of patients.[195–197] Amiodarone may impair sinus node function.[198]

Clinical pharmacology Only limited information is available about the pharmacokinetics of amiodarone. The bioavailability of this drug is estimated to be about 50 percent.[199] One of the metabolites of amiodarone is N-desethyl amiodarone. The antidysrhythmic efficacy of this metabolite is not known. After a single dose of amiodarone, the elimination half-life ranges from 5 to 17 h, with a mean of 7.2 h.[200] However, after chronic oral dosing, the mean elimination half-life appears to be approximately 1 month, with a range of 14 to 52 days.[200–202]

Dosing considerations A loading dose of the drug is mandatory for prompt control of dysrhythmias because of the extraordinarily long half-life of elimination. Eight hundred to 1,400 mg daily may be administered for 1 to 2 weeks prior to maintenance dosing, which ranges from 200 mg 5 days a week to 600 mg/day.[203] Doses above 400 mg/day may be associated with an increase in incidence of long-term adverse effects.

Amiodarone may be given intravenously at a dose of 5 mg/kg over 3 to 5 min. This dose may be repeated in 15 to 30 min followed by a continuous intravenous infusion in glucose and water. There is a physical incompatability of amiodarone with saline.

Indications for use Oral amiodarone can be used to

TABLE 13
Amiodarone

Pharmacology:
  Bioavailability 50 percent
  Half-life 14 to 52 days
Dosing:
  Intravenous loading dose 5 to 10 mg/kg
  Oral loading dose 800 to 1,400 mg/day for 1 to 2 weeks
  Oral maintenance dose 200 to 400 mg/day
Uses:
  Paroxysmal atrial fibrillation
  Paroxysmal supraventricular tachycardia
  Wolff-Parkinson-White syndrome
  Ventricular dysrhythmias
Adverse effects:
  Hypotension
  Sinus node dysfunction
  Hyperthyroidism of hypothyroidism
  Corneal microdeposits
  Photosensitivity
  Tremor, ataxia, peripheral neuropathy
  Potentiates warfarin effect
  Interaction with digoxin, quinidine

treat a wide spectrum of dysrhythmias in children as well as in adults.[204] It is useful for the prevention of recurrent supraventricular and ventricular dysrhythmias.[205,206] The range of drug efficacy includes prevention of recurrent atrial fibrillation and recurrent paroxysmal supraventricular tachycardia in patients who do not have WPW syndrome as well as in those who have an accessory bypass tract.[205,206] It is successful in preventing recurrent ventricular tachycardia in 70 to 80 percent of patients with this condition, including many who have been refractory to conventional antidysrhythmic drugs.[206–209] There is one case report of the effectiveness of this drug in the management of the long Q-T syndrome,[210] although it can also increase the Q-T interval and cause torsade de pointes.[211,212]

Induction of ventricular tachycardia with electrophysiologic stimulation during therapy does not appear to predict efficacy. In general, if the dysrhythmia cannot be induced during chronic therapy, it is unlikely that the dysrhythmia will recur spontaneously. However, induction of the dysrhythmia during therapy does not mean that the dysrhythmia will spontaneously recur.[213,214]

There is still little published information about the efficacy of intravenous amiodarone for treatment of life-threatening dysrhythmias; preliminary reports indicate that it may be highly effective for both supraventricular and ventricular dysrhythmias.[215–218]

Adverse effects Adverse cardiovascular effects have been noted primarily after intravenous infusion of the drug, particularly after rapid intravenous injections. Hypotension has occurred, and several deaths have been reported.[205] After chronic oral dosing, severe sinus bradycardia or sinus arrest may occur that may require insertion of an implanted pacemaker if the drug is to be continued.[219]

Alterations of thyroid function, either hypothyroidism or hyperthyroidism, occur in about 2 to 4 percent of the patients and may require discontinuation of the drug or appropriate therapy. Ophthalmologic side effects consist of corneal microdeposits that have been found to impair vision. Patients may complain of a halo around lights, and this effect appears to be dose-related. Cutaneous photosensitivity may appear in 3 to 10 percent of patients taking the drug. This complication may be diminished or prevented by the liberal use of sunscreen. The incidence of neurologic complications have not been well defined but include tremor, ataxia, and peripheral neuropathy. This complication appears to be dose-related. An increase in hepatic transferases (1.5 to 4 times normal) is not uncommon (8 of 70 patients).[220]

A recently reported complication consists of pneumonitis and pulmonary fibrosis that can be sufficiently severe to cause cardiopulmonary decompensation and death. It may be reversed by corticosteroid therapy and discontinuation of the drug.[221]

Amiodarone potentiates the anticoagulant effect of sodium warfarin and may lead to serious bleeding.[222] It also can increase serum digoxin levels, resulting in clinical evidence of digitalis intoxication.[223] Recent reports indicate that it may cause an increase in quinidine[224] and aprindine[225] plasma concentrations and that these interactions are clinically significant.[224]

REFERENCES

1 White, P. D. and Donovan, H.: "Hearts—Their Long Follow-Up." W. B. Saunders Co., Philadelphia, 1967. p. 250.

1a Hinkle, L. E., Carver, S. T., and Stevens, M.: The Frequency of Asymptomatic Disturbances of Cardiac Rhythm and Conduction in Middle-Aged Men, *Am. J. Cardiol.,* 24:629, 1969.

2 Chiang, B. N., Perlman, L. V., Ostrander, L. D., Jr., et al.: Relationship of Premature Systoles to Coronary Heart Disease and Sudden Death in the Tecumseh Epidemiologic Study, *Ann. Intern. Med.,* 70:1159, 1969.

3 Tominoga, S., and Blackburn, H.: Prognostic Importance of Premature Beats Following Myocardial Infarction. Experience in the Coronary Drug Project, *J.A.M.A.,* 233:1116, 1973.

4 Ruberman, W., Weinblatt, E., Goldberg, J. D., et al.: Ventricular Premature Beats and Mortality after Myocardial Infarction, *N. Engl. J. Med.,* 297:750, 1977.

5 Moss, A. J., Davis, H. T., DeCamilla, J., et al.: Ventricular Ectopic Beats and Their Relation to Sudden and Non-Sudden Cardiac Death after Myocardial Infarction, *Circulation,* 60:998, 1979.

6 Savage, D. D., Seides, S. F., Maron, B. J., et al.: Prevalence of Arrhythmias during 24 Hour Electrocardiographic Monitoring and Exercise Testing in Patients with Obstructive and Non-Obstructive Hypertrophic Cardiomyopathy, *Circulation,* 59:866, 1979.

7 Segal, J. P., Stapleton, J. F., McClellan, J. R., et al.: Idiopathic Cardiomyopathy: Clinical Features, Prognosis, and Therapy, *Curr. Probl. Cardiol.,* 3:1, 1978.

8 Cohen, L. S., Buccino, R. A., Morrow, A. G., et al.: Recurrent Ventricular Tachycardia and Fibrillation Treated with a Combination of Beta-Adrenergic Blockade and Electrical Pacing, *Ann. Intern. Med.,* 66:945, 1967.

9 Kastor, J. A., DeSanctis, R. W., Harthorne, J. W., et al.: Transvenous Atrial Pacing in the Treatment of Refractory Ventricular Irritability, *Ann. Intern. Med.,* 66:939, 1967.

10 DeFrancis, N. A., and Giordano, R. P.: Permanent Epicardial Atrial Pacing in the Treatment of Refractory Ventricular Tachycardia, *Am. J. Cardiol.,* 22:742, 1968.

11 Moss, A. J., Rivers, R. J., Griffith, L. S. C., et al.: Transvenous Left Atrial Pacing for the Control of Recurrent Ventricular Fibrillation, *N. Engl. J. Med.,* 278:928, 1968.

12 Moss, A. J., and Rivers, R. J.: Termination and Inhibition of Recurrent Tachycardias by Implanted Pervenous Pacemakers, *Circulation,* 50:942, 1974.

13 Ruskin, J. N., Garan, H., Poulin, F., et al.: Permanent Radiofrequency Ventricular Pacing for Management of Drug Resistant Ventricular Tachycardia, *Am. J. Cardiol.,* 46:317, 1980.

14 Mirowski, M., Reid, P. R., Mower, M. M., et al.: Termination of Malignant Ventricular Arrhythmias with an Implanted Automatic Defibrillator in Human Beings, *N. Engl. J. Med.,* 303:322, 1980.

15 Ricks, W. B., Winkle, R. A., Shumway, N. E., et al.: Surgical Management of Life-Threatening Ventricular Arrhythmias in Patients with Coronary Artery Disease, *Circulation,* 56:38, 1977.

16 DeSoyza, N., Murphy, M. L., Bissett, J. K., et al.: Ventricular Arrhythmia in Chronic Stable Angina Pectoris with Surgical or Medical Treatment, *Ann. Intern. Med.,* 89:10, 1974.

17 Josephson, M. E., Harken, A. H., and Horowitz, L. N.: Endocardial Excision: A New Surgical Technique for the Treatment of Recurrent Ventricular Tachycardia, *Circulation,* 60:1430, 1979.

18 Horowitz, L. N., Harken, A. H., Kastor, J. A., et al.: Ventricular Resection Guided by Epicardial and Endocardial Mapping for Treatment of Recurrent Ventricular Tachycardia, *N. Engl. J. Med.,* 302:589, 1980.

19 Josephson, M. E., Caracta, A. R., Ricciutti, M. A., Lau, S. H., and Damato, A. N.: Electrophysiologic Properties of Procainamide in Man, *Am. J. Cardiol.,* 33:596, 1974.

20 Manion, C. V., Lalka, D., Baer, D. T., et al.: Absorption Kinetics of Procainamide in Humans, *J. Pharm. Sci.,* 66:981, 1977.

21 Koch-Weser, J., and Klein, S. W.: Procainamide Dosage Schedules, Plasma Concentrations, and Clinical Effects, *J.A.M.A.,* 215:1454, 1971.

22 Koch-Weser, J.: Pharmacokinetics of Procainamide in Man, *Ann. N.Y. Acad. Sci.,* 179:370, 1971.

23 Koch-Weser, J.: Antiarrhythmic Prophylaxis in Ambulatory Patients with Coronary Heart Disease, *Arch. Intern. Med.,* 129:763, 1972.

24 Graffner, C., Johnsson, G., and Sjogren, J.: Pharmacokinetics of Procainamide Intravenously and Orally as Conventional and Slow-Release Tablets, *Clin. Pharmacol. Ther.,* 17:414, 1975.

25 Giardina, E. G. V., Dreyfuss, J., Bigger, J. T., Jr., et al.: Metabolism of Procainamide in Normal and Cardiac Subjects, *Clin. Pharmacol. Ther.,* 19:339, 1976.

26 Gibson, T. P., Matusik, J., and Matusik, E.: Acetylation of Procainamide in Man and Its Relationship to Isonicotinic Acid Hydrazide Acetylation Phenotype, *Clin. Pharmacol. Ther.* 17:395, 1975.

27 Reidenberg, M. M., Drayer, D. E., Levy, M., et al.: Polymorphic Acetylation of Procainamide in Man, *Clin. Pharmacol. Ther.,* 17:722, 1975.

28 Drayer, D. E., Lowenthal, D. T., Woosley, R. L., et al.: Cumulation of *N*-Acetylprocainamide, an Active Metabolite of Procainamide, in Patients with Impaired Renal Function, *Clin. Pharmacol. Ther.,* 22:63, 1977.

29 Giardina, E. G. V., Heissenbuttel, R. H., and Bigger, J. T., Jr.: Intermittent Intravenous Procainamide to Treat Ventricular Arrhythmias, *Ann. Intern. Med.,* 78:183, 1973.

30 Fremstad, D., Dahl, S., Jacobsen, S., et al.: A New Sustained-Release Tablet Formulation of Procainamide, *Eur. J. Clin. Pharmacol.,* 6:251, 1973.

31 Giardina, E. G. V., Fenster, P. E., Bigger, J., Jr., et al.: Efficacy, Plasma Concentrations and Adverse Effects of a New Sustained Release Procainamide Preparation, *Am. J. Cardiol.,* 46:855, 1980.

32 Koch-Weser, J.: Clinical Application of the Pharmacokinetics of Procainamide, *Cardiovasc. Clin.,* 6:63, 1974.

33 Atkinson, A. J., Jr., Lee, W. K., Quinn, M. L., et al.: Dose-Ranging Trial of *N*-Acetylprocainamide in Patients with Premature Ventricular Contractions, *Clin. Pharmacol. Ther.,* 21:575, 1975.

34 Roden, D. M., Reele, S. B., Higgins, S. B., et al.: Antiarrhythmic Efficacy, Pharmacokinetics and Safety of *N*-Acetylprocainamide in Human Subjects, *Am. J. Cardiol.,* 46:463, 1980.

35 Koch-Weser, J., Klein, S. W., Foocanto, L. L., et al.: Antiarrhythmic Prophylaxis with Procainamide in Acute Myocardial Infarction, *N. Engl. J. Med.,* 281:1253, 1969.

36 Lima, J. J., Goldfarb, A. L., Conti, D. R., et al.: Safety and Efficacy of Procainamide Infusions, *Am. J. Cardiol.,* 43:98, 1979.

37 Greenspan, A. M., Horowitz, L. N., Spielman, S. R., et al.: Large Dose Procainamide Therapy for Ventricular Tachyarrhythmia, *Am. J. Cardiol.,* 46:453, 1980.

38 McCord, M. C., and Taguchi, J. T.: A Study of the Effect of Procaine Amide Hydrochloride in Supraventricular Arrhythmias, *Circulation,* 4:387, 1951.

39 Miller, G., Weinberg, L., and Pick, A.: The Effect of Procaine Amide in Clinical Auricular Fibrillation and Flutter, *Circulation,* 6:41, 1952.

40 Fenster, P. E., Comess, K. A., Marsh, R., Katzenberg, C., and Hager, W. D.: Conversion of Atrial Fibrillation to Sinus Rhythm by Acute Intravenous Procainamide Infusion, *Am. Heart J.,* in press.

41 Sellers, T. D., Campbell, R. W. F., Bashore, T. M., and Gallagher, J. G.: Effects of Procainamide and Quinidine Sulfate in the Wolff-Parkinson-White Syndrome, *Circulation,* 55:15, 1977.

41a Wellens, H. J. J., Bar, F. W., Dassen, W. R. M., Brugada, P., Vanagt, E. J., Farre, J.: Effect of Drugs in the Wolff-Parkinson-White Syndrome. *Am. J. Cardiol.,* 46:665, 1980.

42 Blomgren, S. E., Condemi, J. J., and Vaughan, J. H.: Procainamide-Induced Lupus Erythematosus. Clinical and Laboratory Observations, *Am. J. Med.,* 52:338, 1972.

43 Tan, E. M.: Drug-Induced Autoimmune Disease, *Fed. Proc.,* 33:1894, 1974.

44 Woosley, R. L., Drayer, D. E., Reidenberg, M. M., et al.: Effect of Acetylator Phenotype on the Rate at Which Procainamide Induces Antinuclear Antibodies and with the Lupus Syndrome, *N. Engl. J. Med.,* 298:1157, 1978.

45 Heissenbuttel, R. H., and Bigger, J. T.: The Effect of Oral Quinidine on Intraventricular Conduction in Man, *Am. Heart J.,* 80:453, 1970.

46 Greenblatt, D. J., Pfeifer, H. J., Ochs, H. R., et al.: Pharmacokinetics of Quinidine in Humans after Intravenous, Intramuscular and Oral Administration, *J. Pharmacol. Exp. Ther.,* 202:365, 1977.

47 Covinsky, J. O., Russo, J., Kelly, K. L., et al.: Relative Bioavailability of Quinidine Gluconate and Quinidine Sulfate in Healthy Volunteers, *J. Clin. Pharmacol.,* 19:261, 1979.

48 Palmer, K. H., Martin, B., Bagget, B., et al.: The Metabolic Fate of Orally Administered Quinidine Gluconate in Humans, *Biochem. Pharmacol.,* 18:1845, 1969.

49 Drayer, D. E., Restivo, K. and Reidenberg, M. M.: Specific Determinations of Quinidine and $(3S)$-3-Hydroxyquinidine in Human Serum by High-Pressure Liquid Chromotography, *J. Lab. Clin, Med.,* 90:816, 1977.

50 Powell, J. R., Fenster, P. E., Hager, W. D., et al.: Dose Dependence and Time Course of the Digoxin-Quinidine Interaction, *Clin. Pharmacokinet.,* in press.

51 Fenster, P. E., Powell, J. R., Hager, W. D., et al.: Digitoxin-Quinidine Interaction: Pharmacokinetic Evaluation, *Ann. Intern. Med.,* 93:698, 1980.

52 Greenblatt, D. J., Pfeifer, J. H., Ochs, H. R., et al.: Pharmacokinetics of Parenteral Quinidine in Humans, *Clin. Pharmacol. Ther.,* 21:105, 1977.

53 Josephson, M. E., Caracta, A. R., Lau, S. J., Gallagher, J. J., and Damato, A. N.: Electrophysiologic Evaluation of Disopyramide in Man, *Am. Heart J.,* 86:771, 1973.

54 Hinderling, P. H., and Garrett, E. R.: Pharmacokinetics of the Antiarrhythmic Disopyramide in Healthy Humans, *J. Pharmacokinet. Biopharm.* 4:199, 1976.

55 Dubetz, D. K., Brown, N. N., Hooper, W. D., et al.:

Disopyramide Pharmacokinetics and Bioavailability, *Br. J. Clin. Pharmacol.*, 6:279, 1978.

56 Bryson, S. M., Whiting, B., and Lawrence, J. R.: Disopyramide Serum and Pharmacologic Effect Kinetics Applied to the Assessment of Bioavailability, *Br. J. Clin. Pharmacol.*, 6:409, 1978.

57 Cunningham, J. L., Shen, D. D., Shudo, I., et al.: The Effects of Urine pH and Plasma Protein Binding on the Renal Clearance of Disopyramide, *Clin. Pharmacokinet.*, 2:373, 1977.

58 Smith, W. S., Vismara, L., Kalmansohn, R. B., et al.: Clinical Studies of Norpace, *Angiology*, 26 (suppl. 1):124, 1975.

59 Heel, R. C., Brogden, R. N., Speight, T. M., et al.: Disopyramide: A Review of Its Pharmacological Properties and Therapeutic Use in Treating Cardiac Arrhythmias, *Drugs*, 15:331, 1978.

60 Vismara, L. A., Vera, Z., Miller, R. R., et al.: Efficacy of Disopyramide Phosphate in the Treatment of Refractory Ventricular Tachycardia, *Am. J. Cardiol.*, 39:1027, 1977.

61 Hartel, G., Louhija, A., and Konttinen, A.: Disopyramide in the Prevention of Recurrence of Atrial Fibrillation after Electroconversion, *Clin. Pharmacol. Ther.*, 15:551, 1974.

62 Luoma, P. V., Kujala, P. A., Juustila, H. J., et al.: Efficacy of Intravenous Disopyramide in the Termination of Supraventricular Arrhythmias, *J. Clin. Pharmacol.*, 18:293, 1978.

63 Hulting, J., and Rosenhamer, G.: Hemodynamic and Electrocardiographic Effects of Disopyramide in Patients with Ventricular Arrhythmias, *Acta Med. Scand.*, 199:41, 1976.

64 Jensen, G., Sigurd, B., and Uhrenholt, A.: Hemodynamic Effects of Intravenous Disopyramide in Heart Failure, *Eur. J. Clin. Pharmacol.*, 8:167, 1975.

65 Podrid, P. J., Schoenberger, A., and Lown, B.: Congestive Heart Failure Caused by Oral Disopyramide, *N. Engl. J. Med.*, 302:614, 1980.

66 Southworth, J. L., McKusick, V. A., Peirce, E. C., and Rawson, F. L., Jr.: Ventricular Fibrillation Precipitated by Cardiac Catheterization, *J.A.M.A.*, 143:717, 1950.

67 Likoff, W.: Cardiac Arrhythmias Complicating Surgery, *Am. J. Cardiol.*, 3:427, 1959.

68 Rosen, K. N., Lau, S. H., Weiss, M. B., and Damato, A. N.: The Effect of Lidocaine on Atrioventricular and Intraventricular Conduction in Man, *Am. J. Cardiol.*, 25:1, 1970.

69 Lichstein, E., Chadda, K. D., and Jupta, P. K.: Atrioventricular Block with Lidocaine Therapy, *Am. J. Cardiol.*, 31:277, 1973.

70 Josephson, M. E., Caracta, A. R., Lau, S. H., Gallagher, J. J., and Damato, A. N.: Effects of Lidocaine on Refractory Periods in Man, *Am. Heart J.*, 84:778, 1972.

71 Roos, J. C., and Dunning, A. J.: Effects of Lidocaine on Impulse Formation and Conduction Defects in Man, *Am. Heart J.*, 89:686, 1975.

72 Engel, T. R., Soly, K. L., Meister, S. G., and Frankl, W. S.: Effect of Lidocaine on Right Ventricular Muscle Refractoriness, *Clin. Pharmacol. Ther.*, 19:515, 1976.

73 Bigger, J. T., Jr., and Heissenbuttel, R. H.: The Use of Procainamide and Lidocaine in the Treatment of Cardiac Arrhythmias, *Prog. Cardiovasc. Dis.*, 11:515, 1969.

74 de Boer, A. G., Breimer, D. D., Mattie, H., Pronk, J., and Gubbens-Stibbe, J. M.: Rectal Bioavailability of Lidocaine in Man: Partial Avoidance of "First Pass" Metabolism, *Clin. Pharmacol. Ther.*, 26:701, 1979.

75 Routledge, P. A., Shand, D. G., Barchowsky, A., Wagner, G., and Stargel, W. W.: Relationship between Alpha 1-Acid Glycoprotein and Lidocaine Disposition in Myocardial Infarction, *Clin. Pharmacol. Ther.*, 30:154, 1981.

76 Narang, P. K., Crouthamel, W. G., Carliner, N. H., and Fisher, M. L.: Lidocaine and Its Active Metabolites, *Clin. Pharmacol. Ther.*, 24:654, 1978.

77 Burney, R. G., DiFazio, C. A., Peach, M. J., Petrie, K. A., and Sylvester, M. J.: Anti-Arrhythmic Effects of Lidocaine Metabolites, *Am. Heart J.*, 88:765, 1974.

78 Halkin, H., Meffin, P., Melmon, K. L., and Rowland, M.: Influence of Congestive Heart Failure on Blood Levels of Lidocaine and Its Active Monodeethylated Metabolite, *Clin. Pharmacol. Ther.*, 17:659, 1975.

79 Melmon, K. L., Rowland, M., Sheiner, L., and Trager, W.: Clinical Implications of the Disposition of Lidocaine in Man: A Multidisciplinary Study. In D. S. Davies and B. N. C. Prichard (eds.), "Biological Effects of Drugs in Relation to Their Plasma Concentrations," University Park Press, Baltimore, 1973, p. 107.

80 LeLorier, J., Grenon, D., Latour, Y., et al.: Pharmacokinetics of Lidocaine after Prolonged Intravenous Infusion in Uncomplicated Myocardial Infarction, *Ann. Intern. Med.*, 87:700, 1977.

81 Thomson, P. D., Melmon, K. L., Richardson, J. A., et al.: Lidocaine Pharmacokinetics in Advanced Heart Failure, Liver Disease, and Renal Failure in Humans, *Ann. Intern. Med.*, 78:499, 1973.

82 Ochs, H. R., Carstens, G., and Greenblatt, D. J.: Reduction in Lidocaine Clearance During Continuous Infusion and by Coadministration of Propranolol, *N. Engl. J. Med.*, 303:373, 1980.

83 Feely, J., Wilkinsen, G. R., McAllister, C. B., and Wood, A. J. J.: Increased Toxicity and Reduced Clearance of Lidocaine by Cimetidine, *Ann. Intern. Med.*, 96:592, 1982.

84 Harrison, D. C.: Should Lidocaine Be Administered to

All Patients after Acute Myocardial Infarction, *Circulation,* 58:581, 1978.

85 Lie, K. I., Wellens, H. J., van Capelle, F. J., and Durrer, D.: Lidocaine in the Prevention of Primary Ventricular Fibrillation: A Double-Blind, Randomized Study of 212 Consecutive Patients, *N. Engl. J. Med.,* 291:1324, 1974.

86 Wyman, M. G., and Hammersmith, L.: Comprehensive Treatment Plan for Prevention of Primary Ventricular Fibrillation in Acute Myocardial Infarction, *Am. J. Cardiol.,* 33:661, 1974.

87 DeSilva, R. A., Lown, B., Hennekens, C. H., and Casscells, W.: Lignocaine Prophylaxis in Acute Myocardial Infarction: An Evaluation of Randomised Trials, *Lancet,* 2:855, 1981.

88 Valentine, P. A., Frew, J. L., Mashford, M. L., and Sloman, J. G.: Lidocaine in the Prevention of Sudden Death in the Pre-Hospital Phase of Acute Infarction, *N. Engl. J. Med.,* 291:1327, 1974.

89 Lie, K. I., Liem, K. L., and Durrer, D.: A Double-Blind Randomized Study of Intramuscular Lidocaine in Preventing Primary Ventricular Fibrillation, *Am. J. Cardiol.,* 39:275, 1977.

90 Castellanos, A., Ferreiro, J., Pefkaros, K., Rozanski, J. J., Moleiro, F., and Myerburg, R. J.: Effects of Lignocaine on Bidirectional Tachycardia and on Digitalis-Induced Atrial Tachycardia with Block, *Br. Heart J.,* 48:27, 1982.

91 Ribner, H. S., Isaacs, E. S., and Frishman, W. H.: Lidocaine Prophylaxis against Ventricular Fibrillation in Acute Myocardial Infarction, *Prog. Cardiovasc. Dis.,* 21:287, 1979.

92 Boura, A. L. A., and Green, A. F.: The Actions of Bretylium: Adrenergic Neuron Blocking and Other Effects, *Br. J. Pharmacol.,* 14:536, 1959.

93 Leveque, P. E.: Antiarrhythmic Action of Bretylium, *Nature* 207:203, 1965.

94 Waxman, M. B., and Wallace, A. G.: Electrophysiologic Effects of Bretylium Tosylate on the Heart, *J. Pharmacol. Exp. Ther.,* 183:264, 1972.

95 Touboul, P., Porte, J., Huerta, F., and Delahaye, J. P.: Etude des Proprietes electrophysiologiques du tosylate de bretylium chez l'homme, *Arch. Mal. Coeur,* 69:503, 1976.

96 Singh, B. N., and Hauswirth, O.: Comparative Mechanisms of Action of Antiarrhythmic Drugs, *Am. Heart J.,* 87:367, 1974.

97 Anderson, J. L., Patterson, E., Wagner, J. G., Stewart, J. R., Behm, H. L., and Lucchesi, B. R.: Oral and Intravenous Bretylium Disposition, *Clin. Pharmacol. Ther.,* 28:478, 1980.

98 Bernstein, J. G., and Koch-Weser, J.: Effectiveness of Bretylium Tosylate against Refractory Ventricular Arrhythmias, *Circulation,* 45:1024, 1972.

99 Bacaner, M. B.: Treatment of Ventricular Fibrillation and Other Acute Arrhythmias with Bretylium Tosylate, *Am. J. Cardiol.,* 21:530, 1968.

100 Sanna, G., and Arcidiacono, R.: Chemical Ventricular Defibrillation of the Human Heart with Bretylium Tosylate, *Am. J. Cardiol.,* 32:982, 1973.

101 Cervoni, P., Ellis, C. H., and Maxwell, R. A.: The Antiarrhythmic Action of Bretylium in Normal, Reserpine Pretreated, and Chronically Denervated Dog Hearts, *Arch. Int. Pharmacodyn. Ther.,* 190:91, 1971.

102 Allen, J. D., Pantridge, J. F., and Shanks, R. G.: Effects of Lignocaine, Propranolol and Bretylium on Ventricular Fibrillation Threshold, *Am. J. Cardiol.,* 28:555, 1971.

103 Heissenbuttel, R. H., and Bigger, J. T.: Bretylium Tosylate: A Newly Available Antiarrhythmic Drug for Ventricular Arrhythmias, *Ann. Intern. Med.,* 91:229, 1979.

104 Koch-Weser, J.: Bretylium, *N. Engl. J. Med.,* 300:473, 1979.

105 Zipes, D. P., and Fischer, J. C.: Effects of Agents which Inhibit the Slow Channel on Sinus Node Automaticity and Atrioventricular Conduction in the Dog., *Circ. Res.,* 34:184, 1974.

106 Husaini, M. H., Kurasnicka, J., Ryden, L., and Holmberg, S.: Action of Verapamil on Sinus Node, Atrioventricular and Intraventricular Conduction, *Br. Heart J.,* 35:734, 1973.

107 Heng, M. K., Singh, B. N., Roche, A. H. G., Norris, R. M., and Mercer, C. J.: Effects of Intravenous Verapamil on Cardiac Arrhythmias and on the Electrocardiogram, *Am. Heart J.,* 90:487, 1975.

108 Spurrell, R. A. J., Krikler, D. M., and Sowton, G. E.: Concealed Bypasses of the Atrioventricular Node in Patients with Paroxysmal Supraventricular Tachycardia Revealed by Intracardiac Electrical Stimulation and Verapamil in Man, *Am. J. Cardiol.,* 33:590, 1974.

108a Gulamhusein S., Ko, P., Carruthers, S. G., Klein, G. J.: Acceleration of the Ventricular Response During Atrial Fibrillation in the Wolff-Parkinson-White Syndrome After Verapamil. *Circulation,* 65:348, 1982.

109 Schomerus, M., Spiegelhalder, B., Stieren, B., et al.: Physiological Disposition of Verapamil in Man, *Cardiovasc. Res.,* 10:605, 1976.

110 Singh, B. N., Collett, J. T., and Chew, C. Y. C.: New Perspectives in the Pharmacologic Therapy of Cardiac Arrhythmias, *Prog. Cardiovasc. Dis.,* 22:243, 1980.

111 Waxman, H. L., Myerburg, R. J., Appel, R., et al.: Verapamil for Control of Ventricular Rate in Paroxysmal Supraventricular Tachycardia and Atrial Fibrillation or Flutter, *Ann. Intern. Med.,* 94:1, 1981.

112 Schramroth, L., Krikler, D. M., and Garrett, C.: Immediate effects of Intravenous Verapamil in Cardiac Arrhythmias, *Br. Med. J.,* 1:660, 1972.

140

113 Heng, M. K., Singh, B. N., Roche, A. H. G., et al.: Effects of Intravenous Verapamil on Cardiac Arrhythmias and on the Electrocardiogram, *Am. Heart J.*, 4:487, 1975.

114 Belhassen, B., Rotmensch, H. R., and Laniado, S.: Response of Recurrent Sustained Ventricular Tachycardia to Verapamil, *Br. Heart J.*, 46:679, 1981.

115 Wu, D., Kou, H. C., and Hung, J. S.: Exercise-Triggered Paroxysmal Ventricular Tachycardia, *Ann. Intern. Med.*, 95:410, 1981.

116 Harris, A. S., and Kokernot, R. H.: Effects of Diphenylhydantoin Sodium (Dilantin Sodium) and Phenobarbital Sodium upon Ectopic Ventricular Tachycardia in Acute Myocardial Infarction, *Am. J. Physiol*, 163:505, 1950.

117 Mosey, L., and Tyler, M. D.: Effect of Diphenylhydantoin Sodium (Dilantin), Procaine Hydrochloride, Procainamide Hydrochloride and Quinidine Hydrochloride upon Ouabain-Induced Ventricular Tachycardia in Unanesthetized Dogs, *Circulation*, 10:65, 1954.

118 Conn, R. D.: Diphenylhydantoin Sodium in Cardiac Arrhythmias, *N. Engl. J. Med.*, 272:277, 1965.

119 Mercer, E. N., and Osborne, J. A.: The Current Status of Diphenylhydantoin in Heart Disease, *Ann. Intern. Med.*, 67:1084, 1967.

120 Helfant, R. H., Seuffert, G. W., Patton, R. D., et al.: The Clinical Use of Diphenylhydantoin (Dilantin) in the Treatment and Prevention of Cardiac Arrhythmias, *Am. Heart J.*, 77:315, 1969.

121 Dreifus, L. S., and Watanabe, Y.: Current Status of Diphenylhydantoin, *Am. Heart J.*, 80:709, 1970.

122 Atkinson, A. J., Jr., and Davison, R.: Diphenylhydantoin as an Antiarrhythmic Drug, *Ann. Rev. Med.*, 25:99, 1974.

123 Damato, A. N., Berkowitz, W. D., Patton, R. D., and Lau, S. H.: The Effect of Diphenylhydantoin on Atrioventricular and Intraventricular Conduction in Man, *Am. Heart J.*, 79:51, 1970.

124 Caracta, A. R., Damato, A. N., Josephson, M. E., et al.: Electrophysiological Properties of Diphenylhydantoin, *Circulation*, 47:1234, 1973.

125 Rosati, R. A., Alexander, J. A., Schaal, S. F., et al.: Influence of Phenytoin on Electrophysiological Properties of the Canine Heart, *Circ. Res.*, 21:757, 1967.

126 Gugler, R., Manion, C. V., and Azarnoff, D. L.: Phenytoin: Pharmacokinetics and Bioavailability, *Clin. Pharmacol. Ther.*, 19:135, 1975.

127 Lund, L., Lunde, P. K., Rane, A., Borga, O., and Sjoqvist, F.: Plasma Protein Binding, Plasma Concentrations and Effects of Diphenylhydantoin in Man, *Ann. N.Y. Acad. Sci.*, 179:723, 1972.

128 Odar-Cederlof, I., Lunde, P., and Sjoqvist, F.: Abnormal Pharmacokinetics of Phenytoin in a Patient with Uremia, *Lancet*, 2:831, 1970.

129 Glazko, A. J., Chang, T., Baukema, J., et al.: Metabolic Disposition of Diphenylhydantoin in Normal Human Subjects Following Intravenous Administration, *Clin. Pharmacol. Ther.*, 10:498, 1969.

130 Lunde, P. K. M., Rane, A., Yaffee, S. J., et al.: Plasma Protein Binding of Diphenylhydantoin in Man: Interaction with Other Drugs and the Effects of Temperature and Plasma Dilution, *Clin. Pharmacol. Ther.*, 11:846, 1970.

131 Bigger, J. T., Jr., Schmidt, D. H., and Kutt, H.: Relationship between the Plasma Level of Diphenylhydantoin Sodium and Its Cardiac Antiarrhythmic Effects, *Circulation*, 38:363, 1968.

132 Buchanan, R. A., Kinkel, A. W., Goulet, J. R., et al.: The Metabolism of Diphenylhydantoin (Dilantin) Following Once Daily Administration, *Neurology*, 22:126, 1972.

133 Sohn, Y. J., Raines, A., Standert, F. T., and Levitt, B.: The Effect of Diphenylthiohydantoin (DPTH) on Digitalis-Induced Cardiac Arrhythmia, *Arch. Int. Pharmacodyn. Ther.*, 179:434, 1969.

134 Mathur, K. S., Wahal, P. K., and Seth, H. C.: Response of Digitalis-Induced Cardiac Arrhythmias to Diphenylhydantoin Sodium (Dilantin Sodium)—An Experimental Study in Dogs, *J. Assoc. Physicians India*, 17:147, 1969.

135 Hilmi, K. I., and Regan, T. J.: Relative Effectiveness of Antiarrhythmic Drugs in Treatment of Digitalis-Induced Ventricular Tachycardia, *Am. Heart J.*, 76:365, 1968.

136 Bigger, J. T., Jr., and Strauss, H. C.: Digitalis Toxicity: Drug Interactions Promoting Toxicity and the Management of Toxicity, *Semin. Drug Treatment*, 2:147, 1972.

137 Rumack, B. H., Wolfe, R. R., and Gilfrich, H.: Phenytoin (Diphenylhydantoin) Treatment of Massive Digoxin Overdose, *Br. Heart J.*, 36:405, 1974.

138 Helfant, R. H., Lau, S. H., Cohen, S. I., and Damato, A. N.: Effects of Diphenylhydantoin on Atrioventricular Conduction in Man, *Circulation*, 36:686, 1967.

139 Gillis, R. A., McClellan, J. R., Sauer, T. S., and Standerdt, F. G.: Depression of Cardiac Sympathetic Nerve Activity by Diphenylhydantoin, *J. Pharmacol. Exp. Ther.*, 179:599, 1971.

140 Crampton, R.: Preeminence of the Left Stellate Ganglion in the Long Q-T Syndrome, *Circulation*, 59:769, 1979.

141 Moss, A. J., and Schwartz, P. J.: Delayed Depolarization (QT or QTU Prolongation) and Malignant Ventricular Arrhythmias, *Mod. Concepts Cardiovasc. Dis.*, 51:85, 1982.

142 Stone, N., Klein, M. D., and Lown, B.: Diphenylhydantoin in the Prevention of Recurring Ventricular Tachycardia, *Circulation*, 43:420, 1971.

143 Garson, A., Gillette, P. C., and McNamara, D. G.: Treatment of Chronic Ventricular Dysrhythmias in the Young, *Pediatr. Cardiol.*, 1:172, 1980.

144 Garson, A., Jr.: Evaluation and Treatment of Chronic Ventricular Dysrhythmias in the Young, *Cardiovasc. Rev. Rep.,* 2:1164, 1981.

145 Collaborative Group: Phenytoin after Recovery from Myocardial Infarction, Controlled Trial in 568 Patients, *Lancet,* 2:1055, 1971.

146 Peter, T., Ross, D., Duffield, A., et al.: Effect on Survival after Myocardial Infarction of Long-Term Treatment with Phenytoin, *Br. Heart J.,* 40:1356, 1978.

147 Rosen, M., Lisak, R., and Rubin, I. L.: Diphenylhydantoin in Cardiac Arrhythmias, *Am. J. Cardiol.,* 20:674, 1967.

148 Koch-Weser, J.: Antiarrhythmic Prophylaxis in Ambulatory Patients with Coronary Heart Disease, *Arch. Intern. Med.,* 129:763, 1972.

149 Roos, J. C., Paalman, A. C. A., and Dunning, A. J.: Electrophysiologic Effects of Mexiletine in Man, *Postgrad. Med. J.,* 53 (suppl. 1):92, 1977.

150 Prescott, L. F., Clements, J. D., and Pottage, A.: Absorption, Distribution, and Elimination of Mexiletine, *Postgrad. Med. J.,* 53 (suppl. 1):50, 1977.

151 Campbell, N. P. S., Kelly, J. G., Adgey, A. A. J., et al.: Mexiletine in Normal Volunteers, *Br. Clin. Pharmacol.,* 6:372, 1978.

152 Talbot, R. G., Clark, R. A., Nimmo, J., Neilson, J. M. M., Julian, D. G., Prescott, L. F.: Treatment of Ventricular Arrhythmias with Mexiletine, *Lancet,* 2:399, 1973.

153 Beckett, A. H., and Chidomere, E. C.: The Distribution, Metabolism and Excretion of Mexiletine in Man, *Postgrad. Med. J.,* 53 (suppl. 1):60, 1977.

154 Kiddie, M. A., Kaye, C. M., Turner, P., et al.: The Influence of Urinary pH on the Elimination of Mexiletine, *Br. J. Clin. Pharmacol.,* 1:229, 1974.

155 Dresse, A.: Plasma Kinetics of Mexiletine in Normal Subjects and in Patients with Renal Insufficiency: Single Intravenous Administration, in E. Sandoe, D. G. Julian, and J. W. Bell, (eds.), "Management of Ventricular Tachycardia—Role of Mexiletine," Excerpta Medica, Oxford, 1978, p. 286.

156 Campbell, N. P. S., Kelly, J. G., Adgey, A. A. J., et al.: The Clinical Pharmacology of Mexiletine, *Br. J. Clin. Pharmacol.,* 6:103, 1978.

157 Pottage, A.: Oral Dosage Schedules for Mexiletine, *Postgrad. Med. J.,* 53 (suppl. 1):155, 1977.

158 Achuff, S. C., Campbell, R. W. F., Pottage, A., et al.: Mexiletine in the Prevention of Ventricular Arrhythmias in Acute Myocardial Infarction, *Postgrad. Med. J.,* 53 (suppl. 1):163, 1977.

159 Merx, W., Henning, B., Franken, G., et al.: Mexiletine in Acute Myocardial Infarction, in E. Sandoe, D. G. Julian, and J. W. Bell (eds.), "Management of Ventricular Tachycardia—Role of Mexiletine," Excerpta Medica, Oxford, 1978, p. 472.

160 Campbell, N. P. S., Pantridge, J. F., and Adgey, A. A. J.: Long Term Oral Antiarrhythmic Therapy with Mexiletine, *Br. Heart J.,* 40:796, 1978.

161 Talbot, R. G., Julian, D. G., and Prescott, L. F.: Long Term Treatment of Ventricular Arrhythmias with Oral Mexiletine, *Am. Heart J.,* 91:58, 1976.

162 Campbell, R. W. F., Dolder, M. A., Prescott, L. F., et al.: Comparison of Procainamide and Mexiletine in Prevention of Ventricular Arrhythmias after Acute Myocardial Infarction, *Lancet,* 2:1257, 1975.

163 Podrid, P. J., and Lown, B.: Mexiletine for Ventricular Arrhythmia, *Am. J. Cardiol.,* 47:895, 1981.

164 DiMarco, J. P., Garan, H., and Ruskin, J. N.: Mexiletine for Refractory-Ventricular Arrhythmias: Results Using Serial Electrophysiologic Testing, *Am. J. Cardiol.,* 47:131, 1981.

165 Heger, J. J., Natel, S., Rinkenberger, R. L., and Zipes, D. P.: Mexiletine Therapy in 15 Patients with Drug Resistent Ventricular Tachycardia, *Am. J. Cardiol.,* 45:627, 1980.

166 Lalka, D. M., Meyer, B., Duce, B., et al.: Kinetics of the Antiarrhythmic Lidocaine Congener, Tocainide, *Clin. Pharmacol. Ther.,* 19:757, 1976.

167 Winkle, R. A., Meffin, P. J., Fitzgerald, J. W., et al.: Clinical Efficacy and Pharmacokinetics of a New Orally Effective Antiarrhythmic, Tocainide, *Circulation,* 54:884, 1976.

168 Harrison, D. C., Meffin, P. H., and Winkle, R. A.: Clinical Pharmacokinetics of Antiarrhythmic Drugs, *Prog. Cardiovasc. Dis.,* 20:217, 1977.

169 McDevitt, D. G., Nies, A. S., Wilkinson, G. R., et al.: Antiarrhythmic Effects of a Lidocaine Congener, Tocainide, in Man., *Clin. Pharmacol. Ther.,* 19:396, 1976.

170 Bastian, B. C., MacFarlane, P. W., McLaughlin, J. H., et al.: A Prospective Randomized Trial of Tocainide in Patients Following Myocardial Infarction, *Am. Heart J.,* 100:1017, 1980.

171 Ryden, L., Arnman, K., Conradson, T. B., et al.: Prophylaxis of Ventricular Tachyarrhythmias with Intravenous and Oral Tocainide in Patients with and Recovering from Acute Myocardial Infarction, *Am. Heart J.,* 100:1006, 1980.

172 Winkle, R. A., Meffin, P. J., and Harrison, D. C.: Long Term Tocainide Therapy for Ventricular Arrhythmias, *Circulation,* 57:1008, 1978.

173 Ryan, W., Engler, R., LeWinter, M., et al.: Efficacy of a New Oral Agent (Tocainide) in the Acute Treatment of Refractory Ventricular Arrhythmias, *Am. J. Cardiol.,* 43:285, 1979.

174 DeBianco, R., Fletcher, R. D., Cohen, A. I., et al.: Treatment of Frequent Ventricular Arrhythmia with Encainide: Assessment Using Serial Ambulatory Electrocardiograms, Intracardiac Electrophysiologic Studies, Treadmill Exercise Rests, and Radionuclide Cineangiographic Studies, *Circulation,* 65:1134, 1982.

175 Roden, D. M., Reele, S. B., Higgins, S. B., et al.: Total Suppression of Ventricular Arrhythmias by Encainide, *N. Engl. J. Med.,* 302:877, 1980.

176 Winkle, R. A., Peters, F., Kates, R. E., et al.: Clinical Pharmacology and Antiarrhythmic Efficacy of Encainide in Patients with Chronic Ventricular Arrhythmias, *Circulation,* 64:290, 1981.

177 Mason, J. W., and Peters, F. A.: Antiarrhythmic Efficacy of Encainide in Patients with Refractory Recurrent Ventricular Tachycardia, *Circulation,* 63:670, 1981.

177a Duff, H. J., Roden, D. M., Dawson, A. K., Oates, J. A., Smith, R. F., Woosley, R. L.: Comparison of the Effects of Placebo and Encainide on Programmed Electrical Stimulation and Ventricular Arrhythmia Frequency. *Am. J. Cardiol.,* 50:305, 1982.

178 Seipel, L., Abendroth, R. R., and Breithardt, G.: Elektrophysiologische Effekte des neuen Antiarrhythmikums flecainid (R818) beim menschen, *Z. Kardiol.,* 70:524, 1981.

179 Hellestrand, K., Nathan, A., Bexton, R., and Camm, J.: Electrophysiology of the Antiarrhythmic Agent, Flecainide Acetate. Ninth World Congress of Cardiology, Moscow, June 20–26, 1982.

180 Conard, G. J., Carlson, E. L., Froth, J. W., and Ober, R. E.: Human Plasma Pharmacokinetics of Flecainide Acetate (R818), a New Antiarrhythmic, Following Single, Oral and Intravenous Doses, *Clin. Pharmacol. Ther.,* 25:218, 1979. (Abstract.)

181 Conard, G. J., Carlson, E. L., and Ober, R. E.: Binding of Flecainide Acetate (R818) to Human Plasma Protein in Vitro, 31st National Meeting of the American Pharmaceutical Association, Orlando, Florida, 1981.

182 Hodges, M., Haugland, J. M., Granrud, G., et al.: Suppression of Ventricular Ectopic Depolarization by Flecainide Acetate, a New Antiarrhythmic Agent, *Circulation,* 65:879, 1982.

183 Duff, H. J., Roden, D. M., Maffucci, R. J., et al.: Suppression of Resistant Ventricular Arrhythmias by Twice Daily Dosing with Flecainide, *Am. J. Cardiol.,* 48:1133, 1981.

184 Anderson, J. L., Stewart, J. R., Perry, B. A., et al.: Oral Flecainide Acetate for the Treatment of Ventricular Arrhythmias, *N. Engl. J. Med.,* 305:473, 1981.

185 Orning, O. M.: Electrophysiologic Effects of Flecainide Acetate in Arrhythmias, Eighth World Congress of Cardiology, Tokyo, 1978.

186 Manz, M., Steinbeck, G., and Luderitz, B.: Wirkung von Lorcainid (R15889) auf Sinusknotenfunktion und intrakardiale Erregungsleitung, *Z. Kardiol.* (Suppl.) 5:53, 1978.

187 Bar, F. W., Farre, J., Ross, D., et al.: Electrophysiological Effects of Lorcainide, a New Antiarrhythmic Drug, *Br. Heart J.,* 45:292, 1981.

188 Ng, C. K., Gstottner, M., and Gmeiner, R.: Intracardiac Electrophysiological Effects of Lorcainide in Man, *Eur. J. Clin. Pharmacol.,* 15:241, 1979.

189 Jahnchen, E., Bechtold, H., Kasper, W., et al.: Lorcainide: I. Saturable Presystemic Elimination, *Clin. Pharmacol. Ther.,* 26:187, 1979.

190 Meinertz, T., Kasper, W., Kersting, F., Just, H., Bechtold, H., and Jahnchen, E.: Lorcainide: II. Plasma Concentration Effect Relationship, *Clin. Pharmacol. Ther.,* 26:196, 1979.

191 Keefe, D. L., Peters, F., and Winkle, R. A.: Randomized Double-Blind Placebo Controlled Crossover Trial Documenting Oral Lorcainide Efficacy in Suppression of Symptomatic Ventricular Tachyarrhythmias, *Am. Heart J.,* 103:511, 1982.

192 Amery, W. K., Heykants, J. J. P., Xhonneux, R., et al.: Lorcainide (R15889): A First Review, *Acta Cardiol.,* 36:207, 1981.

193 Breithardt, G., Seipel, L., and Abenbroth, R. R.: Klinisch-Elekrophysiologische Untersuchung zur Wirkung von Lorcainid bei Patienten mit ventrikularen Tachykardien, *Z. Kardiol.,* 70:530, 1981.

194 Coutte, R., Fontaine, G., Frank, R., Dragodanne, C., Phanthuc, H., and Facquet, J.: Etude electrocardiologique des effets de l'amiodarone sur la conduction intracardiaque chez l'homme, *Ann. Cardiol. Angeiol. (Paris),* 25:543, 1976.

195 Wellens, H. J. J., Lie, K. I., Bar, F. W., et al.: Effect of Amiodarone in the Wolff-Parkinson-White Syndrome, *Am. J. Cardiol.,* 38:189, 1976.

196 Rasmussen, V., and Berning, J.: Effects of Amiodarone in the Wolff-Parkinson-White Syndrome, *Acta Med. Scand.,* 205:31, 1979.

197 Rowland, E., and Krikler, D. M.: Electrophysiological Assessment of Amiodarone in Treatment of Resistant Supraventricular Arrhythmias, *Br. Heart J.,* 44:82, 1980.

198 Touboul, R., Atallah, G., Gressard, A., and Kirkorian, G.: Effect of Amiodarone on Sinus Node in Man, *Br. Heart J.,* 42:573, 1979.

199 Haffajee, C., Lesko, L., Canada, A., and Alpert, J. S.: Clinical Pharmacokinetics of Amiodarone, *Circulation,* 64 (suppl. 4):263, 1981. (Abstract.)

200 Kannan, R., Nademanee, K., Hendrickson, J. A., Rostami, H. J., and Singh, B. N.: Amiodarone Kinetics after Oral Doses, *Clin. Pharmacol. Ther.,* 31:438, 1982.

201 Andreasen, F., Agerbaek, H., Bjerregaard, P., and Gotzsche, H.: Pharmacokinetics of Amiodarone after Intravenous and Oral Adminstration, *Eur. J. Clin. Pharmacol.,* 19:293, 1981.

202 Harris, L., McKenna, W. J., Rowland, E., Story, G. C. A., Krikler, D. M., and Holt, D. W.: Plasma Amiodarone and Desethyl Amiodarone Levels in Chronic Oral Therapy, *Circulation,* 64 (suppl. 4):263, 1981. (Abstract.)

203 Rakita, L., and Sobol, S. M.: Amiodarone Treatment

for Refractory Arrhythmias: Dose-Ranging and Importance of High Initial Dosage, *Circulation,* 64 (suppl. 4):263, 1981. (Abstract.)

204 Coumel, P., and Fidelle, J.: Amiodarone in the Treatment of Cardiac Arrhythmias in Children: 135 Cases, *Am. Heart J.,* 100:1063, 1980.

205 Marcus, F. I., Fontaine, G. H., Frank, R., and Grosgogeat, Y.: Clinical Pharmacology and Therapeutic Applications of the Antiarrhythmic Agent, Amiodarone, *Am. Heart J.,* 101:480, 1981.

206 Kaski, J. C., Girotti, L. A., Messuti, H., Rutitzky, B., and Rosenbaum, M. B.:Long-Term Management of Sustained, Recurrent, Systematic Ventricular Tachycardia with Amiodarone, *Circulation,* 64:273, 1981.

207 Podrid, P. J., and Lown, B.: Amiodarone Therapy in Symptomatic, Sustained Refractory Atrial and Ventricular Tachyarrhythmias, *Am. Heart J.,* 101:374, 1981.

208 Ward, D. E., Camm, A. J., Spurrell, R. A.: Clinical Antiarrhythmic Effects of Amiodarone in Patients with Resistant Paroxysmal Tachycardias, *Br. Heart J.,* 44:91, 1980.

209 Nademanee, K., Hendrickson, J. A., Cannom, D. S., Goldreyer, B. N., and Singh, B. N.: Control of Refractory Life-Threatening Ventricular Tachyarrhythmias by Amiodarone, *Am. Heart J.,* 101:759, 1981.

210 Bashour, T., Jokhadar, M., and Cheng, T. O.: Effective Management of the Long Q-T Syndrome with Amiodarone, *Chest,* 79:704, 1981.

211 McComb, J. M., Logan, K. R., Khan, M. M., Geddes, J. S., and Adgey, A. A. J.: Amiodarone-Induced Ventricular Fibrillation, *Eur. J. Cardiol.,* 11:381, 1980.

212 Keren, A., Tzivoni, D., Gottlieb, S., Benhorin, J., Stern, S.: Atypical Ventricular Tachycardia (Torsade de Pointes) Induced by Amiodarone, *Chest,* 81:384, 1982.

213 Heger, J. J., Prystowsky, E. N., Jackman, W. M., et al.: Clinical Efficacy and Electrophysiology of Amiodarone during Long-Term Therapy for Recurrent Ventricular Tachycardia or Ventricular Fibrillation, *N. Engl. J. Med.,* 305:539, 1981.

214 Hamer, A. W., Finerman, W. B., Jr., Peter, T., and Mandel, W. J.: Disparity between the Clinical and Electrophysiologic Effects of Amiodarone in the Treatment of Recurrent Ventricular Tachyarrhythmias, *Am. Heart J.,* 102:992, 1981.

215 Chapman, J. R., and Boyd, M. J.: Intravenous Amiodarone in Ventricular Fibrillation, *Br. Med. J.,* 282:951, 1981.

216 Gomes, J., Kang, P., Behl, A., Lyons, J., and El-Sherif, N.: Intravenous Amiodarone: A Potent and Effective Drug for Atrial Ventricular Nodal Reentrant Paroxysmal Tachycardia, *Circulation,* 64 (suppl. 4):317, 1981. (Abstract.)

217 Installe, E., Schoevaerdts, J. C., Gadisseux, D. H., Charles, S., and Tremouroux, J.: Intravenous Amiodarone in the Treatment of Various Arrhythmias Following Cardiac Operations, *J. Thorac. Cardiovasc. Surg.,* 81:302, 1981.

218 Waleffe, A., Mary-Rabine, L., Legrand, V., Demoulin, J. C., and Kulbertus, H. E.: Combined Mexiletine and Amiodarone Treatment of Refractory Recurrent Ventricular Tachycardia, *Am. Heart J.,* 100:788, 1980.

219 McGovern, B., Garan, H., and Ruskin, J. N.: Sinus Arrest during Treatment with Amiodarone, *Br. Med. J.,* 284:160, 1982.

220 Harris, L., McKenna, W. J., Rowland, E., Holt, D. W., and Krikler, D. M.: Amiodarone Therapy: Unwanted Effects, *Br. Heart J.,* 47:192, 1982. (Abstract.)

221 Sobol, S. M., and Rakita, L.: Pneumonitis and Pulmonary Fibrosis Associated with Amiodarone Treatment: A Possible Complication of a New Antiarrhythmic Drug, *Circulation,* 65:819, 1982.

222 Hamer, A., Peter, T., Mandel, W. J., Scheinman, M. M., and Weiss, D.: The Potentiation of Warfarin Anticoagulation by Amiodarone, *Circulation,* 65:1025, 1982.

223 Moysey, J. O., Jaggarao, N. S. V., Grundy, E. N., and Chamberlain, D. A.: Amiodarone Increases Plasma Digoxin Concentration, *Br. Med. J.,* 282:58, 1981.

224 Tartini, R., Steinbrunn, W., Kappenberger, W. L., and Meyer, U. A.: Dangerous Interaction Between Amiodarone and Quinidine, *Lancet,* 2:1327, 1982.

225 Southworth, W., Friday, K. J., and Ruffy, R.: Possible Aprindine-Amiodarone Interaction, *Am. Heart J.,* in press.

JAMES E. DOHERTY, M.D.

The current use of digitalis glycosides continues to place the drugs digoxin, digitoxin, and digitalis leaf eighth, sixteenth, and twenty-third, respectively, on the list of prescriptions written in the United States in 1980. Thus there is little doubt that most physicians continue to believe that these drugs are useful. I believe that current practices reflect conservative views of physicians prescribing drugs. The use of more definite indications and smaller doses and, recognition of the role of pharmacokinetics and drug interactios will be stressed in this article.

INDICATIONS FOR DIGITALIS GLYCOSIDES

There are only two indications for digitalis glycosides: (1) congestive heart failure and (2) arrhythmias. Heart failure of virtually any etiology may be managed with digitalis, with reservations annotated later in this section. Arrhythmias, particularly atrial, in the presence of heart failure yield very well to management with digitalis.

Congestive Heart Failure

Digitalis is useful in either right or left ventricular failure as well as in combined right and left ventricular failure. In years past, "full digitalizing doses" were recommended for congestive failure of any etiology. This was often taken to mean prescription of increasing amounts of drug until cardiac or extracardiac signs of toxicity appeared, as suggested by Withering[1] in his treatise on the foxglove. One, of course, then either discontinued the drug until the next bout of congestive failure appeared (as was the custom for a time in Europe)[2] or "backed off" and, when toxic manifestations abated, restarted a "maintenance" dose of the drug. The relatively high morbidity and mortality associated with digitalis toxicity in hospitalized cardiac patients has been emphasized by Beller et al.,[3] and the wisdom of this approach today is doubtful.

Since the demonstration that the response to digitalis does seem to be dose-related until toxicity intervenes, we should adopt the principle that "optimum" doses may not be maximum tolerated doses of the drug. A small dose does improve cardiac performance.

With these principles in mind, the glycosides may be used in small doses in disease states in which intoxication is greatly feared and with justifiable hope of benefit when given in conjunction with powerful diuretics.

It has recently been suggested that digitalis is really not necessary for management of congestive heart failure.[4,5] This view has been in and out of vogue for nearly 200 years and will gain some adherents during the current swing of opinion. I choose to believe that beginning with Withering[1] and continuing to Arnold et al.[6] and Beeson,[7] we have learned what Withering stated in a letter to Hall Jackson in 1786: "I am more and more convinced that digitalis, under judicious management, is one of the mildest...medicines we have and one of the most efficacious.... It is not necessary to produce nausea or any other disturbances in the system."

Few doubt the value of digitalis in supraventricular arrhythmia[8,9] and atrial fibrillation, where chronotropic effect is so important. Congestive heart failure associated with myocardial infarction, where the toxic dose is 60 percent of the usual toxic dose, may be managed with smaller doses with the hope of benefit. Similarly, patients with cor pulmonale and heart failure,[10] myxedema,[11] shock, or cardiomyopathies may be given the benefit of small doses of digitalis without fear of intoxication.

Patients with renal failure and the often associated heart failure present real problems, and dosage adjustment is determined by the particular glycoside used. All these will be discussed later in the section entitled Problems with Digitalis Treatment.

Cardiac Arrhythmia

The consensus of opinion holds that digitalis glycosides usually are the best agents for control of the ventricular rate in atrial fibrillation or flutter. It should be appreciated, however, that larger than "usual" doses may be necessary to block the atrioventricular node to produce optimum ventricular rates. Particular problems may be noted in patients with hyperthyroidism (where rates may be better controlled with propranolol or reserpine) and in pheochromocytoma (where phentolamine may be preferred).

It should be remembered that propranolol or beta blocking agents will not prevent thyroid storm, and although beta blockers relieve symptoms of thyrotoxicosis, specific antithyroid treatment must be given concomitantly.

*From the Departments of Medicine and Pharmacology, University of Arkansas for Medical Sciences, and the Little Rock Veterans Administration Medical Centers, Little Rock, Arkansas.

Dosage Guide

Table 1 outlines average doses of the digitalis glycosides. Remember that optimum doses for a particular patient may *not* be average. Pediatric patients usually tolerate larger doses (per kilogram of body weight) than adults without toxicity. Elderly patients tolerate less because of reduced renal functional capacity and a smaller, lean body mass.[12]

Bioavailability

Bioavailability (biological availability) is a term designed to describe the ability of a drug to reach its receptor site in the appropriate tissue, where it can produce the desired therapeutic effect. The fact that this was a problem with the digitalis glycosides was not generally recognized until Lindenbaum et al.[13] discovered strikingly different digoxin blood levels in patients receiving different brands of digoxin. Since digoxin is not completely absorbed, this is more of a problem with digoxin than with digitoxin.[14]

The differences in bioavailiability of digoxin preparations are related to differences in particle size of the preparation and the effect of particle size on dissolution in the stomach and upper small intestine, where most of the digoxin absorption takes place.[15]

Bioavailability is no longer a real problem in the United States. It should be stated, though, that all the different products are not equally bioavailable. Reputable brands are still more predictably bioavailable from one lot to the next.

The new gelatin capsule of digoxin will increase bioavailability slightly, but probably not enough to be of importance clinically.[16–18]

PHARMACOKINETICS OF DIGITALIS GLYCOSIDES
Digoxin

Digoxin (12-hydroxydigitoxin) has become the most popular glycoside for clinical use since its introduction 50 years ago. Its preference by clinicians in the United States is shown by the fact that in 1980 (the most recent year available), it was the eighth most frequently clinician-prescribed drug.

The pharmacokinetic behavior of digoxin has been extensively studied by radioactive tracer techniques using tritium(radiohydrogen)-labeled digoxin. These studies show that there are important kinetic differences between the various routes of administration of digoxin: oral, intramuscular, and intravenous.

SERUM TURNOVER AFTER ORAL ADMINISTRATION

A composite graph of the serum digoxin concentrations of 12 patients following a single oral dose of tritium-labeled digoxin is shown in Fig. 1. It should be noted that digoxin in this instance was given in an alcoholic solution or on a sucrose cube from which the alcohol had been allowed to evaporate. The figure used for absorption, then, represents this form of administration rather than that following a Lanoxin brand tablet.

Note that an early peak serum level was demonstrated at 45 to 60 min after oral administration, and digoxin radioactivity was demonstrable 6 min after administration. Two exponential functions can be derived from the oral tritiated digoxin serum disappearance curve. The first of these is attributed to distribution and binding of the glycoside and has a half-

TABLE 1
Usual doses of digitalis glycosides

Drug	Oral			Parenteral
	Rapid digitalization (24 h)	**Slow digitalization**	**Maintenance**	
Digoxin	0.5 mg 0.25 mg 4 hourly × 4 if necessary (do not exceed 2.0 mg)	0.125 to 0.50 mg daily × 7	0.125 mg to 0.5 daily	1.0 mg to 1.5 mg in divided doses in 24 h
Digitoxin	1.2 to 1.6 mg divided doses	0.15 mg daily × 30	0.15 mg daily	1.0 to 1.6 mg in divided doses in 24 h
Lanatoside C	Not recommended	Not recommended	Not recommended	0.8 mg initially; 0.2 mg 2 hourly to total 1.6 mg in 24 h
Digitalis leaf	Not recommended	0.1 g daily × 30	0.1 g daily	Not recommended

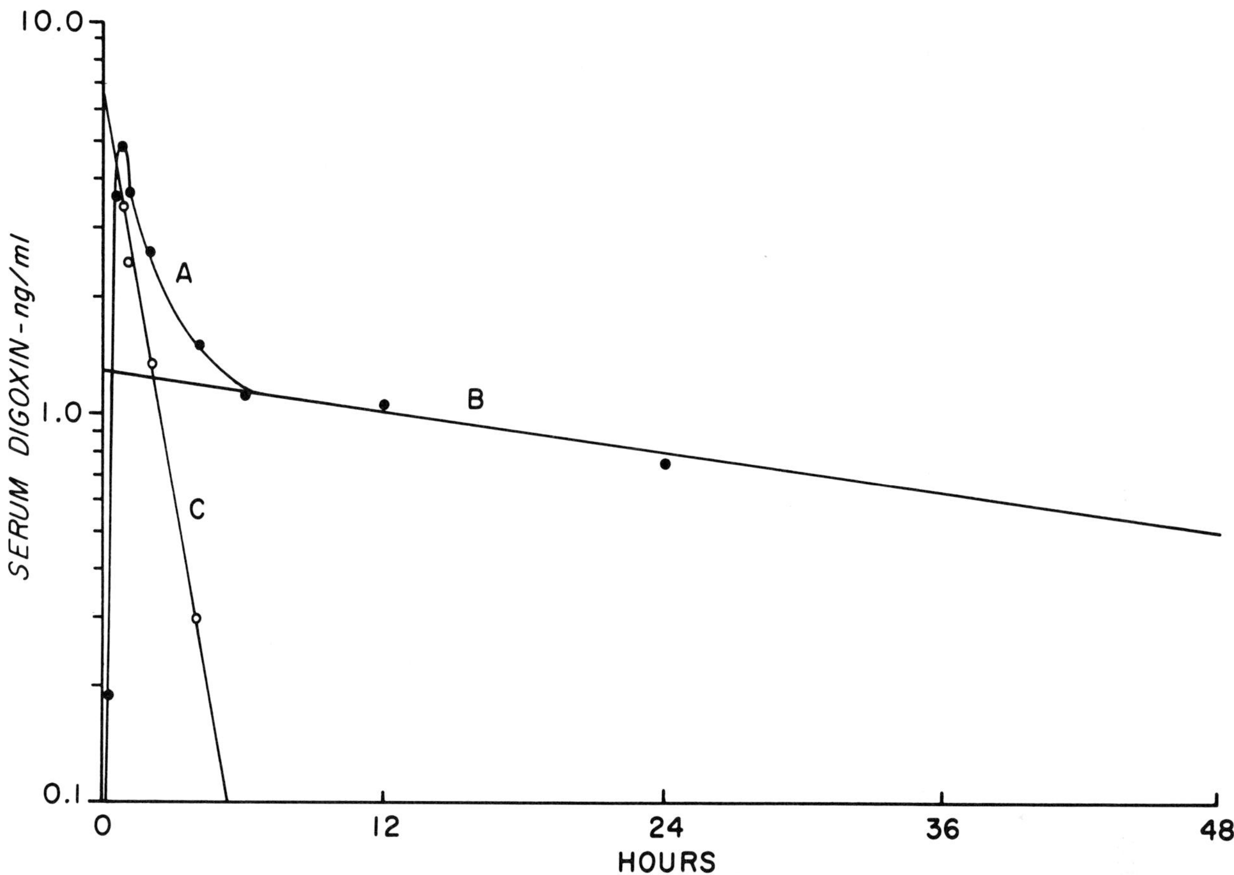

FIGURE 1 Composite (12 patients) serum concentration of digoxin following oral administration. Serum concentration is plotted on the vertical axis and time is plotted on the horizontal axis on a semilogarithmic scale. Although studies were continued for 7 days, only the first 2 days are shown in order to demonstrate the important early differences in the serum turnover curves. Note that serum concentration reaches a peak 45 to 60 min after being given. Line *B* is the best straight line that can be drawn back to zero time, representing the dominant half-life of digoxin of 31.3 h, and is associated with metabolism and excretion of the glycoside. Line *C* is derived by subtracting line *B* from the descending limb of curve *A,* thus eliminating metabolism and excretion from their exponential function, which now should represent distribution and binding of the glycoside to the tissue. Line *C* has a half-life of 60 min. (*From J. E. Doherty, W. H. Perkins, and G. K. Mitchell, Arch. Intern. Med., 108:351, 1961. Used with permission.*)

life of 60 min; the second represents the dominant half-life and is related to metabolism and excretion (primarily the latter) of tritiated digoxin and has a half-life of 31.3 h. It is of interest that the distribution and binding half-life correlates well with the beginning onset of action (inotropic effort) of digoxin seen in human subjects given digoxin orally.

The dominant half-life appears to parallel the disappearance of pharmacologic activity as the drug is withdrawn and is consistent with the terms *short-acting* or *short duration of action* when applied to digoxin. Digoxin excretion by this route of administration is primarily in the urine, and 7-day excretion of the drug by this route of administration is shown in Fig. 2, together with excretion by the other routes of administration.[19]

SERUM TURNOVER AFTER INTRAMUSCULAR ADMINISTRATION

When tritiated digoxin was given as a single dose intramuscularly to 10 patients, a somewhat different composite serum turnover curve was recorded and is reproduced in Fig. 3.

Note that intramuscular administration revealed a serum half-life similar to that with oral administration, although the peak serum concentration occurred later than in the oral study, as did the serum digoxin plateau (indicating a later serum-tissue equilibration of digoxin by this route). It is noted that two exponential functions are also observed after intramuscular administration that are similar to those seen after oral administration. The first exponential function is again related to tissue

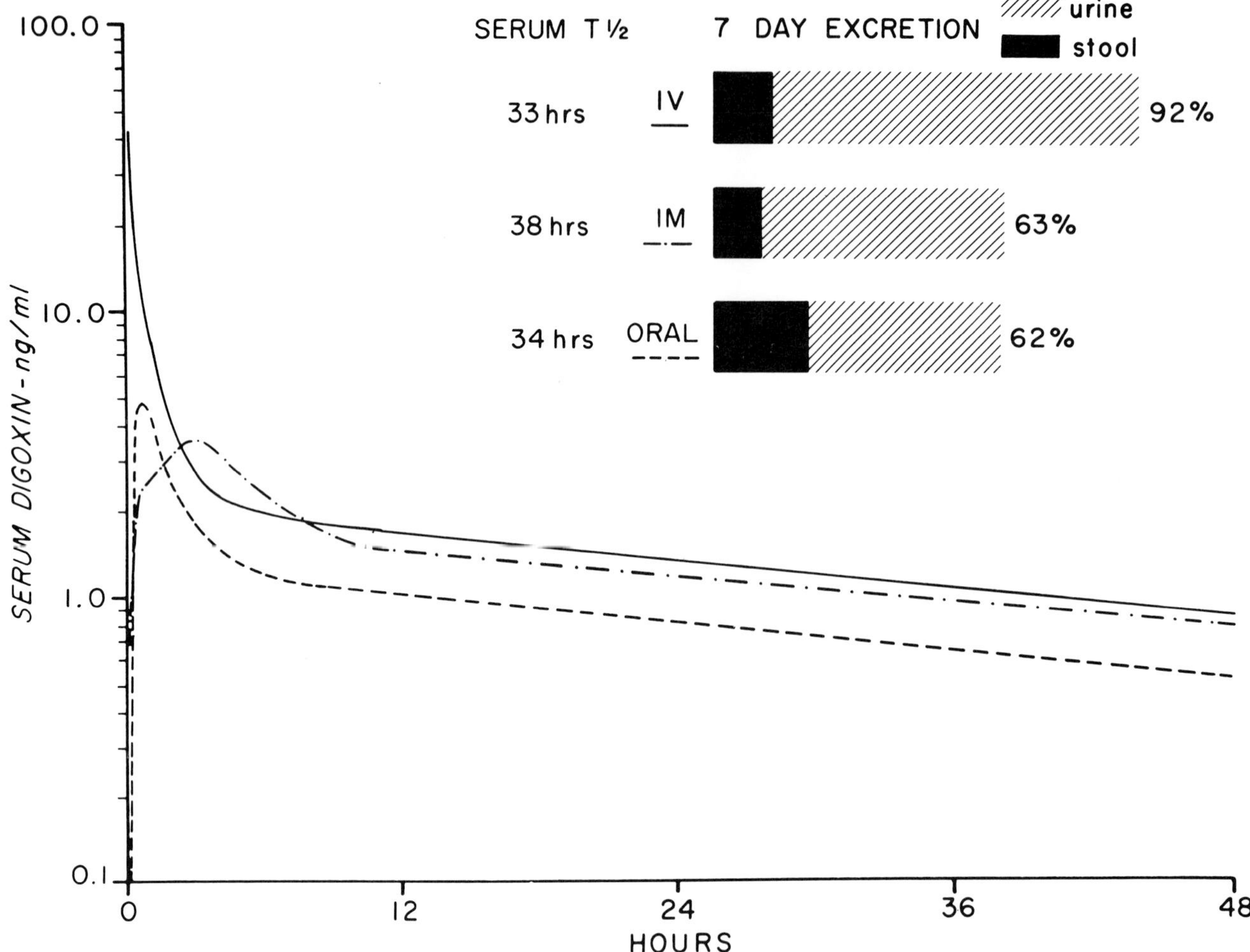

FIGURE 2 Comparative composite serum levels of digoxin and 7-day excretion rates after oral, intramuscular, and intravenous administration. The serum curves in the preceding figure are shown as comparative serum concentration to illustrate the important early differences in serum concentration by the various routes of administration (see text). Excretion rates shown are for the patients with normal renal function and clearly show major route of excretion to be the kidney, regardless of the route of administration. (*From J. E. Doherty, J. Arkansas Med. Soc., 66:120, 1969. Used with permission.*)

distribution and binding and has a half-life of 100 min. The second exponential function represents the dominant half-life of 38 h (mean) for this group of patients, statistically not different from the oral study. However, the distribution and binding half-life is about twice as long by the intramuscular route as it is following oral administration. This could be related to two factors: (1) the tritiated digoxin given orally was in an alcoholic solution, facilitating more rapid distribution and binding to tissue; and (2) the intramuscular (gluteal muscle) route of administration is not as effective in absorbing digoxin (prepared in 40% propylene glycol, 10% ethyl alcohol, and 50% distilled water) as is the gastrointestinal tract. Because the injection is so painful, I do not recommend the intramuscular route for parenteral use.

Excretion of tritiated digoxin by the intramuscular route was again noted to be primarily in the urine as the unchanged glycoside (Fig. 2). Only 10 percent was recovered in the stool of these patients in a 7-day study after a single intramuscular dose of the glycoside.[20]

SERUM TURNOVER AFTER INTRAVENOUS ADMINISTRATION

Studies of 13 patients given a single intravenous dose of tritiated digoxin are reproduced (as before) in Fig. 4, from which it can be seen that there is an early high serum concentration and an earlier serum plateau than after oral or intramuscular administration.

There are three exponential functions in this serum digoxin curve after intravenous administration (in addi-

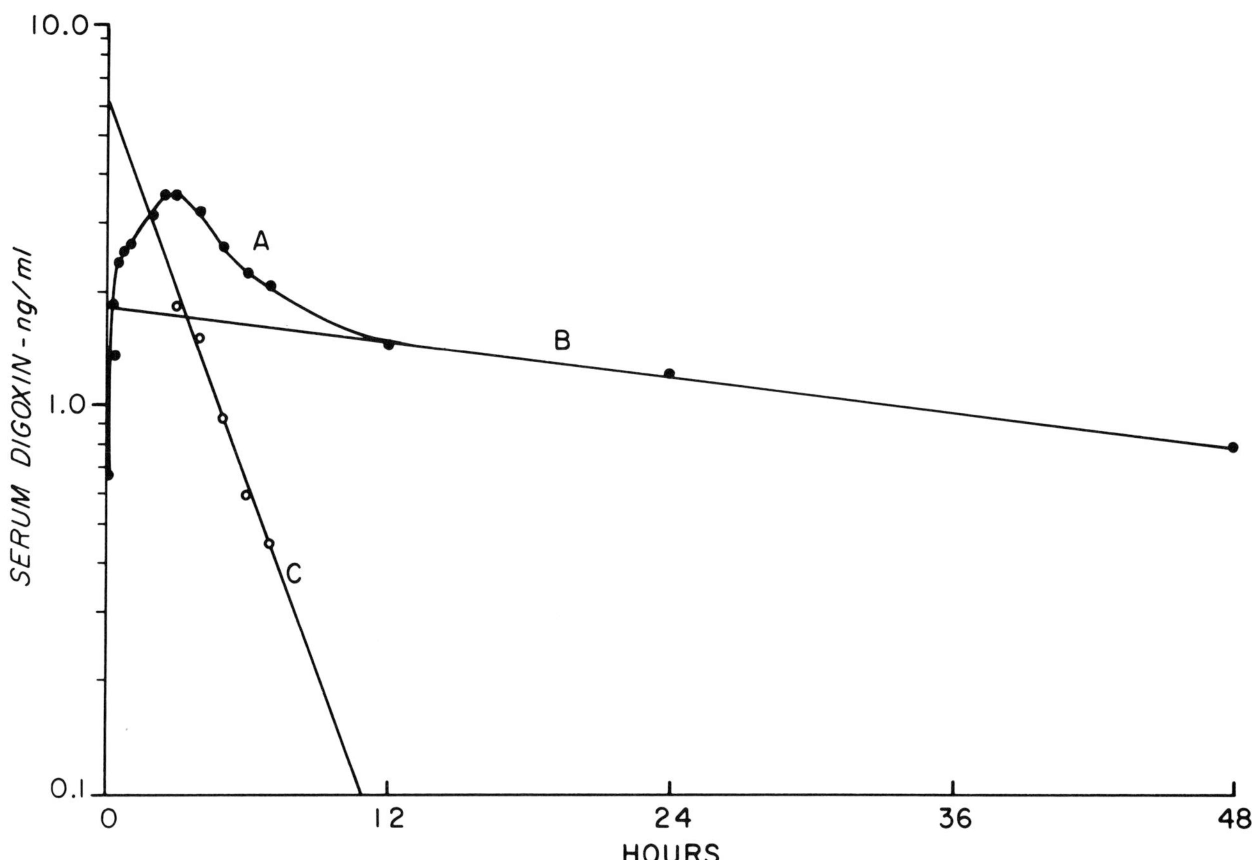

FIGURE 3 Composite (10 patients) serum concentration of digoxin after intramuscular administration. Plotted as described for Fig. 1 with serum concentration on the vertical axis and time on the horizontal. Lines *B* and *C* are derived as on the preceding figure as well. Note that when digoxin is given by the intramuscular route of administration, the peak serum level is later and lower than that by the oral route. The serum plateau is achieved only after about 10 to 12 h compared with 5 to 6 h by the oral route. The dominant half-life (line *B*) is 38 h, and line *C*, representing tissue distribution and binding, is 100 min. (*From J. E. Doherty and W. H. Perkins, Am. J. Cardiol., 15:170, 1965. Used with permission.*)

tion to the oral and intramuscular exponentials shown in the earlier figures) that represent serum distribution and reveal a half-life of 2 min. This rapid early exponential peak is not meaningful because of the variability of blood volume, injection time, cardiac output, and so forth. It is not indicated in Fig. 4 for these reasons.

The second exponential function represents tissue distribution and binding and has a half-life of 30 min, which is a much faster time than that following the oral or intramuscular routes. The third exponential function has a half-life of 33 h and represents metabolism and excretion of digoxin and is not significantly different from that observed after oral and intramuscular administration. Urine excretion in 7 days amounted to 75 percent of the administered dose. Unchanged digoxin was again demonstrated to be the principal excretory product, although small amounts of metabolites were present.[21]

The relative lack of metabolic breakdown of digoxin by the body is of interest because it is somewhat unusual in biologically active pharmaceutical products. This limited metabolic degradation of digoxin may be a product of the relatively short half-life of the compound and the fact that it is one of the major chloroform-soluble metabolic breakdown products of digitoxin, perhaps resisting further metabolism to some degree. The increased polarity of the compound (compared with digitoxin) also probably explains the large quantities of digoxin that are recovered unchanged in the urine.[21] Clark and Kalman[22] report recovery of dihydrodigoxigenin from the urine of a significant number of patients and volunteers. Luchi and Gruber[23] also document the finding of this relatively cardioinactive metabolite from the serum and urine of a patient with unusually large digoxin requirements. We have not identified this metabolite from any patient we studied, probably because it is relatively insoluble in

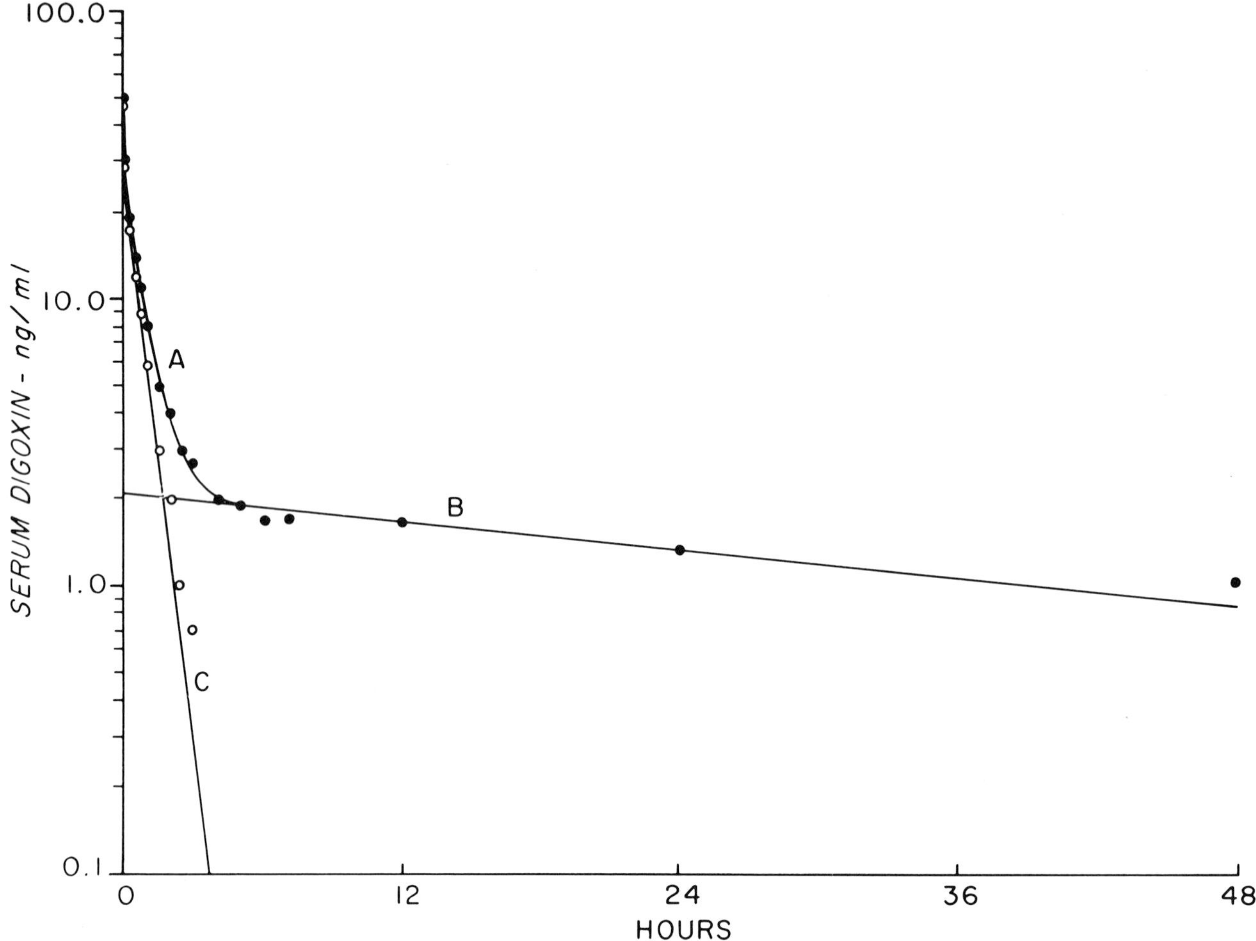

FIGURE 4 Composite (13 patients) serum concentration of digoxin after intravenous administration. The figure is plotted in the same way as Figs. 1 and 3. Note that high initial serum concentration follows intravenous use. A more rapid fall to the serum plateau is achieved than after oral or intramuscular use (note scale is different). Line *B*, the dominant half-life, is 33.1 h and again represents metabolism and excretion of digoxin. Line *C* represents tissue distribution and binding and has a half-life of 30 min (only the first 600 min of a 7-day study are shown). (*From J. E. Doherty and W. H. Perkins, Am. Heart J., 63:528, 1962. Used with permission.*)

chloroform, a prerequisite to extraction by our reported techniques.[24]

SERUM LEVELS AND DIGOXIN ASSAY

The mean dominant serum half-life for all the routes of administration was 34 h. Figure 2 illustrates the differences in the early portion of the digoxin turnover curves given by differenet routes of administration and the serum level of digoxin. The highest serum levels of digoxin are present after intravenous administration, followed by the intramuscular and then the oral route. Figure 2 also demonstrates the importance of the appropriate time for obtaining a serum sample for a serum digoxin level after administration of the drug by various routes. One must wait until the equilibration plateau is achieved to obtain a meaningful measure of that present in the myocardium. Thus one should wait 2 to 4 h after intravenous dose, 8 to 10 h after intramuscular dose, and 5 to 6 h after an oral dose to obtain samples for digoxin assay.

ABSORPTION

Absorption of digoxin was calculated using a formula adapted from one devised by Okita.[25] The formula combined the data noted earlier with that obtained from 6 patients studied with biliary fistula following cholecystectomy.[26] It was determined that digoxin in alcoholic solution, or alcoholic solution dried on a sucrose cube, was 80 to 85 percent absorbed by the gastrointestinal tract; 6.8 percent underwent an enterohepatic recycling. A later study[27] showed up to 10 percent absorption from the stomach. Figure 5 summarizes this data by means of a kinetic diagram showing the serum half-life ($T\frac{1}{2}$), absorption, enterohepatic recycling, and excretion of digoxin.

It should be appreciated that absorption of the tablet form of digoxin is slightly less than this, which approximates that of the elixir.[14] Digoxin from the tablet is 60 to 75 percent absorbed in its present manufactured form.

A new formulation of digoxin, more or less the elixir of digoxin used for infant dosage, has been incorporated into a gelatin capsule and has somewhat improved absorption over the tablet form.[16–18] I feel that there is little to be gained by the modest increase in absorption of this product. Generally, recommended doses will be about 15 to 20 percent smaller than conventional doses because of increased absorption. I suggest continued use of conventional digoxin (Lanoxin) until further experience is gained with this new product, should it be introduced.

EXCRETION

Seven-day excretion of tritiated digoxin by the several routes of administration are also shown in Figs. 2 and 5. Regardless of the route of administration, the major organ of excretion is the kidney—most digoxin being recovered as unchanged digoxin in the urine. The

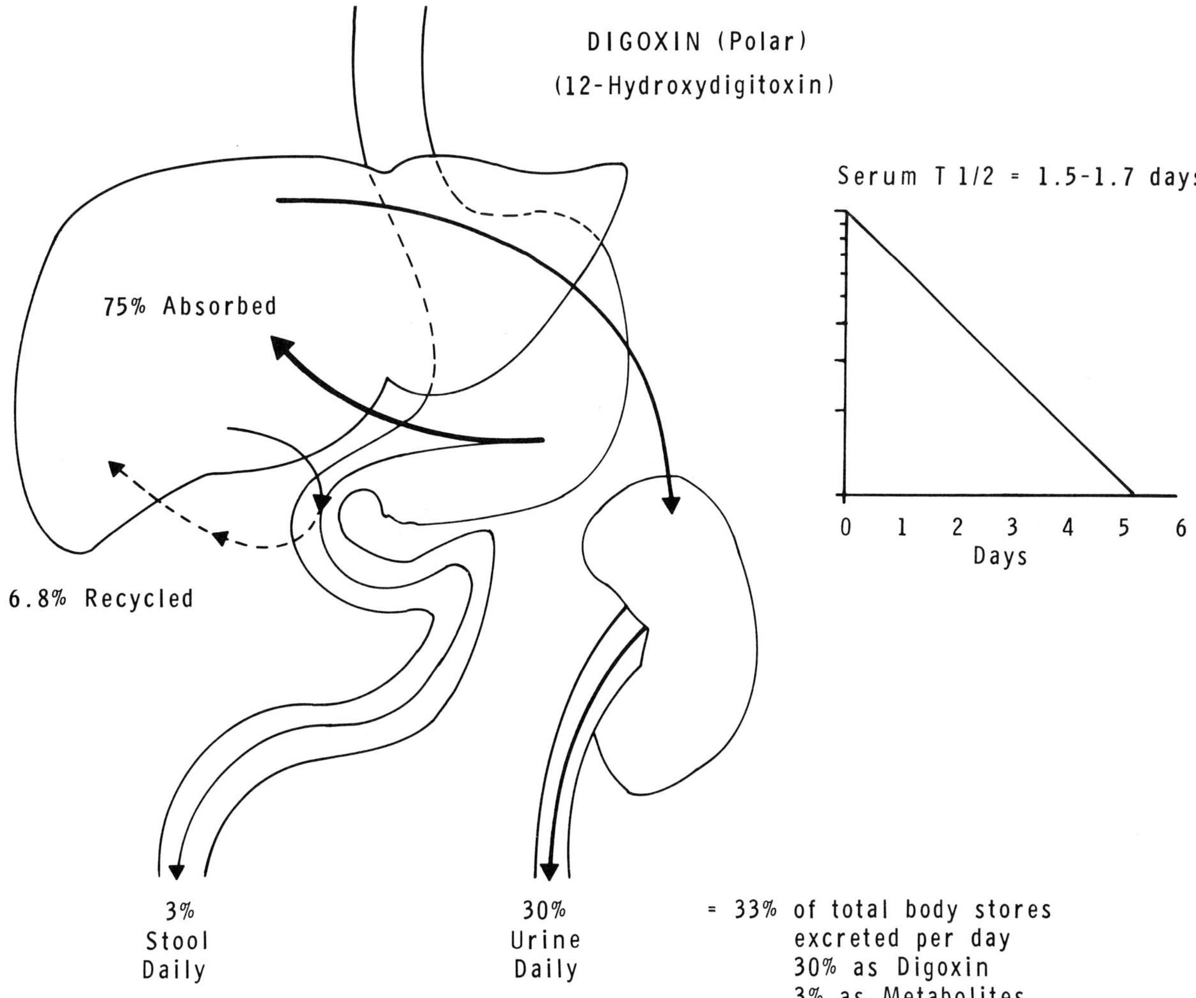

FIGURE 5 Kinetic diagram for digoxin. Diagrammatically shown are absorption, excretion, and metabolism of this glycoside under circumstances of congestive heart failure and relative normal renal and thyroid function and without electrolyte disturbances or hypoxia. (*From J. E. Doherty, W. H. Hall, M. L. Murphy, and O. W. Beard, Chest, 59:433, 1971. Used with permission.*)

larger amount present in the urine after intravenous administration is due to the fact that larger amounts are excreted in the first 24 h after the dose, when serum levels are highest following intravenous use. Between 10 and 20 percent may be recovered from the stool, depending on the route of administration, following a single-dose tracer label. More digoxin is recovered from the stool on maintenance therapy with digoxin.

Lanatoside C: Deslanoside

Lanatoside C is another derivative of the *Digitalis lanata* group (digoxin is the most frequently used one), and it still enjoys popularity, particularly for parenteral use.

ABSORPTION

Clinical studies of many years ago revealed very poor absorption of the drug when administered orally.[28] These were confirmed by radioisotope labeling studies,[29] which show lanatoside C to be only 10 to 40 percent absorbed by the oral route.

EXCRETION

There is very little protein binding (like digoxin) in this respect, and excretion appears to be mostly as deslanoside (80 percent) and its principal metabolite (digoxin), accounting for 17 percent in the urine.[29]

PHYSIOLOGIC HALF-LIFE

The dominant physiologic half-life of the drug determined by noninvasive systolic time intervals[30] is 36 h. Figure 6 illustrates the effect of injecting deslanoside intravenously, with the systolic time intervals expressed as the change in the ejection time index. Note that increasing doses (up to 1.6 mg) increased this physiologic measurement of pharmacologic effect. Because of the similar half-life, if one chooses initial intravenous digitalization with this glycoside, the better-absorbed digoxin may be substituted in usual maintenance doses without difficulty. This is well shown in Fig. 7.

Note that the rate of disappearance of the effect on the ejection time index is nearly identical to that of digoxin. The quabain and digitoxin physiologic half-lives are also shown in this figure and are plotted as previously described.

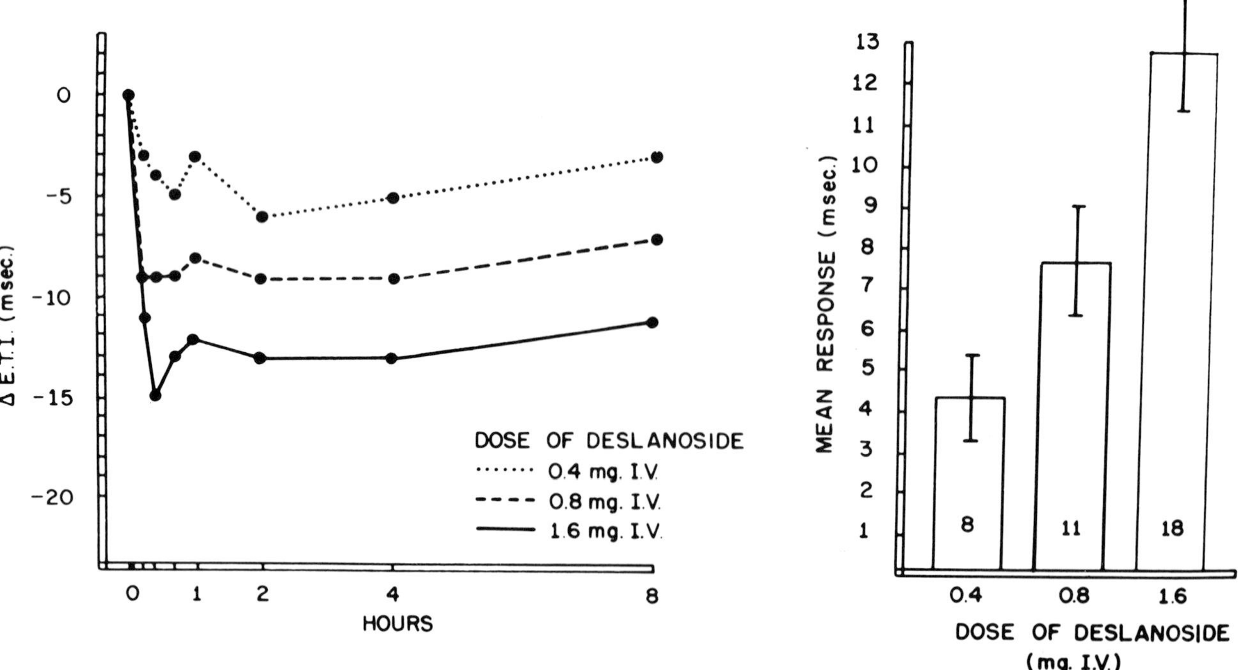

FIGURE 6 Effect of deslanoside C on the systolic time intervals. A loading dose was administered and ejection time index calculated thereafter. Note rapidity of onset of action after intravenous use. Note also that the dose-related response in small doses is effective in induction of intropic response. (*From A. M. Weissler, J. R. Snyder, C. D. Schoenfeld, and S. Cohen, Am. J. Cardiol., 17:768, 1966. Used with permission.*)

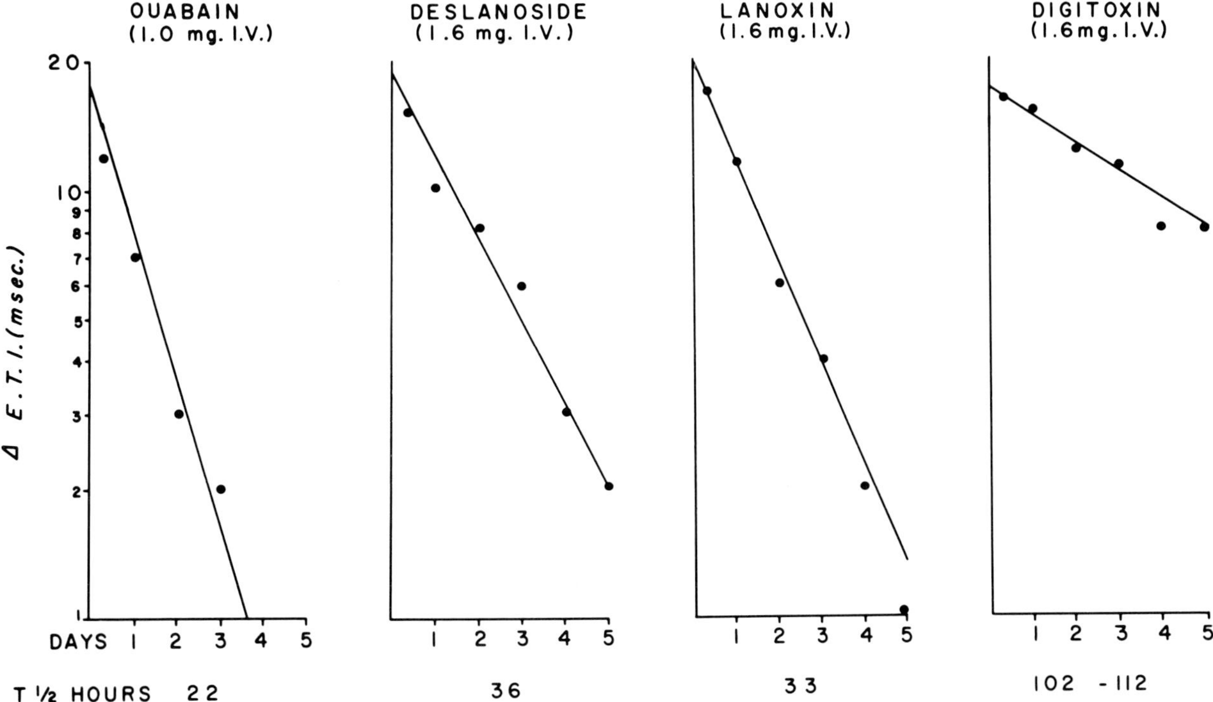

FIGURE 7 Physiologic half-life of ouabain, lanatoside C, digoxin, and digitoxin. The ejection time index is plotted vertically, time horizontally. The change in the ejection time index induced by these glycosides was observed as the drug was stopped and the disappearance of the effect was measured against time. The respective physiologic half-lives observed were ouabain, 22 h; lanatoside C, 36 h; digoxin, 33 h; and digitoxin, 102 to 112 h. (*From Weissler et al., Am. J. Cardiol., 17:768, 1966. Used with permission.*)

A kinetic diagram showing absorption, excretion, serum half-life, and metabolic disposition of deslanoside is presented in Fig. 8; it is self-explanatory and is plotted as in Fig. 5.

Digitoxin

Digitoxin is a purified glycoside, formerly the most popular glycoside, that has now given way to digoxin in the United States.

ABSORPTION

Digitoxin is found in both *Digitalis purpurea* and *lanata* and is available in all parts of the world. It is about 90 percent absorbed by oral routes of administration. Studies with radiocarbon-labeled digitoxin by Okita et al.[31,32] and those with tritiated digitoxin by Beermann et al.[33] supplement the clinical studies of Batterman et al.[28] and Lukas[34] in the definition of digitoxin metabolism.

After absorption from the stomach, duodenum, and proximal jejunum, digitoxin is avidly (90 to 97 percent) bound to serum albumin.[34–36] This property probably accounts for the higher blood levels of digitoxin, the latter being only about 20 percent protein-bound. Serum levels of digitoxin are usually 20 to 25 ng/ml in the well-digitalized patient.

Digitoxin is less preferentially distributed to tissue than digoxin[32,37] and is almost totally metabolized prior to excretion as cardioinactive metabolites. About 8 percent of the total dose is hydrolyzed to digoxin, however, and this, of course, follows the usual pattern of digoxin excretion. Table 2 illustrates the possibilities for metabolism and the interrelationships between digitoxin and digoxin. Both glycosides are inactivated through progressive loss of the sugar (digitoxose) portion of the molecule.

PHYSIOLOGIC HALF-LIFE

The physiologic half-life of digitoxin is shown in Fig. 6, as determined by Weissler[30] utilizing systolic time intervals. The figures for half-life obtained at 102 to 116 h are compatible with those of the therapeutic long-acting glycoside.[34]

EXCRETION

Excretion ultimately takes place by way of the kidney, by elimination in the urine of cardioinactive breakdown products of digitoxin. A smaller amount appears in the stool.[31] Although enterohepatic recycling of digitoxin is about 27 percent in the dog,[37] it has not yet been measured in human beings, but it may well approach this figure.

153

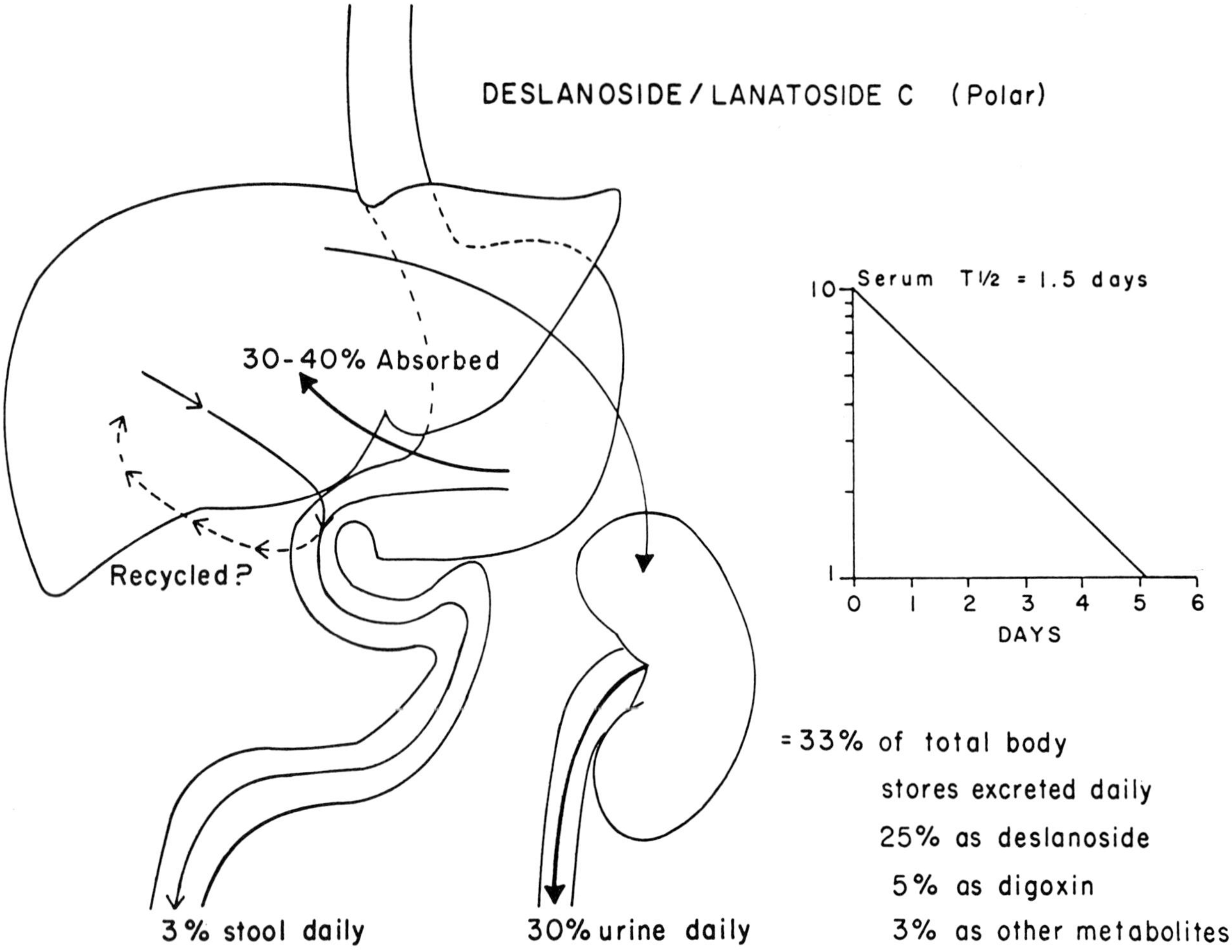

FIGURE 8 A kinetic diagram for lanatoside C (deslanoside). Depicted as the preceding diagrams for digoxin and digitoxin. Note the similarity to the kinetics of digoxin. (Digoxin is a major metabolite of lanatoside C). Poor absorption limits the oral use of this glycoside. One may digitalize parenterally with lanatoside C and begin maintenance with digoxin without "adjustment" if this is desired. (*From J. E. Doherty and J. J. Kane, Drugs, 6:182, 1973. Used with permission.*)

TABLE 2
Metabolities of digitalis

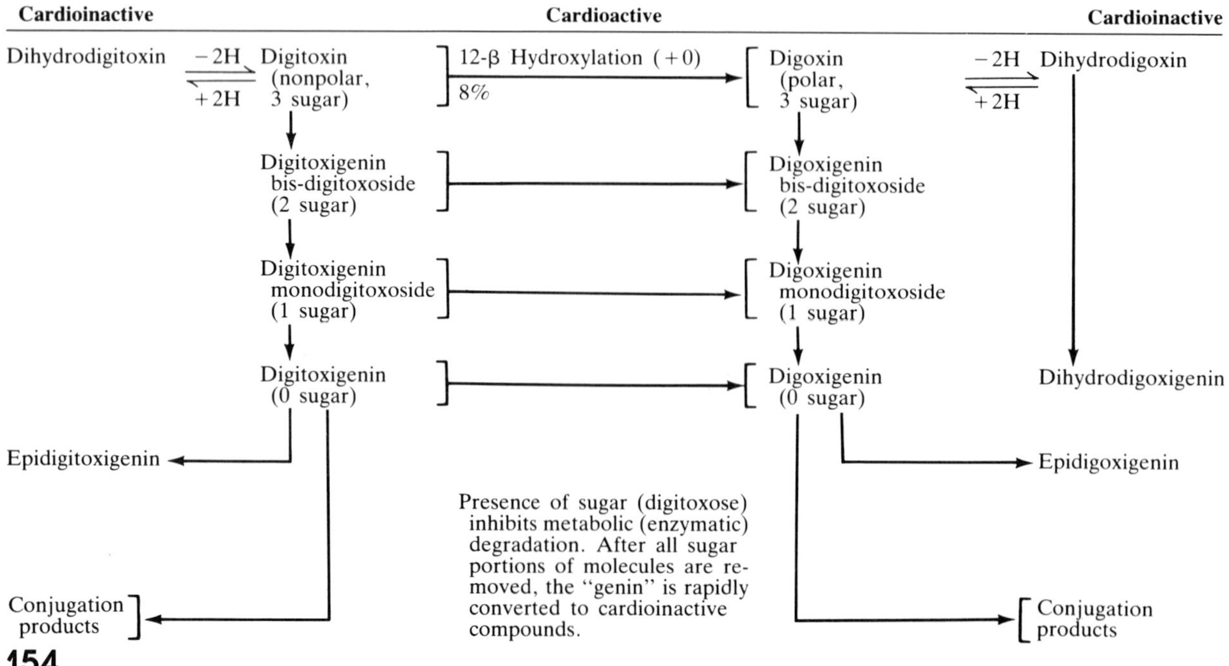

154

A kinetic diagram for digitoxin is shown in Fig. 9. Important features are nearly complete absorption and metabolic degradation for excretion. The long half-life of the drug (5 to 7 days) is well shown graphically.

Digitalis Leaf

The kinetics of digitalis leaf are not well defined because of the multiplicity of cardioactive ingredients present in the crude leaf preparation. The long duration of action appears to favor the principal glycoside of the leaf, digitoxin, as the most important determinant of its cardioactive properties. One should be very cautious about this conclusion, though, because glycoside content of the foxglove plant varies with local climatic conditions. Biological assay may yield consistent cardioactive content but also may yield variable duration of action because of the "mixed bag" of glycosides. Crude digitalis leaf is not recommended for this reason. Should an approximation of pharmacokinetics be desired, interchange with digitoxin is suggested, with the reservations outlined earlier being very important.

SPECIAL PROBLEMS WITH DIGITALIS TREATMENT
Renal Failure

Digoxin excretion is compromised by renal insufficiency. Digoxin is excreted primarily by the kidney in the urine,[38–40] and dosage must be reduced in the presence of renal failure.

Digitoxin, however, has been reported to be metabolized to 12-hydroxydigitoxin (digoxin) in renal insufficiency, and its overall half-life is not significantly changed, because the digoxin half-life is prolonged to near that of digitoxin in the presence of renal failure.[37] Lukas[34] believes digitoxin to be the best drug in renal failure because its half-life does not seem to change.

The most important determinant of the dominant half-life of digoxin is renal function, which is dependent on the functional integrity of both kidneys (Fig. 10). The best index of digoxin excretion is creatinine clearance, plotted in Fig. 11A against digoxin clearance. Although not completely unity, because of some tubular digoxin secretion, it is near enough to allow for reliable estimates of digoxin clearance.

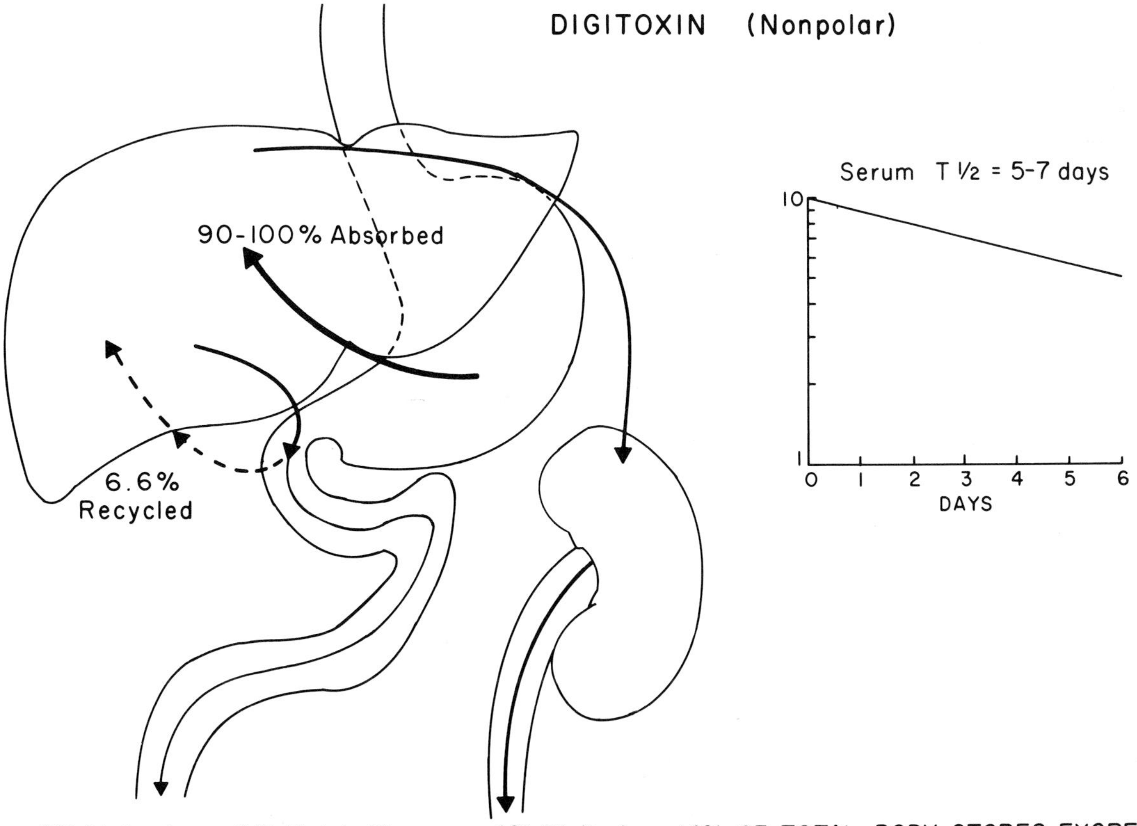

FIGURE 9 A kinetic diagram for digitoxin. Note the long half-life of 5 to 7 days and the extensive amount metabolized for ultimate excretion in the urine. (*From J. E. Doherty et al.: Chest, 59:433, 1971. Used with permission.*)

A more frequently determined index of renal functional capacity is the blook urea nitrogen (BUN) level. Figure 11B plots the BUN level against digoxin clearance in the same patients. Although the result is not as significant, it is reliable, particularly if prerenal azotemia is not present. The higher the BUN level, the less digoxin is cleared by the kidney. Generally, a BUN level of 50 mg per 100 ml should suggest a reassessment of digoxin dosage because of the reduction in excretion.

As peritoneal and hemodialysis have become an accepted and appropriate treatment in the management of renal failure and drug intoxication, the effect of dialysis on digoxin kinetics should be mentioned. Figure 12 illustrates a serum turnover study on a patient undergoing hemodialysis. Note the very modest clearance of digoxin across the artificial kidney and recovery of only 2 percent of the administered dose (0 time) in the dialysate bath.[41] Similar findings are present with peritoneal dialysis. Dialysis is not therefore an effective means for promoting excretion of digoxin and does not change dosage requirements of the drug, nor is it effective in management of digitalis toxicity.

Thyroid Disease

Differences in serum levels of digoxin have been noted in patients with thyroid disease, and an associated lack of therapeutic activity or toxicity has been observed.[42] Patients with myxedema have higher serum levels and patients with hyperthyroidism have lower serum levels of digoxin for comparable doses of the drug based on body weight. This is shown in Fig. 13 and is plotted in the same way as the previously shown serum turnover curves.

An appreciation of the renal plasma clearance of digoxin helps explain these differences (Fig. 14). Since there is no significant difference in the amount excreted in the two states, if the serum level is lower, such as in hyperthyroid patients, a higher rate of plasma clear-

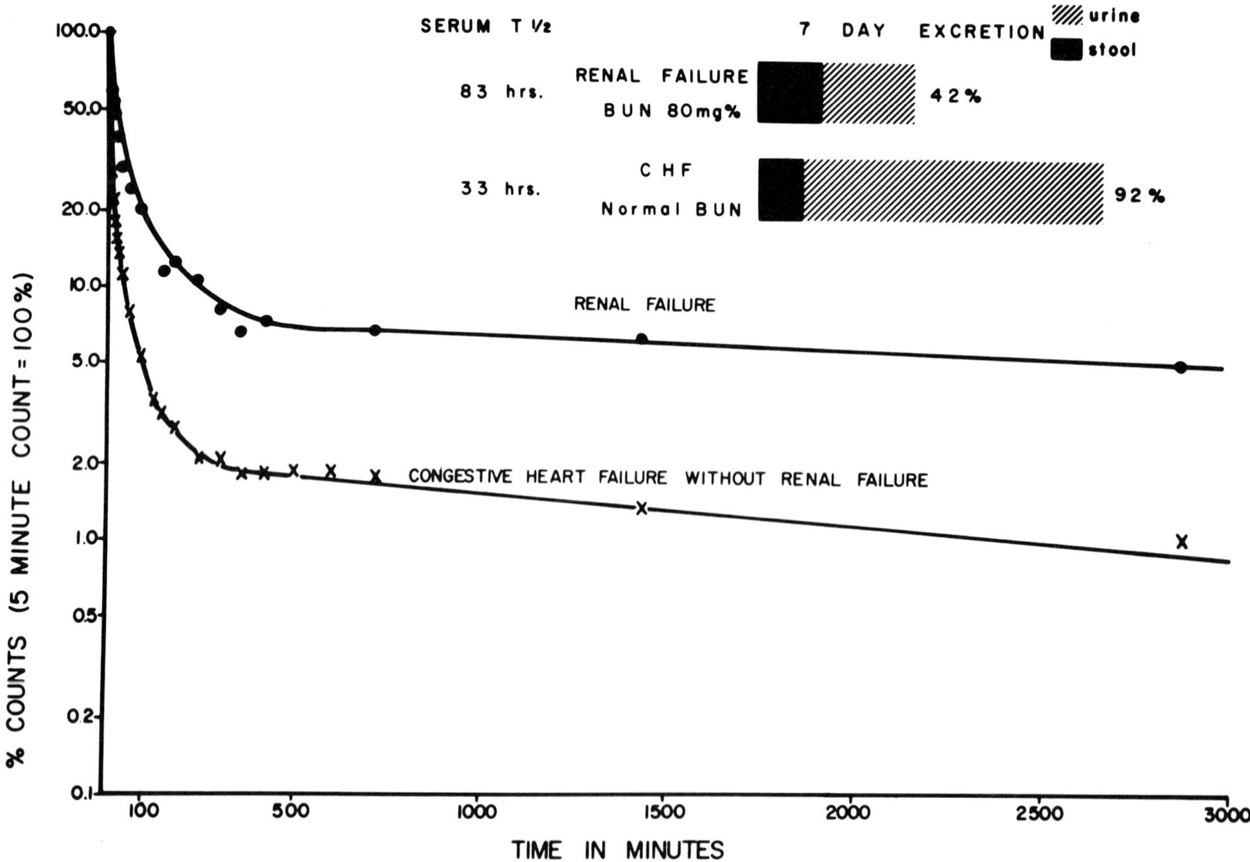

FIGURE 10 Comparative serum concentration and excretion of tritiated digoxin in patients with renal failure (●) and with congestive heart failure (CHF) and "normal" renal function (x). The serum concentration is plotted on the left vertical axis as a percentage of the 5-min specimen; time is shown on the horizontal semilogarithmic scale. Seven-day excretion is shown at upper right. Note the reduced digoxin excretion in patients with renal failure, together with higher serum levels and prolonged dominant half-life, in comparison with normal patients. BUN = blood urea nitrogen level. (*From J. E. Doherty, J. Arkansas Med. Soc., 66:121, 1969. Used with permission.*)

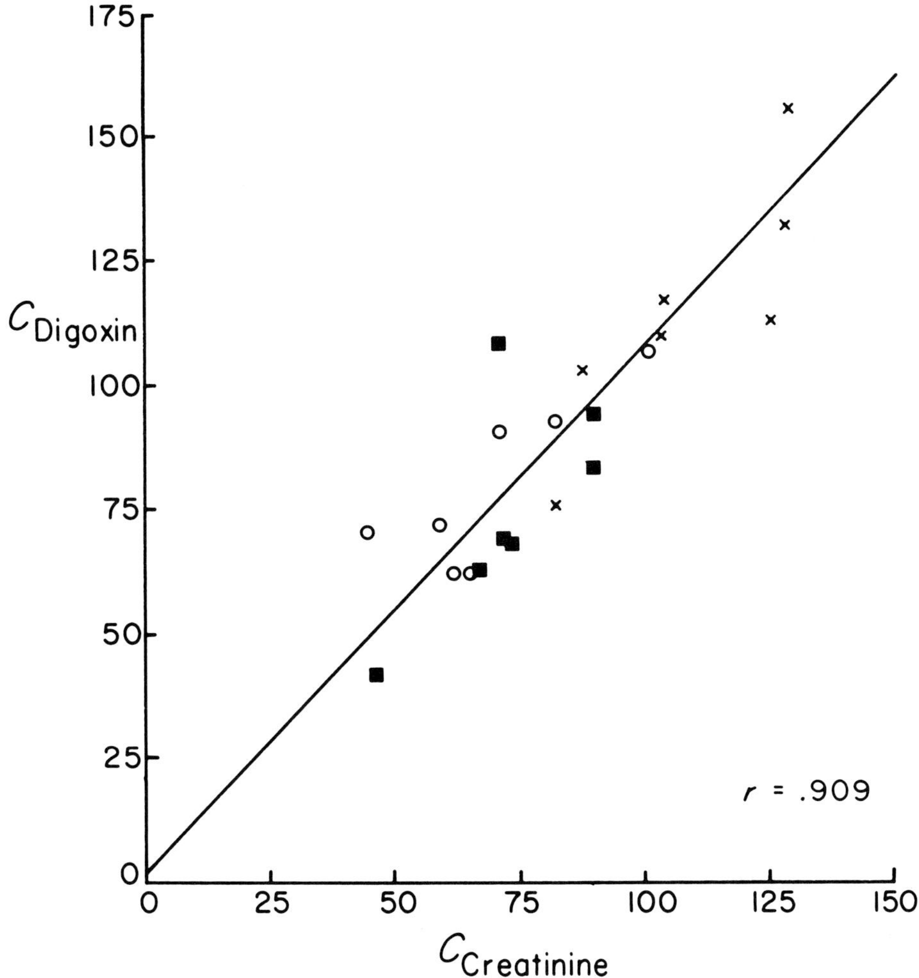

Fig. 11 A

FIGURE 11 (*A*) The relationship of creatinine clearance to digoxin clearance (in milliliters per minute) in donors before (x) and after (o) unilateral nephrectomy and in recipients (■) of these kidneys. The correlation coefficient, r = 0.909, is highly significant. Creatinine clearance is directly related to digoxin clearance. (*From J. E. Doherty, W. J. Flanigan, and G. V. Dalrymple, Am. J. Cardiol., 29:470, 1972. Used with permission.*) (*B*, p. 158) Relationship of the blood urea nitrogen (BUN) level to the clearance of digoxin. The BUN levels are plotted in milligrams per 100 ml on the vertical axis and the clearance of digoxin in milliliters per minute on the horizontal axis on a semilogarithmic scale. Note that the higher the BUN levels, the lower the digoxin clearance (*From J. E. Doherty, Ann. Intern. Med., 79:229, 1973. Used with permission.*)

ance is present (i.e., hypermetabolism). However, there is a lower rate of plasma clearance in myxoedema (i.e., hypometabolism), when serum levels are higher.

Elderly Patients

Ewy et al.[12] showed that digoxin tolerance and excretion were compromised in the elderly subject. This appeared to be related to two major factors: (1) modest diminution in digoxin renal clearance in the elderly, and (2) reduction in lean body mass in this group of patients. The dose of digoxin in the elderly should therefore be smaller than in younger patients.

Figure 15 illustrates the disposition of digoxin in a patient 5.5 h after being given 1.0 mg of tritium-labeled digoxin. A postmortem examination revealed digoxin in the tissues as shown. This demonstrates that although there is not a great deal of digoxin per gram of skeletal muscle, it constitutes 40 percent of body weight, and it is the major depot of digoxin in the human subject. Since lean body mass in the elderly consists of largely skeletal muscle and even this is reduced, this reservoir for digoxin in elderly patients is

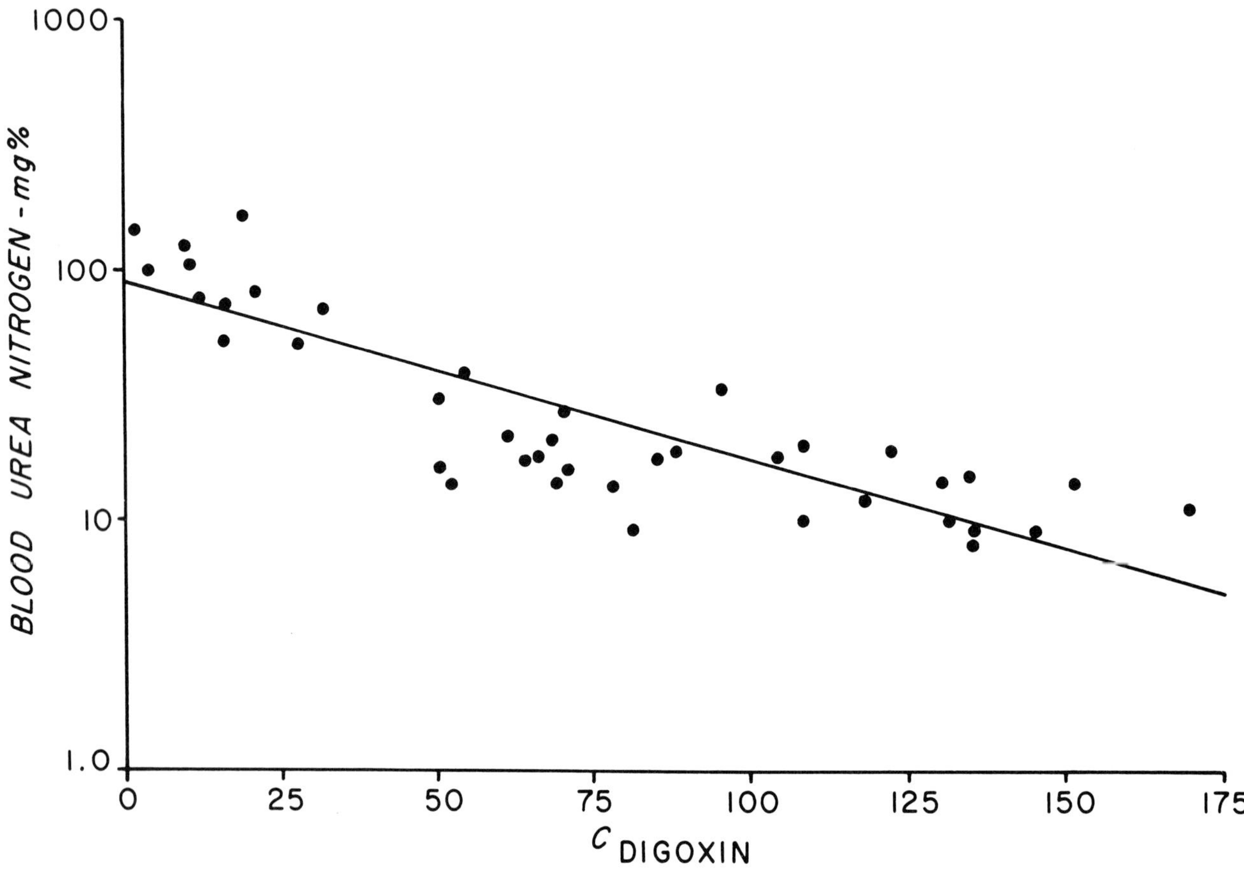

Fig. 11 B

contracted, which helps explain the need for reduced dosage.

Obese Patients

Obese patients require the same amount of digoxin to produce similar blood levels before and after weight reduction. Digoxin dosage in obesity should, therefore, be based on lean body weight and not on total body weight. In contrast to digoxin, which is water-soluble digitoxin is lipid-soluble, and its dosage may be assumed to be more closely related to total body weight in obesity.[43]

Pulmonary Heart Disease

Hypoxia appears to predispose to sensitivity to digitalis. Since there is no increase in serum levels of digitalis glycosides in the toxic patient with hypoxia, one must conclude that toxicity is related to changes in arterial blood gas tensions and pH. Control of the ventilatory dysfunction, then, appears of greater importance than digitalis dosage in this situation.

Figure 16 indicates appearance of digitalis toxicity in a patient with cor pulmonale after an intravenous dose of digoxin. The toxic arrhythmia was present with a normal serum level of digoxin.

It should be noted that immediately after receiving the bolus injection, the cardiac tissues are exposed to potentially toxic amounts of digoxin but require some time to accumulate enough of the drug to result in manifestations of toxicity. The half-life of early disappearance for intravenously administered digoxin is about 30 min,[21] so at 2 h, enough may have accumulated in this patient to account for the arrhythmia that was manifest.

This patient did receive a rather modest dose of digoxin, had normal excretion and slightly increased turnover time (half-life of 58 h), was only moderately hypercarbic and hypoxic, had normal electrolytes, and still manifested toxicity to digitalis. A modest degree of right-sided heart failure was present, and ST-T changes present on the electrocardiogram were of a nonspecific

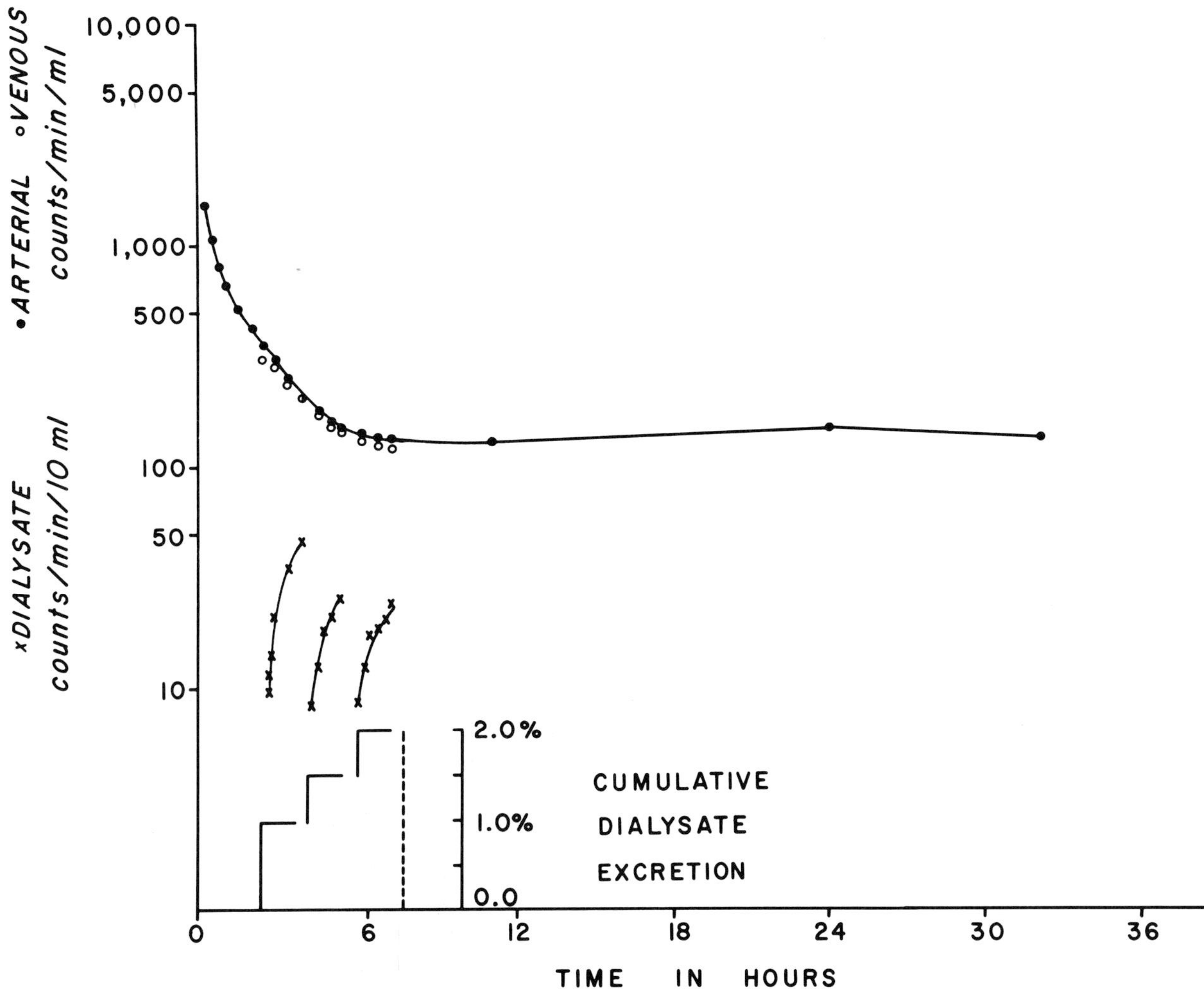

FIGURE 12 Serum levels and recovery of digoxin during hemodialysis. Digoxin concentration is plotted on the vertical axis, time on the horizontal. The arteriovenous difference during hemodialysis and dialysate concentration of digoxin in three exchanges are shown. Dialysate excretion is expressed as a percentage of the total administered dose. (*From G. L. Ackerman, J. E. Doherty, and W. J. Flanigan, Ann. Intern. Med., 68:718, 1967. Used with permission.*)

nature. The arrhythmia was not symptomatic and disappeared 2 h later without treatment.

Electrolyte Disturbances

The current use of effective and very powerful diuretics makes electrolyte disturbances an important area. Excretion of potassium, magnesium, and chloride are important determinants of digitalis action, particularly potassium. Because digitalis toxic arrhythmias may appear with hypokalemia (so common with diuretic therapy) at normal serum glycoside levels, potassium supplementation is advised for patients on daily diuretics. Potassium supplements should not be given when using the potassium "sparing" diuretics amiloride, triamterene, and spironolactone unless potassium is carefully monitored.

Myocardial Infarction

Morris et al.[44] showed that farm pigs were made digitalis toxic after experimentally induced myocardial infarction at 60 percent of the toxic dose before infarction. This information supports the concept of smaller (usually one-half) doses of digitalis in patients with recent infarction. The knowledge that even small amounts of the digitalis glycosides have beneficial inotropic effects is reassuring in this problem area for the administration of digitalis.

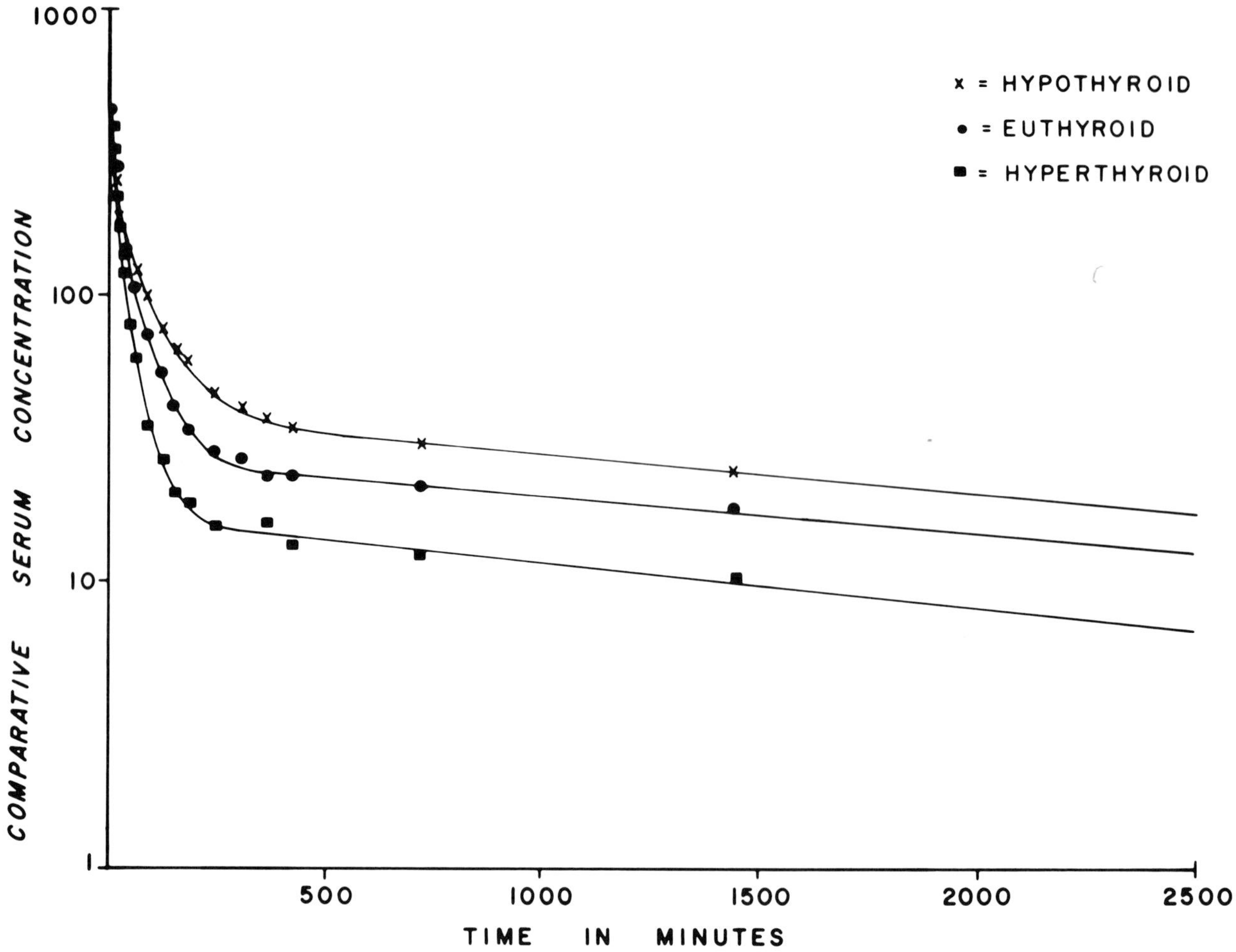

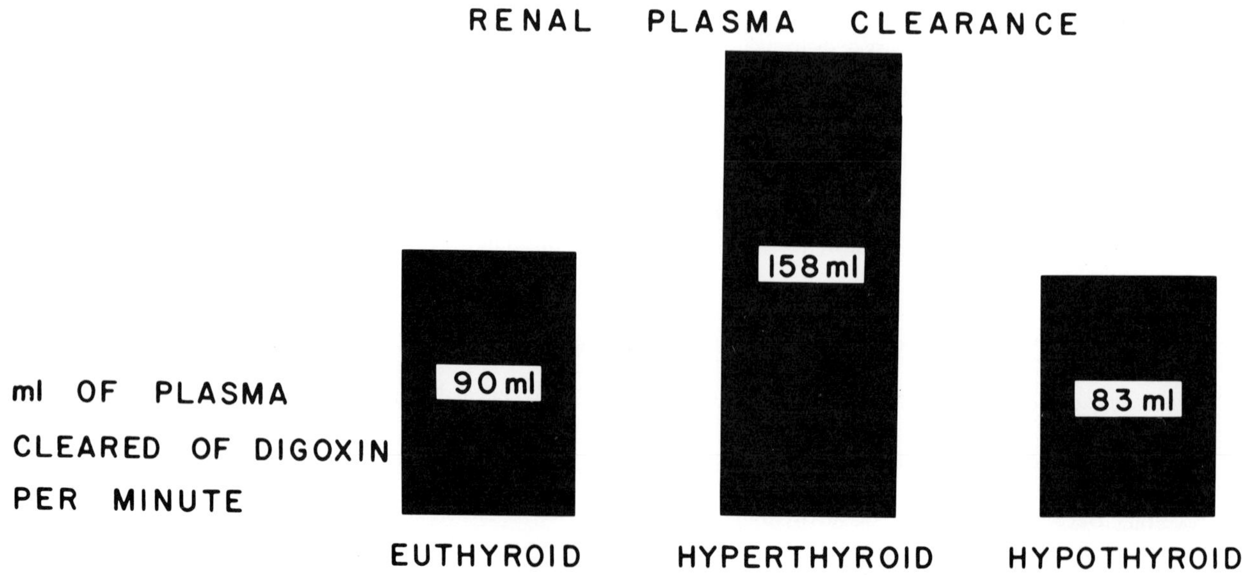

FIGURE 13 Digoxin serum turnover and thyroid disease. Comparative composite serum digoxin turnover in hyperthyroid (●), euthyroid (p), and hypothyroid (x) patients. The comparative serum concentration is plotted on a semilogarithmic scale on the vertical axis, time in minutes on the horizontal axis. Note that serum digoxin levels are highest in patients with myxoedema, intermediate in the euthyroid state, and lowest in hyperthyroidism. (*From J. E. Doherty and W. H. Perkins, Ann. Intern. Med., 64:489, 1966. Used with permission.*)

FIGURE 14 Renal plasma clearance of digoxin in euthyroid, hyperthyroid, and hypothyroid patients. Please consult text for explanation of these obvious differences. (*From J. E. Doherty and W. H. Perkins, Ann. Intern. Med., 64:489, 1966. Used with permission.*)

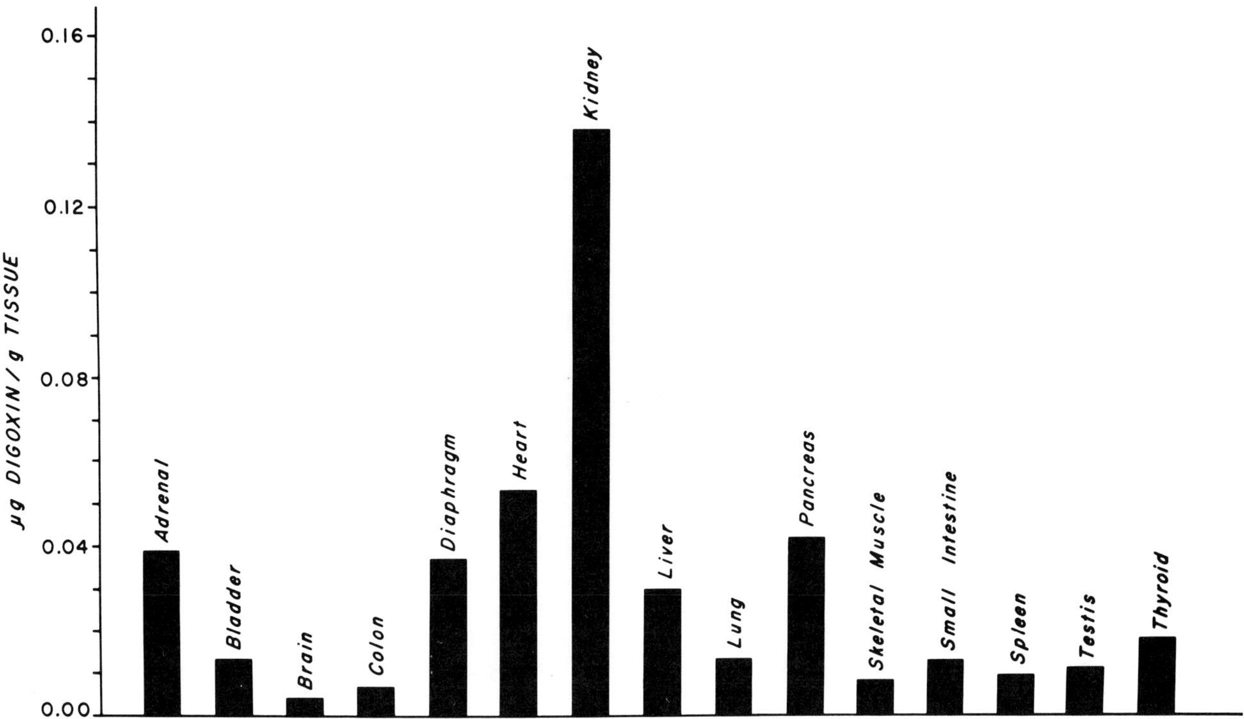

FIGURE 15 Tissue digoxin in a patient who received 1.0 mg of tritium-labeled digoxin 5.5 h before death. Note kidney concentration, the major organ of excretion, and that in heart, diaphragm, and liver. See text for comment regarding skeletal muscle. (*From J. E. Doherty, W. H. Perkins, and W. J. Flanigan, Ann. Intern. Med., 66:116, 1967. Used with permission.*)

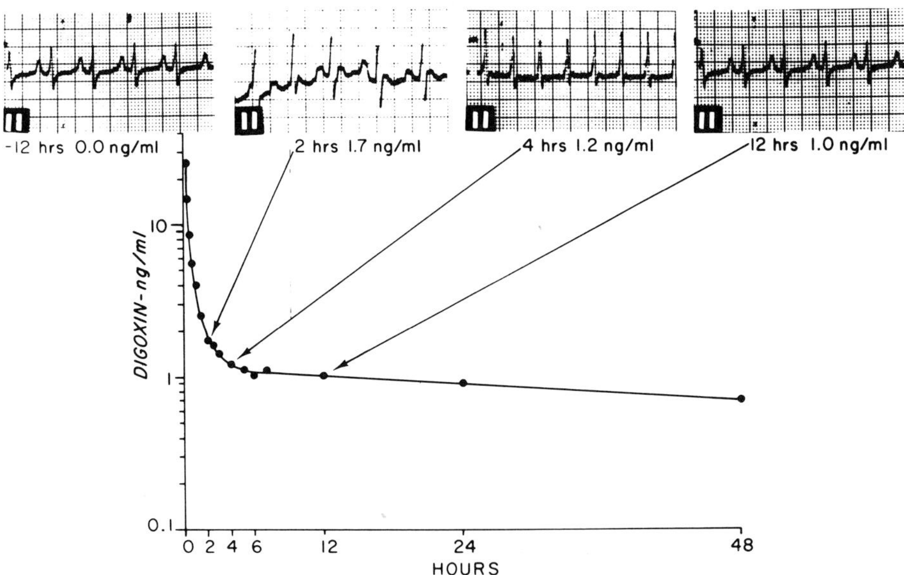

FIGURE 16 Tritiated digoxin serum turnover in cor pulmonale. Digoxin concentration in nanograms per milliliter on horizontal axis (logarithmic scale) and time in hours on the vertical axis. An intravenous dose of 0.75 mg tritiated digoxin was given at zero time, and concentration in the serum is plotted thereafter. PAT with block appeared at 2 h after drug was given at a serum concentration of 1.7 ng/ml and disappeared when a concentration of 1.2 ng/ml was present at 4 hours after the drug was given. Dominant serum half-life was 58 h (normal range is usually 17 to 48 h). Arrows indicate onset and offset of arrhythmia. (*From J. E. Doherty, et al., Drugs, 13:142, 1977. Used with permission.*)

DIGITALIS INTOXICATION

Most of the figures quoted regarding the incidence of digitalis toxicity catalogues hospitalized patients taking the drugs, a group more likely to be having therapeutic problems than outpatients. In the Little Rock Veterans Administration Medical Center, where there is a fairly large group of elderly patients, 26 percent of patients on medical service were taking digitalis and only 6 percent were deemed to be toxic using clinical findings and radioimmunoassay for serum levels. Even fewer patients are seen with toxicity in the outpatient clinics. These smaller figures represent the present trend toward lesser toxicity. This is felt to be a product of improved knowledge of indications for digitalis, smaller doses for digoxin, and appreciation of special situations that may predispose to toxicity. "Suspicion" is the watchword for prevention (Table 3).

Extracardiac Symptoms of Digitalis Intoxication

In a prospective study of digitalis intoxication, the incidence of gastrointestinal symptoms was found to be no different in the toxic patients compared with that in the nontoxic patients.[3] In 1969, a large-scale accidental intoxication of 179 patients occurred in Holland.[45] Fatigue was the most common noncardiac symptom described and was present in 95 percent of the 179 patients. Eighty-two percent expressed a feeling of muscular weakness and difficulty in walking and raising the arms. There were varying degrees of CNS disturbance in 65 percent of the patients, which included mental confusion, hallucinations, restlessness, insomnia, apathy, and drowsiness. Twelve patients (7 percent) had a transient but overt psychosis. Anorexia and nausea were present in about 80 percent, and abdominal pain was reported in 65 percent of the patients. Visual complaints were also very common. Hazy vi-

TABLE 3
Patients in whom digitalis toxicity should be suspected

   1 Any change in rhythm
   2 Presence of renal insufficiency
   3 Electrolyte disturbances
   4 Hypothyroidism
   5 Visual symptoms
   6 Elderly patients
   7 Headache
   8 Psychotic symptoms
   9 Pulmonary disease
   10 Recent myocardial infarction

SOURCE: From *J. Am. Med. Wom. Assoc.*, 33:191, 1978. Used with permission.

sion, difficulty in reading, and alteration of the color of objects was reported in 95 percent. Visual aberrations, such as photophobia, glittering, and seeing moving spots, balls, and various colored flames, were also distinctly common. All patients had difficulty in red-green perception.

The extremely high incidence of extracardiac symptoms in this group of patients occurred as a result of a dose of digitoxin given over a prolonged period that was three times higher than the usually prescribed dose. It should be emphasized that these gastrointestinal, central nervous system, and visual disturbances are helpful if present and elicited but do not always precede the more serious manifestations of digitalis toxicity, the cardiac arrhythmias.

Recent studies from our laboratories indicate there are significant concentrations of digoxin present in canine peripheral nervous tissue, particularly sympathetic ganglia.[46] The time course of accumulation of digoxin in the sympathetic nervous system suggests very early increases in these areas that, after some 10 days, tend to equilibrate with other areas. Increased sympathetic nerve traffic has been noted with digitalis administration. These findings support the hypothesis that some toxic (and perhaps inotropic) activity of digitalis may be neurally mediated.

Cardiac Digitalis Toxicity

Disorders of cardiac rhythm are often the first, and sometimes the only, manifestation of digitalis intoxication. Arrhythmias and conduction disturbances are present in up to 80 percent of patients who exhibit toxicity.[47] The probable mechanisms by which digitalis causes arrhythmias may be a result of alterations of impulse formation or conduction, or both. It should not be surprising that digitalis can cause almost every known arrhythmia, and it is quite common for one patient to demonstrate multiple arrhythmias.

To begin a discussion of digitalis-induced arrhythmias, it should be noted that there are several rhythms that are seldom associated with an excess of digitalis. These are Mobitz type II AV block, parasystole, multifocal atrial tachycardia, and atrial flutter or atrial fibrillation with a rapid ventricular response.[48–50] Although there are reports in the literature of each of these occurring with digitalis therapy, they are distinctly uncommon.

Digitalis-induced arrhythmias may be divided into three general categories: the ventricular arrhythmias, the supraventricular arrhythmias, and arrhythmias associated with disturbances of AV conduction or heart block.

Management of Digitalis Intoxication

An algorithm I have found useful in approaching the problems of decision when arrhythmias are encountered with the possibility of digitalis toxicity is reproduced in Fig. 17. This should assist in the early management of digitoxicity.

Many arrhythmias that occur as a result of digitalis intoxication can be managed effectively by stopping the drug. Discontinuing the digitalis preparation should be coupled with a reasonable period of monitoring to determine if there are arrhythmias present that require a specific therapy or intervention. Arrhythmias that should be treated or suppressed would include ventricular tachycardia, junctional tachycardia, or atrial tachycardia if rate is a problem; very frequent PVCs; and very slow rhythm. One must also evaluate factors that affect the excretion of the digitalis preparation, such as renal function, and look for other reversible conditions that might decrease the tolerance to digitalis, such as hypoxia or electrolyte or pH disturbances.

There is no ideal or specific drug for digitalis intoxication. Such a drug, if it existed, should have the following characteristics: it should increase sinoatrial rate by cholinergic blockade; ectopic atrial rhythms should be suppressed; reentrant rhythms, utilizing the AV node and ventricular tissue, should be abolished; and finally, the drug should decrease automaticity in the bundle of His and the Purkinje fibers.[48]

POTASSIUM

One reason that digitalis intoxication is said to have increased is the widespread use of powerful diuretics and the consequent production of hypokalemia in many patients. Potassium is one of the drugs for digitalis-induced arrhythmias characterized by disturbances in impulse formation.

Arrhythmias caused by alteration in conduction (heart block) should not be treated with potassium, because of the direct effect of potassium in slowing conduction through the myocardial and Purkinje tissue.[49,50] Digitalis and potassium have a synergistic

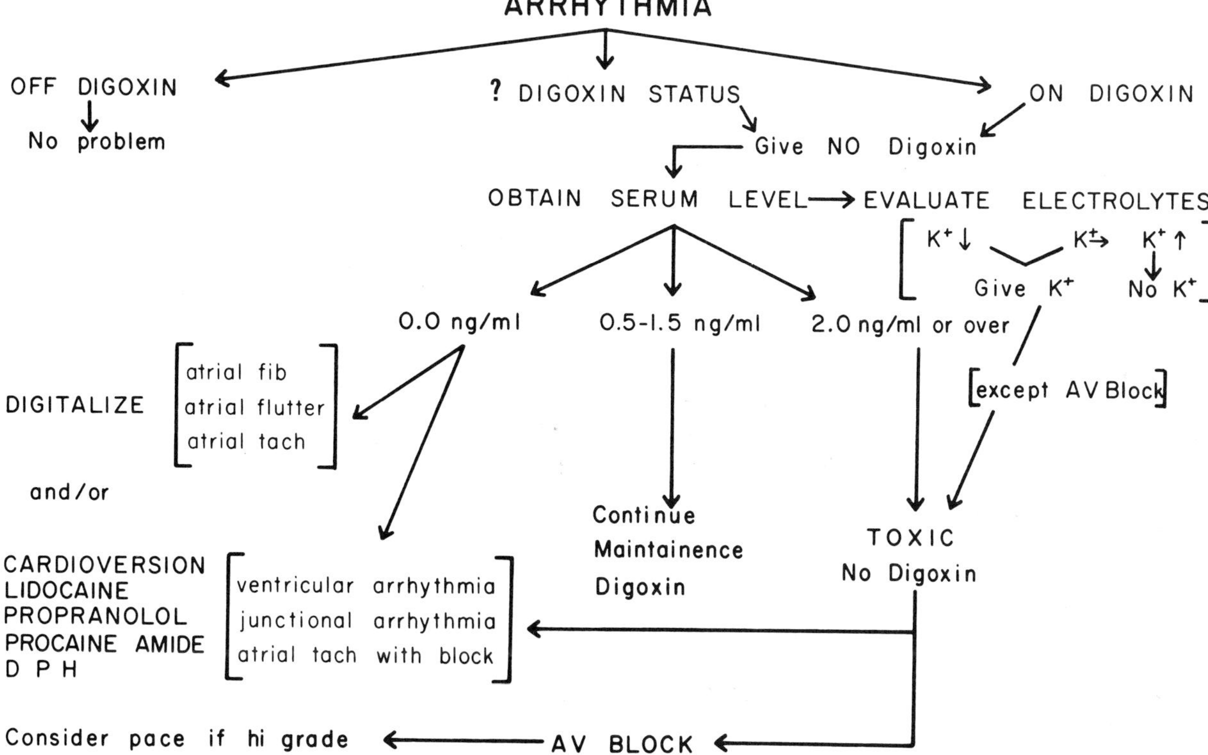

FIGURE 17 Algorithm for arrhythmia related to digoxin therapy. This is a guideline to management, and when used with clinical judgment, it can assist in management of arrhythmias related to digitalis intoxication through use of serum level measurements. (*From J. E. Doherty, Serum Digitalis Level—Practical Value, in E. Chung (ed.), "Controversy Cardiology," Springer-Verlag, New York, 1976, pp. 77–84. Used with permission.*)

effect in the depression of conduction, and giving K^+ in this circumstance could lead to a higher degree of block.

It should be noted that a normal serum potassium does not necessarily indicate a normal total-body potassium. In the presence of digitalis intoxication, potassium may be administered (cautiously), even in the face of normal serum values.

Potassium is effective in abolishing premature ventricular contractions and other ventricular arrhythmias caused by digitalis and may also be effective in the treatment of atrial tachycardia with block.[48] Besides AV block, an obvious contraindication to giving potassium is renal dysfunction with hyperkalemia or a tendency to retain potassium.

Potassium can be given orally or intravenously to treat digitalis toxicity. Oral doses of 20 to 40 mEq three to four times a day should reverse potassium deficit in most patients. This may be accompanied by epigastric pain or discomfort. If the patient is being monitored in the intensive care unit and having ventricular arrhythmias, then intravenous potassium chloride is the preferred route for initial potassium therapy. No more than 120 to 160 mEq of potassium chloride should be mixed in 1 liter of I.V. fluid. Amounts larger than this may be accompanied by marked pain and discomfort along the site of injection. It also has been recommended that potassium should not be infused through central venous lines because there is a theoretical risk of cardiac arrest. Most ventricular arrhythmias that will respond to potassium will do so after 40 mEq is given during the first hour or two. The plasma potassium should be monitored frequently during this initial phase of potassium replacement.

A recent observation of importance when giving potassium intravenously is that extracellular potassium levels may be decreased by intravenous glucose.[48] This occurs because glucose drives potassium into the cell. This could theoretically increase digitalis sensitivity and worsen the arrhythmia. Potassium, therefore, should be given in normal or one-half normal saline. Again, it should be pointed out that potassium should not be given if disturbances of conduction or heart block are present. A saline load should be avoided, of course, if heart failure is a problem.

LIDOCAINE

Lidocaine is now considered to be the current drug of choice for control of ventricular arrhythmia secondary to digitalis intoxication. It is more effective than either procainamide or quinidine and does not affect conduction in the AV node or cause significant depression of myocardial function. Lidocaine is, however, not as effective in abolishing the junctional tachycardias associated with digitalis.

If lidocaine is used, it should be administered in bolus doses of 50 to 100 mg intravenously, depending on the urgency of the ventricular arrhythmia, and then a therapeutic blood level should be maintained with a 2 to 4 mg/min I.V. drip. The great advantage of lidocaine over other antiarrhythmic drugs is its short duration of action. In the event that the arrhythmia worsens, then the pharmacologic effect of any lidocaine administered will be dissipated within 15 to 20 min. By the same token, the short half-life means continuing administration of the drug to maintain blood levels in an effective range.

PHENYTOIN

Phenytoin (diphenylhydantoin) is similar to lidocaine in its effect on the action potential and cardiac tissue. Although there are reports of myocardial depression secondary to intravenous doses of the drug, this effect is probably less pronounced and more transient than that of quinidine or procainamide. Phenytoin is particularly useful for ventricular arrhythmias caused by digitalis.

If phenytoin is used, it should be given initially intravenously in a loading dose of 50 mg/min to a total dose of 5 mg per kilogram of body weight. At this point, if a beneficial effect is seen, the patient may be started on 100 mg orally every 4 to 6 h. It should be remembered when giving phenytoin intravenously that its diluent will not mix with any other intravenous fluids and must be injected directly. Once the arrhythmia ceases to be a problem (usually 1 to 2 days after digoxin is discontinued, provided renal function is normal), then the oral phenytoin may be discontinued.

QUINIDINE, PROCAINAMIDE, AND DISOPYRAMIDE

Although these drugs will abolish ventricular arrhythmia secondary to digitalis, and also may be effective in treating atrial tachycardia, their own toxic effects make them less desirable as a treatment for digitalis intoxication. For example, these drugs may cause a worsening of AV block, severe depression of the sinoatrial node, and depression of conduction in the His and Purkinje systems. They also have an adverse effect on myocardial contractility, although usually minor in clinically used doses unless overt heart failure is present. The digoxin-quinidine interaction must also be considered. This will be discussed in depth later.

PROPRANOLOL, METAPROLOL, NADOLOL, AND ACEBUTOLOL (BETA BLOCKERS)

Although highly effective in abolishing both atrial tachycardia with block and ventricular arrhythmias induced by digitalis, the undesirable side effects of these drugs make their use hazardous in this setting. Asystole after intravenous injection in the treatment of digitalis arrhythmia is a significant problem.[48] Another difficulty is a depression of myocardial contractility. This is due to both the beta-adrenergic receptor blocking activity of propranolol (and the other beta blockers) and a direct myocardial depressant action. Since most patients on digitalis have an impaired hemodynamic status to begin with, the chance of worsening heart failure with propranolol makes this drug of doubtful value in the treatment of digitalis-induced arrhythmias.[51] However, I have seen little beta blocker–induced heart failure.

BRETYLIUM TOSYLATE

Bretylium tosylate has no role in digitalis toxicity. Bretylium causes increased automaticity (phase 4 depolarization) similar to digitalis, and together their effects may be additive and arrhythmogenic.

ANTIDIGOXIN ANTIBODIES

The development of antidigoxin antibodies for use in radioimmunoassay immediately suggests the use of these antibodies to counteract and control digitalis intoxication owing to the drug.[52,53] Although still experimental and only available for life-threatening toxicity, antidigoxin antibodies in the form of a FAB fragment of the original antibody molecule have been shown to be effective in reversing digitalis intoxication owing to both digoxin and digitoxin[54] and may ultimately gain more widespread application for toxicity. The use of the FAB fragment results in an antibody digoxin complex that is small enough to allow for almost immediate renal excretion and mobilization of depot digoxin from tissue, and it is without cardioactive properties. Although a rigid experimental protocol must be followed, antibodies for truly life-threatening toxicity are available from our laboratory in Little Rock (and from Dr. Thomas W. Smith, Brigham and Women's Hospital, Boston, Mass.).

ELECTRICAL THERAPY

Cardioversion Since serious ventricular arrhythmias may occur following dc countershock with normal doses of digitalis, most clinicians prefer to use medical management for the tachyarrhythmias induced by digitalis. Obviously, if medical management fails and/or the vital signs are unstable because of the tachyarrhythmia, cardioversion is indicated and never withheld for fear of "further toxicity."

Pacing The indication for temporary transvenous pacing in digitalis intoxication is that of slow heart rate that has produced hemodynamic change. Additionally, pacing is indicated for control of ventricular arrhythmia when it is felt that an increase in the basic heart rate will suppress the ventricular arrhythmia. Since refractoriness of the AV node is produced by digitalis, ventricular pacing is preferred.

Prevention of Digitalis Intoxication
DOSAGE

The primary considerations in the prevention of digitalis intoxication involve the selection of a lower maintenance dose and a maintenance dose that is compatible with the patient's renal function and lean body weight.

Marcus[55] has shown that it is not necessary to give a loading dose of digitalis in order to obtain therapeutic serum levels and concludes that the usual loading dose may be accompanied by a higher incidence of intoxication. Thus, in most circumstances, it is advisable to begin the patient on a maintenance dose knowing that within 6 days or so, a stable blood and tissue concentration will be reached (Fig. 18). Measurement of the serum levels to assess the adequacy of a maintenance dose is possible and helpful in many circumstances, even though results vary between laboratories and rigid quality control is needed to measure billionths of a gram, a factor seldom considered today in most laboratories.

SERUM LEVELS

In 100 patients on digoxin studies in our laboratory, there was a significant difference ($p = 0.0005$) in serum levels of patients who manifested toxicity compared with those who did not (Fig. 19). The optimal serum concentration appears to range between 0.5 and 2.5 ng/ml. Levels over 3.0 ng/ml almost always represent toxicity. These figures are slightly different from those quoted by most laboratories. Monitoring your own area is recommended. Rigid laboratory standards must be maintained if accurate results are to be attained.

SALIVARY ELECTROLYTES

Salivary electrolyte determinations have been suggested as a method of detecting or monitoring for

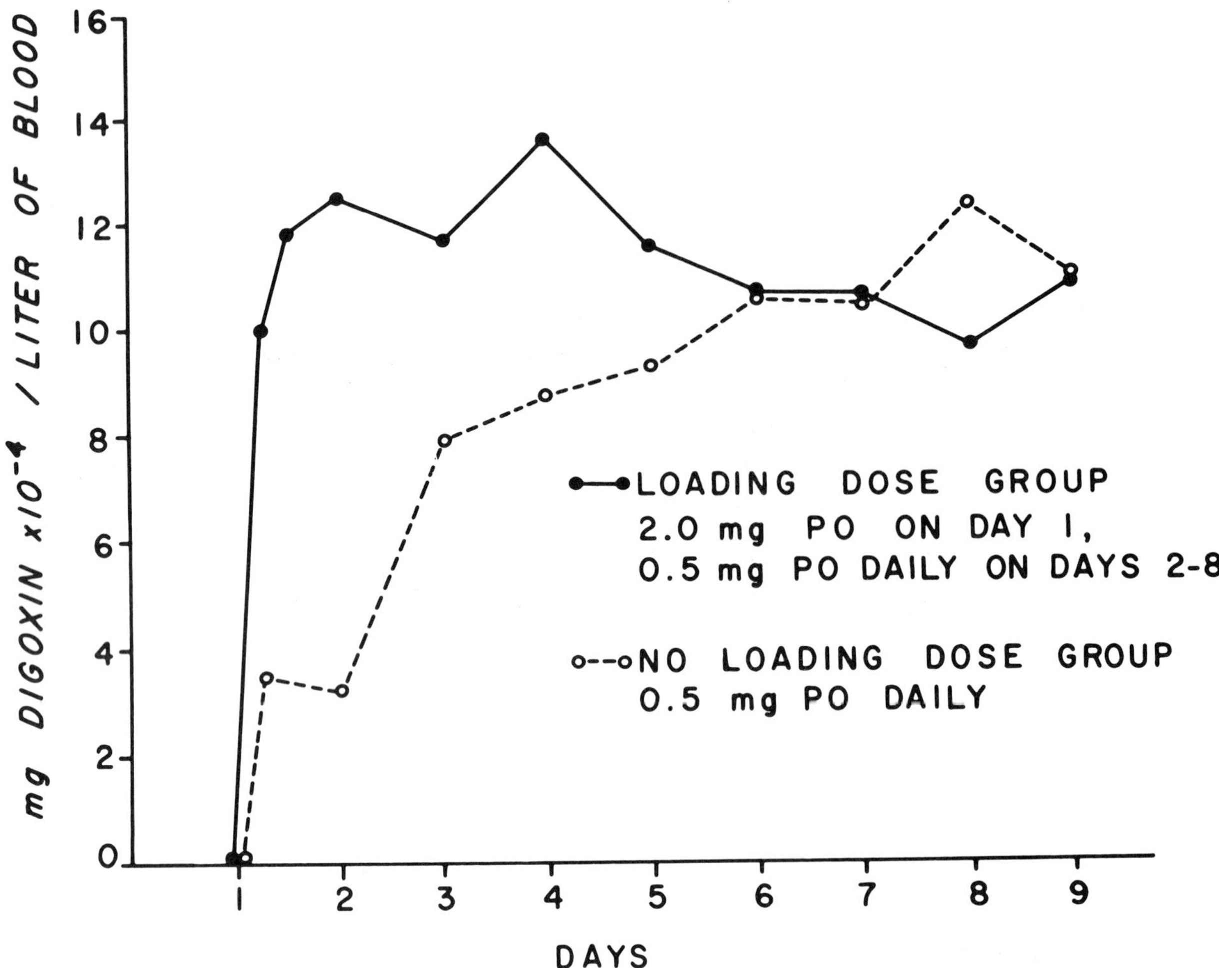

FIGURE 18 Digitalization without a loading dose. Serum concentration of digoxin is plotted on the vertical axis, time on the horizontal. Closed (•) represents patients given 2.0 mg of tritiated digoxin in a single loading dose orally with resulting blood levels. Open circles (o) represent the same patients given 0.5 mg of tritiated digoxin daily for 9 days. Note similar blood level of digoxin at sixth day. (*From Marcus, F. I., Burkhalter, L., Cuccia, C., et al.: Circulation, 34:865, 1966. Used with permission.*)

digitalis toxicity.[56,57] However, studies by Gould[58] and myself[59] do not indicate significant correlation of digitalis intoxication with the potassium and calcium salivary product described by Wotman (Fig. 20). We do not recommend salivary electrolyte determinations to monitor for or confirm the presence of digitalis toxicity.

POTASSIUM SUPPLEMENTATION

Routine replacement of potassium washed out with potent diuretics is an important consideration in the prevention of intoxication. Serum potassium should be monitored, and replacement of excessive losses in the urine is recommended.

DRUG INTERACTIONS WITH DIGITALIS GLYCOSIDES

Drug interactions have received the increasing attention of the medical profession, and those relating to the digitalis glycosides need to be placed in perspective.

I have chosen to divide drug interactions into those which are desirable and those which are undesirable.[60] It appears that most observers tend to create the impression that all interactions are undesirable and harmful. This is not the case.

Desirable Interactions of Other Drugs with Digitalis Glycosides

ANTIARRHYTHMIC AGENTS

Both of Hoffman's group I (propranolol, quinidine, procainamide, disopyramide, bretylium) and group II (phenytoin and lidocaine) tend to increase the negative resting potential of transmembrane action potential on phase 4 in the myocardial cell.[61] This effect is in opposition to that of digitalis, which tends to create and perpetuate arrhythmias, i.e., tends to decrease phase 4 resting potential, thereby bringing this potential closer to threshold and the establishment of automatic rhythms, particularly in the Purkinje fibers.[62] This is a desirable interaction and explains the effective use of

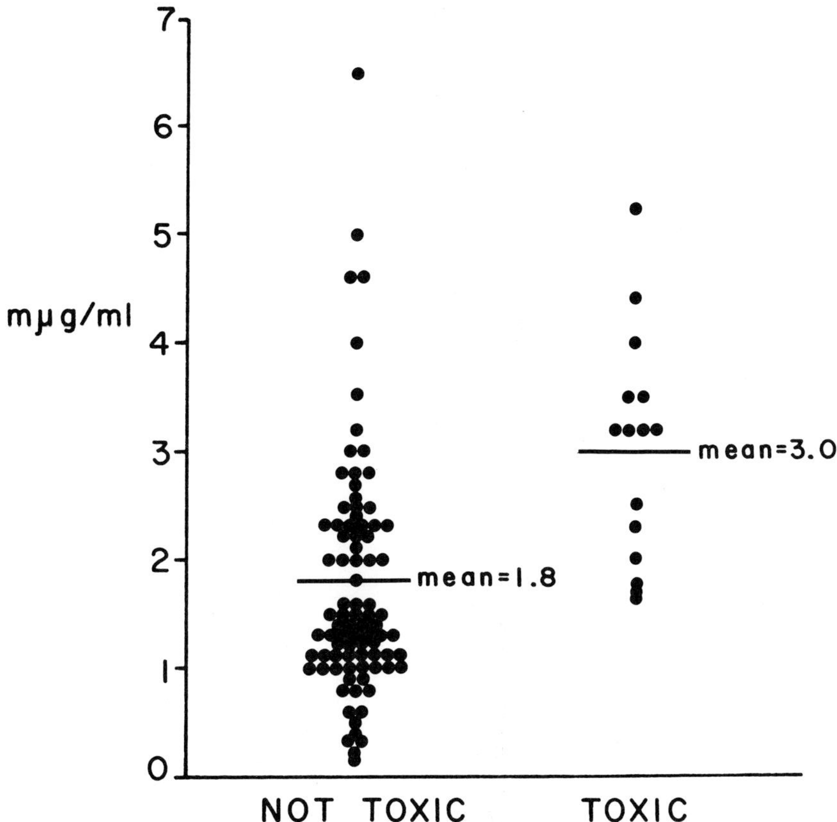

FIGURE 19 One hundred consecutive digoxin blood levels. Difference between groups is highly significant ($p < 0.0005$), but there is considerable overlap. (*From J. E. Doherty, Ann. Intern. Med., 79:299, 1973. Used with permission.*)

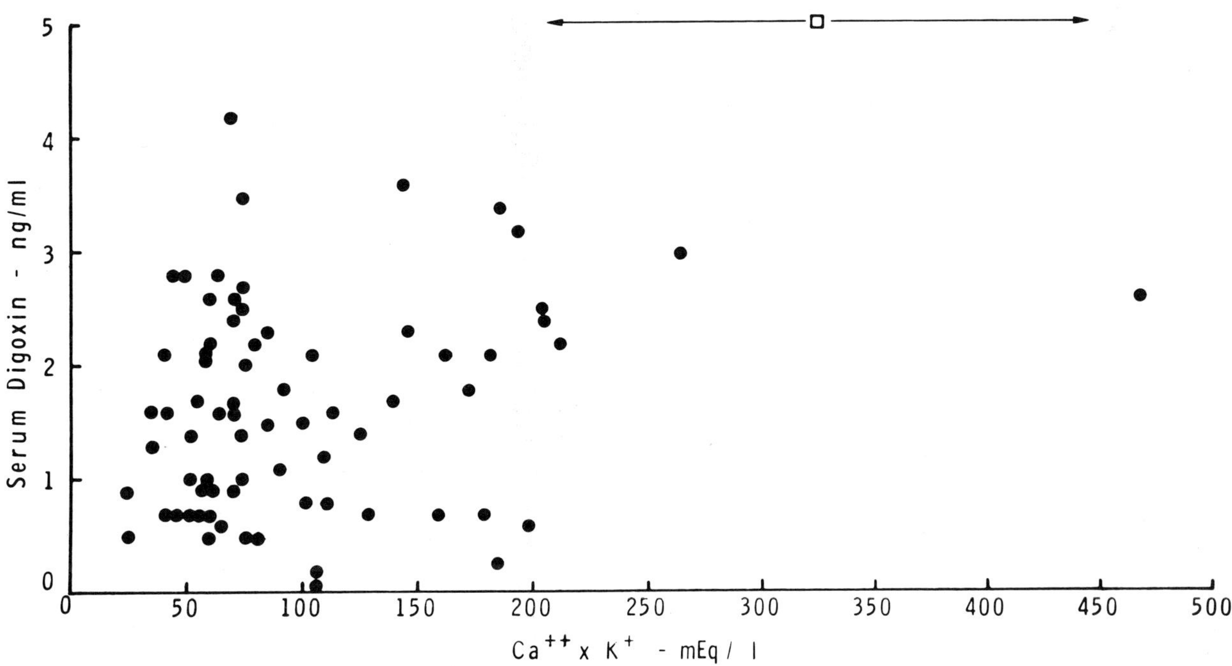

FIGURE 20 Relationship of the salivary electrolytes (calcium $\times$ potassium milliequivalents per liter of product) to serum levels of digoxin in 79 patients. The open square bounded by arrows indicates the mean and the range of patients described by Wotman as toxic. No correlation with serum level of digoxin by radioimmunoassay is apparent. (*From J. E. Doherty, J.A.M.A., 226:1228, 1973. Used with permission.*)

these agents in digitalis-induced arrhythmia. An exception to this rule for the group I agents is bretylium tosolate. It increases spontaneous phase 4 depolarization and thus should not be used when digitalis is "on board."[63]

In addition, digitalis glycosides tend to favor development of reentrant rhythms by reducing the effective refractory period. This effect is reversed by the group I drugs (procainamide, disopyrimide, and propranolol), and these agents are effective in management of such digitalis-induced rhythms through this mechanism.

The group II antiarrhythmic drugs (lidocaine and phenytoin) are also effective against the reentrant rhythms but through an opposite effect. These agents may enhance conduction through an area affected by unidirectional block through further shortening of the action potential duration and effective refractory period and prevent reentry in this fashion.[62]

BETA-ADRENERGIC RECEPTOR STIMULATING DRUGS

A few drugs that have beta-adrenergic receptor stimulator properties may enhance or increase inotropic response with digitalis. These are isoepinephrine, norepinephrine, and epinephrine. Norepinephrine and epinephrine are also alpha-adrenergic receptor stimulators and may increase heart work through vasoconstriction more than any effect they have on contractile performance. They may also induce arrhythmias. Isopropylepinephrine causes an increase in heart rate as well as having a profound inotropic effect that adds to digitalis. It, too, may provoke arrhythmia. Glucagon, dopamine, and dobutamine also have positive inotropic effects that may be additive to that of digitalis.

Undesirable Drug Interactions with Digitalis

ANTIARRHYTHMIC DRUGS

The drugs in the antiarrhythmic group have another undesirable property as well—that of a negative inotropic effect. This effect is generally minor in usual clinical doses for all these agents except propranolol, in which its pronounced beta-adrenergic receptor blocking effects may overcome the positive inotropic effect of the digitalis glycosides and result in a serious problem with the increasing heart failure. The group I drugs (quinidine, procainamide, and propranolol) also

produce AV block, which may be additive, particularly in large doses, to that induced by digitalis.

In addition, quinidine is included in this group because of the recently noted digoxin-quinidine interaction.[64–68] Gold et al.[69] cautioned against use of quinidine and digitalis years ago, and current data seem to bear out this observation.

When quinidine is added to digoxin as a therapeutic maneuver, the serum digoxin level rises two to three times in a dose-related fashion[70] and falls when digoxin is discontinued. About 90 percent of patients experience this phenomenon, and about 50 percent of these may experience adverse effects, often gastrointestinal. Some patients have developed what appears to be cardiotoxicity with ectopic rhythms, and so forth.

We developed a canine model to study this phenomenon and found digoxin levels increased in brain tissue with concomitant quinidine therapy while actually falling in heart tissue.[71] This suggests that toxicity (if present) may be neurally mediated. These findings lend credence to the neural mediation of many of the observed effects of digitalis suggested by Gillis and Quest.[72] Localization of digoxin in the area postrema of the medulla of digitoxic cats by Somberg and Smith[73] also supports the concept of neural mediation of toxicity.

Because of this interaction and uncertainties that still are not resolved, it is prudent to reduce the dose of digoxin to one-half that previously well tolerated when quinidine is given simultaneously. Because the rise in serum level is a result of redistribution of digoxin "on board," it is better to reduce the dose several days before beginning quinidine to avoid potential bad effects of the combination.

Verapamil[74] and nifedipine[75] have recently been noted to also increase digoxin serum levels but not by as significant numbers as quinidine. These interactions have not been studied as extensively as the quinidine-digoxin interaction, and mechanism of action may not be similar. Caution is advised in using these drugs with digoxin.

DRUGS THAT PRODUCE ELECTROLYTE DISTURBANCES: ANTIHYPERTENSIVE AGENTS

The most common undesirable effects are with the diuretic drugs that tend to produce hypokalemia or hypomagnesemia, thus enhancing digitalis action and increasing the risk of digitalis toxicity.

Reserpine and propranolol (used as hypotensive agents) may be responsible for excessive slowing of the heart rate that may be additive to that of digitalis. Propranolol or other beta blockers, as mentioned previously, may also induce AV block that is also additive to that produced by digitalis.

HYPOLIPIDEMIC DRUGS

The bile acid sequestrants colestipol and cholestyramine, which are designed to promote lipoprotein removal, also readily bind with drugs such as digoxin or digitoxin and somewhat inhibit their absorption. Thus a problem may be encountered, particularly if both drugs are ingested simultaneously or taken close together. It is wise to administer digoxin at least 2 h before colestipol or cholestyramine resin.[76,77]

DRUGS THAT ALTER GASTROINTESTINAL TRANSIT TIME

Drugs that tend to increase gastrointestinal transit time (e.g., metoclopramide), thus decreasing the effective absorption time for digoxin, may decrease its absorption. Drugs such as anticholinergics that diminish transit time would tend to increase digoxin absorption, but probably not sufficiently to be a clinical problem.

AN ANTIBIOTIC DRUG INTERACTION WITH DIGOXIN

Lindenbaum and coworkers[78] recently reported that antibiotic changes in bacterial flora alter the metabolism of digoxin to noncardioactive metabolites in human volunteers, thus increasing the amount of digoxin in the serum. Clinical significance of this finding has not been worked out[79,80] and deserves attention. Close scrutiny of more biologically available products—the digoxin in a gelatin capsule (Lanoxicaps)—is needed. As this information is more rapidly and completely absorbed, it may offer some advantage in patient groups likely to receive frequent antibiotic treatment (i.e., those with cor pulmonale owing to bronchitis, renal failure with frequent infections, dialysis, and so forth).

REFERENCES

1 Withering, W.: An Account of Foxglove (1785), in Willius, F. A., and Keys, T. E. (eds.), "Classics in Cardiology," C. V. Mosby, St. Louis, 1941.

2 Luisada, A. A.: Personal communications.

3 Beller, G. A., Smith, T. W., Abelmann, W. H, Haber, E., and Hood, W. B.: Digitalis Intoxication—A Prospective Clinical Study with Serum Level Correlations, *N. Engl. J. Med.*, 284:990, 1971.

4 McHaffie, D., Purcell, H., Mitchell-Heggs, P., and Guz, A.: The Clinical Value of Digoxin in Patients with Heart Failure and Sinus Rhythms, *Q. J. Med.*, 47:401, 1978.

5 Selzer, A.: Digitalis in Cardiac Failure: Do Benefits Justify Risks, *Arch. Intern. Med.*, 141:18, 1981.

6 Arnold, S. B., Byrd, R. C., Meister, W., et al.: Long-term Digitalis Therapy Improves Left Ventricular Function in Heart Failure, *N. Engl. J. Med.*, 303:1443, 1980.

7 Beeson, P. B.: Withering Revisited, *N. Engl. J. Med.*, 303:1475, 1980.

8 Smith, T. W., and Braunwald, E.: "Clinical Use of Digitalis: Cardiac Rhythm Disturbances in Heart Disease," W. B. Saunders, Philadelphia, 1980, p. 526.

9 Shapiro, W.: Digitalis Update, *Arch. Intern. Med.*, 141:17, 1981.

10 Ferrer, M. I., Harvey, R. M., Cathcart, R. T., Webster, C. A., Richards, D. W., and Cournand, A.: Some Effects of Digoxin on the Heart and Circulation in Man: Digoxin in Chronic Cor Pulmonale, *Circulation*, 1:161, 1950.

11 Doherty, J. E., and Perkins, W. H.: Digoxin Metabolism in Hypo- and Hyperthyroidism. Studies with Tritiated Digoxin in Thyroid Disease, *Ann. Intern. Med.*, 64:489, 1966.

12 Ewy, G. A., Kapadia, G. G., Yao, L., Lullin, M., and Marcus, F. I.: Digoxin Metabolism in the Elderly, *Circulation*, 39:449, 1969.

13 Lindenbaum, J., Mellow, M. H., Blackstone, M. O., and Butler, V. P.: Variation in Biologic Availability of Digoxin from Four Preparations, *N. Engl. J. Med.*, 285:1344, 1971.

14 Wagner, J. G., Christensen, M., Sakmar, E., Blair, D., Yates, J. D., Willis, P. W., Sedman, A. J., and Stoll, R. G.: Equivalence Lack in Digoxin Plasma Levels, *J.A.M.A.*, 224:199, 1973.

15 Johnson, B. F., Greer, H., McCrerie, J., Bye, C., and Fowle, A.: Rate of Dissolution of Digoxin Tablets as a Predictor of Absorptions, *Lancet*, 1:1473, 1973.

16 Doherty, J. E., et al.: Gelatin Capsules of Digoxin: A New Formulation, in preparation.

17 Binnion, P. F.: A Comparison of Digoxin Biovailability in Capsule, Tablet and Solution Taken Orally with IV Digoxin, *Clin. Pharmacol. Ther.*, 461, 1978.

18 Lindenbaum, J.: Greater Biovailability of Digoxin Solution in Capsules, *Clin. Pharmacol. Ther.*, 21:278, 1977.

19 Doherty, J. E., Perkins, W. H., and Mitchell, G. K.: Tritiated Digoxin Studies in Human Subjects, *Arch. Intern. Med.*, 108:351, 1961.

20 Doherty, J. E., and Perkins, W. H.: Studies Following Intramuscular Tritiated Digoxin in Human Subjects, *Am. J. Cardiol.*, 15:170, 1965.

21 Doherty, J. E., and Perkins, W. H.: Studies with Tritiated Digoxin in Human Subjects after Intravenous Administrations, *Am. Heart J.*, 63:528, 1962.

22 Clark, D. R., and Kalman, S.: Dihydrodigoxin: A Common Metabolite of Digoxin in Man, *Drug Metab. Dispos.*, 2:148, 1974.

23 Luchi, R. J., and Gruber, J. W.: Unusually Large Digitalis Requirements, *Am. J. Med.,* 45:322, 1968.

24 Gundert-Remy, U., Koch, K., and Hrstka, V.: Chloroform and Polar Metabolites Examined with Different Assays, in G. Bordem and H. J. Dengler (eds.), "Cardiac Glycosides," Springer-Verlag, Berlin, 1978, pp. 28–35.

25 Okita, G. T.: Species Differences in Duration of Action of Digitalis Glycosides, *Fed. Proc.,* 26:1125, 1967.

26 Doherty, J. E., Flanigan, W. J., Murphy, M. L., Bulloch, R. T., Dalrymple, G. L., Beard, O. W., and Perkins, W. H.: Tritiated Digoxin: XIV. Enterohepatic Circulation, Absorption, and Excretion Studies in Human Volunteers, *Circulation,* 42:867, 1970.

27 Hall, W. H., and Doherty, J. E.: Tritiated Digoxin: XVI. Gastric Absorption, *Am. J. Dig. Dis.,* 16:903, 1971.

28 Batterman, R. C., and DeGraff, A. C.: Comparative Study in the Use of the Purified Digitalis Glycosides, Digoxin, Digitoxin and Lanatoside C for the Management of Ambulatory Patients with Congestive Heart Failure, *Am. Heart J.,* 34:663, 1947.

29 Beermann, B.: On the Fate of Orally Administered ^{3}H Lanatoside C in Man, *Eur. J. Clin. Pharmacol.,* 5:11, 1972.

30 Weissler, A. M., Snyder, J. R., Schoenfield, C. D., and Cohen, S.: Assay of Digitalis Glycosides in Man, *Am. J. Cardiol.,* 17:768, 1965.

31 Okita, G.T., Kelsey, F. E., Talso, P. J., Smith, L. B., and Geiling, E. M. K.: Studies on the Renal Excretion of Radioactive Digitoxin in Human Subjects with Cardiac Failure, *Circulation,* 7:161, 1953.

32 Okita, G. T., Kelsey, F. E., Walaszek, E. J., and Geiling, E. M. K.: Biosynthesis and Isolation of Carbon-14 Labelled Digitoxin, *J. Pharmacol. Exp. Ther.,* 110:244, 1954.

33 Beermann, B., Hellstrom, K., and Rosen, A.: Fate of Orally Administered ^{3}H-Digitoxin in Man with Special Reference to the Absorption, *Circulation,* 43:852, 1971.

34 Lukas, D. S.: Some Aspects of Distribution and Disposition of Digitoxin in Man, *Ann. N.Y. Acad. Sci.,* 179:338, 1971.

35 Fawaz, G., and Farah, A.: Study of Digitoxin Binding Power of Serum and Other Soluble Tissue Proteins of Rabbit, *J. Pharmacol. Exp. Ther.,* 80:193, 1944.

36 Rausmussen, K., Jervell, J., Sorstein, L., and Gjerdrum, K.: Digitoxin Kinetics and Patients with Impaired Renal Function, *Clin. Pharmacol. Ther.,* 13:6, 1972.

37 Katzung, B. S., and Meyers, F. S.: Excretion of Radioactive Digitoxin by the Dog, *J. Pharmacol. Exp. Ther.,* 149:257, 1965.

38 Marcus, F. I., Peterson, A. S., Salel, A. F., Scully, J., and Kapadia, G. G.: The Metabolism of Tritiated Digoxin in Renal Insufficiency in Dogs and Man, *J. Pharmacol. Exp. Ther.,* 153:372, 1966.

39 Doherty, J. E., Perkins, W. H., and Wilson, M. C.: Studies with Tritiated Digoxin in Renal Failure, *Am. J. Med.,* 37:536, 1964.

40 Sorstein, L.: The Influence of Renal Function on the Pharmacokinetics of Digitoxin, in O. Storstein (ed.), "Proceedings of the International Symposium on Digitalis," Glydendal Forlag, Oslo, 1973, pp. 158–168.

41 Ackerman, G. L., Doherty, J. E., and Flanigan, W. J.: Peritoneal Dialysis and Hemodialysis of Tritiated Digoxin, *Ann. Intern. Med.,* 67:718, 1967.

42 Doherty, J. E., and Perkins, W. H.: Digoxin Metabolism in Hypo- and Hyperthyroidism. Studies with Tritiated Digoxin in Thyroid Disease, *Ann. Intern. Med.,* 64:489, 1966.

43 Ewy, G. A., Groves, B. M., Ball, M. F., Nimmo, L., Jackson, B., and Marcus, F.: Digoxin Metabolism in Obesity, *Circulation,* 44:810, 1971.

44 Morris, J. J., Taft, C. V., Whalen, R. E., and McIntosh, H. D.: Digitalis and Experimental Myocardial Infarction, *Am. Heart J.,* 77:342, 1969.

45 Lely, A. H., and Van Enter, C. H. J.: Non-Cardiac Symptoms of Digitalis Intoxication, *Am. Heart J.,* 83:149, 1972.

46 Cook, L. S., Doherty, J. E., Straub, K. D., Nash, C. B., and Caldwell, R. W.: Digoxin Uptake into Peripheral Cardiac Nerves: A Possible Mechanism for Antiarrhythmic and Toxic Cardiac Actions, *Am. Heart J.,* 101:58, 1981.

47 Marcus, F. L.: Personal communication, 1981.

48 Bigger, J. T., and Strauss, H. C.: Digitalis Toxicity: Drug Interactions Promoting Toxicity and the Management of Toxicity, *Semin. Drug Treat.,* 2:147, 1972.

49 Mason, D. T., Zelis, R., Lee, G., Hughes, J. L., Spann, J. F., and Amsterdam, E. A.: Current Concepts and Treatment of Digitalis Toxicity, *Am. J. Cardiol.,* 27:546, 1971.

50 Fisch, C., and Knoebel, S. B.: Recognition and Therapy of Digitalis Toxicity, *Prog. Cardiovasc. Dis.,* 13:71, 1970.

51 Ewy, G. A., Marcus, F. I., Fillmore, S. J., and Matthews, N. P.: Digitalis Intoxication—Diagnosis, Management and Prevention, *Cardiovasc. Clin.,* 6:153, 1974.

52 Butler, V. P., Jr., Schmidt, D. H., Smith, T. W., Haber, E., Raynor, B. D., and DeMartini, P.: Effects of Sheep Digoxin-Specific Antibodies and Their Fab Fragments on Digoxin Pharmacokinetics in Dogs, *J. Clin. Invest.,* 59:345, 1977.

53 Lloyd, B. L., and Smith, T. W.: Contrasting Rates of Reversal of Digoxin Toxicity by Digoxin Specific IgG and Fab Fragments, *Circulation,* 58:280, 1978.

54 Smith, T. W., et al.: Reversal of Advanced Digoxin Intoxication with Fab Fragments of Digoxin Specific Antibodies, *N. Engl. J. Med.,* 294:797, 1976.

55 Marcus, F. I., Burkhalter, L., Cuccia, C., Pavlovich, J., and Kapadia, G. G.: Administration of Tritiated Digoxin with or without a Loading Dose, *Circulation,* 34:865, 1966.

56 Wotman, S., Bigger, J. T., Mandel, I. D., and Bartelstone, H. J.: Salivary Electrolytes in the Detection of Digitalis Toxicity, *N. Engl. J. Med.,* 285:871, 1971.

57 Swanson, M., Cacace, L., Chun, G., and Itano, M.: Saliva Calcium and Potassium Concentrations in the Detection of Digitalis Toxicity, *Circulation,* 47:736, 1973.

58 Gould, L., Reddy, C. V. R., and Gomprecht, R. F.: Evaluation of Digitalis Toxicity by Salivary Electrolytes, *N. Engl. J. Med.,* 286:47, 1972.

59 Doherty, J. E.: Salivary Electrolytes and Digitalis Toxicity, *J.A.M.A.,* 226:1228, 1973.

60 Prescott, L. F.: Clinically Important Drug Interactions, *Drugs,* 5:161, 1973.

61 Hoffman, B. F.: The Mechanism of Action of Antiarrhythmic Drugs, in "Clinical Pharmacology of Cardiovascular Drugs," American College of Cardiology, Atlantic City, N.J., April 1970.

62 Mason, D. T., DeMaria, A. N., Amsterdam, E. A., Zelis, R., and Massuni, R. A.: Antiarrhythmic Agents: I. Mechanisms of Action and Clinical Pharmacology, *Drugs,* 5:261, 1973; II. Therapeutic Considerations, *Drugs,* 5:292, 1973.

63 Wit, A. L., Steiner, C., and Damato, A. N.: Electrophysiologic Effects of Bretylium Tosylate on Single Fibers of the Canine Specialized Conduction System and Ventricle, *J. Pharmacol. Exp. Ther.,* 173:344, 1970.

64 Ejvinsson, G.: Effect of Quinidine on Plasma Concentrations of Digoxin, *Br. Med. J.,* 1:279, 1978.

65 Reiffel, J. A., Leahey, E. B., Drusin, R. E., et al.: A Digoxin/Quinidine Adverse Drug Interaction, *Am. J. Cardiol.,* 41:368, 1978.

66 Leahey, E. B., Jr, Reiffel, J. A., Drusin, R. E., et al.: Interaction between Quinidine and Digoxin, *J.A.M.A.,* 240:533, 1978.

67 Hooymans, P. M., and Merkus, F. W. H. M.: Effect of Quinidine on Plasma Concentration of Digoxin, *Br. Med. J.,* 2:1022, 1978.

68 Straub, K. D., Kane, J. J., and Bissett, J. K.: Alteration of Digitalis Binding by Quinidine: A Mechanism of Digitalis-Quinidine: A Mechanism of Digitalis-Quinidine Interaction, *Circulation,* 58 (suppl. 2):58, 1978.

69 Gold, H., Modell, W., and Price, L.: Combined Actions of Quinidine and Digitalis on the Heart: An Experimental Study, *Arch. Intern. Med.,* 50:766, 1932.

70 Hager, W. D., Fenster, P., Mayersohn, M., et al.: Digoxin-Quinidine Interaction: Pharmacokinetic Evaluation, *N. Engl. J. Med.,* 300:1238, 1979.

71 Doherty, J. E., Straub, K. D., Bissett, J., and Murphy, M.: Digoxin-Quinidine Interaction: Increased Digoxin Brain Concentration, *Am. J. Cardiol.,* 45:453, 1980.

72 Gillis, R. A., and Quest, J. A.: The Role of the Nervous System in the Cardiovascular Effects of Digitalis, *Pharmacol. Rev.,* 31:19, 1980.

73 Somberg, J. C., and Smith, T. W.: Localization of Neurally Mediated Arrhythmogenic Properties of Digitalis, *Science,* 204:321, 1979.

74 Somberg, J. C., Wellins, H., Maguire, W., and Miura, D.: Verapamil-Digitalis Interaction: Effect on Cardiac Purkinjie Fibers and Myocardium, *Am. J. Cardiol.,* 49:1025, 1982. (Abstract.)

75 Belz, G. G., Aust, P. E., and Munkes, R.: Digoxin Plasma Concentration and Nefidipine, *Lancet,* 1:844, 1981. (Letter.)

76 Brown, D. D., Juhl, R. P., and Wormer, S. L.: Decreased Bioavailability of Digoxin to Hypocholesterolemic Interventions, *Circulation,* 58:164, 1978.

77 Hall, W. H., Shappell, S. D., and Doherty, J. E.: Effect of Cholestyramine on Digoxin Absorption and Excretion in Man, *Am. J. Cardiol.,* 39:213, 1977.

78 Lindenbaum, J., Rund, D. G., Butler, V. P., et al.: Inactivation of Digoxin by the Gut Flora: Reversal by Antibiotic Therapy, *N. Engl. J. Med.,* 305:789, 1981.

79 Doherty, J. E.: A Digoxin Antibiotic Drug Interaction, *N. Engl. J. Med.,* 305:827, 1981. (Editorial.)

80 George, C. F.: Interactions with Digoxin: More Problems, *Br. Med. J.,* 1:291, 1982. (Editorial.)

The author wishes to acknowledge the expert technical assistance of Jacquelyn Gammill, B.S. (A.S.C.P.), and Joyce Massengill, B.S. (A.S.C.P.), as well as the secretarial assistance of Diane Butler and Faye W. Day.

GORDON A. EWY, M.D.

The sufferer who frustrates a keen therapist by failing to improve is always in danger of meeting primitive human behavior disguised as treatment.

THOMAS F. MAIN, 1911–
The Ailment[1]

Defibrillation is technically the arrest of fibrillation of cardiac muscle (either atrial or ventricular) with restoration of normal rhythm.[1a] By convention, the term *defibrillation* refers to the electrical termination of ventricular fibrillation, and the term *cardioversion* refers to the synchronized electrical termination of tachydysrhythmias other than ventricular fibrillation.[2–4] During cardioversion, the electric discharge is synchronized with the R wave of the electrocardiogram to avoid inducing ventricular fibrillation by inadvertantly delivering the shock during the vulnerable period of ventricular repolarization.[2–4]

The era of electric cardioversion was initiated two decades ago when Zoll and Linenthal used alternating current (ac) precordial shocks to terminate refractory ventricular tachycardia.[5] This era may have been short-lived had not the work of Lown and others followed, demonstrating the superiority and safety of a direct-current (dc) capacitor discharge through an inductance coil (Fig. 1) for the reversion of both atrial and ventricular tachycardias.[2,3,6–12] Using dc synchronized shock, the technique of cardioversion was applied to almost all supraventricular tachyrhythmias.[6–12] The initial enthusiasm for electric cardioversion was such that many considered the mere presence of atrial fibrillation or atrial flutter as an indication for cardioversion.

Over the ensuing years, this enthusiasm waned. Although nearly every tachyrhythmia could be cardioverted, in many, sinus rhythm was short-lived.[13] In some of the early series, less than 30 percent of the patients cardioverted from atrial fibrillation maintained sinus rhythm longer than 1 year.[13] Another unexpected result was that cardioversion would occasionally terminate an atrial tachycardia only to uncover long periods of asystole or extreme sinus bradycardia.[3] The sick sinus syndrome was thus discovered.[3] Based on these findings, stricter guidelines were defined and patients were more carefully selected for cardioversion.[2,3]

INDICATIONS FOR CARDIOVERSION
Atrial Fibrillation and Atrial Flutter

The rationale for cardioversion of atrial fibrillation and atrial flutter is based on the premise that the initiating mechanism of the dysrhythmia is different from the sustaining mechanism.[2,3] If the initiating mechanism is no longer present and the sustaining mechanism is broken, sinus rhythm can resume. Therefore, every effort must be made to eliminate the initiating and predisposing factors prior to elective cardioversion. Patients with heart failure, thyrotoxicosis, electrolyte or acid-base abnormalities, and pulmonary infections, infarction, or embolism should first be treated and stabilized. Patients with significant mitral valve disease may need to have the lesion surgically corrected prior to cardioversion. Those who are in or who develop atrial fibrillation in the perioperative period should not be cardioverted until the fourth or fifth postoperative week.[3] Patients with treated thyrotoxicosis should undergo elective cardioversion if spontaneous reversion has not occurred by 3 months.[14]

It has long been appreciated that the duration of atrial fibrillation and left atrial size are among the major factors that determine how long sinus rhythm will be maintained following successful cardioversion.[3] In the study by Henry and associates, patients with rheumatic mitral or aortic valvular disease or patients with asymmetric septal hypertrophy with left atrial

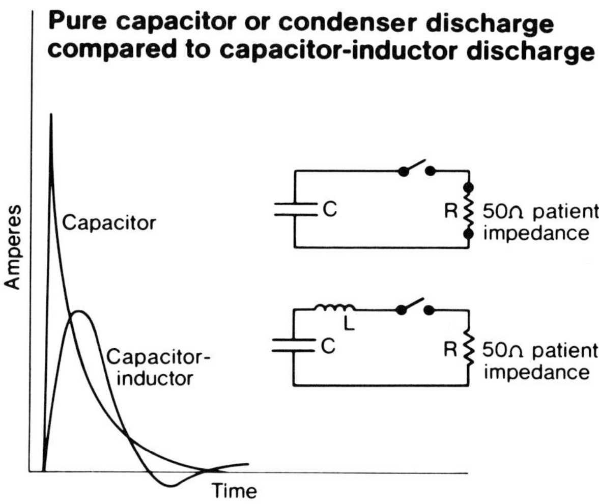

FIGURE 1 Graphic illustration of the waveforms of a pure capacitor or condenser discharge and a capacitor-inductor defibrillator discharge. C - capacitor; R - impedance; L - inductor. (*From G. A. Ewy, Cardiac Arrest and Resuscitation: Defibrillators and Defibrillation, in W. P. Harvey (ed.), "Current Problems in Cardiology," Year Book Medical Publishers, Chicago, 1978, p. 14. Used with permission.*)

*From the Section of Cardiology, University of Arizona College of Medicine, and the Arizona Health Sciences Center, Tucson, Arizona.

diameters (determined by M-mode echocardiography) greater than 4.5 cm did not maintain sinus rhythm longer than 6 months following cardioversion.[15] Ewy and associates confirmed that the left atrial diameter correlated with the patient's response to therapy[16] (Fig. 2). Patients with rheumatic mitral disease and left atrial diameters greater than 5.5 cm were most likely to have persistent atrial fibrillation (Fig. 2). The large overlap indicates that factors other than left atrial diameter are also important. Ewy and coworkers also found that the

relationship between left atrial size and the response to therapy held in patients with idiopathic atrial fibrillation as well,[16] but they found that patients with idiopathic atrial fibrillation had a smaller left atrial diameter in each therapeutic response group (Fig. 3). In this study, patients with idiopathic atrial fibrillation and a left atrial diameter greater than 4.5 cm were most likely to have persistent atrial fibrillation. The physician may want to use the results of these studies as guidelines in determining whether or not cardioversion should be attempted.

In many patients, the initiating factor(s) cannot be removed and therefore cardioversion should not be attempted. The patient's prefibrillatory electrocardiogram must be reviewed for evidence of the sick sinus

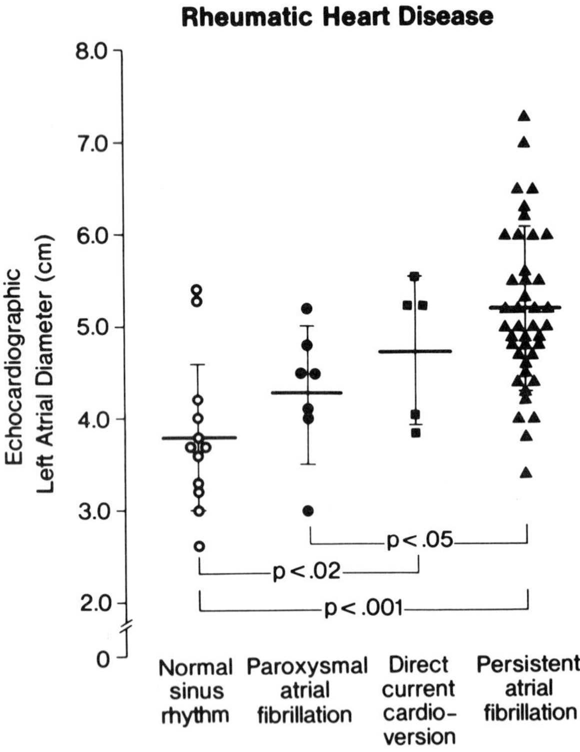

FIGURE 2 The left atrial diameters (determined by M-mode echocardiography) of patients with rheumatic heart disease and predominant mitral valve involvement plotted against their response to therapy. Patients were designated as having *paroxysmal atrial fibrillation* if their dysrhythmia converted to sinus rhythm either spontaneously or following the administration of digitalis or digitalis and quinidine. Patients who failed to convert with digitalis and quinidine (maximal dose of quinidine was 300 mg four times a day) but who responded to synchronized dc shock and remained in sinus rhythm for more than 3 months were placed in the *dc cardioversion* group. Patients were considered to have persistent atrial fibrillation if they either failed to respond to dc cardioversion or if they reverted to atrial fibrillation within 3 months in spite of maintenance therapy with digitalis and quinidine. (*From G. A. Ewy, L. Ulfers, D. Hager, R. A. Rosenfeld, W. R. Roeske, and S. Goldman, Response of Atrial Fibrillation to Therapy: Role of Etiology and Left Atrial Diameter, J. Electrocardiol., 13:119, 1980. Used with permission.*)

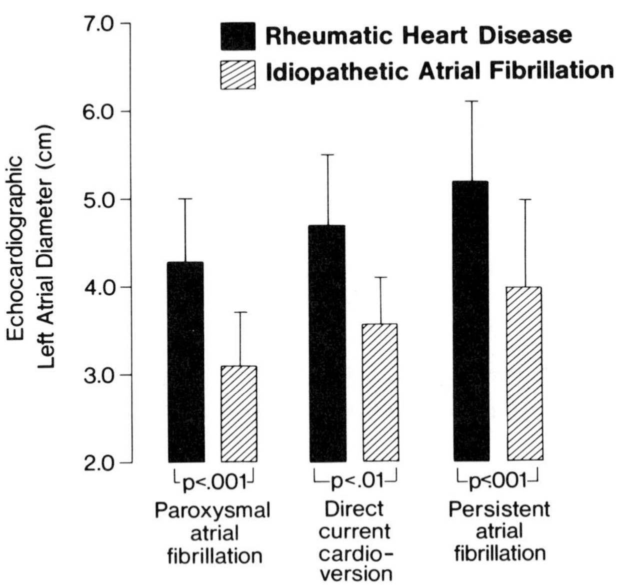

FIGURE 3 Left atrial diameters (determined by M-mode echocardiography) of patients with rheumatic heart disease and predominant mitral valve disease and patients with idiopathic atrial fibrillation plotted against the response of the patient to therapy. Patients were designated as having *paroxysmal atrial fibrillation* if their dysrhythmia converted to sinus rhythm either spontaneously or following the administration of digitalis or digitalis and quinidine. Patients who failed to convert with digitalis and quinidine (maximal dose of quinidine was 300 mg four times a day) but who responded to synchronized dc countershock and remained in sinus rhythm for more than 3 months were placed in the *dc cardioversion* group. Patients were considered to have persistent atrial fibrillation if they either failed to respond to dc cardioversion or if they reverted to atrial fibrillation within 3 months in spite of maintenance therapy with digitalis and quinidine. (*From G. A. Ewy, L. Ulfers, D. Hager, R. A. Rosenfeld, W. R. Roeske, and S. Goldman, Response of Atrial Fibrillation to Therapy: Role of Etiology and Left Atrial Diameter, J. Electrocardiol., 13:119, 1980. Used with permission.*)

TABLE 1
**Relative contraindications to cardioversion in patients
with atrial fibrillation**

Atrial fibrillation of prolonged duration (i.e., generally longer
than 1 year.)
Markedly enlarged left atrium. In general, patients with
rheumatic mitral or aortic valve disease or with asymmetric
septal hypertrophy with a left atrial diameter (LAD) greater
than 5.5 cm and patients with idiopathic atrial fibrillation
with a left atrial diameter greater than 4.5 cm.
Atrial fibrillation in any setting where the initiating factor
(acute left ventricular failure, pneumonia, pulmonary embolism, thyrotoxicosis, tight mitral stenosis, and so forth) is still
present.
Atrial fibrillation that is recurrent in spite of adequate
maintenance antidysrhythmic therapy.
Atrial fibrillation that is a rescue or escape rhythm of the sick
sinus syndrome.

syndrome, another contraindication to cardioversion.
The relative contraindications to cardioversion are
listed in Table 1. Rarely, a patient with atrial fibrillation will have a very rapid ventricular response that is
unresponsive to drugs. In these patients, it is sometimes
necessary to consider oblation of the atrioventricular
node and insertion of a permanent pacemaker. A new
technique of interrupting atrioventricular conduction
by delivering "defibrillation" shocks of 200 watt-
seconds (Ws) via an appropriately placed transvenous
His-bundle recording catheter has been successfully
used by Scheinman and associates[19] and by Gallagher
and coworkers.[20]

Paroxysmal Supraventricular Tachycardia

Cardioversion is seldom indicated in patients with
paroxysmal supraventricular tachycardia (PSVT).[17]
This reentrant dysrhythmia usually responds to vagal
maneuvers or drugs.[21] If simple vagal maneuvers fail,
verapamil may well be the drug of choice.[22] If intravenous verapamil is used, 5 to 10 mg is given over a 2-min
period. The dose may be repeated in 30 min. Because
of its negative inotropic effect, verapamil should not be
used in patients who haves recently received intravenous beta-adrenergic blockers and must be used with
extreme caution in patients with impaired ventricular
function. Adverse electrophysiologic effects of
verapamil can be counteracted by isoproterenol.[23]

Patients in whom the tachycardia is causing ischemia
or hemodynamic embarrassment who do not respond
to vagal maneuvers or drugs are candidates for urgent
electrocardioversion. Care must be exercised in patients with supraventricular tachycardia who are receiving digitalis because supraventricular tachycardias

unresponsive to the vagal maneuvers and drugs may be
secondary to digitalis excess. In this setting, cardioversion may be hazardous; death has been reported
following cardioversion in patients with digitalis-
induced supraventricular tachyrhythmias. Repetitive
atrial tachycardia (Parkinson-Papp syndrome) is
another tachydysrhythmia that should not be cardioverted because of its repetitive nature.[24]

Ventricular Tachycardia

The treatment of tachydysrhythmias depends on the
patient's response. An occasional patient can tolerate
ventricular tachycardia for days without apparent distress, while others develop profound hemodynamic
embarrassment soon after the onset of the tachydysrhythmia. Ventricular tachycardia associated with
shock or acute myocardial infarction should be cardioverted if the dysrhythmia does not immediately
respond to intravenous antidysrhythmic medications
such as lidocaine.

Extremely rapid ventricular tachycardia can have a
sinusoidal appearance—like ventricular flutter. Synchronization is *not* recommended in this form of
ventricular tachycardia because it is difficult to distinguish the QRS from the T wave.

CONSIDERATIONS PRIOR TO CARDIOVERSION
Anticoagulation

If the patient is a candidate for cardioversion, the next
step is to determine whether or not to use anticoagulation. Anticoagulation is not recommended prior to the
cardioversion of PSVT or ventricular tachycardia.
Anticoagulation does not appear to be necessary in
patients with normal cardiac output and recent-onset
(documented to be within hours) atrial fibrillation. The
author recommends anticoagulation in all other patients with atrial fibrillation. In the nonrandomized
study by Bjerkelund and Orning,[25] systemic emboli
occurred in 11 of 209 patients not receiving anticoagulation and in only 2 of 228 patients receiving anticoagulation. Embolism occurred as long as 6 months following
cardioveresion.[25] Without anticoagulation, the reported incidence of systemic emboli varies. With mitral
valve disease the incidence is 1.5 to 3 percent.[26] There
appears to be a consensus that anticoagulation is
indicated in patients with a history of previous systemic
embolism; most cardiologists anticoagulate patients
with mitral stenosis prior to cardioversion. The question is whether or not patients with atrial fibrillation but
without rheumatic mitral valve disease should receive

prophylactic anticoagulation. There is no prospective randomized study to answer this question. Even though the incidence of embolism is low, one millet-seed-sized clot to the middle cerebral artery can drastically change the entire life of an individual.

Lown and associates state that anticoagulation prior to cardioversion is theoretically unnecessary in patients with acute atrial fibrillation if the duration of atrial fibrillation is less than 1 week.[4] They emphasize, however, that many patients who are aware that they have experienced a change in rhythm underestimate the time of onset of atrial fibrillation.[4] Therefore, these investigators routinely anticoagulate patients for a period of 3 weeks prior to cardioversion and for 1 month thereafter.[4] It has been our policy to anticoagulate patients for at least 2 weeks prior to elective cardioversion. Using anticoagulation, the author has not, to date, had an embolic complication in any patient cardioverted. Anticoagulation is continued for at least 6 months after cardioversion. This procedure is followed not only because of the finding that postcardioversion embolic events occur up to 6 months after cardioversion,[25] but also because patients successfully cardioverted not infrequently revert to atrial fibrillation without being aware of this change in rhythm.

Digitalis

Lown originally recommended that digoxin be discontinued 2 to 3 days and digitoxin be discontinued 5 to 6 days prior to cardioversion.[3] This recommendation was sound because of the difficulty in diagnosing digitalis excess in the presence of atrial fibrillation and because of the recent observations of the marked increase in serum digitalis levels that occur with just one dose of quinidine.[27] Lown no longer recommends that digitalis be discontinued when cardioverting patients with atrial fibrillation.[4] This change in recommendation[4,28] should not be interpreted as a lack of respect for the danger of the combination of excess digitalis and countershock; it is potentially dangerous to apply a precordial shock in the presence of digitalis intoxication.[9] This danger can be avoided if the serum potassium and digoxin levels are monitored and the electrocardiogram of the patient in atrial fibrillation is carefully analyzed for subtle signs of digitalis excess prior to cardioversion.[29] The dose of digoxin should be decreased to one-half prior to beginning quinidine because quinidine doubles the serum digoxin level.[27]

Quinidine or Procainamide

There are several reasons why quinidine or procainamide should be administered prior to attempted cardioversion.[18] The first is that a significant number of patients will revert to normal sinus rhythm with digitalis and quinidine or procainamide therapy, thus saving the patient the discomfort, anxiety, and expense of electric cardioversion. The second reason is that quinidine will reduce the energy or strength of the shock required for electric cardioversion.[4] In addition, quinidine will occasionally revert fibrillation to flutter, a rhythm requiring much lower energy levels for cardioversion. Finally, it is important but not mandatory to determine whether the patient can tolerate maintenance quinidine therapy after cardioversion. Fully one-third of patients cannot tolerate quinidine therapy, predominantly because of gastrointestinal side effects. If the patient cannot tolerate quinidine, either disopyramide or procainamide might be used for maintenance therapy. It should be noted that disopyramide is not very effective for reversion of atrial fibrillation, but it is useful in helping to maintain sinus rhythm.[30] Because of its negative inotropic effects, disopyramide should not be administered to patients with poor ventricular function.[31] Procainamide is not an ideal drug for long-term antidysrhythmic therapy because a lupus-like syndrome occurs in 10 to 30 percent of such patients.[32,33] Procainamide (PA) is metabolized to *N*-acetylprocainamide (NAPA) by acetylation.[34,35] Several studies have suggested that subjects who are genetically "slow acetylators" have a higher risk of developing the lupus-like syndrome. One recent study suggests that the plasma NAPA/PA ratio, when determined 3 hours after an oral dose of procainamide at steady state, is predictive of developing antinuclear antibodies and the likelihood of developing the lupus-like reaction.[36,37] In patients in whom this ratio was less than 0.85 (slow acetylators), antinuclear antibodies developed after 2.9 months compared with 7.3 months for patients with a ratio greater than 1.0 (rapid acetylators).[36] These same investigators found that procainamide-induced lupus syndrome occurred at a mean duration of therapy of 12 months in slow acetylators and 54 months in rapid acetylators.[36] This type of information suggests that while procainamide might be an effective antidysrhythmic agent for short-term therapy, its long-term use is fraught with unwanted reactions.

There have been several recommended ways of administering quinidine to attempt drug reversion of atrial fibrillation or flutter. DeSilva, Lown, and their associates recommend a daily dose of 300 mg four times a day for 24 to 48 h prior to cardioversion.[4] Bigger's approach is to give quinidine sulfate 400 mg every 6 h for 2 days prior to cardioversion.[30] Since this dose may be excessive in the small, elderly patient, our approach, if quinidine is to be used, is to give quinidine sulfate 200 mg orally every 6 h on the first day. On the second day, this dose is increased to 300 mg every 6 h. The electrocardiogram is closely followed and incremental doses are not given if the QRS width increases by 25 percent. On the third day, the patient is kept fasting, except for another 300- or 400-mg dose of quinidine given early in the morning. Elective cardioversion is then performed 4 to 6 h later if the patient's rhythm has not reverted to normal. This schedule allows for a gradual increase in the quinidine blood levels during the precardioversion period. Following cardioversion, the patient is placed on maintenance therapy of 200 or 300 mg of quinidine sulfate given orally four times a day. For convenience, quinidine is given with each meal and at bedtime. It is seldom necessary to have the patient set the alarm for 6 A.M. and midnight for routine maintenance quinidine therapy. The maintenance dose should be guided by blood levels and the patient's response. The dose should be increased in patients who have frequent premature atrial contractions because these are harbingers of recurrent atrial fibrillation or flutter.

Another approach to reversion of atrial fibrillation has been used by Fenster and associates at the University of Arizona.[38] Procainamide is administered intravenously, at a rate of 10 to 20 mg/min to a total dose of 10 mg/kg. This technique produces a steadily rising blood concentration of procainamide to therapeutic levels in 25 to 40 min. If the patient's rhythm is not reverted to sinus, one can immediately proceed with electric cardioversion rather than wait the 2 or 3 days that might be necessary when quinidine is used. In Fenster's initial report, 12 of 19 patients reverted to sinus rhythm during procainamide infusion.[38] Five received the full dose and failed to convert. In one patient the infusion was terminated prematurely because of the development of ventricular tachycardia and in another because of the development of new bifascicular block; both these patients had acute myocardial infarction.[38] In this preliminary study, intravenous procainamide was most effective in patients with recent-onset atrial fibrillation and prevented the necessity for cardioversion. This technique may not be advisable in the setting of an acute myocardial infarction.[38]

TECHNIQUE OF CARDIOVERSION

Cardioversion as well as drug reversion of dysrhythmias should be carried out in a well-equipped intensive care area so that the patient can be monitored and observed by a medically trained staff. In this way, dysrhythmias can be promptly treated and more serious complications avoided. Intravenous access is obtained. All drugs and equipment necessary for cardiopulmonary resuscitation should be on hand, including the capability for emergency temporary pacing. The cardioversion procedure should be fully explained to the patient to allay anxiety, since the amount of energy required for cardioversion is related to the level of the patient's agitation and unease.[4] There should be a minimum of personnel and activity in the room, and every effort should be made to ensure the physical comforts of the patient.

Anesthesia

Initial sedation is provided by giving 5 mg diazepam orally 1 to 2 h before the procedure. Intramuscular injections of sedatives should be avoided in anticoagulated patients. Diazepam may also be used for anesthesia. A three-way stopcock is placed between the short intravenous catheter and the intravenous tubing so that the diazepam can be injected directly into the bloodstream. Diazepam will precipitate in most intravenous solutions, but will usually reconstitute in the bloodstream. This precipitation can be avoided if the drug is administered directly into the vein. A 2- to 5-mg dose of diazepam is given intravenously every 2 to 3 min until the patient is asleep or unresponsive to verbal commands. If the circulation time is slow, the interval between doses should be longer. Occasionally, a patient who is extremely anxious or who has been taking tranquilizers may require higher doses of diazepam. The average dose of diazepam required is 15 mg.[4] If the patient requires more than 50 mg and is still not completely sedated, morphine sulfate may be administered and the cardioversion shock delivered or an anesthesiologist should be called. Physicians not familiar with the use of diazepam should have a qualified anesthesiologist to administer an appropriate anesthetic. The incidence of patient recall of the procedure is higher when diazepam is used than when anesthetics such as methohexital are used.

Synchronization

The major danger of transthoracic electric discharge is the induction of ventricular fibrillation by improper synchronization. This can occur when the patient's electrocardiogram has an extremely prominent T wave. The monitor lead that best displays the largest R wave and the least prominent T wave should be selected for synchronization.

Electrode Paddle Position

Lown has shown that it takes less energy to cardiovert patients with atrial fibrillation when the anteroposterior paddle position is used in contrast to the anterolateral paddle position.[3,7] Kerber and associates recently reported on the influence of electrode paddle location on success rates of cardioversion.[39] Using 100 Ws delivered energy, they found no difference in the success rate when anteroanterior electrode paddle placement was used compared with anteroposterior placement.[39] The author still uses the anteroposterior electrode paddle position for elective cardioversion. If these are not available, anterolateral paddle placement is effective. Firm pressure is necessary to ensure uniform electrode contact, as well as to expel excess air from the lungs. Inflated lungs increase transthoracic impedance and decrease the success of electric shocks.[40]

Transthoracic Impedance

Defibrillation and cardioversion success is predicated on an appropriate current density through a critical mass of the cardiac chamber to be defibrillated or cardioverted. When the same amount of energy is stored on the capacitor of a defibrillator, the delivered electric current density depends on the impedance or resistance (Fig. 4). Every effort must be made to ensure a low-impedance pathway for the current flow from the defibrillator and the heart. The lower the impedance, the higher the delivered current. There are several factors known to influence the transthoracic impedance to dc defibrillation discharge (Table 2). At the time of cardioversion, the controllable factors are correct electrode position, heavy electrode paddle pressure, and the application of an effective electrode-skin interface.[41] The electrode paddles must be completely

TABLE 2
Factors influencing transthoracic impedance or resistance to discharge

Shock strength
Electrode paddle size
Interface between electrode and skin
Number of previous shocks
Time interval between previous shocks
Phase of ventilation
Chest size
Electrode paddle pressure

SOURCE: From G. A. Ewy, Cardioversion, in G. A. Ewy and R. Bressler (eds.), "Cardiovascular Drugs and the Management of Heart Disease," Raven Press, New York, 1982, p. 427. Used with permission.

covered with a conductive paste, particularly along the edges, to reduce the likelihood of skin burns. Certain defibrillator pads also may be effective.

Energy Settings

Ninety-five percent of patients with atrial fibrillation are cardioverted when 200 Ws or joules (J) of stored energy are discharged from the capacitor of the dc defibrillator.[4] This is equivalent to a delivered energy of about 150 Ws.[29] Lown has noted that the amount of energy required to cardiovert atrial fibrillation is related to the amplitude of the fibrillatory waves: the larger the "f" waves, the less the energy that is required. Ewy[42] observed that another determinant of

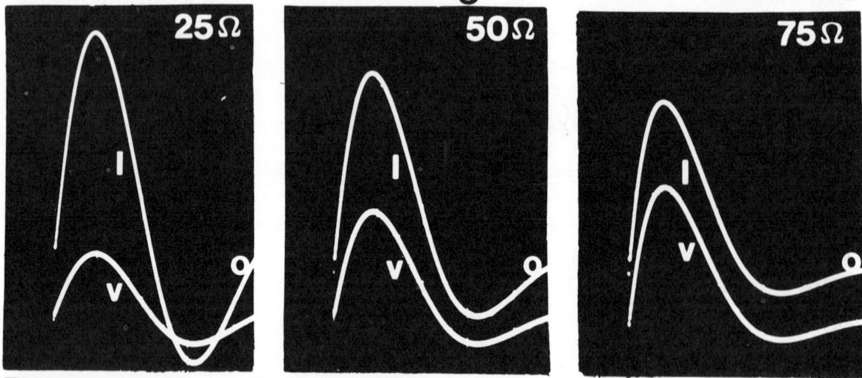

FIGURE 4 Effect of resistance or impedance on voltage (V) and current (I) waveforms. The defibrillator or cardioverter capacitor was charged to 100 Ws for each discharge. Note that the lower the resistance, the higher the delivered current.

TABLE 3
Cardioversion in human beings: importance of transthoracic impedance*

| | Cardioverted | | |
Characteristics	Yes (13 patients)	No (13 patients)	Significance
Weight, kg	75 + 13	75 + 13	N.S.
Chest diameter, cm	22 + 12	24 + 2	N.S.
Impedance	50 + 12	59 + 10	$p > 0.05$

*Results following an initial 100-ws (stored energy) dc discharge.

SOURCE: From G. A. Ewy, Cardioversion, in G. A. Ewy and R. Bressler (eds.), "Cardiovascular Drugs and the Management of Heart Disease," Raven Press, New York, 1982, p. 427. Used with permission.

success is the transthoracic impedance or resistance (Table 3): the higher the resistance, the less the delivered current. Therefore, to deliver an equivalent amount of electric current to a patient with a higher transthoracic impedance, more energy must be discharged.

Lown and associates report that 200 Ws (stored energy) converts 95 percent of patients with atrial fibrillation.[3] Ewy[42] found that an initial stored energy dose of 100 Ws was effective in only 50 percent of patients with atrial fibrillation (Table 3). Therefore, the recommended initial shock strength is 200 Ws of stored (150 Ws delivered) energy for cardioversion of atrial fibrillation.

Less energy is required to cardiovert atrial flutter. Lown reports a 97 percent success rate with an average of 25 Ws in over 200 patients cardioverted from atrial flutter.[4] When cardioverting atrial flutter, very low energy shocks are not recommended because a very low energy discharge given at any time in the cardiac cycle can convert atrial flutter to fibrillation. If the resultant atrial fibrillation does not spontaneously revert to sinus rhythm, much higher energy doses are required. The author recommends an initial shock strength of about 25 Ws. If this is not successful, a 50-Ws synchronized discharge is given. For ventricular tachycardia, low-energy shocks of 10 Ws or less are usually sufficient.[4]

Time Interval between Shocks

The time interval between shocks should be longer than 3 min. Myocardial damage is greater when the same amount of energy from sequential shocks is delivered at 1-min intervals and much less when this interval is increased to 3 min.[43] In addition, approximately 2 percent of patients with atrial fibrillation will not convert to sinus rhythm immediately after the electric discharge but will do so within several seconds to minutes. This is presumed to be due to the fact that a critical mass of the atrium has been depolarized with the shock and that atrial fibrillation cannot be self-sustaining in the small remaining mass of non-depolarized tissue.[44]

Monitor Electrocardiogram

Monitoring lead V^1 after each discharge will assist in defining the resumption of sinus rhythm. This is important, because immediately following cardioversion, the P waves may be small and irregular with frequent premature atrial contractions, leading a casual observer to misinterpret the rhythm as continuing atrial fibrillation. If there is any question, a standard 12-lead electrocardiogram should be recorded.

Change Unit to Defibrillator

Immediately after the shock, the synchronize switch is turned off, changing the unit back to a defibrillator. This precaution is taken in the unlikely event that the patient develops ventricular fibrillation. If one attempts to defibrillate a patient in ventricular fibrillation and the unit is still synchronized, the unit will not discharge because the circuit will be waiting to synchronize on a sharp spike of an electrocardiographic QRS complex.

Monitor Patient

The patient should remain in the intensive care area for at least 1 h after the procedure, and longer if the patient is not fully awake. If frequent premature atrial depolarizations occur, additional antidysrhythmic medication should be considered. Maintenance therapy with oral antidysrhythmic medication is begun.

REFERENCES

1 Main, T. F.: The Ailment, *Br. J. Med. Psych.*, 30:129, 1957.

1a *Stedman's Medical Dictionary*, 22d ed., Williams & Wilkins, Baltimore, 1972, p. 327.

2 Lown, B., Perlroth, M. G., Bey, S. K., et al.: "Cardioversion" of Atrial Fibrillation. A Report on the Treatment of 65 Episodes in 50 Patients, *N. Engl. J. Med.*, 269:325, 1963.

3 Lown, B.: Electrical Reversion of Cardiac Arrhythmias, *Br. Heart J.*, 29:469, 1967.

4 DeSilva, R. A., Graboys, T. B., Podrid, P. J., and Lown, B.: Cardioversion and Defibrillation, *Am. Heart J.*, 100:881, 1980.

5 Zoll, P. M., and Linenthal, A. J.: Termination of Refractory Tachycardia by External Countershock, *Circulation*, 25:596, 1962.

6 Lown, B., Bey, S. K., Perlroth, M. C., and Abe, T.: Comparative Studies of Ventricular Vulnerability to Fibrillation, *J. Clin. Invest.*, 42:953, 1963.

7 Lown, B., Kleiger, R. and Wolff, G.: The Technique of Cardioversions, *Am. Heart J.*, 67:282, 1964.

8 Lown, B.: "Cardioversion" of Arrhythmias (II), *Mod. Concepts Cardiovasc. Dis.*, 33:869, 1969.

9 Lown, B., Kleiger, R., and Williams, B. J.: Cardioversion and Digitalis Drugs: Changed Threshold to Electric Shock in Digitalized Animals, *Circ. Res.*, 17:519, 1965.

10 Kleiger, R., and Lown, B.: Cardioversion and Digitalis: II. Clinical Studies, *Circulation*, 33:878, 1966.

11 Lown, B., Bey, S. K., Perlroth, M. G., and Abe, T.: Cardioversion of Ectopic Tachyarrhythmias, *Am. J. Med. Sci.*, 246:257, 1963.

12 Guiney, T. C., and Lown, B.: Electrical Conversion of Atrial Flutter to Atrial Fibrillation. Flutter Mechanism in Man, *Br. Heart J.*, 34:1215, 1972.

13 Killip, T., III: Indications for Cardioversion, In L. E. Meltzer and J. R. Kitchell (eds.), "Current Concepts of Cardiac Pacing and Cardioversion," Charles Press, Bowie, Md., 1971, p. 273.

14 Nakazawa, H. K., Sakurai, K., Momotani, N., Hamada, N., and Ito, K.: Timing of Cardioversion Application in Thyrotoxic Atrial Fibrillation, *Circulation*, 62 (suppl. 3):296, 1980. (Abstract.)

15 Henry, W. L., Morganroth, J., Pearlman, A. S., et al.: Relation between Echocardiographic Determined Left Atrial Size and Atrial Fibrillation, *Circulation*, 53:273, 1976.

16 Ewy, G. A., Ulfers, L., Hager, D., Rosenfeld, R. A., Roeske, W. R., and Goldman, S.: Response of Atrial Fibrillation to Therapy: Role of Etiology and Left Atrial Diameter, *J. Electrocardiol.*, 13:119, 1980.

17 Vassaux, C., and Lown, B.: Cardioversion of Supraventricular Tachycardias, *Circulation*, 39:791, 1969.

18 Rabbino, M. D., Likoff, W., and Dreifus, L. S.: Complications and Limitations of Direct Current Counter Shock, *J.A.M.A.*, 190:417, 1964.

19 Gonzalez, R., Scheinman, M. M., Margaretten, W., and Rubinstein, M.: Closed-Chest Electrode Catheter Technique for His Bundle Ablation in Dogs, *Am. J. Physiol.*, 241:H283, 1981.

20 Gallagher, J. J., Svenson, R. H., Kasell, J. H., et al.: Catheter Technique for Closed-Chest Ablation of the Atrioventricular Conduction System, *N. Engl. J. Med.*, 306:194, 1982.

21 Waxman, M. B., Wald, R. W., Sharma, A. D., Huerta, F., and Cameron, D. A.: Vagal Techniques for Termination of Paroxysmal Supraventricular Tachycardia, *Am. J. Cardiol.*, 46:655, 1980.

22 Rinkenberger, R. L., Prystowsky, E. N., Heger, J. J., Troup, P. J., Jackman, W. M., and Zipes, D. P.: Effects of Intravenous and Chronic Oral Verapamil Administration in Patients with Supraventricular Tachyarrhythmias, *Circulation*, 62:996, 1980.

23 Krikler, D.: Verapamil in Cardiology, *Eur. J. Cardiol.*, 2:3, 1974.

24 Parkinson, J., and Papp, C.: Repetitive Paroxysmal Tachycardia, *Br. Heart J.*, 9:241, 1947.

25 Bjerkelund, C., and Orning, O. M.: An Evaluation of DC Shock Treatment of Atrial Arrhythmias, *Acta Med. Scand.*, 184:481, 1968.

26 Abernathy, W. S., and Willis, P. W., III: Thromboembolic Complications of Rheumatic Heart Disease, in W. Likoff (ed.), "Cardiovascular Clinics. Valvular Heart Disease," F. A. Davis, Philadelphia, 1973, p. 131.

27 Hager, W. D., Fenster, P., Mayersohn, M., et al.: Digoxin-Quinidine Interaction: Pharmacokinetic Evaluation, *N. Engl. J. Med.*, 300:1238, 1979.

28 Ditchey, R. V., and Karliner, J. S.: Safety of Electrical Cardioversion in Patients without Digitalis Toxicity, *Ann. Intern. Med.*, 95:676, 1981.

29 Kastor, J. A., and Yurchak, P. M.: Recognition of Digitalis Intoxication in the Presence of Atrial Fibrillation, *Ann. Intern. Med.*, 67:1045, 1967.

30 Bigger, J. T., Jr.: Management of Arrhythmias, in: E. Braunwald (ed.), "Heart Disease: A Textbook of Cardiovascular Medicine," W. B. Saunders, Philadelphia, 1980, pp. 708, 724.

31 Podrid, P. J., Schoenberger, A., and Lown, B.: Congestive Heart Failure Caused by Oral Disopyramide, *N. Engl. J. Med.*, 302:614, 1980.

32 Blomgren, S. E., Condemi, J. J., and Vaughan, J. H.: Procainamide-Induced Lupus Erythematosus: Clinical and Laboratory Observations, *Am. J. Med.*, 52:338, 1972.

33 Tan, E. M.: Drug-Induced Autoimmune Disease, *Fed. Proc.,* 33:1894, 1974.

34 Gardina, E.-G. V., Dreyfuss, J., Bigger, J. T., Jr., Shaw, J. M., and Schreiber, E. C., Metabolism of procainamide in Normal and Cardiac Subjects., *Clin. Pharmacol. Ther.,* 19:399, 1976.

35 Gaffner, C., Johnsson, G., and Sjorgren, J.: Pharmacokinetics of Procainamide Intravenously and Orally as Conventional and Slow Release Tablets, *Clin. Pharmacol. Ther.,* 17:414, 1975.

36 Woosley, R. L., Drayer, D. E., Reidenberg, M. M., Nies, A. S., Carr, K., and Oates, J. A.: Effect of Acetylator Phenotype on the Rate at Which Procainamide Induces Antinuclear Antibodies and the Lupus Syndrome, *N. Engl. J. Med.,* 298:1157, 1978.

37 Reidenberg, M. M., Drayer, D. E., Levy, M., et al.: Polymorphic Acetylation of Procainamide in Man, *Clin. Pharmacol. Ther.,* 17:722, 1975.

38 Fenster, P. E., Comess, K. A., Marsh, R., Katzenberg, C., Hager, W. D.: Conversion of Atrial Fibrillation to Normal Sinus Rhythm by Acute Procainamide Infusion, *Am. Heart J.,* in press.

39 Kerber, R. E., Jensen, S. R., Grayzel, J., Kennedy, J., and Hoyt, R.: Elective Cardioversion: Influence of Paddle-Electrode Location and Size on Success Rates and Energy Requirements, *N. Engl. J. Med.,* 305:658, 1981.

40 Ewy, G. A., Hellman, D. A., McClung, S., and Taren, D.: Influence of Ventilation Phase on Transthoracic Impedance and Defibrillation Effectiveness, *Crit. Care Med.,* 8:164, 1980.

41 Ewy, G. A.: Cardiac Arrest and Rescusitation: Defibrillators and Defibrillation, in W. P. Harvery (ed.), "Current Problems in Cardiology," Year Book Medical Publishers, Chicago, 1978, p. 22.

42 Ewy, G. A.: Influence of Paddle-Electrode Location and Size on Success of Cardioversion, *N. Engl. J. Med.,* 306:174, 1982.

43 Dahl, C. F., Ewy, G. A., Warner, E. D., and Thomas, E. D.: Myocardial Necrosis from Direct Current Counter Shock, *Circulation,* 50:956, 1974.

44 Garrey, W. E.: The Nature of Fibrillatory Contractions of the Heart—Its Relation to Tissue Mass and Form, *Am. J. Physiol.,* 33:397, 1914.

Method and Magic in Myocardial Preservation[*]

ROBERT A. GUYTON, M.D.

> But when the black and mortal blood of man
> Has fallen to the ground before his feet, who
> then can sing spells to call it back again?
>
> *AGAMEMNON*[1]

The prevention of damage to the myocardium during open heart surgery has been the focus of a massive investigational effort over the last quarter century. The task was precisely defined by Melrose in 1955: "The unhurried correction of cardiac abnormalities under direct vision.... A most valuable contribution... would be made if the heart could be arrested and restarted at will suffering no damage during periods of arrest and cessation of coronary blood flow."[2] The investigation has been fruitful, but to this day, the magic, perfect poison and the more magic, perfect antidote remain elusive.

Early Cardioplegia

Melrose et al. found that potassium citrate injected into the aortic root of dogs led to rapid and reversible cardiac arrest.[2] Their studies stimulated the application of chemical cardiac arrest in patients with potassium citrate[3] and acetyl choline.[4] Unfortunately, the sequelae of these early "preservation" solutions were found to be worse than the sequelae of simple ischemic cardiac arrest.[5–7]

The Decade of Hypothermic Ischemic Arrest

There followed a decade of cardiac surgery utilizing simple ischemic cardiac arrest. The tolerance of the heart to ischemic arrest was enhanced by hypothermia, either by the use of surface cooling, systemic cooling by cardiopulmonary bypass, local irrigation of the pericardial cavity,[8] or perfusion hypothermia by intracoronary injection of cold solutions.[9] However, clinical results remained unsatisfactory. Extensive and irreversible myocardial damage after open heart surgery was recognized,[10–12] and the search again went out for the magic poison.

*From the Department of Surgery, Cardiothoracic Research Laboratory, Carlyle Fraser Heart Center, Crawford W. Long Memorial Hospital, Emory University School of Medicine, Atlanta, Georgia.

Less Damaging Cardioplegic Solutions

During the decade of ischemic arrest in the United States, investigation continued in continental Europe into infusion solutions that might allow cardiac arrest and recovery. Two major solutions were developed, one based on low sodium concentrations, no calcium, and procaine,[13,14] and the second based on a high magnesium concentration and procaine.[15–17] In Great Britain and in the United States, a resurgence of interest in potassium cardioplegia was led by Gay and Ebert,[18] Tyers et al.,[7] and Hearse et al.[19,20] In the subsequent decade the widespread use of cardioplegic myocardial protection has been a major contributing factor in a dramatic improvement in results after open heart surgery.[21–26]

BASIC CONCEPTS OF MYOCARDIAL PROTECTION
Ischemia and Necrosis

Studies of myocardial ischemia have defined ultrastructural changes that occur with irreversible damage[27] and "explosive" alterations in cellular electrolytes and volume with reperfusion.[28,29] The search for a marker of impending necrosis has focused primarily on high-energy phosphate levels.[10,30–32] Even a short period of ischemia (12 to 15 min) can cause high-energy phosphate depletion, which can last as long as 3 days.[33,34] A certain level of high-energy phosphate depletion is consistent with cellular recovery, but further depletion is associated with eventual necrosis.[32,35,36] The primary target of most techniques of myocardial preservation is this energy deficit that occurs during ischemia: the difference between the energy necessary for the myocyte to retain its cellular integrity and the energy available to the myocyte.

Decreasing Energy Requirements
THE CENTRAL ROLE OF HYPOTHERMIA

As the myocardium is cooled, oxygen consumption is dramatically reduced.[14,37,38] The heart may fibrillate as it is cooled, but as the temperature falls below 25°C, the vigor of fibrillation decreases to the extent that the fibrillating heart has a lower oxygen consumption than the beating empty heart[37,39] (Fig. 1).

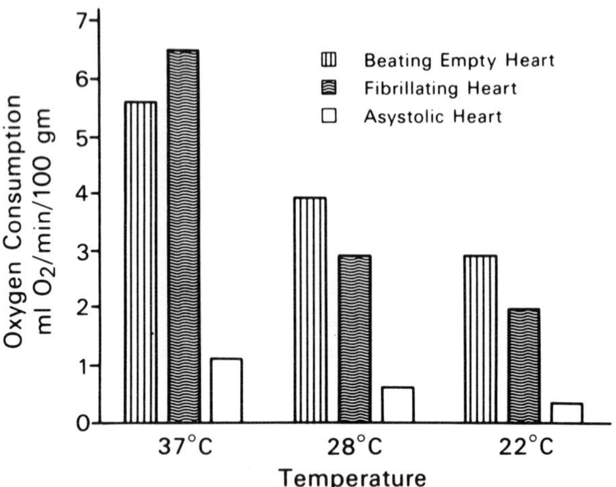

FIGURE 1 Oxygen consumption is decreased by progressive hypothermia in the beating empty heart, the fibrillating heart, and the chemically arrested heart. Constructed from data presented in Buckberg et al.[37]

ASYSTOLE

The goal of chemically induced asystole is the dedication of available energy to the preservation of cellular integrity. Asystole has been repeatedly shown to lead to a decrease in oxygen consumption beyond that caused by hypothermia[14,18,37,40,41] (Fig. 1). Chemically induced asystole has been achieved by a high potassium concentration, a low sodium concentration, a high magnesium concentration, procaine, tetrodotoxin, calcium channel blockers, and acetyl choline.[2,4,14,16,18,42–45]

Increasing Energy Supply
ANAEROBIC METABOLISM

During the period of ischemic arrest, the myocyte can use anaerobic metabolism as an inefficient method of producing high-energy phosphates, utilizing available glycogen stores or substrates provided by intermittent infusion of cardioplegic solution. Unfortunately, this mode of energy production is not only inefficient, it is quickly inhibited by the accumulation of end products. These end products, particularly lactic acid, may themselves be damaging to cellular metabolism.

AEROBIC METABOLISM

Hypothermia and asystole dramatically reduce myocardial oxygen consumption such that at least a portion of the oxygen deficit can be supplied by interval infusion of blood or oxygenated crystalloid solutions.[46,47] This method allows preservation of high-energy phosphates and, in turn, cellular integrity.

Minimizing the Sequelae of Energy Deficit
MEMBRANE STABILIZATION

Loss of lipoprotein membrane integrity is one of the earliest visible markers of eventual cellular necrosis.[27,32] Attempts have been made to use membrane-stabilizing agents such as steroids and procaine as a method of preventing subsequent necrosis.

CALCIUM CHANNEL BLOCKERS

The very rapid accumulation of calcium by subcellular organelles, in particular, mitochrondria, has been identified as an early component of cellular injury with reperfusion after ischemia.[27,29,32] Calcium channel blockers have been utilized in an effort to prevent this accumulation.[47–52]

MANIPULATION OF THE REPERFUSING SOLUTION

Because such dramatic changes occur within the first few minutes of reperfusion, it has been thought that the cell is particularly susceptible to further metabolic injury during this time.[28,29] Reperfusing solutions have been modified several ways. A more alkaline pH may provide more optimal conditions for cellular repair. Maintaining asystole during the first portion of reperfusion may allow a greater proportion of the early oxygen supply to be utilized for cellular repair. Replenishment of lost metabolites, particularly those involved in the replenishment of high-energy phosphate levels, has been attempted to encourage quick cellular recovery.[31,53–55]

EXPERIMENTAL PROBLEMS
Species Differences

Several species have been used extensively in the development of myocardial preservation techniques. An isolated, working rat heart model has been used to determine the optimal composition of cardioplegic solutions. However, there are problems with the extrapolation of these data to human beings. All isolated heart models have been severed from neural influences and from the effect of noncoronary collateral

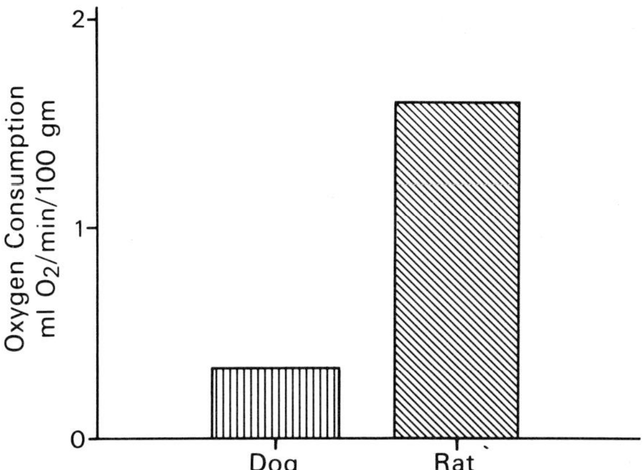

FIGURE 2 The oxygen consumption of the chemically arrested rat heart at 14°C is more than five times the oxygen consumption of the chemically arrested dog heart at 15°C.[38,57]

flow.[56] In addition, the rat heart certainly has a different metabolic rate than large mammal hearts. The oxygen consumption of the arrested rat heart is several times the oxygen consumption of the arrested dog heart at similar hypothermic temperatures[37,57] (Fig. 2). Finally, the rat is unusually susceptible to low magnesium levels and to ischemic contracture.[58] As one attempts to simulate the clinical situation by using larger mammals, one finds that each experiment becomes expensive, both in time and money. The demonstration of differences in a good technique of myocardial preservation and a very good technique of myocardial preservation may require a large number of these expensive preparations because of animal-to-animal variation. One promising model has been developed that involves the infusion of one solution into one region of the dog's heart and a second solution into the second region, allowing comparison of two different solutions within a single animal.[59]

Setting the Experimental Stage

Because of the expense of large animal preparations, a common practice is the manipulation of experimental conditions to exaggerate the consequences of the intervention to be studied. Early studies of potassium cardioplegia used normothermia or only moderate hypothermia to exaggerate the benefits of chemically induced asystole.[60] The first studies of blood cardioplegia compared cold blood cardioplegia with intermittent ischemic arrest rather than comparing blood cardioplegia with cold crystalloid cardioplegia.[46] Experimental stage setting is no problem in itself, but the experimental conditions are often not sufficiently em-

phasized, and the reader and subsequent reviewers may have difficulty remembering the context in which the result was obtained.

Negative Results

The statement "No statistically significant differences were observed between the two groups studied" unfortunately is often interpreted by the reader (and sometimes by the author) to mean that there is no difference between the two groups studied. However, the fact of the matter is often that the investigational technique or the number of experiments is inadequate to detect a difference between the two groups. This statement is particularly common in clinical studies in which experimental control is impossible.[61,62]

Variety of Experimental Methods

A wide variety of experimental end points are available to the investigator. Both global and regional function can be assessed. Ultrastructural studies can demonstrate differences in subcellular structures.[27,63–65] High-energy phosphate levels can be determined.[30,31] Preservation of the metabolic function of the mitochondria and the sarcoplasmic reticulum can be assessed.[66,67] Coronary blood flow can be determined by radioactive microspheres. Intramyocardial P_{CO_2} and P_{O_2} can be determined by mass spectrometry,[60,68] and moment-to-moment intracellular metabolic changes can be determined by nuclear magnetic resonance.[69–71] These new techniques offer the investigator the opportunity to develop more sensitive methods for distinguishing between cardioplegic techniques.

Human Studies

Because of the wide variety of pathologic conditions presented to the cardiac surgeon, patient-to-patient variation is a major problem in the evaluation of cardioplegic techniques in human beings. Experimental protocols cannot be rigidly standardized. The more sensitive investigational techniques are invasive. Myocardial biopsies are required for ultrastructural or biochemical studies.[64,65,72–74] Studies of ventricular dimensions in the perioperative period require fixation of ultrasonic transducers in the heart or to the surface of the heart.[75,76] Coronary sinus sampling involves the placement of a catheter directly into the coronary sinus.[74,77] Noninvasive techniques, such as serial enzyme determinations, gated blood pool scanning, and technetium pyrophosphate scans, lack specificity and sensitivity. A method that may improve the sensitivity of invasive or noninvasive monitoring is the application of stress to the heart (such as volume loading or pacing) in the early postoperative period. The response to stress is then used as a measurement of functional reserve.[77–80]

PREPARATION OF THE HEART FOR ISCHEMIC ARREST

Hemodynamic Preparation

CORONARY PERFUSION AND CARDIOPULMONARY BYPASS

In a careful study of the appearance of the MB band of creatine kinase, it was found that this enzyme appeared in the blood in 18 percent of cardiac surgical patients prior to the institution of cardiopulmonary bypass.[81] Failure to devote proper attention to oxygen supply and demand during the induction of anesthesia and preparation for bypass can clearly cause myocardial damage. With the institution of cardiopulmonary bypass, an additional burden is placed on the diseased coronary circulation. Coronary stenoses that are not detrimental under normal circumstances may become significant with cardiopulmonary bypass.[82–84] A decrease in perfusion pressure to 40 to 60 torr less than prebypass levels may lead to subendocardial ischemia even in the absence of coronary stenosis.[85] Hemodilution decreases the vasodilation reserve of the heart and, in combination with coronary stenoses, leads to ischemia in normal dog hearts and more severe ischemia in hypertrophied dog hearts.[86,87] Myocardial cooling decreases coronary vasodilatory capacity[38,88] and causes ischemia in dogs when the perfusion pressure is lowered to 50 torr from 100 torr.[89] Fibrillation during cardiopulmonary bypass can lead to ischemia in normal hearts[39,90,91] and in acutely and chronically colateralized regions.[91,92] Perfusion pressure should be maintained at prebypass levels with a mean perfusion pressure of at least 75 to 80 torr as the heart is being cooled.

VENTRICULAR DISTENSION

Elevation of preload reduces blood flow to the inner layers of the heart and may be particularly deleterious in vasodilated hearts[93] or during ventricular fibrillation.[39,94] Ventricular distension should be avoided before arrest for any prolonged length of time. During the cardioplegic arrest interval, ventricular distension does not affect subsequent myocardial recovery.[94]

Pharmacologic Preparation

PROPRANOLOL

The metabolic rate of the heart prior to cardioplegic arrest determines, in part, the oxygen consumption of the heart during arrest[57] and the subsequent recovery of the myocardium. Isoproterenol pretreatment is detrimental to myocardial recovery,[95] as is an elevated left ventricular dP/dt prior to ischemic arrest.[96] Pretreatment with propranolol leads to improved functional and metabolic recovery after arrest.[44,51,97]

CORTICOSTEROIDS

Corticosteroids have been shown to protect lysosomal membranes in dogs with permanent coronary artery ligation, but reperfusion of ischemic myocardium may eliminate this benefit.[98,99] Corticosteroids have led to improved recovery after 1 h of ischemic arrest with topical hypothermia,[100] but this effect was not confirmed in dogs undergoing cardioplegic arrest with perfusion hypothermia.[95] Benefit of pretreatment with steroids or of use of steroids as an additive to cardioplegic solutions has not been demonstrated.[101,102]

CALCIUM CHANNEL BLOCKERS

Pretreatment with lidoflazine and nifedipine improves cardiac tolerance to ischemic arrest either alone[52] or as an adjunct to cold cardioplegic arrest.[103,104]

GLUCOSE LOADING

Elevation of glycogen levels by glucose loading may provide more substrate for anaerobic metabolism during the ischemic period. The arterial glucose level and the myocardial glycogen level have been found to correlate with postischemic function.[96,105] In patients, glucose loading prior to cardiopulmonary bypass led to improved myocardial glycogen levels after arrest and decreased operative morbidity.[105,106]

HYPOTHERMIA: THE FIRST PRIORITY

Hypothermia in Theory

Myocardial hypothermia has been shown to reduce oxygen consumption in the beating heart, in the fibrillating heart, and in the chemically arrested heart.[37–39,56] In addition to reducing the energy requirement of the myocyte, hypothermia may decrease the rate of degradive processes that lead to myocardial necrosis.

Hypothermia in Practice

A reduction in the temperature of the myocardium reduces the damage caused by ischemic arrest in all experimental models. There is better preservation of high-energy phosphate levels, better preservation of ultrastructure, improved postarrest regional and global function, and better short- and long-term survival of the animal.[66,94,107–109] Although a short period of chemical cardioplegia with normothermia may be well tolerated, it is clear that the combination of hypothermia with cardioplegia is superior to either modality of protection alone.[58,67,94,110–114]

Perfusion Hypothermia

Local irrigation of the pericardium combined with systemic hypothermia leads to myocardial cooling that is sufficient to allow survival after most cardiac procedures.[8] However, Tyers and colleagues found improved tolerance of ischemic arrest with perfusion hypothermia, that is, injection of cold Ringer's lactate solution into the aortic root. This allows rapid, uniform cooling in animal hearts with normal coronary vasculature.[9]

The Heterogeneous Nature of Clinical Cardioplegia

Early studies of perfusion hypothermia and cardioplegia largely ignored an important feature of the clinical situation: The coronary circulation is usually diseased or the ventricle is hypertrophied with variable coronary resistances in different myocardial regions. Hypothermia, hemodilution, cardiopulmonary bypass, and decreased perfusion pressure all may exacerbate the differences in regional vascular resistance caused by hypertrophy or coronary stenoses.[82,83,86,87,89,115,116] Perfusion hypothermia with experimental coronary stenoses and in human beings with coronary artery disease is distinctly heterogeneous.[116–119] In clinical situations, a variation in myocardial temperatures of 10°C is not uncommon.[107,117,118] In an animal model, with temporary occlusion of the circumflex artery during perfusion hypothermia, the left anterior descending regional temperature decreased from 25°C to less than 10°C, while the circumflex region cooled only a few degrees.[103,104,116] The heterogeneous nature of perfusion

hypothermia makes it necessary to develop techniques that will allow cooling of areas of the heart which are the most difficult to perfuse. These efforts have followed three major pathways: infusion at higher pressures, colder and colder solutions, and perfusion hypothermia through each distal anastomosis as it is completed.

Infusion of Cardioplegia at Higher Pressures

When a proximal coronary stenosis is superimposed on a myocardial vascular region, vasodilation of the distal vessels in that region may be sufficient to allow adequate coronary flow. However, if aortic pressure is subsequently reduced, hypoperfusion results, beginning in the subendocardium and progressing to the subepicardium as pressure in the distal vascular bed progressively decreases.[120] By increasing the cardioplegia infusion pressure in the aortic root, the proximal resistance of coronary stenoses and collateral vessels may be accommodated, allowing adequate pressure in the distal coronary microvasculature. The danger of this technique is that the higher pressure used in the aortic root will be transmitted directly to some distal vascular beds that are not "protected" by a proximal coronary vascular resistance. These "unprotected" regions will be exposed to high pressures and high flows of the cardioplegic solution.

What Infusion Pressure Is Too High?

In attempting to determine the safe range of coronary perfusion pressures (with blood) during cardiopulmonary bypass for aortic valve replacement, Brown et al.[121] found that a pressure of 160 torr was damaging to the heart compared to a pressure of 100 torr. Progressively increasing cardioplegia infusion pressures have been examined, using two pressures in a single heart by separate perfusion of the left anterior descending and circumflex regions. As the infusion pressure was increased, no damage was detected at 50, 100, or 150 torr. An increase in infusion pressure to 200 torr caused regional functional deterioration and accumulation of myocardial water[119] (Fig. 3). Although others have suggested that low infusion pressures should be used to limit edema formation,[122,123] this study found no water accumulation with a pressure of 150 torr.[119] Cardioplegia infusion pressures as high as 150 torr are safe. These higher pressures may allow better perfusion of the myocardium distal to coronary stenoses.[124]

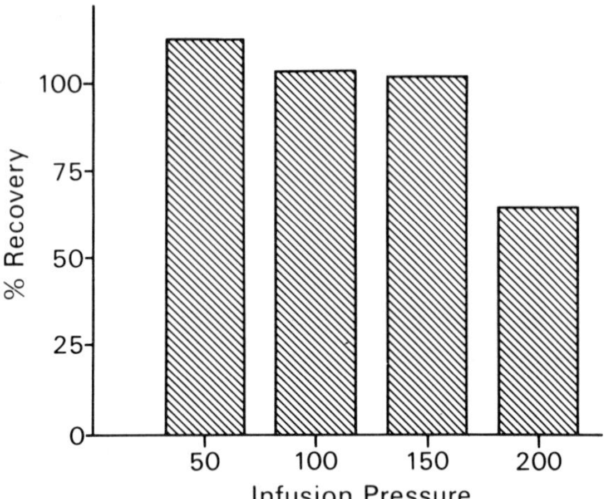

FIGURE 3 As cardioplegia infusion pressure is increased, there is excellent recovery of myocardial function until a pressure above 150 is utilized.[119]

Colder and Colder Solutions

Since perfusion of the heart is necessarily heterogeneous, it would seem reasonable to use a very cold solution so that those regions of the heart receiving only a small volume of the solution could be cooled to acceptable levels. However, again this means that other regions of the heart will be exposed to large volumes of these very cold solutions.[119]

How Cold Is Too Cold?

Tyres and colleagues,[109] using a working rat heart model, studied single-dose noncardioplegic intracoronary perfusion hypothermia. They found that infusion temperatures of 4°C, when followed by reperfusion, led to functional and metabolic deterioration compared with infusion temperatures of 10 to 15°C. Myocardial damage has been found to occur with prolonged exposure to ice slush.[125] Benthancourt and Laks[107] found that hearts preserved in a crystalloid low-pressure perfusion system for 24 h at 4°C developed marked edema and compliance changes.[107] Grieppe et al.[126] suggested that hearts being stored for transplantation were better preserved when perfused with normal saline at 15°C than at 24 or 4°C. Despite these early observations, there is considerable evidence to suggest that myocardial temperatures as cold as 4°C are not damaging. Harlan et al.[127] found excellent recovery of rat hearts infused with 5°C cardioplegia solution and subsequently maintained at 5°C by external cooling for 300 min of ischemia. Shragg et al.,[128] using constant perfusion hypothermia at 0.5°C, found excellent recovery of rat hearts after 2 h of cold perfusion. Swanson et

al.[129] found excellent preservation of isolated canine hearts at 4°C. Engelman et al.[130] found very good recovery in pig hearts with myocardium cooled to 8°C by a combination of cold cardioplegia and local cooling. Reitz et al.[131] have demonstrated functional recovery of dog hearts preserved for 24 h at 4°C. In a study of heterogeneous cardioplegia, some regions in dog hearts were as cold as 4°C. There was no difference in functional recovery between myocardial regions cooled to less than 8°C.[119] The infusion of large volumes of very cold (0 to 2°C) cardioplegic solutions in a situation that leads to heterogeneous cardioplegia is not damaging to those regions which are unprotected by proximal coronary stenoses.[119]

Perfusion Hypothermia after Each Distal Coronary Anastomosis

As each distal coronary anastomosis is completed, one has the opportunity to infuse cold cardioplegic solution into the distal vascular bed. This can be performed by either direct infusion into the vein graft or by performing proximal anastomoses first, allowing perfusion through the graft from the aortic root after completion of each anastomosis.[132,133] Daggett and colleagues[134] have carried this concept one step further in patients. They have used temperature mapping of the myocardium after the first aortic root infusion of cardioplegia to determine which region of the myocardium was least cold. The distal anastomosis in this region was then performed first, allowing early infusion of cold cardioplegic solution into the most vulnerable myocardial region.

Frequency and Volume

Numerous studies have demonstrated the benefit of multidose cardioplegic infusion over single-dose techniques.[42,60,63,80] Repeated infusions of cardioplegic solutions not only will keep the myocardium cold but will also allow washout of metabolites.[135] A single, lengthy arrest period is superior to multiple, shorter periods with intermittent reperfusion.[136,137] The infusion of large volumes of cardioplegic solution is not hazardous, unless the cardioplegic solution itself is cytotoxic or damaging.[119,138] In lengthy procedures, as much as 3 or 4 liters of cardioplegic solution may be utilized.[138,139]

Systemic Hypothermia and Local Irrigation

Systemic hypothermia prior to perfusion hypothermia allows the heart to cool uniformly and provides additional protection for those regions of the heart which cannot be easily cooled by perfusion hypothermia. After perfusion hypothermia has been accomplished, systemic hypothermia decreases the rate of rewarming.[140] Because of the heterogeneous nature of perfusion hypothermia, local irrigation may contribute importantly to the cooling of poorly perfused myocardial regions. Local irrigation may also prevent rewarming of the myocardium during the ischemic arrest period.[141]

CARDIOPLEGIA: THE MAGIC SOLUTION
The Basic Solution
FIRST, DO NO HARM

Cardioplegic solutions have varying degrees of toxicity.[142] The cardioplegic solutions developed in Europe during the 1960s had a composition greatly different from that of extracellular fluid. Hearse and colleagues[143,144] found that the efficacy of these solutions depended on the rate and volume of administration. Cardioplegic solutions similar in composition to extracellular fluid were not so dependent on delivery techniques. Since the clinical situation forces heterogeneous cardioplegia with large volumes in some regions and small volumes in other regions, it is important that variable infusion rates and volumes not greatly affect the efficacy of protection. Hearse et al.[145] also found that additives to cardioplegic solutions such as procaine and lidocaine have dose-response curves with a maximum effect at a certain concentration and deleterious effects at higher concentrations. Additives that are beneficial in low doses may be toxic in higher doses. Again, caution should be exercised, since delivery to the myocardium is heterogeneous. The first requirement of a good cardioplegic solution is that it can be infused in large volumes without any resulting damage to the myocardium. Cardioplegic solutions that simulate the composition of extracellular fluid seem to meet this requirement.[138,144]

ASYSTOLE

Chemical asystole can be achieved by a number of different methods. Early studies demonstrated the benefit of adding chemical asystole to simple hypothermia.[7,14,111–113] The oxygen consumption of the arrested hypothermic heart is lower than the oxygen consumption of the beating or fibrillating hypothermic heart at similar temperatures[11,14,18,37](Fig. 1). Recently, the suggestion was made that perfusion hypothermia was

sufficient and that chemical asystole was not a necessary addition to myocardial protection.[108,146–149] Subsequent work has soundly refuted this suggestion.[59,112–114,150] When perfusion hypothermia is compared with perfusion hypothermia plus hyperkalemia in a single dog heart (infusing the two solutions into two different regions of the same heart), a dramatic difference is easily demonstrated in regional functional recovery.[59] After the heart is initially arrested, it may not be so important to have a high potassium concentration in subsequent infusions of cardioplegia.[151]

THE OPTIMAL POTASSIUM CONCENTRATION

In an analysis of the damage caused by Melrose's original solution, Tyers identified high potassium concentrations as a major problem. With ultrastructure as the end point, studies in rats have revealed a potassium concentration of 25 to 30 mEq to be optimal.[152] In studies of in vivo pig hearts, Rousou et al.[153] found the optimal potassium concentration for ATP preservation to be 15 mEq/liter. Jelnick et al.[154] studied cold blood cardioplegic solutions with increasing levels of potassium. They found little evidence for damage from higher levels of potassium, and they attributed this lack of damage to the fact that the myocardium was very cold. The clinical problem with infusion of large quantities of potassium is perioperative arrhythmias. Ellis et al.[151] found excellent myocardial preservation in patients with either high or low potassium solutions but found fewer arrhythmias with low potassium solutions. A potassium concentration of 15 to 25 mEq/liter in the initial infusion solution seems to be optimal.

AN ALKALINE SOLUTION

There is general agreement that ischemic arrest is better tolerated if the acid milieu that is the consequence of anaerobic metabolism can be prevented or at least delayed.[155] For this reason, cardioplegic solutions are mildly alkaline, with a pH of 7.6 to 7.8. An advantage of one buffering system over another has not been demonstrated.

CALCIUM CONCENTRATION

When isolated rat hearts are perfused with a calcium-free perfusate and then reperfused with a solution containing calcium, rapid calcium accumulation can occur in cell organelles with markedly diminished myocardial function.[143,156] This "calcium paradox" may be inhibited by a calcium channel blocker or hypothermia.[157] However, in intact animals the calcium paradox has not been a problem. It may be that the rat is more susceptible to this phenomenon than larger mammals or that noncoronary collateral flow may prevent very low calcium levels in large, intact mammals.[56,158] The addition of calcium to crystalloid hyperkalemic cardioplegic solutions is not necessary.[158]

Osmotic and Oncotic Pressure

OSMOTIC PRESSURE

The osmotic pressure of a cardioplegic solution should be slightly hyperosmolar. Hypoosmolar solutions may exacerbate cellular swelling, and extremely hyperosmolar solutions may cause cellular dehydration and damage.[7,159,160]

ONCOTIC PRESSURE

Most early crystalloid cardioplegic solutions contained no plasma. Buckberg and colleagues[159] have advocated the addition of plasma or mannitol to cardioplegic solutions to help prevent myocardial edema. They demonstrated that with 10-min cardioplegic arrest intervals, myocardial water content was higher with solutions that did not contain plasma or mannitol than it was with solutions that did contain plasma or mannitol. However, with reperfusion, these differences disappeared.[159] If the myocardium is well protected and there is no ischemic damage, myocardial water content after reperfusion does not increase with crystalloid cardioplegic solutions that contain neither plasma nor mannitol.[119] If there is myocardial damage, increased myocardial water content is to be expected.[29,161]

Oxygen Delivery and Blood Cardioplegia

When high-energy phosphates became identified as a marker for impending cellular necrosis, considerable effort was made to maintain energy levels within the cells during the cardioplegic arrest. The use of cold, oxygenated blood as a vehicle for hyperkalemic cardioplegic arrest was suggested. Better preservation of high-energy phosphates with this technique has been demonstrated.[47] Functional recovery in both experimental and clinical models seems at least as good as that provided by crystalloid cardioplegia.[22] The one exception to this may be situations in which cardioplegia cannot be uniformly and regularly delivered.[162,163] In addition to the use of blood as a vehicle for hyperkalemia, Buckberg[22] has proposed the alkalinization of the blood solution and the addition of citrate to lower the calcium concentration. Recently,

the capacity of blood cardioplegia to provide oxygen to the heart has been questioned, since the oxyhemoglobin dissociation curve is shifted far to the left by hypothermia.[38] The use of oxygenated crystalloid solution as an alternative to blood cardioplegia has been suggested.[47]

Other Additives

GLUCOSE

Glucose-insulin-potassium infusion seems to be beneficial in acute myocardial infarction, but with the profound hypothermia provided by most cardioplegia techniques, the anaerobic production of high-energy phosphates does not seem to be important. The addition of glucose to hypothermic, hyperkalemic cardioplegic solutions has not been shown to be helpful unless the experimental stage has been set by glycogen depletion or induction of diabetes.[164–167] The addition of glutamate, a Krebs-cycle intermediate, may help preserve high-energy phosphate levels with crystalloid cardioplegia.[168]

PROCAINE

The addition of procaine to hyperkalemic crystalloid cardioplegic solutions has been found to be useful, but this benefit is diminished when profound hypothermia is utilized.[63,95,169,170] Elevated doses of procaine may be harmful.[145]

MAGNESIUM

Elevated levels of magnesium seem important to the preservation of myocardial function in rats, but not in rabbits.[58,71,171] The addition of magnesium to clinical solutions is of uncertain importance.

CALCIUM CHANNEL BLOCKERS

Calcium channel blockers (nifedipine, lidoflazine, diltiazam, and verapamil) have shown promise as additives to cardioplegic solutions. These additives have been shown to prevent calcium paradox, to decrease the accumulation of calcium in subcellular compartments, to decrease myocardial necrosis, and to improve postarrest myocardial function.[43,49,50,104,172–179] These benefits have been demonstrated with some experimental stage setting and are diminished when profound hypothermia is employed with hyperkalemic cardioplegic arrest.[180] Perhaps the most useful role of these agents will be as adjuncts to cardioplegia, administering the drug prior to cardioplegic arrest at a time when the intact coronary circulation can allow delivery of the drug to those regions of the myocardium which are difficult to perfuse with cardioplegic solutions.[51,52,103,104]

MANIPULATION OF THE REPERFUSATE

Oxygen Supply during Reperfusion

After ischemic arrest, myocardial damage may increase local coronary vascular resistance (by direct damage to the vasculature or by tissue swelling around the vasculature),[161,181–186] and oxygen extraction from blood may be impaired.[111,187,188] Regional myocardial blood flow may be further impaired by ventricular distension during reperfusion, and ventricular decompression is important during this critical period.[189] Reperfusion hemorrhage, once greatly feared, has now been shown to be the consequence of severe ischemia. Hemorrhage is not the cause of extension of ischemic damage during reperfusion.[190,191] As the myocardium recovers or deteriorates during reperfusion, high-energy phosphate levels may deteriorate further[192] or improve,[36] tissue swelling may increase[193] or decrease,[107] and compliance may increase[53] or decrease.[194]

Resting the Heart

After a period of ischemic or cardioplegic arrest, tolerance to the ischemic injury is enhanced by "resting" the heart on cardiopulmonary bypass for a period of time prior to asking it to resume the work of perfusing the rest of the body. This presumably allows energy supplies to be dedicated to cellular repair rather than draining energy supplies for external mechanical work.[53]

Chemical Asystole during Reperfusion

Buckberg and colleagues[53,54] have suggested that maintaining asystole during the early period of reperfusion will further reduce the oxygen requirement of the heart for mechanical purposes and allow improved recovery (demonstrated with normothermic ischemic arrest in dogs). When a less severe insult was created by hypothermic cardioplegic arrest, the benefits of asystole during reperfusion could not be demonstrated.[195]

An Alkaline Reperfusate

Buckberg and colleagues[53,63,196] have also demonstrated that reperfusion with an alkaline reperfusion solution enhances recovery after ischemic injury, presumably by reversing the metabolic acidosis that has occurred during the ischemic period and providing a better situation for metabolic recovery.

Substrate Enhancement

High-energy phosphate levels in severely injured myocardial tissues continue to decline with reperfusion, and the products of high-energy phosphate degradation can be recovered from the coronary sinus. The limiting factor in the recovery of cells may be in part the availability of the precursors of high-energy phosphates for the restoration of these compounds.[34] The addition of adenosine plus an inhibitor of adenosine diaminase has led to the enhancement of ATP return after ischemic arrest.[31] Carnitine infusion can cause elevation of ATP levels in regional ischemia.[55] The addition of a Krebs-cycle intermediate, L-glutamate, may lead to improved recovery of damaged myocardium.[54]

Calcium Availability

The degree of ischemic contracture after ischemic injury depends in part on the availability of the calcium ion in the early reperfusion period.[197] Contracture can be diminished if calcium concentration is lowered or a calcium channel blocker is added at the onset of contracture.[35,48,53]

Elevated Oncotic Pressure of the Reperfusate

Edema is not only the consequence of ischemic injury, but it may increase vascular resistance and cause further damage to the myocardium.[120,161,183–186,198] Elevation of oncotic pressure in the reperfusion solution has been proposed as one method of decreasing myocardial edema. One convenient method of achieving this is the addition of mannitol to the reperfusate. Mannitol improves myocardial contractility and collateral flow even in the absence of ischemic injury. When added to the reperfusate after ischemic injury, it can significantly decrease myocardial water content, increase regional blood flow, and improve functional recovery.[185,198–201]

The Optimal Reperfusion Pressure

Engelman et al.[202] found that a reperfusion pressure of 100 torr was deleterious to the heart when repeated episodes of ischemia were followed by temporary reperfusion. However, when reperfusion was permanent, no difference between 50 and 100 torr was demonstrated. Todd and colleagues[203] found that a reperfusion pressure of 95 to 100 torr led to better recovery of contractility and compliance than a pressure of 50 to 60 torr. Magee et al.[204] reported that a reperfusion pressure of 80 torr was superior to 50 torr. Although it has been suggested that reperfusion injury may be decreased by hypotension during the early reperfusion period,[53] there is little hard evidence to support this suggestion.

THE SEQUELAE OF CARDIOPLEGIC ARREST

The Characteristics of Damaged Regions after Inadequate Cardioplegic Protection

Ischemic arrest leads to decreased contractility and decreased compliance of damaged regions.[193,205] Studies of heterogeneous cardioplegic arrest have shown that regional protection is heterogeneous. Regions with good cardioplegic protection may have well-preserved contractility but decreased compliance, and regions with poor cardioplegic protection have both decreased contractility and compliance.[60,206,207] The compliance changes with good cardioplegic protection are variable in different experimental models.[63,130,194,207] In addition to a change in the slope of the relationship between muscle length and intracavitary distending pressure, there appears to be a change in the resting length of the muscle such that for a given left atrial pressure, segment length is longer after cardioplegic arrest than it was prior to cardioplegic arrest.[207] In general, cardioplegia seems to attenuate the decreased compliance that follows ischemic arrest in animals and human beings.[46,75,76,194,207,208] The addition of calcium channel blockers may further attenuate this change in compliance.[48,176,207] Neither pressure loading nor volume loading seems to have a deleterious effect on the function of damaged regions after cardioplegic arrest.[207]

How Long Is Cardioplegic Protection Safe?

In animal studies, crystalloid hypothermic hyperkalemic cardioplegic arrest provides very good preservation of myocardial function for periods at least as long as 2 h and in some instances as long as 3 h.[22,104,130,208,209] Similar time intervals have been well tolerated in patients with both crystalloid and blood cardioplegia.[138,139,210] However, it has been demonstrated that preservation of global pump function does not necessarily reflect preservation of regional function.[207] Chronic studies in animals surviving ischemic arrest and cardioplegic arrest have demonstrated fibrosis of the left ventricle in an alarming percentage of specimens.[211,212] In animals and patients, survivors of induced cardiac arrest may have diminished cardiac function 6 months later.[213,214] The surgeon may be happy when his or her patient is weaned from cardiopulmonary bypass with a low filling pressure and good global contractility, but this certainly does not guarantee that there is not severe regional damage and that subsequent scarring will not occur.[207]

TODAY'S METHOD AND MAGIC

There is method in today's cardioplegic protection as theoretical considerations continually advance new ideas to be tested. However, our understanding of the mechanisms of cellular damage remains so incomplete that much of our knowledge is empirical. It is evident that the heart needs to be in good metabolic condition prior to the institution of arrest. Oxygen delivery should be as high as possible and oxygen consumption should be decreased if possible (and certainly not elevated) at the time of arrest. Myocardial hypothermia is the first priority of any cardioplegic delivery technique. The optimal cardioplegic solution may be a blood- or crystalloid-based solution simulating the composition of the fluid that normally perfuses the myocardium with the addition of potassium to provide chemical asystole. Repeated infusions of solution maintain myocardial hypothermia and wash out accumulated metabolites during cardioplegic arrest. Blood cardioplegia or oxygenated crystalloid cardioplegia may provide an advantage in the delivery of oxygen to the myocardium during this period. The benefits of additives other than potassium to the cardioplegic solution seem to be attenuated by profound hypothermia. Calcium channel blockers do seem to show promise in the pretreatment of the myocardium prior to arrest, as an additive to the cardioplegic solution and in preventing damage during reperfusion. Reperfusion of the myocardium should be normotensive, and the work output required of the heart during this period should be minimized.

With current techniques, clinically damaging deterioration of myocardial function during open heart surgery has become a rare event. However, because of the heterogeneous nature of clinical cardioplegic protection, regional damage may occur and does occur without apparent global deterioration. The challenge posed by Melrose in 1955 remains. The search continues for the magic poison and the magic antidote.

REFERENCES

1 Fitts, D. (ed.): Aeschylus: Agamemnon, in "Greek Plays in Modern Translation," The Dial Press, New York, 1947, p. 36.

2 Melrose, D. G., Dreyer, B., Bentall, H. H., and Baker, J. B. E.: Elective Cardiac Arrest, *Lancet*, 2:21, 1955.

3 Effler, D. B., Knight, H. F., Jr., Groves, L. K., and Kolff, W. J.: Elective Cardiac Arrest for Open-Heart Surgery, *Surg. Gynecol. Obstet.*, 105:407, 1957.

4 Lam, C. R., Gahagan, T., Mota, C., and Green, E.: Induced Cardiac Arrest (Cardioplegia) in Open Heart Surgical Procedures, *Surgery*, 73:7, 1957.

5 Willman, V. L., Cooper, T., Zafiracopoulos, P., and Hanlon, C. R.: Depression of Ventricular Function Following Elective Cardiac Arrest with Potassium Citrate, *Surgery*, 46:792, 1959.

6 Waldhausen, J. A., Braunwald, N. S., Bloodwell, R. D., Cornell, W. P., and Morrow, A. G.: Left Ventricular Function Following Elective Cardiac Arrest, *J. Thorac. Cardiovasc. Surg.*, 39:799, 1960.

7 Tyers, G. F. O., Todd, G. J., Niebauer, I. M., Manley, N. J., and Waldhausen, J. A.: The Mechanism of Myocardial Damage Following Potassium Citrate (Melrose) Cardioplegia, *Surgery*, 78:45, 1975.

8 Shumway, N. E., Lower, R. R., and Stoffer, R. C.: Selective Hypothermia of the Heart in Anoxic Cardiac Arrest, *Surg. Gynecol. Obstet.*, 109:750, 1959.

9 Tyers, G. F. O., Hughes, H. C., Jr., Todd, G. J., et al.: Protection from Ischemic Cardiac Arrest by Coronary Perfusion with Cold Ringer's Lactate Solution, *J. Thorac. Cardiovasc. Surg.*, 67:411, 1974.

10 Katz, A. M., and Tada, M.: The "Stone Heart" and Other Challenges to the Biochemist, *Am. J. Cardiol.*, 39:1073, 1977.

11 Cooley, D. A., Reul, G. J., and Wukasch, D. C.: Ischemic Contracture of the Heart: "Stone Heart," *Am. J. Cardiol.*, 29:575, 1972.

12 Sturm, J. T., Bossart, M. I., Holub, D. A., Milam, J. D., and Norman, J. C.: Ultrastructural Analyses of Stone Heart Syndrome at Onset and Six Days Later Following Total Support of the Circulation with a Partial Artificial Heart or Left Ventricular Assist Device (ALVAD), *Cardiovasc. Disc.*, 6:29, 1979.

13 Reidemeister, J. C., Heberer, G., and Bretschneider, H. J.: Induced Cardiac Arrest by Sodium and Calcium Depletion and Application of Procaine, *Int. Surg.*, 47:535, 1967.

14 Bretschneider, H. J., Hubner, G., Knoll, D., Lohr, B., Nordbeck, H., Spieckermann, P. G.: Myocardial Resistance and Tolerance to Ischemia: Physiological and Biochemical Basis, *J. Cardiovasc. Surg.*, 16:241, 1975.

15 Kirsch, U., Rodewald, G., and Lalmar, P.: Induced Ischemic Arrest. Clinical Experience with Cardioplegia in Open-Heart Surgery, *J. Thorac. Cardiovasc. Surg.*, 63:121, 1972.

16 Kalmar, P., Bleese, N., Doring, V., et al.: Induced Ischemic Cardiac Arrest. Clinical and Experimental Results with Magnesium-Aspartate-Procaine Solution (Cardioplegin), *J. Cardiovasc. Surg.*, 16:470, 1975.

17 Althaus, J., and Senn, A.: Clinical Experience with the Bretschneider-Cardioplegia in Aortic Valve Replacement, *J. Cardiovasc. Surg.*, 12:463, 1971.

18 Gay, W. A., Jr., and Ebert, P. A.: Functional, Metabolic, and Morphologic Effects of Potassium-Induced Cardioplegia, *Surgery*, 74:284, 1973.

19 Hearse, D. J., Stewart, D. A., and Chain, E. B.: Recovery from Cardiac Bypass and Elective Cardiac Arrest. The Metabolic Consequences of Various Cardioplegic Procedures in the Isolated Rat Heart, *Circ. Res.*, 35:448, 1974.

20 Hearse, D. J., Stewart, D. A., and Braimbridge, M. V.: Cellular Protection during Myocardial Ischemia. The Development and Characterization of a Procedure for the Induction of Reversible Ischemic Arrest, *Circulation*, 54:193, 1976.

21 Marrin, C. A. S., Spotnitz, H. M., and Bregman, D.: "Myocardial Preservation," Year Book Medical Publishers, Chicago, 1981, p. 479.

22 Buckberg, G. D.: A Proposed "Solution" to the Cardioplegic Controversy, *J. Thorac. Cardiovasc. Surg.*, 77:803, 1979.

23 Kirklin, J. W., Conti, V. R., and Blackstone, E. H.: Prevention of Myocardial Damage during Cardiac Operations, *N. Engl. J. Med.*, 301:135, 1979.

24 Adams, P. X., Cunningham, J. N., Jr., Trehan, N. K., Brazier, J. R., Reed, G. E., and Spencer, F. C.: Clinical Experience Using Potassium-Induced Cardioplegia with Hypothermia in Aortic Valve Replacement, *J. Thorac. Cardiovasc. Surg.*, 75:564, 1978.

25 Stiles, Q. R., and Kirklin, J. W.: Myocardial Preservation Symposium, *J. Thorac. Cardiovasc. Surg.*, 82:870, 1981.

26 Tyers, G. F. O., Manley, N. J., Williams, E. H., Shaffer, C. W., Williams, D. R., and Kurusz, M.: Preliminary Clinical Experience with Isotonic Hypothermic Potassium-Induced Arrest, *J. Thorac. Cardiovasc. Surg.*, 74:674, 1977.

27 Jennings, R. B., and Hawkins, H. K.: Ultrastructural Changes of Acute Myocardial Ischemia, in Wildenthal (ed.), "Degradative Processes in Heart and Skeletal Muscle," Elsevier/North-Holland Biomedical Press, Amsterdam, 1980, p. 295.

28 Jennings, R. B., Sommers, H. M., Kaltenbach, J. P., and West, J. J.: Electrolyte Alterations in Acute Myocardial Ischemic Injury, *Circ. Res.*, 14:260, 1964.

29 Whalen, D. A., Jr., Hamilton, D. G., Ganote, C. E., and Jennings, R. B.: Effect of a Transient Period of Ischemia on Myocardial Cells: I. Effects on Cell Volume Regulation, *Am. J. Pathol.*, 74:381, 1974.

30 Engelman, R. M., Rousou, J. H., Longo, F., Auvil, J., and Vertrees, R. A.: The Time Course of Myocardial High-Energy Phosphate Degradation during Potassium Cardioplegic Arrest, *Surgery*, 86:138, 1979.

31 Foker, J. E., Einzig, S., Wang, T., and Anderson, R. W.: Adenosine Metabolism and Myocardial Preservation. Consequences of Adenosine Catabolism on Myocardial High-Energy Compounds and Tissue Blood Flow, *J. Thorac. Cardiovasc. Surg.*, 80:506, 1980.

32 Reimer, K. A., Jennings, R. B., and Hill, M. L.: Total Ischemia in Dog Hearts, In Vitro: 2. High Energy Phosphate Depletion and Associated Defects in Energy Metabolism, Cell Volume Regulation, and Sarcolemmal Integrity, *Circ. Res.*, 49:901, 1981.

33 Kloner, R. A., DeBoer, L. W. V., Darsee, J. R., et al.: Prolonged Abnormalities of Myocardium Salvaged by Reperfusion, *Am. J. Physiol.*, 241:H591, 1981.

34 Swain, J. L., Sabina, R. L., McHale, P. A., Greenfield, J. C., Jr., and Holmes, E. W.: Prolonged Myocardial Nucleotide Depletion after Brief Ischemia in the Open-Chest Dog, *Am. J. Physiol.*, 242:H818, 1982.

35 Hearse, D. J., Garlick, P. B., and Humphrey, S. M.: Ischemic Contracture of the Myocardium: Mechanisms and Prevention, *Am. J. Cardiol.*, 39:986, 1977.

36 Wright, R. N., Levitsky, S., Holland, C., and Feinberg, H.: Beneficial Effects of Potassium Cardioplegia during Intermittent Aortic Cross-Clamping and Reperfusion, *J. Surg. Res.*, 24:201, 1978.

37 Buckberg, G. D., Brazier, J. R., Nelson, R. L., Goldstein, S. M., McConnell, D. H., and Cooper, N.: Studies of the Effects of Hypothermia on Regional Myocardial Blood Flow and Metabolism during Cardiopulmonary Bypass: I. The Adequately Perfused Beating, Fibrillating, and Arrested Heart, *J. Thorac. Cardiovasc. Surg.*, 73:87, 1977.

38 Chitwood, W. R., Jr., Sink, J. D., Hill, R. C., Wechsler, A. S., and Sabiston, D. C., Jr.: The Effects of Hypothermia on Myocardial Oxygen Consumption and Transmural Coronary Blood Flow in the Potassium-Arrested Heart, *Ann. Surg.*, 190:106, 1979.

39 Buckberg, G. D., and Hottenrott, C. E.: Ventricular Fibrillation. Its Effect on Myocardial Flow, Distribution, and Performance, *Ann. Thorac. Surg.*, 20:76, 1975.

40 Raffa, J., Mavroudis, C., Trunkey, D. D., and Ebert, P. A.: The Effects of Hypothermia and Cardioplegia on Cardiac Intracellular Membrane Potentials, *J. Surg. Res.*, 26:58, 1979.

41 Brandt, B., III, Richardson, J. V., O'Bryan, P., and Ehrenhaft, J. L.: Intramyocardial Electrical and Metabolic Activity during Hypothermia and Potassium Cardioplegia, *Ann. Thorac. Surg.*, 31:117, 1981.

42 Engelman, R. M., Auvil, J., O'Donoghue, M. H., and Levitsky, S.: The Significance of Multidose Cardioplegia and Hypothermia in Myocardial Preservation during Ischemic Arrest, *J. Thorac. Cardiovasc. Surg.*, 75:555, 1978.

43 Magee, P. G., Flaherty, J. T., Bixler, T. J., et al.: Comparison of Myocardial Protection with Nifedipine and Potassium, *Circulation*, 60 (suppl. 1):151, 1979.

44 Vouhe, P. R., Helias, J., and Grondin, C. M.: Myocardial Protection through Cold Cardioplegia Using Diltiazem, a Calcium Channel Blocker, *Ann. Thorac. Surg.*, 30:342, 1980.

45 Tyers, G. F. O., Todd, G. J., Niebauer, I. M., Manley, N. J., and Waldhausen, J. A.: Effect of Intracoronary Tetrodotoxin on Recovery of the Isolated Working Rat Heart from Sixty Minutes of Ischemia, *Circulation*, 49 and 50 (suppl. 2):175, 1974.

46 Follette, D. M., Mulder, D. G., Maloney, J. V., Jr., and Buckberg, G. D.: Advantages of Blood Cardioplegia over Continuous Coronary Perfusion or Intermittent Ischemia. Experimental and Clinical Study, *J. Thorac. Cardiovasc. Surg.*, 76:604, 1978.

47 Engelman, R. M., Rousou, J. H., Dobbs, W., Pels, M. A., and Longo, F.: The Superiority of Blood Cardioplegia in Myocardial Preservation, *Circulation*, 62 (suppl. 1):62, 1980.

48 Nayler, W. G., Yepez, C. E., and Poole-Wilson, P. A.: The Effect of β-Adrenoceptor and Ca^{2+} Antagonist Drugs on the Hypoxia-Induced Increase in Resting Tension, *Cardiovasc. Res.*, 12:666, 1978.

49 Clark, R. E., Ferguson, T. B., West, P. N., Shuchleib, R. C., and Henry, P. D.: Pharmacological Preservation of the Ischemic Heart, *Ann. Thorac. Surg.*, 24:307, 1977.

50 Clark, R. E., Christlieb, I. Y., Henry, P. D., et al.: Nifedipine: A Myocardial Protective Agent, *Am. J. Cardiol.*, 44:825, 1979.

51 Naylor, W. G., Ferrari, R., and Williams, A.: Protective Effect of Pretreatment with Verapamil, Nifedipine and Propranolol on Mitochondrial Function in the Ischemic and Reperfused Myocardium, *Am. J. Cardiol.*, 46:242, 1980.

52 Flameng, W., Daenen, W., Borgers, M., et al.: Cardioprotective Effects of Lidoflazine during 1-Hour Normothermic Global Ischemia, *Circulation*, 64:796, 1981.

53 Lazar, H. L., Buckberg, G. D., Manganaro, A. J., et al.: Reversal of Ischemic Damage with Secondary Blood Cardioplegia, *J. Thorac. Cardiovasc. Surg.*, 78:688, 1979.

54 Lazar, H. L., Buckberg, G. D., Manganaro, A. J., and Becker, H.: Myocardial Energy Replenishment and Reversal of Ischemic Damage by Substrate Enhancement of Secondary Blood Cardioplegia with Amino Acids during Reperfusion, *J. Thorac. Cardiovasc. Surg*, 80:350, 1980.

55 Folts, J. D., Shug, A. L., Koke, J. R., and Bittar, N.: Protection of the Ischemic Dog Myocardium with Carnitine, *Am. J. Cardiol.*, 41:1209, 1978.

56 Brazier, J., Hottenrott, C., and Buckberg, G.: Noncoronary Collateral Myocardial Blood Flow, *Ann. Thorac. Surg.*, 19:426, 1975.

57 Lochner, W., Arnold, G., and Muller-Ruchholtz, E. R.: Metabolism of the Artificially Arrested Heart and of the Gas-Perfused Heart, *Am. J. Cardiol.,* 22:299, 1968.

58 Bersohn, M. M., Shine, K. I., and Sterman, W. D.: Effect of Increased Magnesium on Recovery from Ischemia in Rat and Rabbit Hearts, *Am. J. Physiol.,* 242:H89, 1982.

59 Guyton, R. A., Jacobs, M. L., Fowler, B. N., Greffin, G. A., O'Keefe, D. D., and Daggett, W. M.: Regional Myocardial Protection: Use of a New Method to Compare Cold Potassium Cardioplegia with Hypothermic Coronary Perfusion, *Circulation,* 62 (suppl. 1):126, 1980.

60 Lucas, S. K., Elmer, E. B., Flaherty, J. T., et al.: Effect of Multiple-Dose Potassium Cardioplegia on Myocardial Ischemia, Return of Ventricular Function, and Ultrastructural Preservation, *J. Thorac. Cardiovasc. Surg.,* 80:102, 1980.

61 Lolley, D. M., Fay, J. R., III, Myers, W. O., Sautter, R. D., and Sheldon, G.: Is Reperfusion Injury from Multiple Aortic Cross-Clamping a Current Myth of Cardiac Surgery?, *Ann. Thorac. Surg.,* 30:110, 1980.

62 Bulkley, B. H.: The Reperfusion Injury of Cardiac Operation: Separating Myths from Realities, *Ann. Thorac. Surg.,* 30:103, 1980.

63 Follette, D., Fey, K., Mulder, D., Maloney, J. V., Jr., and Buckberg, G. D.: Prolonged Safe Aortic Clamping by Combining Membrane Stabilization, Multidose Cardioplegia, and Appropriate pH Reperfusion, *J. Thorac. Cardiovasc. Surg.,* 74:682, 1977.

64 Balderman, S. C., Bhayana, J. N., Binette, P., Chan, A., Gage, A. A., and Adler, R. H.: Perioperative Preservation of Myocardial Ultrastructure and High-Energy Phosphates in Man, *J. Thorac. Cardiovasc. Surg.,* 82:860, 1981.

65 Schaper, J., Schwarz, F., Kittstein, H., et al.: The Effects of Global Ischemia and Reperfusion on Human Myocardium: Quantitative Evaluation by Electron Microscopic Morphometry, *Ann. Thorac. Surg.,* 33:116, 1982.

66 Sink, J. D., Pellom, G. L., Currie, W. D., Chitwood, W. R., Jr., Hill, R. C., and Wechsler, A. S.: Protection of Mitochondrial Function during Ischemia by Potassium Cardioplegia: Correlation with Ischemic Contracture, *Circulation,* 60 (suppl. 1):158, 1979.

67 Gillette, P. C., Pinsky, W. W., Lewis, R. M., et al.: Myocardial Depression after Elective Ischemic Arrest. Subcellular Biochemistry and Prevention, *J. Thorac. Cardiovasc. Surg.,* 77:608, 1979.

68 Schaff, H. V., Dombroff, R., Flaherty, J. T., et al.: Effect of Potassium Cardioplegia on Myocardial Ischemia and Post Arrest Ventricular Function, *Circulation,* 58:240, 1978.

69 Flaherty, J. T., Weisfeldt, M. L., Hollis, D. P., Schaff, H. V., Gott, V. L., and Jacobus, W. E.: Mass Spectrometry and Phosphorus-31 Nuclear Magnetic Resonance Demonstrate Additive Myocardial Protection by Potassium Cardioplegia and Hypothermia during Global Ischemia, in M.

Tajuddin, B. Bhatia, H. H. Siddiqui, and G. Rona (eds.), "Advances in Myocardiology," Vol. 1, University Park Press, Baltimore, 1980, p. 487.

70 Flaherty, J. T., Weisfeldt, M. L., Bulkley, B. H., Gardner, T. J., Gott, V. L., and Jacobus, W. E.: Mechanisms of Ischemic Myocardial Cell Damage Assessed by Phosphorus-31 Nuclear Magnetic Resonance, *Circulation,* 65:561, 1982.

71 Pernot, A. C., Ingwall, J. S., Menasche, P., et al.: Limitations of Potassium Cardioplegia during Cardiac Ischemic Arrest: A Phosphorus-31 Nuclear Magnetic Resonance Study, *Ann. Thorac. Surg.,* 32:536, 1981.

72 Flameng, W., Borgers, M., Daenen, W., et al.: St. Thomas Cardioplegia versus Topical Cooling: Ultrastructural and Biochemical Studies in Humans, *Ann. Thorac. Surg.,* 31:339, 1981.

73 Juggi, J. S., Saw, H. S. and Ganendran, A.: Effect of Potassium-Induced Cardioplegia in Hypothermia on Myocardial Energy, Ammonium, and Intermediary Metabolism in Man, in "Advances in Myocardiology," Vol. 2, University Park Press, Baltimore, 1980, p. 501.

74 Schachner A., Siegel, J. H., Schimert, G., et al.: Does Potassium Potentiate Profound Hypothermic Cardioplegia for Myocardial Preservation?, *Surgery,* 84:94, 1978.

75 Chitwood, W. R., Jr., Hill, R. C., Sink, J. D., Kleinman, L. H., Sabiston, D. C., Jr., and Wechsler, A. S.: Measurement of Global Ventricular Function in Patients during Cardiac Operations Using Sonomicrometry, *J. Thorac. Cardiovasc. Surg.,* 80:724, 1980.

76 Slack, J. D., Zeok, J. V., Cole, J. S., et al.: Influence of Potassium Cardioplegia versus Ischemic Arrest on Regional Left Ventricular Diastolic Compliance in Humans, *Ann. Thorac. Surg.,* 31:214, 1981.

77 Hilton, J. D., Weisel, R. D., Baird, R. J., et al.: The Hemodynamic and Metabolic Response to Pacing after Aortocoronary Bypass, *Circulation,* 64 (suppl. 2):48, 1981.

78 Mangano, D. T., Van Dyke, D. C., and Ellis, R. J.: The Effect of Increasing Preload on Ventricular Output and Ejection in Man, *Circulation,* 62:535, 1980.

79 Arom, K. V., Grover, F. L., and Trinkle, J. K.: Does Cardioplegic Arrest Compromise Long-Term Left Ventricular Function?, *Ann. Thorac. Surg.,* 29:539, 1980.

80 Weisel, R. D., Goldman, B. S., Lipton, I. H., Teasdale, S., Mickle, D., and Baird, R. J.: Optimal Myocardial Protection, *Surgery,* 84:812, 1978.

81 Delva, E., Maille, J. G., Solymoss, B. C., Chabot, M., Grondin, C. M., and Bourassa, M. G.: Evaluation of Myocardial Damage during Coronary Artery Grafting with Serial Determinations of Serum CPK MB Isoenzyme, *J. Thorac. Cardiovasc. Surg.,* 75:467, 1978.

82 Engelman, R. M., Spencer, F. C., Boyd, A. D., and Chandra, R.: The Significance of Coronary Arterial Stenosis during Cardiopulmonary Bypass, *J. Thorac. Cardiovasc. Surg.,* 70:869, 1975.

83 Sink, J. D., Hill, R. C., Chitwood, W. R., Jr., Abriss, R., and Wechsler, A. S.: Effects of Phenylephrine on Transmural Distribution of Myocardial Blood Flow in Regions Supplied by Normal and Collateral Arteries during Cardiopulmonary Bypass, *J. Thorac. Cardiovasc. Surg.,* 78:236, 1979.

84 Miyamoto, A. T. M., Robinson, L., Matloff, J. M., and Norman, J. R.: Perioperative Infarction. Effects of Cardiopulmonary Bypass on Collateral Circulation in an Acute Canine Model, *Circulation,* 58 (suppl. 1):147, 1978.

85 Khuri, S. F., Brawley, R. K., O'Riordan, J. B., Donahoo, J. S., Pitt, B., and Gott, V. L.: The Effect of Cardiopulmonary Bypass Perfusion Pressure on Myocardial Gas Tensions in the Presence of Coronary Stenosis, *Ann. Thorac. Surg.,* 20:661, 1975.

86 Kleinman, L. H., Yarbrough, J. W., Symmonds, J. B., Wechsler, A. S., and Sabiston, D. C., Jr.: Pressure-Flow Characteristics of the Coronary Collateral Circulation during Cardiopulmonary Bypass. Effects of Hemodilution, *J. Thorac. Cardiovasc. Surg.,* 75:17, 1978.

87 Anderson, H. T., Kessinger, J. M., McFarland, W. J., Jr., Laks, H., and Geha, A. S.: Response of the Hypertrophied Heart to Acute Anemia and Coronary Stenosis, *Surgery,* 84:8, 1978.

88 Archie, J. P., and Kirklin, J. W.: Effect of Hypothermic Perfusion on Myocardial Oxygen Consumption and Coronary Resistance, *Surg. Forum,* 24:186, 1973.

89 McConnell, D. H., Brazier, J. R., Cooper, N., and Buckberg, G. D.: Studies of the Effects of Hypothermia on Regional Myocardial Blood Flow and Metabolism during Cardiopulmonary Bypass: II. Ischemia during Moderate Hypothermia in Continually Perfused Beating Hearts, *J. Thorac. Cardiovasc. Surg.,* 73:95, 1977.

90 Brazier, J. R., Cooper, N., McConnell, D. H., and Buckberg, G. D.: Studies of the Effects of Hypothermia on Regional Myocardial Blood Flow and Metabolism during Cardiopulmonary Bypass: III. Effects of Temperature, Time, and Perfusion Pressure in Fibrillating Hearts, *J. Thorac. Cardiovasc. Surg.,* 73:102, 1977.

91 Kleinman, L. H., and Wechsler, A. S.: Pressure-Flow Characteristics of the Coronary Collateral Circulation during Cardiopulmonary Bypass. Effects of Ventricular Fibrillation, *Circulation* 58:233, 1978.

92 Schaff, H. V., Ciardullo, R. C., Flaherty, J. T., and Gott, V. L.: Development of Regional Myocardial Ischemia Distal to a Crtical Coronary Stenosis during Cardiopulmonary Bypass: Comparison of the Fibrillating vs. the Beating Nonworking States, *Surgery,* 83:57, 1978.

93 Ellis, A. K., and Klocke, F. J.: Effects of Preload on the Transmural Distribution of Perfusion and Pressure-Flow Relationships in the Canine Coronary Vascular Bed, *Circ. Res.* 46:68, 1980.

94 Lucas, S. K., Gardner, T. J., Elmer, E. B., Flaherty, J. T., Bulkley, B. H., and Gott, V. L.: Comparison of the Effects of Left Ventricular Distention during Cardioplegic-Induced Ischemic Arrest and Ventricular Fibrillation, *Circulation,* 62 (suppl. 1):42, 1980.

95 Kay, H. R., Levine, F. H., Fallon, J. T., et al.: Effect of Cross-Clamp Time, Temperature, and Cardioplegic Agents on Myocardial Function after Induced Arrest, *J. Thorac. Cardiovasc. Surg.,* 76:590, 1978.

96 Butchart, E. G., McEnany, M., Strich, G., Sbokos, C., and Austen, W. G.: The Influence of Prearrest Factors on the Preservation of Left Ventricular Function during Cardiopulmonary Bypass, *J. Thorac. Cardiovasc. Surg.,* 79:812, 1980.

97 Magee, P. G., Gardner, T. J., Flaherty, J. T., Bulkley, B. H., Goldman, R. A., and Gott, V. L.: Improved Myocardial Protection with Propranolol during Induced Ischemia, *Circulation,* 62 (suppl. 1):49, 1980.

98 Spath, J. A., Jr., and Barsotti, R. J.: Blood Flow and Ultrastructure in Ischemic Myocardium of Cats Given Dexamethasone, *Am. J. Physiol.,* 242:H55, 1982.

99 Hoffstein, S., Weissmann, G., and Fox, A. C.: Lysosomes in Myocardial Infarction: Studies by Means of Cytochemistry and Subcellular Fractionation, with Observations on the Effects of Methylprednisolone, *Circulation,* 53 (suppl. 1):34, 1976.

100 Fey, K., Follette, D., Livesay, J., et al.: Effects of Membrane Stabilization on the Safety of Hypothermic Arrest after Aortic Cross-Clamping, *Circulation,* 56 (suppl. 2):143, 1977.

101 Kirsh, M. M., Behrendt, D. M., and Jochim, K. E.: Effects of Methylprednisolone in Cardioplegic Solution during Coronary Bypass Grafting, *J. Thorac. Cardiovasc. Surg.,* 77:896, 1979.

102 Goldman, R. A., Schaff, H. V., Flaherty, J. T., et al.: Failure of Methylprednisolone to Protect Myocardial Function or Prevent Myocardial Edema Following Ischemic Cardiac Arrest, *J. Surg. Res.,* 24:477, 1978.

103 Kates, R. B., Dorsey, L. M., Kaplan, J., Hatcher, C. R., Jr., and Guyton, R. A.: Pretreatment with Lidoflazine, a Calcium-Channel Blocker: A Useful Adjunct to Heterogeneous Cold Potassium Cardioplegia, *J. Thorac. Cardiovasc. Surg.,* in press.

104 Guyton, R. A., Dorsey, L. M., Colgan, T. K., and Hatcher, C. R., Jr.: Calcium Channel Blockade as an Adjunct to Heterogeneous Cardioplegia, *Ann. Thorac. Surg.,* in press.

105 Lolley, D. M., Ray, J. F., III, Myers, W. O., Sautter, R. D., and Tewksbury, D. A.: Importance of Preoperative Myocardial Glycogen Levels in Human Cardiac Preservation. Preliminary Report, *J. Thorac. Cardiovasc. Surg.,* 78:678, 1979.

106 Salerno, T. A., Wasan, S. M., and Charrette, E. J. P.: Glucose Substrate in Myocardial Protection, *J. Thorac. Cardiovasc. Surg.,* 79:59, 1980.

107 Bethencourt, D. M., and Laks, H.: Importance of Edema and Compliance Changes during 24 Hours of Preservation of the Dog Heart, *J. Thorac. Cardiovasc. Surg.,* 81:440, 1981.

108 Ellis, R. J., Pryor, W., and Ebert, P. A.: Advantages of Potassium Cardioplegia and Perfusion Hypothermia in Left Ventricular Hypertrophy, *Ann. Thorac. Surg.,* 24:299, 1977.

109 Tyers, G. F. O., Williams, E. H., Hughes, H. C., and Todd, G. J.: Effect of Perfusate Temperature on Myocardial Protection from Ischemia, *J. Thorac. Cardiovasc. Surg.,* 73:766, 1977.

110 Sunamori, M., Trout, R. G., Kaye, M. P., and Harrison, C. E., Jr.: Quantitative Evaluation of Myocardial Ultrastructure Following Hypothermic Anoxic Arrest, *J. Thorac. Cardiovasc. Surg.,* 76:518, 1978.

111 Nelson, R. L., Goldstein, S. M., McConnell, D. H., Maloney, J. V., Jr., and Buckberg, G. D.: Improved Myocardial Performance after Aortic Cross-Clamping by Combining Pharmacologic Arrest with Topical Hypothermia, *Circulation,* 54 (suppl. 3):11, 1976.

112 Rosenfeldt, F. L., Hearse, D. J., Cankovic-Darracott, S., and Braimbridge, M. V.: The Additive Protective Effects of Hypothermia and Chemical Cardioplegia during Ischemic Cardiac Arrest in the Dog, *J. Thorac. Cardiovasc. Surg.,* 79:29, 1980.

113 Hearse, D. J., Stewart, D. A., and Braimbridge, M. V.: The Additive Protective Effects of Hypothermia and Chemical Cardioplegia during Ischemic Cardiac Arrest in the Rat, *J. Thorac. Cardiovasc. Surg.,* 79:39, 1980.

114 Behrendt, D. M., and Jochim, K. E.: Effect of Temperature of Cardioplegic Solution, *J. Thorac. Cardiovasc. Surg.,* 76:353, 1978.

115 Mundth, E. D., Goel, I. P., Morgan, R. J., McEnany, M. T., and Austen, W. G.: Effect of Potassium Cardioplegia and Hypothermia on Left Ventricular Function in Hypertrophied and Nonhypertrophied Hearts, *Surg. Forum,* 26:257, 1975.

116 Heineman, F. W., MacGregor, D. C., Wilson, G. J., and Ninomiya, J.: Regional and Transmural Myocardial Temperature Distribution in Cold Chemical Cardioplegia. Significance of Critical Coronary Arterial Stenosis, *J. Thorac. Cardiovasc. Surg.,* 81:851, 1981.

117 Landymore, R. W., Tice, D., Trehan, N., and Spencer, F.: Importance of Topical Hypothermia to Ensure Uniform Myocardial Cooling During Coronary Artery Bypass, *J. Thorac. Cardiovasc. Surg.,* 82:832, 1981.

118 Hilton, C. J., Teubl, W., Acker, M., et al.: Inadequate Cardioplegic Protection with Obstructed Coronary Arteries, *Ann. Thorac. Surg.,* 28:323, 1979.

119 Johnson, R. E., Dorsey, L. M., Moye, S. J., Hatcher, C. R., Jr., and Guyton, R. A.: Cardioplegia Infusion: The Safe Limits of Pressure and Temperature, *J. Thorac. Cardiovasc. Surg.,* 83:813, 1982.

120 Guyton, R. A., McClenathan, J. H., Newman, G. E., and Michaelis, L. L.: Significance of Subendocardial S-T Segment Elevation Caused by Coronary Stenosis in the Dog. Epicardial S-T Segment Depression, Local Ischemia and Subsequent Necrosis, *Am. J. Cardiol.,* 40:373, 1977.

121 Brown, A. H., Baimbridge, M. V., Niles, N. R., Gerbode, F., and Aguilar, M. J.: The Effect of Excessively High Perfusion Pressures on the Histology, Histochemistry, Birefringence, and Function of the Myocardium, *J. Thorac. Cardiovasc. Surg.,* 58:655, 1969.

122 Steiner, D., Bleese, N., Doring, V., and Riesner, K.: Prevention of Edema during Coronary Perfusion with Cardioplegic Solution, *Thoraxchir. Vask. Chir.,* 25:235, 1977.

123 Bleese, N., Doring, V., Kalmar, P., et al.: Intraoperative Myocardial Protection by Cardioplegia in Hypothermia. Clinical Findings, *J. Thorac. Cardiovasc. Surg.,* 75:405, 1978.

124 Molina, J. E., Gani, K. S., and Voss, D. M.: Pressurized Rapid Cardioplegia versus Administration of Exogenous Substrate and Topical Hypothermia, *Ann. Thorac. Surg.,* 33:434, 1982.

125 Speicher, C. E., Ferrigan, L., Wolfson, S. K., Jr., Yalav, E. H., and Rawson, A. J.: Cold Injury of Myocardium and Pericardium in Cardiac Hypothermia, *Surg. Gynecol. Obstet.,* 114:659, 1962.

126 Griepp, R. B., Stinson, E. G., Angell, W. W., Dong, E., Jr., and Shumway, N. E.: Hypothermic Preservation of the Canine Heart, *Transplant. Proc.,* 6:315, 1974.

127 Harlan, B. J., Ross, D., MacManus, Q., Knight, R., Luber, J., and Starr, A.: Cardioplegic Solutions for Myocardial Preservation. Analysis of Hypothermic Arrest, Potassium Arrest, and Procaine Arrest, *Circulation,* 58 (suppl. 1):114, 1978.

128 Shragge, B. W., Digerness, S. B., and Blackstone, E. H.: Complete Recovery of the Heart Following Exposure to Profound Hypothermia, *J. Thorac. Cardiovasc. Surg.,* 81:455, 1981.

129 Swanson, D. K., Dufek, J. H., and Kahn, D. R.: Improved Myocardial Preservation at 4°C, *Ann. Thorac. Surg.,* 30:519, 1980.

130 Engelman, R. M., Levitsky, S., O'Donoghue, M. J., and Auvil, J.: Cardioplegia and Myocardial Preservation during Cardiopulmonary Bypass, *Circulation,* 58 (suppl. 1):107, 1978.

131 Reitz, B. A., Brody, W. R., Hickey, P. R. and Michaelis, L. L.: Protection of the Heart for 24 hr. with Intracellular (High K^+) Solution and Hypothermia, *Surg. Forum,* 25:149, 1974.

132 Vander Salm, T. J., Okike, O. N., Cutler, B. S., Paraskos, J. A., Ferulo, J., and Daggett, W.: Improved Myocardial Preservation by Improved Distribution of Cardioplegic Solutions, *J. Thorac. Cardiovasc. Surg.,* 83:767, 1982.

133 Becker, H., Vinten-Johansen, J., Buckberg, G. D., Follette, D. M., and Robertson, J. M.: Critical Importance of Ensuring Cardioplegic Delivery with Coronary Stenoses, *J. Thorac. Cardiovasc. Surg.,* 81:507, 1981.

134 Daggett, W. M., Jacocks, A., Coleman, W. S., Johnson, R. G., Lowenstein, E., and Vander Salm, T. J.: Myocardial

Temperature Mapping. Improved Intraoperative Myocardial Preservation, *J. Thorac. Cardiovasc. Surg.*, 82:883, 1981.

135 Walls, J. T., Nasser, F. N., Baron, D. W., Tinker, J. H., and Harrison, C. E., Jr.: Beneficial Effects of Multidose Coronary Artery Washout during Elective Cardiac Arrest and Cardiopulmonary Bypass. Biochemical and Hemodynamic Evaluation, *J. Thorac. Cardiovasc. Surg.*, 83:772, 1982.

136 Engelman, R. M., Rousou, J. H., O'Donoghue, M. J., Longo, F., and Dobbs, W. A.: A Comparison of Intermittent and Continuous Arrest for Prolonged Hypothermic Cardioplegia, *Ann. Thorac. Surg.*, 29:217, 1980.

137 Roberts, A. J., Abel, R. M., Alonso, D. R., Subramanian, V. A., Paul, J. S., and Gay, W. A., Jr.: Advantages of Hypothermic Potassium Cardioplegia and Superiority of Continuous versus Intermittent Aortic Cross-Clamping, *J. Thorac. Cardiovasc. Surg.*, 79:44, 1980.

138 Catinella, F. P., Cunningham, J. N., Jr., Adams, P. X., Snively, S. L., Gross, R. I., and Spencer, F. C.: Myocardial Protection with Cold Blood Potassium Cardioplegia during Prolonged Aortic Cross-Clamping, *Ann. Thorac. Surg.*, 33:228, 1982.

139 Engelman, R. M., Rousou, J. H., Vertrees, R. A., Rohrer, C., and Auvil, J.,: Safety of Prolonged Ischemic Arrest Using Hypothermic Cardioplegia, *J. Thorac. Cardiovasc. Surg.*, 79:705, 1980.

140 Grover, F. L., Fewel, J. G., Ghidoni, J. J., and Trinkle, J. K.: Does Lower Systemic Temperature Enhance Cardioplegic Myocardial Protection?, *J. Thorac. Cardiovasc. Surg.*, 81:11, 1981.

141 Ochsner, J. L.: Adequacy of Myocardial Protection, *Ann. Thorac. Surg.*, 28:305, 1979.

142 Carpentier, S., Murawsky, M., and Carpentier, A.: Cytotoxicity of Cardioplegic Solutions: Evaluation by Tissue Culture, *Circulation*, 64 (suppl. 2):90, 1981.

143 Jynge, P., Hearse, D. J., de Leiris, J., Feuvray, D., and Braimbridge, M. V.: Protection of the Ischemic Myocardium. Ultrastructural, Enzymatic, and Functional Assessment of the Efficacy of Various Cardioplegic Infusates, *J. Thorac. Cardiovasc. Surg.*, 76:2, 1978.

144 Jynge, P., Hearse, D. J., and Braimbridge, M. V.: Protection of the Ischemic Myocardium. Volume-Duration Relationships and the Efficacy of Myocardial Infusates, *J. Thorac. Cardiovasc. Surg.*, 76:698, 1978.

145 Hearse, D. J., O'Brien, K., and Braimbridge, M. V.: Protection of the Myocardium during Ischemic Arrest. Dose-Response Curves for Procaine and Lignocaine in Cardioplegic Solutions, *J. Thorac. Cardiovasc. Surg.*, 81:873, 1981.

146 Ellis, R. J., Mangano, D. T., Van Dyke, D. C., and Ebert, P. A.: Protection of Myocardial Function Not Enhanced by High Concentrations of Potassium during Cardioplegic Arrest, *J. Thorac. Cardiovasc. Surg.*, 78:698, 1979.

147 Ellis, R. J., Pryor, W., and Ebert, P. A.: Advantages of Potassium Cardioplegia and Perfusion Hypothermia in Left Ventricular Hypertrophy, *Ann. Thorac. Surg.*, 24:299, 1977.

148 Grover, F. L., Fewel, J. G., Ghidoni, J. J., Arom, K. V., and Trinkle, J. K.: Is Potassium a Necessary Component of Cardioplegic Solutions?, *J. Surg. Res.*, 29:62, 1980.

149 Tucker, W. Y., Ellis, R. J., Mangano, D. T., Ryan, C. J. M., and Ebert, P. A.: Questionable Importance of High Potassium Concentrations in Cardioplegic Solutions, *J. Thorac. Cardiovasc. Surg.*, 77:183, 1979.

150 Mavroudis, C., and Ebert, P. A.: Effects of High Potassium Cardioplegia and Hypothermia on Myocardial Compliance and Distribution of Water and Potassium: II. The Hypertrophied Canine Heart, *Surgery*, 85:662, 1979.

151 Ellis, R. J., Mavroudis, C., Gardner, C., Turley, K., Ullyot, D., and Ebert, P. A.: Relationship between Atrioventricular Arrhythmias and the Concentration of K^+ Ion in Cardioplegic Solutions, *J. Thorac. Cardiovasc. Surg.*, 80:517, 1980.

152 Gharagozloo, F., Bulkley, B. H., Hutchins, G. M., et al.: Potassium-Induced Cardioplegia during Normothermic Cardiac Arrest. Morphologic Study of the Effect of Varying Concentrations of Potassium on Myocardial Anoxic Injury, *J. Thorac. Cardiovasc. Surg.*, 77:602, 1979.

153 Rousou, J. H., Engelman, R. M., Dobbs, W. A., and Lemeshow, S.: The Optimal Potassium Concentration in Cardioplegic Solutions, *Ann. Thorac. Surg.*, 32:75, 1981.

154 Jellinek, M., Standeven, J. W., Menz, L. J., Hahn, J. W., and Barner, H. B.: Cold Blood Potassium Cardioplegia. Effects of Increasing Concentrations of Potassim, *J. Thorac. Cardiovasc. Surg.*, 82:26, 1981.

155 Becker, H., Vinten-Johansen, J., Buckberg, G. D., et al.: Myocardial Damage Caused by Keeping pH 7.40 during Systemic Deep Hypothermia, *J. Thorac. Cardiovasc. Surg.*, 82:810, 1981.

156 Jynge, P., Hearse, D. J., and Braimbridge, M. V.: Myocardial Protection during Ischemic Cardiac Arrest. A Possible Hazard with Calcium-Free Cardioplegic Infusates, *J. Thorac. Cardiovasc. Surg.*, 73:848, 1977.

157 Ashraf, J., Onda, M., Benedict, J. B., and Millard, R. W.: Prevention of Calcium Paradox-Related Myocardial Cell Injury with Diltiazem, a Calcium Channel Blocking Agent, *Am. J. Cardiol.*, 49:1675, 1982.

158 Jacocks, M. A., Weiss, M., Guyton, R. A., et al.: Regional Myocardial Protection during Aortic Cross-Clamp Ischemia in Dogs: Calcium-Containing Crystalloid Solutions, *Ann. Thorac. Surg.*, 31:454, 1981.

159 Foglia, R. P., Steed, D. L., Follette, D. M., DeLand, E., and Buckberg, G. D.: Iatrogenic Myocardial Edema with

Potassium Cardioplegia, *J. Thorac. Cardiovasc. Surg.,* 78:217, 1979.

160 Levitsky, S., Mullin, E. D., Sloane, R. E., et al.: Effects of Hyperosmotic Perfusate on Extended Preservation of the Heart, *Circulation,* 43 and 44 (suppl. 1):124, 1971.

161 DiBona, D. R., and Powell, W. J., Jr.: Quantitative Correlation between Cell Swelling and Necrosis in Myocardial Ischemia in Dogs, *Circ. Res.,* 47:653, 1980.

162 Cunningham, J. N., Jr., Adams, P. X., Knopp, E. A., et al.: Preservation of ATP, Ultrastructure, and Ventricular Function after Aortic Cross-Clamping and Reperfusion, *J. Thorac. Cardiovasc. Surg.,* 78:708, 1979.

163 Takamoto, S., Levine, F. H., LaRaia, P. J., et al.: Comparison of Single-Dose and Multiple-Dose Crystalloid and Blood Potassium Cardioplegia during Prolonged Hypothermic Aortic Occlusion, *J. Thorac. Cardiovasc. Surg.,* 79:19, 1980.

164 Clancy, P. E., Slater, A. D., Brandt, D., and Kirsh, M. M.: Substrate Cardioplegia during Hypothermic Arrest in the Alloxan Diabetic Dog, *Ann. Thorac. Surg.,* 31:558, 1981.

165 Salerno, T. A., and Chiong, M. A.: Cardioplegic Arrest in Pigs. Effects of Glucose-Containing Solutions, *J. Thorac. Cardiovasc. Surg.,* 80:929, 1980.

166 Hearse, D. J., Stewart, D. A., and Braimbridge, M. V.: Myocardial Protection during Ischemic Cardiac Arrest. Possible Deleterious Effects of Glucose and Mannitol in Coronary Infusates, *J. Thorac. Cardiovasc. Surg.,* 76:16, 1978.

167 Salerno, T. A., and Chiong, M. A.: Cardioplegic Arrest in Pigs. Effects of Glucose-Containing Solutions, *J. Thorac. Cardiovasc. Surg.,* 80:929, 1980.

168 Engelman, R. M., Dobbs, W. A., Rousou, J. H., and Meeran, M. K.: Myocardial High-Energy Phosphate Replenishment during Ischemic Arrest: Aerobic versus Anaerobic Metabolism, *Ann. Thorac. Surg.,* 33:453, 1982.

169 Bixler, T. J., Gardner, T. J., Flaherty, J. T., Goldman, R. A., and Gott, V. L.: Effects of Procaine-Induced Cardioplegia on Myocardial Ischemia, Myocardial Edema, and Postarrest Ventricular Function. A Comparison with Potassium-Induced Cardioplegia and Hypothermia, *J. Thorac. Cardiovasc. Surg.,* 75:886, 1978.

170 Nishi, T., Guilmette, J. E., and Wakabayashi, A.: Experimental Evaluation of Myocardial Preservation Techniques: V. A Membrane-Stabilizing Agent, Procaine Hydrochloride, *Ann. Thorac. Surg.,* 30:349, 1980.

171 Hearse, D. J., Stewart, D. A., and Braimbridge, M. V.: Myocardial Protection during Ischemic Cardiac Arrest. The Importance of Magnesium in Cardioplegic Infusates, *J. Thorac. Cardiovasc. Surg.,* 75:877, 1978.

172 Robb-Nicholson, C., Currie, W. D., and Wechsler, A. S.: Effects of Verapamil on Myocardial Tolerance to Ischemic Arrest, *Circulation,* 58 (suppl. 1):119, 1978.

173 Magovern, G. J., Dixon, C. M., and Burkholder, J. A.: Improved Myocardial Protection with Nifedipine and Potassium-Based Cardioplegia, *J. Thorac. Cardiovasc. Surg.,* 82:239, 1981.

174 Clark, R. E., Christlieb, I. Y., Spratt, J. A., et al.: Myocardial Preservation with Nifedipine: A Comparative Study at Normothermia, *Ann. Thorac. Surg.,* 31:3, 1981.

175 Pinsky, W. W., Lewis, R. M., McMillin-Wood, J. B., et al.: Myocardial Protection from Ischemic Arrest: Potassium and Verapamil Cardioplegia, *Am. J. Physiol.,* 240:H326, 1981.

176 Henry, P. D., Shuchleib, R., Davis, J., Weiss, E. S., and Sobel, B. E.: Myocardial Contracture and Accumulation of Mitochondrial Calcium in Ischemic Rabbit Heart, *Am. J. Physiol.,* 233(6):H677, 1977.

177 Clark, R. E., Christlieb, I. Y., Ferguson, T. B., et al.: The First American Clinical Trial of Nifedipine in Cardioplegia. A Report of the First 12 Month Experience, *J. Thorac. Cardiovasc. Surg.,* 82:848, 1981.

178 Henry, P. D., Shuchleib, R., Borda, L. J., Roberts, R., Williamson, J. R., and Sobel, B. E.: Effects of Nifedipine on Myocardial Perfusion and Ischemic Injury in Dogs, *Circ. Res.,* 43:372, 1978.

179 Clark, R. E., Christlieb, I. Y., Ferguson, T. B., et al.: Laboratory and Initial Clinical Studies of Nifedipine, Calcium Antagonist for Improved Myocardial Preservation, *Ann. Surg.,* 193:719, 1981.

180 Johnson, R. G., Jacocks, M. A., Aretz, T. H., et al.: Comparison of Myocardial Preservation with Hypothermic Potassium and Nifedipine Arrest, *Circulation,* submitted for publication.

181 Kay, H. R., Levine, F. H., Fallon, J. T., et al.: Correlation of Patterns of Subendocardial Reperfusion and Left Ventricular Performance after Ischemia, *Ann. Thorac. Surg.,* 31:233, 1981.

182 Chitwood, W. R., Jr., Hill, R. C., Kleinman, L. H., and Wechsler, A. S.: The Effects of Intermittent Ischemic Arrest on the Perfusion of Myocardium Supplied by Collateral Coronary Arteries, *Ann. Thorac. Surg.,* 26:535, 1978.

183 Leaf, A.: Cell Swelling, A Factor in Ischemic Tissue Injury, *Circulation,* 48:455, 1973. (Editorial.)

184 Cobb, F. R., McHale, P. A., and Rembert, J. C.: Effects of Acute Cellular Injury on Coronary Vascular Reactivity in Awake Dogs, *Circulation,* 57:962, 1978.

185 Willerson, J. T., Watson, J. T., Hutton, I., Templeton, G. H., and Fixler, D. E.: Reduced Myocardial Reflow and Increased Coronary Vascular Resistance Following Prolonged Myocardial Ischemia in the Dog, *Circ. Res.,* 36:771, 1975.

186 Zelis, R., Lee, G., and Mason, D. T.: Influence of Experimental Edema on Metabolically Determined Blood Flow, *Circ. Res.,* 34:482, 1974.

187 Nelson, R. L., Goldstein, S. M., McConnell, D. H., Maloney, J. V., Jr., and Buckberg, G. D.: Studies of the Effects of Hypothermia on Regional Myocardial Blood Flow and Metabolism during Cardiopulmonary Bypass: V. Profound Topical Hypothermia during Ischemia in Arrested Hearts, *J. Thorac. Cardiovasc. Surg.*, 73:201, 1977.

188 Lucas, S. K., Kanter, K. R., Schaff, H. V., Elmer, E. B., Glower, D. D., Jr., and Gardner, T. J.: Reduced Oxygen Extraction during Reperfusion: A Consequence of Global Ischemic Arrest, *J. Surg. Res.*, 28:434, 1980.

189 Lucas, S. K., Schaff, H. V., Flaherty, J. T., Gott, V. L., and Gardner, T. J.: The Harmful Effects of Ventricular Distention during Postischemic Reperfusion, *Ann. Thorac. Surg.*, 32:486, 1981.

190 Higginson, L. A. J., White, F., Heggtveit, H. A., Sanders, T. M., Bloor, C. M., and Covell, J. W.: Determinants of Myocardial Hemorrhage after Coronary Reperfusion in the Anesthetized Dog, *Circulation*, 65:62, 1982.

191 Fishbein, M. C., Y-Rit, J., Lando, U., Kanmatsuse, K., Mercier, J. C., and Ganz, W.: The Relationship of Vascular Injury and Myocardial Hemorrhage to Necrosis after Reperfusion, *Circulation*, 62:1274, 1980.

192 Coughlin, T. R., Levitsky, S., O'Donoghue, M., et al.: Evaluation of Hypothermic Cardioplegia in Ventricular Hypertrophy, *Circulation*, 60 (suppl. 1):164, 1979.

193 Gaasch, W. H., Bing, O. H. L., Pine, M. B., et al.: Myocardial Contracture during Prolonged Ischemic Arrest and Reperfusion, *Am. J. Physiol.*, 235(6):H619, 1978.

194 Ellis, R. J., Mangano, D. T., Van Dyke, D. C., and Ebert, P. A.: Hypothermic Potassium Cardioplegia Preserves Myocardial Compliance, *Surgery*, 86:810, 1979.

195 Standeven, J. W., Jellinek, M., Menz, L. J., Hahn, J. W., and Barner, H. B.:Cold-Blood Potassium Cardioplegia. Evaluation of Glutathione and Postischemic Cardioplegia, *J. Thorac. Cardiovasc. Surg.*, 78:893, 1979.

196 Follette, D., Fey, K., Livesay, J., Maloney, J. V., Jr., and Buckberg, G. D.: Studies on Myocardial Reperfusion Injury: I. Favorable Modification by Adjusting Reperfusate pH, *Surgery*, 82:149, 1977.

197 Greene, H. L., and Weisfeldt, M. L.: Determinants of Hypoxic and Posthypoxic Myocardial Contracture, *Am. J. Physiol.* 232(5):H526, 1977.

198 Powell, W. J., Jr., DiBona, D. R., Flores, J., Frega, N., and Leaf, A.: II. Consequences of Myocardial Ischemia. Effects of Hyperosmotic Mannitol in Reducing Ischemic Cell Swelling and Minimizing Myocardial Necrosis, *Circulation*, 53 (suppl. 1):45, 1976.

199 Tranum-Jensen, J., Janse, M. J., Fiolet, J. W. T., Krieger, W. J. G., D'Alnoncourt, C. N., and Durrer, D.: Tissue Osmolality, Cell Swelling, and Reperfusion in Acute Regional Myocardial Ischemia in the Isolated Porcine Heart, *Circ. Res.*, 49:364, 1981.

200 Lucas, S. K., Gardner, T. J., Flaherty, J. T., Bulkley, B. H., Elmer, E. B., and Gott, V. L.: Beneficial Effects of Mannitol Administration during Reperfusion after Ischemic Arrest, *Circulation*, 62 (suppl. 1):34, 1980.

201 Weisfeldt, M. L., Scully, H. E., Selden, R., Bello, A. G., Powell, W. J., Jr., and Daggett, W. M.: Effect of Mannitol on the Performance of the Isolated Canine Heart after Fibrillatory Arrest, *J. Thorac. Cardiovasc. Surg.*, 66:290, 1973.

202 Engelman, R. M., Levitsky, S., and Wyndham, C. R. C.: Optimal Conditions for Reperfusion during Cardiopulmonary Bypass, *Circulation*, 56 (suppl. 2):148, 1977.

203 Todd, E. P., Koster, J. K., Utley, J. R., et al.: The Effect of Coronary Perfusion Pressure on Recovery of Myocardial Function Following Normothermic Ischemia, *J. Surg. Res.*, 22:667, 1977.

204 Magee, P. G., Gardner, T. J., Bulkley, B. H., Goldman, R. A., and Gott, V. L.: Importance of Early Post Ischemic Reperfusion Pressure on Left Ventricular Preservation, *Surg. Forum*, 29:272, 1978.

205 Pirzada, F. A., Ekong, E. A., Vokonas, P. S., Apstein, C. S., and Hood, W. B., Jr.: Experimental Myocardial Infarction: XIII. Sequential Changes in Left Ventricular Pressure-Length Relationships in the Acute Phase, *Circulation*, 53:970, 1976.

206 Grondin, D. M., Helias, J., Vouhe, P. R., and Robert, P.: Influence of a Critical Coronary Artery Stenosis on Myocardial Protection through Cold Potassium Cardioplegia, *J. Thorac. Cardiovasc. Surg.*, 82:608, 1981.

207 Dorsey, L. M., Colgan, T. K., Silverstein, J. I., Hatcher, C. R., Jr., and Guyton, R. A.: Alterations in Regional Myocardial Function after Heterogeneous Cardioplegia, submitted for publication.

208 Cunningham, J. N., Jr., Abbas, J. S., Adams, P. X., Nathan, I., Klugman, I., and Spencer, F. C.: Constant-Pressure Aortic Root Perfusion versus Cardioplegia and Hypothermia. Comparison of Methods of Myocardial Protection, *J. Thorac. Cardiovasc. Surg.*, 77:496, 1979.

209 Grover, F. L., Fewel, J. G., Schrank, K. P., Ghidoni, J. J., Arom, K. V., and Trinkle, J. K.: Effects of Various Periods of Cold Potassium Cardioplegic Arrest Upon Myocardial Contractility and Metabolism, *J. Surg. Res.*, 28:328, 1980.

210 Akins, C. W., Buckley, M. J., Austen, W. G., Daggett, W. M., and Levine, F. H.: Myocardial Protection with Hypothermia and Potassium Cardioplegia during Operation for Ascending Aortic Aneurysms, *J. Thorac. Cardiovasc. Surg.*, 79:700, 1980.

211 Schraut, W. H., Kampman, K., Lamberti, J. L., et al.: Myocardial Protection from Permanent Injury during Aortic Cross-Clamping: Effectiveness of Pharmacological

Cardiac Arrest Combined with Topical Cardiac Hypothermia, *Ann. Thorac. Surg.,* 31:225, 1981.

212 Brody, W. R., Reitz, B. A., Andrews, M. J., et al.: Long-Term Morphologic and Hemodynamic Evaluation of the Left Ventricle after Cardiopulmonary Bypass. A Comparison of Normothermic Anoxic Arrest, Coronary Artery Perfusion, and Profound Topical Cardiac Hypothermia, *J. Thorac. Cardiovasc. Surg.,* 70:1073, 1975.

213 Ellis, R. J., Gertz, E. W., Wisneski, J., and Ebert, P. A.: Mild Ventricular Dysfunction Following Cold Potassium Cardioplegia, *Circulation,* 60:(suppl. 1):147, 1979.

214 Herman, S. D., Alonso, D. R., Gay, W. A., Jr., and Ebert, P. A.: Physiologic Observations of the Heart Six Months after Ischemic Normothermic Cardioplegia, *Surgery,* 81:462, 1977.

Use of Streptokinase in Coronary Thrombosis[*]

DETLEF G. MATHEY, M.D., JOCHEN SCHOFER, M.D.,
HANS-JOACHIM KREBBER, M.D., KARL-HEINZ KUCK, M.D.,
VOLKMAR TILSNER, M.D., RICHARD MONTZ, M.D., WALTER
BLEIFELD, M.D., and GEORGE RODEWALD, M.D.

The heart is deceitful above all things, and desperately corrupt; who can understand it?

JEREMIAH 17:9

In most cases, transmural myocardial infarction is caused by coronary artery occlusion consisting of an arteriosclerotic plaque with an acute thrombus superimposed. Although coronary thrombosis was found in most patients who died after an acute myocardial infarction,[1] there has been considerable debate regarding its etiologic significance. Some investigators believe that coronary thrombosis is a consequence of infarction rather than its cause and of little significance. Their view is supported by the fact that a thrombus was not found in every patient, particularly not in those who died suddenly within 1 h of the onset of symptoms, where the incidence of occlusive thrombosis was reported to be only 31 percent.[2] Moreover, autoradiographic studies of human coronary thrombi suggest that thrombus formation may occur after the infarct, since ^{131}I-labeled fibrinogen given within 10 h after the onset of symptoms was found in the entire length of the thrombus at autopsy in 4 of 5 patients. With longer time intervals, only parts or none of the thrombus contained detectable radioactivity.[3]

Coronary angiography in patients with acute myocardial infarction in connection with intracoronary thrombolysis, however, has left no doubt that coronary artery thrombosis is a consistent and pathophysiologically important finding in acute myocardial infarction. The intriguing question, however, of which sequence of different mechanisms leads to the occlusion has remained unclear. According to a plausible but unproven hypothesis, acute coronary occlusion may represent an abnormal variant of the mechanisms normally responsible for hemostasis: an intimal lesion caused by plaque rupture with or without subintimal hemorrhage induces platelet aggregation, which in turn causes constriction of the arterial wall by release of mediator substances and thrombosis, in order to seal the lesion. Histologically, coronary thrombosis has always been found in connection with the subintimal layers of the arterial wall.[4,5]

*From the Departments of Cardiology and Cardiovascular Surgery, University Hospital Eppendorf, Hamburg, West Germany.

Since coronary thrombosis represents an important factor of acute coronary occlusion in the early stage of acute myocardial infarction, it appears to be logical therapy to abolish the thrombus in order to reestablish coronary blood flow. Streptokinase, a catabolic by-product of group C β-hemolytic streptococci, has been extensively used to lyse arterial and venous thrombi.[6] It activates the body's fibrinolytic system by combining with plasminogen to form an activator complex which then transforms plasminogen into plasmin. Plasmin lyses fibrin. Many attempts have been made to document the efficacy of intravenous streptokinase in patients with acute myocardial infarction. However, without coronary angiography, its effect on coronary thrombosis has remained unclear. Until very recently, an improvement in coronary and peripheral microcirculation was still considered the main mechanism by which streptokinase may exert a favorable effect on the acute infarct,[7] and it is for this reason that patients with symptoms of myocardial infarction of up to 12 h or even longer were still thought to be suitable for intravenous streptokinase therapy. Since we now know that intravenous streptokinase may also lyse coronary thrombi and that myocardial necrosis is often completed within 3 or 4 h, a great number of these patients were probably subjected to futile streptokinase therapy. Nevertheless, a lower mortality rate of 15.6 percent in the treated group versus 30.6 percent in the control group was found in a selected group of patients.[8]

By intracoronary thrombolysis it was demonstrated for the first time that coronary thrombi can be rapidly lysed with streptokinase, resulting in recanalization of the occluded coronary artery.[9–11] Although in some earlier experimental and clinical studies similar observations had been made, no particular attention was paid to them,[12,13] whereas the most recent papers were met with great interest by cardiologists many of whom are enthusiastically using this new method. This, however, should not distract from the fact that intracoronary thrombolysis is still an investigational procedure, which leaves many important questions unanswered. For example, it is not known whether a significant portion of ischemic myocardium is preserved by intracoronary thrombolysis and, if so, up to what time after the onset of symptoms salvage of myocardium can be expected. It is also unclear how rethrombosis after successful thrombolysis can be prevented. The complications of the methods are not fully understood; in particular, the significance of myocardial hemorrhage, which is likely to follow reperfusion, is unknown. Controlled studies are needed to determine the effect of intracoronary thrombolysis on short- and long-term mortality rates.

Although intracoronary thrombolysis has the potential of changing our mode of therapy of acute myocardial infarction fundamentally, a final decision on its value cannot be given at the moment. This paper, however, indicates that infarct size can be limited by early recanalization, as evidenced by new ^{201}Tl uptake and an improvement in left ventricular wall motion in the area of the infarct in the majority of patients. It is also shown that early bypass surgery following intracoronary lysis effectively prevents reinfarction. However, autopsy findings suggest that the time period available for intracoronary thrombolysis is limited and that even within the first few hours after the onset of symptoms large transmural infarcts with myocardial hemorrhage may occur.

STREPTOKINASE APPLICATION AND ASSESSMENT OF SALAVAGED MYOCARDIUM

Streptokinase can be infused either selectively via catheter into the occluded coronary artery or intravenously. In our opinion, the selective application has several advantages: The total dosage needed for intracoronary thrombolysis is one-quarter or less than that used for intravenous application, resulting in a local streptokinase concentration that is about twenty times higher than that during intravenous infusion. Since it is known from experimental[13] and clinical[14] studies that the time of clot lysis and the concentration of streptokinase are closely correlated, a more rapid and effective lysis is expected after intracoronary streptokinase application. Obviously, the risk of bleeding is lower after an intracoronary infusion. Angiographic control, which is only possible in connection with intracoronary streptokinase application, allows us to evaluate the effects of thrombolysis step by step and to adjust the dosage and the duration of the infusion to the individual requirements of the patient. Only during intracoronary streptokinase administration is it feasible to include other measures of recanalization, such as guide-wire recanalization, intracoronary nitroglycerin, superselective streptokinase infusion, and subsequent transluminal coronary angioplasty (PTCA). Finally, independent of the mode of streptokinase application, coronary angiography is needed to determine the degree of residual stenosis after thrombolysis as well as

the anatomy of the noninvolved coronary arteries, particularly in those patients in whom bypass surgery or PTCA have to be performed, in order to prevent reinfarction.

Intracoronary Streptokinase Application

PATIENT SELECTION AND PREPARATION

Since the method of intracoronary thrombolysis has been introduced only recently, the indications are not equally accepted by all investigators. There is general agreement, however, that the method should be restricted to patients with early transmural acute myocardial infarction with typical chest pain and ST elevation. Patients with a history of recent gastrointestinal bleeding or stroke or patients more than 70 years of age are usually excluded from streptokinase therapy. Patients with unstable angina or subendocardial infarction do not benefit from thrombolysis, since no coronary thrombus is present in most of them.[15]

There is great uncertainty at the moment as to what time after the onset of chest pain patients should still be accepted. Among investigators, this time period ranges from 3 to 18 h.[9–11,16] Continued chest pain is considered an indication for late thrombolysis by some. We restrict the time period to 3 h, since experimental and autopsy findings suggest that the likelihood of limiting infarct size is low after this period of time.[17–22]

Patients are prepared for intracoronary thrombolysis with a central intravenous line. Blood samples are withdrawn for hemoglobin, electrolytes, enzyme, thrombin time, fibrinogen, and blood group determinations, but the results are not waited for. A 12-lead ECG is recorded. Informed consent is obtained from the patient and relatives and, if possible, from the attending physician as well. Within 30 to 45 min after admission, the patient is transferred to the catheterization laboratory.

INTRACORONARY THROMBOLYSIS

In the catheterization laboratory, a no. 8 French introducer sheet is placed in the femoral artery and the arterial pressure is monitored continuously. A no. 7 French Judkins catheter is advanced through the introducer sheet and in case intracoronary thallium-201 scintigraphy is performed, the nonaffected coronary artery being visualized first. The initial contrast injections are performed carefully to avoid arrhythmias or hypotension. Diatrizoate sodium and meglumine diatrizoate are used as contrast media. The "infarct vessel" is then opacified. It consistently shows an occlusion.[23] A streptokinase infusion of 250,000 units diluted in 500 ml of 0.9% saline is given into the ostium of the occluded coronary artery at an initial infusion rate of 4000 to 6000 units per minute.

After the artery begins to open, the infusion rate is reduced to 2000 units per minute and continued for at least 45 min. In most cases, a total dosage of 250,000 to 350,000 units is not exceeded.[24] If the infarct vessel remains occluded after 15 to 30 min, we attempt guide-wire recanalization using a 0.032-in Teflon-coated guide wire with movable core. If not easily successful, a superselective streptokinase infusion is started. For this purpose, the coronary catheter is changed to a no. 8 French "high-high" flow Judkins coronary catheter with untapered tip. Through this catheter, a no. 2.5 French Ganz reperfusion catheter is advanced into the occluded artery up to the occlusion.[10] For the left anterior descending and the circumflex coronary arteries, preshaped catheters are available (Fig. 1). Under repeat injections through the guiding catheter using a Y connector, the position of the tip of the reperfusion catheter is repeatedly checked. It should remain just in front of the occlusion. Streptokinase is then infused via the reperfusion catheter at the same dosage.

CONCOMITANT THERAPY

Prior to coronary angiography, a pacing catheter is placed via the femoral vein in the right ventricle for management of arrhythmias during the procedure. Then 10,000 units of heparin is given as a bolus intravenously after all catheters have been placed. Infusions with dopamine, lidocaine, nitroglycerin, and potassium are kept ready for immediate use. Instrumentation and medication for orotracheal intubation and mechanical ventilation must be available. After intracoronary thrombolysis, all catheters are pulled back into the abdominal aorta or the inferior vena cava and left there for another 12 to 24 h to avoid bleeding from the puncture sites.

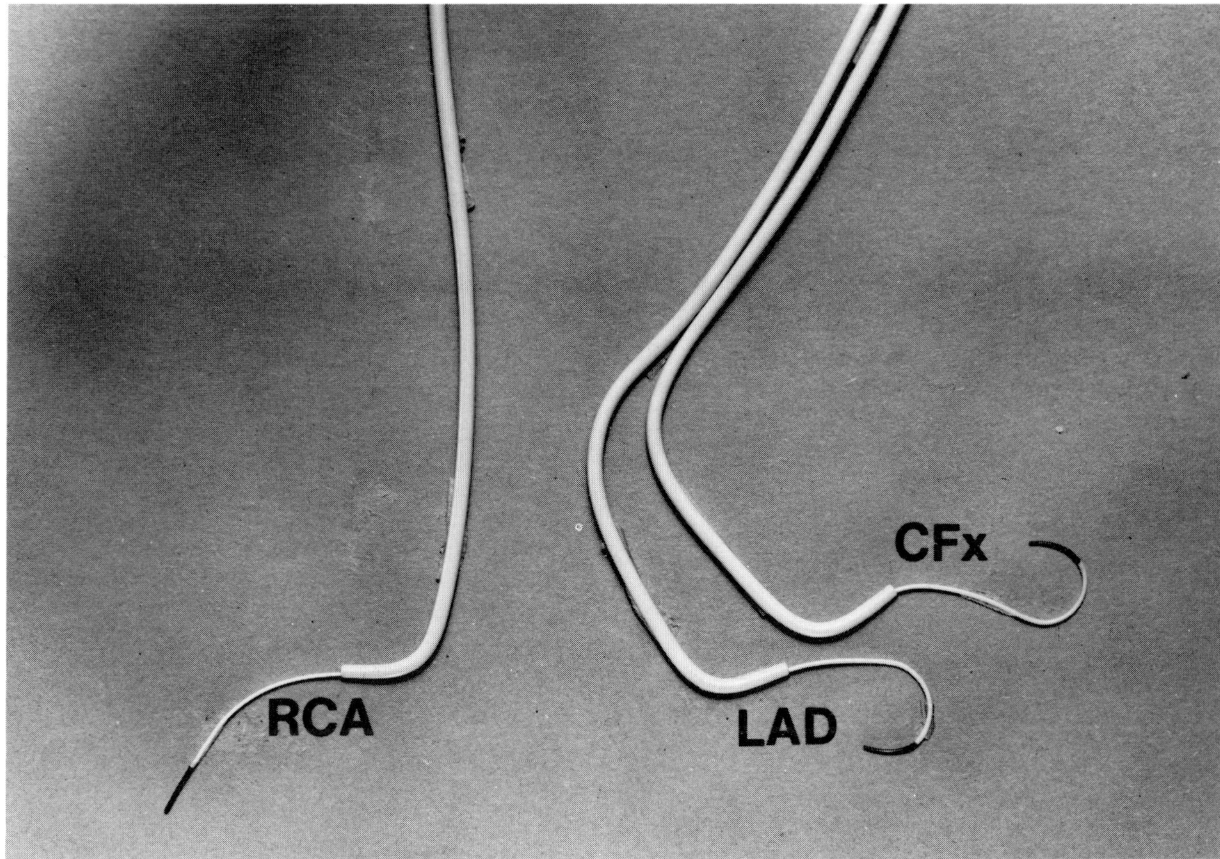

FIGURE 1 Preshaped Ganz reperfusion catheters for superselective streptokinase infusion. RCA = right coronary artery; LAD = left anterior descending coronary artery; CFX = circumflex coronary artery.

Assessment of Salvaged Myocardium

Parallel to the procedure of intracoronary thrombolysis itself, its effects on the ischemic myocardium have to be determined in the individual patient. Analysis of left ventricular wall motion in the area of ischemia from an acute and follow-up contrast cine-angiogram probably represents the best method of determining the potential benefit of intracoronary thrombolysis, whereas measurements of global left ventricular ejection fraction are too insensitive and may even be misleading for reasons outlined later. Since mechanical function recovers only slowly from severe ischemia, the full extent of myocardial salvage can be detected only 2 weeks after the infarct.[25] Therefore, we can obtain the acute left ventricular angiogram immediately after intracoronary thrombolysis knowing that it will still reflect the whole degree of left ventricular dysfunction and thus avoid the time delay and risk of a contrast injection before intracoronary thrombolysis.

However, owing to the slow recovery of mechanical function after reperfusion, left ventricular angiography does not provide an immediate answer to the question of whether jeopardized myocardium was preserved. For this purpose, intracoronary myocardial scintigraphy with ^{201}Tl and ^{99m}Tc pyrophosphate has proved useful. Compared with intravenous ^{201}Tl application, the intracoronary route has the advantage of producing high-quality images with little background activity. A second ^{201}Tl injection immediately after intracoronary thrombolysis can thus be performed in order to determine the acute change in ^{201}Tl defect size following intracoronary thrombolysis. After repeat intravenous ^{201}Tl injections, such an evaluation would be difficult because of the high background activity usually present in rest images after intravenous injection. The evaluation of ^{201}Tl redistribution after a single intravenous injection (which may require up to 24 h) or ^{201}Tl reinjection after 24 h are alternative approaches, but they do not provide the immediate result.[16,26] Obviously, an intracoronary ^{201}Tl scintigram shows unphysiologic distribution of the radionuclide in the left ventricular myocardium owing to different supply areas of the left and right coronary artery. Thallium-201 reinjection after thrombolysis causes further inhomogeneity within the perfusion bed of the injected coronary artery. For this reason, intracoronary ^{201}Tl scintigrams cannot be evaluated quantitatively. However, they do give an immediate answer as to whether or not ^{201}Tl is taken up in the area of the initial defect.

In addition to intracoronary ^{201}Tl scintigraphy, which is being used by several investigators,[27–29] we introduced intracoronary ^{99m}Tc pyrophosphate scintigraphy immediately after successful thrombolysis to further delineate the area of necrosis and thereby

Summary of 132 patients with acute myocardial infarction (chest pain less than 3 h)*

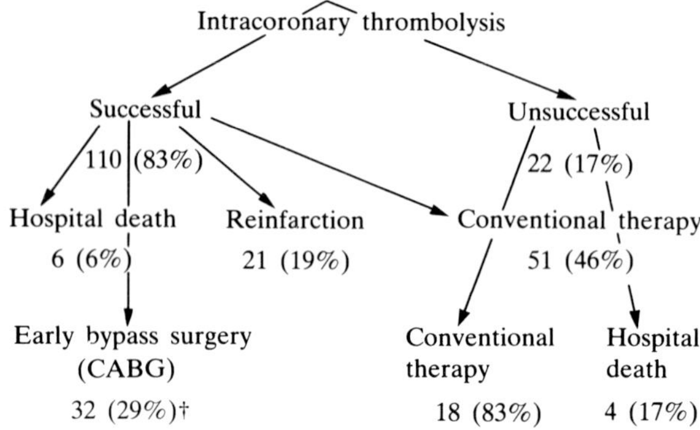

*One hospital death owing to septicaemia

†Authors' cumulative experience with intracoronary thrombolysis and postthrombolytic hospital course. At present, after realizing the high reinfarction rate under conventional postthrombolytic therapy and after the introduction of intracoronary myocardial scintigraphy, the rate of early bypass surgery has increased to about 50 percent of the successfully recanalized patients.

enhance the predictive value of myocardial scintigraphy during intracoronary thrombolysis.[30] Our present protocol is summarized in Table 1. It should be emphasized that intracoronary thrombolysis is not at all delayed by this approach. Scintigraphy is performed on the catheterization table using a mobile gamma camera while streptokinase is being infused.

EFFECTS OF STREPTOKINASE
The Infarct Vessel

In about 80 percent of the patients with transmural acute myocardial infarction, a complete occlusion of a major coronary artery is found within the first 4 h of the onset of symptoms; in 20 percent the occlusion is subtotal.[23] The acute nature of the occlusion is often characterized by a blunt, irregular margin with dye retention after the injection in the area proximal to the occlusion.[11,31] A typical example is shown in Fig. 2. The retention of dye may be absent when nearby branches maintain a runoff of the contrast medium.

An intracoronary infusion of 4,000 to 6,000 units of streptokinase per minute opens the occluded coronary artery in more than 80 percent of patients after an average infusion time of 30 min (range 5 to 60 min).[24] A typical example is shown in Fig. 3. During the initial phase of reopening, contrast filling of the artery may be

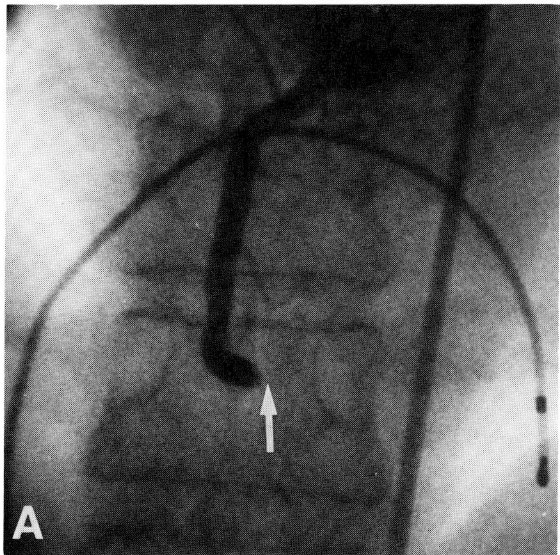
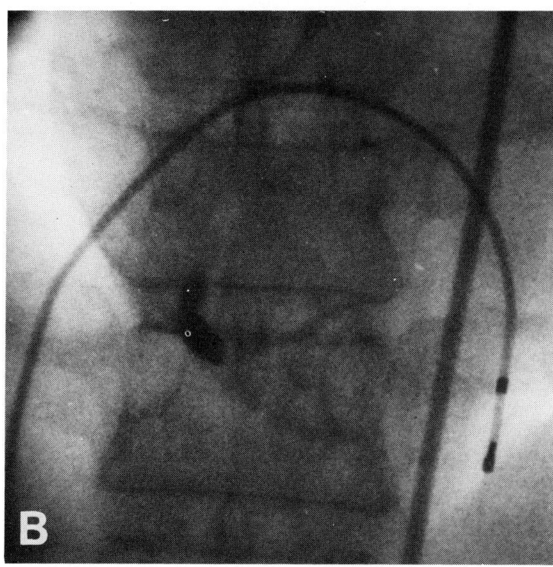

FIGURE 2 (*A*) Acute occlusion of the right coronary artery. Retention of contrast medium in the area proximal to the occlusion (*B*).

markedly delayed, and occasionally, there may be stasis of dye distal to the occlusion, indicating a low perfusion pressure (Fig. 4). At this point in time, the acute thrombus is best seen in the area just behind the stenosis. It appears as an oval-shaped filling defect that is surrounded by contrast medium. Rarely, embolization occurs during a contrast injection, causing a new distal occlusion that may or may not be successfully lysed. In some cases, we observed that the contrast injection itself opened the artery, probably owing to the mechanical effect of the injection and/or the hyperosmolarity of the contrast medium. After the occluded coronary artery has opened, the intracoronary infusion of streptokinase is continued for at least another 45 min, until the thrombus has completely disappeared and the previously occluded artery fills promptly and completely.

In about 20 percent of patients, an ostial infusion of streptokinase fails to open the occluded coronary artery. From the initial angiogram, it is difficult to predict which patient is likely to suffer such failure. Patients with a complete distal occlusion and a long retention column of contrast medium in front of the occlusion are likely to belong to this group, since no significant streptokinase concentration can be achieved at the thrombus. Another unfavorable situation represents a left anterior descending artery occlusion at the bifurcation of the left coronary artery. Under these circumstances, the intracoronary streptokinase infusion may be drained away into the circumflex system.

In case no recanalization is achieved within 15 to 30 min, guide-wire recanalization is attempted (Fig. 5). In only less than half the attempts made can the occlusion be passed and some antegrade flow be reestablished. Subsequent intracoronary streptokinase infusion is very likely to result in successful thrombolysis of the remaining clot. In case guide-wire recanalization also fails, a superselective streptokinase infusion is attempted (Fig. 6).

In our experience, an intracoronary injection of nitroglycerin (0.5 mg) has not been found useful in patients with acute myocardial infarction. In only 2 of 50 patients was reopening of the left anterior descending artery achieved.[11] In both patients, an acute thrombus became visible and could be resolved with intracoronary streptokinase. In view of this low success rate, we no longer recommend the routine use of intracoronary nitroglycerin.

A significant arteriosclerotic stenosis remains after intracoronary thrombolysis in more than 90 percent of patients.[24] In patients under the age of 40 years, the degree of residual stenosis may be slightly lower than in older patients. Some preliminary evidence indicates that the degree of residual stenosis may further decrease with time by about 10 percent.[32]

Only very preliminary data are available concerning the effects of intravenous streptokinase on the occluded coronary artery using coronary angiography for evaluation. According to Schröder et al.,[33] 500,000 units of intravenous streptokinase opens the infarct vessel in 45 percent of patients with total coronary occlusion. In a more recent study by Schwarz et al.,[34] the success rate was only 6 of 16 patients, although 1.5 million units of streptokinase were given intravenously within 90 min,

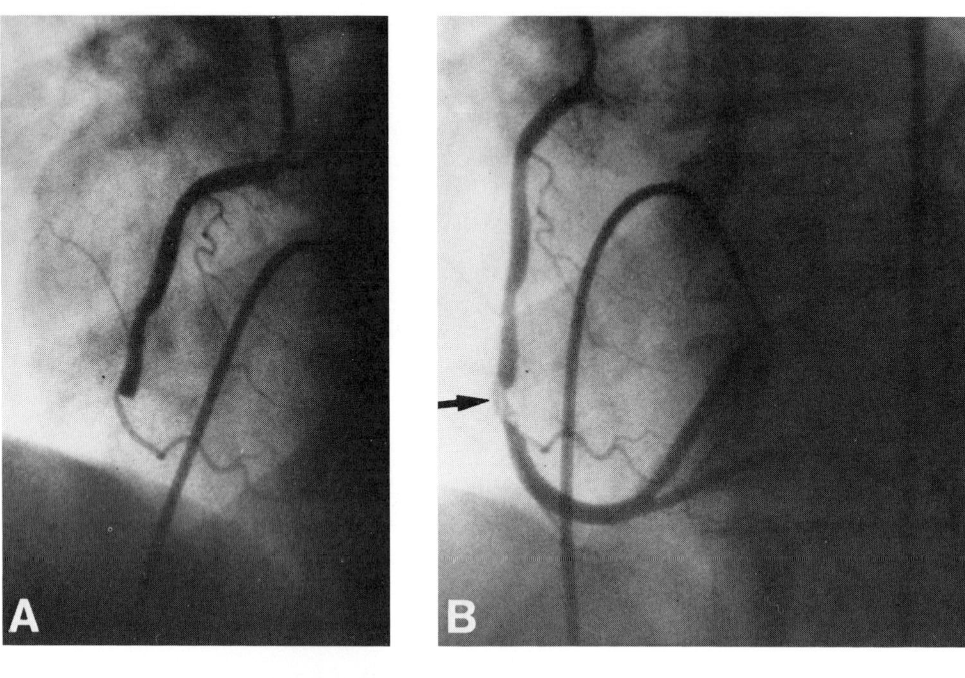

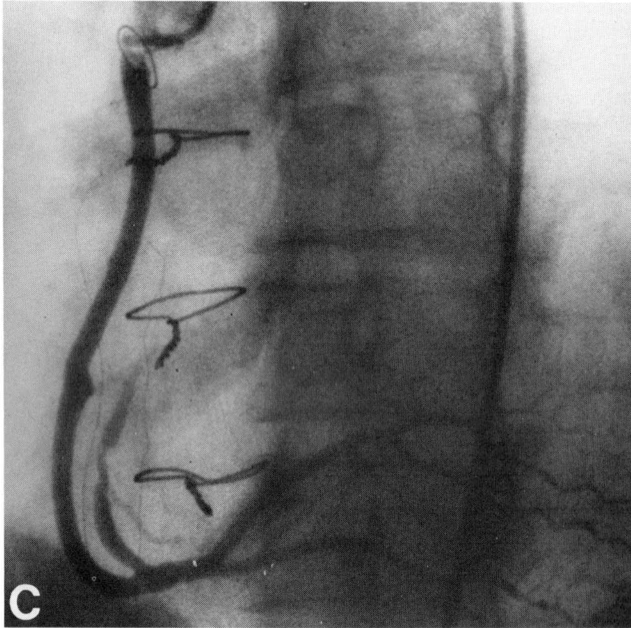

FIGURE 3 (*A*) Right coronary artery occlusion in acute inferior myocardial infarction. (*B*) Opening after intracoronary thrombolysis with a high-grade residual senosis at the site of the previous occlusion. (*C*) The stenosis was bypass grafted on the day of intracoronary thrombolysis.

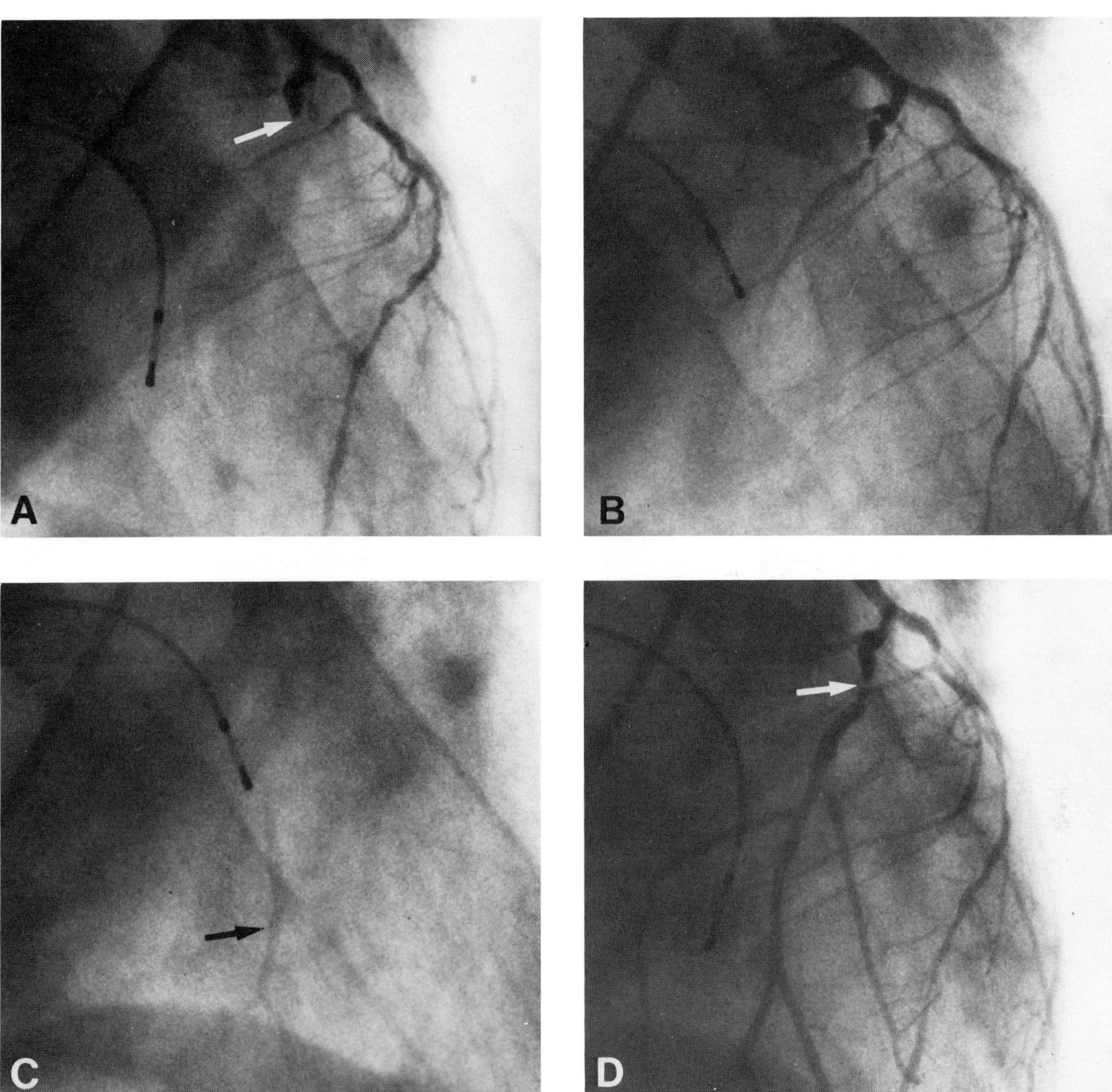

FIGURE 4 Acute circumflex coronary artery occlusion (*A*), gradual opening with delayed filling (*B*), and stasis of dye (*C*). Prompt and complete filling after further intracoronary thrombolysis (*D*).

whereas according to Neuhaus et al.,[35] recanalization was achieved in 67 percent of patients after intravenous streptokinase infusion.

Symptoms, Hospital Mortality, Follow-Up Data

Clinically, intracoronary thrombolysis is always associated with significant relief of angina within 5 to 10 min after opening of the artery, independent of the functional result of recanalization in terms of infarct size. It is rare for reperfusion arrhythmias to aggravate anginal symptoms initially. Following successful intracoronary thrombolysis, the condition of the patient is surprisingly stable, unless reinfarction occurs. In a nonrandomized, retrospective study, hospital mortality was found to be 5.4 percent in successfully recanalized patients, but 24 percent in unsuccessful cases. Death after successful lysis was due to reinfarction in 5 of 7 patients.[36] Our own experience of hospital course in 132 patients with acute myocardial infarction (chest

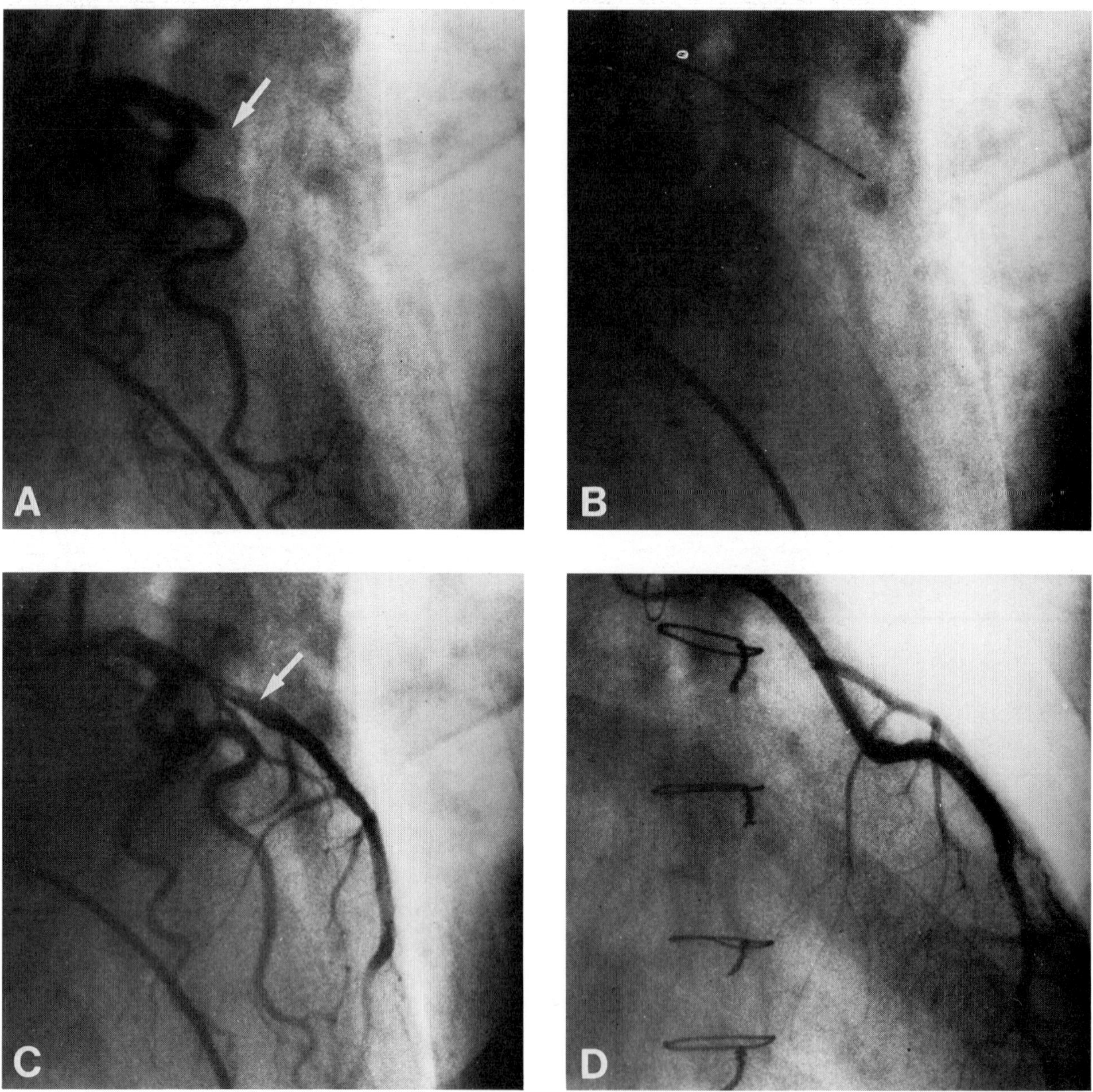

FIGURE 5 (*A* and *B*) Guide-wire recanalization in a patient with proximal LAD occlusion. (*C*) The thrombus that became visible after recanalization was lysed and the residual stenosis bypass-grafted (*D*).

pain less than 3 h) undergoing intracoronary thrombolysis is summarized in Table 1.

So far, no follow-up data have been reported. In our series, no significant differences in mortality, symptoms, arrhythmias, and exercise testing were found 1 year after intracoronary thrombolysis among patients not recanalized, successfully recanalized, and successfully recanalized and bypass grafted. However, definite conclusions on long-term prognosis, mortality, and morbidity can only be expected from the randomized studies that are currently being carried out at several centers.

Left Ventricular Function

The mechanical function of the left ventricular is closely correlated with its blood supply. A reduction in regional blood flow is followed by a decrease in

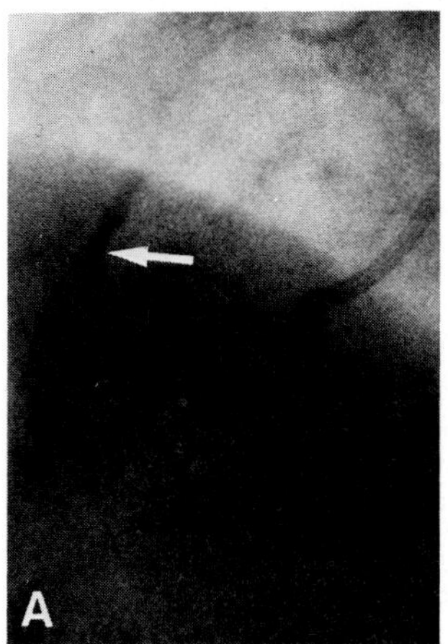
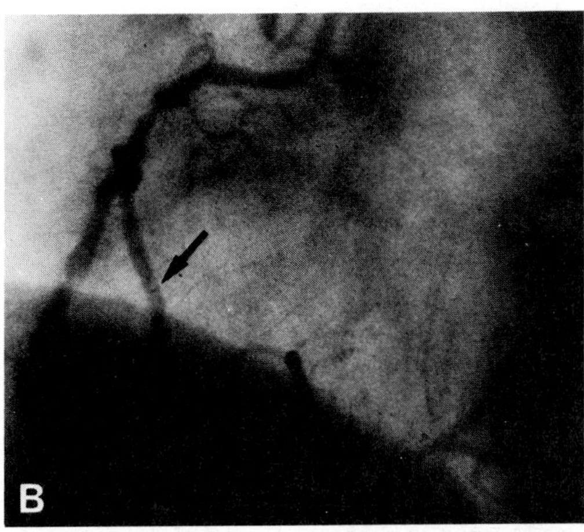

FIGURE 6 Superselective streptokinase infusion in the presence of a large right ventricular branch (*B*, black arrow) through which the streptokinase was drained away not reaching the thrombus in a high enough concentration during ostial streptokinase infusion.

shortening and thickening of the corresponding myocardial segment.[37] Complete interruption of flow causes systolic bulging with thinning of the left ventricular wall. Whereas these changes occur almost immediately after the reduction in coronary flow, the recovery of mechanical function following reperfusion is very slow, even after short periods of coronary occlusion.[38] This is probably due to the deprivation of high-energy phosphates and their time-dependent resynthesis. With increasing duration of coronary occlusion, irreversible myocardial injury occurs, progressing from the subendocardial to subepicardial layers. In dogs, myocardial necrosis was 38 ± 4 percent after 40 min of occlusion with subsequent reperfusion 57 ± 7 percent after 3 h 71 ± 7 percent after 6 h and 85 ± 5 percent after 24 h.[39] Similar observations had been made by other investigators as well.[40] Since dogs are known to have a good collateral circulation, such experimental data that suggest that reperfusion after several hours of occlusion may still be beneficial cannot easily be extrapolated to human beings. To study the effects of reperfusion in the absence of collaterals, similar experiments were carried out in baboons, and these showed that after 4 h of coronary occlusion, reperfusion no longer resulted in a reduction of infarct size, whereas after 2 h of reperfusion, infarct size was limited to 50 percent.[41] These experiments suggest that in the absence of collaterals, a significant portion of ischemic myocardium may survive 2 or 3 h of coronary occlusion and benefit from subsequent reperfusion. In view of these studies, it appears to be prudent at the moment to restrict intracoronary thrombolysis to patients whose infarct is no older than 3 h, although large interindividual differences in the development of a complete infarct exist, particularly in patients with long-standing coronary artery disease and a well-developed collateral circulation.

There is no doubt that measurements of mechanical function provide the most useful and convincing evidence for evaluation of the effects of intracoronary thrombolysis on infarct size. So far, global left ventricular ejection fraction has been used almost exclusively for this purpose because of its ease of determination and the possibility of measuring it noninvasively. In several studies, an improvement in global ejection fraction was found in successfully recanalized patients,[11,42,43] whereas after unsuccessful thrombolysis, ejection fraction did not change or deteriorate. Improvement in ejection fraction after successful intracoronary thrombolysis, however, was not present in every patient and was attributed to the duration of symptoms and/or the existence of collaterals.[43,44] Since acute myocardial infarction means regional injury to the myocardium, global ejection fraction may not necessarily reflect changes in regional function, particularly not when a compensatory increase in wall motion of the nonischemic segment occurs. In order to determine whether regional left ventricular wall motion improves after successful intracoronary thrombolysis and whether such improvement is also reflected in changes in global ejection fraction, we analyzed regional wall motion in 38 patients in whom we could obtain an "acute" left ventricular contrast cineangiogram immediately after recanalization and a follow-up angiogram at the time of hospital discharge (Fig. 7). The angiograms were coded and analyzed "blindly" by independent investigators.* Wall motion

*We gratefully acknowledge the cooperation of Florence H. Sheehan, M.D., and Harold T. Dodge, M.D., from the University of Washington, Seattle, who performed the angiographic analyses.

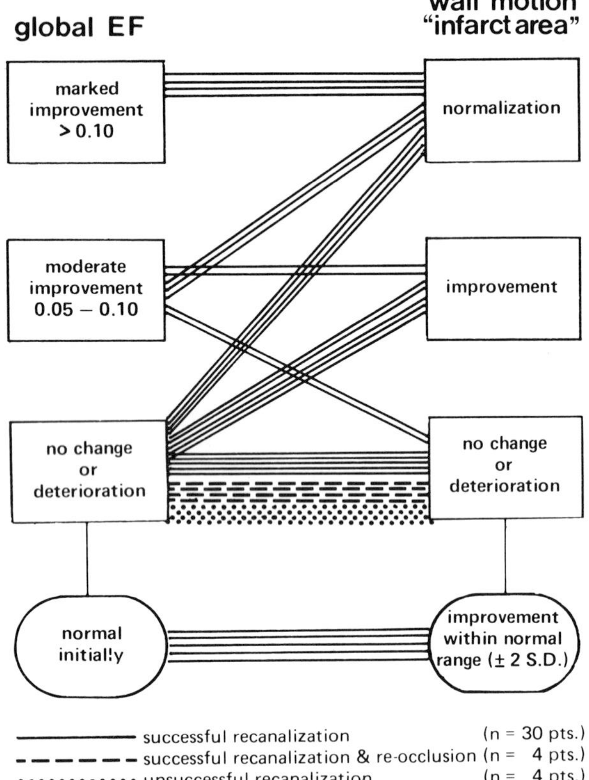

FIGURE 7 The changes in global left ventricular ejection fraction (left column) are compared with those in regional wall motion in the infarct area (right column). Measurements were made from an acute and follow-up contrast cine-angiogram (2 to 4 weeks later). In the majority of cases, regional wall motion normalized or improved, suggesting a reduction in infarct size. No change or deterioration in regional wall motion was often associated with reocclusion or unsuccessful thrombolysis. Note that global ejection fraction did not indicate improvement or normalization in regional wall motion in 12 of 18 patients.

was computed along 100 equally spaced chords constructed between the margins of the end-diastolic and end-systolic images and perpendicular to a line midway between these two images, as illustrated in Fig. 8 and as previously described.[45] The images were not realigned. The changes in chord length during systole were normalized using the area ejection fraction. This normalization enables a comparison of the segmental chord length changes among the different patients, as well as comparisons with normal values for this method, which were expressed as standard deviations from the normal mean (Fig. 8). Regional wall-motion data thus obtained were compared with global ejection fraction measured from the same RAO 30° angiograms.

Using this method of wall-motion analysis, we

compared the wall motion of the ischemic area in the acute angiogram with that at follow-up. According to the change in wall motion in the ischemic area, the patients were classified into the three categories: normalization, improvement, and no change or deterioration. *Normalization* means an abnormal wall motion initially on the infarct area of less than -2 standard deviations from normal that became normal (± standard deviations) at follow-up. *Improvement* was defined as a change of more than 10 standard deviations toward normal. *No change or deterioration* was defined as a change of less than 10 standard deviations.

Five patients with a normal left ventricular ejection fraction (>55 percent) on the initial study and only a slight reduction in regional wall motion (still falling within the ± standard deviation range and further improving until follow-up) were regarded as a separate group. All 5 patients had an inferior infarct with scintigraphic involvement of the right ventricle.

According to the preceding criteria, regional wall

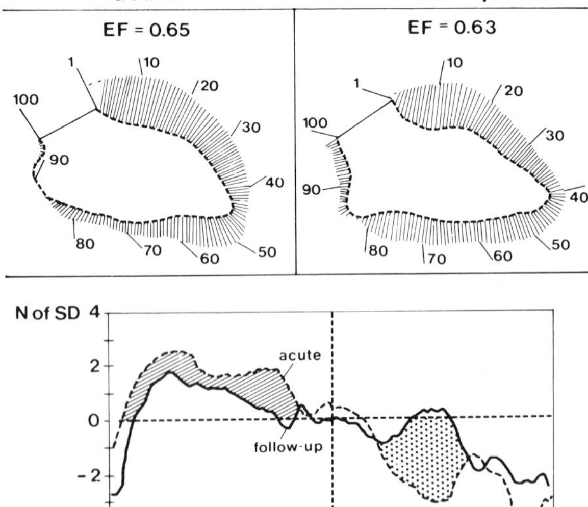

FIGURE 8 Left ventricular contrast angiogram in a patient with acute inferior myocardial infarction. Acutely, the inferior wall is hypokinetic and the anterior wall hyperkinectic. At follow-up, the inferior wall is less hypokinetic and the anterior wall less hyperkinetic, resulting in a global ejection fraction that is not significantly different from that during the acute stage, although wall motion in the infarct area has markedly improved. In the lower pannel, the patient's wall motion is expressed in number of standard deviations from normal (= zero line). The hatched area represents the reduction in hypercontractility in the anterior wall; the dotted area, the reduction in hypokinesis.

motion became normal in 11 of 38 patients and improved in 7 (Fig. 7). Including the 5 patients whose wall motion was only slightly reduced initially, a normal or improved wall motion at follow-up was seen in 61 percent of our successfully recanalized patients, in all of whom the duration of symptoms was no longer than 3 h. In 15 patients, regional wall motion remained unchanged or deteriorated. Four of these 15 patients had a reinfarction owing to reocclusion of the same artery between the first and second angiogram, and in 4 others, intracoronary thrombolysis was unsuccessful. In our opinion, these data indicate that a significant amount of ischemic myocardium was preserved by intracoronary thrombolysis in the majority of patients. Since we do not have a control group describing the natural course of regional wall motion after acute myocardial infarction, our results cannot be regarded as definite proof. However, in view of the fact that reinfarction or unsuccessful thrombolysis was associated with no change or deterioration in regional wall motion, we consider an improvement or normalization of wall motion a consequence of reperfusion rather than spontaneous change.

It is interesting and important to note that global left ventricular ejection fraction did not reflect improvement or normalization in regional wall motion in 12 of 18 patients owing to the hypercontractile behavior of the nonischemic parts of the left ventricle (Fig. 7). This is illustrated in an individual patient with inferior acute myocardial infarction.

Initially, there was hypokinesia of the inferior wall and a hypercontractile motion of the nonischemic anterior wall (Fig. 8). At follow-up, wall motion had improved in the infarct area and the anterior wall was no longer as much hypercontractile as during the acute stage (Fig. 8). Therefore, left ventricular ejection fraction did not reflect the improvement in regional wall motion in this patient. From Fig. 7 it is quite evident that in general, global left ventricular ejection fraction is a poor and often misleading parameter for the evaluation of intracoronary thrombolysis.

The question arises as to how the different results in regional wall motion after successful intracoronary thrombolysis can be explained. Figure 9 shows that the time intervals from the onset of chest pain to opening of the infarct vessel for those patients whose wall motion became normal is slightly shorter than in those patients in whom wall motion only slightly improved or did not change, but there was significant overlap of the individual values. Although we usually visualized the nonaffected coronary artery first, no significant collaterals to the infarct vessel were visualized in those patients whose wall motion normalized or improved. Theoretically, two other factors may be of importance. First, the onset of symptoms may not coincide with the onset of complete and permanent coronary occlusion in all patients, and second, there may be a difference in myocardial oxygen demand in the ischemic myocardial segment. Further investigations are needed to clarify these points and to develop new methods to determine prior to intracoronary thrombolysis whether or not a patient will benefit from the procedure.

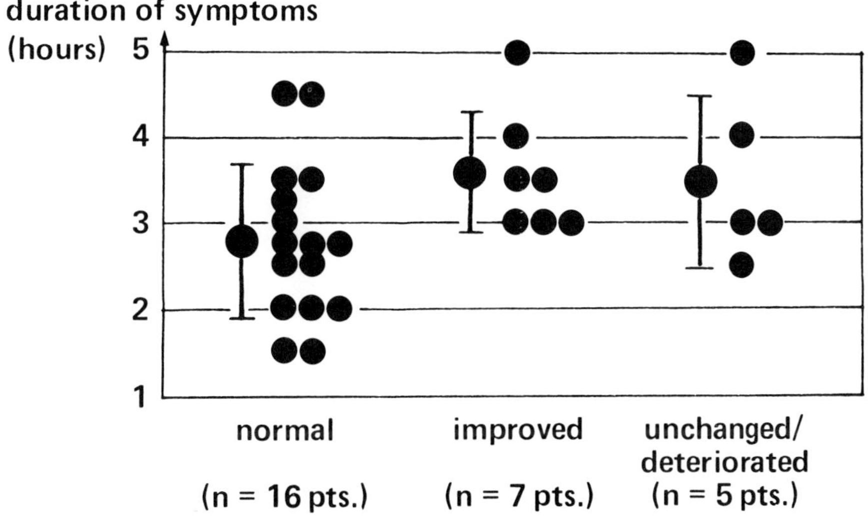

FIGURE 9 The duration from the onset of symptoms until reopening of the infarct vessel is plotted against the late functional result. There was a tendency toward a shorter duration of symptoms in patients whose wall motion was normal at follow-up, but a significant overlap of the individual values was found between the three groups.

Improvement in mechanical function after intracoronary thrombolysis became particularly apparent in some patients with cardiogenic shock.[46] In 4 of 6 patients with cardiogenic shock at the time of intracoronary thrombolysis, reversal of shock was achieved. All 4 patients had an inferior myocardial infarction in the presence of a dominant right coronary artery and were recanalized within 3 h, whereas the 2 unsuccessful patients had large anterior infarcts and were recanalized only after 4.5 h. Possibly the right ventricle was involved in the 4 patients with inferior infarction and it recovered more rapidly and completely from ischemia than the left ventricle did.

Intracoronary Myocardial Scintigraphy

At the moment, intracoronary myocardial scintigraphy with thallium-201 and technetium-99m pyrophosphate is probably the best and most feasable method to determine immediately after successful thrombolysis whether ischemic myocardium was preserved and a special postthrombolytic therapy has to be instituted. Only if there is evidence that infarct size was significantly limited is there an indication for early bypass surgery or PTCA. For reasons outlined earlier, we consider the intracoronary thallium-201 application superior to an intravenous injection. The initial ^{201}Tl defect prior to intracoronary thrombolysis is considered to represent the "area at risk." Its change after successful thrombolysis and intracoronary ^{201}Tl reinjection represents the amount of salvaged myocardium.

The protocol and preliminary scintigraphic results in 13 successfully recanalized patients are summarized in Tables 2 and 3. In 5 other patients in whom intracoronary thrombolysis failed, no change in defect size was noted. In 5 of 13 successfully recanalized patients, a large defect completely disappeared after ^{201}Tl reinjection into the reopened coronary artery. An example is shown in Fig. 10. In 2 patients with inferior myocardial infarction, no significant left ventricular defect was

TABLE 2
Intracoronary myocardial scintigraphy with thallium-201 and technetium-99m pyrophosphate (protocol)

Coronary angiography

↓

Intracoronary ^{201}Tl (0.3 to 0.5 mCi) into right and left coronary artery

↓

First scintigraphy during intracoronary thrombolysis

↓

Intracoronary ^{201}Tl (0.3 to 0.5 mCi) and ^{99m}Tc pyrophosphate (5 mCi) into infarct vessel 20 to 30 min after intracoronary thrombolysis

↓

Second scintigraphy (dual ^{201}Tl and ^{99m}Tc pyrophosphate)

↓

Left ventricular angiogram

seen prior to thrombolysis, but there was significant involvement of the right ventricle. The right ventricular defect disappeared after successful thrombolysis. In 3 patients, new ^{201}Tl uptake was noted after successful intracoronary thrombolysis, but a large residual defect in the center of the infarct remained (Fig. 11). In 3 patients, no change in ^{201}Tl defect size was found despite recanalization of the infarct vessel.

Myocardial ^{201}Tl uptake is generally thought to reflect the viability of the myocardium, since uptake depends on an active transport across the cell membrane. Whether new ^{201}Tl uptake after intracoronary thrombolysis also represents myocardial viability of the reperfused myocardium has not been clarified so far.[47]

TABLE 3
Preliminary scintigraphic results in 13 successfully recanalized patients

No. of patients	Change in left ventricular wall motion	Left ventricular ^{201}Tl after thrombolysis
2	None, but normal initially	No left ventricular defect initially
5	Normalization	Substantial reduction in defect size in 4 patients Questionable left ventricular defect initially in 1 patient
3	Improvement	Substantial reduction in defect size in 1 patient Little change in 1 patient No change in 1 patient
3	No change	No change

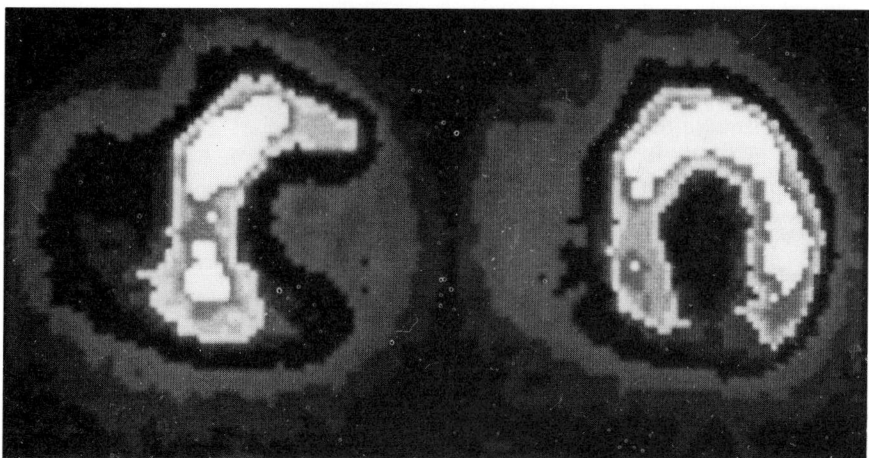

FIGURE 10 Intracoronary ^{201}Tl scintigram in a patient with LAD occlusion. Prior to successful intracoronary thrombolysis a large defect of the anterolateral wall was found that completely disappeared after recanalization and intracoronary ^{201}Tl reinjection.

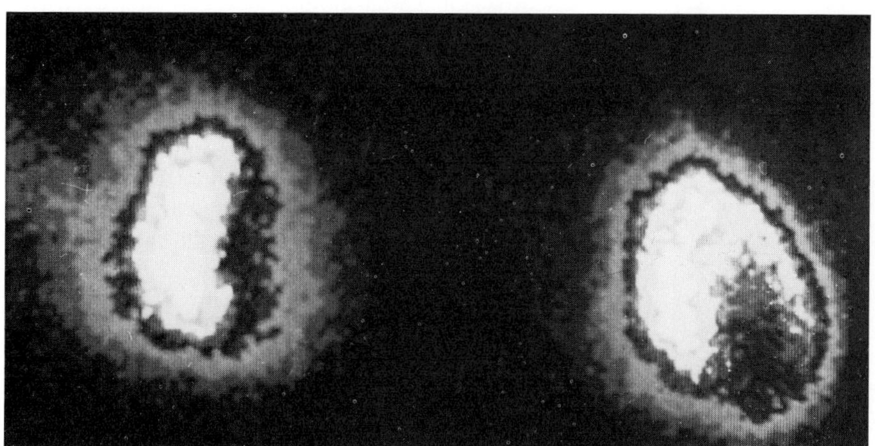

FIGURE 11 Intracoronary ^{201}Tl scintigram in a patient with proximal LAD occlusion. Before intracoronary thrombolysis, a large defect of the anterior, apical, and inferior left ventricular wall was seen. After thrombolysis and intracoronary ^{201}Tl reinjection into the infarct vessel, there is new ^{201}Tl uptake, but a large residual defect in the center of the infarct remains.

We addressed this question by comparing the acute change in ^{201}Tl defect size with the change in regional left ventricular wall motion between the acute and follow-up contrast cine-angiograms.[29] These results are also summarized in Table 2.

In most patients, there was a good correlation between the acute change in ^{201}Tl defect size and the change in regional left ventricular wall motion. In patients in whom regional wall motion in the infarct area had normalized at the time of follow-up, a large initial defect disappeared after thrombolysis, whereas in patients with no change in ^{201}Tl defect size, left ventricular wall motion remained unchanged or deteriorated. The correlation was less obvious in the 3 patients who only showed improvement in regional wall motion. One of these patients had significant new ^{201}Tl uptake in the area of the initial defect. In this patient, intracoronary ^{201}Tl scintigraphy has to be considered false positive. It is very interesting to note that in this patient, intracoronary ^{99m}Tc pyrophosphate given at the time of ^{201}Tl reinjection after successful thrombolysis did not only accumulate in the area of the residual ^{201}Tl defect but also in the area of new ^{201}Tl uptake (Fig. 12). We explain such ^{201}Tl and ^{99m}Tc pyrophos-

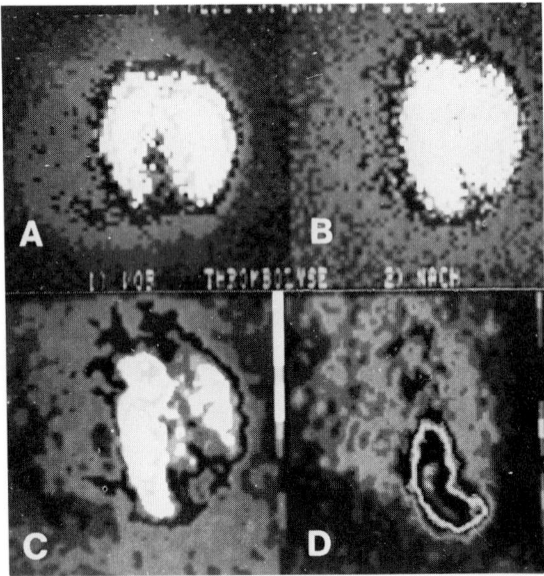

FIGURE 12 (*A*) Thallium-201 defect in the lower part of the interventricular septum. (*B*) New thallium-201 uptake in infarct area after intracoronary thrombolysis. (*C*) Substraction thallium-201 image indicating where new thallium-201 uptake has taken place. (*D*) Intracoronary technetium-99m pyrophosphate scintigram obtained 15 min after thrombolysis with technetium-99m pyrophosphate accumulation in the area of new thallium-201 uptake.

phate overlap by the proximity of ischemic but viable and necrotic myocardial cells in the same region of the left ventricular wall.

Thus, we may conclude that intracoronary myocardial scintigraphy with ^{201}Tl predicts myocardial salvage immediately after intracoronary thrombolysis in most cases. Additional intracoronary ^{99m}Tc pyrophosphate scintigraphy may enhance the predictive value. Therefore, intracoronary myocardial scintigraphy is a good basis for postthrombolytic therapy.

Electrocardiography

To determine whether the effect of successful intracoronary thrombolysis on infarct size is reflected by ECG criteria, we compared the QRS abnormalities with the change in regional left ventricular shortening fraction that occurred in the infarct area between the acute and the follow-up contrast cine-angiograms 2 to 4 weeks later. As ECG criteria we used the presence or absence of an abnormal Q wave in the lead of maximal ST elevation as well as a QRS scoring system that was recently described and evaluated by Wagner et al.[48] for the estimation of infarct size. According to the change in regional wall shortening fraction, two groups of patients could be distinguished. Group A consisted of 17 successfully recanalized patients in whom regional shortening fraction did not change significantly, with an average of 0.21 acutely versus 0.20 at follow-up. Group B consisted of 12 successfully recanalized patients in whom regional wall motion markedly improved from 0.20 acutely to 0.37 at follow-up ($p < 0.005$). The QRS changes in these two groups are summarized in Table 4. Thus in both groups abnormal Q waves were present prior to intracoronary thrombolysis in about a third of the patients and therefore do not preclude marked improvement in regional wall motion. The development of new Q waves, however, was associated with persistent reduction in regional wall motion.

Serum Creatinine Kinase Levels

Serum levels of creatinine kinase and its isoenzyme CK-MB rise after intracoronary thrombolysis in almost all patients. Already in the very beginning of intracoronary thrombolysis, it has been noted that the rise in serum creatinine kinase and CK-MB levels is more rapid after successful thrombolysis, with an early peak 10 to 18 h (average 14 h) after the onset of chest pain. However, in patients whose infarct vessel remains occluded, serum creatinine kinase level rises more slowly, reaching its peak value after 21 to 26 h (average 23 h).[33] A typical example of a serum creatinine kinase curve after successful thrombolysis as compared with a curve of a patient with permanent coronary occlusion is

TABLE 4
The QRS changes in groups A and B (see text)

Group		Abnormal Q wave	QRS score
A ($n = 17$)	Acute	7 of 17 patients	2.8
	Follow-up	14 of 17 patients	5.2
B ($n = 12$)	Acute	4 of 12 patients	2.4
	Follow-up	5 of 12 patients	3.7

given in Fig. 13. Washout of creatinine kinase following successful thrombolysis is seen as responsible for this difference in the curves. Not only the shape of the serum creatinine kinase curve is different after successful intracoronary thrombolysis, but also the total amount of creatinine kinase released is greater because of the washout phenomenon. It has been suggested that the time of peak serum creatinine kinase level can be used as indirect, noninvasive evidence of whether or not reperfusion has taken place. However, the sensitivity and specificity of this approach remain to be determined. It is not unlikely that the degree of the residual stenosis after thrombolysis affects the speed of creatinine kinase washout.

These differences in creatinine kinase kinetics after intracoronary thrombolysis make it difficult to use serum creatinine kinase level as an index of infarct size or myocardial salvage after intracoronary thrombolysis. When the change in regional wall motion, which was determined according to the method described earlier, is compared with peak creatinine kinase level in patients who were successfully recanalized and had no reinfarction, this becomes obvious (Fig. 14). We found no correlation between peak creatinine kinase level and the change in wall motion, which is expressed as the difference in standard deviations between the acute and follow-up left ventricular cine-angiograms that reflect the change in the degree of dysfunction as well as the

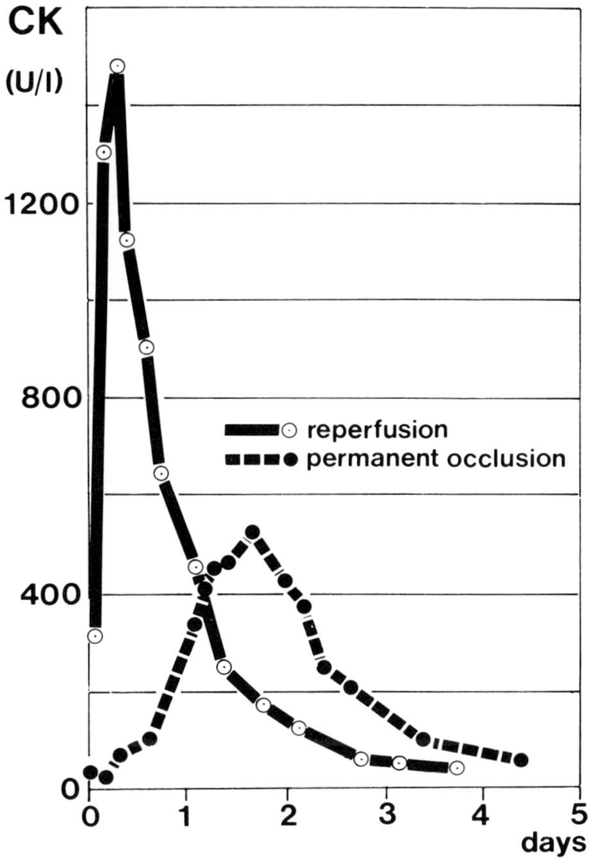

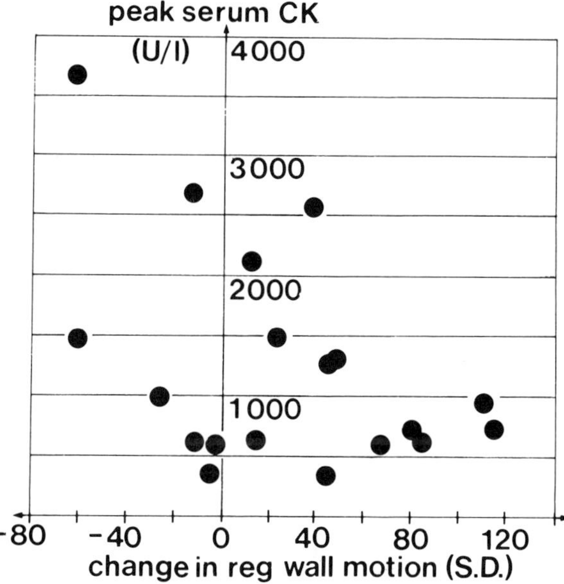

FIGURE 13 Note the early peak in the creatinine kinase serum curve in a patient who underwent successful thrombolysis as compared with a patient with permanent coronary occlusion.

FIGURE 14 Lack of correlation between change in regional wall motion in infarct area (abscissa) and peak serum creatinine kinase level.

area of the left ventricle involved. This lack of correlation is probably mainly due to the fact that the "area of risk," depending on the perfusion bed of the occluded coronary artery and the amount of myocardium salvaged, may vary from patient to patient. For instance, in the presence of a small but complete infarct, peak serum creatinine kinase level may rise to 1000 units per liter after successful intracoronary thrombolysis with no change in regional wall motion at follow-up, whereas in the presence of a large "area at risk," the same peak creatinine kinase value may be associated with significant salvage of ischemic myocardium and improvement in wall motion.

COMPLICATIONS

With regard to complications, all studies performed so far have to be considered as pilot studies. Only large, randomized trials can show the true incidence and significance of the complications of intracoronary or systemic thrombolysis. Up to this time, a number of complications, such as bleeding, reperfusion arrhythmias, reinfarction, and myocardial hemorrhage, have been observed.

Bleeding Complications

Although a systemic fibrinolytic effect on intracoronary streptokinase infusion with a reduction in plasma fibrinogen to less than 100 mg/dl is observed after an average intracoronary streptokinase dosage of 100,000 units,[49] in a series of 232 patients, serious bleeding complications (cerebral or gastrointestinal) were noted in only 2 patients.[24] Cerebral bleeding occurred in an 81-year-old female patient, and gastrointestinal bleeding occurred in a patient who suffered from severe vomiting prior to intracoronary thrombolysis. In the latter patient, bleeding could be controlled by substituting fibrinogen. Bleeding from puncture sites is the most frequent bleeding complication, and such bleeding resulted in blood transfusions in 7.4 percent of patients. Bleeding from puncture sites was significantly associated with fibrinogen levels below 100 mg/dl and independent of the additional heparin therapy.[36]

Reperfusion Arrhythmias

Serious ventricular arrhythmias, i.e., ventricular tachycardia and/or fibrillation, may be observed during coronary artery occlusion as well as after reperfusion. When their occurrence is coincident with the time of opening of the infarct vessel and no arrhythmias were present prior to this time, we call them *reperfusion arrhythmias*. According to the literature, their incidence ranges from 5 to 22 percent.[9–11,28]. Most frequently, idioventricular tachycardia with a rate of 70 to 110 beats per minute has been observed. It usually causes a reduction in systolic arterial pressure of about 20 mm Hg owing to the lack of atrial contribution, which may be serious if the patient's blood pressure is already low. Rarely, anginal symptoms are aggravated by idioventricular tachycardia. In most cases, no therapy is needed.

The mechanism underlying reperfusion ventricular arrhythmias is not known at the moment. Idioventricular tachycardia is usually considered focal in origin, and the observation of different types of idioventricular tachycardia with different rates in the same patient (Fig. 15) is considered focal in origin. However, we also found that reperfusion idioventricular tachycardia can be interrupted either by ventricular extrastimuli or by spontaneous premature ventricular beats, which would be more typical of a reentry mechanism. Recently, Corr et al.[51] suggested that an increase in alpha receptor density in the ischemic myocardium may be responsible for reperfusion arrhythmias. In the experience of these investigators, alpha blockade with intravenous phentolamine prevented reperfusion arrhythmias in dogs. An intracoronary injection of 100 µg of phentolamine given after opening of the infarct vessel also reduced the incidence of reperfusion arrhythmias significantly.[52]

In 4 of our patients we observed substained ventricular tachycardia with a rate of 130 to 180 beats per minute. In our experience, reperfusion ventricular tachycardia could be briefly interrupted for one or two beats by ventricular extrastimuli, but it immediately

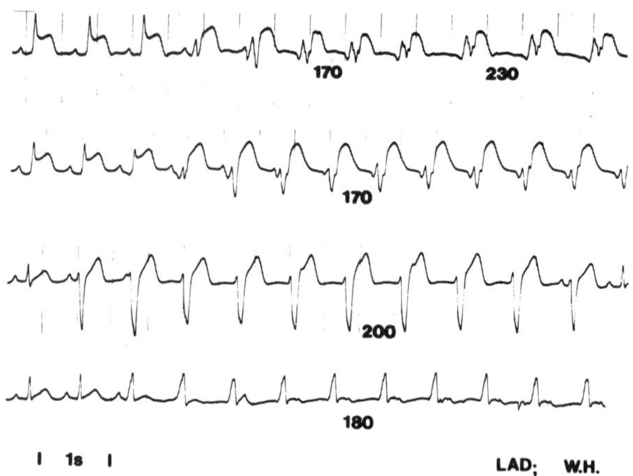

FIGURE 15 Reperfusion idioventricular tachycardias of different morphologies and rates. Note the reduction of ST elevation after intracoronary thrombolysis.

recurred thereafter. Therefore, electric cardioversion was not performed as a therapeutic measure. Reperfusion ventricular tachycardia did not respond to intravenous lidocaine. Experimentally, intracoronary lidocaine given superselectively into the infarct vessel has been found to be effective.[50] It should, however, not be injected into the ostium of the affected coronary artery because of its negative inotropic effects. Intravenous ajmaline or encainide proved to be useful in our patients by lowering the ventricular rate or abolishing the tachycardia completely.

Ventricular fibrillation was observed in 10 percent of our patients during the early stage of reperfusion, occasionally in connection with a contrast coronary injection. Defibrillation has always been successful in restoring a normal sinus rhythm.

Reperfusion arrhythmias also may be observed in those patients in whom intracoronary thrombolysis initially failed but late opening of the infarct vessel occurred because of the residual systemic fibrinolytic effect. We observed late reperfusion in a patient with left anterior descending artery occlusion that did not open at the time of intracoronary thrombolysis. Ten hours later, however, repeat episodes of ventricular tachycardia and fibrillation suddenly occurred, resulting in irreversible cardiogenic shock despite immediate resuscitation. Postmortem angiography revealed a patent left anterior descending artery and a hemorrhagic anterior myocardial infarction, indicating that reperfusion had taken place and that the patient's death was probably related to late reperfusion arrhythmias.

Reinfarction

According to the literature, the reinfarction rate during the initial hospital period after intracoronary thrombolysis ranges from 0 to 26 percent.[9,10,36] Different methods of postthrombolytic therapy may partly account for these large differences. In addition, the success of intracoronary thrombolysis itself is an important factor. Only when ischemic myocardium is preserved in the first place will reinfarction with typical symptoms, ECG changes, and creatinine kinase elevation occur. When intracoronary thrombolysis does not limit infarct size, reocclusion will be silent.

In our experience, reinfarction occurred in 15 percent of patients during the first days in the coronary care unit and in 4 percent thereafter on the general ward. In all cases of reinfarction where we performed a second attempt at intracoronary thrombolysis, reinfarction was caused by thrombolytic reocclusion of the infarct vessel. In only two-thirds of the attempts was the second intracoronary thrombolysis effective in reopening the artery. Insufficient anticoagulation has been accused of being the cause of early reocclusion,

but no data have been reported to clearly prove this point. We observed thrombotic reocclusion within a short time after intracoronary thrombolysis, when a full heparin effect and a systemic fibrinolytic effect were still present.

Myocardial Hemorrhage

Myocardial hemorrhage has been repeatedly observed after intravenous streptokinase therapy.[53] Its significance is not known. In 5 of our patients who underwent successful intracoronary thrombolysis and died in cardiogenic shock without prior reinfarction 1 to 18 days after the infarct, an autopsy was performed in order to determine the size of the infarct and whether or not myocardial hemorrhage was present.[22] The time interval from the onset of symptoms to reperfusion was less

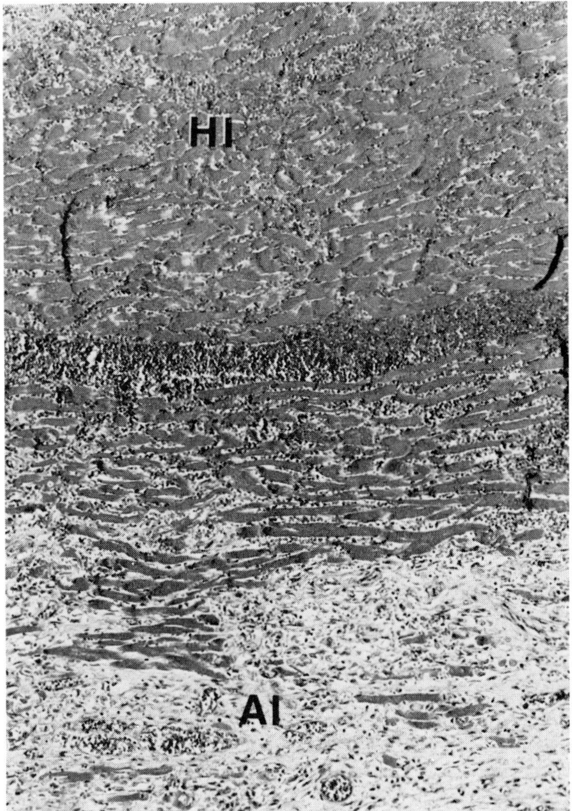

FIGURE 16 Histologic specimen from the margin of an anemic (AI) and hemorrhagic infarct (HI) in a patient who died 18 days after the onset of myocardial infarction. Whereas in the anemic infarct area the necrotic muscle fibers are almost completely replaced by typical granulation tissue, no signs of repair were found in the hemorrhagic infarct.

than 3.5 h in all 5 patients. Creatinine kinase level on admission was still normal, and the electrocardiogram showed marked ST elevation with no Q waves. At autopsy, the infarct vessel was patent in all 5 patients and a large transmural infarct (average area 40 ± 16 cm^2) was found that was completely hemorrhagic in 4 of the 5 patients, leaving only a small anemic border zone. Myocardial hemorrhage was confined to the area of necrosis with no evidence of cardiac rupture. Histologically, the hemorrhage infarct consisted of an eosinophilic coagulation necrosis of the cardiac muscle fibers, which were separated by fresh hemorrhage. The patient who died 18 days after the acute infarct had both types of infarction—an anemic infarct in the area of a severly stenotic left anterior descending artery and a hemorrhagic infarct in the area of an occluded and reperfused circumflex coronary artery. There were signs of advanced repair in the anemic infarct area with replacement of the necrotic muscle fibers by typical granulation tissue, whereas in the hemorrhagic infarct no signs of repair were found (Fig. 16). This suggests that infarct healing may be delayed by myocardial hemorrhage.

POSTTHROMBOLYTIC THERAPY

In view of a 20 to 25 percent reinfarction rate after intracoronary thrombolysis and a high-grade residual stenosis, a special postthrombolytic therapy should be instituted in those patients in whom the infarct was definitely limited in size in order to prevent reinfarction from rethrombosis. In principle, three methods are available: medical therapy, percutaneous transmural coronary angioplasty (PTCA), and early bypass surgery.

Medical Therapy

In a series of 119 patients who underwent successful intracoronary thrombolysis, reocclusion occurred despite medical therapy in 26 percent.[36] In 17 of the 25 patients more than 20,000 units of heparin was infused per day, and in addition to heparin, 8 of the 25 patients had also 1 g intravenous aspirin acutely and another 9 patients had additional aspirin acutely and chronically. Our own patients also received intravenous nitroglycerin as well as nifedipine, 10 to 20 mg four times per day, in order to prevent reocclusion from coronary artery spasm. As mentioned earlier, our reinfarction rate is not significantly different from that observed by Merx et al.[36] These data, therefore, suggest that heparin, aspirin, nitroglycerin, and nifedipine cannot prevent reinfarction in about 20 to 25 percent of patients.

Percutaneous Coronary Angioplasty (PTCA)

Since in most cases a significant arteriosclerotic stenosis remains after successful intracoronary thrombolysis, PTCA could be one way of reducing the tendency of thrombotic reocclusion by reducing the degree of stenosis. However, new intimal lesions caused by PTCA increase the risk of rethrombosis. The preliminary experience available at this time does not allow one to draw any definite conclusions.[54,55] A patient infarct vessel at the time of follow-up angiography does not necessarily indicate that the artery has remained permanently patent. Only when infarct size is limited by intracoronary thrombolysis does reocclusion become clinically apparent by causing reinfarction.

Since such evidence is not given in the studies performed so far, it is very difficult to exclude intermittent, silent reocclusion. In our own limited experience with PTCA performed immediately after intracoronary thrombolysis, thrombotic reocclusion occurred within the first few days in 4 of 5 patients. We feel that the clinical experience with PTCA in patients with chronic arteriosclerotic stenoses cannot simply be extrapolated to patients in whom the underlying stenosis has caused recent coronary artery thrombosis.

Early Bypass Surgery (CABG) following Intracoronary Thrombolysis

At the moment, we prefer early bypass surgery after successful intracoronary thrombolysis, where *successful* means not only reopening of the occluded artery but also a marked reduction in the ^{201}Tl defect size as judged from the intracoronary scintigram. In a cooperative study, we reviewed our preliminary experience with early bypass surgery following intracoronary thrombolysis in 34 patients.[56] These patients represent a subgroup out of 188 successfully recanalized patients. On the average, opening of the infarct vessel was achieved within 2.6 h in these patients and was followed by early bypass surgery after an interval of 3.6 ± 1.2 days. In 8 patients, early bypass surgery was performed on the day of intracoronary thrombolysis. There were no bleeding complications at the time of surgery, which was uncomplicated in all 34 patients. The indications for early bypass surgery in these patients were recurrent angina in 7 patients, 1 high-grade remaining stenosis in 12 patients, a remaining stenosis and other stenoses in 13 patients, and a remaining stenosis and recurrent coronary artery spasm in 2 patients.

As far as the surgical procedure is concerned, effective myocardial protection is of utmost importance. In the ischemic and reperfused area, energy-rich phosphates are depleted, and their resynthesis takes up to 3 days, a time period during which the heart is very sensitive to another ischemic injury. Early bypass surgery following intracoronary thrombolysis implies such an ischemic stress to the reperfused area and could easily lead to a perioperative myocardial infarction unless effective myocardial protection is achieved.[57,58]

After surgery, 29 of these 34 patients were studied again. The patency rate of the graft to the infarct vessel was 83 percent and for the grafts to the other coronary arteries, the rate was 87 percent. Regional left ventricular injection fraction in the ischemic segment markedly improved after surgery from 17 to 40 percent (Fig. 17). There was no difference between patients with a patent and an occluded graft to the infarct vessel, indicating that the improvement in all motion was exclusively due to intracoronary thrombolysis.

So far, we have followed up the 34 patients for more than 1 year. There was one late death. This patient, a 51-year-old man in whom both bypass grafts were occluded, died suddenly 4 months following surgery. Another 28-year-old patient with coronary artery spasm in whom the left anterior descending artery graft was occluded had a nonfatal reinfarction 3 months after surgery. One patient had occasional mild angina, and 31 patients were completely asymptomatic.

The main purpose of early bypass surgery following successful intracoronary thrombolysis is to reduce the risk of reinfarction. As reported earlier, the reinfarction rate after thrombolysis is 20 to 25 percent. In the operated patients, reinfarction was observed in only 1 of the 34 patients. The frequency of angina following acute transmural myocardial infarction is reported to be 35 percent. After recanalization, angina was the indication for acute early bypass surgery in 7 of the 34 patients. Following intracoronary thrombolysis and bypass surgery, only 1 of the 34 patients had mild angina. Thus early bypass surgery appears to be a safe and effective method of preventing reinfarction after successful intracoronary thrombolysis.

MISCELLANEOUS INDICATIONS FOR INTRACORONARY STREPTOKINASE INFUSION

Recently, we have found that acute coronary artery occlusion complicating PTCA could be reopened by an intracoronary streptokinase infusion.[59] According to the NIH registry, acute coronary occlusion occurred in 5 percent of patients during PTCA, requiring emergency bypass surgery. In 38 percent of these patients, a transmural myocardial infarction could not

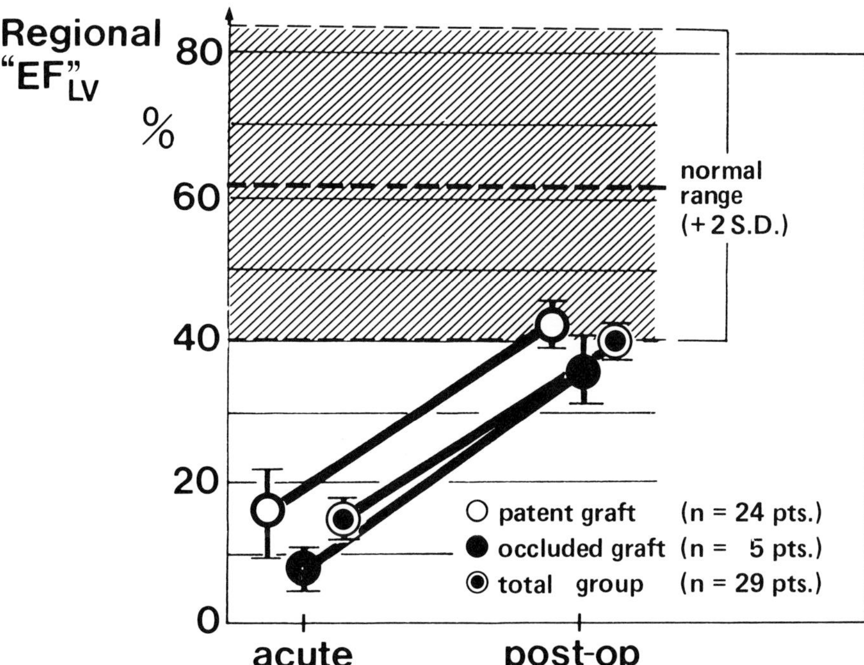

FIGURE 17 Marked improvement in regional ejection fraction in infarct area after intracoronary thrombolysis and early bypass surgery independent of whether the graft to the infarct vessel was occluded or not.

222

be prevented despite surgery, because the time interval between the occlusion and surgery was too long. In an attempt to reestablish flow early after occlusion, we infused 2,000 units of streptokinase per minute into the occluded coronary artery in 3 patients in whom we observed acute coronary occlusion during PTCA. In all 3 patients, the artery was opened within a few minutes. Then, emergency bypass surgery was performed. Postoperative angiography revealed no wall-motion abnormalities in the area of the occluded, reopened, and bypass-grafted artery. Thus reinfarction was prevented in these 3 patients.

Another potential indication for intracoronary streptokinase infusion is the acute thrombotic occlusion of an aortocoronary bypass graft, as reported by Rentrop et al.[60] However, there may be a significant risk of bleeding within the first week after bypass surgery when a total dosage of 100,000 units of streptokinase is exceeded. Moreover, it is probably very difficult to keep the reopened graft patent.

CONCLUSIONS

Reviewing the first 3 years of intracoronary thrombolysis with streptokinase in patients with transmural acute myocardial infarction, there is no doubt that in more than 80 percent of patients the acutely occluded coronary artery can be reopened. In this paper, evidence in terms of regional wall motion and myocardial scintigraphy is presented that demonstrates that infarct size is significantly limited by successful thromboylsis in the majority of patients whose symptoms did not last longer than 3 h. However, there are considerable interindividual differences in the rapidity with which a complete infarct develops, and even within 3 h irreversible necrosis may be completed. Future investigations should be directed toward determining, prior to intracoronary thrombolysis, which patient will benefit from the method and for whom it will be too late. At the moment, we determine myocardial salvage immediately after thrombolysis by intracoronary myocardial scintigraphy with ^{201}Tl and ^{99m}Tc pyrophosphate, which predicts the late functional results.

Since a high-grade arteriosclerotic stenosis remains after intracoronary thrombolysis with a risk of reinfarction in the range of 20 to 25 percent, a special postthrombotic therapy has to be instituted to prevent reinfarction. In our experience, only early bypass surgery has proved effective and safe in this regard.

Among the complications of intracoronary thrombolysis, myocardial hemorrhage deserves further attention, in particular its influence on infarct healing. The full extent of complications as well as the long-term benefits of intracoronary thrombolysis can be expected only from the randomized trials that are at present being carried out at several institutions.

REFERENCES

1 Chandler, A. B., Chapman, I., Erhardt, W. C., Roberts, L. R., et al.: Coronary Thrombosis in Myocardial Infarction. Report of a Workshop on the Role of Coronary Thrombosis in the Pathogenesis of Acute Myocardial Infarction, *Am. J. Cardiol.*, 34:823, 1974.

2 Baroldi, G., Falzi, G., and Mariani, F.: Sudden Coronary Death. A Postmortem Study in 208 Selected Cases Compared to 97 "Control" Subjects, *Am. Heart J.*, 98:20, 1979.

3 Erhardt, L. R., Unge, G., and Boman, G.: Formation of Coronary Arterial Thrombi in Relation to Onset of Necrosis in Acute Myocardial Infarction in Man. A Clinical and Autoradiographic Study, *Am. Heart J.*, 91:592, 1976.

4 Friedman, M., and van den Bovenkamp, G. J.: The Pathogenesis of a Coronary Thrombus, *Am. J. Pathol.*, 48:19, 1966.

5 Horie, T., Sekigudi, M., and Hirosawa, K.: Coronary Thrombosis in Pathogenesis of Acute Myocardial Infarction. Histopathological Study of Coronary Arteries in 108 Necropsied Cases Using Serial Section, *Br. Heart J.*, 40:153, 1978.

6 Verstraete, M.: Biochemical and Clinical Aspects of Thrombolysis, *Semin. Hematol.*, 15:35, 1978.

7 Ehrly, A. M.: "Rheological Changes Due to Fibrinolytic Therapy, Hemodilution: Theoretical Basis and Clinical Application," Karger, Basel, 1972, pp. 289–297.

8 European Cooperative Study Group for Streptokinase Treatment in Acute Myocardial Infarction: Streptokinase in Acute Myocardial Infarction, *N. Engl. J. Med.*, 301:798, 1979.

9 Rentrop, P., Blanke, H., Karsch, K. R., Kaiser, H., Köstering, H., and Leitz, K.: Selective Intracoronary Thrombolysis in Acute Myocardial Infarction and Instable Angina Pectoris, *Circulation*, 63:307, 1981.

10 Ganz, W., Buchbinder, N., Marcus, H., et al.: Intracoronary Thrombolysis in Evolving Myocardial Infarction, *Am. Heart J.*, 101:4, 1981.

11 Mathey, D. G., Kuck, K. H., Tilsner, V., Krebber, H. J., and Bleifeld, W.: Nonsurgical Coronary Artery Recanalization in Acute Transmural Myocardial Infarction, *Circulation*, 63:489, 1981.

12 Boucek, R. J., and Murphy, W. P.: Segmental Perfusion of the Coronary Arteries with Fibrinolysis in Man Following a Myocardial Infarction, *Am. J. Cardiol.*, 6:525, 1960.

13 Moschos, C. B., Burke, W. M., Lehan, P. H., Vedewurtel, H. A., and Regan, T. J.: Thrombolytic Agents and Lysis of Coronary Artery Thrombosis, *Cardiovasc. Res.*, 4:228, 1970.

14 Boyles, P. W., Meyer, W. H., Graff, J., Ashley, C. C., and Ripic, R. G.: Comparative Effectiveness of Intravenous and Intraarterial Fibrinolysin Therapy, *Am. J. Cardiol.*, 6:439, 1960.

15 Vetrovec, G. W., Cowley, M. J., Overton, B. A., and Richards, D. W.: Intracoronary Thrombus in Syndromes of Unstable Myocardial Ischemia, *Am. Heart J.*, 102:1202, 1981.

16 Reduto, L. A., Freund, G. G., Gacta, J. M., Smalling, R. W., Lewis, B., and Gould, K. L.: Coronary Artery Reperfusion in Acute Myocardial Infarction: Beneficial Effects of Intracoronary Streptokinase on Left Ventricular Salvage and Performance, *Am. Heart J.*, 102:1168, 1981.

17 McNamara, J. J., Smith, G. T., Suehiro, G. T., et al.: Myocardial Viability after Transient Ischemia in Primates, *J. Thorac. Cardiovasc. Surg.*, 68:248, 1974.

18 Blumenthal, M. R., Wang, H., and Liu, L. M. P.: Experimental Coronary Artery Occlusion and Release, *Am. J. Cardiol.*, 36:225, 1975.

19 Puri, P. S.: Contractile and Biochemical Effects of Coronary Reperfusion after Extended Periods of Coronary Occlusion, *Am. J. Cardiol.*, 36:244, 1975.

20 Costantini, C., Corday, E., Lang, T., et al.: Revascularization after 3 Hours of Coronary Arterial Occlusion: Effects on Regional Cardiac Metabolic Function and Infarct Size, *Am. J. Cardiol.*, 36:368, 1975.

21 Marthur, V. S., Guinn, G. A., and Burris, W. H.: Maximal Revascularization (Reperfusion) in Intact Conscious Dogs after 2 to 5 Hours of Coronary Occlusion, *Am. J. Cardiol.*, 36:252, 1975.

22 Mathey, D. G., Klöppel, G., Kuck, K. H., Beil, U., Schofer, J.: Transmural, Hemorrhagic Infarction Following Intracoronary Streptokinase: Clinical, Angiographic and Autoptical Findings, *Circulation*, 64 (suppl. 4):194, 1981.

23 De Wood, M. A., Spores, J., Notske, R., et al.: Prevalence of Total Coronary Occlusion during the Early Hours of Transmural Myocardial Infarction, *N. Engl. J. Med.*, 303:897, 1980.

24 Rutsch, W., Schartl, M., Mathey, D. G., et al.: Percutaneous Transluminal Coronary Recanalization: Procedure, Results and Acute Complications, *Am. Heart J.*, 102:1178, 1981.

25 Baugham, K. L., Maroko, P. R., and Vatner, S. F.: Effects of Coronary Artery Reperfusion on Myocardial Infarct Size and Survival in Conscious Dogs, *Circulation*, 63:317, 1981.

26 Schuler, G., Schwarz, F., Hofmann, M., et al.: Left Ventricular Performance and Myocardial Perfusion Following Recanalization of Occluded Coronary Arteries, *Circulation*, 64 (suppl. 4):106, 1981.

27 Maddahi, J., Ganz, W., Ninomiya, K., et al.: Myocardial Salvage by Intracoronary Thrombosis in Evolving Acute Myocardial Infarction: Evaluation Using Intracoronary Injection of Thallium-201, *Am. Heart J.*, 102:664, 1981.

28 Markis, J. E., Malagold, M., Parker, A., et al.: Myocardial Salvage after Intracoronary Thrombolysis with Streptokinase in Acute Myocardial Infarction: Assessment by Intracoronary Thallium-201, *N. Engl. J. Med.*, 305:777, 1981.

29 Schofer, J., Mathey, D. G., Kuck, K. H., Montz, R., Bleifeld, W.: Early Assessment of Salvaged Myocardium after Coronary Artery Recanalization by Sequential Intracoronary Thallium-201 Scintigraphy, *Am. J. Cardiol.*, 49:962, 1982.

30 Schofer, J., Mathey, D. G., Stritzke, P., Montz, R., Kuck, K. H., and Bleifeld, W.: Early Assessment of Salvaged Myocardium after Coronary Artery Recanalization by Intracoronary Tl-201 and Tc-99m Scintigraphy, "European Society of Cardiology, Working Group, Vienna, April 1–3, 1982," p. 5. (Abstract book.)

31 Vetrovec, G., Cowley, M., Overton, H., and Richardson, D.: Intracoronary Thrombus: Angiographic Features in Acute Myocardial Infarction and Unstable Angina Pectoris, *Circulation*, 64 (suppl. 4):162, 1981.

32 Karsch, K., Blanke, H., Pichard, A., et al.: Changes in the Degree of Stenosis of the Infarct Vessel Following Intracoronary Streptokinase, *Circulation*, 64 (suppl. 4):107, 1981.

33 Schröder, R., Biamino, G., and v. Leitner, E. R.: Intravenous Short-Time Thrombolysis in Acute Myocardial Infarction, *Circulation*, 64 (suppl. 4):10, 1981.

34 Schwarz, F., et al.: Personal communication (Heidelberg).

35 Neuhaus, K. L., Tebbe, U., Sauer, G., Kreuzer, H., and Köstering, H.: Determinanten der Frührekanalisation durch intravenöse Streptokinase-Infusion beim akuten Herzinfarkt, *Zeitschr. f. Kardiol.* 71:149, 1982.

36 Merx, W., Dörr, R. Rentrop, P., et al.: Evaluation of the Effectiveness of Intracoronary Streptokinase Infusion in Acute Myocardial Infarction: Postprocedure Management and Hospital Course in 204 Patients, *Am. Heart J.*, 102:1181, 1981.

37 Stowe, D., Mathey, D. G., Moores, W., et al.: Segment Stroke Work and Metabolism Depend on Coronary Flow in the Pig, *Am. J. Physiol.*, 234(5):H597, 1978.

38 Heyndrick, G. R., Millard, K. W., McRitchie, R., Maroko, P. K., and Vatner, S. F.: Regional Myocardial Functional and Electrophysiological Alterations after Brief Coronary Artery Occlusion in Conscious Dogs, *J. Clin. Invest.*, 56:978, 1975.

39 Reimer, K. A., Lowe, J. E., Rasminssen, M. M., and Jennings, R. B.: The Wave Front of Ischemic Cell Death, *Circulation*, 56:786, 1977.

40 Ginks, W. R., Syberg, H. O., Maroko, P. R., Corell, J. W., Sobel, B. E., and Ross, J.: Coronary Artery Reperfusion: Reduction of Myocardial Infarct Size at 1 Week after the Coronary Occlusions, *J. Clin. Invest.*, 51:2717, 1972.

41 Geary, G. G., Smith, G. T., and McNamara, J. J.: Extent of Myocardial Salvage by Early Coronary Artery Reperfusion in the Absence of Signifikant Collaterals in Baboons, *Circulation,* 64 (suppl. 4):98, 1981.

42 Reduto, L. A., Freund, G. C., Gaeta, J., Killingsworth, B., Nussey, G., and Gould, K. L.: Thallium Redistribution Following Intracoronary Streptokinase in Acute Myocardial Infarction: Relation to Changes in Left Ventricular Performance, *Circulation,* 64 (suppl. 4):33, 1981.

43 Rentrop, P., Merx, W., Mathey, D. G., Blanke, H., Rutsch, W., and Karsch, K. R.: Functional Results of Streptokinase Reperfusion in Relation to Collaterals and Duration of Symptoms, *Circulation,* 64 (suppl. 4):194, 1981.

44 Mehmel, H. C., Schwarz, F., Schuler, H. et al.: The Functional Result of Intracoronary Streptokinase Therapy after Myocardial Infarction May Be Determined by Collaterals, *Circulation,* 64 (suppl. 4):194, 1981.

45 Sheehan, F. H., Bolson, E. L., Dodge, H. T., and Mitten, S.: Center Line Method—Comparison with Other Methods for Measuring Regional Left Ventricular Motion, *Comput. Biol. Med.,* in press.

46 Mathey, D. G., Kuck, K. H., Remmecke, J., Tilsner, V., and Bleifeld, W.: Transluminal Recanalization of Coronary Artery Thrombosis: A Preliminary Report of Its Application in Cardiogenic Shock, *Eur. Heart J.,* 1:207, 1980.

47 Horowitz, S. F., Karsch, K. R., Driesman, M. H., et al.: Intracoronary Thrombolysis with Streptokinase in Acute Myocardial Infarction, *N. Engl. J. Med.,* 306:300, 1982. (Letter.)

48 Wagner, G. S., Freye, C. J., Palmeri, S. T., et al.: Evaluation of a QRS Scoring System for Estimating Myocardial Infarct Size, *Circulation,* 54:342, 1982.

49 Cowley, M., Hastillo, A., Vetrovec, G., and Hess, M. L.: Fibrinolytic Effects of Low Dose Intracoronary Streptokinase Administration in Acute Myocardial Infarction, *Circulation,* 64 (suppl. 4):10, 1981.

50 Geft, I. L., Peter, T., Mercier, Y. C., Lando, H., Kanmatsuse, K., and Ganz, W.: Successful Prevention and Treatment of Reperfusion Ventricular Tachycardia with Intracoronary Lidocaine, *Circulation,* 64 (suppl. 4):319, 1981.

51 Corr, P. B., and Witkowski, F. X.: Potential Electrophysiological Mechanisms for Dysrhythmias Associated with Reperfusion of Ischemic Myocardium, *Circulation,* in press.

52 Williams, L. T., Guerrero, J. L., Leinbach, R. C., and Gold, H. K.: Prevention of Reperfusion Dysrhythmias by Selective Coronary Alpha Adrenergic Blockade, *Am. J. Cardiol.,* 49:1047, 1981.

53 Schachenmayer, W., and Haferkamp, O.: Der hämorrhagische Herzinfarkt, *Dtsch. Med. Wochenschr.,* 97:1172, 1972.

54 Hartzler, G. O., Rutherford, B. D., and McConahay, D. R.: Percutaneous Coronary Angioplasty with or without Prior Streptokinase Infusion for Treatment of Acute Myocardial Infarction, *Am. J. Cardiol.,* 49:1033, 1982.

55 Meyer, J., Merx, W., Schmitz, H. J., et al.: Percutaneous Transluminal Coronary Angioplasty (PTCA) Immediately after Intracoronary Streptolysis of Transmural Myocardial Infarction, *Circulation,* in press.

56 Mathey, D. G., Rodewald, G., Rentrop, P., et al.: Intracoronary Streptokinase Thrombolytic Recanalization and Subsequent Surgical Bypass of Remaining Arteriosclerotic Stenosis in Acute Myocardial Infarction: Complementary Combined Approach Effecting Reduced Infarct Size Preventing Reinfarction and Improving Left Ventricular Function, *Am. Heart J.,* 102:1194, 1981.

57 Bleese, N., Döring, V., Kalmar, P., Pokar, H., Polonius, M.-J., Steiner, D., and Rodewald, G.: Intraoperative Myocardial Protection by Cardioplegia in Hypothermia, *J. Thorac. Cardiovasc. Surg.,* 75:405, 1978.

58 Krebber, H.-J., Mathey, D. G., Kuck, K. H., Kalmar, P., and Rodewald, G.: Management of Evolving Myocardial Infarction by Intracoronary Lysis and Subsequent Aortocoronary Bypass, *J. Thorac. Cardiovasc. Surg.,* 83:186, 1982.

59 Mathey, D. G., Schofer, J., Krebber, H.-J., and Bleifeld, W.: Reopening of Coronary Artery Occlusion Following PTCA by Intracoronary Streptokinase Prevents Myocardial Infarction, *Am. J. Cardiol.,* 49:916, 1982.

60 Rentrop, P., Blanke, H., Karsch, K. R., Köstering, H., Oster, H., and Leitz, H.: Recanalization of an Acutely Occluded Aortocoronary Bypass by Intragraft Fibrinolysis, *Circulation,* 62:1123, 1980.

Diagnosis and Management of Intraventricular Conduction Disorders[*]

JAMES J. HEGER, M.D., and CHARLES FISCH, M.D.

Intraventricular conduction disorders are electrocardiographic manifestations of delay or failure of conduction in one or more of the bundle branches or specialized conducting fascicles. As a result of localized conduction delay or block, ventricular depolarization loses its normal synchrony. This discussion presents the electrocardiographic manifestations and clinical significance of the individual intraventricular conduction disorders and selected clinical aspects of management of patients who have intraventricular conduction disorders.

ANATOMIC CONSIDERATIONS

Conduction of the cardiac impulse from the arteriovenous junction to the ventricular myocardium proceeds through the intraventricular conduction system, comprised of the main bundle branches and the fascicles and terminating at the Purkinje fiber–muscle cell junction. Diseases may affect the intraventricular conduction system at any site and may produce a variety of electrocardiographic abnormalities and cardiac arrhythmias, many of which have major clinical importance. Disorders of intraventricular conduction are usually manifest as conduction block in one or more fascicles. Some of the anatomic and physiologic factors that predict vulnerability of a particular fascicle to a conduction block include the location, structure, and vascular supply of the fascicle.

The penetrating portion of the arteriovenous bundle, or bundle of His, traverses the fibrous skeleton of the heart and in normal hearts provides the sole muscular connection between atria and ventricle. The arteriovenous bundle is 2 to 3 cm long, arises from the arteriovenous node, and is encased in a vascular and fiber sheath as it courses anteriorly and somewhat superiorly to reach the junction of the membranous and muscular septum in the ventricle.[1] By its proximity to the membranous septum, the arteriovenous bundle may be affected by congenital defects of the membranous septum or, more commonly, following surgical repair of these defects. Likewise, since the noncoronary cusp of the aortic valve is adjacent to the arteriovenous bundle, calcific aortic valve disease, infective endocarditis with ring abscess, and aortic dissection may produce abnormalities in arteriovenous

conduction. This portion of the arteriovenous conduction system has a dual vascular supply from the anterior and posterior descending coronary arteries, so the arteriovenous bundle is less likely to be directly affected by ischemic events.

The bundle of His generally does not have a discrete bifurcation, but rather gives off fine strands that form the left bundle branch, while the right bundle branch arises more as a direct continuation. The right bundle is a thin, compact structure that courses intramyocardially through the upper portions of the muscular septum before reaching the subendocardium on the right side of the septum. A main portion of the right bundle extends to the base of the anterior papillary muscle of the right ventricle.

The left bundle is a broad structure that fans out in the subendocardium on the left side of the septum. Two major branches, anterior and posterior fascicles, extend to the anterosuperior and posteroinferior papillary muscles, respectively. The anterior fascicle remains in the subendocardial layer of the septum, while the left posterior fascicle courses away from the septum along the inflow region of the left ventricle.

Vascular supply of the distal portions of the bundle of His, the right bundle, and the left anterior fascicle is through branches of the anterior descending coronary artery. The left posterior fascicle has a dual vascular supply from both anterior and posterior descending coronary arteries and thus is less vulnerable to ischemic events as compared with the right bundle and left anterior fascicle.

TYPES OF BLOCK

The estimated prevalence associated with HV prolongation of various types of intraventricular conduction disorders is given in Table 1.

Left Anterior Fascicular Block (LAFB)

Conduction block in the anterior fascicle of the left bundle results in a characteristic electrocardiographic pattern whereby activation of myocardium is first posterior or interior and then spreads superiorly. The initial QRS vector is directed inferiorly, producing small, 0.02-s Q waves in leads I and aV_L and small R waves in leads II, III, and aV_F. The remainder of the QRS vector represents depolarization of the anterior

[*]From the Krannert Institute of Cardiology, the Department of Medicine, Indiana University School of Medicine, and the Veterans Administration Hospital, Indianapolis, Indiana.

TABLE 1
Chronic intraventricular conduction disorders: estimated prevalence and association with HV prolongation

Intraventricular conduction disorder	Estimated prevalence in normal population*	Incidence of prolonged HV interval†
LAFB	0.9–1.4%	30%
LPFB	0.1%	40%
RBBB	0.3–0.4%	30–50%
LBBB	0.1%	60–90%
Bifascicular block	0.1%	
RBBB and LAFB		60–90%
RBBB and LPFB		80–100%

*From Ref. 3.
†From Ref. 17.

and superior myocardium of the left ventricle and is directed superiorly and leftward, producing R waves in leads I and aV_L and deep S waves in leads II, III, and aV_F. The mean QRS vector in left anterior fascicular block is leftward and superior. The electrocardiographic criteria for left anterior fascicular block are the following: (1) mean QRS axis is leftward, beyond negative 45°; (2) limb leads demonstrate an initial Q wave in lead I and a deep S wave in lead III; (3) the precordial leads also reflect the altered sequence of myocardial depolarization with QS complexes in right precordial leads and RS complexes in left precordial leads.[2]

Left anterior fascicular block is the most common form of intraventricular conduction disorder. While frequently indicating disease of the left ventricle, left anterior fascicular block has been estimated to be present in 0.9 to 1.4 percent of populations that have no evidence of clinical heart disease.[3] The most common forms of cardiac disease associated with left anterior fascicular block are ischemic heart disease, systemic hypertension, congestive cardiomyopathy, and aortic valve disease. Left anterior fascicular block may accompany acute myocardial infarction and usually indicates extensive necrosis of the intraventricular septum.

Left anterior fascicular block is important in electrocardiographic diagnosis because it may simulate or conceal the manifestations of myocardial infarction. With left anterior fascicular blocks, precordial leads may demonstrate small QS complexes in right precordium or RS complexes in all precordial leads, simulating anterior infarction. The correct diagnosis of left anterior fascicular block may be resolved by recording the precordial leads one interspace lower on the chest wall. When left anterior fascicular block accompanies acute anterior myocardial infarction, the expected Q waves in the precordial leads may be converted to RS complexes as a result of the fascicular block. With inferior infarction, the diagnostic Q waves in leads II,

III, and aV_F may be converted to RS complexes in the presences of left anterior fascicular block. Serial ECG records are often necessary for correct diagnosis.

Left Posterior Fascicular Block (LPFB)

In left posterior fascicular block, activation of the posterior and inferior segments of the left ventricle is delayed, while initial myocardial activation precedes through the anterior fascicle. The initial QRS vector is leftward and superior, while the mean and terminal vector shifts rightward and inferiorly. These changes in sequence of depolarization produce a mean QRS vector of more than +110° with RS complexes in leads I and aV_L and QR complexes in leads II, III, and aV_F.

Isolated left posterior fascicular block is uncommon, and its diagnosis is almost never made from a single electrocardiogram but is rather based on a clinical-electrocardiographic correlation of serial tracings. To diagnose left posterior fascicular block, it is first necessary to exclude other causes of right axis deviation, namely, right ventricular enlargement, chronic obstructive lung disease, vertical heart, and lateral myocardial infarction. Left posterior fascicular block is most often accompanied by block in another fascicle, either the right bundle or left anterior fascicle.

Right Bundle Branch Block (RBBB)

In right bundle branch block the QRS is prolonged beyond 0.11 s. The initial 0.06 to 0.08 s, representing left ventricular activation, is unaffected by right bundle branch block, but the terminal 0.04 s, representing delayed activation from the blocked right bundle, is directed rightward and anteriorly. These changes produce the characteristic terminal S wave in leads I, aV_L

and V_{5-6} with an RSR' pattern in lead V_1. The mean QRS axis, which is determined from the initial 0.08 s of the QRS, is usually normal.

Right bundle branch block may occur with normal hearts and is stated to have an incidence of 0.3 percent in a clinically normal population.[3] Heart diseases of ischemic, rheumatic, and hypertensive etiologies and cor pulmonale are the most common causes of right bundle branch block in the adult. In the Framingham Study, right bundle branch block developed in 70 of over 5,000 patients during an 18-year observation. Hypertension was the most common associated condition. Once right bundle branch block occurred, the risk of subsequent cardiac events was increased compared with the group without bundle branch block, since one-third developed manifestations of coronary artery disease during follow-up.[4]

Isolated right bundle branch block may develop acutely during anterior myocardial infarction or acute pulmonary embolism. While the latter is often transient, during acute infarction the appearance of right bundle branch block accompanies a large infarction often associated with heart failure. Right bundle branch block may presage further conduction abnormalities, since 40 percent of these patients develop bifascicular or trifascicular block.[5]

Bifascicular Block

Bifascicular block indicates there is conduction delay in two of the three fascicles of the conduction system. The term *bifascicular block* is usually applied when the electrocardiogram demonstrates right bundle branch block with either left anterior fascicular block or left posterior fascicular block or when there is complete left bundle branch block.

Right Bundle Branch Block and Left Anterior Fascicular Block

In right bundle branch block and left anterior fascicular block, the QRS is prolonged to at least 0.11 s. The initial 0.06-s QRS vector is a result of left anterior fascicular block, so there is a left-axis shift in the frontal plane with initial Q in lead I and terminal S in leads II, III, and aV_F. The terminal 0.05-s vector of the QRS, which results from right bundle branch block, is directed rightward and anteriorly. The mean QRS vector, determined from the initial QRS portion is oriented leftward and superiorly. Precordial leads in right bundle branch block and left anterior fascicular block show the pattern of RSR' in lead V_1 and wide terminal S wave in lead V_6.

Bifascicular block is rarely found in the absence of heart disease, with perhaps less than 0.1 percent incidence in a clinically normal population.[3] Right bundle branch block with left anterior fascicular block is most commonly associated with ischemic heart disease. Since the right bundle and left anterior fascicle derive vascular supply from the left anterior descending coronary artery, conduction block in both fascicles may occur during infarction involving the anterior interventricular septum. Other conditions associated with right bundle branch block with left anterior fascicular block are congestive cardiomyopathy and aortic valve disease, particularly calcific aortic stenosis. Occasionally right bundle branch block with left anterior fascicular block occurs in patients thought to have primary disease of the conduction system without other evidence of organic heart disease. Lenegre's disease is a sclerodegenerative process that affects the conduction system but spares the remainder of the heart and usually is manifest in patients aged 40 to 60 years.[6] More prevalent in older age groups is Lev's disease, which produces sclerosis and calcification of the entire cardiac skeleton, including the arteriovenous annulus and the conduction system.[7] Both may present as bifascicular conduction block which then progresses to complete heart block, although this sequence appears to occur more frequently with Lenegre's disease.

Congenital heart diseases associated with right bundle branch block with left anterior fascicular block are endocardial cushion defects, ventricular septal defects, and following surgical repair of tetralogy of Fallot. The long-term prognosis in patients who have conduction disorders following surgical repair of congenital heart disease remains to be defined. Late postoperative sudden death does occur in some of these patients owing to either ventricular tachyarrhythmias or the development of complete heart block.[8]

Right Bundle Branch Block and Left Posterior Fascicular Block

Combined conduction block in the right bundle and left posterior fascicle is an uncommon electrocardiographic finding, as noted by Rosenbaum, who collected only 29 such cases over a 10-year period.[2] In this conduction disorder the electrocardiogram displays the typical findings of right bundle branch block, in which the terminal QRS vector is delayed and directed anteriorly and rightward, and this is accompanied by the changes of left posterior fascicular block, in which the initial QRS vector is rightward and inferior. The resulting ECG pattern in the frontal plane is a right-axis deviation to at least $+110°$, an S_1Q_3 pattern, and terminal conduction delay. In the precordial leads there may be an initial Q wave in lead V_1 and persistent S waves in the left precordial leads. As with isolated left posterior fascicular block, the diagnosis of right bundle branch block with left posterior fascicular block is made after correlating clinical and electrocardiographic findings, and in most cases the diagnosis rests on the availability of serial electrocardiographic tracings that show progression from normal conduction to bifascicular block.

The presence of right bundle branch block and left posterior fascicular block nearly always indicates heart disease with ischemic heart disease, congestive cardiomyopathy, and primary conduction system disease being the most common causes. Right bundle branch block with left posterior fascicular block is of particular clinical importance because it often is a precursor of high-degree arteriovenous heart block (usually other components of the conduction system are diseased by the time left posterior fascicular block is manifest).

Left Bundle Branch Block (LBBB)

Left bundle branch block may be due to block in the common bundle or a combined block in both the left anterior and left posterior fascicles. Electrocardiographic features of left bundle branch block are QRS prolongation to 0.11 s or more, broad R waves without initial Q waves in leads I, aV_L, and left precordial leads, and initial, small R waves with deep S waves in right precordial leads. QRS complexes are often notched or slurred. Characteristically, secondary ST and T wave changes are produced by the direction of repolarization vectors in a manner opposite that from the main QRS vector. The frontal plane QRS axis in left bundle branch block may be normal or leftward. It has been argued that left-axis deviation in left bundle branch block may represent more severe conduction disease or left-sided heart disease. However, in pathologic electrocardiographic correlations, no significant difference was found in left ventricular weight, coronary anatomy, or infarct location among cases of left bundle branch block and either left or normal axis.[9]

Left bundle branch block may be found in 0.1 to 0.7 percent of clinically normal individuals, but usually it is seen in association with heart disease, which includes ischemic heart disease, hypertension, congestive and hypertrophic cardiomyopathy, and aortic valve disease.[3] Often left bundle branch block occurs in association with other electrical abnormalities of the sinus node, arteriovenous node, and His-Purkinje system.[10]

In the Framingham population of 5,177 patients observed for over 18 years, 55 patients had new onset of left bundle branch block during the observation period.[4] Most had hypertension as an underlying cause, and during follow-up, 20 percent developed new symptoms of coronary heart disease and 20 percent had developed heart failure. Therefore, it appears that the presence of either right or left bundle branch block may actually presage the development of clinical heart disease in a significant number of individuals.

Trifascicular Block

The concept of trifasicular block is useful in understanding the pathophysiologic abnormalities of intraventricular conduction, but the term itself is nonspecific. It is more correct to specify the exact conduction pattern when interpreting the electrocardiogram rather than use the term *trifascicular block*. *Trifascicular block* refers to conduction delay or block or a combination of delay and block in all three fascicles, and trifascicular block may be complete, incomplete, or intermittent. *Complete trifascicular block* is equivalent to complete heart block with the site of block located distal to the bundle of His. This is the type of complete heart block that occurs during acute anterior myocardial infarction and occurs spontaneously in most adult patients who develop heart block. *Incomplete trifascicular block* refers to complete block in two fascicles and incomplete block or conduction delay in the remaining fascicle. A common manifestation is bifascicular block with prolonged P-R interval, the latter suggesting conduction delay in the remaining fascicle. In many cases, however, P-R prolongation represents delay in the arteriovenous node and not below the bundle of His, so diagnosis of trifascicular block from the electrocardiogram alone is inferential. *Intermittent trifascicular block* is manifest by the electrocardiogram when there is alternating conduction block in all three fascicles, often in the form of alternating bundle branch block. Alternation may occur during successive QRS complexes in one tracing or in successive tracings performed at different times. Intermittent trifascicular block indicates significant disease of the conduction system and is often a precursor of complete heart block.

MANAGEMENT OF INTRA-VENTRICULAR CONDUCTION DISORDERS (IVCD)

The management of patients manifesting intraventricular conduction disorders is based on the clinical state in which block occurs and the known natural history of the conduction disturbance. The prime consideration in management of such disorders is the recognition of those forms which are likely to develop complete heart block and thereby result in cardiac asystole or ventricular fibrillation.

Intraventricular Conduction Disorders in Acute Myocardial Infarction (see Table 2)

The onset of intraventricular conduction disorders during acute myocardial infarction identifies a group of patients who have an increased mortality. However, the presence of intraventricular conduction disorders may be a marker of increased risk, not by being a precursor of complete heart block, but rather by being a marker for development of left ventricular failure. New onset of bundle branch block or bifascicular block occurs in about 13 percent of cases of acute myocardial infarction, and a mortality rate when cardiogenic shock does not precede the intraventricular conduction disorder is about 28 percent which compares to an average mortality in patients without such disorders of 12 percent.[5]

Patients who develop new bifascicular block, particularly when associated with P-R interval prolongation, are at highest risk of subsequent appearance of high-degree arteriovenous block.[11] Management centers around the need for temporary pacemaker insertion. When intraventricular conduction disorders complicate acute myocardial infarction, the majority of deaths are due to left ventricular failure, in which case the prognosis is not altered by pacemaker therapy. However, a number of patients who have new-onset bundle branch block and bifascicular block will develop high-degee arteriovenous block, and over one-quarter of these die as a result of heart block.[5] Therefore, it is reasonable to recommend temporary prophylactic pacemaker insertion in patients who have the new onset of bundle branch block or bifascicular block during myocardial infarction, particularly if this is not accompanied or preceded by severe heart failure. Preexisting stable bundle branch block or bifascicular block is not an indication for temporary pacing.

TABLE 2
Recommended management of new intraventricular condition disorders during acute myocardial infarction

Disorder	Temporary pacemaker*	Permanent pacemaker*
LAFB	–	–
LPFB	–	–
RBBB	+	–
LBBB	+	–
RBBB plus LAFB	+	–
RBBB plus LPFB	+	–
Bifascicular block plus high-degree arteriovenous block	+	+

*+ = pacemaker recommended; – = pacemaker not recommended

Patients who have new-onset bundle branch block and survive the acute infarction have an increased mortality and increased risk of sudden death and left ventricular failure during follow-up, with most of the deaths resulting from ventricular fibrillation.[12,13] In the absence of accompanying high-degree arteriovenous block during acute myocardial infarction, permanent pacemaker implantation is not recommended for the long-term treatment of patients who develop bundle branch block during acute infarction. For patients who have developed bundle branch block and have had transient arteriovenous block during the infarction, permanent pacing had been recommended, but a distinct improvement in survival has not been established because of the small number of patients studied to date.[8]

Intraventricular Conduction Disorders in the Chronic Setting

The clinical significance of chronic intraventricular conduction disorders not associated with acute infarction derives from the association of such disorders with significant underlying heart disease. The presence of intraventricular conduction disorders may precede development of high-degree arteriovenous block with subsequent syncope or sudden death.

Several ongoing studies have examined the prognosis of patients who have chronic bundle branch block or bifascicular block. Rates for sudden death and cardiac mortality are higher for patients with bifascicular block and bundle branch block as compared with control population, but death is usually due to ventricular tachyarrhythmias or progression of the underlying heart disease.[8] During long-term follow-up, spontaneous second- or third-degree arteriovenous block occurs in 2 to 3 percent of patients who have bundle branch block or bifascicular block.[14,15] A group of patients who are at increased risk to develop high-degree arteriovenous block is able to be identified by finding a prolonged HV interval at electrophysiologic study, progressive HV prolongation at repeat study, or infra-Hisian block at paced atrial rates of greater than 130 per minute.[15,16] However, even with this group there is a low overall incidence of subsequent arteriovenous block. Therefore, pacemaker insertion is not recommended for asymptomatic patients who have bundle branch block or bifascicular block.

In symptomatic patients (syncope, presyncope) who have intraventricular conduction disorders and documented second- or third-degree arteriovenous block, permanent pacemaker therapy is recommended. For patients who have unexplained recurrent syncope or presyncope and bundle branch block, it is reasonable to recommend permanent pacemaker therapy once other cardiac and noncardiac causes of syncope have been evaluated. For many patients in this category, intracardiac electrophysiologic study is suggested to investigate the integrity of arteriovenous conduction and to test for the presence of bradyarrhythmia and tachyarrhythmia once noninvasive studies, including long-term ECG recordings, have failed to establish a cause for the symptoms.

ROLE OF ELECTROPHYSIOLOGIC STUDY

Originally introduced as a method to record depolarization of the His bundle, the intracardiac electrophysiologic study provides more precise information to assess the integrity of arteriovenous conduction in patients who have intraventricular conduction disorders. For example, data from the electrophysiologic study can determine if a prolonged PR interval with bifascicular block is due to prolonged arteriovenous nodal conduction or to conduction delay in the remaining intraventricular fascicle.[17] The latter finding suggests an increased risk for development of high-degree arteriovenous block. The ability to record His-Purkinje depolarization has added greatly to the understanding of the mechanisms and prognosis of arteriovenous conduction disorders. However, as indicated earlier, the benefit for the individual patient in terms of prescribing specific therapy is less clear. Only a very few patients who have bivascicular block and prolonged HV interval will develop high-degree arteriovenous block, and furthermore, arteriovenous block may occur in the presence of a normal HV interval. Therefore, electrophysiologic study is not indicated for the asymptomatic patient who has intraventricular conduction disorders. Electrophysiologic study appears to be indicated to help evaluate and manage patients who have such disorders with recurrent unexplained syncope or presyncope, with transient arteriovenous block, or with transient trifascicular block.

REFERENCES

1 Rossi, L.: "Histopathology of Cardiac Arrhythmias," 2d ed., Casa Editrice Ambrosiana, Milan, 1979, p. 16.

2 Rosenbaum, M. B.: The Hemiblocks: Diagnostic Criteria and Clinical Significance, *Mod. Concepts Cardiovasc. Dis.,* 39:141, 1970.

3 Barrett, P. A., Peter, C. T., Swan, H. J. C., Singh, B. N., and Mandel, W. J.: The Frequency and Prognostic Significance of Electrocardiographic Abnormalities in Clinically Normal Individuals, *Prog. Cardiovasc. Dis.,* 23:299, 1981.

4 Schneider, J. F., Thomas, H. E., Jr., Sorlie, P., Kreger, B. E., McNamara, P. M., and Kannel, W. B.: Comparative Features of Newly Acquired Left and Right Bundle Branch Block in the General Population: The Framingham Study, *Am. J. Cardiol.,* 47:931, 1981.

5 Hindman, M. C., Wagner, G. S., JaRo, M., et al.: The Clinical Significance of Bundle Branch Block Complicating Acute Myocardial Infarction: I. Clinical Characteristics, Hospital Mortality and One Year Follow-Up, *Circulation,* 58:679, 1978.

6 Lenegre, J.: Etiology and Pathology of Bilateral Bundle Branch Block in Relation to Complete Heart Block, *Prog. Cardiovasc. Dis.,* 6:409, 1964.

7 Lev, M.: Anatomic Basis of Atrioventricular Block, *Am. J. Med.,* 37:742, 1964.

8 Fisch, G. R., Zipes, D. P., and Fisch, C.: Bundle Branch Block and Sudden Death, *Prog. Cardiovasc. Dis.,* 23:187, 1981.

9 Havelda, C. J., Sohi, G. S., Flowers, N. C., Horan, L. G.: The Pathologic Correlates of the Electrocardiogram: Complete Left Bundle Branch Block, *Circulation,* 65:445, 1982.

10 Barrett, P. A., Yamaguchi, I., Jordan, J. L., Mandel, W. J.: Electrophysiological Factors of Left Bundle Branch Block, *Br. Heart J.,* 45:594, 1981.

11 Hindman, M. C., Wagner, J. S., JaRo, M., et al.: The Clinical Significance of Bundle Branch Block Complicating Acute Myocardial Infarction: II. Indications for Temporary and Permanent Pacemaker Insertion, *Circulation,* 58:689, 1978.

12 Lie, K. I., Liem, K. L., Schuilenburg, R. M., David, G. K., and Durrer, D.: Early Identification of Patients Developing Late In-Hospital Ventricular Fibrillation After Discharge from the Coronary Care Unit, *Am. J. Cardiol.,* 41:674, 1978.

13 Hauer, R. N. W., Lie, K. I., Liem, K. L., and Durrer, D.: Long-Term Prognosis in Patients with Bundle Branch Block Complicating Acute Anteroseptal Infarction, *Am. J. Cardiol.,* 49:1581, 1982.

14 Dhingra, R. C., Wyndham, C., Amat y Leon, F., et al.: Incidence and Site of Atrioventricular Block in Patients with Chronic Bifascicular Block, *Circulation,* 59:238, 1979.

15 Dhingra, R. C., Palileo, E., Strasberg, B., et al.: Significance of the H-V Interval in 517 Patients with Chronic Bifascicular Block, *Circulation,* 64:1265, 1981.

16 Peters, R. W., Scheinman, M. M., Dhingra, R., et al.: Serial Electrophysiologic Studies in Patients with Chronic Bundle Branch Block, *Circulation,* 65:1480, 1982.

17 Narula, O. S.: Intraventricular Conduction Defects: Current Concepts and Clinical Significance, in O. S. Narula (ed), "Cardiac Arrhythmias: Electrophysiology, Diagnosis and Management," Williams & Wilkins, Baltimore, 1979, pp. 124–127.

Supported in part by the Herman C. Krannert Fund, and by Grants HL-06308, HL-18795, and HL-07182 from the National Heart, Lung and Blood Institute of the National Institutes of Health, U.S. Public Health Service, and the American Heart Association, Indiana Affiliate.

Mechanical Cardiac Assistance[*]

SPYRIDON D. MOULOPOULOS, M.D.

When mechanical failure (pump failure) develops in a
dynamic hydraulic system, such as the human blood
circulation system, the first logical thought in terms of
treatment should be "mechanical" help. In fact, exsan-
guination has been a procedure honored for centuries
by which one parameter, namely, the circulating blood
volume, is affected in such cases. Beyond this attempt,
contemporary therapeutic approaches have sought in
the past only chemical means to help the heart.

The impetus for the use of mechanical cardiac
assistance developed only after it was shown that the
circulation can be maintained by an external pump
during brief periods of time in order to perform
corrective surgery on the heart.[1] The lack of essential
progress in the pharmaceutical treatment of myocardial
failure has enhanced the use of mechanical devices
during the last decades. Furthermore, experimental
attempts to construct a pump that could totally replace
the damaged heart have significantly contributed to the
field of assistance by developing new techniques and
equipment.[2]

Thus the contribution of mechanical means may not
be as significant today in support of the failing heart as
"medical" treatment, but some progress has been
made, and the first results of this approach are apparent in the clinical field.

THE NEED FOR MECHANICAL CARDIAC ASSISTANCE

One can envision the use of mechanical cardiac assistance in a series of clinical situations in which adequate
perfusion of peripheral organs cannot be maintained by
a failing heart, even when it is supported by conventional treatment. Offering the missing energy required
by the circulatory system may be useful in two types of
conditions. In acute, short-lasting deficiency of the
systematic circulation, as appears, for example, during
acute valvular regurgitation, acute myocardial infarction, rupture of the interventricular septum, or a
chorda tendina, temporary supplementation of the
heart function using an external energy source may be

*From the Department of Therapeutics, University of Athens Medical
School, and the National University, Athens, Greece.

life-saving, until the situation improves such that the
heart can be self-sufficient again, following healing of
the pathologic lesions, readjustment of the remaining
healthy myocardium, surgical corrective procedures,
metabolic milieu restoration, and so forth.

However, there are patients in low output failure
who are gradually deteriorating and no medical treatment is helping because of irreversible damage to a
large percentage (above 40 percent) of the myocardial
mass. These patients would require a chronic assist
device to permanently supplement the deficient heart
function by offering the missing amount of energy to
the system.

PRINCIPLES OF MECHANICAL CARDIAC ASSISTANCE

Several principles have been used in the attempt to
mechanically assist the heart.

The first principle originated in the extracorporeal
circuits technique. If blood could be withdrawn from
the venous side or the left atrium and pumped into the
systemic network, a part or all of the load could be
taken off the ventricles. A second energy source, a
mechanical pump, would thus be connected in parallel
to the heart.

The disadvantages of the "bypass" techniques based
on this principle are (1) the left-sided heart cavities are
not easily accessible, (2) venous blood requires oxygenation before being rendered back into the systemic
circulation, (3) blood is handled in an extracorporeal
circuit, and (4) the resistance to the left ventricle
remains the same/or may even increase while the
preload is reduced. Beyond certain limits (see Quantitation of Mechanical Cardiac Assistance), this may be
detrimental to heart function.

The second principle consists of mechanically compressing the ventricular myocardium, thus helping it to
expel the blood. Techniques based on this principle are
mainly used for short periods of time, usually on the
order of seconds or minutes, although attempts have
been made to employ such compressing techniques in
permanent pulsating devices. Most of these longer-
term techniques require a thoracotomy, however, and
traumatic lesions to the heart and adjacent structures
may result.

The third principle is an ingenious conception.[3,4]
Counterpulsation is the term used to indicate that an
external energy source will operate (pump) in the
arterial part of the circulation during heart diastole and
utilize the systolic period to withdraw blood. Thus one

cannula is used both to withdraw and propel blood.[3] The left ventricle faces a low resistance during the ejection phase, since at that time the outside pump is in the negative operating stage. Pumping during diastole does not counteract the ventricle, since the aortic valve is closed. In addition, it helps diastolic filling of the coronary network and propels the blood toward the periphery. Counterpulsation is thus, in a way, doubling "systole" within the same cardiac cycle.

The disadvantages of this technique are that the mechanical assistance, in order to be efficient, requires a minimum of operation of the ventricle and a minimum of diastolic period length. It does not operate efficiently if the heart has a very low output or a very fast rate, especially if the rhythm is irregular. The drawback of handling blood outside the body has been eliminated[5] by the use of an air chamber in the aorta, operating in the same way as the outside-the-body counterpulsating pump.

The "copulsation" principle is a variation of counterpulsation that consists of pumping during systole.[6] This may have the advantage of increasing systolic and diastolic perfusion pressures, mainly toward the coronary arteries, but it may induce an increase in resistances, potentially detrimental to the failing left ventricle. A nonpulsatile obstruction of the descending aorta has also been tried, with the intent to increase coronary perfusion via an increase in mean "central" aortic pressure.[7]

A fourth principle has recently been suggested.[8] Preload increases, as in volume loading, may have a positive effect on output, according to Starling's law of the heart, up to a certain limit, determined by the heart's condition and the effects of stasis in the lungs. On the other side, increasing the afterload, as in copulsation, may result in a positive inotropic effect, but the increase in resistance does not allow this effect to be profitable in augmenting output. However, if the preload or the afterload is increased only for a brief fraction of diastole or systole (60 to 80 ms), one may achieve the profitable effect and practically avoid the disadvantages.[8]

The short-term increase in afterload may result in positive inotropy, while the integrated systolic resistance may not be substantially increased. A similar, brief end-diastolic preload increase can be considered as a magnified "atrial kick," while at the same time, the integral of diastolic pressures in the venous side of the pulmonary circulation may not be significantly affected. Exaggerated (but brief) diastolic preload increases, larger than those tolerated by the ventricle operating within the limitations of the "law of the heart," may be expected to increase the output by overdistending the ventricle and optimizing the operation of normally non or less-working myocardial elements. Reorientation of fibers may be another way to optimize performance by this assistance technique.

Combining the preceding principles has also been suggested. Bypass techniques have been applied using selectively diastolic pumping. Brief preload increase has been combined with early systolic copulsation.

QUANTITATION OF MECHANICAL CARDIAC ASSISTANCE

In any system that is in need of assistance there is an optimal amount of help above and below which the assistance may be either inadequate or even injurious, in that it may hinder the full development of the existing capabilities of the system. The blood circulation is no exception. Experimental evidence suggests that the optimal assistance quantity is the one providing around 40 percent of the total output of the left ventricle.[9] Offering more than this part of the ventricle's load leads to a reduction of ventricular output.

At this point, some investigators argue that one could possibly assist the heart by taking over as much of its load as possible and let the myocardium "rest." However, there is very little clinical evidence that "resting" of the heart is advantageous in finally improving its function in the long run. This view is not based on solid scientific evidence, but rather on the common belief that one can be stronger following a period of rest. Reducing or increasing the heart's activity may have different effects under different conditions. Therefore, as far as the immediate effect of circulatory assistance is concerned, one should prefer to use it in such a quantity that the ventricular activity is optimized, i.e., that the ventricle ejects the maximal quantity of blood with an acceptable (harmless to the lungs) inflow pressure. A complete takeover of the ventricular action by a pump for a period of time may be useful, mainly in specific cases in which the blood chemistry or other cardiac and/or extracardiac causes are impeding heart function and time is needed for their correction. Detailed studies are lacking as to the quantitative optimization of assistance in view of its corrective effect on long-term heart activity.

METHODS
Cardiac Massage

Compressing the left ventricle between the thumb and the other fingers at a rate of 40 to 60 compressions per minute was first tried during open heart operations. Thereafter, the so-called open chest cardiac massage was used in many dying or already dead patients as a last attempt to save them.

It was not until 1960 that closed chest cardiac massage was suggested as a method by which an elementary output could be maintained by mechanical means.[10] If the heart is adequately compressed between the anterior and posterior chest wall by the palm of one hand, helped by the other hand, producing an excursion of the anterior chest wall on the order of 5 cm against a nonmovable posterior wall, the brain and coronary circulation can be maintained for a few minutes (maximal massage time up to 6 h). During this period, the heart, if in fibrillation, may defibrillate automatically or after an electric shock. If the heart is in asystole, a pacemaker can be inserted and maintain an electrically stimulated rhythm until other conditions can be met.

It is important to consider that such mechanical assistance requires some training of the personnel and a change to operator every 5 minutes, so that he or she will not get tired and reduce the applied pressure. Machines utilizing a moving piston that compresses the chest were not proven more efficient than human operators under the circumstances of this emergency procedure.

Precordial Thump

Precordial thump is the mechanical treatment for arrhythmias. The method is well known as a first attempt during an Adams-Stokes episode. It is less well known as a method for the termination of ventricular paroxysmal tachycardia.[11] The method also can be used in converting ventricular tachycardia refractory to the usual treatment, especially in acute myocardial infarction cases.

Optimization of Circulating Blood Volume

Besides the heart's pumping activity and the peripheral vascular network resistances, the circulating blood volume is today an easily accessible mechanical parameter of the circulatory system. Bleeding as a technique to reduce (overabundant) blood has in fact been used since ancient times. Leaches and phlebotomies were readily and indiscriminately applied to many patients during the Middle Ages. Indirect techniques to induce a reduction in blood volume without losing precious blood elements have also been tried. Laxatives and diminished fluid intake may reduce blood volume through dehydration. Modern potent diuretics offer a faster action and are used to treat both acute and chronic preload increase.

Increasing the circulating blood volume in order to optimize heart action and peripheral perfusion can be tried in chronic situations through increased intake of fluid and electrolytes and under more urgent conditions by intravenous or intraarterial infusion of blood or other compatible fluids. Learning to exploit volume loading to bring ventricular pumping to an optimal maximum by following wedged pulmonary pressure changes has offered a strictly mechanical way of assisting a damaged heart, usually during the course of an acute myocardial infarction. As a matter of fact, this technique acquainted physicians with the concept that the heart can be helped not only by unloading and rest, but also by loading, provided one can optimize the load.

Counterpulsation Techniques

Diastolic counterpulsation can be achieved using several methods, both invasive and noninvasive.

EXTERNAL COUNTERPULSATION (INVASIVE)

The first approach was the use of a positive-pressure pump with a blood chamber connected to a cannula inserted through the femoral artery into the aorta.

The pump is synchronized to the R wave of the patient's electrocardiogram by means of an electric amplifier with an adjustable delay circuit. The pump withdraws blood from the aorta during ventricular systole and injects it back during diastole, that is, between the closure of the aortic valve and the beginning of the next systole. Actually, since termination of pump ejection occurs before the end of diastole and the pump starts "sucking," the aortic end-diastolic pressure is lowered (Fig. 1) because of "bleeding" in the aorta, and the next ventricular systole faces a reduced aortic impedance. Heparinization is necessary. The amount of blood moved during each cycle depends on the capcity of the pump's blood chamber and the diameter and length of the cannula. Two cannulas have also been used in the two femoral arteries to increase the amount of blood.

In another modification of the technique,[12] one femoral cannula was used to withdraw the blood and a second cannula was inserted and forwarded to the root of the aorta in order to achieve the highest diastolic pressure as close to the ostia of the coronary arteries as possible (Fig. 2).

EXTERNAL COUNTERPULSATION (NONINVASIVE)

Application of the counterpulsation principle was tried in a noninvasive technique.[13] Airtight cuffs were applied to the lower half of the body[14] or, preferably, to

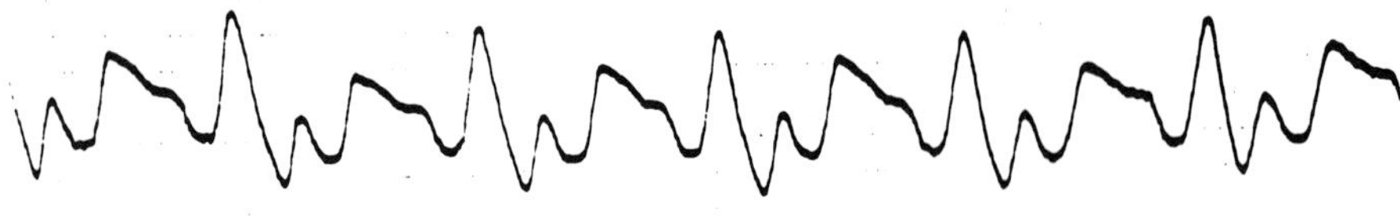

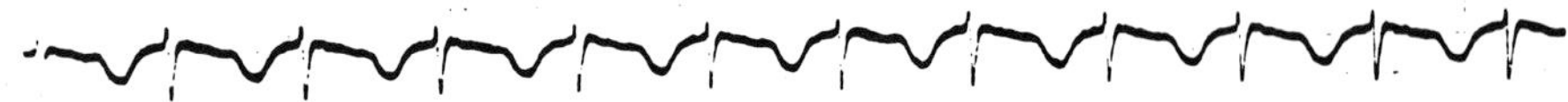

FIGURE 1 ECG (lower tracing) and aortic pressure (upper tracing). A second wave every second beat in the pressure tracing is due to the intraaortic balloon activity. Note the lower end-diastolic pressure.

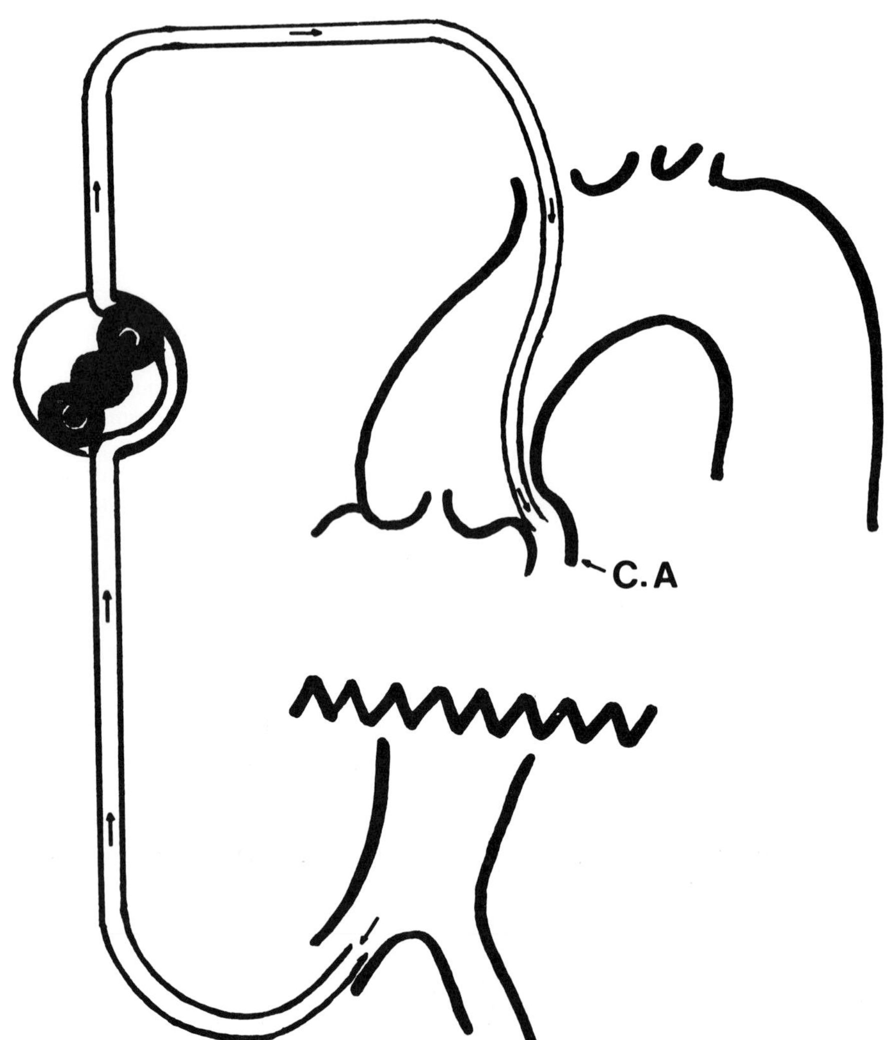

FIGURE 2 External, invasive aorta-to-coronary artery counterpulsation.

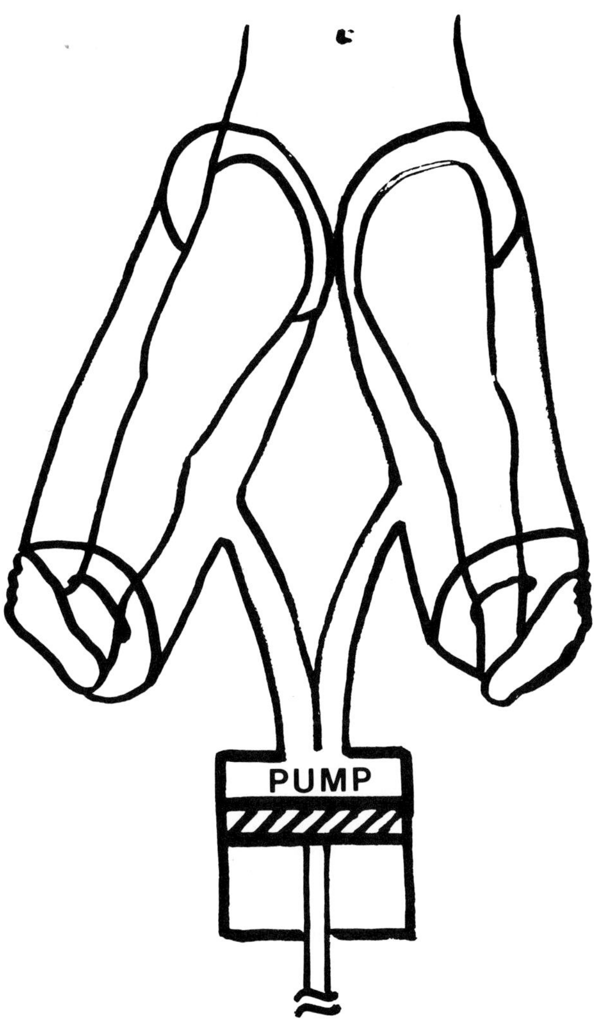

FIGURE 3 Airtight cuffs around both legs for external counterpulsation.

the lower legs[13] (Fig. 3). A pump synchronized with the R wave of the ECG is used to inflate the cuffs during diastole in an attempt to counterpulsate. The cuffs are deflated during systole, and resistances in the area are presumably reduced. It appears that it is difficult with this technique to substantially reduce the end-diastolic pressure in the aorta, despite the production of a diastolic pressure wave. Moreover, the technique may be painful. This technique has also been applied as copulsation in increasing peripheral resistance or in propelling the blood out of the peripheral veins. Recently, periodical compression of the lower half of the body has been used to improve circulation by increasing right atrial pressure following a Fontane operation.[15]

THE INTRAAORTIC BALLOON

A plastic air chamber mounted on a catheter is inserted into the descending aorta. It is inflated during diastole and deflated before the beginning of the next systole. Counterpulsation is thus effected within the aorta[5] (Fig. 4).

Technique The commercially available balloons are 30 and 40 cm long. They are made of polyurethane and are inflatable but not distensible. They are mounted on an F 7 to 12 catheter.

The balloon is inserted in one of two ways, either surgically or percutaneously. The common femoral artery is surgically isolated and an incision is made in it while the artery is temporarily ligated on both sides of the incision. The balloon, after being dipped in a lubricating solution, is slipped through the incision toward the aorta (Fig. 5). A 10-mm Dacron graft passed around the balloon before the insertion is then sutured around the incision in the femoral artery. The ligatures around the artery are then loosened and the blood is allowed to circulate to the extremity. Care is taken so that with the loosening of each ligature a small amount of blood is allowed to flow out through the graft. Thus any thrombi will not be directed toward the periphery and embolize smaller vessels. A ligature is then put around the graft on the catheter.

The choice between the left or right artery for insertion of the balloon is based on palpatory proof of a patent artery. Some authors prefer to have an aortogram before deciding, so that they can avoid iliofemoral obstructive disease or marked degrees of tortuosity of the external or common iliac artery.[16] This is practical in some situations, but in others it may unduly delay the procedure. In an effort to overcome insertion difficulties and inherent complications, a separate central lumen has been incorporated in the standard balloon to be used for several purposes.[16] It could be connected to a pressure transducer and indicate an obstacle when the pressure wave is damped. It could be used to inject a radiopaque medium and help differentiate between occlusive disease and tortuosity. It can also serve as a passageway for a guide wire. In case of difficulty of insertion, a guide wire can thus be introduced and manipulated beyond the tortuous area. The balloon can then be advanced over the wire. In surgical patients, a graft can be sutured directly on the aorta and be used for balloon insertion. The rate of complications in such situations is reported to be much lower.

Percutaneous insertion of the balloon is also possible.[17–19] It can be done on the basic principle of the Sedlinger technique by providing the catheter balloon with a second airtight lumen for the guide wire, by

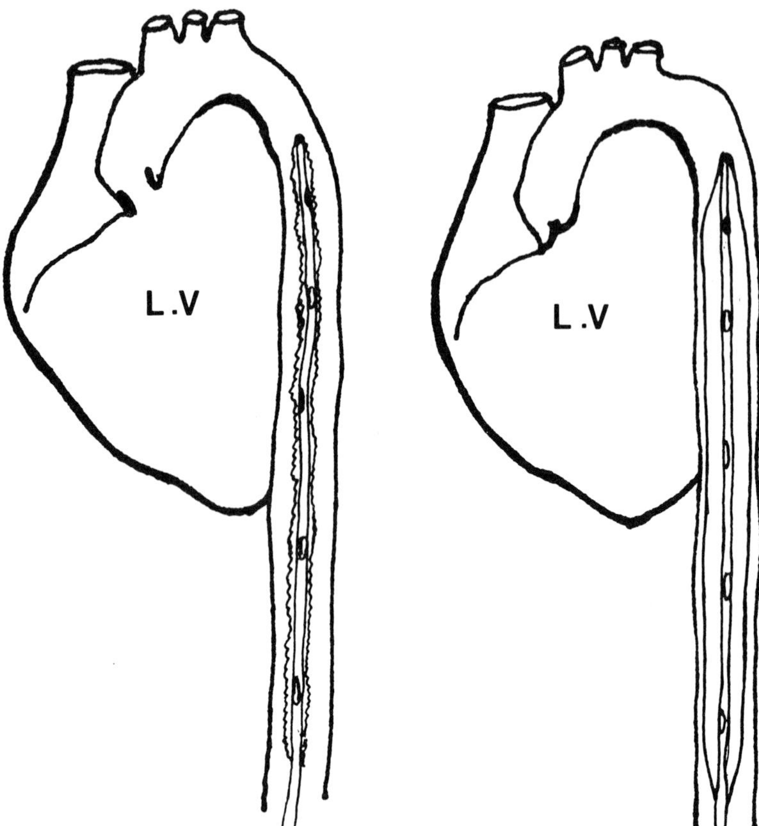

FIGURE 4 Inflated (right) and deflated balloon in the descending aorta.

having the guide wire come out of the catheter before the proximal attachment side of the balloon, or by replacing the catheter inside the balloon with a wire to hold it in place.

Currently, one commercially available set employs a sheath that is inserted over a guide wire. A long (15 in) sheath that reaches the aorta is preferred by some authors, who claim that it virtually eliminates insertion failures.[17] The balloon is folded around the catheter and the air is sucked out so that it stays in that form while it is threaded through the sheath. The balloon is forwarded so that the tip approaches the aortic arch. This is done either by radioscopy of the opaque catheter, by simply measuring the necessary insertion length before the procedure, or by aortography if a central separate lumen is available.[15] Actually, it has not been proven that any position of the balloon is preferable, but it is advisable to clear the balloon away from the lowest and narrowest part of the aorta and the outlets of the renal arteries.

Heparinization of the patient is necessary, despite the fact that new, less thrombogenic materials are used for balloon construction. A miniheparinization scheme has been used in the immediate postoperative period.

The equipment to operate the balloon includes a safety chamber. Pressure from the pump of over 300 mm Hg is exercised around this chamber and not on the intraaortic balloon itself. Thus, in case of balloon leak, only the amount of gas that is contained in it and the catheter can escape into the circulation. For that very rare eventuality, filling the balloon with CO_2 is also recommended.

The pumping system is activated preferably by the amplified voltage of the R wave of any electrocardiographic lead. The deflection with the highest voltage is chosen for triggering. The peak of an arterial pressure wave obtained by catheterization from the patient has also been used. The use of central aortic pressure obtained through a central lumen of the balloon catheter has recently been advocated.

The delay between the triggering signal and the activation of the pump can be regulated. The length of inflation of the balloon can also be adjusted. Prompt inflation at the desired time is necessary. Prompt deflation, which is more difficult to achieve, is secured in commercial equipment by the operation of a suction pump.

Beyond all manipulations necessary, the most im-

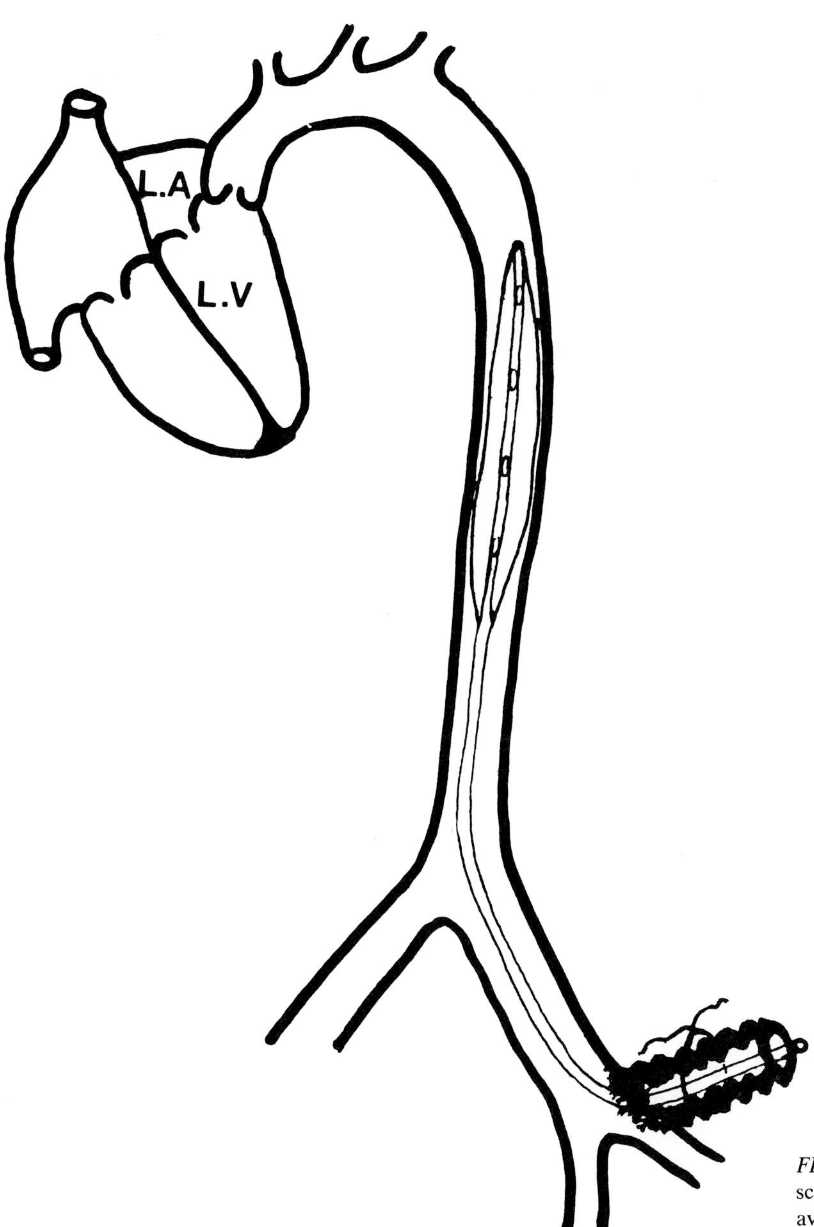

FIGURE 5 The intraaortic balloon in the descending aorta. A short Dacron graft is used to avoid obstruction of flow to the leg.

portant is the positioning of the balloon wave within a cardiac cycle between two recorded pressure waves. The balloon-produced wave should start following the dicrotic notch of the autochthonous pressure wave and end before the beginning of the upstroke of the next pressure wave. The height of the balloon wave, under proper pumping conditions, is usually equal to or larger than the arterial pressure wave, and the end-diastolic pressure is significantly lowered during pumping. If these conditions are not met, positioning of the balloon pumping wave within the cardiac cycle is the first item to be checked. In view of some divergence between

what is happening in the aorta around the balloon and what is read in a peripheral artery pressure tracing, because of the time required for the waves to cover the distance, it is advisable that the recording arterial pressure catheter be pushed as close to the ascending aorta as possible.

It is also recommended that the equipment be tested before operation; the batteries should be charged and working properly. Suddenly stopping the pumping because of equipment failure during the phase of effective assistance may be harmful. A sharp increase in resistance to the heart is thus produced and a drop in diastolic pressure is unfavorable to the coronary circulation.

The main difficulty during insertion in approximately 20 to 30 percent of patients is the inability to pass the balloon through the arteries into the aorta. Tortuous arteries or those mostly obstructed or stenosed by atherosclerotic plaques are responsible. If this is the case, one should try the artery on the other side. It has been mentioned that use of the guide wire during percutaneous or surgical insertion facilitates introduction under such conditions.

The most frequent problem during operation of the device is noise interference with the triggering signal and the necessity to change the settings as soon as the rate of the heart is significantly changed. Irregular heart activity does not help, because changes in heart cycle length require an automatic beat-to-beat readjustment in all pumping characteristics, which is not possible with all equipment currently available. Rechecking proper electrode contact and choosing the lead with the highest voltage will help prevent pumping to noise. R wave discriminating devices have also been tried.

When pumping is started, it is performed at a 1:4 beat ratio, in order to make certain that pumping occurs with the proper timing within the cardiac cycle. When everything is secure, 1:1 pumping can be applied.

Although modern equipment includes several safety devices, the procedure should be closely followed and a general checkup by an experienced person should be carried out hourly. Such a check should include verification of proper wave positioning. A check on the air volume in the balloon is also necessary because of changes that sometimes occur as a result of leaks at the valves. Repositioning of the ECG electrodes is also indicated because the paste soon dries out or the water of the wetpads evaporates and proper contact is not achieved. Such minor operational details, if not properly dealt with, can lead to frustrating difficulties. Pedal pulses should also be checked to discover possible emboli.

When it is decided to cease pumping, a ratio of 1:2 is first applied for a few hours and then a ratio of 1:4 is used in order to secure the ability of the heart to take over. When the balloon is taken off, both sides of the arteries are allowed to bleed for 1 to 2 s to eject potential emboli. The artery is sutured, or in the case of percutaneous insertion, the side is compressed for up to 60 min, preferably with a mechanical clamp, to achieve hemostasis. In case the pedal pulses are not palpable, a Fogarty catheter thrombectomy is performed.

Hemodynamic effects The aortic pressure tracing shows a second wave produced by the balloon expansion. The proper position of the second wave is in the diastolic phase. The second wave may be higher than the aortic pressure wave, indicating adequate and probably necessary pumping.

The mean aortic pressure does not change immediately following the initiation of pumping, because the increase in diastolic pressure is neutralized by the fall in systolic aortic and end-diastolic pressures. However, with general improvement in the patient's condition, there is a significant increase in mean aortic pressure.[20] This is particularly evident in patients with deep shock and a low mean aortic pressure before pumping.

The systemic artery systolic pressure remains unchanged or is reduced at the initiation of pumping. Later it increases to acceptable levels. The systemic venous pressure is lowered during pumping. The same is true for the pulmonary artery wedge pressure (from 20 ± 2 to 15 ± 2 mm Hg,[16] from 22 ± 5 to 17 ± 2 mm Hg[20]).

The left ventricular systolic pressure changes correspondingly to the changes in aortic systolic pressure. Facing lower systemic resistances, the left ventricle may show a reduction in systolic pressure until changes in contractility and venous return lead to an increase during the phase of improvement.[21] The left ventricular end-diastolic pressure is reduced.

The stroke index increases by 49 percent in patients who respond to treatment.[22] Similar figures are given for cardiac index by other authors[19] [from 1.7 ± 0.5 to 2.5 I/(min·m^2)]. The stroke work index was found to increase by 90 percent.[22] The total systemic resistance falls[22] (from 2.055 ± 206 to $1,471 \pm 514$ dyn·s/cm^5).

An increase in coronary flow was noted.[23,24] Experimental evidence indicates that the coronary flow may increase up to 40.9 ± 8.6 percent if the prepumping value is less than 50 ml/min per 100 g of left ventricle.[20]

An increase of coronary flow through ischemic areas has been ascertained.[25,26] In refractory angina, an increase in coronary sinus flow was observed during counterpulsation, but the increase involved only the ischemic region.[23] The oxygen consumption required for an increased stroke work is minimized by the reduction of peripheral resistance faced by the left ventricle. The ratio of availability to need of oxygen is reduced.[27] Oxygen delivery to the ischemic region was found selectively increased.[23]

Myocardial contractility measured experimentally with the mx dp/dt/P or with left ventricular function curves was found to increase.[28] There is some evidence that myocardial compliance may be reduced during pumping.[28] End-systolic and end-diastolic left ventricular volumes were found to diminish during pumping.[25]

A decrease in ventricular asynergy was noted,[29] while other investigators,[30] using multigated cardiac blood pool imaging, found an improvement in function of the marginally ischemic region. A significant reduction in infarct size was also found in experimental animals following delayed balloon pumping. The heart rate is not affected directly by the balloon pumping.[22]

Hemodynamic changes are usually apparent within 10 to 20 min from the initiation of pumping. They are more obvious within the first 12 h and show a peak improvement at a mean of 25 h.[20] Besides the general improvement in the patient's condition, the increase in urinary output (Fig. 6) usually seen within the first hour of pumping is probably the best indicator of a favorable hemodynamic effect. The fluid infusion must therefore be modified following pumping, according to urinary output and pulmonary wedge pressure changes.

It should be noted that hemodynamic measurements involving parameters in the aorta have to be performed after the end of the procedure or while temporarily stopping the pumping. The second wave in the aorta is an "unnatural" occurrence, and one should be particularly careful in using accepted procedures and calculations of normally measured hemodynamic parameters.

On the basis of experimental and clinical hemodynamic studies, some suggestions can be made as to the

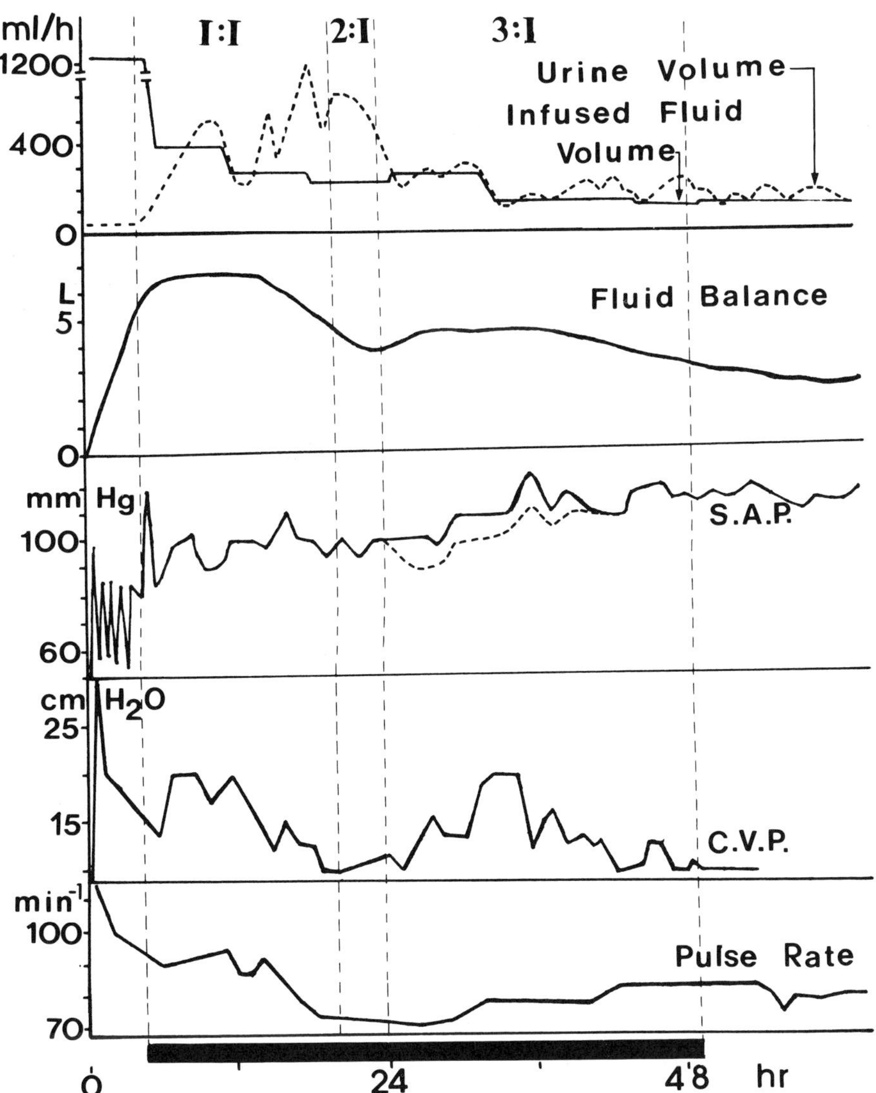

FIGURE 6 Compiled data from a patient in cardiogenic shock following acute myocardial infarction. The black line indicates the period of pumping in the aorta at a 1:1, 2:1, and 3:1 ratios (see top of the diagram). Notice the rise in urinary output and systolic aortic pressure and a drop in central venous pressure. The dotted line on the S.A.P. row indicates systolic arterial pressure for the beat without pumping.

mechanism of action of intraaortic balloon counterpulsation. Most investigators agree that a reduction in peripheral resistance may be helpful in cardiogenic shock. However, when intraaortic pumping is compared with sodium nitroprusside infusion, a functional improvement occurs with pumping that is out of proportion to that of systolic unloading alone.[31,32] Therefore, besides the flow resistance, the diastolic augmentation helps to improve heart function, presumably through better diastolic irrigation of tissues and in particular of the ventricular myocardium. The increase in coronary flow, especially through the ischemic regions, the reduction of the supply and demand ratio, the optimization of myocardial compliance, and the decrease in ventricular asynergy[29] may be contributing, albeit intertwined, mechanisms that account for the clinical improvement that is so obvious in most patients following initiation of intraaortic pumping. The reduction in infarct size has also been suggested by experimental data,[33] with intraaortic counterpulsation instituted as long as 3 h after coronary occlusion.

Clinical indications Intraaortic counterpulsation was conceived for "pump failure" syndrome. The most frequently helped patient today is the surgical patient following open heart surgery whose heart is not ready to take over and perform adequately when the heart-lung machine is switched off.[34]

Some surgeons prefer to have the balloon inserted in advance in some or in most of their patients. The balloon has proven very helpful during coronary and left ventricular catheterization in patients with unstable angina who are candidates for emergency revascularization. Patients with severe coronary heart disease who have to undergo a serious operation on other organs have been placed under demand counterpulsation.

In cardiology, the main indication remains cardiogenic shock that is not responding to conventional treatment in acute myocardial infarction. Patients with acute infarction who are anuric for more than 1 to 2 h, despite an optimally high central venous or pulmonary artery pressure and the lack of important arrhythmias, are already in a practically lethal, nonreversible cardiogenic shock. There is no doubt that they represent candidates for assistance.

Some clinicians have been using the intraaortic balloon under less strict criteria. Impending shock has been accepted by some as an indication, with the argument that the response might be more favorable at this stage than after it develops into irreversible shock. Other investigators have even suggested the use of intraaortic counterpulsation in all myocardial infarctions, with the intend to limit the infarction area. They report that this was achieved in some cases with anterior wall infarctions.[29]

Other indications are acute left ventricular failure owing to rupture of the intraventricular septum or to acute mitral regurgitation. Left ventricular failure under the influence of beta blocking drugs is a clear indication, since counterpulsation may help the patient survive until the effect of the drugs is gone. Pulmonary edema, mainly owing to coronary heart disease, may respond to this type of assistance. Ventricular tachycardias, irreversible with the usual treatment, may respond to pumping.[35,36] Noncardiac surgical procedures in cardiac patients have been carried out with the support of an intraaortic balloon pump.[37]

In view of the fact that the technique is invasive, time-consuming, and expensive (some units estimate that the use of the intraaortic balloon increases hospital costs threefold for both surviving and nonsurviving patients,[34] mainly because of the longer hospitalization time), as well as the fact that the number of long-term survivors is limited, several attempts were made to more accurately assess the candidates and predict which of them would profit most. Lorente et al.[35] selected an extensive list of variables, including hemodynamic data, prior to balloon insertion. On the basis of the data, they suggested that a satisfactory prediction of short-term survival was feasible. One hesitates at present to accept strict criteria for the selection of patients, because the condition of cardiogenic shock is not well studied as yet and many uncontrollable or even unknown factors may interfere with the outcome. It is therefore suggested that the technique be used in every patient with acute myocardial infarction and cardiogenic shock, until sufficient data are collected to allow a more discriminative approach.

Pulmonary artery counterpulsation Intrapulmonary artery pumping to relieve right-sided heart failure was tested experimentally in 1970.[38] The large compliance of the pulmonary artery and the small volume of the main artery plus one of the branches pointed to a reduced possibility for adequate hemodynamic changes. Miller and associates[39] used an aortic-sized balloon and pumped it into a Dacron tubular graft that was anastomosed to the main pulmonary artery. The technique is applicable during open heart operations and has helped in the removal from the heart-lung machine of a patient with signs of acute right-sided heart failure.

Counterindications There is no absolute counterindication to intraaortic counterpulsation except in the case of aortic regurgitation and aortic aneurysm. Atherosclerotic lesions of the aorta or the iliac and femoral arteries, as well as fast irregular rhythms, present difficulties in the application of the technique rather than clear counterindications. Age is not a counterindication. However, it may increase the possibility of insertion difficulties. Presumably, though, intraaortic counterpulsation should be more effective when the aortic compliance is reduced by atheromatosis. However, the end result is, for obvious reasons, poor in patients above 70 years of age, or even above 60.[39]

Complications One should draw the attention of the operator in aortic counterpulsation to a complication that may not be apparent and may lead to undesired effects that are thought to be due to the patient's deteriorating condition. The position of the balloon wave should be in diastole and not override systole, because then it would increase the systolic impedance to the heart. Estimating the balloon wave position from pressure tracings obtained from small peripheral arteries may sometimes lead to erroneous conclusions, becuase of the time delay between the origin of the aorta and a peripheral artery. Central aortic pressure tracings may be used to trigger the balloon pump, especially if such tracings can be recorded from a catheter inside the balloon catheter.

The major reported complication is ischemia of the leg in whose main artery the balloon was inserted. It is observed in 10 to 20 percent of patients, no matter whether grafting or a percutaneous technique is used. It may very rarely lead even to amputation of the leg.

Aortic dissection is a complication infrequently reported in clinical cases but seen more often in postmortem material. Wound infection at the insertion site is not frequently seen. Hematomas owing to heparinization have been reported.

Rupture of the balloon has been reported by several authors, but this has been uneventful. Embolism of peripheral arteries or the kidney has been seen.[24]

Autopsy material from patients dying following counterpulsation shows a 36 percent (16 of 45) incidence of complications related to the balloon. The material of the study is, of course, selective and cannot mirror the total incidence of complications.[40] However, the study attributes most of the complications to the insertion of the device and provides evidence that some of the complications are not suspected during the clinical observation.

Results It is estimated that over 120,000 patients have undergone intraaortic balloon counterpulsation. Unfortunately, there is no national registry or a large cooperative study to evaluate the results. Data in the literature can only be compiled by specific indication for which the balloon was used and taking into consideration the use of other treatment and the specific condition of the patient at that moment. So-called control studies consider as a control group "similar" patients not treated with the balloon or patients who were candidates for counterpulsation but insertion of the balloon could not be achieved. It is obvious that matching patients is extremely difficult. The fact that in some series, such as ours, no patient considered for intraaortic counterpulsation survived if the treatment was denied by the relatives or if the balloon could not be inserted is a strong argument for the beneficial effect, but it still cannot replace the irrefutable proof of a properly controlled series.

Postoperative use of the balloon has been made extensively in patients who cannot be "weaned off" the cardiopulmonary bypass following open heart operations. Under these circumstances, successful application is reported to be up to 75 percent. However, the percentage of patients discharged from the hospital ranges between 35 and 54 percent. Patients with valve replacement (especially aortic) have a higher mortality. Age below 70 does not seem to be a factor affecting the results. Although there are no control series in these cases, the inability to disconnect a patient from cardiopulmonary bypass beyond a certain period of time is equivalent to death. Therefore, the use of the balloon in such situations is beneficial, especially when the main help consists of "buying" time, so that chemical or metabolic abnormalities can be corrected whenever possible and the heart can recover.

The effect of the preoperative use of the balloon is much more difficult to evaluate. It is being instituted for unstable angina in order to help the patient undergo catheterization and angiography or to improve and maintain the hemodynamic status until an emergency bypass procedure can be undertaken. There are reports that indicate a lower mortality in patients treated with counterpulsation,[42,43] as well as a lower incidence of perioperative infarction[43] (3 versus 23 percent) in patients operated on for left main artery stenosis.

The use of intraaortic counterpulsation in postinfarction cardiogenic shock is undertaken either as an autonomous procedure, in cases of failing medical treatment, or as a preparatory step for emergency revascularization. The survival (and hospital discharge) of patients with acute myocardial infarction and cardiogenic shock considered irreversible has been reported as varying between 13 and 30 percent.[24,29] This may be a relatively small improvement in mortality statistics, but occasional patients can undoubtedly be saved. Much better results are obtained if a surgical procedure follows the first favorable results of counterpulsation. In large series, aggressive treatment with early balloon insertion (within 1 to 6 h following the appearance of shock) at a patient age of less than 60 years achieved a survival rate of 65 percent[44] or even 79 percent.[41]

There is an increase in survival rate in recent years,[44] probably owing to a better selection of patients and experience in handling the counterpulsation technique. The results are not as favorable in patients with overt left-sided heart failure and pulmonary edema. In a small controlled series of 30 patients with 11 undergoing pumping, no difference in survival rate was found.[45] The occurrence of pulmonary edema in patients while on the pump has been observed.

The preventive use of balloon counterpulsation in acute anterior myocardial infarction, where 5 of 11 patients preserved the R waves,[29] has been disputed[24] on grounds of the acceptability of the complication rate of the balloon in patients with the low (6 percent) mortality rate of uncomplicated acute myocardial infarction.

Modifications and related techniques Several investigators tried to improve the efficiency of intra-aortic counterpulsation. They have added a second small balloon distally to the long one in order to hinder the flow to the periphery and promote the flow toward the coronary arteries. An umbrella-shaped construction was used for the same purpose. There is not sufficient evidence that any of these techniques offers a substantial advantage.

The use of a balloon to produce a pulsatile flow during extracorporeal circulation instead of the continuous flow was thought to be advantageous by some surgeons. Connecting the pumping system to a small digital device in order to operate the equipment only when a hemodynamic parameter, such as the average wedge pulmonary pressure, rises above a preset level has been suggested but not put in clinical use.[46]

The use of the intraaortic balloon without the pumping equipment connected to an outside chamber with a pressure in the system slightly above the aortic diastolic pressure has increased the cardiac output by 7 to 30 percent.[47] With this setup, the "compliance" of the aorta is increased and a small diastolic wave appears. The technique may be potentially useful for chronic support in cases requiring limited assistance.

LEFT VENTRICULAR BYPASS

Assistance methods based on the principle of bypassing the left ventricle are used mainly in postoperative patients (Fig. 7). Small pumps have been constructed to withdraw the blood from the left atrium or the left ventricle and pump it into the aorta, and less frequently, from the right atrium to the pulmonary artery. Temporary biventricular bypass has also been reported in postoperative patients. Cannulation of the left-sided heart cavities and the aorta is done with the help of Dacron grafts sutured on their walls. An experimental approach suggested the use of a single double-lumen cannula that could be inserted either through the carotid artery[48] or through the apex of the heart.[49]

Bypass pumps require two valvular systems to maintain the correct direction of blood flow. If the pump is connected to the aorta only, it does not require valves, provided the pumping is synchronized with the ventricular contraction. Such pumps have been implanted in calfs for periods of up to many months and in patients for as long as 1 week.[50] They are taken off as soon as the ventricle is able to function adequately.

The pumping devices are driven by external sources of energy, usually electromechanical.[51] Experimentation continues with other sources, such as electrohydraulic, thermal, and nuclear, in an attempt to derive an autonomous implantable source or one that can be implanted and charged through the intact skin.

Sporadic applications of permanent biventricular bypass with excision of the heart have been carried out in terminal patients, with the intent to keep the patients alive until a suitable transplantation donor is available.

OTHER ASSISTANCE TECHNIQUES

A multitude of mechanical assistance techniques have been devised. Some of them were utilized in a small number of patients. Others remained at the experimental stage. They are catalogued here in order to indicate the amount of research in this direction.

Among noninvasive techniques, besides external counterpulsation, the ballistocardiogram-triggered movement of the whole body was suggested in order to promote flow and relieve the left ventricle.[2] Pulsatile positive pressure applied through an endotracheal tube on the lungs was used to affect the filling of the left ventricle.[2]

Among invasive techniques not requiring a thoracotomy, the following are mentioned: First, the extracorporeal system with an oxygenator was used in a small number of patients to relieve the ventricles and the lungs in cases of heart failure.[52] The blood was drawn from venous cannulas and pumped into the arterial system. The system cannot be used for long periods of time, and the results have been disappointing. Second, a left ventricular bypass can be achieved using a pump to circulate the blood from the left atrium (cannulated with a venous catheter piercing the atrial septum) to a peripheral artery.[53] Third, cannulation of the left ventricle via the brachial artery can be used to relieve the ventricle and pump the blood in a peripheral artery during ventricular fibrillation. Fourth, narrowing or periodically occluding the coronary sinus venosus

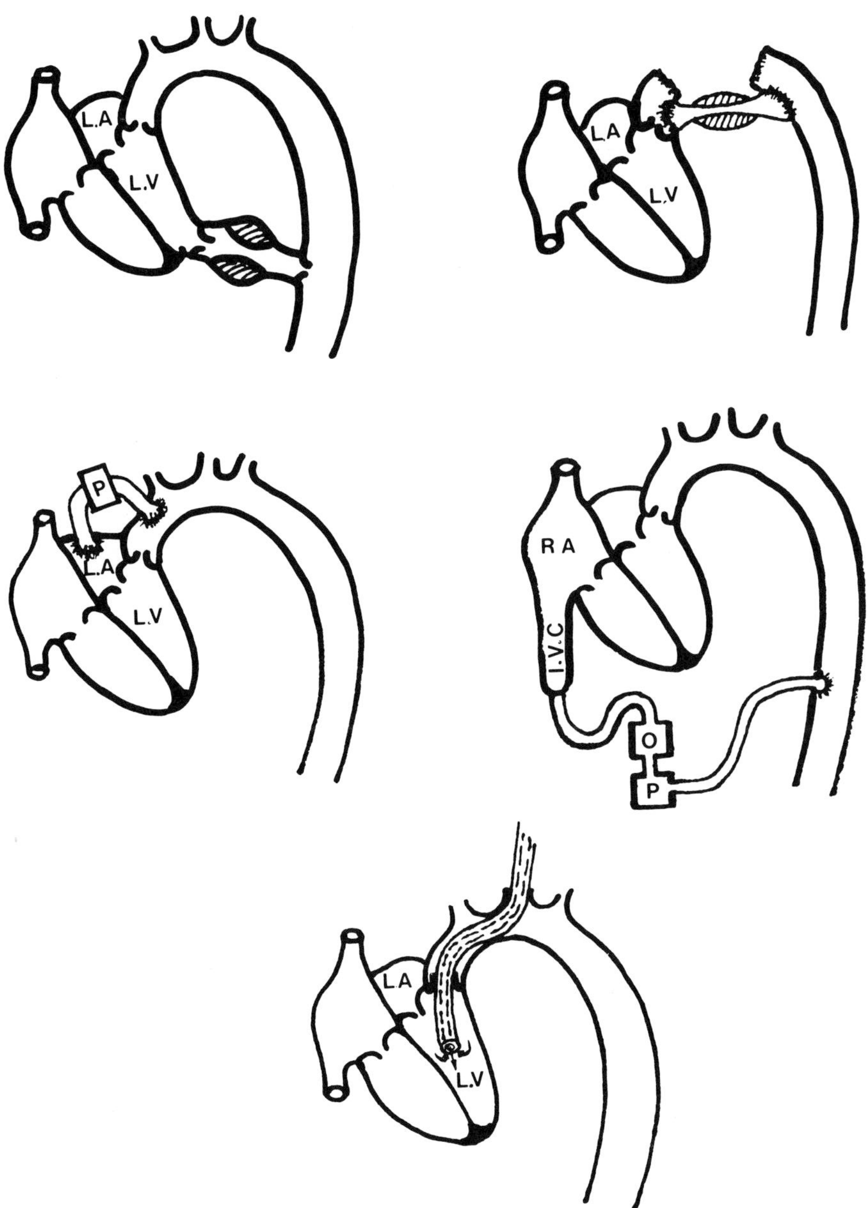

FIGURE 7 Assistance techniques: ventriculoaortic (upper row, left), aortoaortic (upper row, right), atrioaortic (middle row), and ventriculoventricular (lower row).

may help diverting more blood flow to ischemic areas of the myocardium.[2] Finally, pumping air into the pericardial sac in a pulsatile way has been attempted[54] in order to assist the ventricles (pneumomassage).

Among the methods requiring thoracotomy, the following are mentioned briefly: First, the Anstadt cup[55] is an air chamber fitted around the ventricles and inflated simultaneously with ventricular contraction. The method has been tried in a number of patients, but the results have not encouraged further application. Second, compression of the aorta, properly timed, has been attempted with an air-chamber sleeve or a para-aortic balloon. Lastly, brief end-diastolic pumping, for 50 to 80 ms, with an air-pressure pump connected to the apex of the ventricle may increase the cardiac output.[8] The blood volume "injected" into the ventricle is withdrawn at the beginning of the isometric phase of ventricular contraction.

REFERENCES

1 Gibbon, I.: Artificial Maintenance of Circulation during Experimental Occlusion of Pulmonary Artery, *Arch. Surg.,* 34:1115, 1937

2 Kolff, W. J., Moulopoulos, S. D., Kwan-Gett, C. S., and Kralios, A.: Mechanical Assistance to the Circulation. The Principle and the Methods, *Prog. Cardiovasc. Dis.,* 12:243, 1969.

3 Harken, D. E.: Assisted Circulation, "3d World Congress of Cardiology," Brussels, 1958.

4 Claus, R. H., Birtwell, W. C., Albertal, G., et al.: Assisted Circulation: I. The Counterpulsator, *J. Thorac. Cardiovasc. Surg.,* 41:447, 1961.

5 Moulopoulos, S., Topaz, S., and Kolff, W.: Diastolic Balloon Pumping with CO_2 in the Aorta. Mechanical Assistance to the Circulation, *Am. Heart J.,* 63:669, 1962.

6 Donald, D. E., and McGoon, D. C.: Circulatory Support by Left Ventricular Balloon Pump, *Circulation,* 43:96, 1971.

7 Kuhn, L. A., Gruber, F. L., and Frankel, A.: Hemodynamic Effects of Balloon Obstruction of the Abdominal Aorta and Superior Vena Cava–Distal Aorta Shunting in Dogs with Myocardial Infarction and Shock, *Am. J. Cardiol.,* 7:218, 1961.

8 Moulopoulos, S. D., Stamatelopoulos, S., Petrou, P., Saridakis, N., Yannopoulos, N., and Jarvic, R.: Left Intraventricular Pseudoaugmentation. A New Principle of Mechanical Assistance, *Trans. Am. Soc. Artif. Intern. Organs,* 10:65, 1981.

9 Moulopoulos, S. D., Anthopoulos, L. P., Stamatelopoulos, S. F., and Boufas, D. G.: Optimal Changes in Stroke Work during Left Ventricular Bypass, *J. Appl. Physiol.,* 24:12, 1973.

10 Jude, J. R., Kouwenhoven, W. B., and Knickerbocker, G. G.: Cardiac Arrest: Report of Application of External Cardiac Massage on 118 Patients, *J.A.M.A.,* 178:1063, 1961.

11 Pennington, J. E., Taylor, J., and Lown, B.: Chest Thump for Reverting Ventricular Tachycardia, *N. Engl. J. Med.,* 283:1192, 1970.

12 Jocobey, J. A., Taylor, W. J., Smith, G. T., Gorlin, R., and Harken, D. E.: A New Therapeutic Approach to Acute Coronary Occlusion, *Surg. Forum.,* 12:225, 1961.

13 Birtwell, W., Giron, F., Soroff, H., Roiz, V., Collins, J., and Deterling, R.: Support of the Systemic Circulation and Left Ventricular Assist by Synchronous Pulsation of Extramural Pressure, *Trans. Am. Soc. Artif. Intern. Organs,* 11:43, 1965.

14 Dennis, C.: External Counterpulsation as a Means to Reduce the Work of the Left Ventricle. In Mechanical Devices to Assist the Failing Heart, *Proc. Natl. Acad. Sci.,* 1966.

15 Heck, H., and Doty, D.: Assisted Circulation by Phasic External Lower Body Compression, *Circulation,* 64 (suppl. 2):118, 1981.

16 Lundell, D. C., Hammond, G. L., Geha, A. S., Laks, H., and Wolfson, S.: Randomized Comparison of the Modified Wire-Guided and Standard Intraaortic Balloon Catheters, *J. Thorac. Cardiovasc. Surg.,* 81:297, 1981.

17 Vignola, A. P., Swaye, S. P., and Gosselin, I. A.: Guidelines for Effective and Safe Percutaneous Intraaortic Balloon Pump Insertion and Removal, *Am. J. Cardiol.,* 48:660, 1981.

18 Bregman, D., and Casarella, W. I.: Percutaneous Intraaortic Balloon Pumping: Initial Clinical Experience, *Ann. Thorac. Surg.,* 29:153, 1980.

19 Subramanian, V. A.: Percutaneous Intraaortic Balloon Pumping, *Ann. Thorac. Surg.,* 29:102, 1980.

20 Dunkman, W. B., Leinbach, R. C., Buckley, M. J., et al.: Clinical and Hemodynamic Results of Intraaortic Balloon Pumping and Surgery for Cardiogenic Shock, *Circulation,* 46:465,1972.

21 Powell, W. J., Dagget, W. M., Magro, A. E., et al.: Effects of Intraaortic Balloon Counterpulsation on Cardiac Performance, Oxygen Consumption and Coronary Blood Flow in Dogs, *Circ. Res.,* 26:713, 1970.

22 Ehrich, D. A., Biddle, T. L., Kronenberg, M. W., and Yu, P. N.: The Hemodynamic Response to Intraaortic Balloon Counterpulsation in Patients with Cardiogenic Shock Complicating Acute Myocardial Infarction, *Am. Heart J.,* 93:274, 1977.

23 Whittle, J. L., Feldman, R. L., Pepine, C. J., et al.: Effects of Intraaortic Balloon Pumping on Regional and Total Coronary Flow in Patients with Coronary Disease, *Am. J. Cardiol.,* 43:395, 1980. (Abstract.)

24 Sheidt, S.: Preservation of Ischemic Myocardium with Intraaortic Balloon Pumping: Modern Therapeutic Intervention or Primum Non Nocere?, *Circulation,* 58:211, 1978.

25 Limet, R. R., Roos, N. J., and Hipera, I.: Effects of Intraaortic Balloon Counterpulsation on the Distribution of Coronary Blood Flow in Experimental Ischemic Left Ventricular Failure, *J. Cardiovasc. Surg.,* 13:305, 1972.

26 Cox, J. L., Pass, H. I., Anderson, R. W., Wehslen, A. S., Aoldham, H. N., Sabiston, D. C.: Augmentation of Coronary Collateral Blood Flow in Acute Myocardial Infarction, *Surg. Forum,* 26:238, 1975.

27 Braunwald, E., Covell, J. W., Maroko, P. R., and Ross, J., Jr.: Effects of Drugs and Counterpulsation on Myocardial Oxygen Consumption: Observations on the Ischemic Heart, *Circulation,* 39 (suppl. 4):220, 1969.

28 Moulopoulos, S. D., Stamatelopoulos, S., Zakopoulos, N., and Yannopoulos, C.: Intraaortic Balloon Pumping Corrects Myocardial Contractility Reduced by Propranolol, "5th World Congress of Cardiology," Vol. 2, 1978, p. 534.

29 Leinbach, R., Gold, H., Harper, R., Buckley, M., and Austen, G.: Early Intraaortic Balloon Pumping for Anterior Myocardial Infarction without Shock, *Circulation*, 58:204, 1978.

30 Sasayama, S., Osakada, G., and Takahashi, M.: Effects of Intraaortic Balloon Counterpulsation on Regional Myocardial Function during Acute Coronary Occlusion in the Dog, *Am. J. Cardiol.*, 43:59, 1979.

31 Moulopoulos, S. D.: Die Klinische Bedeutung der assistierten Zirkulation für die Behandlung des Herzversagens, "Verhandlungen der Deutschen Gesellschaft für innere Medizin, Wiesbaden, W. Germany, April 26–30, 1981," J. F. Bergmann Verlag, München, 1981.

32 Hill, R. C., Sink, J. D., Chitwood, R. W., et al.: Effects of Intraaortic Balloon Diastolic Augmentation and Nitroprusside on Postoperative Regional Left Ventricular Function, *Am. J. Cardiol.*, 45:432, 1980 (Abstract).

33 Roberts, A. J., Alonso, D. R., Combes, J. R., et al.: Role of Delayed Intraaortic Balloon Pumping in Treatment of Experimental Myocardial Infarction, *Am. J. Cardiol.*, 41:1202, 1978.

34 Downing, T. P., Miller, D. C., Stinson, E. B., et al.: Therapeutic Efficacy of Intraaortic Balloon Pump Counterpulsation. Analysis with Concurrent "Control" Subjects, *Circulation*, 64 (suppl. 2):108, 1981.

35 Lorente, P., Gourgon, R., Beaufils, P., et al.: Multivariate Statistical Evaluation of Intraaortic Counterpulsation in Pump Failure Complicating Acute Myocardial Infarction, *Am. J. Cardiol.*, 46:124, 1980.

36 Culliford, D. T., Madden, M. R., Isom, O. W., Glassman, E.: Intraaortic Balloon Counterpulsation. Refractory Ventricular Tachycardia, *J.A.M.A.*, 239:431, 1978.

37 Kaplan, J., Craver, J., Jones, E., and Sumpter, R.: The Role of Intraaortic Balloon in Cardiac Anesthesia and Surgery, *Am. Heart J.*, 98:580, 1979.

38 Kralios, A., Zwart, H., Moulopoulos, S. D., Gollan, R., Kwan-Gett, C., Kolff, W. J.: Intrapulmonary Artery Balloon Pumping to Assist the Right Ventricle, *J. Thorac. Cardiovasc. Surg.*, 60:215, 1970.

39 Miller, O. C., Moreno-Cabral, R. J., Stinson, E. B., Shinn, J. A., Shumway, N. E.: Pulmonary Artery Balloon Counterpulsation for Acute Right Ventricular Failure, *J. Thorac. Cardiovasc. Surg.*, 80:760, 1980.

40 Isner, J. M., Cohen, S. R., Virmani, R., Lawrinson, N., and Roberts, W. C.: Complications of the Intraaortic Balloon Counterpulsation Device: Clinical and Morphologic Observations in 45 Necropsy Patients, *Am. J. Cardiol.*, 45:280, 1980.

41 Macoviak, J., Stephenson, L. W., Edmunds, L. H., Harken, A., and Macvaugh, H.: The Intraaortic Balloon Pump: An Analysis of Five Years Experience, *Ann. Thorac. Surg.*, 29:451, 1980.

42 Langou, R. A., Geha, R. S., Hammond, L. G., and Cohen, L. S.: Surgical Approach for Patients with Unstable Angina Pectoris: Role of the Response to Initial Medical Therapy and Intraaortic Balloon Pumping in Perioperative Complications after Aortocoronary Bypass Grafting, *Am. J. Cardiol.*, 42:629, 1978.

43 Tahn, S. R., Geha, A S., Hammond, G. L., Cohen, L. S., and Langou, R. A.: Bypass Surgery for Left Main Artery Disease. Reduced Perioperative Myocardial Infarction with Preoperative Intraaortic Balloon Counterpulsation, *Br. Heart. J.*, 43:191, 1980.

44 McEnany, T. M., Kay, H. R., Buckley, M. J., et al.: Clinical Experience with Intraaortic Balloon Pump Support in 728 Patients, *Circulation*, 58 (suppl. 1) 124, 1978.

45 O'Rourke, M. F., Narris, R. M., Campbell, T. J., Chang, V. P., and Sammel, N. L.: Randomized Controlled Trial of Intraaortic Balloon Counterpulsation in Early Myocardial Infarction with Acute Heart Failure, *Am. J. Cardiol.*, 47:815, 1981.

46 Moulopoulos, S. D., Darsinos, J., Stamatelopoulos, S., Elias, C., and Pandis, A.: Automatically Regulated Intraaortic Balloon Pumping as a Method of Assistance to the Circulation, "5th European Congress of Cardiology," 1968.

47 Sideris, D. A., Nanas, J. N., Chrysos, D. N., and Moulopoulos, S. D.: Haemodynamic Effects of Aortic Compliance Changes, *Eur. Heart J.*, in press.

48 Zwart, H. J., Kralios, A. C., Collan, R., and Kolff, W. J.: Transarterial Closed-Chest Left Ventricular (TaCLV)Bypass, *Trans. Am. Soc. Artif. Intern. Organs*, 15:386, 1969.

49 Kralios, A. C., Kwan-Gett, C. S., DeVries, W., and Kolff, W. J.: Transapical Left Ventricular Bypass. *Appl. Eng. Sci.*, 1:179, 1973.

50 Turina, M, Bosio, R., Kragenbühl, C., and Senning, A.: Clinical Application of the Paracorporeal Artificial Heart, S. Hayase (ed.), "8th World Congress of Cardiology," Excerpta Medica, Amsterdam, 1015, 1979.

51 Pierce, W. S., Parr, G. V., Myers, I. L., Pae, W. E., Bull, A. P., and Waldhausen, I. A.: Ventricular Assist Pumping in Patients with Cardiogenic Shock after Cardiac Operation, *N. Engl. J. Med.*, 305:1606, 1981.

52 Moulopoulos, S. D., Topaz, S. R., and Kolff, W. J.: Extracorporeal Assistance to the Circulation, *Trans. Am. Soc. Artif. Intern. Organs*, 8:85, 1961.

53 Dennis, C., Hall, C. P., Moreno, J. R., and Senning, A.: Atrial Septal Puncture for Total Left Heart Bypass, *Acta Chir. Scand.*, 123:267, 1962.

54 Benzini, A., and Parda, P.: The Pneumomassage of the Heart, *Surgery*, 39:375, 1956.

55 Anstadt, G., Blakemore, W., and Baue, A.: A New Instrument for Prolonged Mechanical Cardiac Massage, *Circulation*, 32 (Suppl. 2):43, 1965.

Indications for Surgery for Aortic Valve Disease in Children*

W. DEAN WILCOX, M.D.

In those parts of the world where rheumatic fever prevention and treatment have greatly reduced the incidence of rheumatic heart disease, congenital abnormalities of the aortic valve constitute the most common reason for aortic valve surgery in childhood. The most frequent congenital abnormality of the aortic valve is aortic stenosis, which accounts for 10 to 12 percent of all congenital cardiac malformations. Acquired calcific aortic stenosis such as that seen in later adult life is exceedingly rare in childhood. Aortic insufficiency as an isolated lesion is also a rarity in childhood. Indeed, most accounts of congenital aortic insufficiency in infants and children deal with congenital aortic–left ventricular tunnel rather than incompetence of the aortic valve. In nearly every case of aortic insufficiency in childhood, the abnormality is associated with another, usually more significant, cardiac lesion that predisposes the aortic valve to insufficiency.

The age at which a child presents with symptoms or significant electrocardiographic or radiographic manifestations of aortic valve disease and the timing of surgical intervention are variable and depend primarily on the severity of obstruction or regurgitation. In aortic stenosis, especially, the relationship between the severity of the lesion and the appearance of symptoms and electrocardiographic changes is notoriously unreliable and variable. Most cases of aortic valve abnormality, except those of trivial magnitude, must be considered potential surgical candidates, since the nature of these lesions is one of progression in severity. Although those lesions of trivial magnitude, both obstructive and regurgitant, may remain mild for several years, lesions of moderate degree tend to progress to severe impairment more rapidly. Without surgical intervention, severe aortic stenosis or insufficiency is almost uniformly fatal. Although general guidelines exist to aid in the timing of surgical intervention, each case must be considered individually. The decision to operate is based on repeated careful evaluation of the patient.

Surgical treatment of aortic valve disease must be considered palliative. Presently, there is no way of creating a normal valve from the congenitally malformed structure. The commissures either must be incised or plicated, or the valve must be completely excised and replaced with an exogenous valve. Rarely, the stenotic aortic valve may be a normal-appearing tricuspid valve with a normal annulus that is simply impaired by variable commissural fusion. Most commonly it is a bicuspid or unicuspid unicommisural valve

with an eccentric orifice. The annulus usually exhibits a variable degree of hypoplasia and does not increase in diameter as the child grows. Therefore, growth, with its demand for increasing cardiac output, results in a concomitant increase in the gradient across the restricted aortic valve orifice. Commissurotomy also is limited by the annulus and by the restriction of systolic opening of the valve incident to abnormal leaflet geometry. Following commissurotomy, restenosis and progressive deformity of the leaflets, with thickening and curling of the free margins, are common. This frequently necessitates removal of the native aortic valve and replacement with a prosthesis. Moderate degrees of aortic insufficiency, such as that associated with ventricular septal defect, may be effectively palliated by the use of plicating or reefing sutures in the aortic valve. However, severe aortic insufficiency almost always requires valve replacement. Several prosthetic valves are presently available that are extremely effective and reliable. However, most require life-long anticoagulant therapy and present the limitations or risks[1] of fixed valve orifice, mechanical deterioration, thrombus formation, periprosthetic leak, and infective endocarditis.[2,3] Each obligates valve replacement in almost every instance. In spite of these limitations, appropriately timed surgical intervention and prudent follow-up care have permitted a vastly improved and expanded lifestyle and expectancy in these children. There can be no question as to the effectiveness of surgery in children with significant aortic valve disease.

AORTIC STENOSIS IN INFANCY

Although a murmur may be present from infancy or early childhood in children with congenital aortic stenosis, symptoms and significant changes are usually not present or apparent until later in childhood or adolescence. However, approximately 10 percent of children with isolated aortic stenosis present with manifestations within the first few weeks of life.[4,5] Of these, a small subset presents within the first 2 months of life as desperately ill infants in congestive heart failure, shock, and metabolic acidosis. The infant may be cyanotic as a result of right-to-left shunt through a patent ductus arteriosus. This condition is described as "critical aortic stenosis."[6] These infants usually manifest tachypnea, expiratory grunting, hepatomegaly, hyperactive right ventricular lift, and diminished peripheral pulses. Rales may or may not be present. S_1 is usually normal, and S_2 is diminished. A systolic ejection click is present in over one-half of these patients, and a systolic ejection murmur is audible in most patients.[7] However, depending on the degree of myocardial decompensation, the heart sounds may be diminished and the murmur insignificant or absent. The murmur may also be diminished because of a large left-to-right atrial shunt. Prior to birth, the right ventricle is responsible for 66 percent of the combined ventricular output, and the left ventricle 33 percent.[8] After birth, with expansion of the lungs, the entire right ventricular output goes to the lungs, returning to the left atrium and left ventricle and resulting in a 25 percent increase in left ventricular output. This increase in filling volume in the presence of left ventricular outflow obstruction results in an increase in left ventricular end-diastolic and left atrial pressures. The latter encourages left-to-right atrial shunting through a stretched patent foramen ovale. Although this atrial shunt may ameliorate left ventricular failure by reducing the left ventricular preload, it also reduces the left ventricular output, leading to acidosis, a spuriously low gradient across the stenotic aortic valve, and reduced intensity of the murmur.[5] In addition, mitral insufficiency secondary to papillary muscle infarction is not uncommon in these infants.[9] This results in additional reduction in forward flow and an increase in left atrial pressure with a resultant increase in left-to-right atrial shunt and pulmonary venous load.

The chest radiogram reveals an enlarged heart (Fig. 1). Pulmonary vascular markings frequently cannot be appreciated because of the very large cardiac silhouette. Electrocardiographic findings are variable (Fig. 2), but most exhibit RVH with upright T waves in the right precordial leads. ST-segment depression and T wave flattening or inversion may be present in the left precordial leads. Rarely, the electrocardiogram will be normal. On echocardiographic examination, the left ventricle is hypertrophied and frequently exhibits poor contractility (Fig. 3). The aortic valve echo frequently produces multiple linear echoes, decreased systolic excursion, and eccentric diastolic closure (Fig. 4). In some cases, the aortic valve opening may appear nearly normal on the M-mode echocardiogram because, as the valve domes into the aorta and through the narrow echo beam, only the anterior and posterior walls of the valve dome reflect echoes, giving the illusion of a much larger valve diameter than actually exists (Fig. 5).

At cardiac catheterization, the cardiac index is usually reduced and may be as low as 1.0 to 1.5 L/min·m^2).[5,8] Aortic valve area is less than 0.7 cm^2/m^2, indicative of severe aortic stenosis.[10,11] Mixed venous oxygen saturation is decreased, and the arterial pH is usually 7.0 or less. Right-sided heart pressures are frequently increased; those in the right ventricle and pulmonary artery may exceed systemic levels. However, this does not reliably reflect severity of the aortic

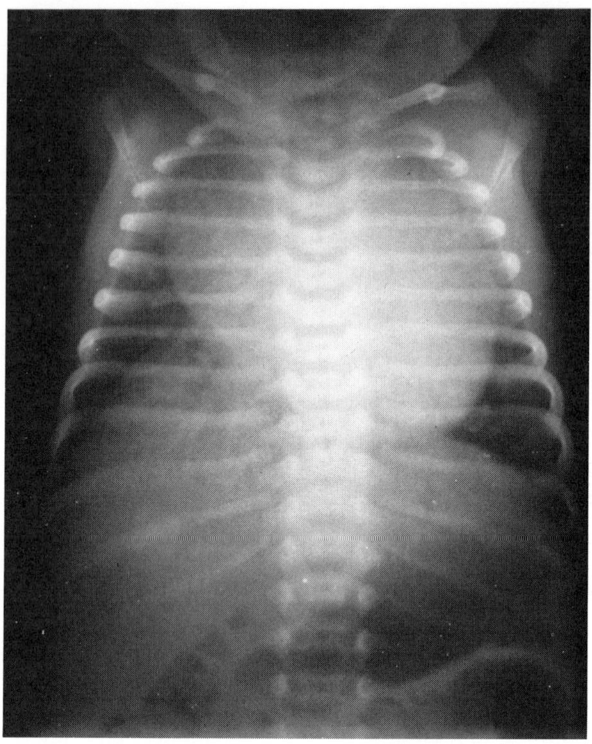

FIGURE 1 Chest radiogram of 6-week-old infant with critical aortic stenosis. The heart occupies approximately 75 percent of the chest, rendering assessment of pulmonary arterial and venous status impossible.

valve obstruction because in some cases the right-sided heart pressures may be normal in the presence of a severe gradient. Pulmonary artery wedge, left atrial, and left ventricular end-diastolic pressures are elevated. Depending on the extent of myocardial failure, left ventricular systolic pressure may be only moderately elevated, spuriously lowering the gradient measured across the aortic valve at the time of catheterization. In the absence of congestive heart failure, the gradient in most of these infants is 60 to 100 mm Hg. Mean aortic pressure is usually normal, but the pulse pressure is greatly diminished. Angiography performed from either the pulmonary artery or the left ventricle usually reveals reduced left ventricular end-diastolic volume. The range of reduction is variable in these infants, extending from marked hypoplasia to nearly normal. This is an important point in evaluating these infants, because the left ventricular end-diastolic volume is a significant indicator of survival after valvotomy. A value less than one-half that found in normal children (42 ± 10 cm^3/m^2)[12] portends a fatal outcome.[4,5,7] The ventricular septum and left ventricular posterior wall are hypertrophied and may exhibit reduced contractility. However, in the presence of

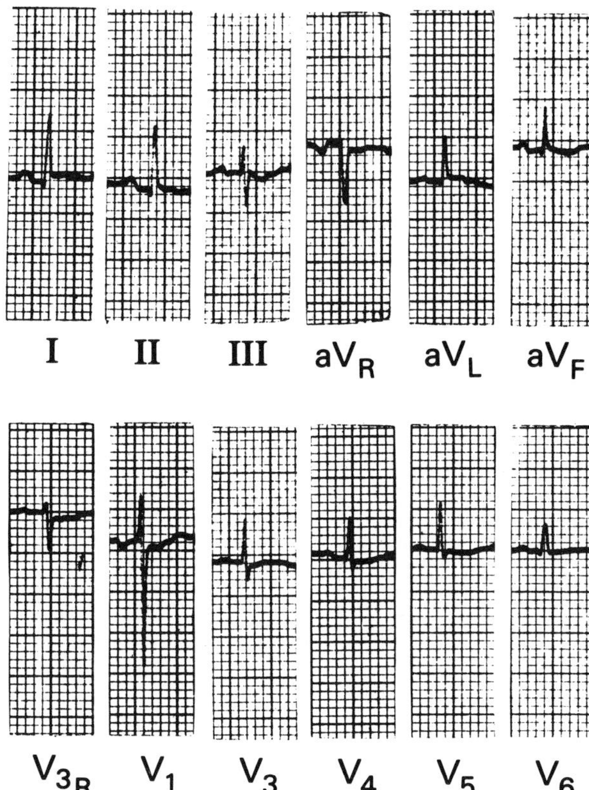

FIGURE 2 Electrocardiogram of same patient as in Fig. 1. Note large S wave in V_1, upright T waves in aV_R and right precordial leads, T wave flattening, and inversion in leads V_{5-6}.

adequate myocardial compensation, the left ventricular cavity may become nearly obliterated during systole. The aortic annulus usually appears hypoplastic and contrast exits the left ventricle in an eccentric jet through the thickened, domed aortic valve. Frequently, the structure and function of the aortic valve are better demonstrated by aortic root angiography (Fig. 6). As contrast fills the area immediately above the aortic valve, leaflet motion and thickness may be appreciated. Location and size of the aortic valve orifice can be assessed by the jet of "undyed" blood from the left ventricle that enters the aortic contrast bolus. The presence and severity of associated aortic insufficiency also can be determined by this technique. The ascending aorta is normal or dilated.

The infant with critical aortic stenosis usually does not survive without surgery for more than a few days after presentation. After establishing the diagnosis and bringing the infant to the best metabolic and hemodynamic status possible under the circumstances, valvotomy under direct vision, using inflow occlusion or cardiopulmonary bypass, must be accomplished.[13–17] It must be remembered that myocardial function in these infants is severely depressed. The congestive failure may improve briefly with digitalis and diuretics, but it cannot be completely controlled until the obstruction is relieved.[7] Therefore, no time should be wasted between establishing the diagnosis and proceeding with valvotomy. At surgery there may be substantial hypoplasia of the annulus, resulting in significant residual obstruction. However, valvotomy permits survival in

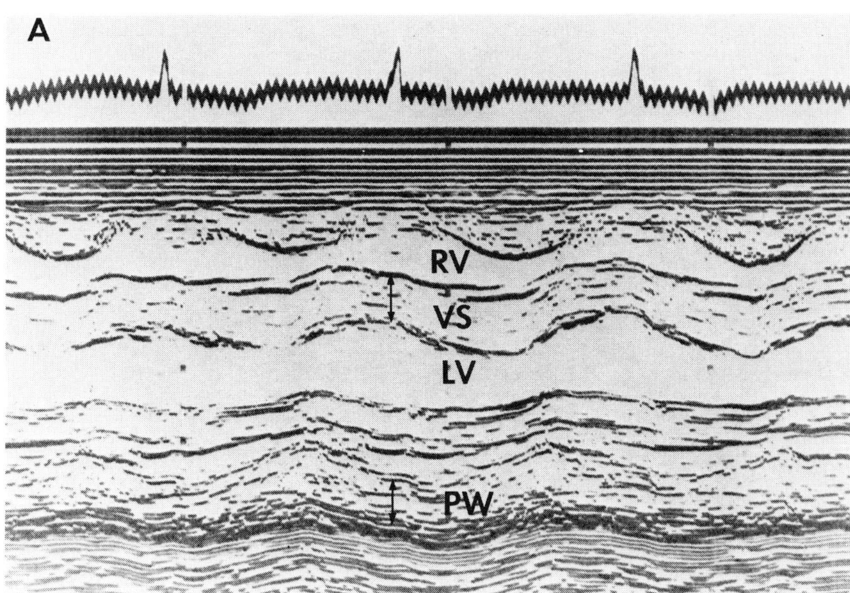

FIGURE 3 M-mode echocardiogram on same patient as in Fig. 1. (*A*) Left ventricular (LV) echogram recorded just below the mitral valve demonstrates concentric left ventricular hypertrophy. Diastolic dimension (arrows) of the ventricular septum (VS) and left ventricular posterior wall (PW) is 7 mm. (*B*, p. 252) Aortic valve echogram appears nearly normal in spite of critical obstruction (see Fig. 5). Other abbreviations: RV = right ventricle; RVOT = right ventricular outflow tract; Ao = aorta; LA = left atrium.

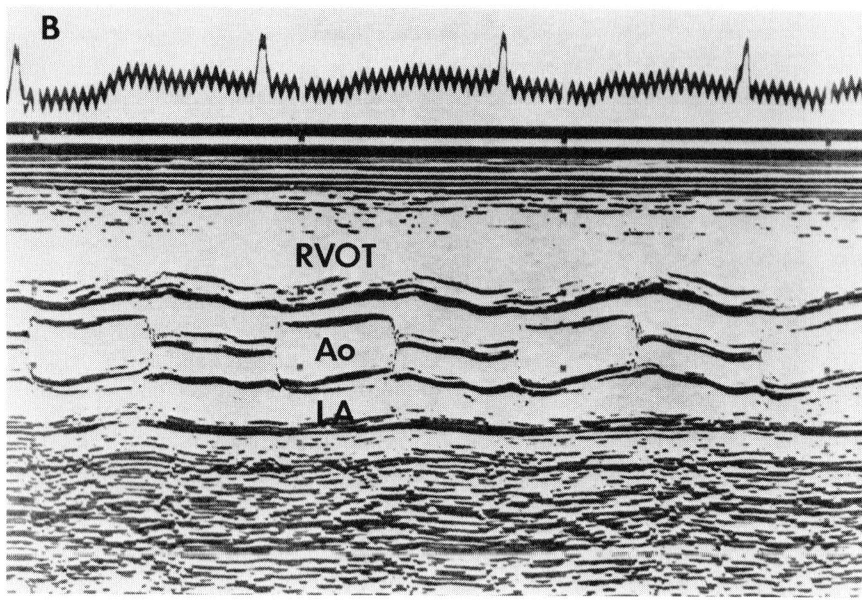

many of these infants to an age at which more effective valvotomy or valve replacement may be performed. The postoperative function of the aortic valve is related to the extent of the valvotomy. With more extensive commissurotomy, there is a lower postoperative gradient, but a high incidence of mild to moderate aortic insufficiency. These patients usually do not require repeat valvotomy or aortic valve replacement as early as infants who have a more limited valvotomy with lower incidence of aortic insufficiency and higher residual gradient.[7,16] Even with surgery, the early mortality rate is very high in infants who require valvotomy before 2 months of age.[5,7] This probably reflects a combination of problems, including the

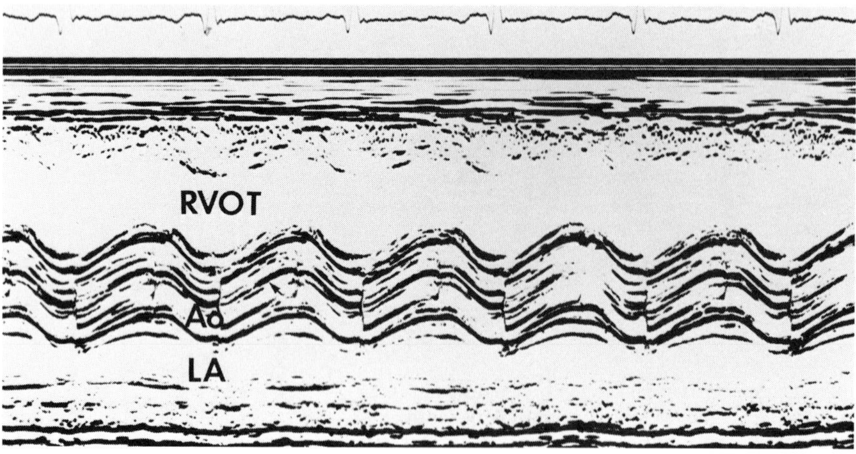

FIGURE 4 Aortic valve echogram on infant with severe aortic stenosis demonstrating multiple systolic and diastolic echoes, including a central systolic echo (small arrow).

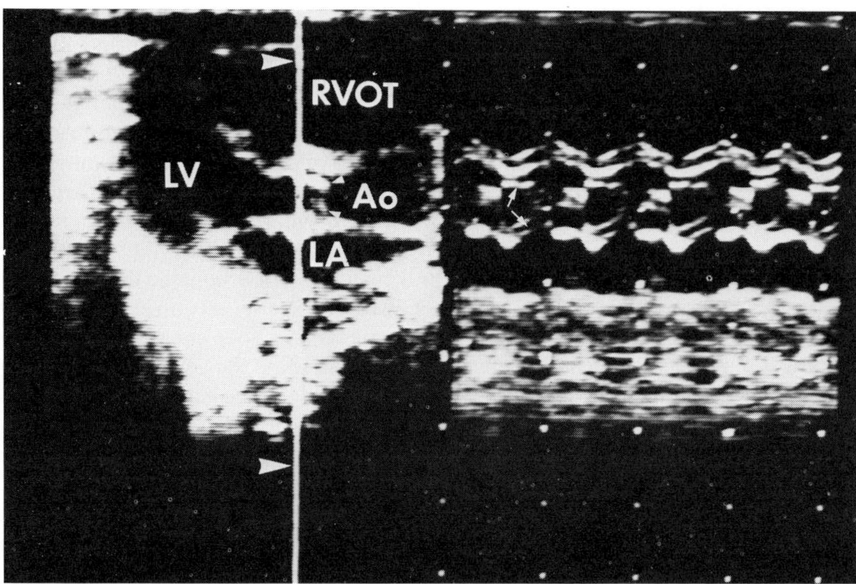

FIGURE 5 Split-image two-dimensional and M-mode echocardiogram on same infant as in Fig. 3, directing the M-mode beam (large arrowheads) through the aortic valve (small arrowheads). As the aortic valve dome passes through the M-mode beam into the aorta, only the anterior and posterior walls of the dome reflect echoes recorded on the M-mode (small arrowheads).

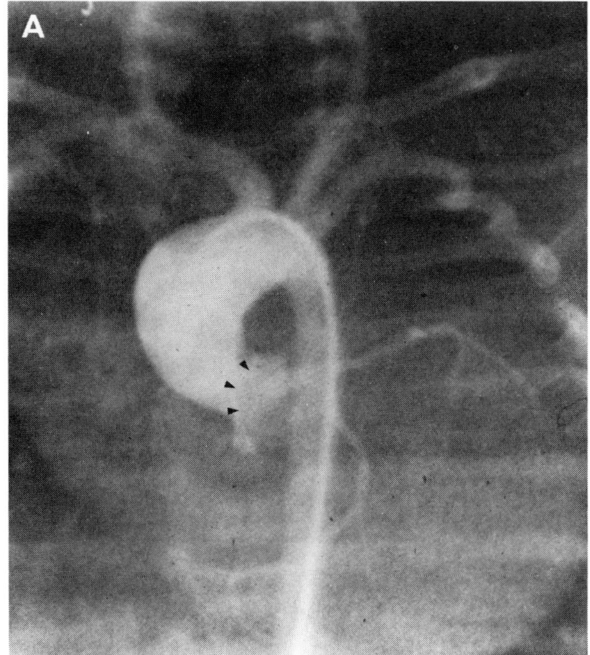

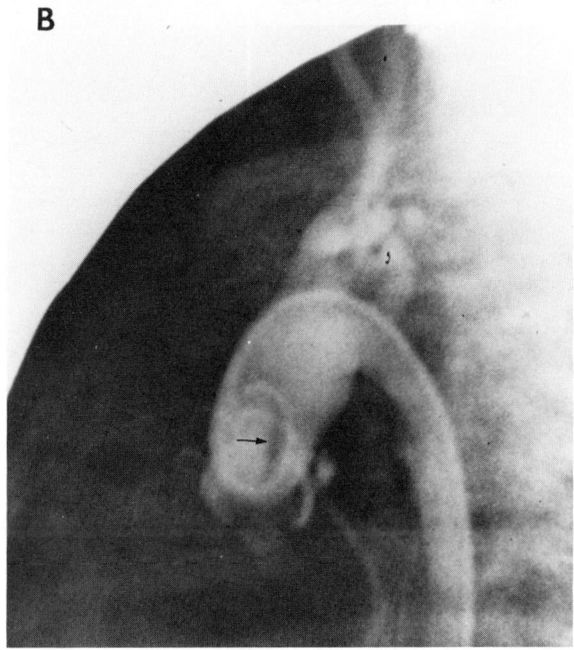

FIGURE 6 Anteroposterior (*A*) and lateral (*B*) projections of aortic root angiogram in infant with critical aortic stenosis demonstrating systolic doming of the aortic valve (small arrowheads) into the aorta and narrow jet (arrow) of "undyed" blood being ejected from the left ventricle through the stenotic valve orifice. Same patient as is Fig. 3.

metabolic changes associated with prolonged shock and acidosis, impaired left ventricular function incident to myocardial hypertrophy, subendocardial ischemia, myocardial or papillary muscle necrosis, and endocardial fibroelastosis. At autopsy, small left ventricular size, endocardial fibroelastosis, and severe dysplasia of the aortic valve are frequent findings.[7]

A second group of infants presents a bit later, from 2 to 6 months of age. At the time of initial evaluation, they usually have mild symptoms or no symptoms at all. The presence of a harsh grade 4/6 systolic ejection murmur is usually the reason for referral of these infants and is the most striking finding on physical examination. S_1 may be normal or increased in intensity, S_2 is usually normal, and an ejection click is present in nearly every case. The click is usually best heard at the mid-left sternal border radiating toward the apex, but in some cases it is heard only at the apex. Peripheral pulses may be diminished in magnitude. Systolic blood pressure is usually normal, but the diastolic pressure is elevated, resulting in a narrow pulse pressure.[7] The lungs are free of rales, and the liver edge is generally palpable 1.0 to 1.5 cm below the right costal margin. Chest radiogram reveals an en-

larged heart, but there is rarely evidence of pulmonary venous distension. The electrocardiogram usually reveals left ventricular hypertrophy (Fig. 7). There may be ST-segment depression and T wave flattening in the left precordial leads. A large Q wave is often present in leads I, aV_L and V_{5-6}. An occasional patient may have pure right ventricular hypertrophy; rarely, the electrocardiogram will be normal. The echocardiogram in these infants demonstrates concentric left ventricular hypertrophy and, usually, good contractility (Fig. 8). Aortic valve closure is usually eccentric. Frequently there are multiple diastolic echoes emanating from the aortic valve. However, in some the aortic valve opening may appear normal. At cardiac catheterization, the cardiac output is usually normal. Pulmonary artery wedge, left atrial, and left ventricular end-diastolic pressures are almost always elevated. Right-sided heart pressures may be increased as well. The gradient across the aortic valve is usually 50 to 65 mm Hg; these infants require early valvotomy.

Those infants in the older age group who exhibit evidence of congestive failure when seen initially usually respond well to anticongestive measures and may be managed medically for a short time. However, they

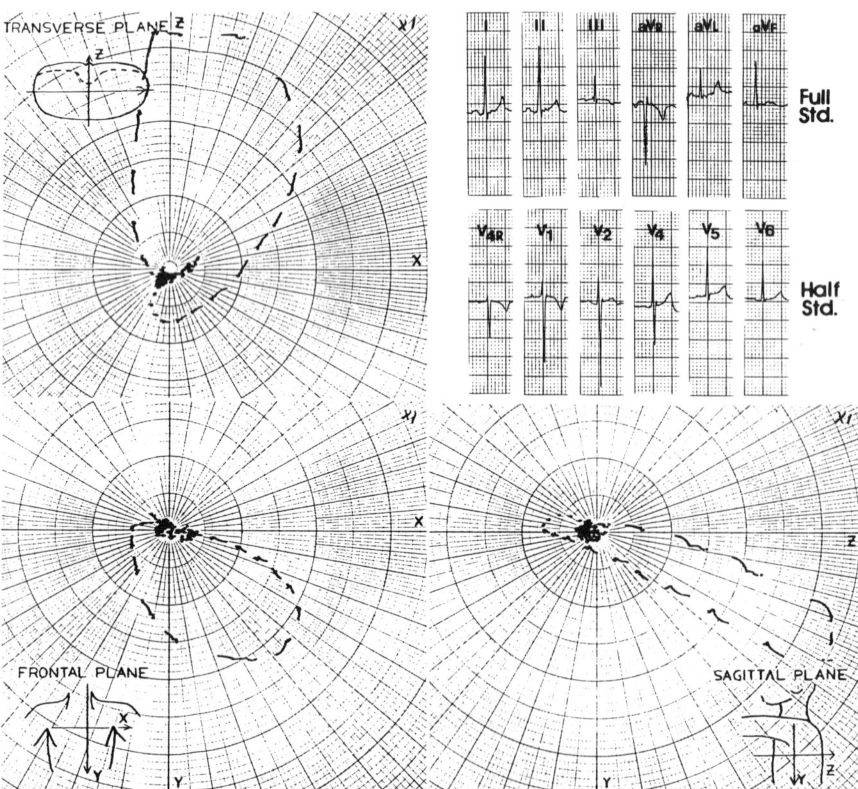

FIGURE 7 Vectorcardiogram and electrocardiogram of 5-month-old infant with severe aortic stenosis demonstrating left ventricular hypertrophy but no ST or T changes suggestive of myocardial ischemia.

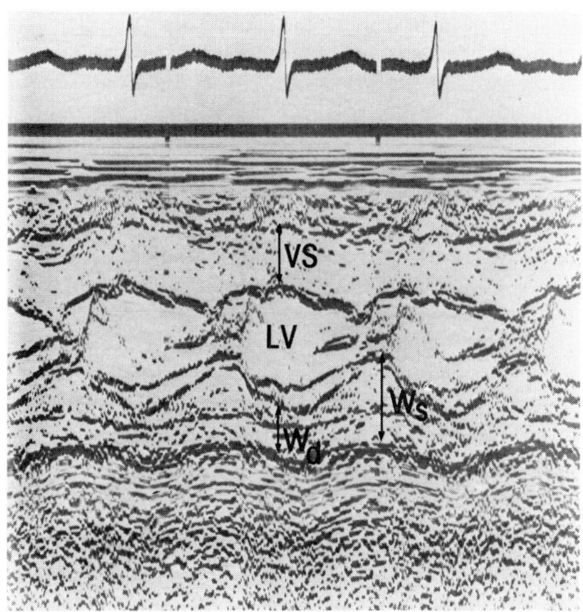

FIGURE 8 M-mode echocardiogram of same patient as in Fig. 3 demonstrating marked concentric left ventricular hypertrophy and brisk contractility, with nearly complete obliteration of the left ventricular cavity during systole. Abbreviations: W_d = diastolic left ventricular posterior wall thickness; W_s = systolic left ventricular posterior wall thickness.

almost always require surgery within a few weeks. Therefore, surgery should be scheduled as soon as congestive failure is brought under reasonable control.[7] With the improved intra- and postoperative management that has evolved over the past few years, prognosis has improved dramatically for these infants.[16] Valvotomy improves congestive failure and reduces the gradient in most cases, with a low incidence of hemodynamically significant aortic insufficiency. The electrocardiogram improves and cardiac enlargement decreases in most cases. Infants with gradients above 50 mm Hg, normal heart size on chest x-ray, and no evidence of congestive failure may be followed closely to permit growth and technically easier surgery. Progressive cardiomegaly, echocardiographic evidence of increasing left ventricular hypertrophy, ST-segment depression or T wave flattening or inversion in left precordial leads, or the onset of congestive failure constitute indications for immediate valvotomy. Surgery cannot be delayed for more than a few months in most of these infants, because continued growth demands increased cardiac output, thereby increasing the gradient across the stenotic aortic valve.[18] To compensate, the myocardium rapidly hypertrophies; the coronary blood flow becomes inadequate, leading to myocardial ischemia and infarction.[19,20]

AORTIC STENOSIS IN CHILDREN

The majority of children with aortic stenosis are asymptomatic, even in the presence of severe obstruction. The electrocardiogram, chest x-ray, and clinical findings are not reliable predictors of severity.[21] The peak systolic gradient across the aortic valve and calculated aortic valve area[10,11] have been heavily relied upon to assess the need for surgical intervention, especially in asymptomatic patients. A gradient of less than 50 mm Hg is considered evidence of mild obstruction; one between 50 and 75 mm Hg, moderate; and a gradient greater than 75 mm Hg represents severe obstruction. The aortic valve area (AVA) is also derived from cardiac catheterization data according to the Gorlin[10] formula:

$$AVA = \frac{\dfrac{C.O.}{SEP \times HR}}{44.5 \times \sqrt{LV_s - Ao_s}}$$

where C.O. is cardiac output, SEP is the systolic ejection period, and HR is the heart rate per minute. The result of the numerator in the equation is aortic valve flow (AVF). LV_s and Ao_s are mean systolic pressures in the left ventricle and aorta derived from measuring the respective pressure tracings with a planimeter. Bache et al.[11] have derived a simpler method in which the denominator employs the difference between the peak systolic pressures in the left ventricle (LV) and aorta (Ao):

$$AVA = \frac{AVF}{37.8 \times \sqrt{(LV - Ao) + 10}}$$

Results using the two equations are very similar. The normal aortic valve area is 2.0 cm^2/m^2 or greater. A valve area between 1.2 and 2.0 cm^2/m^2 represents mild stenosis; 0.7 to 1.2 cm^2/m^2, moderate; and less than 0.7 cm^2/m^2, severe.[22,23] While the gradient and aortic valve area determinations do not take into account the adequacy of coronary blood flow and myocardial function, they do permit quantitative estimate of obstruction and are widely used for that purpose as a guide to timing surgical intervention and assessing the surgical result.

The child with severe aortic stenosis, i.e., a gradient greater than 75 mm Hg or aortic valve area less than 0.7 cm^2/m^2, should have immediate relief of the obstruction. Persistence of severe obstruction results in a cascading sequence of myocardial compromise—progressive left ventricular hypertrophy and decrease in diastolic compliance lead to increased left ventricular end-diastolic pressure. The ensuing reduction in diastolic gradient between the aorta and left ventricle impairs myocardial blood flow and oxygen delivery. This has been demonstrated by Lewis et al.[22] using

256

myocardial oxygen supply/demand ratio.[24] Myocardial oxygen supply is derived by multiplying the area between the aortic and left ventricular pressure curves during diastole, the *diastolic pressure time index* (DPTI), by the arterial oxygen content (C). Myocardial oxygen demand is the area beneath the left ventricular pressure curve during systole, the *systolic pressure time index* (SPTI) (Fig. 9). The ratio DPTI $\times$ (C/SPTI) expresses adequacy of coronary blood flow relative to myocardial oxygen demands. Values less than 10 have been shown experimentally in animals to be associated with reduced subendocardial blood flow.[20,25] Myocardial oxygen demands are met first by coronary vasodilatation. After maximum dilatation occurs, subendocardial blood flow becomes pressure-dependent and is determined by the relationship among coronary arterial diastolic pressure, left ventricular intramural pressure, and diastolic time.[19] Lewis et al.[22] also demonstrated that children with a calculated aortic valve area less than 0.7 cm²/m² and a heart rate below 100 beats per minute maintain DPTI $\times$ (C/SPTI) above 10, but at heart rates above 100, the ratio falls, becoming consistent with subendocardial ischemia, and is usually associated with T wave changes on the electrocardiogram. The result of inadequate coronary

blood flow in these patients is myocardial ischemia and fibrosis,[26] which further compromise left ventricular function, predisposing to progressive myocardial impairment[27] and sudden death,[28–31] even when exercise restriction is faithfully observed.

Children with moderate aortic stenosis, gradient 50 to 75 mm Hg, or a calculated aortic valve area of 0.7 to 1.2 cm²/m² and symptoms of fatigue, dyspnea, angina, or syncope should also have immediate operation. Progressive myocardial impairment and sudden death are significant risks in these children, just as they are for children with severe obstruction.

For those children with an obstruction of moderate degree, no symptoms, and a normal electrocardiogram and chest x-ray, the role and timing of surgical intervention are less well defined. Most children in this category are followed medically and restricted from most competitive sports and isometric exercises. The extent of restriction is based on judgment and cannot be completely objective.[32] Patient compliance is a substantial problem in management. In following these patients, one must assume that the obstruction will become more severe. Aortic stenosis is a progressive disorder, even in early childhood. Friedman et al.[33] and Cohen et al.[23] have demonstrated a significant increase

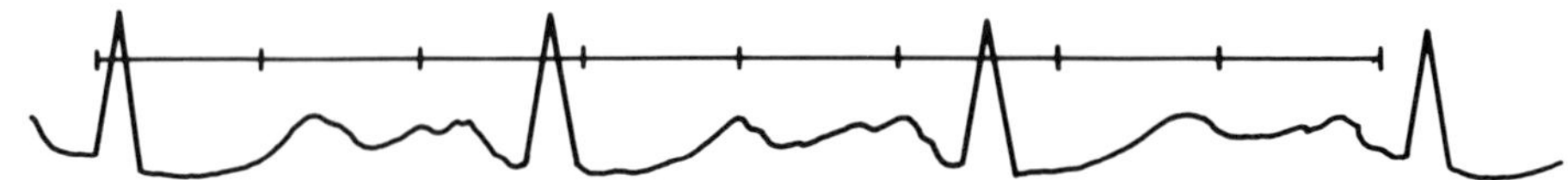

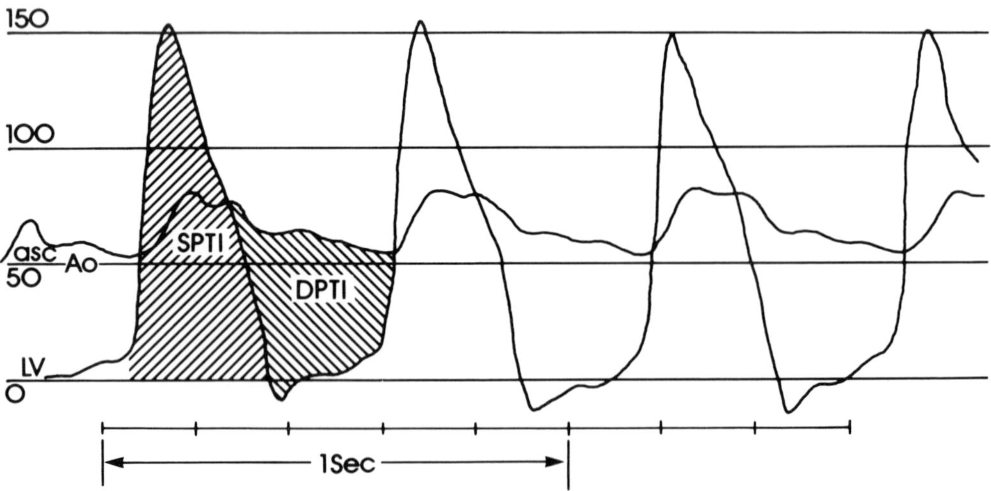

FIGURE 9 Left ventricular pressure tracing superimposed on ascending aorta pressure tracing at similar R-R interval in a 14-year-old boy with an aortic valve gradient of 65 mm Hg, a calculated aortic valve area of 1.3 cm²/m², and a DPTI $\times$ (C/SPTI) of 13 (see text).

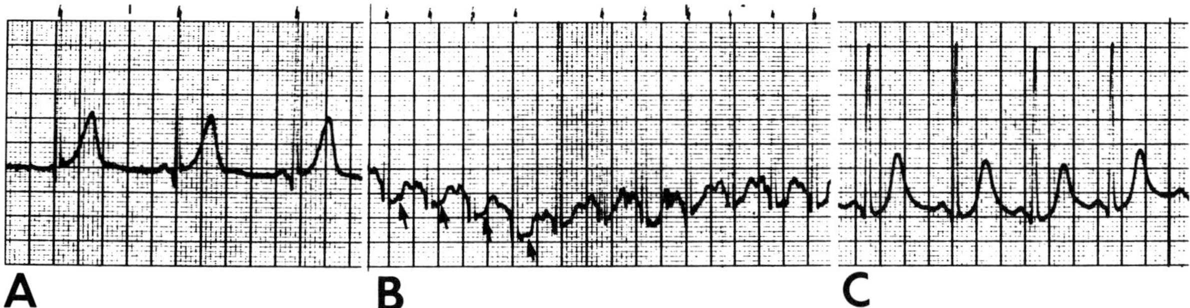

FIGURE 10 Exercise electrocardiogram lead V_5 from an 11-year-old boy with aortic stenosis and no previous aortic valve surgery. (*A*) Resting tracing after hyperventilation, normal ST segment. (*B*) After 2 min at 800 KPM, significant ST-segment depression occurs (arrows). (*C*) Two minutes after discontinuation of exercise, ST segment has reverted to normal.

in gradient over a 5- to 7-year period in 80 percent of children presenting initially with mild obstruction. A full 50 percent of these patients had progressed to severe obstruction requiring surgery. Although the aortic orifice may become smaller in some patients,[34] it appears to be relatively constant in most. Growth of the child leads to an increase in the gradient because of increased stroke volume in proportion to the systolic ejection period.[18] Poor correlation between progression of the obstruction and clinical or electrocardiographic manifestations[21] necessitates cardiac catheterization every 5 to 7 years in asymptomatic children with mild to moderate obstruction.[33] Even this is not optimum, because the gradient progresses more rapidly in some patients than in others, and patients who have no manifestations at rest may have evidence of myocardial ischemia during activity.[22] In this context, exercise testing has provided a valuable noninvasive method for detecting progression in severity in this group of patients. Halloran[35] and Chandramouli et al.[36] demonstrated a consistent relationship between an aortic valve gradient greater than 50 to 55 mm Hg and significant ST-segment depression on exercise electrocardiogram (Fig. 10), distinguishing those patients whose gradients had progressed to a moderate or severe obstruction. Whitmer et al.[37] have found ST-segment depression at maximum exercise in approximately 75 percent of children with a resting gradient greater than 30 mm Hg. In contradistinction to adults with coronary artery disease, the ST-segment changes in children with aortic stenosis return to the pre-exercise profile immediately after exercise is discontinued. Exercise-induced ST-segment depression resolves after effective surgical relief of the obstruction. This suggests that most children whose obstruction is more than very mild experience subendocardial ischemia at exercise.[18,19,22,24] Riopel et al.[38] and Alpert et al.[39] have demonstrated an abnormal systolic blood pressure response to exercise in children with aortic stenosis. The latter found a close correlation between

an increase in the systolic pressure from resting to peak exercise of less than 35 mm Hg and a resting aortic gradient greater than 50 mm Hg, providing additional evidence of progression in severity.

The child whose initial resting gradient at cardiac catheterization is less than 50 mm Hg should undergo exercise testing as a part of the annual clinical reevaluation. The appearance of significant ST-segment depression and/or abnormal systolic blood pressure response indicates that the gradient has progressed beyond the mild degree, and repeat cardiac catheterization should be performed to establish the gradient and assess the functional status of the left ventricle. Most of these children will require early surgical intervention.

Echocardiography has provided a new and important noninvasive dimension in assessing aortic stenosis. M-mode echographic imaging of the left ventricle has proven very helpful in monitoring the progress of ventricular changes both preoperatively and postoperatively. The extent of left ventricular hypertrophy is determined by wall stress, with wall thickness increasing in proportion to the ventricular pressure load until systolic wall stress is normalized. Based on this principle, formulas have been derived for estimating the left ventricular peak systolic pressure from echocardiographic systolic measurements of the posterior wall (W_s) and ventricular cavity (D_s)[40–42] (Fig. 11). By subtracting the brachial artery systolic blood pressure obtained with a standard sphygmomanometer and stethoscope, the gradient may be estimated. The shortening fraction of the transverse diameter of the left ventricle also reflects the degree of obstruction. Expressed as the difference between the end-diastolic and peak systolic dimensions of the left ventricle, divided by the end-diastolic dimension.

$$\frac{D_d - D_s}{D_d}$$

a shortening fraction of less than 40 percent almost always indicates an aortic valve gradient of less than 45

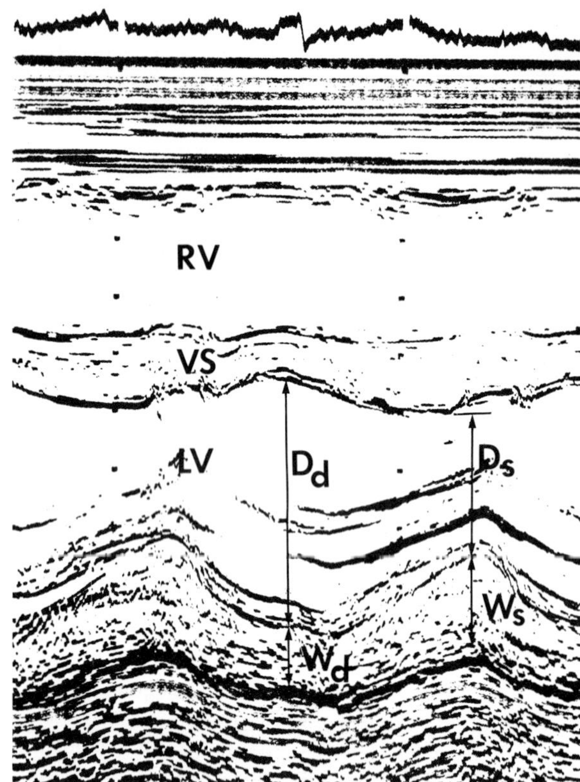

FIGURE 11 M-mode echocardiogram on a 14-year-old boy with aortic stenosis and previous valvotomy in infancy. Using the equation left ventricular peak systolic pressure = 225 × (W_s/D_s), the predicted pressure was 150 mm Hg.[40] Shortening fraction of the left ventricle, $(D_d - D_s)/D_d$, was 43 percent.[41] At catheterization, left ventricular pressure was 150 mm Hg, ascending aortic pressure was 85 mm Hg, and the gradient was 65 mm Hg.

mm Hg.[43] The echocardiographic estimate of severity has some limitations,[44] however, and is not valid in the presence of congestive heart failure, cardiomyopathy, mitral insufficiency, or aortic insufficiency of more than mild degree.

Echocardiographic imaging of the stenotic aortic valve is of limited value in assessing aortic stenosis. Ideally, the M-mode echocardiogram of the stenotic aortic valve should demonstrate increased density of the aortic cusp echoes, multiple diastolic echoes, a central systolic echo, and in most cases, an eccentric closure line (Fig. 4). It is rare that all are seen in a given patient and not infrequent that none is detected.[45] Two-dimensional techniques have permitted better assessment of aortic valve motion and are more sensitive in detecting the presence of aortic stenosis than M-mode, but they permit no better assessment of severity[46,47] (Fig. 12).

As with all noninvasive techniques to date, exercise testing and echocardiography fall short of providing accurate determination of severity of the obstruction. However, the information they do provide regarding ventricular hypertrophy and subendocardial ischemia have added significantly to our understanding of the myocardial response to aortic stenosis. The exercise electrocardiogram has enabled more prudent timing of follow-up catheterization and surgery. The role and timing of surgical intervention in those patients with gradients in the moderate, or 50 to 75 mm Hg, range, no resting symptoms, and minimal or no electrocardiographic changes have been redefined substantially as a result of exercise testing. The demonstration of significant ST-segment depression with exercise in a patient in this group is an indication for early surgical relief of the obstruction.

REOPERATION FOR AORTIC STENOSIS

The surgical treatment of aortic stenosis must be considered palliative.[48–51] Although relief of the obstruction as a result of valvotomy is dramatic in most cases, restenosis occurs frequently (Fig. 13). This is usually associated with thickening of the valve leaflets and curling and retraction of the free margins. The resultant valve deformity frequently results in aortic insufficiency, adding volume overload of the left ventricle to the preexisting pressure overload. Even in the absence of significant aortic insufficiency, effective relief of restenosis by valvotomy may be difficult to achieve. Therefore, the need for subsequent aortic valve replacement must be realistically entertained. In addition, aortic valve replacement does not constitute the ultimate solution to this problem. Prosthetic valves have fixed orifices; continued growth of the child may render the valve orifice inadequate, necessitating replacement with a larger valve. For these reasons, both the initial and subsequent operations on the stenotic aortic valve are usually delayed for as long as safely possible in the child with a less than severe obstruction. However, even ideal planning of aortic valve replacement from the standpoint of growth does not eliminate the possibility of subsequent replacement. Although prosthetic valve technology has improved tremendously over the past 20 years, mechanical malfunction is still a potential problem, as are prosthetic valve thrombus, periprosthetic leak, and prosthetic valve endocarditis.[52] The indications for reoperation for aortic stenosis are similar in many respects to those for initial operation. Clinical and laboratory evidence of severe obstruction or moderate obstruction in the presence of symptoms or exercise-induced ST-segment changes are indications for immediate operation. These

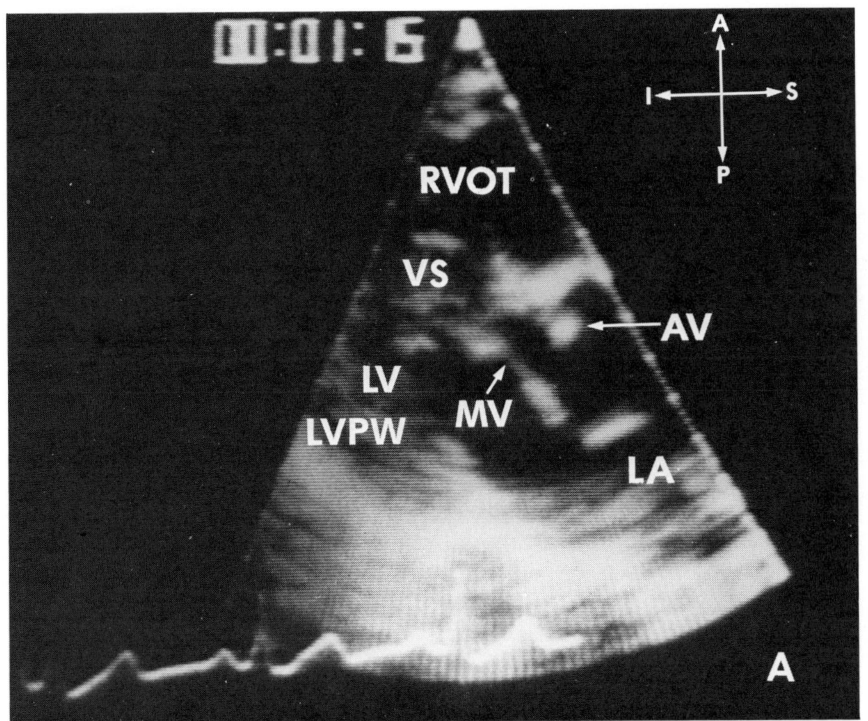

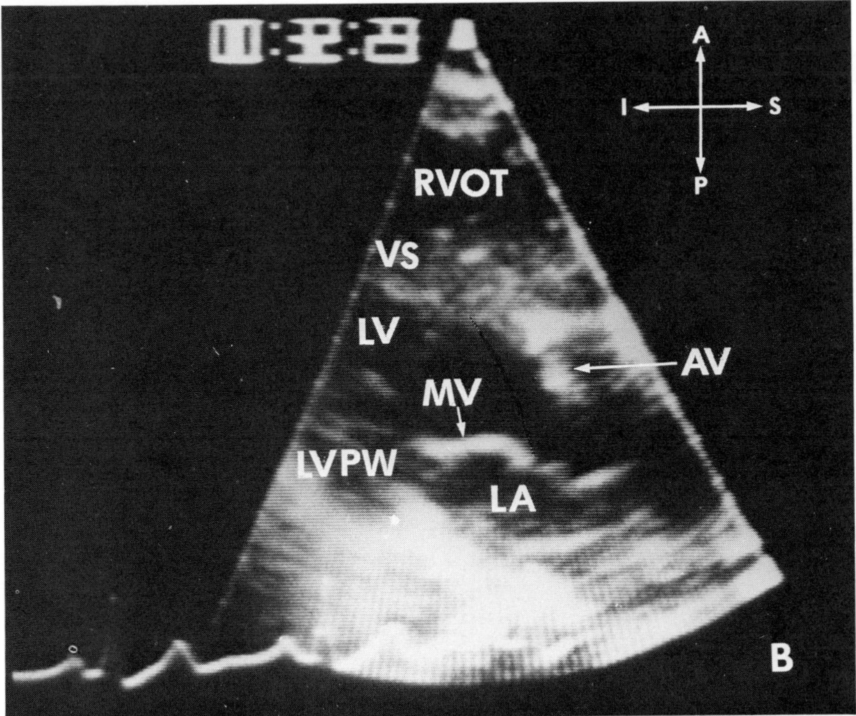

FIGURE 12 Two-dimensional echocardiographic frames from same patient as in Fig. 11. (*A*) Left parasternal long-axis view of left ventricular outflow tract during diastole demonstrating thickened aortic valve. (*B*) Same projection during systole demonstrating immobility of the thickened aortic valve. (*C*, page 260) Left parasternal short-axis view of the aorta demonstrating bicuspid aortic valve (arrows). (*D*, p. 260) Left parasternal long-axis view of left ventricle at end-systole demonstrating marked left ventricular hypertrophy nearly obliterating the left ventricular cavity. Abbreviations: A = anterior; P = posterior; I = inferior; S = superior; R = right; L = left; MV = mitral valve; AV = aortic valve; LA = left atrium; LVPW = left ventricular posterior wall; RVOT = right ventricular outflow tract; VS = ventricular septum.

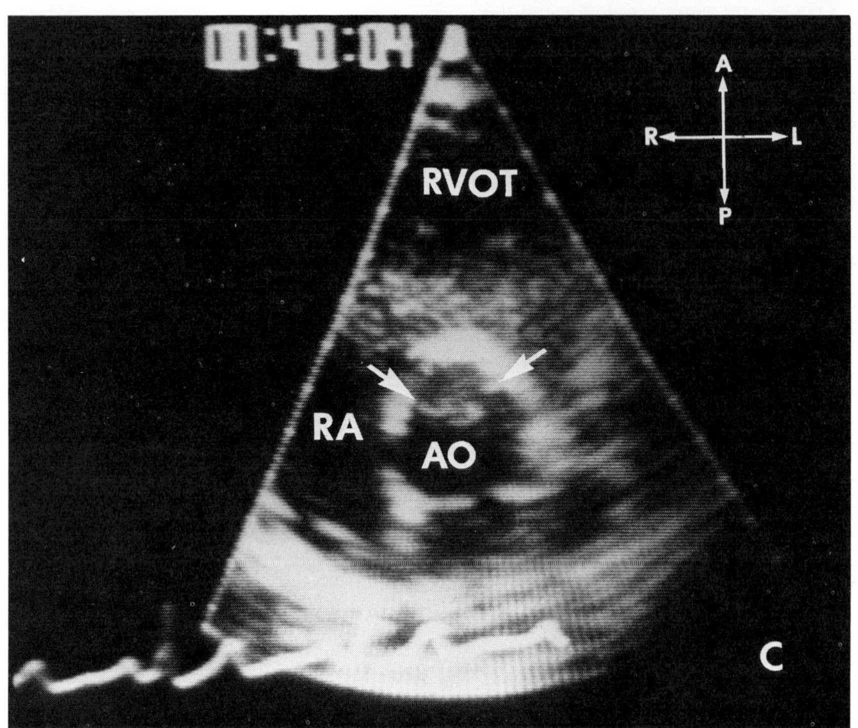

RVOT
A
R
L
P
RA
AO
C

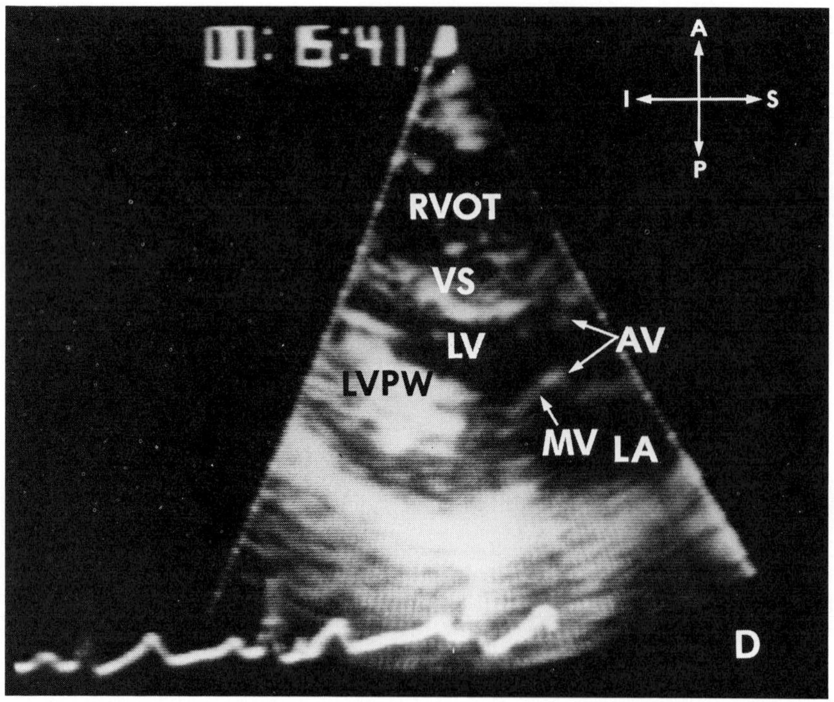

A
I
S
P
RVOT
VS
LV
AV
LVPW
MV
LA
D

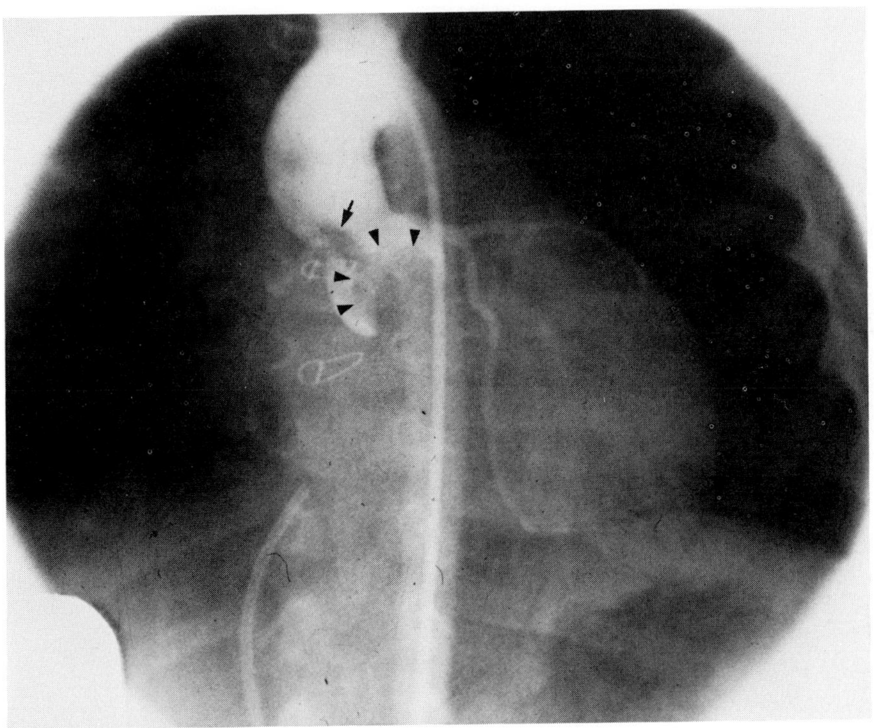

FIGURE 13 Aortic root angiogram demonstrating severe restenosis in a child who underwent valvotomy in infancy. Note doming of the aortic valve (arrowheads) and narrow jet of "undyed" blood (arrow) from the stenotic valve orifice.

patients are at risk of sudden death. In addition, the left ventricle has been functioning under a chronically increased pressure load, resulting in ventricular hypertrophy (Fig. 14). The addition of myocardial ischemia resulting from a progressively increasing gradient predisposes the myocardium to infarction and fibrosis, leading to poor postoperative function. A special case must be made for the patient in whom significant aortic insufficiency has developed (Fig. 15). In these patients there may be a moderate gradient, or less, across the valve because the ventricular dilatation associated with aortic insufficiency prevents progressive increase in the left ventricular peak systolic pressure as the stenosis becomes more severe. However, the combination of volume and pressure overload in the left ventricle results in elevation of the left ventricular end-diastolic pressure and decrease in the cardiac index.[50] Mild degrees of aortic insufficiency in association with aortic stenosis may be well tolerated for many years, and the need for reoperation is dictated solely by the status of the stenosis. Moderate and severe degrees of aortic insufficiency in association with aortic stenosis are not well tolerated, however, and lead to relatively early cardiac enlargement (Fig. 16), left ventricular hypertrophy with ST-segment changes (Fig. 17), and symptoms. The latter may not be a prominent part of the patient's history and may be denied completely. Because of the insidious manner in which decreased exercise capacity occurs, mild degrees of fatigue and dyspnea may not be appreciated by the adolescent. It is frequently only after aortic valve replacement and

dramatic improvement in their functional capacity that they are aware of symptoms present preoperatively. Generally, the child with moderate aortic stenosis and moderate or severe aortic insufficiency with cardiac enlargement on the chest x-ray and left ventricular hypertrophy on the electrocardiogram should have the aortic valve replaced. The relationship between preoperative heart size and postoperative survival has been demonstrated quite clearly in adults.[53,54] It seems logical that the same relationship would prevail in the adolescent and young adult.

Obviously, any infant or child with aortic stenosis requires careful, life-long follow-up and periodic reassessment of aortic valve and left ventricular functional status. Counseling of the child and family to this end must be realistic and honest and commence at the time the diagnosis is first made.

AORTIC INSUFFICIENCY

Most accounts of congenital aortic insufficiency in children are concerned with congenital aortic–left ventricular tunnel, a fistulous communication outside the aortic valve annulus. These patients may also have central aortic valve insufficiency secondary to dilatation of the aortic annulus. True congenital aortic insufficiency rarely occurs as an isolated lesion in children, and when it does, it is almost invariably the result of a bicuspid aortic valve. Most commonly, aortic insuffi-

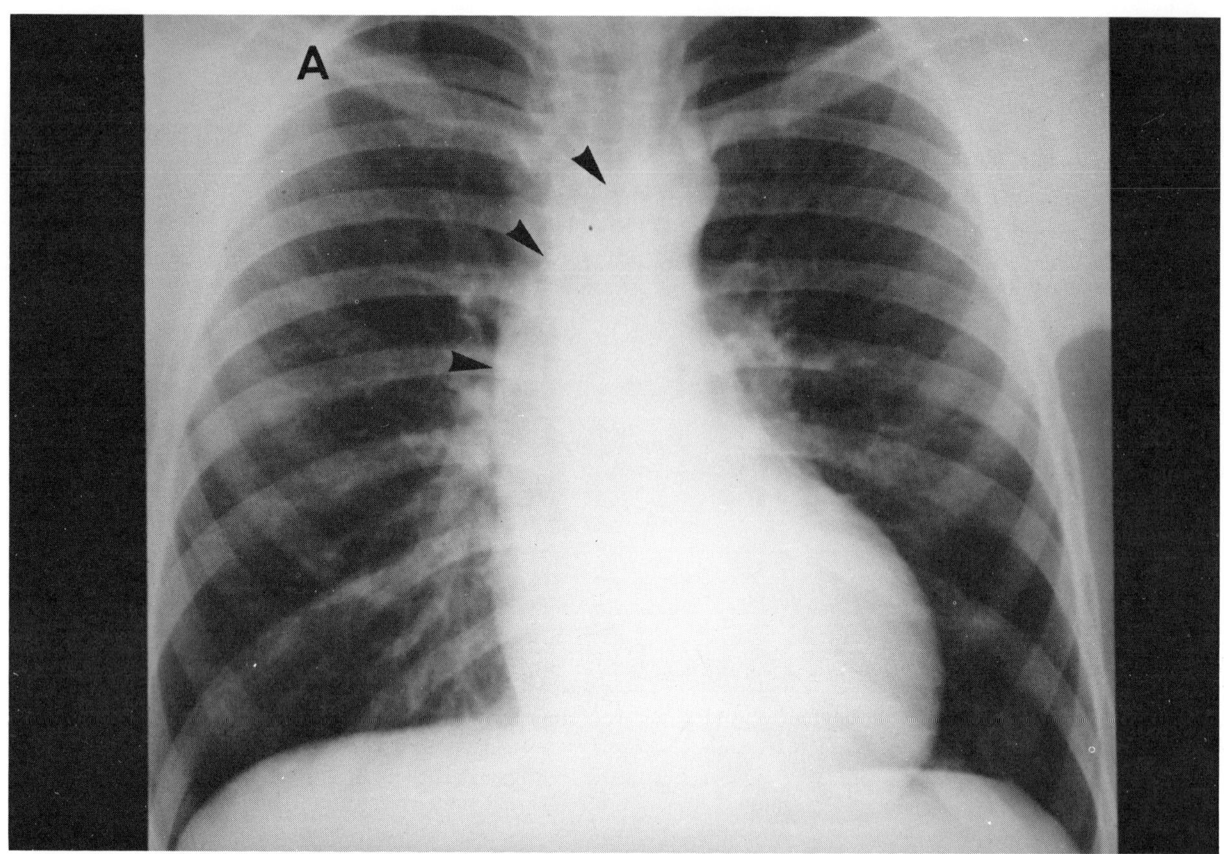

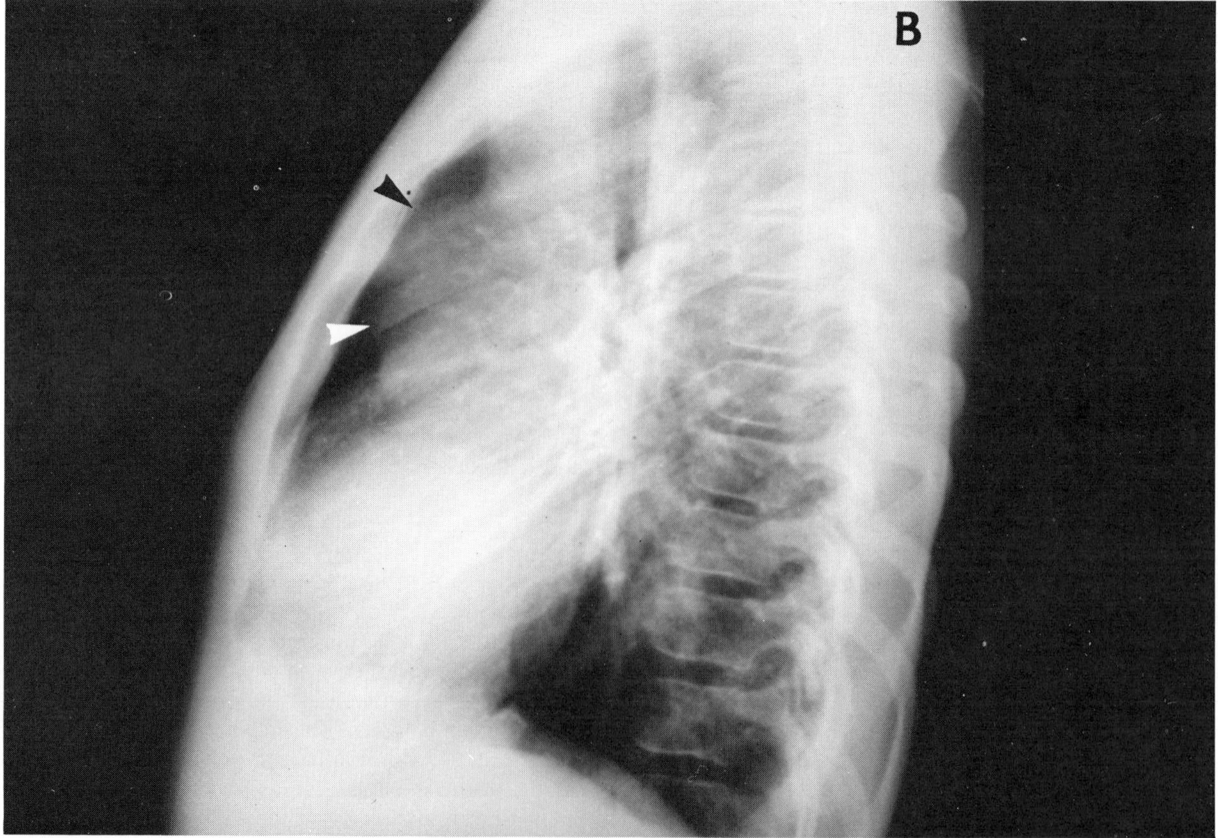

FIGURE 14 (*A*) Posteroanterior and (*B*) lateral chest radiogram of 14-year-old boy with restenosis of aortic valve demonstrating left ventricular hypertrophy and dilated ascending aorta (arrowheads).

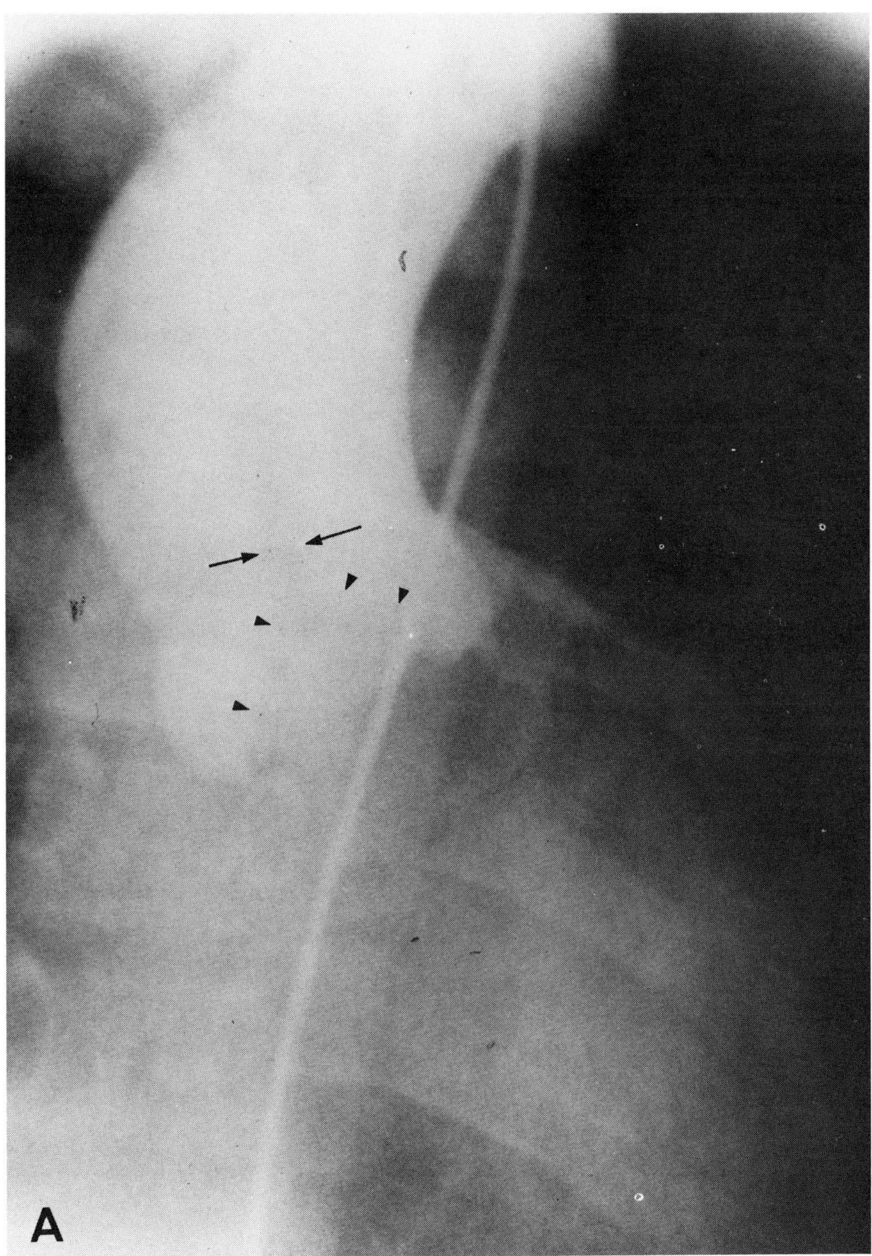

FIGURE 15 Aortic root angiogram on a 15-year-old boy who had aortic valvotomy in early childhood. (*A*) Upon injection of contrast medium into the dilated ascending aorta, doming of the aortic valve (arrowheads) and jet of "undyed" blood (arrows) are faintly imaged. (*B*, p. 264) Subsequent diastolic frame demonstrates aortic regurgitation completely filling the dilated, hypertrophied left ventricle.

ciency occurs as a complicating feature in association with other more significant cardiac abnormalties or diseases (Table 1). In those parts of the world where rheumatic fever remains a prevalent health problem, rheumatic heart disease is the most common cause of aortic insufficiency in childhood. Classification of se-

verity is more subjective than that for aortic stenosis, with most being characterized as mild or severe. In mild aortic insufficiency, the patient is asymptomatic, the heart is not enlarged on chest x-ray, and there is no LVH on the ECG. The diastolic murmur is grade 2/6 or less, and the pulse pressure is normal. Severe aortic

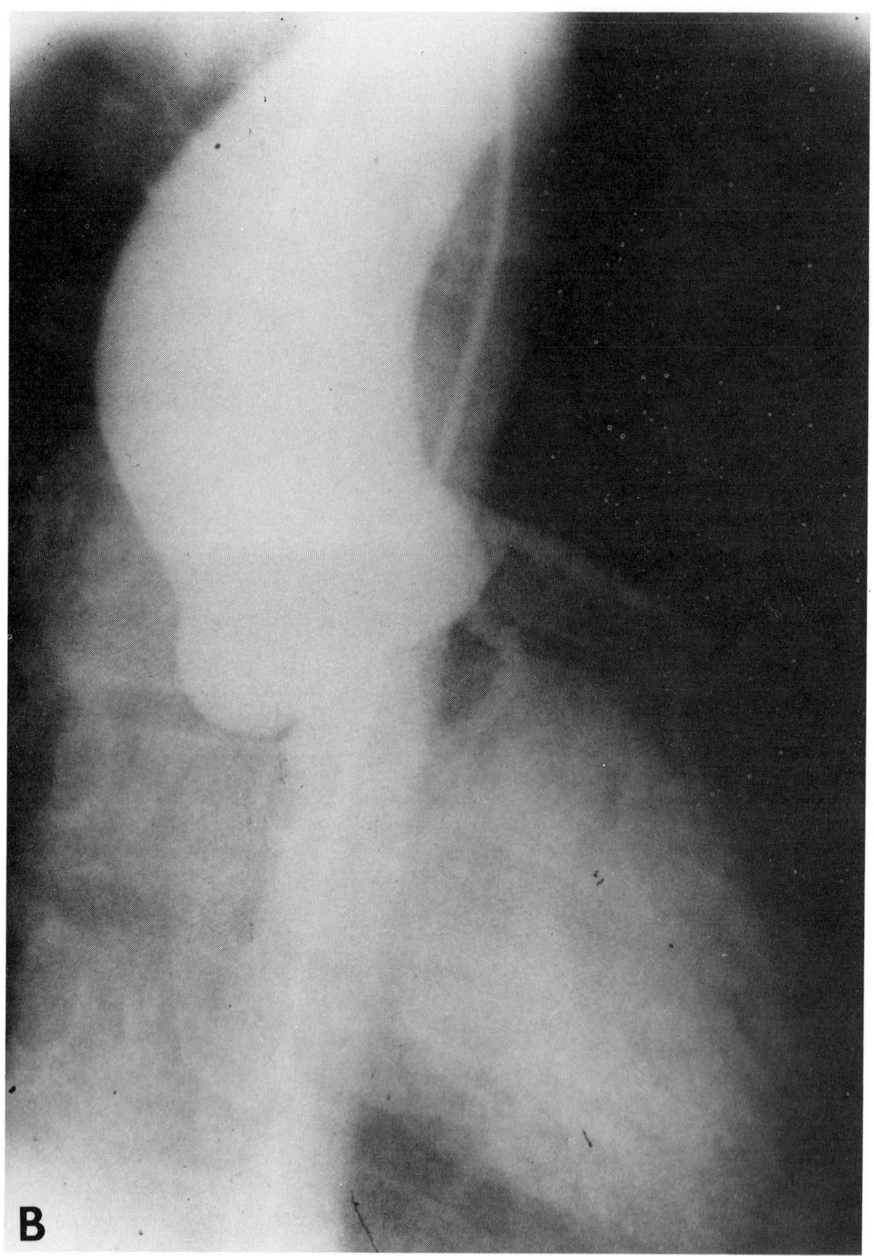

insufficiency is associated with a grade 3 to 4/6 diastolic regurgitant murmur and frequently an Austin-Flint murmur. The pulse pressure is wide, greater than one-half the systolic pressure, and it may approach or equal the systolic pressure. Heart size is increased, and the electrocardiogram reflects left ventricular hypertrophy. With increasing grades of severity, the cardiac enlargement becomes more marked and ST-segment and T wave changes appear in the left precordial leads of the electrocardiogram. Symptoms are a relatively late occurrence.

Chronic aortic insufficiency of significant magnitude may be well tolerated for a long period of time,[55] and cardiac function demonstrates a normal response to exercise.[32,56] However, as the insufficiency and cardiac enlargement progress, the resting left ventricular end-diastolic pressure falls to normal levels, the ejection fraction decreases, and there is an abnormally low increase in cardiac index in response to exercise. The decision to operate is based primarily on the presence of progressive cardiac enlargement, wide pulse pressure, and left ventricular hypertrophy. These are

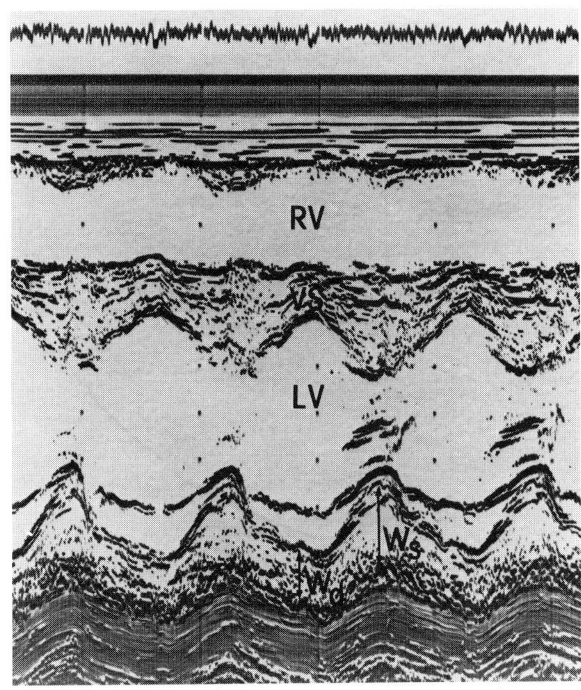

FIGURE 16 M-mode echocardiogram from same patient as in Fig. 15 revealing marked dilatation and concentric hypertrophy of the left ventricle.

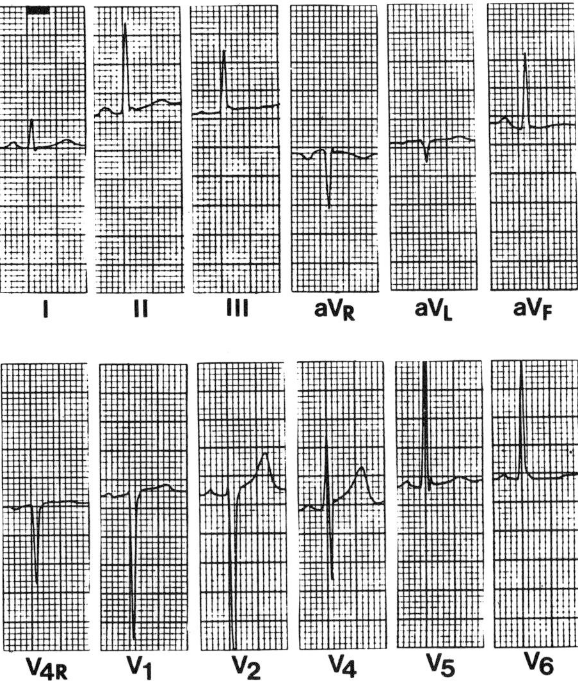

FIGURE 17 Electrocardiogram from same patient as in Figs. 15 and 16 exhibiting left ventricular hypertrophy and T wave flattening in leads aV$_f$ and V$_6$.

TABLE 1
Causes of aortic insufficiency in children

Bicuspid aortic valve—rarely causes significant insufficiency in childhood
In association with aortic stenosis:
  A Isolated aortic valve stenosis
  B Discrete subaortic stenosis
  C Supravalve aortic stenosis
In association with ventricular septal defect
Aortic–left ventricular tunnel
Sinus of Valsalva aneurysm
Infective endocarditis, usually in congenitally abnormal valve:
  A Bicuspid aortic valve
  B Aortic stenosis
  C Prolapsed aortic leaflet in VSD
Rheumatic heart disease
Complex congenital heart disease:
  A Truncus arteriosus
  B Pulmonary atresia
  C Tetralogy of Fallot
  D L-transposition of great arteries
Trauma
Connective-tissue disorders:
  A Marfan's syndrome
  B Osteogenesis imperfecta
  C Ehlers-Danlos syndrome
Mucopolysaccharidosis:
  A Hurler's syndrome
  B Morquio's syndrome
  C Scheie's syndrome

associated with a very high risk of rapid deterioration if the insufficiency is not relieved.[57,58] Once cardiac enlargement has reached massive proportions and congestive heart failure has occurred, prognosis for good postoperative performance is poor.[59,60]

The vast majority of children requiring surgical correction of aortic insufficiency have significant associated aortic stenosis with a thickened, deformed valve that prohibits any realistic hope of effective valvuloplasty. These children require aortic valve replacement. In some patients with aortic insufficiency associated with other cardiac abnormalities, such as ventricular septal defect[61] (Fig. 18) and truncus arteriosus,[62] closure of the septal defect and plication or reefing sutures in the aortic valve improve or arrest progression of the aortic insufficiency. A significant number of these patients will subsequently require aortic valve replacement (Fig. 19).

Acute aortic insufficiency such as that associated with aortic valve endocarditis, trauma, or prosthetic valve malfunction is usually severe and is not tolerated. Hemodynamic deterioration occurs rapidly, necessitating immediate repair or replacement of the aortic valve.[63,64] In patients with aortic valve endocarditis, the status of the infection should have no bearing on the decision to operate. It must be kept in mind that the greatest immediate threat to the patient's life is the

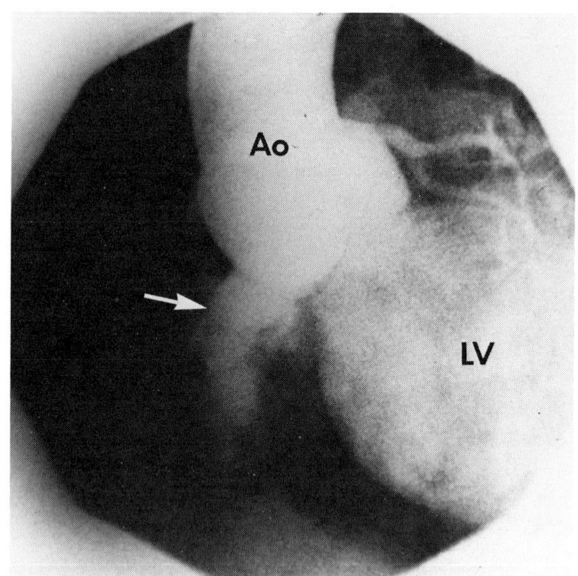

FIGURE 18 Left anterior oblique projection of aortic root angiogram in a 10-year-old boy with ventricular septal defect and aortic insufficiency. Regurgitant contrast medium has filled the left ventricle and is passing across a very high ventricular septal defect (arrow) into the right ventricle.

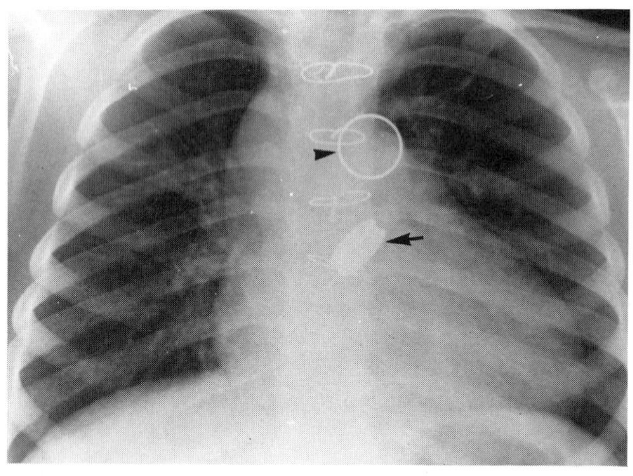

FIGURE 19 Chest radiogram on a 5-year-old patient with persistent truncus arteriosus who underwent correction in infancy utilizing a porcine valved (arrowhead) conduit from right ventricle to pulmonary artery confluence. Subsequent development of severe truncal valve insufficiency necessitated replacement of the truncal valve with a prosthetic valve (arrow).

aortic insufficiency. Excellent results may be achieved from aortic valve replacement in the presence of active infective endocarditis.[65]

Just as with aortic stenosis, aortic valve replacement for aortic insufficiency must be considered palliative.

Continued growth of the child, mechanical malfunction, periprosthetic leak, prosthetic valve endocarditis, or thrombus formation all may necessitate subsequent replacement.[1,3,52,66]

REFERENCES

1 Roberts, W. C.: Complications of Cardiac Valve Replacement: Characteristic Abnormalities of Prostheses Pertaining to Any or Specific Site, *Am. Heart J.,* 103:113, 1982.

2 Wilson, W. R., Jaumin, P. M., Danielson, G. R., Giuliani, E. R., Washington, J. A., II, and Geraci, J. E.: Prosthetic Valve Endocarditis, *Ann. Intern. Med.,* 82:751, 1975.

3 Rossiter, S. J., Stinson, E. B., Oyer, P. E., et al.: Prosthetic Valve Endocarditis: Comparison of Heterograft Tissue Valves and Mechanical Valves, *J. Thorac. Cardiovasc. Surg.,* 76:795, 1978.

4 Keane, J. F., Bernhard, W. F., and Nadas, A. S.: Aortic Stenosis Surgery in Infancy, *Circulation,* 52:1138, 1975.

5 Lakier, J. B., Lewis, A. B., Heymann, M. A., Stanger, P., Hoffman, J. I. E., and Rudolph, A. M.: Isolated Aortic Stenosis in the Neonate: Natural History and Hemodynamic Considerations, *Circulation,* 50:801, 1974.

6 Hastreiter, A. R., Oshima, M., Miller, R. A., Lev, M., and Paul, M. H.: Congenital Aortic Stenosis Syndrome in Infancy, *Circulation,* 28:1084, 1963.

7 Kugler, J. D., Campbell, E., Vargo, T. A., McNamara, D. G., Hallman, G. L., and Cooley, D. A.: Results of Aortic Valvotomy in Infants with Isolated Aortic Valvular Stenosis, *J. Thorac, Cardiovasc. Surg.,* 78:533, 1979.

8 Rudolph, A. M.: "Congenital Diseases of the Heart," Year Book Medical Publishers, Chicago, 1975, p. 8.

9 Moller, J. H., Nakib, A., and Edwards, J. E.: Infarction of the Papillary Muscles and Mitral Insufficiency Associated with Congenital Aortic Stenosis, *Circulation,* 34:87, 1966.

10 Gorlin, R., and Gorlin, S. G.: Hydraulic Formula for Calculation of the Area of Stenotic Mitral Valve, Other Cardiac Valves, and Central Circulatory Shunts, part 1, *Am. Heart J.,* 41:1, 1951.

11 Bache, R. J., Jorgenson, C. R., and Yang, Y.: Simplified Estimation of Aortic Valve Area, *Br. Heart J.,* 34:408, 1972.

12 Graham, T. P.: Left Heart Volume Estimation in Infancy and Childhood. Reevaluation of Methodology and Normal Values, *Circulation,* 43:895, 1971.

13 Hallman, G. L., and Cooley, D. A.: "Surgical Treatment of Congenital Heart Disease," 2d ed, Lea & Febiger, Philadelphia, 1975, pp. 59–62.

14 Coran, A. G., and Bernhard, W. F.: The Surgical Management of Valvular Aortic Stenosis during Infancy, *J. Thorac. Cardiovasc. Surg.,* 58:401, 1969.

15 McGoon, D. C., Geha, A. S., Scofield, E. L., and DuShane J. W.: Surgical Treatment of Congenital Aortic Stenosis, *Dis. Chest,* 55:388, 1969.

16 Keane, J. F., Bernhard, W. F., Casteneda, A. R., and Nadas, A. S.: Course of Survivors Following Valvotomy for Critical Aortic Stenosis in Infancy, *Circulation,* 56 (suppl. 3):103, 1977. (Abstract.)

17 Edmunds, L. H., Wagner, H. R., and Heymann, M. A.: Aortic Valvotomy in Neonates, *Circulation,* 61:421, 1980.

18 Hoffman, J. I. E.: The Natural History of Congenital Isolated Pulmonic and Aortic Stenosis, *Ann. Rev. Med.,* 20:15, 1969.

19 Vincent, W. R., Buckberg, G. D., and Hoffman, J. I. E.: Left Ventricular Subendocardial Ischemia in Severe Valvar and Supravalvar Aortic Stenosis: A Common Mechanism, *Circulation,* 49:326, 1974.

20 Brazier, J., Cooper, N., and Buckberg, G.: The Adequacy of Subendocardial Oxygen Needs, *Circulation,* 48 (suppl. 4):91, 1973.

21 Braunwald, E., Goldblatt, A., Aygen, M. M., Rockoff, S. D., and Morrow, A. G.: Congenital Aortic Stenosis, *Circulation,* 27:426, 1963.

22 Lewis, A. B., Heymann, M. A., Stanger, P., Hoffman, J. I. E., and Rudolph, A. M.: Evaluation of Subendocardial Ischemia in Valvar Aortic Stenosis in Children, *Circulation,* 49:978, 1974.

23 Cohen, L. S., Friedman, W. F., and Braunwald, E.: Natural History of Mild Congenital Aortic Stenosis Elucidated by Serial Hemodynamic Studies, *Am. J. Cardiol.,* 30:1, 1972.

24 Hoffman, J. I. E., and Buckberg, G. D.: The Myocardial Supply: Demand Ratio—A Critical Review, *Am. J. Cardiol.,* 41:327, 1978.

25 Buckberg, G. D., Fixler, D. E., Archie, J. P., and Hoffman, J. I. E.: Experimental Subendocardial Ischemia in Dogs with Normal Coronary Arteries, *Circ. Res.,* 30:67, 1972.

26 Oldershaw, P. J., Brooksby, I. A. B., Davies, M. J., Coltart, D. J., Jenkins, B. S., and Webb-Peploe, M. M.: Correlations of Fibrosis in Endomyocardial Biopsies from Patients with Aortic Valve Disease, *Br. Heart J.* 44:609, 1980.

27 Bailey, I. K., Come, P. C., Kelly, D. T., et al.: Thallium-201 Myocardial Perfusion Imaging in Aortic Valve Stenosis, *Am. J. Cardiol.,* 40:889, 1977.

28 Hohn, A. R., Van Praagh, S., Moore, A. A. D., Vlad, P., and Lambert, E. C.: "Aortic Stenosis—5 Congenital Cardiac Defects," American Heart Association Monograph no. 12, *Circulation,* 31 (suppl. 3):4, 1965.

29 Campbell, M.: The Natural History of Congenital Aortic Stenosis, *Br. Heart J.,* 30:514, 1968.

30 Schwartz, L. S., Goldfischer, J., Sprague, G. J., and Schwartz, S. P.: Syncope and Sudden Death in Aortic Stenosis, *Am. J. Cardiol.,* 23:647, 1969.

31 Glen, R. H., Varghese, J. P., Krovetz, J. L., Dorst, J. P., and Rowe, R. D.: Sudden Death in Congenital Aortic Stenosis, *Am. Heart J.,* 78:615, 1969.

32 Cueto, L., and Moller, J. H.: Haemodynamics of Exercise in Children with Isolated Aortic Valvular Disease, *Br. Heart J.,* 35:93, 1973.

33 Friedman, W. F., Modlinger, J., and Morgan, J. R.: Serial Hemodynamic Observations in Asymptomatic Children with Valvar Aortic Stenosis, *Circulation,* 43:91, 1971.

34 El-Said, G., Galioto, F. M., Mullins, C. E., and McNamara, D. G.: Natural Hemodynamic History of Congenital Aortic Stenosis in Childhood, *Am. J. Cardiol.,* 30:6, 1972.

35 Halloran, K. H.: Telemetered Exercise Electrocardiogram in Congenital Aortic Stenosis, *Pediatrics,* 47:31, 1971.

36 Chandramouli, B., Ehmke, D. A., and Lauer, R. M.: Exercise-Induced Electrocardiographic Changes in Children with Congenital Aortic Stenosis, *J. Pediatr.,* 87:725, 1975.

37 Whitmer, J. T., James, F. W., Kaplan, S., Schwartz, D. C., and Knight, M. J. S.: Exercise Testing in Children before and after Surgical Treatment of Aortic Stenosis, *Circulation,* 63:254, 1981.

38 Riopel, D. A., and Hohn, A. R.: Age Effect on Treadmill Blood Pressure Responses in Aortic Stenosis, *Pediatr. Res.,* 11:399, 1977. (Abstract.)

39 Alpert, B. S., Kartodihardjo, W., Harp, R., Izukawa, T., and Strong, W. B.: Exercise Blood Pressure Response—A Predictor of Severity of Aortic Stenosis in Children, *J. Pediatr.,* 98:763, 1981.

40 Glanz, S., Hellenbrand, W. E., Berman, M. A., and Talner, N. S.: Echocardiographic Assessment of the Severity of Aortic Stenosis in Children and Adolescents, *Am. J. Cardiol.,* 38:620, 1976.

41 Blackwood, R. A., Bloom, K. R., and Williams, C. M.: Aortic Stenosis in Children. Experience with Echocardiographic Prediction of Severity, *Circulation,* 57:263, 1978.

42 Brenner, J. I., Baker, K. R., and Berman, M. A.: Prediction of Left-Ventricular Pressure in Infants with Aortic Stenosis, *Br. Heart J.,* 44:406, 1980.

43 Johnson, G. L., Meyer, R. A., Schwartz, D. C., Korfhagen, J., and Kaplan, S.: Left Ventricular Function by Echocardiography in Children with Fixed Aortic Stenosis, *Am. J. Cardiol.,* 38:611, 1976.

44 Bass, J. L., Einzig, S., Hong, C. Y., and Moller, J. H.: Echocardiographic Screening to Assess the Severity of Congenital Aortic Valve Stenosis in Children, *Am. J. Cardiol.,* 44:82, 1979.

45 Kececioglu-Draelos, Z., and Goldberg, S. J.: Role of M-Mode Echocardiography in Congenital Aortic Stenosis, *Am. J. Cardiol.,* 46:1267, 1981.

46 Weyman, A. E., Feigenbaum, H., Hurwitz, R. A., Girod, D. A., and Dillon, J. C.: Cross-Sectional Echocardiographic Assessment of the Severity of Aortic Stenosis in Children, *Circulation,* 55:773, 1977.

47 DeMaria, A. N., Bommer, W., Joye, J., Lee, G., Bouteller, J., and Mason, D. T.: Value and Limitations of Cross-Sectional Echocardiography of the Aortic Valve in the Diagnosis and Quantification of Valvular Aortic Stenosis, *Circulation,* 62:304, 1980.

48 Shackleton, J., Edwards, F. R., Bickford, B. J., and Jones, R. S.: Long-Term Follow-Up of Congenital Aortic Stenosis after Surgery, *Br. Heart J.,* 34:47, 1972.

49 Jack, W. D., Jr., and Kelly, D. T.: Long-Term Follow-Up of Valvulotomy for Congenital Aortic Stenosis, *Am. J. Cardiol.,* 38:231, 1976.

50 Lawson, R. M., Bonchek, L. I., Menashe, V., and Starr, A.: Late Results of Surgery for Left Ventricular Outflow Tract Obstruction in Children, *J. Thorac. Cardiovasc. Surg.,* 71:334, 1976.

51 Dobell, A. R. C., Bloss, R. S., Gibbons, J. E., and Collins, G. F.: Congenital Valvular Aortic Stenosis. Surgical Management and Long-Term Results, *J. Thorac. Cardiovasc. Surg.,* 81:916, 1981.

52 Wilson, W. R., Danielson, G. K., Giuliani, E. R., and Geraci, J. E.: Prosthetic Valve Endocarditis, *Mayo Clin. Proc.,* 57:155, 1982.

53 Gault, J. H., Covell, J. W., Braunwald, E., and Ross, J., Jr.: Left Ventricular Performance Following Correction of Free Aortic Regurgitation, *Circulation,* 42:773, 1970.

54 Braun, L. O., Kincaid, O. W., and McGoon, D. C.: Prognosis of Aortic Valve Replacement in Relation to Preoperative Heart Size, *J. Thorac. Cardiovasc. Surg.,* 65:381, 1973.

55 O'Rourke, R. A., and Crawford, M. H.: Timing of Valve Replacement in Patients with Chronic Aortic Regurgitation, *Circulation,* 61:493, 1980.

56 Lewis, R. P., Bristow, J. D., and Griswold, H. E.: Exercise Hemodynamics in Aortic Regurgitation, *Am. Heart J.,* 80:171, 1970.

57 Spagnuolo, M., Kloth, H., Taranta, A., Doyle, E., and Pasternack, B.: Natural History of Rheumatic Aortic Regurgitation. Criteria Predictive of Death, Congestive Heart Failure, and Angina in Young Patients, *Circulation,* 44:368, 1971.

58 Smith, H. J., Neutze, J. M., Roche, A. H. G., Agnew, T. M., and Barratt-Boyes, B. G.: The Natural History of Rheumatic Aortic Regurgitation and the Indications for Surgery, *Br. Heart J.,* 38:147, 1976.

59 Henry, W. L., Bonow, R. O., Borer, J. S., et al.: Observations on the Optimum Time for Operative Intervention for Aortic Regurgitation. I. Evaluation of the Results of Aortic Valve Replacement in Symptomatic Patients, *Circulation,* 61:471, 1980.

60 Henry, W. L., Bonow, R. D., Rosing, D. R., and Epstein, S. E.: Observations on the Optimum Time for Operative Intervention for Aortic Regurgitation: II. Serial Echocardiographic Evaluation of Asymptomatic Patients, *Circulation,* 61:484, 1980.

61 Karpawich, P. P., Duff, D. E., Mullins, C. E., Cooley, D. A., and McNamara, D. G.: Ventricular Septal Defect with Associated Aortic Valve Insufficiency, *J. Thorac. Cardiovasc. Surg.,* 82:182, 1981.

62 De Leval, M. R., McGoon, D. C., Wallace, R. B., Danielson, G. K., and Mair, D. D.: Management of Truncal Valvular Regurgitation, *Ann. Surg.*, 180:427, 1974.

63 Wilson, W. R., Danielson, G. K., Giuliani, E. R., Washington, J. A., II, Jaumin, P. M., and Geraci, J. E.: Cardiac Valve Replacement in Congestive Heart Failure Due to Infective Endocarditis, *Mayo Clin. Proc.*, 54:223, 1979.

64 Gersony, W. M., Willerson, W. D., Jr., Johnson, A. F., and Webb, W. R.: Aortic Valvuloplasty during Acute Rheumatic Fever, *J. Thorac. Cardiovasc. Surg.*, 55:598, 1968.

65 Wilson, W. R., Danielson, G. K., Giuliani, E. R., Washington, J. A., II, Jaumin, P. M., and Geraci, J. E.: Valve Replacement in Patients with Active Infective Endocarditis, *Circulation*, 58:585, 1978.

66 Slaughter, L., Morris, J. E., and Starr, A.: Prosthetic Valvular Endocarditis: A 12-Year Review, *Circulation*, 47:1319, 1973.

Ventricular Septal Defect and Surgical Indications for Closure[*]

KENNETH J. DOOLEY, M.D.

Physician, do your best for your patient in judgment and practice. When uncertainty prevails seek council from others and above all do no harm.

HIPPOCRATES

A *ventricular septal defect* is an abnormal communication between the ventricular chambers of the heart that allows the passage of blood from one chamber to the other. The clinical features of this defect were first described in 1879 by Roger,[1] at which time the underlying pathology was described. His description of a heart murmur as a harsh systolic murmur over the fourth left intercostal space has been carried on as the classical description of the defect in its mildest form, known by the term *maladie de Roger.*

The complex of a simple ventricular septal defect associated with elevation of the pulmonary artery pressure and pulmonary vascular resistance, known as *Eisenmenger's complex,* was described by Dalrymple[2] in 1847, and Eisenmenger[3] reported a similar case in 1897. Maude Abbott,[4] in 1932, gathered a number of case records together from the literature and established the use of the term *Eisenmenger's complex.* The hemodynamics of this complex were confirmed by Blount[5] in 1955 and Wood[6] in 1954.

The surgical closure of the ventricular septal defect was first described by Lillehei[7] in 1955 using controlled cross-circulation in order to allow direct visualization of the defect. Since that time, the use of cardiopulmonary bypass and profound hypothermia has advanced the techniques of assisted circulation and allowed for the repair of this defect in young children and infants.

This paper includes an anatomic classification of ventricular septal defect with an embryonic description. The incidence, natural history, and clinical features will be discussed as well as physiologic data. The indications for surgical intervention will be presented with a review of the published results of surgery, including the various methods of surgical intervention. The information in this paper will be limited to the simple ventricular septal defect, with the exception of acquired aortic insufficiency associated with ventricular septal defect. The common atrioventricular communication or endocardial cushion defect will not be reviewed.

EMBRYOLOGY

When one reviews the embryogenesis of the ventricular septum, it is really quite amazing that the ventricular septum is intact as frequently as it is. From the combined embryologic and anatomic standpoint, the ventricular septum is composed of four components: (1) the bulbar septum, (2) the retrocristal septum, (3) the atrioventricular septum (endocardial cushion tissue), and (4) the ventricular sinus portion, or muscular portion (Fig. 1). In order for the ventricular septum to ultimately be intact, it requires the union of all four of these segments at the appropriate time. The ventricular sinus portion of the ventricular septum is formed by an out-pouching of the two ventricular cavities around the bulboventricular foramen, while, at the same time, there is elevation of the papillary muscles from the ventricular free walls and septum. The muscular septum does not grow from the apex of the heart toward the inflow portion, but rather is an out-pouching as just described. The formation of the bulbar septum is the result of fusion of cardiac jelly in the great vessels secondary to flow patterns in these vessels. Their ultimate alignment with the appropriate ventricular chambers then occurs. The inferior fusion of the bulbar septum with the muscular septum and atrioventricular septum then occurs for completion of the fusion, with the final component being closure of the membranous portion of the ventricular septum. The formation of the ventricular septum is occurring at the 5-mm stage of embryonic development, which is approximately the latter part of the fourth week of gestation.[8] Incomplete fusion between the bulbar and muscular septa leads to the formation of type I and type II ventricular defects, while imperfect fusion of the atrioventricular septum with the muscular septum leads to the type III defect. Incomplete or inadequate muscular development in the ventricular septum leads to the formation of type IV defects. The etiology of incomplete fusion and the residual defect is unknown.

ANATOMIC DESCRIPTION

Many attempts have been made at classification of the ventricular septal defect.[9-11] The most commonly accepted classification is that seen in Fig. 1. This classification is divided into four types based on embryologic development of the ventricular septum. Type I is the subpulmonic or supracristal ventricular communication. This defect comprises approximately 8 percent of

[*]From the Department of Pediatrics, Emory University School of Medicine, Atlanta, Georgia.

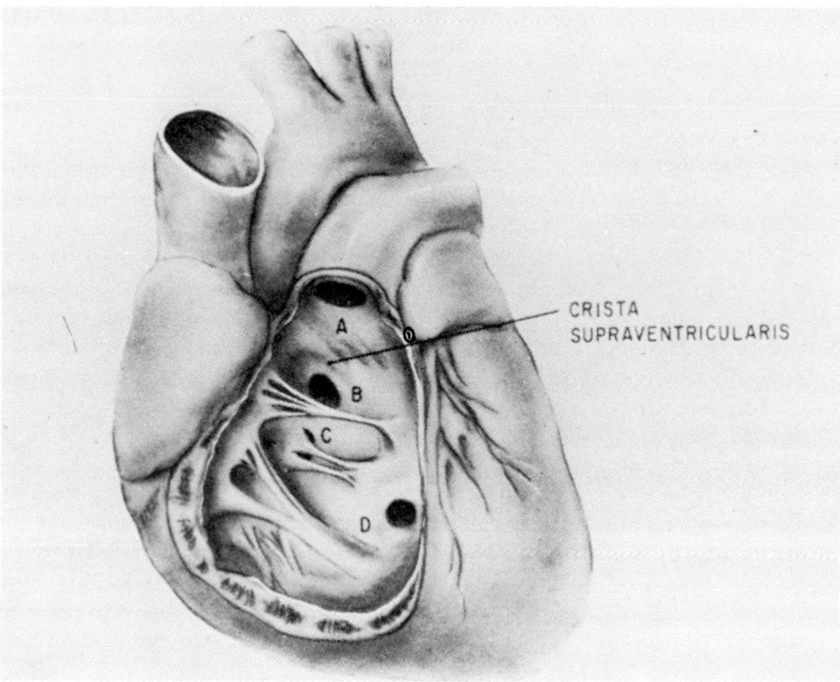

FIGURE 1 (*A*) Bulbar septum or conotruncal septum with supracristal or subpulmonic ventricular defect, type I. (*B*) Retrocristal or membranous septum with membranous ventricular defect, type II. (*C*) Atrioventricular septum with associated defect, type III. (*D*) Ventricular sinus or muscular septum with associated defect, type IV. (*From J. W. Kirklin, H. G. Harshbarger, D. E. Donald, and J. E. Edwards, Surgical Correction of Ventricular Septal Defect: Anatomic and Technical Considerations, J. Thorac. Surg., 33:45, 1957. Slightly modified. Used with permission.*)

ventricular septal defects. The most common form of the ventricular septal defect is the supracristal membranous ventricular defect and lies in the area below the crista supraventricularis and posterior to the papillary muscle of the conus of the tricuspid valve. Seventy-five percent of ventricular defects lie in this region. The third category of defect is that found in the posterior ventricular septum beneath the septal and posterior leaflets of the tricuspid valve. This is the region of the ventricular septum comprised and closed by the endocardial cushions and makes up approximately 4 percent of ventricular defects. The fourth category of defect is that found in the muscular ventricular septum, and this comprises the remainder of the defects. These defects may either be single or multiple, having tortuous channels as they cross the ventricular septum. Of special interest when evaluating the anatomy of the ventricular septum is the position of the aortic valve in relationship to the supracristal ventricular defects. Because of the flow currents through the defect, very often the right, or noncoronary, cusp of the aortic valve may actually be drawn into the defect, giving the impression of small size, but this allows continued distortion and deterioration of the aortic cusp, leading to aortic insufficiency.

In evaluating patients with type III ventricular septal defect, one must also keep in mind the embryology and development of this defect involving the endocardial cushion. These patients may have evidence of a primum atrial septal defect as well as anomalies of the atrioventricular valve.

One must also be keenly aware of the location of the conduction system in dealing with ventricular defects, since it traverses the posterior tricuspid annulus and very often the His bundle and bundle branches are located on the posteroinferior and inferior rims of these defects. This has even greater importance when one is contemplating surgical closure of the defect.

INCIDENCE, NATURAL HISTORY, AND PROGNOSIS OF VENTRICULAR SEPTAL DEFECTS

Incidence

Ventricular septal defects have been long recognized as among the most common congenital cardiac defects. The incidence of ventricular septal defects has varied between 16.6 and 31.3 percent, as referenced in articles by Keith et al.,[12] Nadas and Fyler,[13] Mitchell et al.,[14] Hoffman and Christianson,[15] and Fyler.[16] The defect occurs in approximately 2 per 1,000 live births, and it is estimated to be present in 1 per 1,000 children of school age. There is no differentiation by sex in this defect, and the mode of transmission is thought to be multifactorial. In evaluating the adult population, approximately 10 percent of congenital malformations found in adults are those of ventricular septal defect.[17,18]

Natural History and Prognosis

The natural history of ventricular septal defect, being the most common congenital lesion in children, has been followed quite thoroughly. These patients are fortunate in that the majority of defects will become hemodynamically insignificant as the child grows. The natural history of these defects, as one might expect, is related to the size of the defect and the pulmonary vascular resistance.

Factors that influence the natural history of the ventricular septal defect include congestive heart failure, acquired pulmonic stenosis, acquired pulmonary vascular obstructive disease, and aortic insufficiency. Congestive heart failure is usually the presenting problem in the child who is physically disabled by the congenital defect. The evidence of heart failure usually is recognized between the second and the sixth week of life. Eighty percent of infants who will develop congestive heart failure require medical management by the fourth month of life, and it is very unusual for a child to present with congestive heart failure beyond the eighth month. Late causes of congestive heart failure include associated congenital malformations and other conditions that may be superimposed on the ventricular septal defect, such as infective endocarditis, anemia, thyrotoxicosis, pneumonia, or myocardial disease. Premature infants may present with congestive heart failure earlier in life because of the more rapid regression of pulmonary vascular resistance related to the immaturity of the premature vascular tree.

Spontaneous improvement in the child who has developed congestive heart failure from a ventricular septal defect may have several etiologies. The most common cause for improvement is spontaneous decrease in size or closure of the defect. The development of subpulmonic stenosis would also show improvement in the clinical condition with congestive heart failure, and this occurs in approximately 3 percent of infants and children. Children with supracristal ventricular defects can very often show evidence of improvement as the coronary cusp prolapses into the ventricular defect causing progressive decrease in the lumen of the defect and therefore decrease in size. As this particular condition progresses, eventually the patient will de-

velop evidence of aortic insufficiency, and sometimes the clinician is misled into feeling that the patient may have a ductus arteriosus. The final etiology for evidence of improvement in congestive heart failure is the development of pulmonary vascular obstructive disease. This rarely occurs before 12 months of age and becomes more common as an etiology as time progresses.[19] This phenomenon is often referred to as *Eisenmenger's complex,* and the average age of death of these patients is 33 years, with the causes commonly being related to arrhythmia or acute pulmonary hemorrhage, both usually of sudden onset.[20] In rare instances, a patient may have persistence of the fetal pattern of pulmonary vascular resistance and not present with the clinical findings of a large ventricular septal defect. This can occur in individuals who are living at high altitude and also is frequently seen in patients with Down's syndrome.[21] They do not present with the classical murmur or evidence of congestive heart failure.

Patients not presenting with congestive heart failure very often have small- to modest-sized defects. In the series reported by Alpert et al.,[22] 24 percent of the patients with small defects showed spontaneous closure by 18 months; 50 percent by 4 years; and 75 percent by 10 years. Moderate- and large-sized defects may also become smaller and eventually close, and Blackstone et al.[19] have estimated that approximately 75 percent of patients with defects estimated to be large at 6 months of age would show either closure or enough reduction in size to produce eventual closure by 10 years of age.

When the natural history of the ventricular septal defect is being reviewed, one must keep in mind the ever-present complication of infective endocarditis. The risk of this complication is approximately 10 percent in the first 30 years of life, with the risk increasing six times for the interval between 20 and 30 years of life when compared with the interval between birth and 20 years.[23]

CLINICAL FEATURES AS RELATED TO DEFECT SIZE
Small

As one would expect, the clinical features of the ventricular septal defect are very much related to its size. Infants presenting with small defects are usually referred for evaluation because of the presence of a heart murmur. Most commonly, the systolic murmur is heard on the first examination at approximately 4 weeks of age, but in infants with very tiny defects, the murmur may be heard as early as 24 to 36 h of age. The murmur is loudest near the left lower sternal border. These infants usually have a fairly normal examination with no evidence of congestive heart failure, and their cardiac examination would possibly reveal a faint systolic thrill at the lower left sternal border, but this may be absent. The first and second heart sounds are usually normal, and there is usually no evidence of a diastolic flow murmur.

Moderate

The next group of patients to present is comprised of children with moderate-sized defects. These patients will show evidence of mild growth retardation, mild feeding difficulties with diaphoresis, and some tachypnea. Their clinical examination often shows evidence of mild tachypnea and hepatomegaly. Cardiac examination reveals a slight increase in the left ventricular impulse, a normal first heart sound, and a second heart sound that may show some mild increase in the pulmonic component. Such patients very often have a thrill at the left lower sternal border, and on auscultation, they have a characteristic holosystolic murmur at the left lower sternal border and a middiastolic flow murmur at the apex. The latter murmur is referred to as a *mitral rumble* and is heard most frequently in patients with a shunt ratio of greater than 2:1. These patients very often will need some medical intervention, but the majority of these defects become smaller in size and very often close. Once one is sure of the diagnosis of ventricular septal defect and the child is beyond 4 months of age, there is little likelihood that the child will develop evidence of congestive heart failure, and therefore, the prognosis in this group of patients is usually quite good.

Large

The infant with a large ventricular septal defect, however, presents with a different picture. The history will usually reveal that the child has had rather poor weight gain, poor feeding, excessive sweating, and fatigue. The parents may or may not recognize that the child has evidence of tachypnea and grunting, and not infrequently the child may have had hospitalizations for pulmonary infections. The clinical examination in the large defect usually reveals a child with poor weight gain and obvious lack of subcutaneous fat. The child will be obviously tachypneic, very often with retractions and nasal flaring. On palpation, it may be noted that the child is diaphoretic and the liver and sometimes the spleen are enlarged. Pulses are usually palpable but may be decreased in volume. Precordial examination

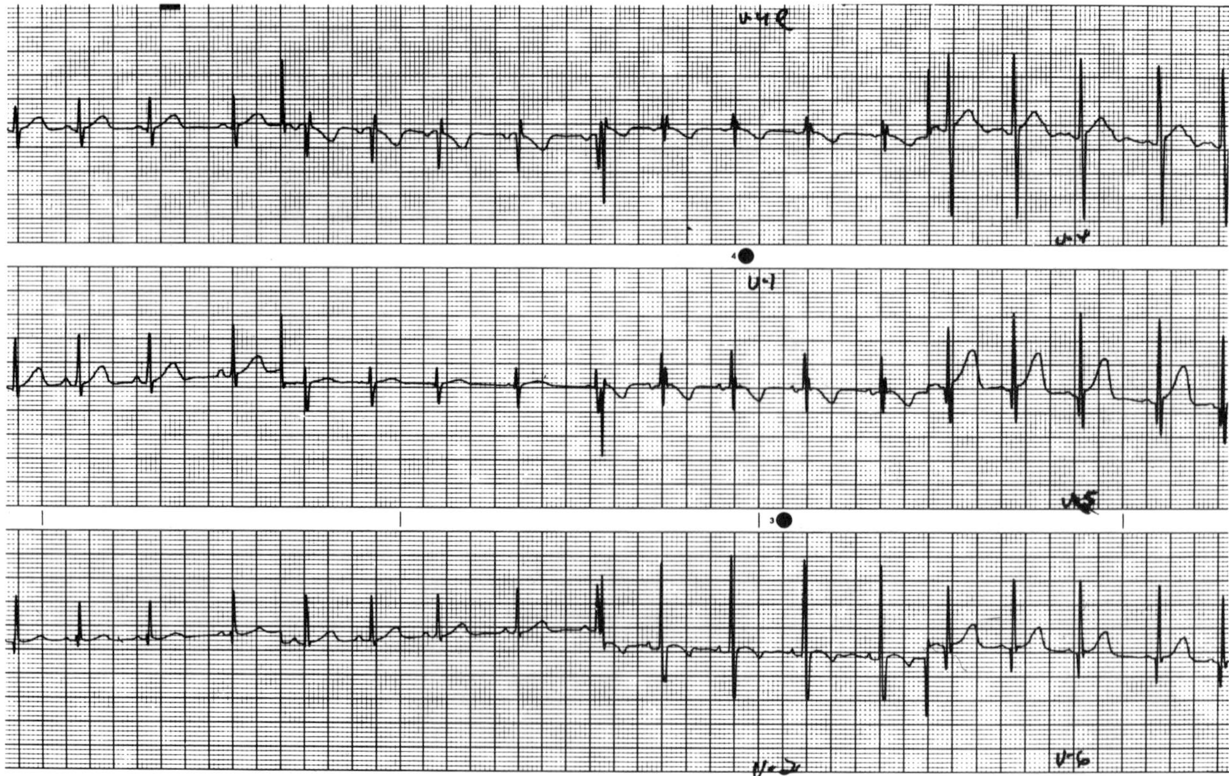

FIGURE 2 ECG in patient with moderate VSD.

will reveal hyperdynamic right and left ventricular impulses associated with palpable thrill along the left sternal border. Auscultation usually reveals a first heart sound with increased intensity and a second heart sound that is split with an increased intensity of the pulmonary component. In these children, it is quite common to find an S_3, best heard at the apex, and, with marked deterioration, an S_4. The murmur is usually of grade IV intensity, holosystolic, and is loudest near the left lower sternal border. A middiastolic rumble of grades II to III in intensity is usually heard at the apex. Examination of the lungs rarely reveals evidence of rales, but it may if there is an associated pulmonary infection.

Evidence of cyanosis or absent or markedly diminished pulses should lead one to suspect associated cardiac defects. Although the child with profound congestive heart failure will appear somewhat ash-gray, oxygen analysis usually reveals that they are not extremely hypoxic, and they respond quite appropriately to the administration of oxygen. It is the child with the large ventricular septal defect that most frequently requires medical intervention and usually surgical intervention. As time progresses, the defect may become smaller in size and the symptomatology improve. However, one must constantly be alert to the possible development of increasing pulmonary vascular resistance, which could lead to pulmonary vascular obstructive disease as well as the development of subvalvar pulmonic stenosis.

LABORATORY DATA
Electrocardiogram

The electrocardiogram in infants with small to moderate ventricular defects usually is quite normal, both in axis and ventricular voltage. As the volume overload of the left ventricle progresses in the moderate- to large-sized defect, there is progressive evidence of left ventricular hypertrophy with evidence of progressively increasing Q waves over the lateral precordium, indicative of volume overload of the ventricle (Fig. 2). It is usually about this time that evidence of left atrial hypertrophy becomes apparent. The child who has persistence of the fetal right ventricular hypertrophy very often will have a very large ventricular defect with pulmonary artery hypertension. The child who acquires right ventricular hypertrophy, however, may be developing either subvalvular pulmonic stenosis or pulmo-

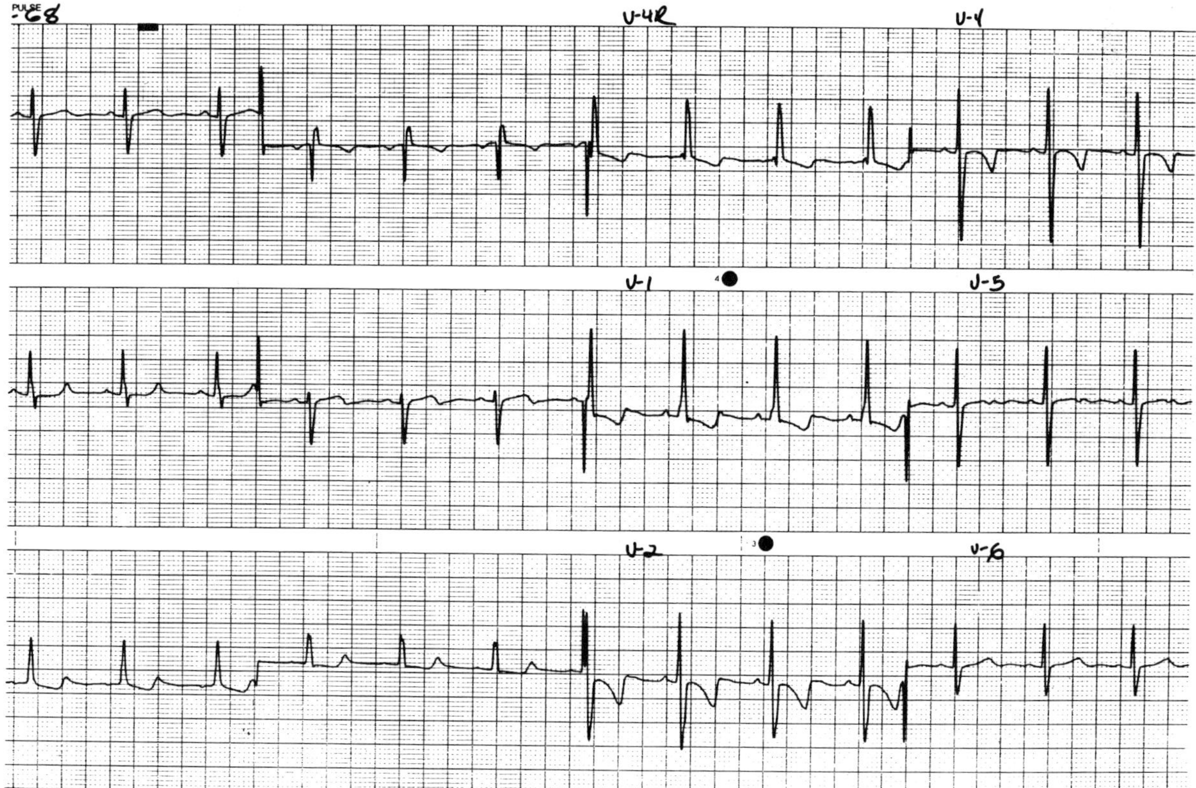

FIGURE 3 ECG in patient with large VSD and right ventricular hypertension.

nary vascular disease, and these entities must be differentiated because their ultimate prognoses are markedly different. The development of right ventricular hypertrophy is often associated with a progressive shift of the QRS axis toward the right (Fig. 3).

Chest Roentgenogram

The child with the small- to moderate-sized ventricular defect very often shows a normal cardiac silhouette and pulmonary vascular markings. As the size and flow increase in the moderate to large defect, the pulmonary vascular markings become more prominent, particularly in the lower lung field, and the cardiac silhouette progressively increases. The lateral plane will very often show a progressive evidence of left atrial enlargement as the flow is increasing. Interstitial edema and true pulmonary edema may be seen in patients with congestive heart failure (Fig. 4). Evidence of an increase in pulmonary vascular flow without left atrial enlargement should lead one to suspect that there is also an atrial communication. Progressive cardiac enlargement can also cause compression of the left main stem bronchus, leading to atelectasis, either partial or complete, and pneumonia. As the defect becomes smaller or pulmonary stenosis develops, the cardiac contour progressively becomes smaller and the pulmonary vascular pattern does not remain as prominent. However, if pulmonary vascular obstruction is occurring, the proximal and main pulmonary arteries usually become quite prominent, indicative of the high pressure reflected in these vessels.

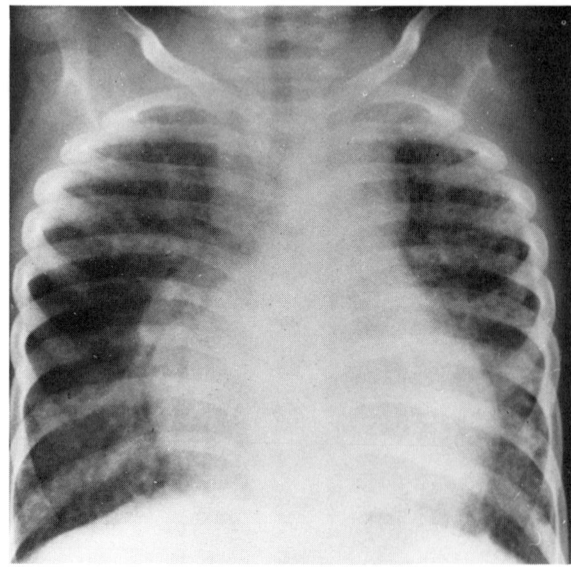

FIGURE 4 Radiograph of child with congestive heart failure and pulmonary hypertension.

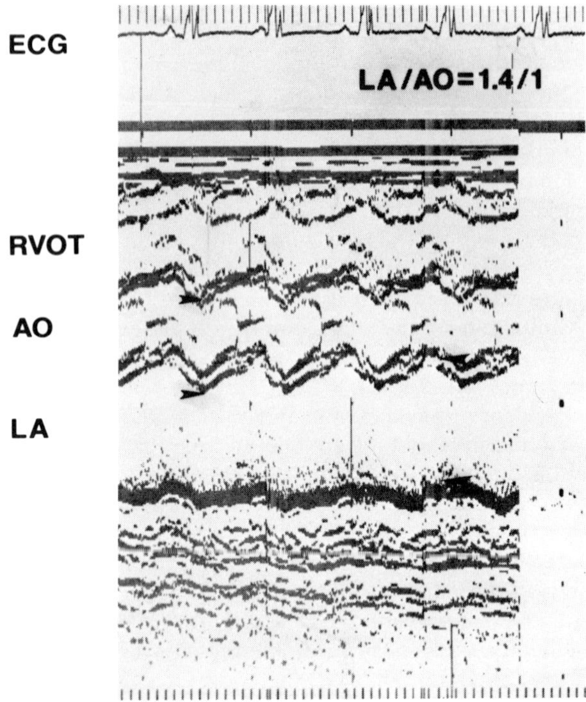

FIGURE 5 Echocardiogram indicating increased left atrial (LA) to aortic (AO) ratio. RVOT = right ventricular outflow tract.

Echocardiogram

The echocardiogram has progressively gained importance in evaluating children with congenital heart disease. Using the two-dimensional echocardiogram for anatomic definition and M-mode imaging for chamber size and function aids significantly in evaluating the physiologic status of the patient. Evidence of an increased left atrial diameter when compared with that of the ascending aorta (Fig. 5) can be used to indicate left atrial volume overload.[24] Measurement of right ventricular pre-ejection period over right ventricular ejection time has been useful in predicting pulmonary artery diastolic hypertension. A ratio of greater than 0.3 is suggestive of pulmonary artery hypertension.[25] The use of two-dimensional echocardiography, needless to say, allows visualization of the larger defects and can often assist in the evaluation of subpulmonic stenosis and aortic overriding and the differentiation of the various types of single ventricle, which may present with findings compatible to a ventricular septal defect.

Radionuclide Angiocardiography[26]

Radioisotopes are progressively becoming a useful tool in the evaluation of the cardiac patient. Not only can volume analysis, cardiac output, and ejection fractions be calculated, but this technique can be used for shunt quantitation.[27] Although this is a somewhat invasive procedure in the fact that the isotope is injected intravenously, it is usually a fairly reliable study, and when combined with previous laboratory studies, it should be quite helpful in guiding the physician as to which patients will require invasive diagnostic procedures.

Cardiac Catheterization

Invasive procedures such as cardiac catheterization should be reserved for those patients who are unresponsive to routine medical management or in whom there is any question as to the accuracy of diagnosis. If one has any doubt as to whether a lesion is a pure ventricular septal defect or not, cardiac catheterization is indicated if one is not totally convinced from noninvasive studies. Cardiac catheterization is divided into two components—anatomic definition and physiologic function. The physiologic component of catheterization should be performed before the volume change created by contrast injections occurs. During a physiologic procedure, completeness of the study is imperative. Oxygen saturations and pressures should be obtained in all the major vessels entering and leaving the heart, as well as in all the heart chambers. It is preferable to be able to measure simultaneous systemic arterial pressure with systemic venous pressures, but this is not always possible. Information should be obtained that rules out evidence of pulmonic or aortic stenosis, as well as mitral stenosis and coarctation of the aorta. Anatomic definition is achieved by means of angiography. The techniques most frequently used today to outline ventricular septal defects are those of Bargeron et al.[28] and Elliott et al.,[29] and these have the advantage over the direct anteroposterior and lateral projections in the fact that they allow for better definition of the site and size of the ventricular septal defect, which carries a significant amount of information for the surgeon. Defects located in the posterior portion of the ventricular septum are often of the endocardial cushion variety, while very often defects in the anterior muscular septum are only clearly visualized in the right anterior oblique projections. The most useful view for the endocardial cushion (Fig. 6) and membranous type (Fig. 7) of defects is the left anterior oblique with cranial angulation, while the supracristal (Fig. 8) and anterior muscular septal (Fig. 9) defects are best seen in the right anterior oblique projection. One must also be careful to evaluate the coronary arterial anatomy and distribution, as well as to be sure that there is no evidence of a ductus arteriosus associated with the ventricular septal defect.

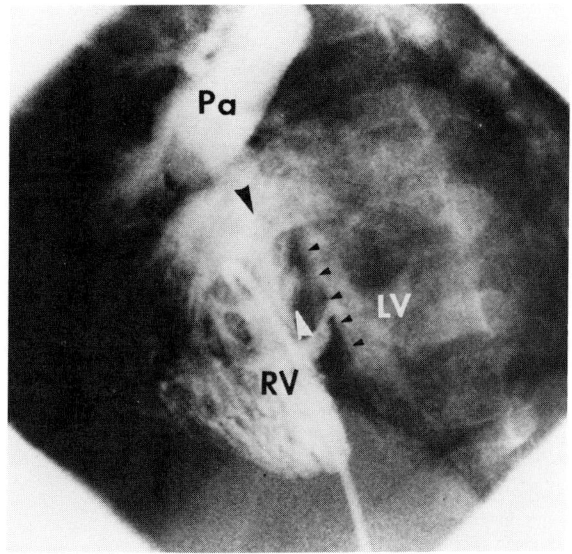

FIGURE 6 Four-chamber view visualizing posterior ventricular septal defect in endocardial cushion defect (large arrows). Anterior septal margins (small arrows). RV = right ventricle; LV = left ventricle; PA = pulmonary artery. (LAO 45° with cranial 45°.)

Accurate anatomic definition is an absolute necessity when evaluating a patient for surgical intervention.

INDICATIONS FOR SURGICAL INTERVENTION

The indications for surgical intervention are based more on the physiologic status of the patient than on the anatomic deformity. The *first* indication for surgical intervention is failure of medical management of congestive heart failure. Such failure usually occurs in infants with large ventricular communications and low pulmonary vascular resistance resulting in large systemic to pulmonary shunts and pulmonary artery hypertension. If the usual measures for control of congestive heart failure, i.e., digitalization, diuretics, and afterload reduction, are unsuccessful, these patients will require surgical intervention to allow them to have appropriate growth and development and not suffer the adverse effects of prolonged chronic congestive heart failure. The *second* indication for early intervention is persistent pulmonary artery hypertension beyond 1 year of age. This group of patients, if left without intervention, will eventually progress to pulmonary vascular disease, and this, in turn, will place them in the inoperable category with a poor prognostic outlook.

Those patients who continue to have a ventricular

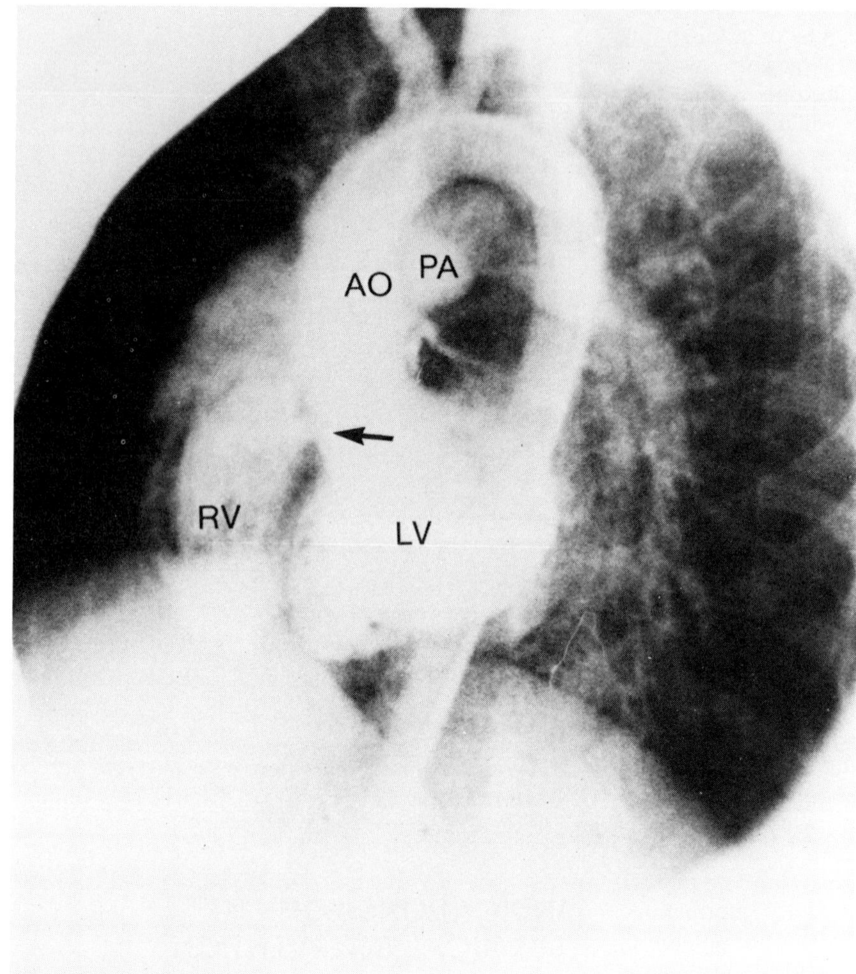

FIGURE 7 Membranous ventricular septal defect (arrow). Ao = aorta; PA = pulmonary artery; RV = right ventricle; LV = left ventricle. (LAO 60° with cranial 15°.)

septal defect beyond the first year of life with a pulmonary artery pressure of less than 50 percent of systemic level and a pulmonary-to-systemic flow ratio of greater than 2:1 require continued observations. Many of these defects will get smaller and eventually close, but very often a decision must be made as to when, and if, elective closure is indicated. It is my feeling that a patient with a pulmonary-to-systemic flow ratio of greater than 2:1 and a pulmonary artery pressure of less than 50 percent of systemic should undergo elective closure before entering school.

A very interesting group of patients is comprised of patients with a supracristal ventricular septal defect (type I) who are at risk of the aortic valve prolapsing into the defect and causing aortic insufficiency (Fig. 10). These patients, even though their shunts do not seem to be of significant size, may actually have large defects, because the cusp of the aortic leaflet (right or noncoronary) very often fills some of the defect, thus making it and the shunt seem smaller. The problem with allowing this to persist is that it causes progressive deterioration and deformity of the aortic valve, which eventually leads to aortic insufficiency.

TYPES OF REPAIR
Palliative Surgery

There are two surgical approaches to treating the patient with a ventricular septal defect. The first is the use of the pulmonary artery banding. This procedure, first described by Dammann et al.,[30] was the mainstay of treatment for young children with ventricular septal

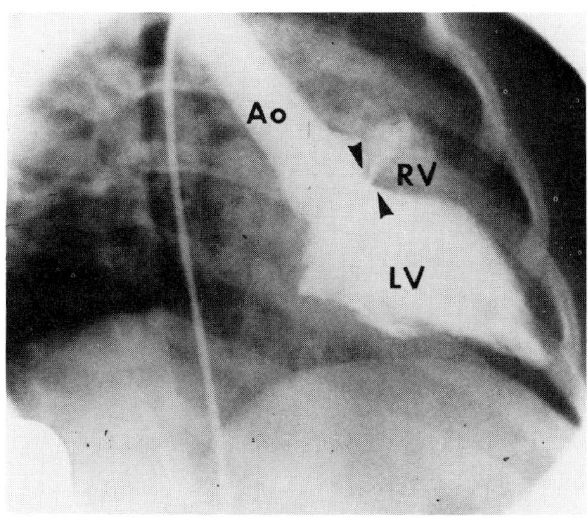

FIGURE 8 Supracristal defect in right anterior oblique projection (arrow). LV = left ventricle; Ao = aorta; RV = right ventricle. (RAO 30°.)

defects for many years. The principle behind the procedure is to produce an obstruction to flow and pressure and thus protect the lungs from these adverse effects. This procedure was used for many years, but in the early 1970s, the age at which total correction could be achieved progressively started to decline to the point where today corrective surgery is performed at almost

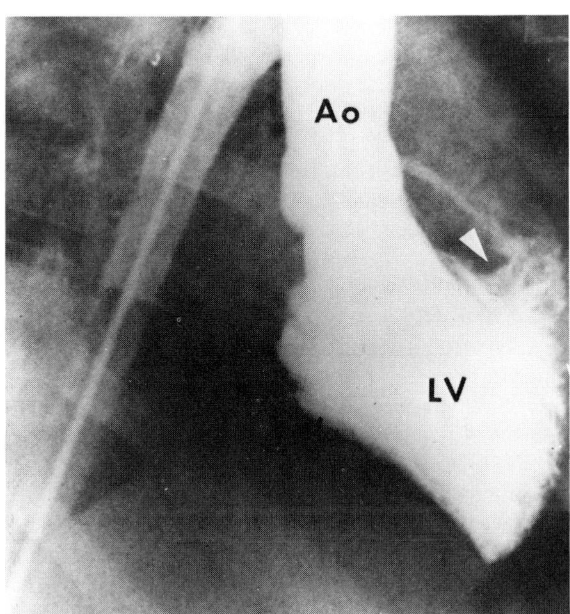

FIGURE 9 Anterior muscular defect in right anterior oblique projection (arrows). LV = left ventricle; Ao = aorta. (RAO 30°.)

any age or weight. Unfortunately, numerous problems with pulmonary artery banding have been reported in several large series.[31–35] These problems involve the structural deformity of the pulmonary arteries and are as follows: First, migration of the pulmonary artery band to the bifurcation of the pulmonary arteries, creating bilateral pulmonary arterial obstruction. This sequela causes considerable difficulty at the time of total repair. Second, erosion of the pulmonary artery band through the pulmonary artery has also been documented. Third, infundibular hypertrophy, particularly of the crista supraventricularis and conotruncal tissue, results in subpulmonary and sometimes subaortic stenosis.[36] Finally, the presence of the pulmonary artery band on the pulmonary outflow tract, if adequate to produce the effects desired, will require surgical intervention for its removal, even if the ventricular septal defect should close.

Although pulmonary artery banding was a very useful surgical procedure in young children with profound heart failure, it is not recommended in children with simple ventricular septal defect. There are, however, indications for the use of a pulmonary artery band in patients who have multiple muscular ventricular septal defects, because the surgical risk of primary closure of these defects in infancy is as high as or higher than that of the combined banding and later closure of the defects.

Corrective Surgery

Total correction by direct closure of the ventricular septal defect, as stated earlier, was first performed by Lillehei.[7] At that time and since, the standard approach to the ventricular septal defect is via a right ventriculotomy in the high right ventricular outflow tract area. This allows good visualization of the subpulmonic and membranous defect.

A more common approach used today is the transatrial approach described by Subramanian[37] and Anderson et al.[38] In this technique, the surgeon approaches the ventricular septal defect by way of the tricuspid annulus, either using traction sutures to draw the tricuspid tissue away from the defect or by removing a portion of the leaflet of the tricuspid valve to allow exposure and, at the completion of ventricular septal defect closure, reattachment of the tricuspid valve to the annulus. This technique is particularly useful in patients with pulmonary artery hypertension because it avoids a ventriculotomy, which is known to interfere with ventricular function in the postoperative period. This technique allows for excellent exposure of type I and type II ventricular defects, and since these are the majority of defects, it allows one to avoid the complications of ventriculotomy in most patients undergoing surgical correction.

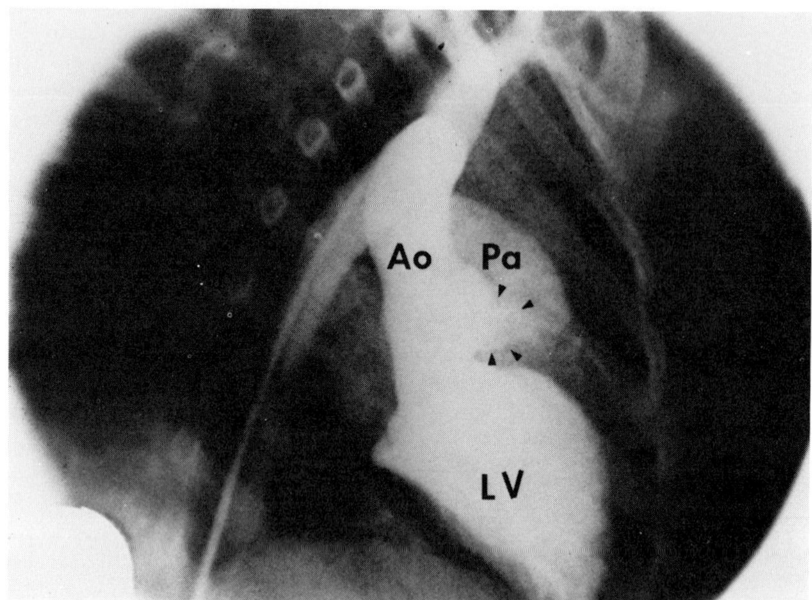

FIGURE 10 Aortic cusp in ventricular septal defect, type I (arrow). Ao = aorta; PA = pulmonary artery; LV = left ventricle. (RAO 30° with cranial 15°.)

The use of profound hypothermia has also made early surgical intervention possible.[39] This allows for a quiet heart and, with the newer cardioplegic solutions, good myocardial perservation.

The approach to multiple muscular ventricular septal defects is usually a combined technique involving both transatrial closure, right ventriculotomy, and possibly even left ventriculotomy. Many operators recommend that patients with ventricular defects that may require left ventriculotomy undergo pulmonary artery banding to allow them to grow, reserving the ventriculotomy for a later age.

SURGICAL RESULTS

Surgical correction of isolated type I and type II ventricular septal defects is presently being accomplished with a low mortality and excellent long-term survival. The past 20 years have brought about considerable improvement in surgical techniques and, in turn, a progressive decrease in the age at which successful repair can be achieved. Numerous articles have been published concerning the optimal age for repair of ventricular septal defects,[19] incremental risk factors and hospital mortality after repair of ventricular septal defects,[40] and comparison of early and late results for closure of ventricular septal defects[41] and postoperative follow-up.[42] The operative mortality rate

from these studies varies from 3 to 36 percent. Age does not seem to be a significant risk factor for surgical correction of the single ventricular septal defect. Blackstone et al.[19] quote a mortality rate of 0 in 50 patients beyond the age of 2 years, and Rein et al.[41] quote a mortality rate of 3 percent in children between 13 days and 18 months of age.

Pulmonary artery banding, which in itself carries a low mortality rate,[43] when combined with the approach of later surgical repair has been quoted to have a mortality rate as high as 19 percent.[44]

The presence of multiple ventricular septal defects carries a much higher mortality than the simple type I and type II defects. Rizzoli et al.[40] give a mortality rate of 31 percent in patients with multiple ventricular septal defects without associated lesions. However, they state that in the past 5 years, this rate has decreased to 7 percent with increasing accuracy in the diagnosis of multiple ventricular septal defects. Their data analysis states that age does not appear to be a significant factor in terms of mortality, but that the presence of trabecular muscular defects does increase the risk. There is still a strong surgical and medical contingent that believes that these patients should undergo pulmonary artery banding prior to total correction and that age definitely plays a part in this decision. It is my personal opinion that unless the surgical results for primary repair of this lesion become more universal, the conservative approach of banding is preferential. Foxx et al.[45] quote a mortality rate of 27 percent for two-stage repair of multiple ventricular septal defects, which includes pulmonary artery banding, and an 18 percent mortality rate in patients corrected beyond 1 year of age by a single procedure. These results are quite good and probably can be improved, but it is the infant with intractable congestive heart failure that must be approached at an earlier age. The identification of multiple ventricular septal defects preoperatively is a significant factor, as pointed out by Kirklin et al.[46] In their series of 29 patients, 14 patients were found to have multiple defects intraoperatively or postoperatively, and 28 percent required reoperation for closure of residual defects.

Pulmonary Hypertension

Surgical closure of ventricular septal defects in patients with pulmonary hypertension has a poorer prognosis than such closure in patients with normal pulmonary pressure and resistance. Published studies by Weidman et al.,[47] Whitman and Ellis,[48] and DuShane et al.[49] show that patients undergoing surgical repair for ventricular septal defects under 2 years of age usually have a normal pulmonary artery pressure and resistance on follow-up. The hospital mortality for patients with elevated pulmonary vascular resistance and pressure is stated to be no greater than that for patients with normal pulmonary resistance.[19] This, however, may be somewhat influenced by the fact that for many years it has been known that there is a very high mortality rate in surgical closure of ventricular septal defects in patients with a pulmonary vascular to systemic vascular resistance ratio of greater than 0.75, and therefore, these patients may be selected out in considering mortality. There is, however, a significant difference in the long-term prognosis for patients surviving surgical intervention. Age at operation has been shown to be directly related to the mean pulmonary artery pressure 5 years after surgery, as was the preoperative pulmonary vascular resistance and mean pulmonary arterial pressure. Five-year survival for patients with high pulmonary vascular resistance and pressure has been stated to be as low as 15 percent. A pulmonary vascular resistance of 4 units or less has a 92 percent probability of surgical cure if operation is performed before 27 months of age, while a pulmonary vascular resistance of 12 units has a probability of 80 percent cure if operated on before 6 months of age.[19] Thus one can very easily conclude that the longer the patient is allowed to have an elevated pulmonary arterial pressure and pulmonary vascular resistance, which has been directly correlated with age,[50] the greater the likelihood of continued and progressive pulmonary vascular changes after surgical intervention.[51,52]

Ventricular Septal Defect with Aortic Insufficiency

The development of aortic insufficiency in association with ventricular septal defect has been very well documented and has led many to recommend early closure of the ventricular septal defect with or without repair of the aortic valve.[53,54] A recent study by Karparwich et al.[55] shows that residual aortic insufficiency was found after surgery in 63 percent of patients. Children less than 5 years of age, even with minimal valvular involvement, exhibited minimal benefit from attempted correction compared with those having surgery in the latter part of the first decade. Closure of the ventricular septal defect with associated valvuloplasty resulted in greater improvement or elimination of the aortic insufficiency as compared with patients having the ventricular septal defect closed alone. One question that has not yet been answered pertains to closure of all type I ventricular septal defects irrespective of size to see if this eliminates the development of aortic insufficiency in this particular type of lesion.

SURGICAL SEQUELA

Experience has taught us that all attempts must be made to prevent residual problems after surgical correction of ventricular septal defect, but unfortunately, in a small percentage of patients there are continued problems.

Residual Defects

Although attempts are made at surgery to be sure there is no evidence of residual defects, many reports indicate that there are defects which are missed at preoperative diagnostic catheterization, very often in the muscular septum, and that on occasion, because of friability of tissues, sutures may be pulled loose. Some defects can be avoided by filling the ventricle via the left ventricular vent before discontinuing bypass. The incidence of residual defects present has been noted to be in the area of 30 percent, and many of these will require further surgical intervention.[56] As long as there is a residual defect, there is the ongoing risk of infectious endocarditis, and for this reason, these patients should continue to follow endocarditis prophylaxis therapy as recommended by the American Heart Association Committee on Rheumatic Fever. The committee also recommends continued endocarditis therapy for patients with successful closure of ventricular septal defects on the premise that the abnormal contour of the surface following patch closure of ventricular septal defect could be a site for endocarditis development.

Postpericardiotomy Syndrome

Although the incidence of this syndrome varies from institution to institution, it has been reasonably well documented and thought to be due to an autoimmune response that develops after cardiotomy. It is a problem that has to be dealt with in the postoperative period, but because it is recognizable by its evidence of fever, fluid retention with progressive congestive heart failure, decreasing myocardial function, and elevation in white count, and because of the fact that it can be adequately treated with aspirin and steroids and is a self-limiting disorder, it will not be discussed further.

Ventricular Function

Postoperative angiographic studies evaluating ventricular volume, ejection fraction, and ventricular mass 2 years after successful closure of ventricular septal defects indicate that there is a reduction in ventricular volume, mass, and ejection fraction. These, however, do not return to normal values, and it is suspected that there may be some depression in contractility that could be related to processes associated with the ventricular hypertrophy, which developed in order to meet the myocardial demands for cardiac output.[57] Whether there is eventual return of these parameters to normal is yet to be determined.

Postoperative Heart Block and Intraventricular Conduction Defects

A variety of conduction disorders may complicate repair of ventricular septal defect. The disorder carrying the worst prognosis is that of complete heart block, but as long as it is recognized in the postoperative period and treated appropriately with pacing, it should be relatively well managed, although the long-term prognosis is somewhat guarded. *Transient* complete heart block in the postoperative period should lead to very careful follow-up of the patient. This is an indication of some injury to the conduction system. Even though it may only be secondary to edema, it may eventually result in fibrotic change in the conduction system, which could lead to sudden death from heart block.[58]

With newer surgical techniques and increased awareness of the conduction system in repairing ventricular defects, the incidence of conduction disturbances has been shown to decrease. The use of the transatrial approach to close ventricular septal defects has been shown to reduce the incidence of right bundle branch block from 78 to 33 percent.[59] The surface electrocardiogram, although very useful in diagnosing conduction disturbances, does not always tell the entire story. Electrophysiologic studies performed on children, after ventricular septal defect repair, who have surface electrocardiographic findings of right bundle branch block and left axis deviation and who go on to develop complete heart block show evidence of the block being distal to the area generating the His potential. Patients with right bundle branch block and a normal axis who develop complete heart block have their block proximal to the area generating the His potential. Many of these patients also show evidence of HV interval prolongation. Of particular interest is the fact that many of these patients had transient complete heart block during the postoperative period.[60] It is therefore of utmost importance that any patient showing evidence of intraventricular conduction disturbances, particularly associated with complete heart block in the postoperative period, be watched very carefully because of the relationship of sudden death with these conduction disturbances. Any history of syncope or suspected arrhythmia should stimulate one to look for evidence of abnormal conduction patterns, and it is my feeling that at the first evidence of syncope, one should very carefully consider insertion of a permanent pacemaker.

SUMMARY

The surgical repair of ventricular septal defect utilizing present-day surgical techniques has reduced the mortality and morbidity for this lesion to a very acceptable level. Elective repair of defects with large flow and low pulmonary artery pressures should be achievable with a mortality of less than 5 percent. Congestive heart failure, failure to thrive, and pulmonary artery hypertension are all indications for early surgical intervention with an excellent long-term prognosis. Aortic insufficiency associated with a ventricular septal defect is an ongoing problem that must be dealt with, particularly in the type I defect and in the small percentage of type II defects. Whether the approach of closure of all type I defects will improve the long-term outlook for this complication is yet to be determined. Postoperative conduction disturbances, particularly complete heart block, carry a guarded prognosis because of their association with sudden death, and any episode of syncope or rhythm disturbances should lead to a thorough evaluation of the cardiac conduction system and, where appropriate, insertion of a permanent pacemaker.

REFERENCES

1 Roger, H.: Recherches cliniques sur la communication congenitale des deux coeurs, par inocclusion du septum interventriculaire, *Bull. Acad. Med. (Paris)*, 8:1074, 1879.

2 Dalrymple: 1847; quoted in ref. 4.

3 Eisenmenger, V.: Die angebosenen Defecte de Kammerscheidewand des Herzens, *Ztsche. f. Klin. Med.*, 32 (suppl. 1), 1897.

4 Abbott, M. E.: Congenital Heart Disease, in "Nelson's Loose-Leaf Medicine," Vol. 4, Thomas Nelson & Son, New York, 1932, p. 207.

5 Blount, S. G., Mueller, H., and McCord, M. C.: Ventricular Septal Defect, *Am. J. Med.*, 18:871, 1955.

6 Wood, P., Magidson, O., and Wilson, P. A. O.: Ventricular Septal Defect, with Note on Acyanotic Fallot's Tetralogy, *Br. Heart J.*, 16:387, 1954.

7 Lillehei, C. W., Cohen, M., Warden, H. E., Ziegler, N. R., and Varco, R. L.: The Results of Direct Vision Closure of Ventricular Septal Defects in Eight Patients by Means of Controlled Cross Circulation, *Surg. Gynecol. Obstet.*, 101:447, 1955.

8 Arey, L. B.: "Developmental Anatomy," 5th ed., W. B. Saunders Co., Philadelphia, 1947, p. 330.

9 Soto, B., Becker, A., Morehaert, A., Lie, J. T., and Anderson, R. H.: Classification of Ventricular Septal Defects, *Br. Heart J.*, 43:332, 1980.

10 Lev, M.: The Pathologic Anatomy of the Ventricular Septal Defect, *Dis. Chest*, 35:533, 1959.

11 Goor, D. A., Lillehei, C. W., Rees, R., and Edwards, J. E.: Isolated VSD; Development Basis for Various Types and Presentation of Classification, *Chest*, 58:468, 1970.

12 Keith, J. D., Rowe, R. D., and Vlad, P.: "Heart Disease of Infancy and Childhood," 3rd ed., The Macmillan Co., New York, 1978.

13 Nadas, A. S., and Fyler, D. C.: "Pediatric Cardiology," 3rd ed., W. B. Saunders Co., Philadelphia, 1972.

14 Mitchell, S. C., Korones, S. B., and Berendes, H. W.: Congenital Heart Disease in 56,109 Births: Incidence and Natural History, *Circulation*, 43:323, 1971.

15 Hoffman, J. I. E., and Christianson, R.: Congenital Heart Disease in a Cohort of 19,502 Births with Long Term Follow-Up, *Am. J. Cardiol.*, 42:641, 1978.

16 Fyler, D. C.: Report of the New England Regional Infant Cardiac Program, *Pediatrics*, 65 (suppl. II):375, 1980.

17 Hoffman, J. I. E., and Rudolph, A. M.: The Natural History of Isolated Ventricular Septal Defect, *Adv. Pediatr.*, 17:57, 1970.

18 Engle, M. A., and Kline, S. A.: Ventricular Septal Defect in the Adult, in W. C. Roberts (ed.), "Congenital Heart Disease in Adults," F. A. Davis Co., Philadelphia, 1979.

19 Blackstone, E. H., Kirklin, J. W., Bradley, E. L., DuShane, J. W., and Applebaum, A.: Optional Age and Results in Repair of Large Ventricular Septal Defects, *J. Thorac. Cardiovasc. Surg.*, 72:661, 1976.

20 Wood, P.: The Eisenmenger Syndrome, *Br. Med. J.*, 2:701, 1958.

21 Blount, S. G., Jr.: Clinical Course in Adults with Ventricular Septal Defect at High Altitude and Sea Level, *Circulation*, 56 (suppl. 1):1, 1977.

22 Alpert, B. S., Cook, D. H., Varghese, P. J., and Rowe, R. D.: Spontaneous Closure of Small Ventricular Septal Defects: 10 Year Follow-Up, *Pediatrics*, 63:204, 1979.

23 Weidman, W. H., Blount, S. G., Jr., DuShane, J. W., Gersony, W. M., Hayes, C. J., and Nadas, A. S.: Clinical Course in Ventricular Septal Defect, *Circulation* 54 (suppl. 1):1, 1977.

24 Silverman, N. H., Lewis, A. B., Heyman, M. A., and Rudolph, A. M.: Echocardiographic Assessment of Ductus Arteriosus Shunt in Premature Infants, *Circulation*, 50:821, 1974.

25 Riggs, T., Mehta, S., Hirschfeld, S., Borkat, G., and Liebman, J.: Ventricular Septal Defect in Infancy: A Combined Vectorgraphic and Echocardiographic Study, *Circulation*, 59:385, 1979.

26 Jones, R. H., Scholz, P. M., and Anderson, P. A. W.: Radionuclide Studies in Patients with Congenital Heart Disease, *Cardiovasc. Clin.*, 10(2):225, 1979.

27 Askenazi, J., Ahnberg, D. S., Korngold, E., LaFarge, C. G., Malty, D. L., and Treves, S.: Quantitative Radionuclide Angiocardiography: Detection and Quantitation of Left to Right Shunts, *Am. J. Cardiol.*, 37:382, 1976.

28 Bargeron, L. M., Elliott, L. P., Soto, B., Bream, P. R., and Curry, G. C.: Axial Cineangiography in Congenital Heart Disease, *Circulation*, 56:1075, 1977.

29 Elliott, L. P., Bargeron, L. M., Bream, P. R., Soto, B., and Curry, G. C.: Axial Cineangiography in Congenital Heart Disease, *Circulation*, 56:1084, 1977.

30 Dammann, J. F., Jr., and Muller, W. H., Jr.: Treatment of Certain Congenital Malformations of the Heart by the Creation of Pulmonic Stenosis to Reduce Pulmonary Hypertension and Excessive Pulmonary Blood Flow, *Surg. Gynecol. Obstet.*, 95:2131, 1952.

31 Goldblatt, A., Bernhard, W. F., Nadas, A. S., et al.: Pulmonary Artery Banding: Indications and Results in Infants and Children, *Circulation*, 32:172, 1965.

32 Stark, J., Aberdeen, E., Waterston, D. J., et al.: Pulmonary Artery Constriction (Banding): A Report of 146 Cases, *Surgery*, 68:808, 1969.

33 Hunt, C. E., Formanck, G., Levine, M. A., et al.: Banding of the Pulmonary Artery: Results in 111 Children, *Circulation*, 43:395, 1971.

34 Dobell, A. R. C., Murphy, D. A., Poirier, N. L., et al.: The Pulmonary Artery after Debanding, *J. Thorac. Cardiovasc. Surg.,* 65:32, 1973.

35 Griepp, E., French, J. W., Shumway, N. R., et al.: Is Pulmonary Artery Banding for Ventricular Septal Defect Obsolete? *Circulation,* 49, 50 (suppl. 2):14, 1974.

36 Freed, M. D., Rosenthal, A., Plauth, W. H., et al.: Development of Subaortic Stenosis after Pulmonary Artery Banding, *Circulation,* 47, 48 (suppl. 3):7, 1973.

37 Subramanian, S.: Primary Definitive Intracardiac Operation in Infants: Ventricular Septal Defects, in J. W. Kirklin (ed.), "Advances in Cardiovascular Surgery," Grune & Stratton, New York, 1973, p. 141.

38 Anderson, R. C., Lellehei, C. W., and Lester, R. G.: Corrected Transportation of the Great Vessels of the Heart: A Review of 17 Cases, *Pediatrics,* 20:626, 1957.

39 Barrett-Boyes, B. G., Simpson, M. J., and Neutze, J. D.: Intracardiac Surgery in Neonates and Infants Using Deep Hypothermia with Surface Cooling and Limited Cardiopulmonary Flows, *Circulation,* 43, 44 (suppl. 1):25, 1971.

40 Rizzoli, G., Blackstone, E. H., Kirklin, J. W., Pacifico, A. D., and Bargeron, L. M.: Incremental Risk Factors in Hospital Mortality Rate after Repair of Ventricular Septal Defect, *J. Thorac. Cardiovasc. Surg.,* 80:494, 1980.

41 Rein, J. G., Freed, M. D., Norwood, W. I., and Castaneda, A. R.: Early and Late Results of Closure of Ventricular Septal Defect in Infancy, *Am. Thorac. Surg.,* 24:19, 1977.

42 Allen, H. D., Anderson, R. C., Noren, G. R., et al.: Postoperative Follow-Up of Patients with Ventricular Septal Defects, *Circulation,* 50:465, 1974.

43 Dooley, K. J., Parisi-Buckley, L., Fyler, D. C., and Nadas, A. S.: Results of Pulmonary Arterial Banding in Infancy, *Am. J. Cardiol.,* 36:484, 1975.

44 McNicholas, K., De Leval, M., Stark, J., Taylor, J. F. N., and Macartney, F. J.: Surgical Treatment of Ventricular Septal Defect in Infancy, *Br. Heart J.,* 41:133, 1979.

45 Foxx, K. M., Patel, R. G., Graham, G. R., Taylor, J. F. N., Stark, J., et al.: Multiple and Single Ventricular Septal Defect: A Clinical and Hemodynamic Comparison. *Br. Heart J.,* 40:141, 1978.

46 Kirklin, J. K., Castaneda, A. R., Keane, J. F., Fellows, K. E., and Norwood, W. I.: Surgical Management of Multiple Ventricular Septal Defects, *Am. Thorac. Surg.,* 24:19, 1977.

47 Weidman, W. H., and DuShane, J. W.: Course of Pulmonary Hypertension Following Surgical Closure of Ventricular Septal Defects, *Adv. Cardiol.,* 2:13, 1974.

48 Whitman, V., and Ellis, N. G.: Pulmonary Hemodynamics after Repair of Left to Right Shunt Lesions Associated with Pulmonary Artery Hypertension, *Prog. Cardiovasc. Dis.,* 17:467, 1975.

49 DuShane, J. W., Krongrad, E., Ritter, D. G., and McGoon, D. C.: Fate of Raised Pulmonary Vascular Resistance after Surgery in Ventricular Septal Defect, in B. S. D. Kidd and R. D. Rowe (eds.), "The Child with Congenital Heart Disease after Surgery," Futura, Mt. Kisco, New York, 1976, pp. 299–312.

50 Clarkson, P. M., Frye, R. L., DuShane, J. W., Bruchell, H. B., Wood, E. H., and Weidman, W. H.: Prognosis for Patients with Ventricular Septal Defects and Severe Pulmonary Vascular Obstructive Disease, *Circulation,* 38:129, 1968.

51 Krongrad, E., Ritter, D. G., Weidman, W. H., McGoon, D. C., and DuShane, J. W.: Long Term Prognosis for Infants with Total Correction of Ventricular Septal Defects, *Am. J. Cardiol.,* 31:143, 1973. (Abstract.)

52 Lueker, R. D., Vogel, J. H. K., and Blount, S. G.: Cardiovascular Abnormalities Following Surgery for Left to Right Shunts. Observations in Atrial Septal Defects, Ventricular Septal Defects and Patent Ductus Arteriosus, *Circulation,* 40:785, 1969.

53 Spencer, F., Doyle, E., Danilowicz, D., Bohnson, H., and Weldon, C.: Long Term Evaluation of Aortic Valvuloplasty for Aortic Insufficiency and Ventricular Septal Defect, *J. Thorac. Cardiovasc. Surg.,* 65:15, 1973.

54 Sommerville, J., Brando, A., and Ross, D.: Aortic Regurgitation with Ventricular Septal Defect. Surgical Management and Clinical Features *Circulation,* 41:317, 1979.

55 Karpawich, P. P., Duff, D. F., Mullins, C. E., Cooley, D. E., and McNamara, D. G.: Ventricular Septal Defect with Associated Aortic Valve Insufficiency. Progression of Insufficiency and Operative Results in Young Children, *J. Thorac. Cardiovasc. Surg.,* 82:182, 1981.

56 Allen, H. D., Anderson, R. C., Noren, G. R., and Moller, J. H.: Postoperative Follow-Up of Patients with Ventricular Septal Defects, *Circulation,* 50:465, 1974.

57 Jarmakani, J. M. M., Graham, T. P., Canent, R. V., and Capp, M. P.: The Effect of Corrective Surgery on Left Heart Volume and Mass in Children with Ventricular Septal Defects, *Am. J. Cardiol.,* 27:254, 1971.

58 Krongrad, E.: Prognosis for Patients with Congenital Heart Disease and Postoperative Intraventricular Conduction Defects, *Circulation,* 57:867, 1978.

59 Hobbins, S. M., Izukawa, T., Radford, D., Williams, W., and Trusler, G. A.: Conduction Disturbances after Surgical Correction of Ventricular Septal Defect by the Atrial Approach, *Br. Heart J.,* 41:289, 1979.

60 Godman, M. J., Roberts, M. B., and Izukawa, T.: Late Postoperative Conduction Disturbances after Repair of Ventricular Septal Defect and Tetralogy of Fallot, *Circulation,* 49:214, 1974.

The Effects of Psychotropic Drugs on the Heart[*]

I. SYLVIA CRAWLEY, M.D., and ROBERT M. KOLODNER, M.D.

When an erroneous hypothesis becomes entrenched and generally accepted, it is transformed into a kind of tenet that no one is allowed to question and investigate; and it then becomes an evil which endures for centuries.

GOETHE[1]

The use of psychotropic drugs is an important part of the armamentarium for the care of patients with psychiatric problems, particularly in the treatment of depression, anxiety, or psychosis. Since these drugs have potentially serious cardiovascular effects in both therapeutic and toxic doses, the prescribing physician must be familiar with these effects in order to provide the necessary pretreatment and follow-up evaluations. The internist or cardiologist may be consulted regarding decisions in specific patients with heart disease or cardiovascular side effects.

Early experience with these agents, the tricyclics and phenothiazines in particular, generated an abhorrence for their use in patients with heart disease. Recent experience suggests that with proper selection of patients and choice of agent, they may be used safely and effectively. The patient with a psychiatric problem should not be unnecessarily denied effective psychotropic therapy because of an existent heart disease, nor should unnecessary risks be taken in the psychotropic treatment of any patient.

It is the purpose of this paper to review the basic pharmacology, therapeutic effectiveness, potential cardiovascular effects, and drug interactions of selected groups of psychotropic drugs. The antidepressants, including the tricyclic agents and monoamine oxidase inhibiters, lithium, and the major tranquillizers, will be discussed. This information should aid the prescribing physician and consultant in providing effective and safe therapy for all patients requiring these psychotropic drugs.

ANTIDEPRESSANTS

In the mid-1950s, two classes of psychotropic medications, tricyclic antidepressants (TCAs) and monoamine oxidase inhibitors (MAOIs), were discovered to have specific antidepressant activity. Research during the past 10 years has helped to improve the effective use of these drugs by defining the diagnostic groups most likely to respond and by documenting the need for adequate dosages to ensure maximum response.[2–7] Only recently have the first of the "second-generation antidepressants" been available in the United States, with a significantly different side-effect profile and a potential for greater safety, particularly in patients with heart disease.[8,9] Lithium carbonate, which also has antidepressant activity, will be discussed later in this paper.

Tricyclic Derivatives

PHARMACOLOGY

The tricyclic antidepressants (TCAs) are based on a 6-7-6 three-ring nucleus and are often separated into secondary and tertiary subgroups based on methylation of the terminal nitrogen on their aliphatic side chain. The TCAs are rapidly and completely absorbed orally and are highly protein-bound in plasma.[10,11] There is a significant first-pass metabolism followed by a slower rate of metabolism and excretion. Tertiary TCAs are partially metabolized to secondary derivatives that retain clinical activity.[10–13] Hydroxylation and glucuronide coupling in the liver account for a major portion of the inactivation,[14] with the half-life of most TCAs ranging from 9 to 93 h, reaching steady-state levels after 1 to 2 weeks of treatment.[10,11] Protriptyline has an unusually long half-life of 54 to 198 h, requiring 4 or more weeks to reach steady-state.[11,15,16]

The pharmacologic actions are similar among all of the TCAs. Variations in the relative activities account for the different side-effect profiles between medications. All these antidepressants have significant affinities for H_1, H_2,[17] muscarinic[18,19] (Table 1) and alpha-adrenergic receptors,[20] causing antihistaminic, anticholinergic, and sympathetic side effects.[21,22] The main therapeutic action has been hypothesized to be related to their bioamine reuptake blockade, with some drugs more active at adrenergic synapses and others at serotonergic synapses.[21] More recently, this theory of antidepressant action has been challenged as a result of the discovery of effective antidepressants that lack either of these actions.[8,23] Alternate hypotheses have been proposed, including alterations in postsynaptic receptor sensitivity,[24] which are also compatible with TCA actions.

[*]From the Departments of Medicine and Psychiatry, Emory University School of Medicine and Atlanta Veterans Administration Medical Center, Atlanta, Georgia.

TABLE 1
Selected psychotropic drugs: Anticholinergic activity*
(in decreasing order)

Protriptyline
Thioridazine†
Amitriptyline
Chlorpromazine†
Imipramine
Doxepin
Nortriptyline
Desipramine
Loxapine†
Trifluoperazine†
Mianserin
Fluphenazine†
Haloperidol†
Molindone†
Tranylcypromine

*Based on muscarinic receptor affinity as assayed by measuring inhibition of H³-QNB (quinuclidinyl benzilate) binding to human caudate receptors.

†Antipsychotics.

CLINICAL USE

Tricyclic antidepressants have been approved by the FDA for use in the treatment of depression and childhood enuresis. The depressive subtypes that are most responsive to treatment by TCAs are those associated with changes in vegetative functions, especially those of the melancholic subtype,[10,25] but patients formerly classified as having neurotic depression may also respond to TCA treatment.[26,27] Patients respond whether they are diagnosed as having major depressive disorder or bipolar disorder, depressed; although the latter may be susceptible to the TCA triggering of a manic episode.[7] Depressed patients with delusions often require the addition of an antipsychotic agent to a TCA or may require electroconvulsive treatment (ECT) for maximum improvement.[25,28] Some researchers have reported correlations between TCA response and neuroendocrine abnormalities,[29] or between particular antidepressants (primarily noradrenergic or serotonergic) and biochemical tests that attempt to distinguish between different depressive subtypes.[30] Such research is still preliminary, however, and clinicians usually select the particular TCA based on history of past treatment, family history of response to a specific TCA, or side-effect profile best suited to the patient's symptoms and medical conditions.[2,31]

Dosage ranges are indicated in Table 2, with an average effective dose of imipramine or amitriptyline being 150 mg/day. Many patients require higher doses to respond because of marked interindividual variations in TCA metabolism, with blood levels of TCAs covering a 30-fold range between individuals on the same oral dose.[10,11] An average starting dose is 50 mg of imipramine or equivalent drug, increasing 25 to 50 mg every 2 or 3 days until the chosen target dose is reached. This is maintained for at least a week before adjusting dosages up or down, unless side effects require an earlier change.[10,25] Antidepressant response usually takes 1 to 2 weeks after a therapeutic dose has been attained. Owing to the long half-life, single daily dosing, usually near bedtime, is equally effective and serves to minimize side effects and improve compliance.[10,32–35] Multiple daily dosing has been suggested in patients with cardiac disease to minimize peak blood levels.[7]

Measurement of TCA blood levels is available at many commercial laboratories. Nortriptyline and imipramine are the TCAs that have the best documentation for a correlation between blood levels and clinical response.[5,12,13,36–38] Nortriptyline appears to have a curvilinear response curve, with poor response at levels that are too low (<50 ng/ml) or too high (>140 ng/ml).

TABLE 2
Antidepressants

Generic name	Trade name	Effective dose range (mg/day)
TCAs: Tertiary		
Amitriptyline	Elavil, Endep, others	50–300
Doxepin	Adapin, Sinequan	50–300
Imipramine	Tofranil, Presamine, others	50–300
Trimipramine	Surmontil	50–300
TCAs: Secondary		
Desipramine	Norpramin, Pertofrane	50–300
Nortriptyline	Aventyl, Pamelor	30–125
Protriptyline	Vivactil	10–60
Newly available antidepressants		
Amoxapine	Asendin	100–600
Maprotiline	Ludiomil	50–300
Trazodone	Desyrel	50–600
Antidepressants not yet available		
Buproprion	Welbutrin	200–600
Mianserin	Bolvidon, Norval	40–120
Nomifensine	Merital	50–200
MAOIs		
Isocarboxazid	Marplan	20–60*
Phenelzine	Nardil	45–90
Tranylcypromine	Parnate	20–60*

*Dosage exceeds FDA-approved limit

In contrast, imipramine has a sigmoid response curve, with most patients needing blood levels (imipramine plus desipramine) of at least 150 ng/ml and minimal additional improvement above 250 ng/ml.[38] The remaining TCAs have not been studied extensively, and a few authors have cautioned against clinical use of blood levels of these medications until more research has been performed.[7,10,11,36,37] Guidelines have been proposed for specific clinical situations in which tricyclic blood levels may be clinically useful.[39–41]

In addition to the approved uses, researchers have reported therapeutic response to TCAs in the following conditions: panic attacks,[42] cataplexy, obsessive-compulsive disorder, phobic disorder, including school phobia, chronic pain, migraine headaches, and minimal brain disorder.[10]

NONCARDIOVASCULAR SIDE EFFECTS

Many of the side effects experienced by patients are related to the anticholinergic, antihistaminic, and alpha-adrenergic blocking actions of the TCAs.[11,18,20,22] Dry mouth and increased sweating are the most common long-term side effects.[43] Sedation and light-headedness, which often bother patients initially or when dosage is increased, usually decrease after several days of therapy.[7,25] Paralytic ileus, an acute crisis in patients with narrow-angle glaucoma, acute urinary retention, seizures, and an allergic reaction with cholestatic jaundice or agranulocytosis are the most serious (and rare) noncardiovascular side effects.[7,10,25] Great caution is necessary when combining TCAs with other medications that have anticholinergic activity owing to the additive interaction that may precipitate untoward side effects.[25]

CARDIOVASCULAR EFFECTS

The cardiovascular side effects of TCAs have been the subject of several recent reviews.[40,44–46] Early reports of serious cardiovascular side effects were case reports that suggested TCAs caused congestive heart failure, myocardial infarction, life-threatening arrhythmias, and sudden death.[47,48] The presence of heart disease became a contraindication to the use of TCAs. More recent studies, although confirming potentially serious cardiac effects of these drugs, have demonstrated their safety in patients with heart disease. The cardiovascular effects to be considered include (1) an increase in heart rate, (2) orthostatic hypotension, (3) electrophysiologic changes both in conduction abnormalities and arrhythmias, and (4) suppressed ventricular function. Published studies report variable effects and inconsistent correlations of blood levels with effects. Interpretation

of the available data is limited by variations in blood levels, dosages, dosage schedules, presence or absence of underlying heart disease, concomitant use of other medications, duration of therapy in which observations were made, inpatient versus outpatient therapy, and age groups treated. The findings in a number of reports (Table 3) will be summarized.[49–68]

Heart rate An increase in heart rate is a consistent effect in all series. Anticholinergic and possible direct chronotropic properties may explain this effect. A weak correlation with blood levels is reported in two studies.[49,63] A heart rate of 100 beats per minute or greater (sinus tachycardia) is probably uncommon with therapeutic doses unless the patient has other reasons for an increase in sinus rate.[64,65] This increase in heart rate is likely to persist with prolonged therapy and may be present as long as 7 days after discontinuing therapy.[50]

Orthostatic hypotension This is not a universal effect; it is reported in only 5 to 20 percent of patients.[67] Peripheral vasodilation (decrease in peripheral resistance), direct alpha-adrenergic blocking effects, and direct myocardial depression are postulated mechanisms of action. The decrease in systolic blood pressure on standing is usually less than 25 mm Hg, although two studies report greater changes.[59,68] There is no good correlation with the dosage or blood levels. It usually becomes manifest early in the course of treatment with low doses and does not progress with higher doses.[59] Doxepin is reported to have a lower incidence of this side effect.[69] A patient with pretreatment orthostatic hypotension is more likely to have significant symptomatic orthostatic hypotension with treatment.[59] A recent study suggests that patients with heart disease who are taking cardiac medications and have left ventricular dysfunction are more likely to develop significant orthostatic hypotension.[67] Patients who have been confined for prolonged periods on a psychiatric ward have a tendency to lower their baseline blood pressure and/or develop orthostatic hypotension, and this may be a factor in some patients.[70,71] Although in some patients the symptoms may resolve with continued therapy, the actual drop in pressure with standing may persist.[51]

Electrocardiographic changes Abnormalities or changes over pretreatment tracings are variable but include prolongation of P-R, QRS, and Q-T$_c$; ST-T wave changes; heart block (bundle branch and AV); and tachyarrhythmias.[46] Although a statistically significant increase in P-R and QRS duration is reported in some studies, they are usually not prolonged to abnormal. A limited number of electrophysiologic studies

TABLE 3
Cardiovascular effects of TCAs

Authors	No. of patients	Age	Heart disease	Drug	Dosage (mg/day)	Blood levels (ng/ml)	Studies
Ziegler et al.[49]	15	18–50	No	Am	75–200	53–114	ECG
Taylor and Braithwaite[50]	8	22–71	No	Nt	25–150	40–170	STIs
Kantor et al.[51]	7	35–71	4 IHD or HHD 6 Abn. ECG	Im	175–400	120–450	ECG, BP, Holter
Vohra et al.[52]	32	19–57	No	20 Nt 8 Do 1 Im 3 Am	150	60–497 (Nt)	ECG, BP, ETT
Vohra et al.[53]	12	N.A.		Nt	150–200	75–490	HBE
Freyschuss et al.[54]	40	20–72	3 HBP	Nt	75–150	20–295	ECG, ETT, BP
Veith et al.[55]	24	39–74	Yes	8 Im 8 Do	10–200 25–300	34–468 21–646	RNA with exercise Holter, ECG, BP
Winsberg et al.[56]	7	7–10	No	Im	5 mg/kg	140–440	ECG
Veith et al.[57]	26	19–57	No	De	200	13–882	ECG
Burgess et al.[58]	24	24–62	No	6 Am 8 Mi 7 Zi 3 No	150 60 200 150	No	BP, STIs, HR
Glassman et al.[59]	44	34–76	5 HBP 14 HD	Im	218–245	"Therapeutic"	BP
Mielke et al.[60]	60	N.A.	No	30 Im 30 Ma	150–300	No	ECG, ETT, BP, ECHO
Raeder et al.[61]	25	61 ± 13				No	ECG, Holter, STIs
Giardina et al.[62]	46	34–76	16 yes 30 No	Im	225 ± 68	220 ± 88	ECG
Ziegler et al.[63]	17	20–65	No	Nt	50–150	131 ± 54	ECG
Reed et al.[64]	12	60–78	6 Abn ECG	Nt	150	90–160	ECG, BP
Rudorfer et al.[65]	14	22–41	No	De	150	201 ± 34	ECG, BP
Hayes et al.[66]	18	42–64	2 HBP	Im Cl	150–200	No	BP
Glassman et al.[67]	45	63 ± 13	30 Yes	Im	3.5 mg/kg	Yes; range not stated	Forearm resistance, RNA, BP
Burckhardt et al.[68]	60	19–81	No	22 Tr 9 Am 16 Ma 4 Mi 7 Im	38–300 45–150 45–150 40 100–250	No	HR, ECG, STIs

Abbreviations: Abn = abnormal; AM = amitriptyline; BP = blood pressure; Cl = clomipramine; De = desipramine; Do = doxepin; ECG = electrocardiogram; ECHO = echocardiogram; ETT = exercise test; HBE = His bundle electrogram; HBP = hypertension; HD = heart disease; HHD = hypertensive heart disease; Holter = ambulatory monitoring; HR = heart rate; IHD = ischemic heart disease; IM = imipramine; MA = maprotiline; Mi = mianserin; Mult = multiple; No = nomifensine; Nt = nortriptyline; RNA = radionuclide angiography; STIs = systolic time intervals; TR = trimipramine; ZI = zimelidine; N.A. = not available.

have documented that the prolongation of P-R and QRS is below the bundle of His.[53] A significant correlation of blood levels with this change in conduction has not been established, but the His bundle studies suggest that a blood level over 200 ng/ml for nortriptyline is more likely to produce an increase in H-V interval.[53,72] Logically, abnormalities will be more likely not only with higher blood levels, but also with overt (or occult) preexisting conduction abnormalities or concomitant administration of other medications with similar electrophysiologic effects.[51,73] Limited studies suggest that doxepin has less effect on cardiac conduction,[53,74] although this may be related to lower plasma levels.[73]

Q-T_c (Q-T interval corrected for heart rate) is inconsistently abnormal and not correlated with blood levels. As with other electrocardiographic abnormalities, it may be enhanced by concomitant drugs, electrolyte abnormalities, or preexisting heart disease. Marked prolongation in association with ventricular ectopy is an especially serious finding.

ST-T wave changes, ST-segment depression, and T wave inversion may occur. Some observations suggest that both the Q-T prolongation and ST-T wave changes may resolve with continued therapy.[68]

The TCAs may be both antiarrhythmic[62] and arrhythmogenic.[2] This quinidine-like effect has been demonstrated to actually reduce the frequency of ventricular premature beats with therapeutic doses, possibly an effect of the drug and not a result of relief of depression.[75] In a recent study, imipramine was used as an effective antiarrhythmic in patients with heart disease and ventricular ectopy.[76] Toxic amounts (see later discussion) may produce life-threatening arrhythmias.

Ventricular function A serious suppression of ventricular function precipitating congestive heart failure was the subject of early reports. These reports are difficult to assess, because unrecognized heart disease or other causes of the heart failure may have been present. More recent studies of the effect of TCAs on ventricular function have utilized systolic time intervals (STIs),[50,61,68] echocardiography,[60] exercise testing,[52,54,60] and nuclear scintigraphy.[55] Most studies utilizing STIs have shown a prolongation of PEP (preejection period) and PEP/LVET (left ventricular ejection time) ratio. The use of STIs to assess ventricular function, however, is open to some criticism.[77] One echocardiographic study of patients without heart disease reported no significant changes.[60] Exercise testing has not demonstrated any deleterious effects on left ventricular function.[52,54,66] A more recent study of patients with pretreatment left ventricular dysfunction demonstrated no deleterious effects on ejection fraction at rest or during exercise as measured by nuclear scintigraphy.[55]

Based on these studies, it would seem that there is minimal if any effect on left ventricular function in patients with normal hearts. Further studies in patients with preexisting left ventricular dysfunction are needed, but preliminary reports suggest that TCAs may be used safely in selected patients.

Sudden death Earlier reports based on drug surveillance programs, primarily with the use of amitriptyline, were contradictory but nevertheless disturbing.[78–80] More appropriate patient evaluation regarding preexisting heart disease and the paucity of reports of sudden death in patients on therapeutic doses have made this an extremely unlikely complication.

TOXICITY

Tricyclic antidepressant overdose is characterized by variable anticholinergic effects, alterations of consciousness, respiratory depression, seizures, and cardiovascular effects.[81–83] For the purposes of this review, only cardiovascular manifestations and management will be highlighted.

The mechanisms of the cardiovascular effects have not been completely elucidated, but they include anticholinergic effects, blockade of catecholamine uptake to the heart and peripheral adrenergic receptors, quinidine-like effects, and depression of myocardial contractility. Although higher blood levels were more frequently associated with serious cardiovascular abnormalities,[84] lower levels do not preclude these problems.[83] A blood level of greater than 1,000 ng/ml and/or a QRS duration of 100 ms or more may be useful in identifying the high-risk patient.[84] There is poor correlation of cardiovascular and central nervous system effects, and either may predominate in any given patient.[83] One study reports that the amount of drug (amitriptyline) taken did not correlate with the electrocardiographic changes.[81]

Sinus tachycardia and hypotension are the most common cardiovascular effects.[85] Myocardial depression as the cause of hypotension may be excluded in some patients with hemodynamic monitoring.[83,85] Peripheral vasodilation, with or without volume depletion, can be a major mechanism of the hypotension.

Death is most often related to the effects on cardiac conduction and the production of arrhythmias. Complete heart block and recurrent ventricular tachycardia are the most ominous.[81] P-R prolongation, supraventricular tachyarrhythmias, and bundle branch blocks occur. Right bundle branch block seems more common than left bundle branch block,[85] Q-T prolongation is common.[85] Ventricular ectopy and/or tachycardia are usually associated with Q-T prolongation.

Treatment Sinus tachycardia does not require therapy in most patients. With severe myocardial dysfunction or myocardial ischemia, slowing of the rate may improve hemodynamics. Physostigmine has been used, but caution is advised in its use.[86] Beta blockers may be used, but only in the context of possible deleterious effects on left ventricular function.[86]

Hemodynamic monitoring can aid in the management of hypotension. With low filling pressures, intravenous fluids may be administered safely. If significant hypotension persists after adequate filling pressures are achieved, dopamine or norepinephrine are most often the recommended first-line agents, but they must be used with caution, and initial doses should be small.[45,46,86] Norepinephrine may exert a fourfold to eightfold increase in vasopressor effect in the presence of TCAs.[87] Indirect sympathomimetic amines are reported to be less effective, because the TCAs block their uptake into the adrenergic neuron.[88]

Ventricular ectopy and ventricular tachycardia are usually associated with Q-T prolongation, and type I antiarrythmics (procainamide, quinidine, and disopyramide) are contraindicated. Lidocaine has been effective in some cases.[85,86] Sodium bicarbonate to achieve an alkaline pH may alleviate arrhythmias and conduction abnormalities associated with a wide QRS. Diphenylhydantoin[89] and physostigmine[90] have been used, but both have potential deleterious effects and should not be considered first-line drugs. A temporary transvenous pacemaker may be used for the treatment of recurrent ventricular tachycardia (overdrive suppression), complete heart block, or severe sinus bradycardia. The value of prolonged efforts at resuscitation, particularly in patients without heart disease, has been emphasized.[91]

The appropriate duration of electrocardiographic monitoring is controversial. A few reports of late arrhythmic complications have recommended prolonged periods of monitoring even without obvious initial cardiac effects, and prolonged elevation of plasma levels has been documented.[92] More recent reports suggest that once the ECG returns to normal, no more than 24 h of additional monitoring is required.[93,94] This guideline is subject to individual variations; i.e., patients who require antiarrhythmic therapy to maintain a normal ECG or who have preexisting heart disease must be monitored for longer periods.

INTERACTIONS WITH CARDIAC DRUGS[45,86,87,95–97] (Table 4)

The antihypertensive effects of guanethidine and clonidine are blocked by TCAs. Alpha-methyldopa and reserpine may be less effective and can even worsen depression. The effect of direct sympathomimetic

TABLE 4
TCAs drug interactions

Antihypertensives:	
Guanethidine	Antihypertensive
Clonidine	effects blocked
Alpha-methyldopa	Variable blood
Reserpine	pressure control; depression
Diuretics	Possible hypotension
Direct sympathomimetic amines:	
Norepinephrine	
Epinephrine	Potentiated
Phenylephrine	
Indirect sympathomimetic amines	Possibly blocked or potentiated
Propranolol	Possible potentiation of myocardial depression
Oral anticoagulants	Potentiated
Narcotics	Possible potentiation
Sedative-hypnotics	Possible potentiation
Type I antiarrhythmics	Possible potentiation of electrophysiologic effects

amines, oral anticoagulants, narcotics, and sedative-hypnotics are potentiated. Propranolol may have additive effects on depression of myocardial function. Type I antiarrhythmics may have an additive electrophysiologic effect, and the dosage should probably be reduced if they are used with the TCAs.

The reader is referred to other sources for more complete information on these and other drug interactions.[97–99]

Newer-Generation Antidepressants (TCA Derivatives and Others)

Amoxapine, a derivative of loxapine, an antipsychotic medication, possesses antidepressant activity in addition to retaining dopamine receptor blocking ability.[9,100,101] It is rapidly absorbed, with peak levels 1 to 2 h after administration, and has a half-life of about 8 h. Two active metabolites have half-lives as long as 30 h.[100,101] Although the three-ring structure of amoxapine is more similar to those of antipsychotic medications than tricyclic antidepressants, its mode of action, onset of therapeutic effect, and side-effect profile resembles those of TCAs when given in comparable therapeutic doses.[101] In addition, amoxapine has been reported to have extrapyramidal side effects due to its dopamine blocking activity. A possible role in the treatment of psychotic depression has been hypothesized but not yet tested.[9,101]

Amoxapine is about one-half as potent as imipramine or amitriptyline. Thus the usual starting dose of amoxapine is 100 to 150 mg/day, given in two or three doses. This may be increased to 200 to 300 mg/day after only a few days. Some patients may require up to 600 mg/day to achieve an adequate response.[100,101] Amoxapine may be given as a single bedtime dose, but it should not exceed 300 mg in any single dose because of reports of seizure activity in patients taking larger single doses.[100,102] Although some studies reported an earlier onset of antidepressant activity than standard TCAs, recent reviews question these claims.[101]

Maprotiline is the only tetracycline antidepressant presently available in the United States. It has a side chain that terminates with a secondary amine.[9,21,26,103] Maprotiline resembles the standard tricyclic antidepressants in its degree of protein binding, metabolism, and activity profile, with less anticholinergic activity than the others. It is slowly but completely absorbed orally with a half-life of up to 48 h.[104]

Maprotiline can be prescribed for the treatment of depression in the manner described for TCAs.[9] A starting dose of one-third to one-half the initial target dose is increased gradually over several days.[26] A single daily (bedtime) dose may be used. Although initial reports suggested a more rapid onset of action than TCAs, recent assessments do not support this claim.[104] Average response time is 2 weeks at therapeutic dosage. Side effects from maprotiline closely resemble those of the TCAs, with the primary difference being fewer, but still significant, anticholinergic effects.[9,104] Maprotiline has not been studied as a treatment for psychiatric disorders other than depression.

Mianserin is a tetracyclic antidepressant synthesized in 1966 that is available in Europe but not in the United States.[8] It is significantly different from maprotiline or TCAs because the fourth ring lies in the same plane as the other three rings, with no aliphatic side chains.[8,9,103,105,106] The action of mianserin on central neurotransmitters remains unclear, possibly through antagonist action on presynaptic alpha-2-adenoreceptors,[21] and this lack of clarity has raised questions regarding former theories of depression and antidepressant actions.[9] Most significantly, mianserin is reported to lack anticholinergic and cardiotoxic side effects, even in cases involving overdose.[8,9,107] The drug is well absorbed orally, with peak blood levels after 2 to 4 h, and it has a half-life of 6 to 12 h.[106]

Mianserin has been effective in either a divided or single bedtime dosage regimen, with an average response time of 2 weeks. The side-effect profile is notable for its lack of anticholinergic symptoms, with a moderate sedative effect being the most prominent complaint.[8,9,105,106]

Trazodone is an antidepressant medication released in the United States in 1982 that is chemically unique among the antidepressants.[8,9,21,108,109] It is a triazolopyridine derivative with a distinct pharmacologic profile, including a lack of anticholinergic and antihistaminic activity and no potentiation of characteristic animal response to L-dopa or methylamphetamine.[8,109,110] Trazodone has serotonergic activity, and this may account for its antidepressant activity.[9,108,109] Peripherally, the drug has antiserotonergic activity.[109] It is absorbed rapidly, with a peak blood level 2 to 4 h after oral doses. The parent molecule has a short half-life of about 4 h, with no active metabolites yet documented in vivo.[21,109]

Trazodone is used in the treatment of depression and is usually given in divided doses owing to its short half-life, although up to half the responders do well on a single bedtime dose.[111] Trazodone may be initiated at 150 mg/day and increased gradually to 400 mg/day for outpatients and 600 mg/day for inpatients.[109,112,113] These doses are often taken with food to decrease gastrointestinal distress. Response time is the same as for TCAs.

This medication is the first antidepressant released for use in the United States that has virtually no anticholinergic side effects.[112–115] In addition, trazodone reduces ocular tone in contrast to the opposite action by TCAs.[109] Drowsiness, lethargy, dizziness, headaches, and nausea are the most frequent side effects reported.[108,109,111–115] Trazodone does not aggravate psychotic symptoms in schizophrenic patients with secondary depression. Trazodone appears to potentiate barbiturates, volatile anesthetics, succinylcholine, and muscle relaxants.[109]

Buproprion is an antidepressant under investigation in the United States. Its unique pharmacologic profile includes no apparent action on CNS neurotransmission of serotonin, norepinephrine, or acetylcholine, while it increases dopamine activity through an unknown mechanism.[8,111] The medication appears to have little toxicity in early studies and a very low level of side effects. Weight loss, insomnia, activation, and sweating are the side effects most often reported.[111] The possibility has also been raised that buproprion may not trigger manic episodes in patients with bipolar disorder and may even be prophylactic for manic episodes in these patients.[8]

Nomifensine is another compound being studied in the United States for its antidepressant properties. The drug is a tetrahydroisoquinolone that enhances both norepinephrine and dopamine transmission.[8,9,21,111] Although nomifensine is reported to have mild anticholinergic activity and less cardiac toxicity, it may have an amphetamine-like action, accounting for reports of a stimulant-like effect with agitation, insomnia, and irritability and an aggravation of schizophrenic symptoms.[8,111] This antidepressant might be useful in the treatment of depressions marked by psychomotor retardation.[110]

CARDIOVASCULAR EFFECTS AND TOXICITY

Amoxapine is reported to have fewer cardiovascular side effects,[100] but since it has potentially the same effects as the TCAs, it should be used with the same caution in patients with heart disease. There are few reported cases of overdose,[116] and any differences from TCAs cannot be assessed.

Maprotiline has the same potential cardiovascular effects in therapeutic and toxic doses as the TCAs.[60] Some studies suggest that it has fewer side effects with less frequent orthostatic hypotension, tachycardia, and ECG changes[117] and that it can be used safely in the elderly.[118] Other studies comparing it with imipramine and other TCAs show no difference.[60,68] Potential effects of overdose are similar to those of TCAs, and management should follow similar guidelines.[117,119] Neither maprotiline nor amoxapine is recommended in the setting of acute myocardial infarction.

Mianserin has few anticholinergic effects, and reported cardiovascular side effects to date are insignificant.[58,120] Orthostatic hypotension and ECG changes are minimal.[121,122] Studies of its use in the elderly or in patients with heart disease are limited and thus not yet proven to be generally safe.[120] In the few reported cases of overdose, no significant cardiovascular effects are described.[74]

Trazodone in animal studies has no effects on intracardiac conduction, although some prolongation of Q-T$_c$ may occur.[123] There have been no reported electrophysiologic studies in humans, but clinical studies have confirmed no ECG changes nor arrhythmogenic properties.[124] Anticholinergic effects are absent. Heart rate and blood pressure may decrease slightly, but orthostatic hypotension is uncommon. Since the pharmacology of trazodone is quite different from that of the TCAs,[125] it may prove to have greater safety in patients with heart disease.[126,127] In the few reported cases of overdose, no cardiovascular effects are described.[126]

Buproprion is reported to have no anticholinergic effects and little effect on norepinephrine or serotonin.[128] The degree of cardiovascular effects and the safety of its use in patients with heart disease have not been adequately studied.

Nomifensine is thought to have fewer cardiovascular side effects, but the available studies are limited.[58,120,128,129] It may cause an increase in heart rate, although its anticholinergic activity is less than with the first-generation TCAs.[120]

Monoamine Oxidase Inhibitors (MAOI)

Iproniazide is an MAOI that was synthesized in an effort to find newer antitubercular drugs. Although it was found to have antidepressant activity in the 1950s, it was removed from clinical use because of rare hepatotoxicity.[7,25,103] The MAOIs have not been used very widely owing to early reports of low efficacy,[130] the concurrent discovery of TCAs, and the experience of severe, and sometimes fatal, hypertensive crises induced by interactions with medications and food.[25,103,131] Only in the past few years has their use increased, as newer studies document both the higher doses needed for clinical improvement and the existence of patients who respond to treatment with MAOIs but not TCAs.[25,131,132]

PHARMACOLOGY

Currently, there are three MAOIs marketed for antidepressant use in the United States, representing two subgroups of medications, hydrazine and nonhydrazine derivatives. Tranylcypromine is a nonhydrazine MAOI that is related to amphetamine derivatives and which has mild stimulant activity. Phenelzine and isocarboxazid are hydrazine MAOIs.[7,25,103] There are conflicting reports regarding the metabolism of these latter drugs. Some researchers claim that they are metabolized by acetylation,[133,134] which has a genetic polymorphism with "fast" and "slow" acetylators in the general population that might affect dosage requirements.[135] Other researchers dispute this hypothesis.[74,136]

Phenelzine is the best studied of the MAOIs,[6,137] but its pharmacokinetics have still not been well defined, with one research group reporting a steady rise in phenelzine blood levels over 6 weeks.[136]

The MAOIs noncompetitively bind to the monoamine oxidase enzymes in the body, inhibiting the enzymatic activity.[136,138] Although these drugs affect the MAO enzymes located in the GI tract, liver, and platelets, their primary therapeutic action is thought to be on the MAO enzymes in the presynaptic terminals in the central nervous system, by preventing the internal degradation of biogenic amine neurotransmitters, affecting both adrenergic and serotonergic neurons.[10,136,138] As the theory of the biochemical basis of depressive disorders undergoes evolution, this explanation of the antidepressant action of the MAOIs has been challenged.[10] The MAO inhibition is irreversible and persists until regeneration of the MAO enzyme, a process that takes up to 2 weeks after the MAOI is discontinued.[138] Thus drug blood levels are less meaningful than with TCAs. A technique of measuring inhibition of platelet MAO activity has been developed to monitor the biochemical effect of the MAOIs,[139] and preliminary research indicates that this technique may be clinically useful for confirming that an adequate dose of MAOI ($\geq$80% inhibition) has been given.[6,131,136,139,140]

CLINICAL USE

The MAOIs are approved for the treatment of depression. Anecdotal experience and several clinical studies suggested that they were more effective in atypical depressions associated with increased somatic concerns and hysteroid and anxiety features.[6,7,25,141–143] In addition, a recent study found phenelzine to be as effective as amitripyline, even in major depressive disorders or neurotic depression.[144,145] The MAOIs are also reported to be highly effective in the treatment of panic disorder and panic attacks[146] and phobic disorder[147,148] and possibly effective in obsessive-compulsive disorders[149] and as adjunctive treatment in posttraumatic stress disorder.[150]

Dosage ranges are given in Table 2. The medications are usually given in two or three divided doses early in the day; because of some activation effects, the MAOIs can cause insomnia if taken near bedtime.[31] They can often be given in full therapeutic doses after only 2 or 3 days.[10] Therapeutic response usually takes 2 or 3 weeks, but it can take up to 6 weeks in some patients.[25,137] Platelet inhibition can be measured by a few commercial laboratories, but the clinical indications and utility have still not been clearly established.[140]

NONCARDIAC SIDE EFFECTS

The most serious and life-threatening side effect of MAOIs is a hypertensive crisis caused by their interaction with a variety of foods and medications (see later discussion).[7,138,151,152]

They have other noncardiac autonomic side effects not related to the hypertensive crises, including dry mouth, urinary hesitancy, delayed ejaculation and orgasm (phenelzine only), constipation, decreased gastrointestinal tone, and blurred vision.[7,25,31,131,138]

CARDIOVASCULAR EFFECTS

Direct cardiovascular effects of the MAOIs in humans appear to be minimal.[95,153] Although the mechanisms of their action on the autonomic nervous system are not completely understood, their effects on the metabolism and release of sympathomimetic amines is responsible for the most serious cardiovascular complication, hypertensive crisis. Based on animal studies, MAOIs may have either a positive or negative ionotropic effect.[154]

Heart rate   Unlike the TCAs, they may produce a decrease in resting heart rate.[153] This effect is usually of no clinical significance, and the mechanism is probably sympatholytic.

Orthostatic hypotension   This is a prominent side effect,[136,153] possible more frequently than with TCAs, and it may be the limiting side effect in MAOI use. The degree of orthostatic drop may increase with continued therapy.[155] One study reports a correlation of the degree of orthostasis with the degree of MAO inhibition.[153] Orthostatic symptoms in the absence of significant orthostatic hypotension have been observed, but other mechanisms for these symptoms have not been explored.[153]

Electrocardiographic changes   Although these effects have not been extensively reported, a shortening of the Q-T$_c$ interval does occur.[153]

Hypertensive crisis   This is the most feared complication of MAOIs. It is characterized by severe hypertension, headaches, and tachycardia.[95] Seizures, coma, intracerebral hemorrhage, hyperpyrexia, hypothermia, or hyperglycemia may also occur.[74] It is precipitated by the interaction of MAOIs with drugs or foods containing indirect-acting sympathomimetic amines.[156,157] Since inhibition of MAO potentiates and prolongs the effects of sympathomimetic amines, their concurrent administration may result in a severe vasopressor effect.[95,156] The indirect sympathomimetic amines (amphetamine, methamphetamine, metaraminol, ephedrine, phenylpropanolamine) produce a greater effect, because MAOIs can increase norepinephrine stores for release by these amines.[95,96] The usual metabolism of ingested tyramine and other pressor amines in foods by intestinal and hepatic MAO is inhibited, and large amounts enter the circulation, resulting in norepinephrine release.[156] MAOIs also potentiate the effect of dopamine, and the administration of this amine or its precursor, L-dopa, is dangerous.[95] Potentiation of the pressor effect of noradrenaline and adrenaline in patients taking MAOIs is probably minimal, unlike the potentiation that occurs with TCAs.[87,95,156] Other drug interactions are listed in Table 5.

Phentolamine or nitroprusside are recommended for the treatment of this hypertensive crisis.[95,155] If beta blockers are to be used for a treatment of supraventricular tachycardias, alpha-adrenergic blockade should be achieved first.[95]

Since the MAO inhibition is irreversible (see earlier discussion), such drug and food interactions should be avoided for at least 2 weeks after discontinuation of therapy. Delayed recovery beyond this time has been reported.[158]

The administration of general anesthesia to patients taking MAOIs is a special management problem requiring a thorough understanding of potential drug interactions.[159]

Patients should be given written instructions on foods to avoid[152,160] (Table 6), and they should be told

TABLE 5
MAOI drug interactions

Antihypertensives:	
Guanethidine	Hypo- or hypertension
Alpha-methyldopa	Hypertension
Hydralazine	Hypotension possible
Reserpine	Hypertension
Diuretics	Hypotension possible
Direct sympathomimetic amines:	
Norepinephrine	
Epinephrine	Mildly potentiated
Phenylephrine	
Indirect sympathomimetic amines:	
Tyramine	
Phenethylamine	
Ephedrine	
Metaraminol	Hypertensive crisis
Amphetamine	
Methylphenidate	
L-Dopa	
Dopamine	
Propranolol	Possible hypertension
Oral anticoagulants	Possible potentiation
Narcotics:	
Meperidine	Hypo- or hypertension, hyperpyrexia
Morphine	Possible potentiation
Sedative-hypnotics	Possible potentiation

TABLE 6
MAOI dietary restrictions

Foods that must be avoided

Beer, wine (particularly Chianti)
Cheese (except cottage and cream cheese)
Smoked or pickled fish (herring)
Beef or chicken liver
Summer (dry) sausage
Fava or broad bean pods (Italian green beans)
Yeast vitamin supplements (brewer's yeast)

Foods that are questionable
(unlikely to cause problems unless consumed in large quantities)

Other alcoholic beverages
Ripe avocado
Ripe fresh banana
Sour cream
Soy sauce (possible individual sensitivity to MSG)
Yogurt

Foods that may be used
(evidence insufficient to support exclusion)

Chocolate
Figs
Meat tenderizers
Raisins
Yeast breads
Coffee, tea, and caffeine-containing beverages

From B. McCabe, and M. T. Tsuang: Dietary consideration in MAO inhibitor regimens, *J. Clin. Psychiatry*, 43:178, 1982. Used with permission.

that no medications other than ASA and acetaminophen should be taken without consulting their physician.

INTERACTION WITH CARDIAC DRUGS[87,95–97] (Table 5)

Most antihypertensive agents are contraindicated with MAOIs. Indirect sympathomimetic amines (see earlier discussion) and meperidine can produce a hypertensive crisis.[95] The effect of direct sympathomimetic amines are mildly potentiated (see earlier discussion). Oral anticoagulants may be potentiated, and sedative-hypnotics should be carefully chosen and dosage reduced.

The reader is referred to other sources for more complete information on these and other drug interactions.[97–99]

LITHIUM

Lithium is the lightest metallic element on the periodic table of the elements.[161] It is administered as a lithium ion in a salt preparation, making it structurally the simplest psychotropic agent yet discovered.[10] Lithium was first used to treat psychiatric patients in 1949 by John Cade in Australia.[162] However, several deaths had resulted from the unregulated use of a lithium salt as a dietary substitute for sodium chloride in the 1940s before its toxicity potential was recognized.[163,164] Thus lithium preparations were not available for treatment of psychiatric patients in the United States until 1970.[161,164]

PHARMACOLOGY

Lithium is usually prescribed as a carbonate or citrate salt.[164,165] Lithium is available as a standard capsule, tablet, or liquid,[165] and as a slow-release tablet that has lower peak levels and can be prescribed in a twice-daily dosage schedule.[166]

Lithium salts are completely absorbed after oral administration, reaching peak levels after 30 min to 2 h for standard preparations[10] and 3 to 5 h for slow-release tablets.[166] Lithium half-life varies considerably from 5 to 40 h,[167,168] with most patients averaging 18 to 24 h.[164] Steady-state levels are achieved in 5 to 7 days.[10,168]

Lithium is not bound to protein in the plasma,[10,164] and it is usually measured as a serum level using a flame photometer or atomic absorption spectro-photometry.[164] Lithium levels to monitor therapy should be tested in the morning, 12 h after the last dose of medication,[168] when the redistribution phase has terminated and the gradual decrease in serum level is due solely to renal excretion.[164]

Lithium is excreted unchanged by the kidneys, with the rate being determined by the renal lithium clearance, accounting for the great variation in dosage requirements.[164,169] Resorption of lithium with sodium occurs primarily in the proximal tubules and is enhanced by sodium-depleted states, increasing the possibility of toxicity.[169]

The mechanism of action by which lithium exerts its psychotropic activity is not well established, although a variety of mechanisms have been proposed, including neurotransmitter alterations, membrane stabilization, and hormonal changes.[10,103,164]

CLINICAL USE

The primary use of lithium preparations is in the acute treatment and prophylaxis of bipolar affective disorder (manic depressive disorder).[161,164] Lithium is the drug of choice for treatment of this disorder, especially for manic episodes,[164] although initially it may be prescribed along with antipsychotics owing to a delayed onset of action.[10] Lithium is an effective agent in preventing or minimizing future relapses in many patients with bipolar disorder. Therapeutic 12-h lithium levels are 0.8 to 1.4 mEq/liter for acute treatment and 0.4 to 1.0 mEq/liter for maintenance.[170] Lithium has a low therapeutic index, with toxicity reported in patients having therapeutic blood levels,[171,172] but more usually occurring in the range of 2.0 to 3.0 mEq/liter.[161] Levels above 3.0 mEq/liter are associated with life-threatening situations.[103,161]

Lithium has been reported to be effective in selected cases for the acute and prophylactic treatment of major depressive disorder and schizoaffective disorder.[10,161,164,173] Preliminary studies have suggested that lithium may be useful in the treatment of uncontrollable aggressive behavior, periodic catatonia, premenstrual tension syndromes, cluster headaches, and alcoholism.[161,164,174]

Lithium is usually prescribed in a three- to four-times daily regimen for standard preparations[10] and twice daily for the slow-release form.[166] The medication is tolerated better when taken with food to avoid gastrointestinal irritation.[10] The dosage needed by an individual patient to reach a therapeutic range can be predicted by the blood level achieved after a single 600-mg dose[175] or by linear extrapolation from the steady-state level reached by a fixed daily dose. Daily lithium dosages range from 600 to 2400 mg to achieve therapeutic effects.[103,164]

NONCARDIAC SIDE EFFECTS

Lithium can cause a spectrum of reversible side effects in most organ systems at therapeutic doses.[164,176,177] The most frequent side effects in patients maintained on therapeutic doses of lithium are tremor, polydipsia, and polyuria.[178] Thyroid abnormalities,[179] gastrointestinal side effects, and weight gain also occur in a smaller, but still significant, number of patients.[176]

Long-term lithium therapy has been associated with morphologic changes in the kidneys.[180] However, these do not seem to lead to progressive azotemia, although they may be associated with a permanent impairment in renal concentrating ability.[181–183] Despite the slight possibility of permanent renal damage, clinicians have consistently concluded that the risk/benefit assessment weighs very strongly in favor of using lithium if the clinical situation is one for which lithium treatment is indicated.[181,183–186]

CARDIOVASCULAR EFFECTS

In the 1940s, lithium chloride was used as a sodium substitute in patients with cardiac or renal disease. Since it was palatable, large quantities were consumed by some patients and toxicity occurred.[187] Although the major toxic symptoms were neurologic, death was attributed to cardiac complications, so the use of lithium in patients with heart disease was considered dangerous. A critical review of these early cases of toxicity and more recent clinical experience fail to substantiate serious cardiovascular complications in most patients.[188] It should be used with caution in patients with renal insufficiency; however, it has been used safely in patients on chronic dialysis.[189]

Heart rate The resting heart rate is not usually affected. A blunting of heart rate response to exercise[190] and mental stress[191] has been observed. Sinus node block with a slow junctional or idioventricular escape rhythm has been reported even with *therapeutic* blood levels.[188] In some cases, coexisting disease of the conduction system was likely. These observations and a limited number of electrophysiologic studies[192–195] imply an effect on sinoatrial node function by either suppression of automaticity or exit block. Since escape rhythms are also slow, automaticity at the junctional and ventricular levels may also be suppressed.[196] Existing sinoatrial node dysfunction may be worsened, and permanent ventricular pacing has been employed so that lithium therapy could be continued.[194,195,197,198]

Electrocardiogram Flattening of T waves is almost universal if all 12 standard ECG leads are monitored.[199,200] Prominent U waves or T wave inversion may occur. Q-T prolongation with therapeutic blood levels is uncommon. Since these ECG changes simulate hypokalemia,[201] they are postulated to result from the replacement of intracellular potassium by lithium.[196,202] These T wave changes are reversible after discontinuing lithium therapy, but they may take up to 2 weeks.[203] Significant ST-segment changes have not been described, except for one instance during anesthesia.[204] Lithium therapy was not associated with ST-segment changes during stress testing in one series of 10 patients.[190] Other ECG changes are uncommon.[188] P-R prolongation, bundle branch block, and complete heart block have been described.[205,206]

Ventricular and supraventricular arrhythmias have not been clearly related to lithium therapy. Some studies have demonstrated an improvement in supraventricular arrhythmias.[190] Precipitation or exacerbation of ventricular premature beats has also been observed.[190,207] Some animal experiments suggest that lithium may have an antiarrhythmic effect.[208]

Ventricular function A significant deleterious effect on ventricular function has not been established. There have been reports of congestive heart failure and myocarditis in patients on lithium therapy, but a causal effect is not obvious.[209] Exercise testing in a small number of patients has shown no impairment of functional capacity.[190] Since chronic hypokalemia is thought to produce myocardial dysfunction,[210] it has been postulated that long-term lithium therapy, by intracellular depletion of potassium, may also result in suppressed myocardial function. Although clinical experience to date has not substantiated this suspicion, further studies are needed.

TOXICITY

Lithium toxicity that develops insidiously begins with prodromal neurological symptoms, which include drowsiness, blurred vision, dizziness, generalized weakness, tinnitus, muscle tremor, and twitching.[176,211] Vomiting and diarrhea are more common in acute toxicity. Hyperreflexia, gross tremor, fasciculations, seizures, and coma may develop.[163,187] Serious cardiovascular complications are uncommon.[212] Sinus bradycardia[197] with a slow junctional or ventricular escape rhythm may occur and can possibly be worsened by concomitant hypokalemia,[213] other medications, or underlying heart disease. T wave changes with U waves and Q-T prolongation occur.[214]

Treatment of lithium toxicity is directed toward enhancement of lithium excretion and supportive care. Electrocardiographic monitoring should be carried out even when cardiac complications are not present initially.

Since the normal rate of renal clearance is slow,

TABLE 7
Lithium drug interactions

Antihypertensives:	
Diuretics	Increased lithium blood levels
Alpha-methyldopa	Possible hypotension
Propranolol $\left.\begin{array}{c} \\ \\ \end{array}\right\}$ Reserpine Digoxin	Possible potentiation of bradycardia

forced diuresis can increase the rate of renal excretion. Mannitol, acetazolamide, sodium bicarbonate, and aminophylline have been used to increase renal clearance of lithium.[215] Appropriate potassium replacement is essential, since hypokalemia may accentuate the cardiac effects. In patients with serious toxicity or impairment of renal function, hemodialysis or peritoneal dialysis is recommended.[189,212,216]

Bradyarrhythmias may require temporary transvenous pacing. The response to intravenous atropine is blunted.[197] Hemodynamic monitoring during volume loading and forced diuresis should be considered in patients suspected of having left ventricular dysfunction.

INTERACTION WITH CARDIAC DRUGS[95–97,176] (Table 7)

The use of thiazide diuretics or dietary sodium restriction may increase lithium blood levels unless the lithium dosage is adjusted.[217] Digoxin, beta blockers, and reserpine may have additive effects on sinoatrial node suppression. Sedative-hypnotics, hydroxyzine, and methyldopa have been reported to have interactions with lithium.[95]

The reader is referred to other sources for more complete information on these and other drug interactions.[97–99,218,219]

ANTIPSYCHOTIC AGENTS

The discovery of the antipsychotic effects of chlorpromazine and reserpine in the early 1950s marked the beginning of a new era in psychiatric treatment. Use of reserpine as an antipsychotic decreased rapidly as clinicians recognized the reliability and safety of chlorpromazine.[10] Previous pharmacologic agents, such as phenobarbital, had provided only nonspecific sedation and had not been effective in reducing the specific symptoms associated with psychotic states. Following the introduction of chlorpromazine, the approach to patients with chronic psychiatric illness shifted from "warehousing" patients in large state hospitals to

TABLE 8
Antipsychotics

Generic name	Trade name	Relative potency*	Adult daily dosage range (mg/day)
Phenothiazines:			
Chlorpromazine	Thorazine, others	100	50–2000
Thioridazine	Mellaril	100	50–800
Mesoridazine	Serentil	50	25–400
Acetophenazine	Tindal	25	40–120
Carphenazine	Proketazine	25	50–400
Triflupromazine	Vesprin	25	50–150
Butaperazine	Repoise	10	5–100
Perphenazine	Trilafon	10	8–64
Piperacetazine	Quide	10	10–160
Trifluoperazine	Stelazine	5	4–60
Fluphenazine	Prolixin, Permitil	2	1–60†
Butyrophenones:			
Haloperidol	Haldol	2	2–100
Dibenzoxazepines:			
Loxapine	Loxitane, Daxolin	10	15–160
Dihydroindolones:			
Molindone	Moban, Lidone	6–10	15–225
Thioxanthenes:			
Chlorprothixene	Taractan	50	75–600
Thiothixene	Navane	5	6–120

*Relative dose necessary to attain therapeutic effect equivalent to 100 mg of chlorpromazine.

†Fluphenazine decanoate and enanthate dosage is 12.5 to 100 mg I.M. every 1 to 4 weeks.

returning most of these patients to community settings.[220,221]

Since that time, a large number of antipsychotic medications representing five different chemical classes have been released for use in the United States[10,103,220] (Table 8). Chlorpromazine has continued to be the standard against which all antipsychotic medications have been compared. Because of the similarities in pharmacologic activity, metabolism, and range of side effects among the available antipsychotic agents,[220] they will be discussed as a group.

PHARMACOLOGY

Antipsychotic medications are available in oral and parenteral forms. Oral doses are erratically absorbed, with a large first-pass metabolism. Peak blood levels usually occur 2 to 4 h after oral doses, although a range of 30 min to 8 h has been reported in some series.[10] Peak and steady-state levels can vary as much as 100-fold between individuals for a given oral dose.[103] Variations in absorption and hepatic metabolism between individuals appear to account for most of the variation in blood levels. Intramuscular administration results in more complete absorption, a threefold to fourfold increase in potency as compared with oral doses,[10] and an earlier peak blood level, after only 20 min to 1 h. Long-acting depot fluphenazine (decanoate or enanthate) is administered parenterally with slow absorption. The gradual release of this medication allows it to be effective when given as infrequently as every 2 to 4 weeks.[222,223] Although not well documented, an individual may metabolize the various antipsychotic medications at different rates, leading to the clinical observation of specific patients responding to one class of antipsychotic and not to another.[10]

The antipsychotic medications are highly protein-bound in the plasma, and they are lipophilic in nature, being concentrated in many tissues including the CNS. The decrease in blood levels following a single dose occurs in two phases: a rapid fall due to redistribution and tissue sequestration followed by a much more gradual decline resulting from hepatic metabolism. The half-life from this second phase averages 15 to 24 h, depending on the chemical class and the specific patient. Because of its concentration in tissues, antipsychotic medication has been detected in excretions up to 18 months after discontinuation.[10]

Blood levels for antipsychotic medications have been studied, but these levels have not consistently been shown to correlate with clinical response.[10,221] The presence of unmeasured active metabolites may partially account for these indeterminate results. A new technique using a radio-receptor assay (which measures dopamine blocking activity in blood samples) looks very promising as a method of determining total antipsychotic activity of the parent molecule and all active metabolites.[224] More research is needed to determine if this technique will have clinical utility.

Most of these antipsychotic medications have several known pharmacologic actions,[103,225,226] including dopamine receptor blockade,[227] alpha-adrenergic receptor blockade,[225,228] and antihistaminic[17] and anticholinergic activity.[18,19] All except for thioridazine have antiemetic activity, which for many years was the basis of animal model screening for potential antipsychotic agents.[221] The most widely accepted hypothesis for the antipsychotic effect of the drugs focuses on the dopamine-blocking action in the mesolimbic pathway of the CNS.[10,221,226]

The relative differences between these drugs with regard to their dopamine receptor blocking activity in the nigrostriatal pathway and their other pharmacologic activities account for the variation in their side-effect profiles.[226]

CLINICAL USE

The primary indication for antipsychotic medications is the treatment of psychotic states, such as those characterized by thought disorders, delusions, or hallucinations.[103,220,221] They are also beneficial for calming states of severe agitation, confusion, and motor restlessness.[103] These symptoms respond even though they may be associated with distinctly different psychiatric conditions, such as schizophrenia, schizoaffective disorder, bipolar disorder, major depressive disorder with psychosis, or organic brain disorders associated with drug, trauma, or neuropathologic etiologies.[10,221] In some cases, the antipsychotic medications are the treatment of choice, while in others, they are adjunctive to more specific treatment aimed at the underlying cause. Antipsychotic drugs are also effective in the treatment of Gilles de la Tourette syndrome.[10,229]

Antipsychotic medication has also been advocated as treatment for less severe psychiatric conditions, such as personality disorders,[230] and nonpsychotic anxiety, or depressive disorder.[231] Caution is advised regarding long-term use of these drugs in such conditions because of the potential for developing tardive dyskinesia.[10,232–234] Nonpsychiatric uses for antipsychotic medications include treatment of intractable hiccoughs, chronic pain, and hyperthermic reactions to anesthesia and as antiemetics.[103]

No replicable difference in efficacy or indications has been demonstrated between the antipsychotic medications.[10,220,221] Thus the clinician should choose the antipsychotic drug to use in a given patient based on the patient's past drug response history, the list of drugs with which the clinician is most familiar, and the side-

effect profile least noxious or dangerous to the patient.[10] Former guidelines regarding the use of sedating drugs in agitated states and less-sedating drugs in apathetic, retarded states are not supported by research, with both types of drugs leading to a normalization of behavior regardless of the presenting symptoms.[10,220,221]

Antipsychotic medication is usually begun in low to moderate dosages and adjusted based on patient response[10,103] (Table 8). In severely agitated patients, a mechanism for rapid treatment has been utilized.[235,236] Although multiple daily doses may be used initially to decrease some of the side effects, once a steady dosage has been reached, single bedtime doses are equally effective and improve patient compliance.[221,237,238] For maintenance therapy, the dosage should be decreased to the lowest effective amount.[220,239] The dosages for response and maintenance vary widely between different individuals owing to differences in rates of metabolism, although a general guideline has been that a dosage equivalent to 400 mg or more chlorpromazine is needed for treatment of acute psychosis.[220] Much lower doses may be effective in treatment of organic brain disorders.[240]

NONCARDIOVASCULAR SIDE EFFECTS

Davis[221] divides the side effects of antipsychotic medication into the following eight categories: (1) autonomic effects, (2) extrapyramidal effects, (3) other central nervous system effects (including sedation), (4) behavioral toxicity, (5) allergic reactions, (6) agranulocytosis, (7) long-term skin and eye effects, and (8) endocrine effects. The most frequent side effects experienced by patients occur in the first three categories.

Autonomic side effects, including dry mouth, blurred vision, and constipation, occur commonly and often subside with continued treatment.[10,221] Retrograde ejaculation is very common with thioridazine.[241] Infrequent effects such as acute urinary retention or paralytic ileus may be lethal.[10]

Extrapyramidal symptoms also occur frequently in patients treated with antipsychotic medications and usually respond to treatment with anti-Parkinson or antihistaminic agents.[221,242,243] Acute dystonias are distressing, short-lived symptoms that may occur within 48 h of initiating or increasing antipsychotic treatment. Akathisia can occur early in the course of treatment and is a subjective feeling of muscle discomfort accompanied by a need to be in constant motion. Patients who experience akathisia complain of an inability to sit or stand still, and the symptoms may be mistaken for psychotic agitation.[103,221] Typical signs of Parkinson's syndrome secondary to antipsychotic medications are indistinguishable from those due to Parkinson's disease. Masked facies, decreased arm movements, akinesia, tremor, and rigidity are among the signs that may occur at variable times during antipsychotic treatment.[221]

Tardive dyskinesia is a side effect that has caused great concern to clinicians and led to more conservative recommendations regarding the use of neuroleptic medications.[10,232,234] Estimates of the frequency with which this sign develops in patients treated with antipsychotic medications vary widely in the literature from 0 to 70 percent.[244] Onset is usually after many years of treatment, although some cases have been reported after only a few months.

Older patients,[244] females, and patients with brain damage seem to be more vulnerable to developing these side effects. Signs are diverse, often including continuous movements of the tongue, lips, and jaw or choreiform movements of the trunk or limbs.[243,245] The pathophysiologic basis is not certain. Although a mechanism of denervation hypersensitivity secondary to dopamine blockade is one of the more popular hypotheses,[103,221,246] recent reviewers suggest that more complex interactions may be involved.[247] Signs of tardive dyskinesia are resistant to treatment, and while these signs are reversible in some patients, they may persist in other patients long after antipsychotic medications have been discontinued.[221,244] Although stopping anti-Parkinson and antipsychotic treatment has been recommended if at all possible, no treatment has been identified as consistently effective.[221,246]

Other CNS effects of antipsychotic medications include lowering the seizure threshold and inducing sedation. The latter is one of the most common effects about which patients complain. As a general guideline, the high-potency, low-dose preparations (haloperidol, trifluoperazine, fluphenazine) cause more extrapyramidal side effects and less sedation than the low-potency drugs. Those medications with intermediate potency tend to produce moderate side effects of both types.[242,248]

CARDIOVASCULAR EFFECTS

As with TCAs, phenothiazines have been reported to cause sudden death, and some pathologic studies have implied that they produce myocardial changes. Patients at risk of these complications of therapy have not been defined. Their action on the autonomic nervous system as well as a direct myocardial effect are possible mechanisms of cardiovascular effects.[249,250]

Heart rate Resting heart rate is usually increased, and rates of 100 beats per minute are not uncommon. Elevated plasma noradrenaline levels have been documented with chlorpromazine.[251]

Orthostatic hypotension The occurrence and severity of orthostatic hypotension are variable.[252,253] Parenteral administration of phenothiazines is more likely to produce supine hypotension and severe orthostatic changes. Oral administration has little effect on supine blood pressure with variable orthostatic changes.[254] Chronic oral administration is associated with lesser effects, even with large doses.[255] Peripheral vasodilitation and reduced systemic vascular resistance contribute to the orthostatic change, and this pharmacologic effect has been utilized in the treatment of patients with heart failure and cardiogenic shock.[256,257]

Electrocardiogram The frequency of electrocardiographic changes is influenced by the drug used and other factors.[258] Some degree of T wave change is described in up to 70 percent of patients.[259] A decrease in amplitude, with or without a change in configuration, is most common. T wave inversion in several to all leads occurs less frequently. These T wave changes are variable in any individual patient and are less frequent in the fasting state.[260,261] They occur more frequently in women.[259] Nitrates, ergotamine, potassium salts,[260] and propranolol have been reported to frequently normalize these changes.[261] These changes are considered benign and are postulated to be related to an intracellular shift of potassium.[262] Thioridazine is reported to produce these changes more frequently than chlorpromazine or trifluoperazine.[263] They usually resolve within 7 days after discontinuing the medication, but they may persist for 2 weeks.[263,264] Q-T prolongation is variable but is probably more common with greater T wave changes (T wave inversion). Bundle branch block, complete heart block, and atrial arrhythmias[265–267] are infrequent. Ventricular tachycardia can occur (see later discussion.)

Ventricular function Early reports implicated phenothiazines in the development of congestive heart failure, acute pulmonary edema, and death. Perivascular and intramyocardial changes[267–269] have been described in patients dying suddenly, but it is not clear whether these changes are specific nor whether they contribute to sudden death or ventricular dysfunction. Prolonged administration of phenothiazines may produce a significant alteration of ventricular function in patients without heart disease.[270] Hemodynamic studies have demonstrated a blunted increase in cardiac output with exercise.[271]

Sudden death There have been a number of reports of sudden death in patients receiving phenothiazines.[272] The use of large doses has been incriminated (3.6 g/day), but in some cases less than 800 mg/day of chlorpromazine was used. Profound peripheral vasodilatation, asphyxia, and seizures have also been proposed mechanisms.[273–275] However, since episodes of heart block, ventricular tachycardia, and ventricular fibrillation have been documented in patients on moderate to large doses, these arrhythmias are likely to be the cause of sudden death. Factors identifying patients at risk have not been defined. Q-T prolongation is a common finding in patients with ventricular tachycardia and/or ventricular fibrillation, and this electrophysiologic effect may provide a mechanism for such arrhythmias and sudden death.[249] Electrophysiologic studies of the effects of phenothiazines in humans are limited.[276] One case report demonstrated that perphenazine facilitated the induction of ventricular tachycardia by the extrastimulus technique. This patient had baseline Q-T prolongation and ventricular extopy.[277] Canine studies suggest a quinidine-like effect that may be both antiarrhythmic and arrhythmogenic.[278–281] Decreased mitochondrial calcium-binding activity has also been reported.[282]

Ventricular tachycardia is frequently unrelenting, associated with Q-T prolongation, and requires special therapeutic consideration (see later discussion). It may occur with usual doses and without premonitory signs. Hypokalemia may facilitate its occurrence.[283]

TOXICITY

Overdose with the phenothiazines produces variable effects on the central and autonomic nervous system and the heart. Seizures, coma, anticholinergic toxicity, hypotension, shock, and life-threatening arrhythmias may occur.[270] In addition to T wave changes and Q-T prolongation,[284] serious cardiac arrhythmias may include complete heart block,[267] ventricular tachycardia,[269,274] and ventricular fibrillation.[277] Marked Q-T prolongation may be present and the ventricular fibrillation may be the torsade de pointes type.[285] Type I antiarrhythmias (quinidine, procainamide, and disopyramide) are not only ineffective but contraindicated. Lidocaine has been used with variable success. Temporary transvenous pacing has been successful[286,287] and should be utilized early in management. Electrolyte abnormalities should be corrected, and other drugs that may prolong the Q-T interval should be discontinued or avoided. Physostigmine has been reported to dramatically correct an idioventricular rhythm with marked intraventricular conduction delay.[288] Its use, however, is not without danger, and the effects on cardiac rhythm are transient, requiring repeated doses.

Hypotension and shock may require intravascular volume expansion and vasopressors. Hemodynamic monitoring may be useful to assess appropriate fluid therapy. Norepinephrine is a recommended vasopressor.[289] Epinephrine should not be used, since it may have no effect or may worsen the hypotension.[275,289] Methoxamine has been used.[274] Shock has been reported to occur when phenothiazines were administered to a patient with pheochromocytoma.[290]

INTERACTION WITH CARDIAC DRUGS[96,97,242,249](Table 9)

The concomitant use of thiazide diuretics may produce hypotension. If hypokalemia occurs, phenothiazine cardiovascular toxicity may be potentiated.[283] The antihypertensive effects of guanethidine and alpha-methyldopa are blocked. The effects of norepinephrine may be potentiated, but epinephrine may cause hypotension. The effects of the indirect sympathomimetic amines are variable. Oral anticoagulants, narcotics, and sedative-hypnotics are potentiated. Haloperidol, an exception, may decrease the effect of oral anticoagulants. Since the antipsychotic agents, particularly chlorpromazine and thioridazine, have electrophysiologic effects similar to those of the type I antiarrhythmics, the combination should probably be avoided.

The reader is referred to other sources for more complete information on these and other drug interactions.[97–99]

TABLE 9
Phenothiazine drug interactions

Antihypertensives:	
Guanethidine	Antihypertensive effect blocked
Alpha-methyldopa	Possible hypotension; haloperidol potentiated
Diuretics	Possible hypotension; hypokalemia may potentiate cardiac toxicity of phenothiazines
Direct sympathomimetic amines:	
Norepinephrine	Variable
Phenylephrine	Variable
Epinephrine	Possible hypotension
Indirect sympathomimetic amines	Potentiated or blocked
Propranolol	Questionable
Oral anticoagulants	Potentiated, except haloperidol, which may block effect
Narcotics	Possibly potentiated
Sedative-hypnotics	Possibly potentiated
Type I antiarrhythmics	Possible potentiation of electrophysiologic effects

USE OF PSYCHOTROPIC AGENTS IN PATIENTS WITH HEART DISEASE

The presence of cardiovascular disease that would predispose to an increased risk with any psychotropic agent requires careful evaluation.[96,291,292] Certain patients are at particular risk from the consequences of an increase in heart rate, orthostatic hypotension, electrophysiologic effects, or suppression of myocardial function that might occur (Table 10). The need for the concomitant use of other medications and the risk of withholding effective psychotropic agents must also be considered.

Tricyclic Derivatives

The TCAs in therapeutic doses almost always produce an increase in heart rate and occasionally cause significant orthostatic hypotension. Potentially serious electrophysiologic effects are rare in patients without heart disease. In patients with heart disease, these effects may become more significant. TCAs are especially hazardous, for example, in patients with *unstable angina pectoris, acute myocardial infarction,* or *severe left ventricular dysfunction.* TCAs should also be avoided in selected patients with cerebrovascular disease. They should be used with caution in patients with *hypertrophic obstructive cardiomyopathy,* especially when a large gradient is provocable; hemodynamically *significant valvular disease,* especially aortic stenosis; and *severe pulmonary hypertension,* whether primary or secondary. The development of orthostatic hypotension in these cases may be dangerous.

For patients who require *antiarrhythmic* or *antihypertensive* therapy, potential drug interactions must be considered. The presence of electrocardiographic abnormalities should be determined prior to treatment.

Q-T prolongation should be evaluated for cause and correction prior to TCA therapy. With *bundle branch block,* especially left, with concomitant heart disease or electrocardiographic evidence of *incomplete trifascicular block,* TCAs should be used cautiously if at all. Although *ventricular ectopy* per se is not a contraindication to their use, the presence of atrial and ventricular ectopy should be carefully assessed prior to TCA therapy.

The most frequently chosen antidepressants for patients with heart disease at the present time include maprotiline, amoxapine, doxepin, norpramine, and nortriptyline. Although a large number of clinical studies in patients with heart disease have not been reported, the available data suggest that these have fewer cardiovascular side effects.[291] Caution is advised, however, since overdose of these antidepressants may still produce significant cardiovascular effects. Nortriptyline may be especially useful, because dosage can be monitored with blood levels. Trazodone seems to have the greatest potential for safety in patients with heart disease, but since it has only recently been released in the United States, further clinical experience is needed. Mianserin is also of special interest, because it is thought to have few cardiovascular effects, even with toxicity, and compared with the TCAs, it has fewer drug interactions.[291]

Monoamine Oxidase Inhibitors

Although the direct cardiovascular effects of the MAOIs is minimal, orthostatic hypotension is a major side effect, and this limits their safe use in patients with cardiac and cerebrovascular disease. The potential consequences of a hypertensive crisis are also greater in these patients. Many antihypertensive agents are contraindicated. The MAOIs should not be used in pa-

TABLE 10
Possible cardiovascular effects of psychotropic drugs

	TCAs	MAOIs	Lithium	Phenothiazines
Heart rate	Increase	Minimal decrease	Blunted response to stress; SB	Increase
Orthostatic hypotension	Yes	Yes	No	Yes
ECG	ST-T changes Increase P-R and QRS; BBB; CHB (prolonged H-V); VPBs decreased or increased	Shortened $Q\text{-}T_c$	ST-T changes; BBB; CHB	ST-T changes; prolonged $Q\text{-}T_c$; BBB; CHB; VPBs; VT
Ventricular function	Possibly suppressed	No effects reported	Possibly suppressed	Possibly suppressed

Abbreviations: BBB = bundle branch block; CHB = complete heart block; SB = sinus bradycardia; VPBs = ventricular premature beats; VT = ventricular tachycardia.

302

tients with significant heart disease without careful consideration of these factors.

Lithium

There are few cardiovascular effects of lithium therapy. Sinoatrial node dysfunction, although uncommon, represents the most significant side effect. Blood levels are helpful, but the occurrence of this complication in the presence of therapeutic levels must be emphasized. Patients who have pretreatment sinus bradycardia or who require cardiac medications that can suppress sinoatrial node function, such as digitalis, beta blockers, and reserpine, have an added risk of this complication. Permanent ventricular pacing has been used to allow continued lithium therapy. Lithium therapy has been continued during acute myocardial infarction,[293] but the combination of lithium therapy and inferior myocardial infarction may require pacemaker therapy.[198] Although the long-term effects of lithium on left ventricular function have not been clarified, its use is not contraindicated in all patients with left ventricular dysfunction.

The use of lithium in patients who have congestive heart failure, who require diuretic therapy or dietary sodium restriction, or who have impaired renal function requires special attention to lithium dosage and blood levels.

Antipsychotics

Like the TCAs, the antipsychotics may produce an increase in heart rate, orthostatic hypotension, and serious ventricular arrhythmias. The significant orthostatic hypotension that can occur with parenteral use must be noted. This side effect with oral use may be minimized with gradually increasing doses. In general, guidelines for their use in patients with heart disease are similar to those outlined for TCAs. Whether serious ventricular arrhythmias occur more frequently with the phenothiazines than with the TCAs is unclear. This complication has been more frequently reported in association with the low-potency phenothiazines (chlorpromazine and thioridazine) than with other antipsychotics. For this reason, the low-potency phenothiazines should be used more cautiously in patients with significant heart disease. For patients who require antiarrhythmic or antihypertensive therapy, potential drug interactions must be considered.

The high-potency phenothiazines[245] (trifluoperazine and fluphenazine) and the butyrophenones, also high-potency,[294] have less frequent cardiovascular effects, since a therapeutic effect can be accomplished with smaller doses. There have been few reports of significant hypotension or arrhythmias with haloperidol.[295,296]

Thiothixene and loxapine are also thought to have less electrocardiographic and hypotensive effects than low-potency phenothiazines, but their use in patients with heart disease has not been extensively reported.[297–299]

REFERENCES

1 Quoted in Schuckit, M., Robins, R., and Feighner, J.: Tricyclic Antidepressants and Monoamine Oxidase Inhibitors, *Arch. Gen. Psychiatry*, 24:509, 1971.

2 Hollister, L. E.: Tricyclic Antidepressants, *N. Engl. J. Med.*, 299:1106, 1168, 1978.

3 Hollister, E.: Treatment of Depression with Drugs, *Ann. Intern. Med.*, 89:78, 1978.

4 Glassman, A. H., Perel, J. M., Shostak, M., Kantor, S. J., and Fleiss, J. L.: Clinical Implications of Imipramine Plasma Levels for Depressive Illness, *Arch. Gen. Psychiatry*, 34:197, 1977.

5 Tricyclic Antidepressant Concentrations and Clinical Response, *Br. Med. J.*, 2:783, 1978. (Editorial.)

6 Robinson, D. S., Nies, A., Ravaris, L., Ives, J. O., and Bartlett, D.: Clinical Pharmacology of Phenelzine, *Arch. Gen. Psychiatry*, 35:629, 1978.

7 Davis, J. M.: Antidepressant Drugs, in H. I. Kaplan, A. M. Freedman, and B. J., Sadock, (eds.), "Comprehensive Textbook of Psychiatry," vol. 3, 3d ed., Williams and Wilkins, Baltimore, 1980, p. 2290.

8 Shopsin, B.: Second Generation Antidepressants, *J. Clin. Psychiatry*, 41:45, 1980.

9 Hollister, L. E.: "Second Generation" Antidepressant Drugs, *Psychosomatics*, 22:872, 1981.

10 Hollister, L. E.: "Clinical Pharmacology of Psychotherapeutic Drugs," Churchill Livingstone, New York, 1978.

11 Peet, M., and Coppen, A.: The Pharmacokinetics of Antidepressant Drugs: Relevance to Their Therapeutic Effects, in E. S., Paykel and A. Coppen, (eds.), "Psychopharmacology of Affective Disorders," Oxford University Press, New York, 1979, p. 91.

12 Risch, S. C., Huey, L. Y., and Janowsky, D. S.: Plasma Levels of Tricyclic Antidepressants and Clinical Efficacy: Review of the Literature. Part 1, *J. Clin. Psychiatry*, 40:4, 1979.

13 Risch, S. C., Huey, L. Y., and Janowsky, D. S.: Plasma Levels of Tricyclic Antidepressants and Clinical Efficacy: Review of the Literature. Part 2, *J. Clin. Psychiatry*, 40:58, 1979.

14 Scoggins, B. A., Maguire, K. P., Norman, T. R., and Burrows, G. D.: Measurement of Tricyclic Antidepressants: II. Applications of Methodology, *Clin. Chem.*, 26:805, 1980.

15 Moody, J. P., Whyte, S. F., MacDonald, A. J., and Naylor, G. J.: Pharmacokinetic Aspects of Protriptyline Plasma Levels, *Eur. J. Clin. Pharmacol.,* 11:51, 1077.

16 Ziegler, V. E., Biggs, J. T., Wylie, L. T., Coryell, W. H., Hanifl, K. M., Hawf, D. J., and Rosen, S. H.: Protriptyline Kinetics, *Clin. Pharmacol. Ther.,* 23:580, 1978.

17 Kanof, P. D., and Greengard, P.: Brain Histamine Receptors as Targets for Antidepressant Drugs, *Nature,* 272:329, 1978.

18 Snyder, S. H., and Yamamura, H. I.: Antidepressants and the Muscarinic Acetylcholine Receptor, *Arch. Gen. Psychiatry,* 34:236, 1977.

19 Tollefson, G. D., Senogles, S. E., Frey, W. H., II, Tuason, V. B., and Nicol, S. E.: A Comparison of Peripheral and Central Human Muscarinic Cholinergic Receptor Affinities for Psychotropic Drugs, *Biol. Psychiatry,* 17:555, 1982.

20 U'Prichard, D. C., Greenberg, D. A., Sheehan, P. P., and Snyder, S. H.: Tricyclic Antidepressants: Therapeutic Properties and Affinity for Alpha-Noradrenergic Receptor Binding Sites in the Brain, *Science,* 199:197, 1978.

21 Iverson, L. L., and Mackay, A. Y. P.: Pharmacodynamics of Antidepressants and Antimanic Drugs in E. S. Paykel and A. Coppen, (eds.), "Psychopharmacology of Affective Disorders," Oxford University Press, New York, 1979, p. 60.

22 Richelson, E.: Tricyclic Antidepressants and Neurotransmitter Receptors, *Psychiatr. Ann.,* 9:186, 1979.

23 Frazer, A., and Mendels, J.: Do Tricyclic Antidepressants Enhance Adrenergic Transmission? *Am. J. Psychiatry,* 134:1040, 1977.

24 Charney, D. S., Menkes, D. B., and Heninger, G. R.: Receptor Sensitivity and the Mechanism of Action of Antidepressant Treatment, *Arch. Gen. Psychiatry,* 38:1160, 1981.

25 Greist, J. H., and Greist, T. H.: "Antidepressant Treatment—The Essentials," Williams and Wilkins, Baltimore, 1979.

26 Van der Velde, C. D.: Maprotiline versus Imipramine and Placebo in Neurotic Depression, *J. Clin. Psychiatry,* 42:138, 1981.

27 Rowan, P. R., Paykel, E. S., and Parker, R. R.: Phenelzine and Amitriptyline: Effects on Symptoms of Neurotic Depression, *Br. J. Psychiatry,* 140:475, 1982.

28 Glassman, A. H., and Roose, S. P.: Delusional Depression: A Distinct Clinical Entity? *Arch. Gen. Psychiatry.* 38:424, 1981.

29 Brown, W. A., and Qualls, C. B.: Pituitary-adrenal Disinhibition in Depression: Marker of a Subtype with Characteristic Clinical Features and Response to Treatment, *Psychiatry Res.,* 4:115, 1981.

30 Maas, J. W.: Biogenic Amines and Depression. Biochemical and Pharmacological Separation of Two Types of Depression, *Arch. Gen. Psychiatry,* 32:1357, 1975.

31 Rosen, H.: "A Clinician's Guide to Affective Disorders," 2d ed., Mnemosyne Publishing Co., Miami, 1981.

32 Mendels, J., and DiGiacomo, J.: The Treatment of Depression with a Single Daily Dose of Imipramine Pamoate, *Am. J. Psychiatry,* 130:1022, 1973.

33 Mendels, J., and Schless, A. P.: Antidepressant Effects of Desipramine Administration in Two Dosage Schedules, *Dis. Nerv. Syst.,* 38:249, 1977.

34 Weise, C. C., Stein, M. K., Pereira-Ogan, J., Csanalosi, I., and Rickels, K.: Amitriptyline Once Daily vs Three Times Daily in Depressed Outpatients, *Arch. Gen. Psychiatry,* 37:555, 1980.

35 Swinyard, E. J.: Principles of Prescription Order Writing and Patient Compliance Instruction, in A. G. Gilman, L. S. Goodman, and A. Gilman, (eds.) "The Pharmacological Basis of Therapeutics," 6th ed., Macmillan Publishing Co., Inc., New York, 1980, p. 1660.

36 Gram, L. F.: Pharmacokinetics and Clinical Response to Tricyclic Antidepressants, *Acta Psychiatr. Scand.,* 61 (suppl. 280):169, 1980.

37 Amdisen, A.: Blood Concentration of Cyclic Antidepressants as a Daily Routine? A Critical Review from the Doorstep of the Clinical Laboratory, *Acta Psychiatr. Scand.,* 61 (suppl. 280):261, 1980.

38 Cole, J. O., and Orsulak, P.: Tricyclic Antidepressant Blood Levels, in J. O. Cole, (ed.), "Psychopharmacology Update," The Collamore Press, Lexington, Mass., 1980, p. 19.

39 Smith, R. C., Chojnacki, M., Hu, R., and Mann, E.: Cardiovascular Effects of Therapeutic Doses of Tricyclic Antidepressants: Importance of Blood Level Monitoring, *J. Clin. Psychiatry,* 41:57, 1980.

40 Hollister, L. E.: Plasma Concentrations of Tricyclic Antidepressants in Clinical Practice, *J. Clin. Psychiatry,* 43:66, 1982.

41 Preskorn, S. H., and Simpson, S.: Tricyclic-Antidepressant-Induced Delirium and Plasma Drug Concentration, *Am. J. Psychiatry,* 139:822, 1982.

42 Klein, D. F., Zitrin, C. M., and Woerner, M.: Antidepressants, Anxiety, Panic, and Phobia, in M. A. Lipton, A. DiMascio, and K. F. Killam, (eds.), "Psychopharmacology: A Generation of Progress," Raven Press, New York, 1978, p. 1401.

43 Ziegler, V. E., Taylor, J. R., Wetzel, R. D., and Biggs, J. T.: Nortriptyline Plasma Levels and Subjective Side Effects, *Br. J. Psychiatry,* 132:55, 1978.

44 Glassman, A. H., and Bigger, J. T., Jr.: Cardiovascular Effects of Therapeutic Doses of Tricyclic Antidepressants. A Review, *Arch. Gen. Psychiatry,* 38:815, 1981.

45 Jefferson, J. W.: A Review of the Cardiovascular Effects and Toxicity of Tricyclic Antidepressants, *Psychosom. Med.,* 37:160, 1975.

46 Marshall, J. B., and Forker, A. D.: Cardiovascular Effects of Tricyclic Antidepressant Drugs: Therapeutic Usage,

Overdose, and Management of Complications, *Am. Heart J.,* 103:401, 1982.

47 Luke, C. M.: Tricyclic Antidepressants and Heart Disease, *N.Z. Med. J.,* 74:345, 1971.

48 Gwynne, J. F.: Tricyclic Antidepressants and Heart Disease, *N.Z. Med. J.,* 74:414, 1971.

49 Ziegler, V. E., Co, B. T., and Biggs, J. T.: Electrocardiographic Findings in Patients Undergoing Amitriptyline Treatment, *Dis. Nerv. Syst.,* 38:697, 1977.

50 Taylor, D. J. E., and Braithwaite, R. A.: Cardiac Effects of Tricyclic Antidepressant Medication. A Preliminary Study of Nortriptyline, *Br. Heart J.,* 40:1005, 1978.

51 Kantor, S. J., Glassman, A. H., Bigger, J. T., Jr., Perel, J. M., and Giardina, E. V.: The Cardiac Effects of Therapeutic Plasma Concentrations of Imipramine, *Am. J. Psychiatry,* 135:534, 1978.

52 Vohra, J., Burrows, G. D., and Sloman, G.: Assessment of Cardiovascular Side Effects of Therapeutic Doses of Tricyclic Anti-Depressant Drugs, *Aust. N.Z. J. Med.,* 5:7, 1975.

53 Vohra, J., Burrows, G., Hunt, D., and Sloman, G.: The Effect of Toxic and Therapeutic Doses of Tricyclic Antidepressant Drugs on Intracardiac Conduction, *Eur. J. Cardiol.,* 3:219, 1975.

54 Freyschuss, U., Sjöqvist, F., Tuck, D., and Asberg, M.: Circulatory Effects in Man of Nortriptyline, a Tricyclic Antidepressant Drug, *Pharmacol. Clin.,* 2:68, 1970.

55 Veith, R. C., Raskind, M. A., Caldwell, J. H., Barnes, R. F., Gumbrecht, G., and Ritchie, J. L.: Cardiovascular Effects of Tricyclic Antidepressants in Depressed Patients with Chronic Heart Disease, *N. Engl. J. Med.,* 306:954, 1982.

56 Winsberg, B. G., Goldstein, S., Yepes, L. E., and Perel, J. M.: Imipramine and Electrocardiographic Abnormalities in Hyperactive Children, *Am. J. Psychiatry,* 132:542, 1975.

57 Veith, R. C., Friedel, R. O., Bloom, V., and Bielski, R.: Electrocardiogram Changes and Plasma Desipramine Levels during Treatment of Depression, *Clin. Pharmacol. Ther.,* 27:796, 1980.

58 Burgess, C. D., Montgomery, S., Wadsworth, J., and Turner, P.: Cardiovascular Effects of Mianserin, Zimelidine and Nomifensine in Depressed Patients, *Postgrad. Med. J.,* 55:704, 1979.

59 Glassman, A. H., Bigger, J. T., Jr., Giardina, E. V., Kantor, S. J., Perel, J. M., and Davies, M.: Clinical Characteristics of Imipramine-Induced Orthostatic Hypotension, *Lancet,* 1:468, 1979.

60 Mielke, D. H., Koepke, R. P., and Phillips, J. H.: A Controlled Evaluation of a Tetracyclic (Maprotiline) and a Tricyclic (Imipramine) Antidepressant and Their Effects on the Heart, *Curr. Therap. Res.,* 25:738, 1979.

61 Raeder, E. A., Burkhardt, D., Neubaurer, H., Walter, R., and Gastpar, M.: Long-Term Tri- and Tetra-Cyclic Antidepressants, Myocardial Contractility, and Cardiac Rhythm, *Br. Med. J.,* 2:666, 1978.

62 Giardina, E. V., Bigger, J. T., Glassman, A. H., Perel, J. M., and Kantor, S. J.: The Electrocardiographic and Antiarrhythmic Effects of Imipramine Hydrochloride at Therapeutic Plasma Concentrations, *Circulation,* 60:1045, 1979.

63 Ziegler, V. E., Co, B. T., and Biggs, J. T.: Plasma Nortriptyline Levels and ECG Findings, *Am. J. Psychiatry,* 134:441, 1977.

64 Reed, K., Smith, R. C., Schoolar, J. C., Hu, R., Leelavathi, D. E., Mann, E., and Lippman, L.: Cardiovascular Effects of Nortriptyline in Geriatric Patients, *Am. J. Psychiatry,* 137:986, 1980.

65 Rudorfer, M. V., and Young, R. C.: Desipramine: Cardiovascular Effects and Plasma Levels, *Am. J. Psychiatry,* 137:984, 1980.

66 Hayes, J. R., Born, G. F., and Rosenbaum, A. H.: Incidence of Orthostatic Hypotension in Patients with Primary Affective Disorders Treated with Tricyclic Antidepressants, *Mayo Clin. Proc.,* 52:209, 1977.

67 Glassman, A. H., Walsh, B. T., Roose, S. P., Rosenfeld, R., Bruno, R. L., Bigger, J. T., and Giardina, E. V.: Factors Related to Orthostatic Hypotension Associated with Tricyclic Antidepressants, *J. Clin. Psychiatry,* 43:35, 1982.

68 Burckhardt, D., Raeder, E., Müller, V., Imhof, P., and Neubauer, H.: Cardiovascular Effects of Tricyclic and Tetracyclic Antidepressants, *J.A.M.A.,* 239:213, 1978.

69 Pinder, R. M., Brogden, R. N., Speight, T. M., and Avery, G. S.: Doxepin Up-to-Date: A Review of Its Pharmacological Properties and Therapeutic Efficacy with Particular Reference to Depression, *Drugs,* 13:161, 1977.

70 Bishop, M. P., Mason, L. B., and Gallant, D. M.: Blood Pressure Abnormalities in Schizophrenic Patients: Some Considerations Relevant to the Clinical Testing of Investigational Drugs, *Curr. Therap. Res.,* 10:315, 1968.

71 Masterton, G., Main, C. J., Lever, A. F., and Lever, R. S.: Low Blood Pressure in Psychiatric Inpatients, *Br. Heart J.,* 45:442, 1981.

72 Burrows, G. D., Vohra, J., Hunt, D., Sloman, J. G., Scoggins, B. A., and Davies, B.: Cardiac Effects of Different Tricyclic Antidepressant Drugs, *Br. J. Psychiatry,* 129:335, 1976.

73 Brennan, F. J.: Electrophysiologic Effects of Imipramine and Doxepin on Normal and Depressed Cardiac Purkinje Fibers, *Am. J. Cardiol.,* 46:599, 1980.

74 Edelstein, E. L.: Antidepressant Drugs, in M. N. G. Dukes, (ed.), "Side Effects of Drugs Annual," vol. 9, Excerpta Medica, Amsterdam, 1980, p. 21.

75 Bigger, J. T., Jr., Giardina, E. V., Perel, J. M., Kantor, S. J., and Glassman, A. H.: Cardiac Antiarrhythmic Effects of Imipramine Hydrochloride, *N. Engl. J. Med.,* 296:206, 1977.

76 Giardina, E. V., and Bigger, T. J., Jr.: Antiarrhythmic Effect of Imipramine Hydrochloride in Patients with Ventricular Premature Complexes without Psychological Depression, *Am. J. Cardiol.*, 50:172, 1982.

77 Lewis, R. P., Rittgers, S. E., Forester, W. F., and Boudoulas, H.: A Critical Review of the Systolic Time Intervals, *Circulation*, 56:146, 1977.

78 Boston Collaborative Drug Surveillance Program: Adverse Reactions to the Tricyclic-Antidepressant Drugs, *Lancet*, 1:529, 1972.

79 Coull, D. C., Crooks, J., Dingwall-Fordyce, I., Scott, A. M., and Weir, R. D.: Amitriptyline and Cardiac Disease. Risk of Sudden Death Identified by Monitoring System, *Lancet*, 2:590, 1970.

80 Moir, D. C., Crooks, J., Cornwell, W. B., O'Malley, K., Dingwall-Fordyce, I., Turnbull, M. J., and Weir, R. D.: Cardiotoxicity of Amitriptyline, *Lancet*, 2:561, 1972.

81 Siddiqu, J. H., Vakassi, M. M., and Ghani, M. F.: Cardiac Effects of Amitriptyline Overdose, *Curr. Therap. Res.*, 22:321, 1977.

82 Callaham, M.: Tricyclic Antidepressant Overdose, *J.A.C.E.P.*, 8:413, 1979.

83 Nicotra, M. B., Rivera, M., Pool, J. L., and Noall, M. W.: Tricyclic Antidepressant Overdose: Clinical and Pharmacologic Observations, *Clin. Toxicol.*, 18:599, 1981.

84 Petit, J. M., Spiker, D. G., Ruwitch, J. F., Ziegler, V. E., Weiss, A. N., and Biggs, J. T.: Tricyclic Antidepressant Plasma Levels and Adverse Effects after Overdose, *Clin. Pharmacol. Ther.*, 21:47, 1977.

85 Langou, R. A., Van Dyke, C., Tahan, S. R., and Cohen, L. S.: Cardiovascular Manifestations of Tricyclic Antidepressant Overdose, *Am. Heart J.*, 100:458, 1980.

86 Preskorm, S. H., and Irwin, H. A.: Toxicity of Tricyclic Antidepressants—Kinetics, Mechanism, Intervention: A Review, *J. Clin. Psychiatry*, 43:151, 1982.

87 Boakes, A. J., Laurence, D. R., Teoh, P. C., Barar, F. S. K., and Benedikter, L. T.: Interactions between Sympathomimetic Amines and Antidepressant Agents in Man, *Br. Med. J.*, 1:311, 1973.

88 Penny, R.: Imipramine Hydrochloride Poisoning in Childhood, *Am. J. Dis. Child.*, 116:181, 1968.

89 Hagerman, G. A., and Hanashiro, P. K.: Reversal of Tricyclic-Antidepressant-Induced Cardiac Conduction Abnormalities by Phenytoin, *Ann. Emerg. Med.*, 10:82, 1981.

90 Nattel, S., Bayne, L., and Ruedy, J.: Physostigmine in Coma Due to Drug Overdose, *Clin. Pharmacol. Ther.*, 25:96, 1979.

91 Orr, D. A., and Bramble, M. G.: Tricyclic Antidepressant Poisoning and Prolonged External Cardiac Massage during Asystole, *Br. Med. J.*, 283:1107, 1981.

92 Spiker, D. G., and Biggs, J. T.: Tricyclic Antidepressants. Prolonged Plasma Levels after Overdose, *J.A.M.A.*, 236:1711, 1976.

93 Pentel, P., and Sioris, L.: Incidence of Late Arrhythmias Following Tricyclic Antidepressant Overdose, *Clin. Toxicol.*, 18:543, 1981.

94 Fasoli, R. A., and Glauser, F. L.: Cardiac Arrhythmias and ECG Abnormalities in Tricyclic Antidepressant Overdose, *Clin. Toxicol.* 18:155, 1981.

95 Risch, S. C., Groom, G. P., and Janowsky, D. S.: Interfaces of Psychopharmacology and Cardiology. Part 1, *J. Clin. Psychiatry*, 42:23, 1981.

96 Risch, S. C., Groom, G. P., and Janowsky, D. S.: The Effects of Psychotropic Drugs on the Cardiovascular System, *J. Clin. Psychiatry*, 43:16, 1982.

97 Gaultieri, C. T., and Powell, S. F.: Psychoactive Drug Interactions, *J. Clin. Psychiatry*, 39:720, 1978.

98 Hansten, P. D.: "Drug Interactions," Lea and Febiger, Philadelphia, 1976.

99 Adverse Interactions of Drugs, *Med. Lett.*, 23:17, 1981.

100 Smith, R. S., and Ayd, F. J., Jr.: A Critical Appraisal of Amoxapine, *J. Clin. Psychiatry*, 42:238, 1981.

101 Lydiard, R. B.: Amoxapine, *Biol. Ther. Psychiatry*, 5:21, 1982.

102 Ragheb, M., Wilson, W. H., Ban, T. A., and Brannen, J. O.: Amoxapine: Once versus Divided Daily Doses in Neurotic and Endogenous Depression, *J. Clin. Psychiatry*, 42:318, 1981.

103 van Praag, H. M.: "Psychotropic Drugs—A Guide for the Practitioner," Brunner/Mazel, Inc., New York, 1978.

104 Maprotiline (Ludiomil)—Another Antidepressant, *Med. Lett.*, 23:58, 1981.

105 Jansen, F. H. J.: Mianserin Differentiated from Tricyclic Antidepressants, *J.A.M.A.*, 240:1339, 1978. (Letter.)

106 Mindham, R. H. S.: Tricyclic Antidepressants and Amine Precursors, in E. S., Paykel, and A. Coppen, (eds.), "Psychopharmacology of Affective Disorders," Oxford University Press, New York, 1979, p. 123.

107 Crome, P., Braithwaite, R., Newman, B., and Montgomery, S.: Choosing an Antidepressant, *Br. Med. J.*, 1:859, 1978. (Letter)

108 Feighner, J. P.: Trazodone, a Triazolopyridine Derivative, in Primary Depressive Disorder, *J. Clin. Psychiatry*, 41:250, 1980.

109 Al-Yassiri, M. M., Ankier, S. I., and Bridges, P. K.: Trazodone—A New Antidepressant, *Life Sci.*, 28:2449, 1981.

110 Taylor, D. P., Hyslop, D. K., and Riblet, L. A.: Trazodone, a new Nontricyclic Antidepressant without Anticholinergic Activity, *Biochem. Pharmacol.*, 29:2149, 1980.

111 Feighner, J. P.: "Psychopharmacology—Update on 2nd and 3rd Generation Antidepressants," presented at the Seventh Annual Scientific Meeting, American Academy of Clinical Psychiatrists, San Diego, Calif., October 1981.

112 Goldberg, H. L., and Finnerty, R. J.: Trazodone in the Treatment of Neurotic Depression, *J. Clin. Psychiatry,* 41:430, 1980.

113 Gershon, S., Mann, J., Newton, R., and Gunther, B. J.: Evaluation of Trazodone in the Treatment of Endogenous Depression: Results of a Multicenter Double-Blind Study, *J. Clin. Psychopharmacol.,* 1 (6, suppl.):39S, 1981.

114 Gershon, S., and Newton, R.: Lack of Anticholinergic Side Effects with a New Antidepressant—Trazodone, *J. Clin. Psychiatry,* 41:100, 1980.

115 Gerner, R., Estabrook, W., Steuer, J., and Jarvik, L.: Treatment of Geriatric Depression with Trazodone, Imipramine, and Placebo: A Double-Blind Study, *J. Clin. Psychiatry,* 41:216, 1980.

116 Goldberg, M. J., and Spector, R.: Amoxapine Overdose: Report of Two Patients with Severe Neurologic Damage, *Ann. Intern. Med.,* 96:463, 1982.

117 Lloyd, A. II.. Practical Considerations in the Use of Maprotiline (Ludiomil) in General Practice, *J. Int. Med. Res.,* 5 (suppl. 4):122, 1977.

118 Ghosh, A. K.: Cardiovascular Effects of Maprotiline, In "New Dimensions in Antidepressants," Excerpta Medica, Amsterdam, 1981.

119 Park, J. Y., and Proudfoot, A. T.: Acute Poisoning with Maprotiline Hydrochloride, *Br. Med. J.,* 1:1573, 1977.

120 Jarvik, L.: Antidepressant Therapy for the Geriatric Patient, *J. Clin. Psychopharmacol.,* 1 (6, suppl.):55S, 1981.

121 Pichot, P., Dreyfus, J. F., and Pull, C.: A Double-Blind, Controlled Multicenter Study Comparing Mianserin and Imipramine, *Br. J. Clin. Pharmacol.,* 5 (suppl. 1):87S, 1978.

122 Burrows, G. D., Davies, B., Hamer, A., and Vohra, J.: Effect of Mianserin on Cardiac Conduction, *Med. J. Aust.,* 2:97, 1979.

123 Gomoll, A. W., and Byrne, J. E.: Cardiovascular Effects of Trazodone in Animals, *J. Clin. Psychopharmacol.,* 1 (6, suppl.):70S, 1981.

124 Ayd Medical Communication: Trazodone: A Unique New Broad Spectrum Antidepressant, *Int. Drug Ther. Newsletter,* 14:33, 1979.

125 Riblet, L. A., and Taylor, D. P.: Pharmacology and Neurochemistry of Trazodone, *J. Clin. Psychopharmacol.,* 1 (6, suppl.):17S, 1981.

126 Himmelhoch, J. M.: Cardiovascular Effects of Trazodone in Humans, *J. Clin. Psychopharmacol.,* 1 (6, suppl.):76S, 1981.

127 Branconnier, R. J., and Cole, J. O.: Effects of Acute Administration of Trazodone and Amitriptyline on Cognition, Cardiovascular Function and Salivation in the Normal Geriatric Subject, *J. Clin. Psychopharmacol.,* 1 (6, suppl.):82S, 1981.

128 Feighner, J. P.: Clinical Efficacy of the Newer Antidepressants, *J. Clin. Psychopharmacol.,* 1 (6, suppl.):23S, 1981.

129 Blackwell, B.: Antidepressant Drugs, in M. N. G. Dukes, (ed.), "Side Effects of Drugs Annual," vol. 10, Excerpta Medica, Amsterdam, 1982, p. 16.

130 Medical Research Council: Clinical Trial of the Treatment of Depressive Illness, *Br. Med. J.,* 1:887, 1965.

131 Tyrer, P.: Clinical Use of Monoamine Oxidase Inhibitors, In E. S. Paykel, and A. Coppen, (eds.), "Psychopharmacology of Affective Disorders," Oxford University Press, New York, 1979, p. 159.

132 Quitkin, F., Rifkin, A., and Klein, D. F.: Monoamine Oxidase Inhibitors, *Arch. Gen. Psychiatry,* 35:749, 1979.

133 Johnstone, E. C., and Marsh, W.: Acetylator Status and Response to Phenelzine in Depressed Patients, *Lancet,* 1:567, 1973.

134 Johnstone, E. C.: The Relationship between Acetylator Status and Inhibition of Monoamine Oxidase. Excretion of Free Drug and Antidepressant Response in Depressed Patients on Phenelzine, *Psychopharmacologia,* 46:289, 1976.

135 Moller, P. W.: Clinical Implications of Acetylator Status, *Drug Ther. (Hosp.),* 4:40, 1979.

136 Robinson, D. S.: Monoamine Oxidase Inhibitors and the Elderly, in A. Raskin, D. S. Robinson, and J. Levine (eds.), "Age and the Pharmacology of Psychoactive Drugs," Elsevier North Holland, Inc., New York, 1981, p. 151.

137 Robinson, D. S., Nies, A., and Ravaris, C. L.: Acute versus Chronic Effects of Monoamine Oxidase Inhibitors in Depressed Patients: The Time Course of MAO Inhibitors, *Proc. Psychopharmacol. Bull.,* 13:50, 1977.

138 Edelstein, E. L.: Antidepressant Drugs, in N. N. G. Dukes, (ed.), "Meyler's Side Effects of Drugs," 9th ed., Excerpta Medica, Amsterdam, 1980, p. 21.

139 Ravaris, C. L., Nies, A., Robinson, D. S., Ives, J. O., Lamborn, K. R., and Korson, L.: A Multi-Dose, Controlled Study of Phenelzine in Depression-Anxiety States, *Arch. Gen. Psychiatry,* 33:347, 1976.

140 Other MAOIs, *Biol. Ther. Psychiatry,* 5:5, 1982.

141 New Look at Monoamine Oxidase Inhibitors, *Br. Med. J.,* 2:69, 1976. (Editorial.)

142 Paykel, E. S., Parker, R. R., Penrose, R. J. J., and Rassaby, E. R.: Depressive Classification and Prediction of Response to Phenelzine, *Br. J. Psychiatry,* 134:572, 1979.

143 Nies, A., and Robinson, D. S.: Comparison of Clinical Effects of Amitriptyline and Phenelzine Treatment, in M. B. H. Youdim, and E. S. Paykel, (eds.), "Monoamine Oxidase Inhibitors—The State of the Art," John Wiley and Sons, Inc., New York, 1981, p. 141.

144 Ravaris, C. L., Robinson, D. S., Ives, J. O., Nies, A., and Bartlett, D.: Phenelzine and Amitriptyline in the Treatment of Depression, *Arch. Gen. Psychiatry*, 37:1075, 1980.

145 Davidson, J. R. T., McLeod, M. N., Turnbull, C. D., and Miller, R. D.: A Comparison of Phenelzine and Imipramine in Depressed Inpatients, *J. Clin. Psychiatry*, 42:395, 1981.

146 Schuckit, M. A.: Current Therapeutic Options in the Management of Typical Anxiety, *J. Clin. Psychiatry*, 42:15, 1981.

147 Tyrer, P., Candy, J., and Kelly, D.: Phenelzine in Phobic Anxiety: A Controlled Trial, *Psychol. Med.*, 3:120, 1973.

148 Rohs, R. G., and Noyes, R.: Agoraphobia: Newer Treatment Approaches, *J. Nerv. Ment. Dis.*, 166:701, 1978.

149 Isberg, R. A.: A Comparison of Phenelzine and Imipramine in an Obsessive-Compulsive Patient, *Am. J. Psychiatry*, 138:1250, 1981.

150 Hogben, G. L., and Cornfield, R. B.: Treatment of Traumatic War Neurosis with Phenelzine, *Arch. Gen. Psychiatry*, 38:440, 1981.

151 McGilchrist, J. M.: Interactions with Monoamine Oxidase Inhibitors, *Br. Med. J.*, 3:591, 1975. (Letter.)

152 Stewart, M. M.: MAOIs and Food—Fact and Fiction, *Adverse Drug Reaction Bull.*, 58:200, 1976.

153 Robinson, D. S., Nies, A., Corcella, J., Cooper, T. B., Spencer, C, and Keefover, R.: Cardiovascular Effects of Phenelzine and Amitriptyline in Depressed Outpatients, *J. Clin. Psychiatry*, 43:8, 1982.

154 Lee, W. C., Shin, Y. H., and Shideman, F. E.: Cardiac Activities of Several Monoamine Oxidase Inhibitors, *J. Pharmacol. Exp. Ther.* 133:180, 1961.

155 Goldberg, L.: Monoamine Oxidase Inhibitors. Adverse Reactions and Possible Mechanisms, *J.A.M.A.*, 190:132, 1964.

156 Sjöqvist, F.: Psychotropic Drugs: 2. Interactions between Monoamine Oxidase Inhibitors and Other Substances, *Proc. R. Soc. Med.*, 58:964, 1965.

157 Rosenbaum, A. H., Maruta, T., and Richelson, E.: Drugs that Alter Mood: 1. Tricyclic Agents and Monoamine Oxidase Inhibitors, *Mayo Clin. Proc.*, 54:335, 1979.

158 Cousins, M. J., and Maltby, J. R.: Delayed Recovery of Sympathetic Transmission Following Ten Years Monoamine Oxidase Inhibition, *Br. J. Anaesth.*, 43:803, 1971.

159 Thornton, J. A.: The Effects of Drug Therapy on the Response to Anaesthetic Agents, in J. A. Thornton, (ed.), "Adverse Reactions to Anaesthetic Drugs," Excerpta Medica, New York, 1981, p. 1.

160 McCabe, B., and Tsuang, M. T.: Dietary Considerations in MAO Inhibitor Regimens, *J. Clin. Psychiatry*, 43:178, 1982.

161 Fieve, R. R.: Lithium Therapy, in H. I. Kaplan, A. M. Freeman, and B. J. Sadock (eds.), "Comprehensive Textbook of Psychiatry," vol. 3, 3d ed., Williams and Wilkins, Baltimore, 1980, p. 2348.

162 Cade, J. F. J.; Lithium Salts in the Treatment of Psychotic Excitement, *Med. J. Aust.*, 36:349, 1949.

163 Corcoran, A. C., Taylor, R. D., and Page, I. H.: Lithium Poisoning from the Use of Salt Substitutes, *J.A.M.A.*, 139:685, 1949.

164 Jefferson, J. W., and Greist, J. H.: "Primer of Lithium Therapy," Williams and Wilkins, Baltimore, 1977.

165 Heiman, M. F., Schwabach, G., and Tubin, J.: Liquid Lithium vs Solid Lithium: An Open, Cross-Over, Pilot Study Comparing Oral Preparations, *Dis. Nerv. Syst.*, 37:9, 1976.

166 Cooper, T. B., Simpson, G. M., Lee, J. H., and Bergner, P. E.: Evaluation of a Slow-Release Lithium Carbonate Formulation, *Am. J. Psychiatry*, 135:917, 1978.

167 Amdisen, A.: Serum Lithium Estimations, *Br. Med. J.*, 2:240, 1975. (Letter.)

168 Amdisen, A.: Monitoring Lithium Dose Levels: Clinical Aspects of Serum Lithium Estimation, in F. N. Johnson (ed.), "Handbook of Lithium Therapy," University Park Press, Baltimore, 1980, p. 179.

169 Thomsen, K.: The Renal Excretion of Lithium, in M. Schou and E. Strömgren (eds.), "Origin, Prevention and Treatment of Affective Disorders," Academic Press, London, 1979, p. 95.

170 Hullin, R. P.: Minimum Serum Lithium Levels for Effective Prophylaxis in F. N. Johnson (ed.), "Handbook of Lithium Therapy," University Park Press, Baltimore, 1980, p. 243.

171 Strayhorn, J. M., and Nash, J. L.: Severe Neurotoxicity Despite Therapeutic Serum Lithium Levels, *Dis. Nerv. Syst.*, 38:107, 1977.

172 Speirs, J., and Hirsch, S. R.: Severe Lithium Toxicity with "Normal" Serum Concentrations, *Br. Med. J.*, 1:815, 1978.

173 Pesecow, E. D., Dunner, D. L., Fieve, R. R., and Lautin, A.: Lithium Prophylaxis of Depression in Unipolar, Bipolar II, and Cyclothymic Patients, *Am. J. Psychiatry*, 139:747, 1982.

174 Rees, W. L.: The Value and Limitations of Lithium Therapy in Psychiatric Disorders, *Psychiatr. Ann.*, 11:172, 1981.

175 Cooper, T. B., Bergner, P.-E. E., and Simpson, G. M.: The 24-Hour Serum Lithium Level as a Prognosticator of Dosage Requirements, *Am. J. Psychiatry*, 130:601, 1973.

176 Amdisen, A., and Schou, M.: Lithium, in M. N. G. Dukes (ed.), "Meyler's Side Effects of Drugs," 9th ed., Excerpta Medica, Amsterdam, 1980, p. 43.

177 Brown, W. T.: The Patterns of Lithium Side-Effects and Toxic Reactions in the Course of Lithium Therapy, in F.

N. Johnson (ed.), "Handbook of Lithium Therapy," University Park Press, Baltimore, 1980, p. 279.

178 Johnston, B. B., Dick, E. G., Naylor, G. J., and Dick, D. A. T.: Lithium Side Effects in a Routine Lithium Clinic, *Br. J. Psychiatry,* 134:482, 1979.

179 Lindstedt, G., Nilsson, L., Wälinder, J., Skott, A., and Öhman, R.: On the Prevalence, Diagnosis, and Management of Lithium-Induced Hypothyroidism in Psychiatric Patients, *Br. J. Psychiatry,* 130:452, 1977.

180 Hestbech, J., Hansen, H. E., Amdisen, A., and Olsen, S.: Chronic Renal Lesions Following Long-Term Treatment with Lithium, *Kidney Int.,* 12:205, 1977.

181 Lippmann, S.: Is Lithium Bad for the Kidneys? *J. Clin. Psychiatry,* 43:220, 1982.

182 Hansen, H. E., Hestbech, J., and Olsen, S.: Renal Function and Renal Pathology in Patients with Lithium-Induced Impairment of Renal Concentrating Ability, *Proc. Eur. Dial. Transplant. Assoc.,* 14:518, 1977.

183 Vestergaard, P.: Renal Side-Effects of Lithium, in F. N. Johnson (ed.), "Handbook of Lithium Therapy," University Park Press, Baltimore, 1980, p. 345.

184 Lithium-induced Nephrotoxicity: A Further Report, *Int. Drug Ther. Newsletter,* 13:25, 1978.

185 Lithium and the Kidney: Grounds for Cautious Optimism, *Lancet,* 2:1056, 1979. (Editorial.)

186 Cole, J. O., Altesman, R. I., Ionescu-Pioggia, M., and Brewster, P. M.: Lithium and the Kidney, in J. O. Cole, (ed.), "Psychopharmacology Update," The Collamore Press, Lexington, Mass., 1980, p. 173.

187 Hanlon, L. W., Romaine, M., III, and Gilroy, F. J.: Lithium Chloride as a Substitute for Sodium Chloride in the Diet, *J.A.M.A.,* 139:688, 1949.

188 Mitchell, J. E., and Mackenzie, T. B.: Cardiac Effects of Lithium Therapy in Man: A Review, *J. Clin. Psychiatry,* 43:47, 1982.

189 Rosenbaum, A. H., Maruta, T., and Richelson, E.: Drugs that Alter Mood. 2. Lithium, *Mayo Cin. Proc.,* 54:401, 1979.

190 Tilkian, A. G., Schroeder, J. S., Kao, J., and Hultgren, H.: Effect of Lithium on Cardiovascular Performance: Report on Extended Ambulatory Monitoring and Exercise Testing before and during Lithium Therapy, *Am. J. Cardiol.,* 38:701, 1976.

191 Belmaker, R. H., Lehrer, R., Ebstein, R. P., Lettik, H., and Kugelmass, S.: A Possible Cardiovascular Effect of Lithium, *Am. J. Psychiatry,* 136:577, 1979.

192 Wilson, J. R., Kraus, E. S., Bailas, M. M., and Rakita, L.: Reversible Sinus-Node Abnormalities Due to Lithium Carbonate Therapy, *N. Engl. J. Med.,* 294:1223, 1976.

193 Wellens, H. J., Cats, V. M., and Düren, D. R.: Symptomatic Sinus Node Abnormalities Following Lithium Carbonate Therapy, *Am. J. Med.,* 59:285, 1975.

194 Hagman, A., Arnman, K., and Ryden, L.: Syncope Caused by Lithium Treatment, *Acta Med. Scand.,* 205:467, 1979.

195 Rector, W. G., Jarzobski, J. A., and Levin, H. S.: Sinus Node Dysfunction Associated with Lithium Therapy: Report of a Case and a Review of the Literature, *Nebr. Med. J.,* 64:193, 1979.

196 Carmeliet, E. E.: Influence of Lithium Ions on the Transmembrane Potential and Cation Content of Cardiac Cells, *J. Gen. Physiol.,* 47:501, 1964.

197 Roose, S. P., Nurnberger, J. I., Dunner, D. L., Blood, D. K., and Fieve, R. R.: Cardiac Sinus Node Dysfunction During Lithium Treatment, *Am. J. Psychiatry,* 136:804, 1979.

198 Wong, K. C.: Tachy-Bradycardia Syndrome Related to Lithium Therapy, *C. M. A. Journal,* 124:1324, 1981.

199 Demers, R. G., and Heninger, G.: Electrocardiographic Changes during Lithium Treatment, *Dis. Nerv. Syst.,* 31:674, 1970.

200 Tilkian, A. G., Schroeder, J. S., Kao, J. J., and Hultgren, H. N.: The Cardiovascular Effects of Lithium in Man. A Review of the Literature, *Am. J. Med.,* 61:665, 1976.

201 Kochar, M. S., Wang, R. I. H., and D'Cunha, G. F.: Electrocardiographic Changes Simulating Hypokalemia during Treatment with Lithium Carbonate, *J. Electrocardiol.,* 4:371, 1971.

202 Keynes, R. D., and Swan, R. C.: The Permeability of Frog Muscle Fibers to Lithium Ions, *J. Physiol.,* 147:262, 1959.

203 Schou, M.: Electrocardiographic Changes during Treatment with Lithium and with Drugs of the Imipramine Type, *Acta Psychiatr. Scand. (suppl. 38),*331, 1962.

204 Pratila, M. G., and Pratilas, V.: ST Depression under Anesthesia in a Patient on Lithium Carbonate, *Mt. Sinai J. Med.,* 46:549, 1979.

205 Jaffe, C. M.: First-Degree Atrioventricular Block during Lithium Carbonate Treatment, *Am. J. Psychiatry,* 134:88, 1977.

206 Azar, I., and Turndorf, H.: Paroxysmal Left Bundle Branch Block during Nitrous Oxide Anesthesia in a Patient on Lithium Carbonate: A Case Report, *Anesth. Analg. (Paris),* 56:868, 1977.

207 Tangedahl, T. N., and Gau, G. T.: Myocardial Irritability Associated with Lithium Carbonate Therapy, *N. Engl. J. Med.,* 387:867, 1972.

208 Horgan, J. H., Ford, G. D., Proctor, J. D., and Wasserman, A. J.: The Effect of Prophylactic and Therapeutic Administration of Lithium on Ventricular Tachyarrhythmia, *Arch. Int. Pharmacodyn. Ther.,* 207:77, 1974.

209 Swedberg, K., and Winblad, B.: Heart Failure as Complication of Lithium Treatment, *Acta Med. Scand.,* 196:279, 1974.

210 Potts, J. L., Dalakos, T. G., Streeten, D. H. P., and Jones, D.: Cardiomyopathy in an Adult with Bartter's Syndrome and Hypokalemia. Hemodynamic Angiographic and Metabolic Studies, *Am. J. Cardiol.,* 40:995, 1977.

211 Schou, M., Amdisen, A., and Trap-Jensen, J.: Lithium Poisoning, *Am. J. Psychiatry,* 125:520, 1968.

212 Hansen, H. E., and Amdisen, A.: Lithium Intoxication, *Q. J. Med.,* 186:123, 1978.

213 Habibzadeh, M. A., and Zeller, N. H.: Cardiac Arrhythmia and Hypopotassemia in Association with Lithium Carbonate Overdose, *South. Med. J.,* 70:628, 1977.

214 Jacob, A. I., and Hope, R. R.: Prolongation of the Q-T Interval in Lithium Toxicity, *J. Electrocardiol.,* 12:117, 1979.

215 Thomsen, K., and Schou, M.: Renal Lithium Excretion in Man, *Am. J. Physiol.,* 215:823, 1968.

216 Brown, E. A., and Pawlikowski, T. R. B.: Lithium Intoxication Treated by Peritoneal Dialysis, *Br. J. Clin. Pract.,* 35:90, 1981.

217 Jefferson, J. W., and Kalin, N. H.: Serum Lithium Levels and Long-Term Diuretic Use, *J.A.M.A.,* 241:1134, 1979.

218 McGennis, A. J.: Lithium Carbonate and Tetracycline Interaction, *Br. Med. J.,* 1:1183, 1978.

219 Frölich, J. C., Leftwich, R., Ragheb, M., Oates, J. A., Reimann, I., and Buchanan, D.: Indomethacin Increases Plasma Lithium, *Br. Med. J.,* 1:1115, 1979.

220 Cavis, J. M., and Garver, D. L.: Neuroleptics: Clinical Use in Psychiatry, in L. L. Iverson, S. D. Iverson, and S. H. Snyder (eds.), "Neuroleptics and Schizophrenia," Plenum Press, New York, 1978, p. 29.

221 Davis, J. M.: Antipsychotic Drugs, in H. I. Kaplan, A. M. Freedman, and B. J. Sadock (eds.), "Comprehensive Textbook of Psychiatry," vol. 3, 3d ed., Williams and Wilkins, Baltimore, 1980, p. 2257.

222 Groves, J. E., and Mandel, M. R.: The Long-Acting Phenothiazines, *Arch. Gen. Psychiatry,* 32:893, 1975.

223 Donlon, T. T., Axelrad, A. D., Tupin, J. P., and Chien, C.-P.: Comparison of Depot Fluphenazines: Duration of Action and Incidence of Side Effects, *Compr. Psychiatry,* 17:369, 1976.

224 Tune, L. E., Creese, I., DePaulo, J. R., Slavney, P. R., Coyle, J. T., and Snyder, S. H.: Clinical State and Serum Neuroleptic Levels Measured by Radioreceptor Assay in Schizophrenia, *Am. J. Psychiatry,* 137:187, 1980.

225 Richelson, E.: Neuroleptics and Neurotransmitter Receptors, *Psychiatr. Ann.,* 10:459, 1980.

226 Peroutka, S. J., and Snyder, S. H.: Relationship of Neuroleptic Drug Effects at Brain Dopamine, Serotonin, Alpha-Adrenergic, and Histamine Receptors to Clinical Potency, *Am. J. Psychiatry,* 137:1518, 1980.

227 Creese, I., Burt, D. R., and Snyder, S. H.: Dopamine Receptor Binding Predicts Clinical and Pharmacological Potencies of Antischizophrenia Drugs, *Science,* 192:481, 1976.

228 Peroutka, S. J., U'Prichard, D. C., Greenberg, D. A., and Snyder, S. H.: Neuroleptic Drug Interactions with Norepinephrine Beta-Receptor Binding Sites in Rat Brain, *Neuropharmacology,* 16:549, 1977.

229 Shapiro, A. K., Shapiro, E., and Wayne, H.: Treatment of Tourette's Syndrome, *Arch. Gen. Psychiatry,* 28:92, 1973.

230 Brinkley, J. R., Beitman, B. D., and Friedel, R. O.: Low-Dose Neuroleptic Regimens in the Treatment of Borderline Patients, *Arch. Gen. Psychiatry,* 36:319, 1979.

231 Fann, W. E., Lake, C. R., and Majors, L. F.: Thioridazine in Neurotic, Anxious, and Depressed Patients, *Psychosomatics,* 15:117, 1974.

232 Gotbetter, S.: Tardive Dyskinesia: A Latent Legal Concern for Psychiatrists, *Leg. Aspects Med. Pract.,* 6:39, 1978.

233 Cancro, R., Davis, J. M., Klawans, H., and Tancredi, L.: Medical and Legal Implications of Side Effects from Neuroleptic Drugs. A Round-Table Discussion, *J. Clin. Psychiatry,* 42:78, 1981.

234 Tardive Dyskinesia, *Br. Med. J.,* 2:1313, 1979. (Editorial.)

235 Carter, R. G.: Psychotolysis with Haloperidol—Rapid Control of the Acutely Disturbed Psychotic Patient, *Dis. Nerv. Syst.,* 38:237, 1977.

236 Stutsky, B. A.: Relative Efficacy of Parenteral Haloperidol and Thiothixene for the Emergency Treatment of Excited and Agitated Patients, *Dis. Nerv. Syst.,* 38:967, 1977.

237 Rivera-Calimlim, L., Nasrallah, H., Strauss, J., and Lasagna, L.: Clinical Response and Plasma Levels: Effect of Dose, Dosage Schedules, and Drug Interactions on Plasma Chlorpromazine Levels, *Am. J. Psychiatry,* 133:646, 1976.

238 Callahan, E. J., Alevizos, P. N., Teigen, J. R., Newman, H., and Campbell, M. D.: Behavioral Effects of Reducing the Daily Frequency of Phenothiazine Administration, *Arch. Gen. Psychiatry,* 32:1285, 1975.

239 Davis, J. M.: Overview: Maintenance Therapy in Psychiatry: I. Schizophrenia, *Am. J. Psychiatry,* 132:1237, 1975.

240 Lipowski, Z. J.: Organic Mental Disorders: Introduction and Review of Syndromes, in H. I. Kaplan, A. M. Freedman, and B. J. Sadock (eds.), "Comprehensive Textbook of Psychiatry," vol. 2, 3d ed., Williams and Wilkins, Baltimore, 1980, p. 1359.

241 Kotin, J., Wilbert, D. E., Verburg, D., and Soldinger, S. M.: Thioridazine and Sexual Dysfunction, *Am. J. Psychiatry,* 133:82, 1976.

242 Korczyn, A. D.: The Major Tranquilizers, in M. N. G. Dukes, (ed.), "Meyler's Side Effects of Drugs," 9th ed., Excerpta Medica, Amsterdam, 1980, p. 76.

243 American College of Neuropsychopharmacology: Neurological Syndromes Associated with Antipsychotic-Drug Use, *N. Engl. J. Med.*, 289:20, 1973.

244 Smith, J. M., and Baldessarini, R. J.: Changes in Prevalence, Severity, and Recovery in Tardive Dyskinesia with Age, *Arch. Gen. Psychiatry*, 37:1368, 1980.

245 Weiner, W. J., Goetz, C. G., Nausieda, P. A., and Klawans, H. L.: Respiratory Dyskinesias: Extrapyramidal Dysfunction and Dyspnea, *Ann. Intern. Med.*, 88:327, 1978.

246 Klawans, H. L.: The Pharmacology of Tardive Dyskinesia, *Am. J. Psychiatry*, 130:82, 1973.

247 Jeste, D. V., and Wyatt, R. J.: Dogma Disputed: Is Tardive Dyskinesia Due to Post Synaptic Dopamine Receptor Supersensitivity? *J. Clin. Psychiatry*, 42:455, 1981.

248 Zavodnick, S.: A Pharmacological and Theoretical Comparison of High and Low Potency Neuroleptics, *J. Clin. Psychiatry*, 39:332, 1978.

249 Risch, S. C., Groom, G. P., and Janowsky, D. S.: Interfaces of Psychopharmacology and Cardiology. Part 2, *J. Clin. Psychiatry*, 42:47, 1981.

250 Rosati, D.: Hypotensive Side Effects of Phenothiazine and Their Management, *Dis. Nerv. Syst.*, 25:366, 1964.

251 Carlsson, C., Dencker, S. J., Grimby, G., Häggendal, J., and Johnsson, G.: Effects of Hemodynamics and Plasma Noradrenaline Levels in Man on Long Term Treatment with Imipramine, Haloperidol and Chlorpromazine, *Eur. J. Clin. Pharmacol.*, 3:163, 1971.

252 Kaplan, N. M.: Hypotension as a Complication of Promazine Therapy, *Arch. Intern. Med.*, 103;219, 1957.

253 Korol, B., Lang, W. J., Brown, M. L., and Gershon, S.: Effects of Chronic Chlorpromazine Administration on Systemic Arterial Pressure in Schizophrenic Patients: Relationship of Body Position to Blood Pressure, *Clin. Pharmacol. Ther.*, 6:587, 1965.

254 Moyer, J. H.: The Pharmacology of Chlorpromazine, *J. Clin. Exp. Psychopathol.*, 16:179, 1955.

255 Blumberg, A. G., Klein, D. F., and Pollack, M.: Effects of Chlorpromazine and Imipramine on Systolic Blood Pressure in Psychiatric Patients: Relationships to Age, Diagnosis and Initial Blood Pressure, *J. Psychiatr. Res.*, 2:51, 1964.

256 Elkayam, U., Rotmensch, H. H., Terdiman, R., Geller, E., and Laniado, S.: Hemodynamic Effects of Chlorpromazine in Patients with Acute Myocardial Infarction and Pump Failure, *Chest*, 72:623, 1977.

257 Gulotta, S. J.: Chlorpromazine in the Treatment of Cardiogenic Shock, *Am. Heart J.*, 80:570, 1970.

258 Nasrallah, H. A.: Factors Influencing Phenothiazine-Induced ECG Changes, *Am. J. Psychiatry*, 135:118, 1978.

259 Huston, J. R., and Bell, G. E.: The Effect of Thioridazine Hydrochloride and Chlorpromazine on the Electrocardiogram, *J.A.M.A.*, 198:16, 1966.

260 Wendkos, M. H.: Cardiac Changes Related to Phenothiazine Therapy, with Special Reference to Thioridazine, *J. Am. Geriatr. Soc.*, 15:20, 1967.

261 Alvarez-Mena, S. C., and Frank, M. J.: Phenothiazine-Induced T-Wave Abnormalities. Effects of Overnight Fasting, *J.A.M.A.*, 224;1730, 1973.

262 Chouinard, and Annabel, L.: Phenothiazine-Induced ECG Abnormalities. Effect of a Glucose Load, *Arch. Gen. Psychiatry*, 34:951, 1977.

263 Ban, T. A., and St. Jean, A.: The Effect of Phenothiazines on the Electrocardiogram, *Can. Med. Assoc. J.*, 91:537, 1964.

264 Dillenkoffer, R. L., George, R. B., Bishop, M. P., and Gallant, D. M.: Electrocardiographic Evaluation of Thiothixene: A Double-Blind Comparison with Thioridazine, *Adv. Biochem. Psychopharmacol.*, 9:487, 1974.

265 Fletcher, G. F., Kazamias, T. M., and Wenger, N. K.: Cardiotoxic Effects of Mellaril: Conduction Disturbances and Supraventricular Arrhythmias, *Am. Heart J.*, 78:135, 1969.

266 Aherwadker, S. J., Efendigil, M. C., and Coulshed, N.: Chlorpromazine Therapy, and Associated Disturbances of Cardiac Rhythm, *Br. Heart J.*, 36:1251, 1974.

267 Kelly, H. G., Fay, J. E., and Laverty, S. G.: Thioridazine Hydrochloride (Mellaril): Its Effects on the Electrocardiogram and a Report of Two Fatalities with Electrocardiographic Abnormalities, *Can. Med. Assoc. J.*, 89:546, 1963.

268 Richardson, H. L., Grauper, K. I., and Richardson, M. E.: Intramyocardial Lesions in Patients Dying Suddenly and Unexpectedly, *J.A.M.A.*, 195:114, 1966.

269 Giles, T. D., and Modlin, R. K.: Death Associated with Ventricular Arrhythmia and Thioridazine Hydrochloride, *J.A.M.A.*, 205:98, 1968.

270 Alexander, C. S., and Nino, A.: Cardiovascular Complications in Young Patients Taking Psychotropic Drugs. A Preliminary Report, *Am. Heart J.*, 78:757, 1969.

271 Carlsson, C., Dencker, S. J., Grimby, G., and Häggendal, J.: Circulatory Studies during Physical Exercise in Mentally Disordered Patients: I. Effects of Large Doses of Chlorpromazine, *Acta Med. Scand.*, 184:499, 1968.

272 Hollister, L. E., and Kosek, J. C.: Sudden Death during Treatment with Phenothiazine Derivatives, *J.A.M.A.*, 192:1035, 1965.

273 Cancro, R., and Wilder, R.: A Mechanism of Sudden Death in Chlorpromazine Therapy, *Am. J. Psychiatry*, 127:368, 1970.

274 Desautels, S., Filteau, D., and St. Jean, A.: Ventricular

Tachycardia Associated with Administration of Thioridazine Hydrochloride (Mellaril): Report of a Case with a Favorable Outcome, *Can. Med. Assoc. J.,* 90:1030, 1964.

275 Leestma, J. E., and Koenig, K. L.: Sudden Death and Phenothiazines, *Arch. Gen. Psychiatry,* 18:137, 1968.

276 Arita, M., and Surawicz, B.: Electrophysiologic Effects of Phenothiazines on Human Atrial Fibers, *Jpn. Heart J.,* 14:398, 1973.

277 Magorien, R. D., Jewell, G. M., Schaal, S. F., and Leier, C. V.: Electrophysiologic Studies of Perphenazine and Protriptyline in a Patient with Psychotropic Drug-Induced Ventricular Fibrillation, *Am. J. Med.,* 67:353, 1979.

278 Descotes, J., Ollagnier, M., Faucon, G., and Evreux, J. Cl.: Study of Thioridazine Cardiotoxic Effects by Means of His Bundle Activity Recording, *Acta Pharmacol. Toxicol.,* 44:370, 1979.

279 Yoon, M. S., Han, J., Dersham, G. H., and Jones, S. A.: Effects of Thioridazine (Mellaril) on Ventricular Electrophysiologic Properties, *Am. J. Cardiol.,* 43:1155, 1979.

280 Arita, M., and Surawicz, B.: Electrophysiologic Effects of Phenothiazines on Canine Cardiac Fibers, *J. Pharmacol. Exp. Ther.,* 184:619, 1973.

281 Madan, B. R., and Pendse, V. K.: Antiarrhythmic Activity of Thioridazine Hydrochloride (Mellaril), *Am. J. Cardiol.,* 11:78, 1963.

282 Kitazawa, M., Sugiyama, S., Ozawa, T., Miyazaki, Y., and Kotaka, K.: Mechanism of Chlorpromazine-Induced Arrhythmia—Arrhythmia and Mitochondrial Dysfunction, *J. Electrocardiol.,* 14:219, 1981.

283 Sydney, M. A.: Ventricular Arrhythmias Associated with Use of Thioridazine Hydrochloride in Alcohol Withdrawal, *Br. Med. J.,* 2:467, 1973.

284 Burda, C. D.: Electrocardiographic Abnormalities Induced by Thioridazine (Mellaril), *Am. Heart J.,* 76:153, 1968.

285 Krikler, D. M., and Curry, P. V. L.: Torsade de pointes, an Atypical Ventricular Tachycardia, *Br. Heart J.,* 38:117, 1976.

286 Tranum, B. L., and Murphy, M. L.: Case Report: Successful Treatment of Ventricular Tachycardia Associated with Thioridazine (Mellaril), *South. Med. J.,* 62:357, 1969.

287 Schoonmaker, F. W., Osteen, R. T., and Greenfield, J. C., Jr.: Thioridazine (Mellaril)-Induced Ventricular Tachycardia Controlled with an Artificial Pacemaker, *Ann. Intern. Med.,* 65:1076, 1966.

288 Weisdorf, D., Kramer, J., Goldbarg, A., and Klawans, H. L.: Physostigmine for Cardiac and Neurologic Manifestations of Phenothiazine Poisoning, *Clin. Pharmacol. Ther.,* 24:663, 1978.

289 Foster, C. A., O'Mullane, E. J., Gaskell, P., and Churchill-Davidson, H. C.: Chlorpromazine. A Study of Its Action on the Circulation in Man, *Lancet,* 2:614, 1954.

290 Lund-Johansen, P.: Shock after Administration of Phenothiazines in Patients with Pheochromocytoma, *Acta Med. Scand.,* 172:525, 1962.

291 Wheatley, D.: "Stress and the Heart," 2d ed., Raven Press, New York, 1981, p. 191.

292 Stimmel, B.: "Cardiovascular Effects of Mood-Altering Drugs," Raven Press, New York, 1979, p. 133.

293 Schwarcz, G., and Lopez-Toca, R.: Continued Lithium Treatment after Myocardial Infarction, *Am. J. Psychiatry,* 139:255, 1982.

294 Brannan, M. D., Riggs, J. J., Hageman, W. E., and Pruss, T. P.: A Comparison of the Cardiovascular Effects of Haloperidol, Thioridazine, and Chlorpromazine HCl, *Arch. Int. Pharmacodyn. Ther.,* 244:48, 1980.

295 Gerl, B.: Clinical Observations of the Side Effects of Haloperidol, *Acta Psychiatr. Scand.,* 40:65, 1964.

296 Mehta, D., Mehta, S., Petit, J., and Shriner, W.: Cardiac Arrhythmia and Haloperidol, *Am. J. Psychiatry,* 136:1468, 1979.

297 Filho, U. V., Caldeira, M. V. V., and Bueno, J. R.: The Efficacy and Safety of Loxapine Succinate in the Treatment of Schizophrenia: A Comparative Study with Thiothixene, *Curr. Therap. Res.,* 18:476, 1975.

298 Ayd, F. J.: Loxapine Update: 1966–1976, *Dis. Nerv. Syst.,* 38:883, 1977.

299 Babayan, E. A., Rudenko, G. M., and Lepakhin, V. K.: Neuroleptics and Antipsychotic Drugs, in M. N. G. Dukes (ed.), "Side Effects of Drugs Annual," vol. 6, Excerpta Medica, Amsterdam, 1982, p. 46.

Heart Disease in South Asia: Experiences in Pakistan[*]

AZHAR M. A. FARUQUI, M.D.

The study of diseases and their varied expressions among different populations allows appreciation of genetic and environmental factors altering the occurrence, frequency, manifestation, and course of the disease process.[1] It can provide epidemiologic data that could prove invaluable in preventive and curative medical efforts. It could also allow international collaborative studies to be designed to test hypotheses in a fashion not possible in a single population.[2–4]

There is very little in the scientific literature about heart disease in the underdeveloped Asian countries.[2] What follows is an attempt to review the scientific literature and available information that exists about cardiovascular diseases in one such South Asian country, Pakistan.

PAKISTAN

Geographic Data

Pakistan is located[5] on a large land mass north of the Tropic of Cancer between latitudes N24 and 37° (Fig. 1). It has an area of 307,374 mi^2 (excluding the disputed territory of Jammu and Kashmir under India's occupation), which is slightly larger than the combined area of the six Great Lakes states of Illinois, Indiana, Michigan, Minnesota, Ohio, and Wisconsin.[6] It is bounded on the west by Iran, on the north by Afghanistan and Russia, on the northeast by China, on the south and southeast by India, and due south by the Arabian Sea. It has six natural regions: the desert areas, the Baluchistan plateau, the western bordering mountains, the Indus Plain, the Submontane plateau, and the northern mountains. The climate is of continental type, with wide variations in daily and seasonal temperatures. The mountains modify the climate in the cold north; the western plateau is somewhat hotter; along the coastline the temperatures remain moderate; while in most of the remaining country the summer is very hot (up to 52°C recorded) and winters are cold (mean of 4°C). Most of the country is very arid, except the northern mountain slopes and the Submontane region,

which have yearly rainfalls of 750 to 900 mm. Cultivation in the Indus plain and the south is mainly by large irrigation networks.

Demographic and Ethnic Data

The country has a population of 83.78 million[7] as opposed to 33.74 million about 30 years ago, when it emerged as an independent state from the colonial British India. Presently, the urban population comprises 28 percent of the total population, compared with 17 percent at the time of independence.[7] Islamabad, in the north, is the present capital city, while the coastline city of Karachi (the country's former capital) is the largest city, with a population of approximately 8 million.[7] There are 18 cities with populations exceeding 100,000.[5] Average population density is 272 per square mile. The country is divided into four administrative provinces of Sind, Punjab, Baluchistan, and Northwest Frontier Province.

The per capita yearly income is about Rs. 2,837 (US$245).[8] Less than 30 percent of males and 20 percent of females are literate.[6] About 10 percent of the literates are without formal education.[5]

The population is a complex mixture of many racial types. Aryans, Persians, Greeks, Pathans (Pushtuns), and Mughals came from the northeast and spread across the Indogangetic Plain, while the Arabs conquered Sind from the sea.[5] There have in addition been waves of migrations across the Indopakistan subcontinent throughout history, especially the mass migration of millions at the time of independence and the separation of Pakistan and India in 1947. Racial types to be seen in Pakistan include the tall, fair-skinned, blue-eyed type; the olive-skinned, fine-boned, hawk-nosed "Iranian" types; smaller, dark-skinned types of "Dravidian" and "Australoid" origin; wheaten-skinned, dark-eyed "Indoaryan" types; short-headed and long-headed Mongoloid peoples; and, in Baluchistan, the broad-headed, stocky-built alpine Europoid types.[5] While attempts to identify racial origins in different regions are somewhat arbitrary, most Pakistanis are of caucasoid stock and, hence, different from the aboriginal peoples in majority in the rest of the Indian subcontinent.[6] About 97 percent of the people of Pakistan are Muslims. Christians contitute 1.4 percent and Hindus 0.5 percent.

Water supply and sewerage systems are inadequate, even in the urban areas, and potable water is available to less than 30 percent of the population. Forty-five percent of the people are below the age of 15, owing to

*From the National Institute of Cardiovascular Diseases Karachi, Pakistan.

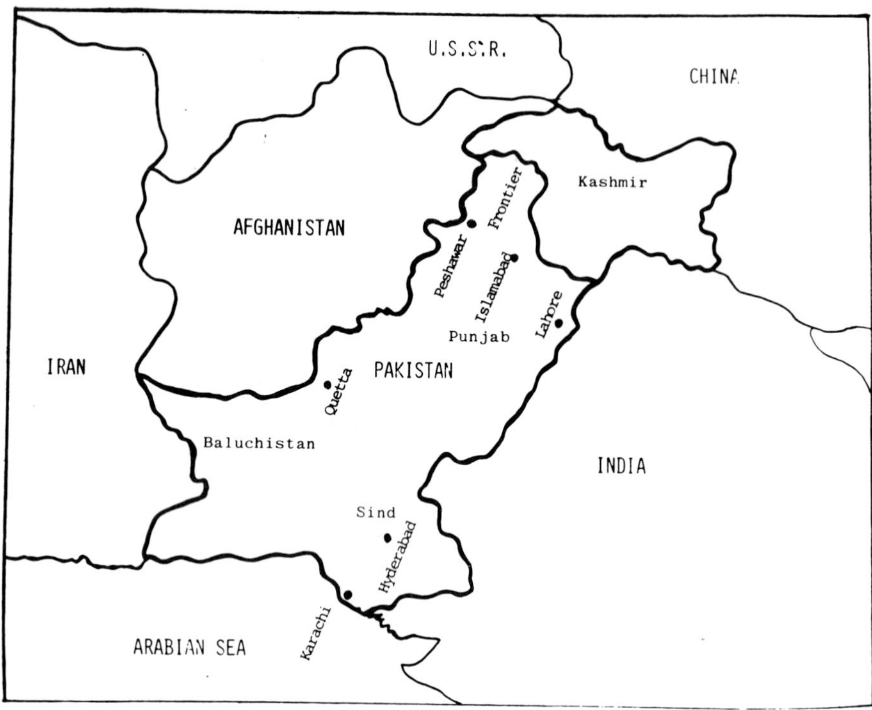

FIGURE 1 Map of Pakistan and its geographic boundaries.

a very high birth rate combined with a decline in infant mortality, which still is among the highest in the world. The average life expectancy at birth in 1971 was 52.9 years for males and 51.8 years for females.[9] Soon after independence, over 30 years ago, the average life expectancy at birth was 33.0 years for males and 34.64 years for females.[10] At last count in 1978 there were 528 hospitals, 3,998 dispensaries (outpatient clinics), 850 maternal and child health centres, 46,092 hospital beds, 19,016 doctors, 4,300 nurses, 1,047 dentists, and 1,800 lay health visitors in the country.[11] Modern medical facilities are few and mostly available only to the urban population, whereas traditional, nonscientific systems of medicine are legal and widely practiced. The author's institution is presently the country's only fully developed facility devoted to the diagnosis and medical and surgical treatment of cardiovascular disorders.

EPIDEMIOLOGY OF CARDIOVASCULAR DISEASES IN PAKISTAN

Sources of Available Data

POPULATION SURVEYS

Large, prospective, well-designed, and reliably conducted surveys for disease incidence and prevalence

rates are difficult to find anywhere in the world.[12] It is therefore not surprising that in a developing country such as Pakistan there is dearth of reliable epidemiologic data regarding the true prevalence and incidence rates of various cardiovascular disorders. There have been from time to time several attempts to study the prevalence of cardiovascular diseases in many population samples.[13–23] However, there is no longitudinal study that has defined the true incidence of these disorders in Pakistan.

HOSPITAL DATA

It is obvious that hospital data are fraught with all kinds of bias shown to be related to factors that control patient selection and referral trends.[24,25] However, in the absence of other reliable data, this source provides information as to occurrence, prevalence, and manifestation of the disease in the selected group sick enough to seek hospital admission. Many such studies are available for review.[26–38]

MORTALITY DATA

In Pakistan, death certificates have not been obligatory and, when issued in the urban communities, are for specific legal or insurance purposes. As such, no reliable mortality figures for the general population exist.

Since there is a customary bias against autopsy, the only autopsy data are from the police surgeon's (coroner's) cases or anatomy departments that include traffic accidents, homicides, suicides, unclaimed bodies, and the like. Yet, this is useful information from the general population, and some of it has been reviewed.[39–42] Some data from life insurance death statistics are available.[43] However, only a small selected fraction of the population carries life insurance.

A special local problem with all studies is the age data. In the past, most births were not recorded. Therefore, particularly in the illiterate rural populations, age determination is mostly guesswork.

Prevalence of Cardiovascular Disorders

ADULT POPULATION SURVEYS

The data from the various population surveys are outlined in Table 1. The best designed and most reliable series is that of Syed et al.[16] According to this series, hypertension is the most common cardiovascular problem in Pakistan, with an overall prevalence of 17.6 percent in the adult population. Ischemic heart disease is the second most common with an overall prevalence of 2.3 percent. Next comes rheumatic heart disease, with a prevalence of 0.6 percent. Congenital heart disease was shown to have a prevalence of 0.17 percent in adults. Cerebrovascular disease and peripheral vascular disease were not particularly looked for by defined and acceptable criteria. However, there was a

prevalence of 0.02 percent for peripheral vascular disease, while no case of cerebrovascular disease was found. Another population survey for major cardiovascular problems was that by Hashmi,[13] which was restricted to males and not randomized by acceptable criteria. This study showed an overall lower incidence in all categories of disease, except for a prevalence of 0.93 percent for cerebrovascular disease. No case of peripheral vascular disease was identified although it was specifically looked for. The other studies have shown various prevalence figures, mostly in selected and biased population samples, and are, as such, not very reliable or applicable to the general population. The study of Syed et al.[16] had a great impact on the thinking and planning of health care in this country, since it proved for the first time the point that earlier hospital-based studies had raised regarding the high prevalence of cardiovascular disorders in Pakistan.[26–29,33] The figures from the study[16] are almost 15 years old, and the general anecdotal impression is that the present prevalence is definitely higher than assessed then. However, if we accept these old figures as true today, then, with an estimated 50 percent of adults in the population, there would be presently 9.06 million adults in Pakistan suffering from cardiovascular disorders. Of this total, there would be 7.3 million suffering from hypertension, almost 1 million suffering from ischemic heart disease, a quarter of a million suffering from rheumatic heart disease, and about 70,000 suffering from congenital heart disease (Fig. 2). Reliable figures for cerebrovascular and peripheral vascular disease are unavailable.

Very interesting facts are provided by the combined data from the two autopsy studies on 225 unselected mediocolegal (coroner's) cases.[40,41] The age of patients

TABLE 1
Prevalence figures per thousand for cardiovascular disorders

Place and year	No. in sample	Age of sample (years)	Sex	HBP*	IHD	RHD	CHD	CRVD	PAD
Rabwah, 1967–1968	1,039	30 and above	Male	163	23	8.6	0.9	N.A.	0.4
(rural)[16]	1,355	30 and above	Female	204	11	5.1	1.4	N.A.	
Karimabad, 1967–1968	839	30 and above	Male	159	47	3.5	1.2	N.A.	N.A.
(urban)[16]	946	30 and above	Male	167	20	6.3	3.2	N.A.	N.A.
Sind, 1963–1964		22–80	Male	102	8	6	0	2	0
(rural and urban)[13]	2,146	(mean 48.5)	only						
Punjab, 1970	5,202†	20–40	Both	41	N.A.	N.A.	N.A.	N.A.	N.A.
(rural and urban)[17]		Over 40	Both	136	N.A.	N.A.	N.A.	N.A.	N.A.
Punjab, 1981	1,110	12–61	Both	56	N.A.	N.A.	N.A.	N.A.	N.A.
(rural and urban)[23]		(mean 33.5)							
Lahore, 1974	322	14–90	Both	236	N.A.	N.A.	N.A.	N.A.	N.A.
(shopkeepers)[19]		(mean 37.1)							

Abbreviations: N.A. = not assessed; HBP = hypertensive disease; IHD = ischemic heart disease; RHD = rheumatic heart disease; CHD = congenital heart disease; CRVD = cerebrovascular disease; PAD = peripheral arterial disease.

*Hypertension defined as BP of 160/95 mm Hg or higher.

†Breakdown of numbers in various age groups not given.

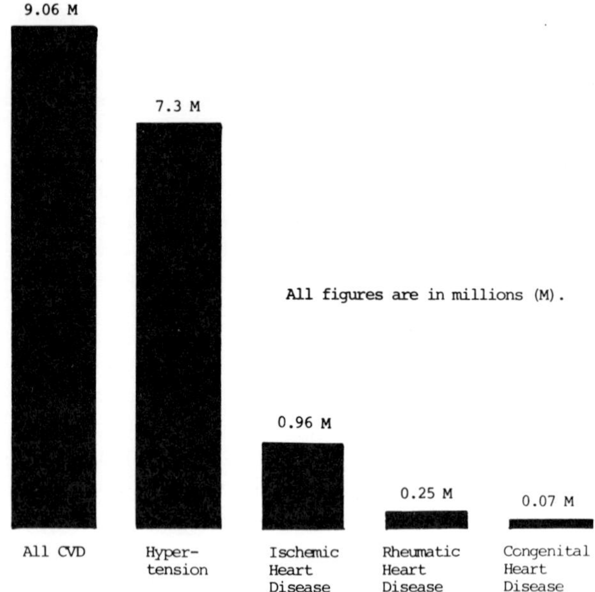

FIGURE 2 Estimated prevalence of major cardiovascular diseases in the Pakistani adult population based on a general population survey.[16]

ranged from 11 to over 70 years. Some degree of atherosclerosis in the aorta was seen in 94.2 percent of patients with 31.6 percent showing complicated plaques (ulcerated, calcified, or thrombosed). The coronary arteries showed involvement in 48.4 percent of patients, with significant narrowing (greater than 50 percent diameter reduction) present in half the involved vessels. Moreover, 12.4 percent of patients showed the presence of myocardial infarction. The youngest patient showing atherosclerosis of the aorta was 16 years old. Patients showing significant coronary lesions were all over 30 years of age, although minor coronary lesions were seen in some teenagers. Of the 22 females, 11 had coronary atherosclerosis, with 4 showing significant narrowing. Most patients showing myocardial infarction were over 40 years old, although in two patients showing myocardial infarction, the ages of the deceased were 25 and 35 years, respectively. In 125 patients, the common carotids and renal arteries were also studied.[41] The common carotid arteries showed atherosclerosis in 93.6 percent of patients, with complicated lesions in 12.8 percent. In 28.8 percent, an atheromatous lesion was seen near the osteum of the renal arteries. No patient showed atheromatous involvement of the distal renal arteries beyond the origin.

It is remarkable how close the figures are in their order of frequency to figures from the United States.[12] The higher overall percentages of prevalence in the United States may well be accounted for by the higher life expectancy (73.2 years)[12] and low birth rate compared with Pakistan, which has a very high birth rate and a lower life expectancy (52.3 years).[9]

SURVEYS IN CHILDREN AND ADOLESCENTS

In the younger population in Pakistan, the surveys have limited themselves to school children. The prevalence

TABLE 2
Prevalence figures per thousand for cardiovascular disorders in school children and adolescents

Place and year	No. in sample	Age of sample (years)	Sex	HBP*	RHD	CHD
Karachi, 1964–1965 (urban)[14]	2,591	5–14	Male	58	N.A.	N.A.
	1,070	5–14	Female	82	N.A.	N.A.
Karachi, 1966 (urban)[15]	4,002	8–14	Both	N.A.	1.8	1.8
Karachi, 1981 (urban)[22]	464	2½–17	Both	13	N.A.	N.A.
Punjab, 1970 (urban and rural)[17]	5,202†	Under 20	Both	15	N.A.	N.A.
Peshawar, 1973–1976 (urban)[18]	17,662	5–15	Both	N.A.	9.0	N.A.
Chitral, 1973–1976 (rural)[18]	2,678	5–15	Both	N.A.	11.0	N.A.
Peshawar, 1976–1977 (urban)[20]	1,656	5–20	Male	16	N.A.	N.A.
	1,681	5–20	Female	13	N.A.	N.A.
Islamabad, 1978–1979 (urban)[21]	15,100	5–15	Both	N.A.	1.52	3.25

Abbreviations: N.A. = not assessed; HBP = hypertensive disease; RHD = rheumatic heart disease; CHD = congenital heart disease.
*Hypertension defined as BP 130/90 mm Hg.
†Breakdown of numbers in various age groups not given.

picture thus painted in a population with less than 30 percent going to school[6] may not be very reliable. However, the data at hand (Table 2) show hypertension as the most common problem, followed by rheumatic heart disease and congenital heart disease. The prevalence rates for rheumatic heart disease vary markedly from a high of 0.9 to 1.1 percent in the rural and poor communities[18] to a low of 0.15 to 0.18 percent in the urban and economically better-off areas.[15,21] The lower figures are comparable with those from more advanced Western and Far Eastern countries.[15,21]

HOSPITAL PREVALENCE DATA

Less than two decades ago, the only data available in Pakistan were hospital admission figures. It was this sort of data[26] that first drew the attention of the medical profession and the general population to the frequency of cardiovascular diseases in Pakistan, which were generally held to be uncommon. The percentage of cardiovascular patients reportedly admitted to the various large medical centers has ranged from 4.6 to 26.7 percent of all admissions.[26–30,33] An interesting facet of these data is the relative frequency of the various cardiovascular disorders in the same hospital at different points in time (Table 3). It can be seen that in the symptomatic population seeking admission to the cardiology departments of various hospitals, ischemic heart disease now ranks as the most frequent cause among all cardiovascular diseases.[26,28,33,34,37] In the most recent data, ischemic heart disease was the most frequent cause for admission even in the females.[37] Rheumatic heart disease, which was the most common cause for admission to the hospital in the older series,[29] is much less conspicuous.[37] A fallacy in all the hospital-based data is that such centers are situated in the major cities and cater mostly to the urban population. Whether these data are at all applicable to the rural population is unknown. Also, as has been mentioned earlier, hospital data may not have any relevance to the disease prevalence in the general population.

While there are no data from population surveys as to the frequency of cerebrovascular disease in the general population, data are available from hospital admissions for cerebrovascular disease.[38] In the neurology department of this large, urban-based hospital, 56 percent of all admissions were due to cerebrovascular accidents.[38] However, again, the relevance of this highly symptomatic population (seeking admission) to the general population is open to question, but these data certainly show that cerebrovascular disease is not uncommon in this population.

MORTALITY RATES

The general mortality rates for the population at large are unknown, and at present there is no reliable system whereby they can be ascertained. While hospital mortality rates are available,[30] it would be totally inappropriate to discuss them or draw any conclusions from them.

A very small segment of the population can afford life insurance. Data from this group of persons living in the relatively affluent city of Karachi,[43] with a total population of greater than 8 million, are summarized in Table 4. It is plain that despite all kinds of bias, the frequency of cardiac deaths is so high that it cannot be ignored and in this group accounts for the majority of deaths. A very striking fact that emerges from these data is the very young age of the deceased.

The only autopsy series that has looked at deaths from natural causes is the one from the Pakistan Armed Forces Institute of Pathology.[42] In this series, out of 917 autopsies of death from natural causes, 27.7 percent were due to cardiac causes, and ischemic heart disease accounted for 88.9 percent of all cardiac deaths. Again, this is a selected group belonging to the army; autopsies were done for one reason or another and the findings are of limited value. However, the findings point to cardiac problems, and in particular, ischemic heart disease, as a very common cause of death.

TABLE 3
Prevalence of cardiovascular disorders in hospital patients

Place and year	Sex	IHD (%)	RHD (%)	HBP (%)	CHD (%)	Miscellaneous (%)
Lahore, 1944–1948	Both	1.7	N.A.	N.A.	N.A.	—
1954–1958[26]	Both	17.9	N.A.	N.A.	N.A.	—
Multan, 1961[29]	Both	N.A.	40.8	N.A.	N.A.	—
Karachi, 1967[34]	Both	41.8	22.2	9.6	2.4	24.0
Karachi, 1981[37]	Male	75.8	7.4	5.5	5.6	5.6
	Female	51.8	22.7	6.8	9.8	8.0

Note: All figures are expressed as percentage of total admissions for cardiovascular problems. Abbreviations: IHD = ischemic heart disease; RHD = rheumatic heart disease; HBP = hypertensive disease; CHD = congenital heart disease; N.A. = not assessed.

TABLE 4
Three-year mortality data*

	Cardiac deaths	Noncardiac deaths†	Death cause unknown
Number	472	351	152
Percent total deaths	48	36	16
Mean age ± S.D. (years)	48.8 ± 8.5	44.0 ± 11.6	43.8 ± 11.8

Note: Data from life insurance policy holders of Karachi from January 1, 1979 to December 31, 1981.[43]

*Total number of effective policies as of December 31, 1981 is 220,496; total deaths in 3 years ending December 31, 1981 is 975.

†Includes deaths from nonnatural causes.

Changing Picture of Cardiovascular Diseases

There was a time in the past when rheumatic fever was believed to occur rarely in this area of the world.[44,45] It was then realized that rheumatic heart disease was the most common cardiac problem in this area of the world.[27,46,47] Presently, this opinion continues to be held, and ischemic heart disease has been described as rare or a relatively minor problem.[48] With all its limitations, the data presented show the frequency of cardiovascular disorders to be high and hypertension and ischemic heart disease to be major problems at present. Rheumatic heart disease is still a significant problem, but it is assuming secondary importance in the adult population surveyed.

SYSTEMIC HYPERTENSION

Systemic hypertension, as seen from the foregoing epidemiologic evidence, is Pakistan's foremost cardiovascular problem, just as it is in most of the world today.[49] Various factors relating to blood pressure and to systemic hypertension have been studied in Pakistan, and some of the observations are summarized below.

Age

While in the Western world there is a definite rise in blood pressure with age,[12,50,51] it has been noted that in certain primitive societies blood pressure fails to rise with age.[52,53] Whether this failure of blood pressure to rise with age is the true biologic "normal" for human beings or whether this refects genetic or acquired differences or a lower life expectancy is these areas is unknown. It is also claimed that change in lifestyle from "primitive" to "modern" seems to cause an elevation in blood pressure.[54,55] In Pakistan, there is a definite tendency toward increases in blood pressure and prevalence of hypertension with age[17,20,23,56] (Table 5). In addition, hypertension remains the most common cardiovascular disorder at all ages (Tables 1 and 2). While the rise of blood pressure with age appears to be more marked for the urban compared with the rural population in Pakistan,[23] the incidence of hypertension is not significantly different between the urban and rural populations.[23,56]

Other Variables

In Western populations, pressures in females are lower than those in males in early and mid-adult life and become higher later on.[50,51] In Pakistan there appears to be a higher overall prevalence of hypertension in the female from childhood[14] through adulthood.[23,56] As in the West, in Pakistan there is a definite relationship to weight and ponderal index.[19,23] The relationship of hypertension to salt intake has not been investigated, although in general the intake of salt and various spices and condiments by Pakistanis is high. Licorice is taken by a segment of the population, but there are no figures on how widespread its use is and its role, if any, in the causation of hypertension. Women on contraceptive pills have higher blood pressures and a higher prevalence of hypertension.[57]

The effect of "hard" versus "soft" water was investigated in one community and found not to be significant.[58] No single study has specifically looked at blood pressure differences between the racial types in Pakistan, but the prevalence of hypertension in the various regions of Pakistan is not remarkably different in the adult population.[13,16,17,23] The highest prevalence

TABLE 5
Prevalence of hypertension in various age groups in Punjab

Age (years)	Percentage of group with hypertension*
15–19	1.5
20–24	3.2
25–29	2.7
30–34	3.8
35–39	6.3
20–39	4.1
40–44	7.7
45–49	12.0
50–59	16.4
60 and above	19.6
Above 40 years	13.6

*Hypertension defined as BP of 160/95 mm Hg or above.[17]

Note: If the definition of hypertension used had been 140/90 mm Hg or above, these figures would have been more than doubled.

(23.6 percent) is reported from a survey of sedentary shopkeepers,[19] while the lowest prevalence (2.0 percent) is reported in the active army commandos.[20] There is evidence of a greater prevalence of hyperlipidemia[59,60] in hypertension compared with control groups.

Secondary Hypertension

As elsewhere, in Pakistan, too, the majority of hypertensives are suffering from "essential" hypertension.[61,62] The percentage of secondary hypertension in different hospital-based reports has varied from 2.3 to 58.3 percent. In one study that looked at 60 consecutive hypertensives below 40 years of age, 38 (58.3 percent) were found to have secondary hypertension, with 10 (28.5 percent) having toxemia of pregnancy, 6 having renal artery stenosis, 16 having various chronic renal

disorders, 1 having coarctation of the aorta, 1 having retroperitoneal fibrosis, and 1 suspected (but not proven) of having an aldosteronoma.[63]

Rare cases of pheochromocytoma have also been reported.[65,66] An unusual cause of hypertension, especially in young adults, is nonspecific (Takayasu type) aortitis. In the author's own experience of 5 fully investigated patients, the renal arteries were involved in only 2 (Fig. 3), and in the other 3 patients there appeared to be a generalized aortic involvement that spared the renal vessels.

Complications and Therapy

Studies that have looked at the prevalence of target organ damage in hypertensives in Pakistan have shown a high rate, ranging from 28.5 to 45.3 percent of all cases worked up.[61,63,65] The reason for this high rate of

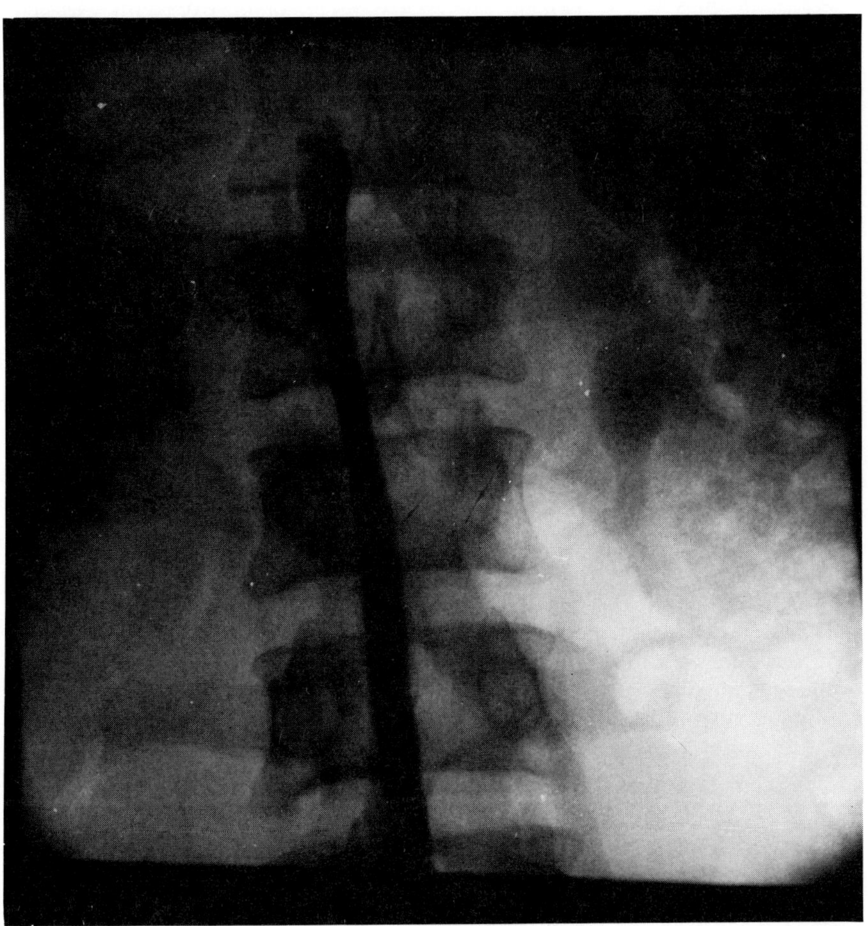

FIGURE 3 Nonspecific (Takayasu-type) aortitis, abdominal aortogram. Note the tapering of the aorta to a thin channel, the involvement of the region of the renal vessels, and the absence of major branches.

end organ damage at presentation appears to be late detection and late referral. The response of hypertension of various grades to the common antihypertensive drugs has been quite satisfactory.[64,68–70] The anecdotal observation that the Pakistani population is excessively sensitive to beta blockers is not borne out by the trials of various beta blockers.[70–73] There are presently no studies available that have looked at the impact on morbidity and mortality of antihypertensive treatment. The patient compliance in the local population has been in general disappointing, with satisfactory follow-up in 15 to 30 percent only.[65,74] A study that looked at the effect of antihypertensive treatment on serum lipids showed a significant rise in total lipids and triglycerides during therapy with methyldopa.[75]

ISCHEMIC HEART DISEASE

The study of ischemic heart disease is for the most part a study of coronary atherosclerosis and its complications. Atherosclerosis occurred in the ancient Egyptians, as shown by study of the Egyptian mummies. It is also known that atherosclerosis occurs in almost all people around the world, including communities in which ischemic heart disease is said to be rare.[76] While atherosclerosis and ischemic heart disease were thought to be rare in this part of the world[48] there is good evidence that the opposite is true. Ischemic heart disease is a major problem in the general population,[13,16] and presently it is the main cause of admission to cardiology units in Pakistan.[26,33,37]

Coronary Atherosclerosis

As seen from the two autopsy studies available,[40,41] coronary atherosclerosis, as seen in Pakistan, is no different in its frequency, distribution, severity, and histology from that in the contemporary Western studies.[77,78] These and other studies laid to rest the suspicion that the atheromatous process in the East and tropics may be a different disease.[48] Fatty streaks were documented in young children, and fibrous plaques as well as complicated lesions were documented in young adults,[40,41] much the same as in young American soldiers killed in Korea.[79]

RISK FACTORS

While the etiology of coronary heart disease remains elusive, the identification in the Western population of risk factors for the development of this disease is a major advance.[80,81] Following the Western lead, attempts to identify risk factors have been made.[16,82]

Smoking Population surveys of various types of smoking habits in Pakistan[82–84] have revealed that 29.5 percent of the urban population regularly smokes. The prevalence of smokers among patients suffering from ischemic heart disease has been stated to range from 61.8 to 83 percent.[82,85,86] The increasing number of smokers in Pakistan[84] makes this an important preventable variable.

Hypertension The general prevalence of hypertension in the adult population of Pakistan is between 10.2 and 17.6 percent[13,16] All case-control studies have identified hypertension as a definite risk factor.[33,82,85,86] In a follow-up of a hypertensive population over 5 years,[74] the most frequent complication was ischemic heart disease.

Diabetes The prevalence of diabetes mellitus in the general population is between 1.89 and 3.8 percent.[16,23] The prevalence of diabetes in the patient population with ischemic heart disease is between 9.0 and 16.8 percent.[26,33,86] Diabetes is a major risk factor, especially since diabetes is a very common problem in Pakistan, with 8.5 to 20 percent of diabetics screened having clinical ischemic heart disease.[87,88]

Hyperlipidemia In the study of normal lipid levels of the Pakistani population, it became obvious that the normal level of cholesterol (mean value around 190 mg) was lower than that of Western populations.[16,26] It was also shown in the case-control studies that hypercholesterolemia was a definite risk factor.[16,82,86,89] For the Pakistani population, therefore, a lower level of serum cholesterol had the risk equivalent of a higher value in the Western population.[89] It appears that in Pakistan the entire normal cholesterol distribution curve[16] is moved leftward about 30 mg/dl from that of the American population.[90] The data on serum triglycerides as a risk factor are controversial.[16,82] There are some data on lipoprotein phenotyping, but the numbers are too small to be meaningful.[59,91] Until very recently, HDL estimations have not been available, and no information on HDL cholesterol is available, except an international collaborative study of HDL cholesterol in young children that shows a lower level of total and HDL cholesterol in Pakistan.[92] A study of lipids in anemias, which are so common in Pakistan, showed low serum cholesterol levels in anemic patients.[93] Interestingly, experimentally induced anemia in animal models failed to bring down serum lipid levels.[94]

Diet The fat content of the Pakistani diet[16,26,33] is between 20.0 and 62.5 g/day (i.e., 10 to 25 percent of total calories) and is lower than the fat content of the Western diet. The ratio of saturated to unsaturated fats varies from 1.04 to 2.67.[16] An important facet of the fat content in the Pakistani diet is the increasing use of Vanaspati Ghee, which is the most popular cooking fat and is obtained by hydrogenation of vegetable oils to make them solid and thereby improve their shelf life, taste, and smell. Vanaspati Ghee contains, on the average, 40 percent palm oil (Table 6) with a high content of palmitic acid (48 percent), which falls among the group of fatty acids with 12 to 16 carbon atoms that is said to be almost exclusively responsible for the cholesterol-raising effect.[95] The hydrogenation process converts the polyunsaturated fatty acids to saturated ones in the presence of the catalyst nickel. While the process requires that all nickel be removed, traces remain in the final product consumed by the public. The effect of trace nickel on the human metabolism remains to be clarified, and its role, if any, in the development of atherosclerosis is conjectural at present. What is definite is the tremendous increase in production of Vanaspati Ghee, from 187 million tons in 1972–1973 to 503.5 million tons in 1980–1981.[96] While there is yet no scientific evidence linking Vanaspati Ghee with coronary heart disease, the consumption in such large amounts of artificially saturated fats cannot but raise suspicion. The effect of "soft" and "hard" water has been studied in a single community and no difference found.[58] Study of trace elements shows interesting observations but has lead to no definite conclusions.[97]

Other risk factors Obesity, ponderal index, and somatotype by themselves are not definite risk factors

TABLE 6
Fatty acid content (percentage) of oils and Vanaspati Ghee

	Palm oil	Cottonseed oil	Soybean oil	Vanaspati GHEE*
Myristic acid ($C_{13}H_{27}COOH$)	0.5	0.6	—	0.2
Palmitic acid ($C_{15}H_{31}COOH$)	48.3	22.9	8.3	21.6
Stearic acid ($C_{17}H_{35}COOH$)	2.9	2.2	5.4	6.6
Oleic acid ($C_{17}H_{33}COOH$)	40.0	24.7	24.9	63.7
Linoleic acid ($C_{17}H_{31}COOH$)	8.3	49.7	52.7	4.5
Linolenic acid ($C_{17}H_{29}COOH$)	—	—	7.9	1.0
Arachidic acid ($C_{19}H_{39}COOH$)	—	—	0.9	2.1

SOURCE: Report Ghee Corporation, Rarachi, Pakistan. Used with permission.

*Fatty acid composition of Vanaspati Ghee based on the average oil blend of palm oil 40 percent, Soybean oil 30 percent, cottonseed oil 30 percent.

in Pakistan.[82,85] As elsewhere in the world, male sex is a major risk factor, with a male:female ratio in the population surveys for ischemic heart disease being 2.3:1.[16] Graying of hair and balding, especially tonsorial balding, are associated with increased risk.[16,85] Serum uric acid has been uniformly higher in small samples of ischemic heart disease patients compared with normal controls.[82,98] Arcus cornealis seems to be a major independent risk factor, especially in the young.[85,99] Earlobe crease also has a statistical significance to risk factor.[100] In the studies examining physical activity, in particular sedentary versus physically active jobs, no definite difference in the groups compared was noted.[82] Comparison of normal controls and coronary heart disease patients revealed decreased fibrinolytic activity and greater generation of thromboplastin.[101] In addition, patients with angina pectoris had decreased fibrinolytic activity and higher fibrinogen values compared with those without angina who had suffered an acute myocardial infarction in the past.[102] Plasma fibrinogen rose with age.[102] No correlation between fibrinolytic activity and cholesterol values was observed.

Comparison of urban and rural populations is deficient. There has not been a prospective study to evaluate the predictive value of the various risk factors identified in the foregoing studies.

Clinical Ischemic Heart Disease

The major manifestations of ischemic heart disease are angina pectoris and myocardial infarction. The mean age at presentation for acute myocardial infarction is about 53 years.[33,34,82] The mode of presentation,[26,34] the types of infarction, the complication rates,[26,34] and the hospital course do not appear to be different from elsewhere in the world. There appear to be two peaks per year in the rate of hospital admission for acute myocardial infarction: one in summer and the other in winter.[26,34,99,103] The inhospital mortality for acute myocardial infarction ranges between 4.5 and 17.8 percent.[34,104,105] The main cause of inhospital mortality is cardiogenic shock.[34] Since defibrillators and monitoring facilities are becoming widespread, inhospital death from primary ventricular fibrillation is decreasing. An interesting innovation was attempted several years ago when defibrillators were expensive and not widely available; the cheaper and widely available electroconclusive therapy (ECT) machine was used successfully for defibrillation.[106] This has, of course, been given up now. Early treadmill testing 2 weeks after an uncomplicated myocardial infarction has been found to be safe[107] and as useful as the exercise test done several weeks later.[108] Lipid levels during the acute infarction are altered and cannot be used as baseline values.[109] Long-term prognosis for various subsets of ischemic heart disease and after acute myocardial infarction has not been studied. Rehabilitation after acute myocardial infarction is very good, with 75 percent of all discharged patients being gainfully employed, and mostly at their previous jobs.[16]

The occurrence rates of Prinzmetal angina,[110] infarction with normal coronary arteriogram,[111] and angina due to nonspecific (Takayasu-type) aortitis[67,112] and syphilis[113] have been documented. Among the post-myocardial infarction complications recorded are Dressler's syndrome,[114,115] papillary muscle rupture,[116] and interventricular septal rupture.[116] In a recent case of mine, a ventricular septal rupture was diagnosed by two-dimensional echocardiography and surgical repair was done as an emergency procedure without cardiac catheterization in view of the rapidly deteriorating condition of the patient. The patient survived the surgery but died 2 weeks later owing to hepatorenal failure.

PAN ANGINA

A peculiar form of angina seen locally has been nicknamed "Pan Angina."[117] *Pan* is a piece of betel leaf that is chewed with tobacco by some people; chewing of tobacco in this form has been shown to precipitate chest pains with ECG changes in angina patients.[117]

CORONARY HEART DISEASE IN THE YOUNG

It has been appreciated right from the early studies in Pakistan[26] that a considerable percentage of acute myocardial infarction cases were very young, with 7.3 to 21 percent[26,33,99,118] of all cases studied being below 40 years of age. Whether this higher percentage of younger adults with infarction reflects a low life expectancy and a larger number of younger people in the population or some other factors is unknown. There are data to suggest that younger patients have a higher percentage of single-vessel disease compared with other patients.[119] An increase in ischemic heart disease in young females also has been noted.[37,112] While there is evidence of increase in female smokers,[84] the birth control pill is not in very common use locally, mainly because of its expense. An interesting case has been reported of a young female aged 35 years with no apparent risk factors who suffered an anteroseptal myocardial infarction and then went on to develop a

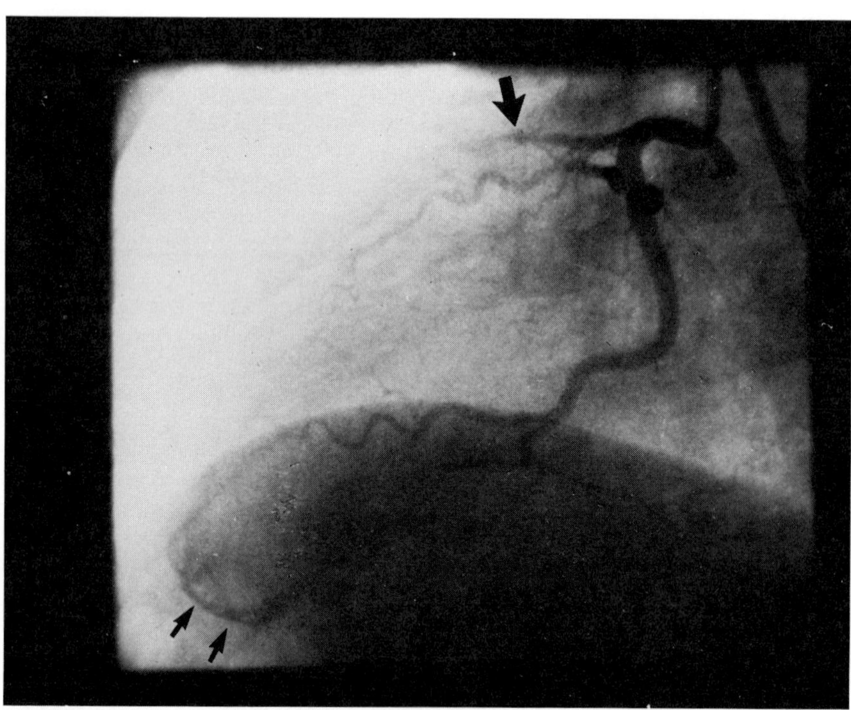

FIGURE 4 Left coronary injection in the 30° right anterior oblique projection in a 35-year-old female with an anteroseptal infarction 6 months prior to this angiogram.[120] Note the totally obstructed left anterior descending coronary artery (large arrow) and the calcification in the apical aneurysm (small arrows).

calcified left ventricular apical aneurysm 6 months later[120] (Fig. 4). Coronary arteriogram showed a single anterior descending obstruction in this woman.[120] The youngest among the author's own cases is an unmarried 21-year-old female who suffered an acute anteroseptal infarction, and coronary arteriography revealed a single anterior descending block. No known risk factors were present in this female. While anecdotal, these case reports point to the occurrence of obstructive coronary atherosclerotic heart disease in young adults, and surprisingly young females as well, in a population previously thought to be relatively free of coronary heart disease.

CORONARY ANGIOGRAPHIC DATA

Coronary angiography has been available only recently in Pakistan.[121] The pattern of coronary arterial anatomy as well as the coronary dominance and pattern of collateral vasculature appears to be no different than in the Western Hemisphere and is in agreement with earlier autopsy work in Pakistan that looked at the coronary anatomy.[39] It is the author's impression that the general size of the major epicardial vessels is smaller in the Pakistani population compared with Western populations. This most likely is related to the smaller size of the average Pakistani compared with the average Westerner[122] and has implications for coronary bypass surgery technique and graft patency. Preliminary data on angiographic anatomy in patients under 40 years of age[119] show a high percentage of isolated anterior descending artery obstruction in those with anteroseptal infarction and double- or triple-vessel disease in those with a prior inferior infarction or angina of effort. Anteroseptal myocardial infarction has been described in a young man with a normal coronary arteriogram.[111]

ELECTROCARDIOGRAPHIC PECULIARITIES

A prospective epidemiologic study[123] of a cross section of the normal population showed a number of ECG abnormalities simulating disease. The most common abnormalities after sinus tachycardia and bradycardia were premature ventricular beats (1.6 percent of sample), early repolarization (Grusin's) pattern (1.6 percent), and persistent juvenile pattern (1.25 percent). Rare cases of atrial premature beats, first-degree heart block, right or left bundle branch blocks, W-P-W syndrome, and isolated left axis deviation were also noted. Nonspecific T wave changes were noted in a large number of cases (19.4 percent). A common pattern seen in healthy young Pakistani women resembles the persistent juvenile pattern with T inversion in most V leads (Fig.5), as well as some ST-segment depression and changes in the inferior limb leads. An interesting group has been described with recurrent ventricular tachycardia (Fig. 6) and a completely normal cardiovascular workup, including coronary arteriograms.[124] The age range of these "patients" is from 17 to 45 years, with all complaining of runs of palpitations. None has required defibrillation, and response of the arrythmias to drugs was poor. The follow-up has ranged from 1 to 4 years, and the arrythmias in these "patients" so far appear to be benign.

Various types of familial as well as isolated cases of Q-T prolongation with or without congenital deafness have been reported in Pakistan.[125,126] Moreover, Q-T prolongation has been noted to occur with prenylamine, which is a popular antianginal drug, and patients have been documented with ventricular tachycardia (torsade de pointes) during treatment with this agent.[126a]

RHEUMATIC HEART DISEASE

Rheumatic heart disease remains Pakistan's main cardiac problem in the younger population (Table 2). The incidence of rheumatic heart disease is much less in the more affluent urban areas of Pakistan, such as Karachi[15] and Islamabad,[21] where the prevalence rate in school children of 1.3 to 1.8 per 1,000 contrasts sharply with the prevalence rate of 9 to 11 per 1,000 in the less developed regions.[18] This marked variation within one country lends support to the claim that the worldwide variation in the prevalence of this disease as well as the dramatic decrease in the developed countries represents mostly the impact of socioeconomic conditions and the environment rather than genetic or racial differences.

Acute Rheumatic Fever

Acute rheumatic fever is responsible for 1.05 to 3.5 percent of all medical and pediatric admissions.[32,127,128] The mean age at first documented attack is about 10 years, with a range of 5 to 22 years. The data show a higher admission rate during cooler months and winter. Only 30 to 40 percent give a definite history of preceding sore throats. Throat culture during the acute phase is reported to grow beta-hemolytic streptococcus in 31 percent.[127] In the general pediatric population, beta-hemolytic streptococcal infections account for 8.3 to 19.7 percent of all sore throats.[129] Manifestations of the acute illness are no different than elsewhere in the

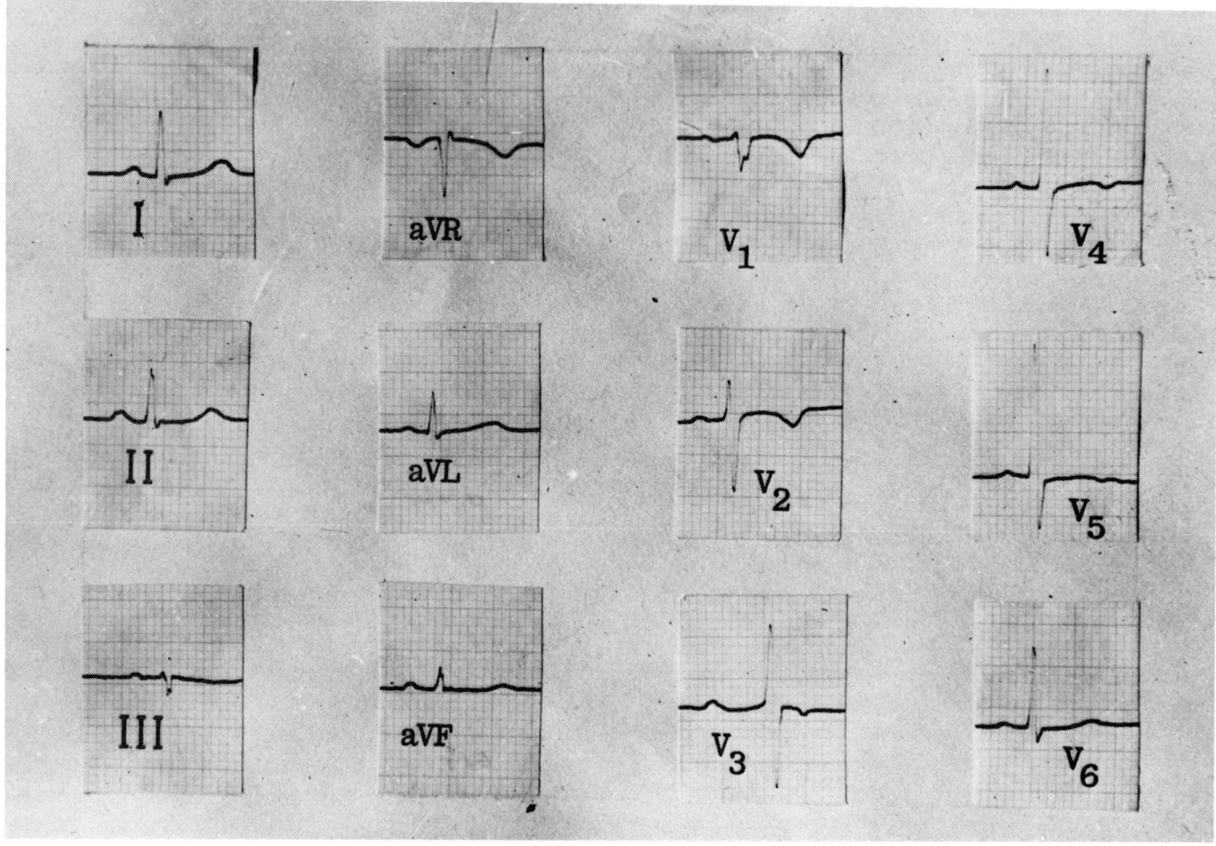

FIGURE 5 Electrocardiogram in a 30-year old female with a normal echocardiogram and coronary arteriogram. The ECG changes represent a commonly seen normal variant pattern in young women. Nonspecific repolarization changes are present in most chest leads.

world. However, Jones criteria appear less useful in this population, because all the major criteria other than carditis are seen less frequently[32] (Table 7). Acute carditis is very frequent, with 65 to 73 percent of acute cases having evidence of carditis.[32,127] The reason for this high incidence may be the simple fact that it is the more seriously ill that seek admission. It is believed by others that the disease may indeed be more serious in the tropics or that malnutrition or other immune differences make the heart more susceptible.[127] Because of the generally darker skin, erythema marginatum is less frequently seen, and both erythema marginatum and subcutaneous nodules are reported in only 1.8 to 3.4 percent.[32] There have been attempts to question the relationship of acute rheumatic fever with beta-hemolytic streptococcal infection.[130] Indirect evidence against this proposition is available from a study of penicillin prophylaxis in a group of patients with documented acute rheumatic fever.[131] There were 30.6 streptococcal infections per 100 patient-years in the subgroup on regular penicillin prophylaxis versus 81.6 infections per 100 patient-years in the subgroup taking prophylaxis irregularly, with the recurrence rate for rheumatic fever being 0.8 per 100 patient-years in the regular group versus 26.6 per 100 patient-years in the irregular group. The lowest recurrence rate of rheumatic fever was with monthly long-acting penicillin injections compared with oral regimens. The mortality from acute rheumatic fever in hospital series [32,127,128] is between 5 and 14 percent and quite high despite what appears to be appropriate and vigorous treatment. A mortality this high resembles that reported decades ago from the West.[132]

Chronic Valvular Disease

The average age at presentation with established chronic rheumatic valvular disease is 25.1 $\pm$ 9.2 years[31] and therefore younger than in the West. The reason for this is unknown, but poor socioeconomic conditions and malnutrition, recurrent rheumatic activity, and

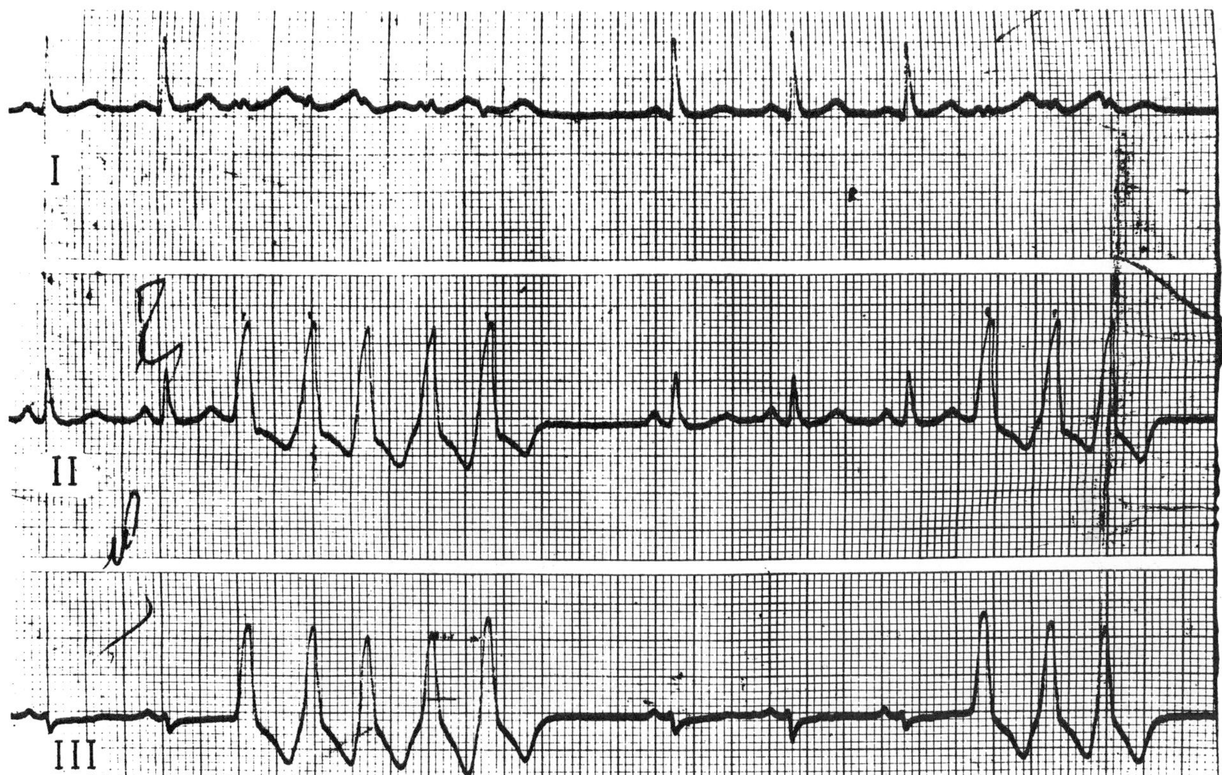

FIGURE 6 Electrocardiogram showing runs of ventricular tachycardia in a young patient with a completely normal workup, including complete left- and right-sided heart catheterization and coronary arteriogram. The ventricular tachycardia in this patient disappears during exercise and reappears after exercise.

poor compliance with penicillin prophylaxis may all have a role. Less than half the patients with established valve disease give a history of definite rheumatic fever[29] that may have been misdiagnosed as one of the other common infectious diseases. Indeed, in one report, 90 percent of patients with valve disease gave a history of "typhoid fever" in childhood.[133] The most frequent valve to be affected is the mitral valve, being involved in 94 to 97 percent of cases.[29,31] Females predominate in patients with mitral disease and males in the group with aortic valve disease. Not only is the natural history abbreviated, but indeed the disease pursues a fulminant course in many, with moderate to severe pulmonary hypertension being present in over 50 percent of patients at surgery.[134] Some of these patients develop severe congestive heart failure and severe right ventricular hypertension and dilatation. On angiography in these cases, one can see the interventricular septum bulging into the left ventricle (Fig. 7*A*) and the left ventricular geometry distorted by this shape change (Fig. 7*B*). In addition, the enlarged right ventricle literally lifts the left ventricle off the diaphragm. All these changes make the assessment of left ventricular function difficult from single-plane angiography, and a biplanar left ventriculogram is important. An interesting feature in the author's personal experience is the very high wedge pressures that some of these patients can tolerate without being in overt pulmonary edema or orthopnea. It is not uncommon to see patients with severe mitral valve disease and reliable mean pulmonary wedge pressures of between 30 and 50 mm Hg lying supine on the catheterization table without difficulty and without bubbling over with pulmonary edema. The mean age of patients operated on for mitral stenosis is 32.5 years, with 44 percent in old NYHA functional classes III and IV at the time of surgery. Aschoff's bodies are found in only 10 percent of excised atrial appendages, but the reason for this low rate has not been established.[135]

THE STENOTIC, BILLOWING MITRAL VALVE

A group of patients has been described who at catheterization reveal, in addition to their mitral stenosis, moderate to severe mitral valve prolapse[136] (Fig. 8). Whether this entity represents a spectrum of rheumatic disease itself or whether, as in this author's

TABLE 7
Acute rheumatic fever: Frequency (percent) of Jones major and minor criteria in various series

Manifestation	Robinson et al.[127]	Rahimtoola et al.[128]	Ilyas et al.[138]
Carditis	73%	64.5%	68%
Arthritis	59%	58.1%	39%
Chorea	6.8%	13.6%	—
Erythema marginatum	3.4%	2.7%	
Subcutaneous nodules	3.4%	1.8%	4%
Arthralgia	14%	—	—
Fever	78%	87.2%	—
History of sore throat	40%	59%	—
Leukocytosis	30%	—	—
Raised ESR	95%	70.9%	—
Positive throat culture	31%	43.6%	—
Raised ASOT (Todd units)	90% (>250)	56.3% (>333)	—

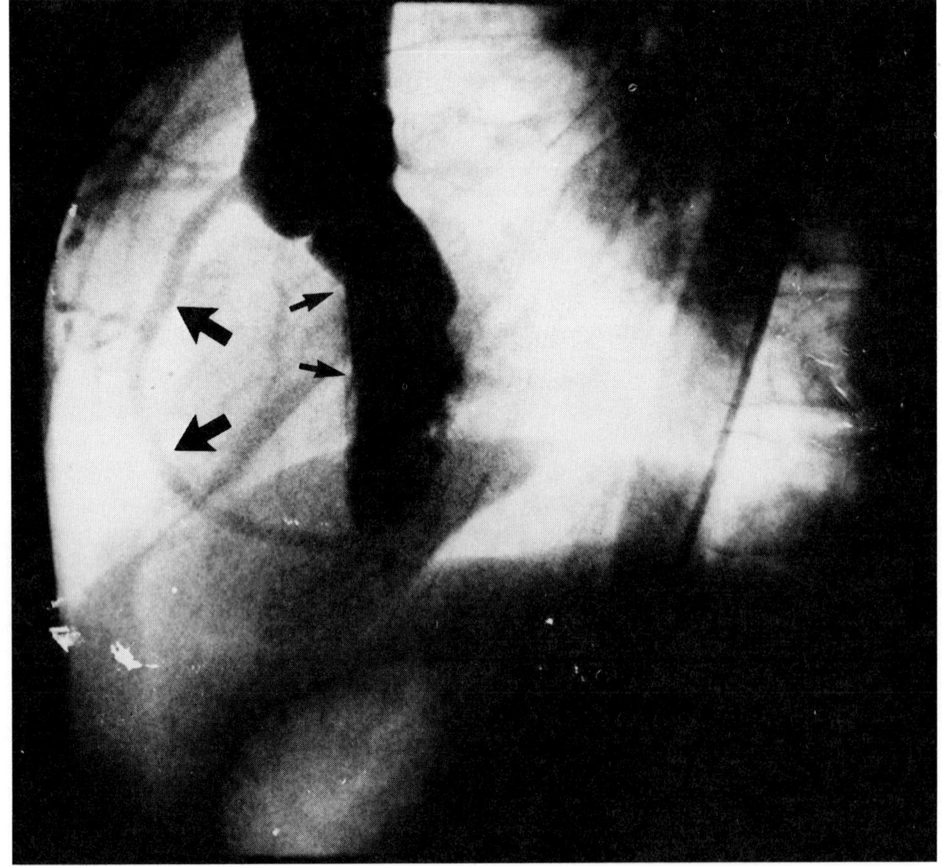

A

Figure 7 (*A*) Left ventriculogram in the 60° left anterior oblique projection. In this young adult with severe mitral stenosis and suprasystemic pulmonary hypertension, the greatly enlarged right ventricle is causing the interventricular septum to bulge (small arrows) into the left ventricle. Also note the large sweep of the right coronary artery, a sign reflecting the enlarged right atrioventricular ring (large arrows) due to right-sided heart dilatation. (*B*, opposite) Left ventriculogram in the 30° right anterior oblique projection in the same patient showing the distortion in shape of the left ventricle caused by the septal bulge. Note the raising of the left ventricular apex in both the left and right anterior oblique views, which is another sign of greatly enlarged right ventricle in these cases.

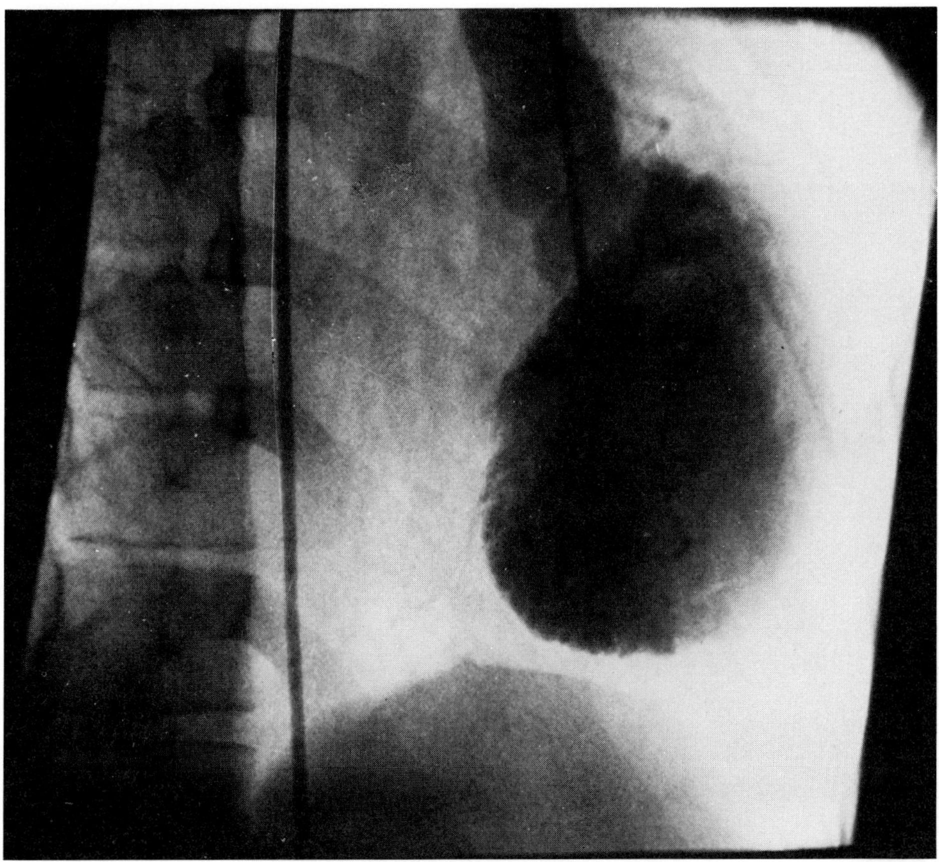

B

belief, it represents rheumatic disease on a myxomatous valve is unknown at present. An as yet unconfirmed observation seems to be a higher incidence of postcommissurotomy mitral regurgitation in these stenotic, billowing valves.

A useful addition to the medical treatment of rheumatic valvular disease, especially those patients with predominant regurgitant valve lesions and those with severe pulmonary hypertension, has been the use of vasodilators.[137] Beneficial hemodynamic effects have been studied at the time of cardiac catheterization and in clinical follow-up. The most useful application of vasodilators has been in the group with advanced disease and failure who seemed inoperable but improved enough to become surgical candidates. Vasodilators also seem to improve the functional class and surgical risk when used preoperatively in those who are surgical candidates. Whether vasodilators will delay the time of surgery when used earlier in the disease is under study.

JUVENILE MITRAL STENOSIS

Juvenile mitral stenosis is a very interesting aspect of rheumatic valvular disease in tropical countries, where it develops under the age of 20 years. In Pakistan, about 30 percent of patients with mitral stenosis are below 20 years of age[138] and 16.3 percent of patients are below 15 years of age.[139] In surgical series, 23 to 40 percent of patients undergoing mitral valvuotomy have been below 20 years of age.[134,140] Indeed, the author has a patient aged 7 years who developed mitral stenosis after definite rheumatic fever at age 3 and 5 years. Not only is mitral stenosis common in juveniles, but a fulminant form of rheumatic valvular lesion is seen with severe valvular damage and predominantly mitral regurgitation starting with the acute episode and continuing and worsening after the febrile phase with rapid development of pulmonary hypertension, severe cardiomegaly, and congestive failure (Fig. 9). These children are severely undernourished and show stunted growth.[139] The condition is nicknamed "rheumatic cachexia" and usually progresses to a fatal outcome. Valve surgery has been attempted in some of these children with a higher mortality, and it is too early to assess the role of surgery in altering the malignant natural history of this group.[141]

NONRHEUMATIC VALVULAR DISEASE

It was not too long ago that all valvular heart disease was thought synonymous with rheumatic heart disease. It was only recently that other etiologies were described.[142] Ever since the availability of echocardiography in Pakistan,[143] there seems to have been an

327

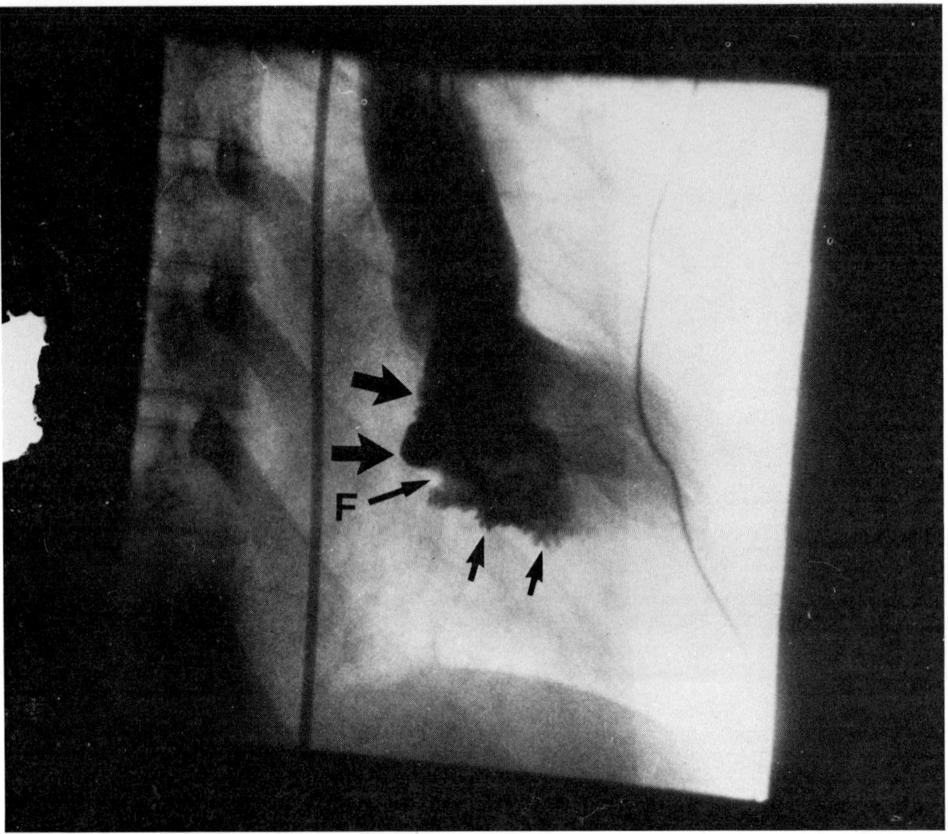

FIGURE 8 A left ventriculogram in the 30° right anterior projection in a patient with tight mitral stenosis. Note the billowing of the mitral valve (large arrows) above the fulcrum (F) in this midsystolic frame. Also note the indentations and roughness in the posterobasal portion of the left ventricle (small arrows), which are commonly seen in cases of rheumatic heart disease.

explosion in the number of nonrheumatic valve cases. Mitral valve prolapse is now recognized to be a very common problem with features no different than those reported from Western studies.[144] Since both mitral valve prolapse and rheumatic heart disease are common problems in this population, it is not surprising to see the two of them coexisting, as seen in the previous discussion about the stenotic, billowing mitral valve. Myxomatous degeneration seems to be the most common cause of isolated aortic regurgitation when the mitral valve is normal, as has been well recognized in the West. Other documented causes of nonrheumatic valvular disease include nonspecific (Takayasu-type aortitis, rheumatoid arthritis, and syphilis.[113]

CONGENITAL HEART DISEASE

There is very little information in this country about congenital heart disease. One reason for this is that rheumatic heart disease has been a bigger cardiac problem in the younger population. The other main reason is the dearth of physicians trained in pediatric cardiology. Until very recently, the lack of sophisticated diagnostic facilities as well as the unavailability of palliative or corrective surgery have also contributed.[145] From surveys of the general population as well as hospital patients it is apparent that congenital heart disease is not less of a problem here than elsewhere in the world.[15,21,37,146] There is no reason to believe that the disease pattern seen here is substantially different from that seen elsewhere in the world[147] (Table 8). The relative frequency of certain lesions and the absence of others is mostly related to whether congenital heart disease is suspected at all and, if suspected, whether the child survives long enough to be seen at an appropriate facility. In the author's own experience and the published data,[146–149] pulmonary valve stenosis, ventricular and atrial septal defect, and patent ductus are the most common acyanotic lesions seen, and among the cyanotic diseases, tetralogy is by far the most common.

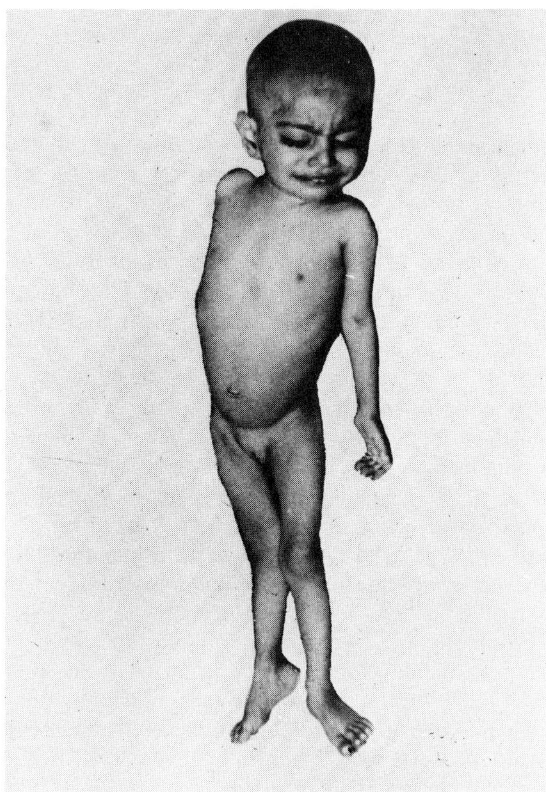

A

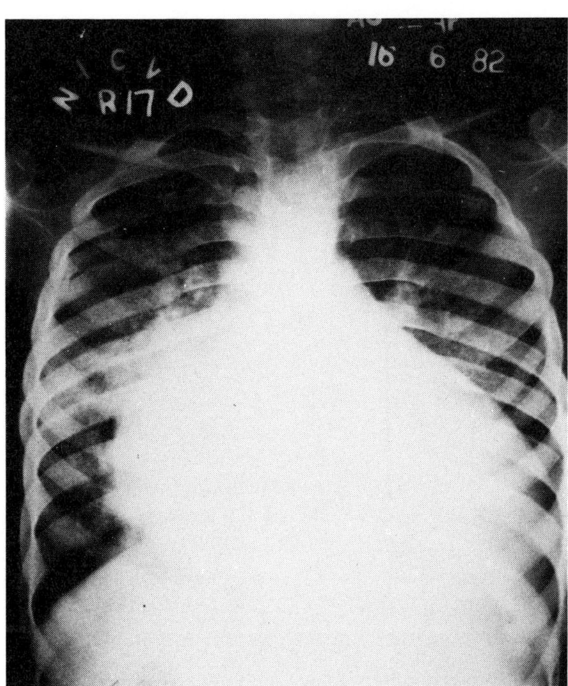

B

FIGURE 9 (*A*) A 7-year-old child showing the stigmata of "rheumatic cachexia" due to severe unremitting rheumatic heart disease. (*B*) The chest x-ray shows severe cardiomegaly and failure despite intensive medical treatment.

Among unusual lesions seen frequently enough to raise doubts as to their increased frequency in this population are supracristal ventricular septal defects. Also not uncommonly seen are aneurysms (ruptured and nonruptured) of the sinus of Valsalva, most of which are probably congenital in etiology.[150] Another interesting problem related to the general trend of late presentation of congenital heart disease is a peculiar presentation of severe (gradients over 80 mm Hg) long-standing pulmonic valve stenosis, as has been documented in other parts of this subcontinent.[130,151] These patients present with congestive heart failure and cardiomegaly (Fig. 10). Most improve postoperatively, although the surgical mortality is high and the long-term postoperative course not yet documented.

CARDIOMYOPATHIES

Cardiomyopathies form an important group of diseases that make up 1.6 percent of all cardiac admissions[37] and are most completely confined to the dilated (congestive) and hypertrophic varieties. The dilated variety is by far the more common and seems to be a disease similar to that elsewhere in the world. A peculiar M-mode echocardiographic feature commonly seen in our patients with dilated cardiomyopathy is apparent aortomitral noncontinuity[152] (Fig. 11). The M-mode echogram shows the anterior mitral leaflet behind and apparently noncontinuous with the posterior aortic wall. No definite explanation for this phenomenon is available, although in some cases the two-dimensional echogram shows a higher location of the mitral leaflets and an angulation behind the aorta, which seems to be the cause of this peculiar phenomenon in M-mode

TABLE 8
Frequency of congenital heart disease

Lesion	No.	Percentage of total
Ventricular septal defect	269	33.0
Tetralogy of Fallot	142	17.0
Rheumatic heart disease	122	15.0
Patent ductus arteriosus	58	7.0
Atrial septal defect	56	6.8
Pulmonary valve stenosis	41	5.0
Aortic valve stenosis	30	3.6
No cardiac lesion	29	3.6
Transposition of great arteries	17	2.0
Miscellaneous*	60	7.0
Total	814	100

Source: Congenital Heart Disease Workup Clinic, National Institute of Cardiovascular Diseases, Karachi, October 1980 to October 1981.

*The miscellaneous group includes cases of total anomalous pulmonary venous return, tricuspid valve atresia, pulmonary valve atresia, pseudotruncus, truncus type I, WPW syndrome, pulmonary incompetence, double-outlet right ventricle, single ventricle, AV canal defects, arteriovenous fistula, situs inversus dextrocardia, coarctation of the aorta, primary pulmonary hypertension, Eisenmenger reaction, systemic hypertension, endocardial fibroelastosis, congestive and hypertrophic cardiomyopathy, myocarditis, mitral valve prolapse, and anomalous origin of the coronary artery.

329

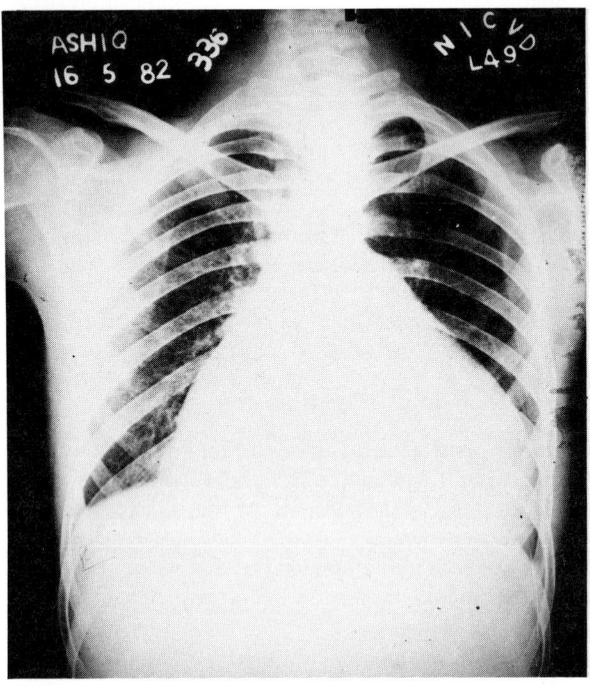

FIGURE 10 A plain chest x-ray (PA view) in a patient with severe pulmonary valve stenosis and a gradient over 100 mm Hg. Note the greatly enlarged heart and an appearance unlike that expected in pulmonary valve stenosis.

recordings. Of all the clinical varieties of dilated cardiomyopathies, the worst prognosis is seen in post-partum cardiomyopathy.[153] In some cases, a relentless and progressive course results in a fatal outcome in a matter of days and weeks. In the author's institution, a number of children have been described as having dilated cardiomyopathy with large hearts and later were found to have advanced hypertensive heart disease.

Hypertrophic cardiomyopathy was rarely diagnosed until echocardiography became available.[143] The autopsy and histologic features are the same as prescribed classically.[42] There seems to be a high prevalence of the nonobstructive, symmetrically hypertrophic form.[154]

None of the African obliterative forms of cardiomyopathies or idiopathic ventricular aneurysms are seen in Pakistan. While eosinophilia, especially severe "tropical eosinophilia," is common in Pakistan, none of these patients develop cardiac problems even after years of follow-up.[155,155a] Isolated cases of endomyocardial fibrosis and endocardial fibroelastosis have been reported at autopsy,[156] but their prevalence in the patient population is unknown.

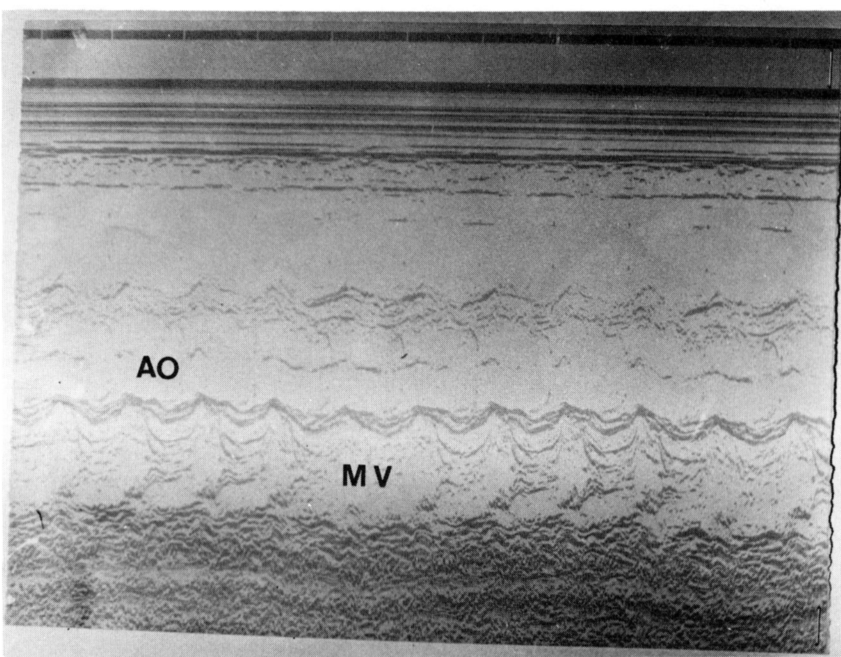

FIGURE 11 An M-mode echogram in a case of dilated (congestive) cardiomyopathy showing apparent aortomitral noncontinuity. Note that the mitral leaflets (MV) are seen behind the aortic root (AO) echos.

MISCELLANEOUS CARDIOVASCULAR AILMENTS

Pericardial Diseases

Tuberculosis of the pericardium is a common cause of both pericardial effusion and constrictive pericarditis.[157–159] The classical teaching that "all constrictive pericarditis is tuberculous in etiology unless proven otherwise" holds true for Pakistan, as would be expected from the high prevalence rate of tuberculosis in the general population[160] (54 percent tuberculin-positive; 1.9 percent with active disease). A significant number of cases of tuberculous pericardial effusion very quickly begin to organize the effusion and, within weeks and months of starting treatment, develop a subacute constrictive phase. Echocardiography shows the pericardial space filled with high-density echos and return of movement in the outer pericardium. This picture is difficult to distinguish from the echogram of classically thickened pericardium in established fibrocalcific constrictive pericarditis. Cardiac catheterization shows the presence of moderately severe constrictive physiology. At surgery, the pericardial cavity is filled with "cheesy" material much more solid than the caseous material of active tuberculosis.[158] Technically, the surgeon finds it much easier to do a complete and safe pericardiectomy in these cases than in the late fibrocalcific cases. It also appears that the patient response and improvement after surgery are more rapid and complete. Further work and data collection in this group are underway to prove these initial impressions. A radiologic and echographic feature noted in the majority of cases with significant constriction is the presence of left atrial enlargement in the absence of gradient across the mitral valve.[161,162] A rare and unusual cause of a serious and fulminant type of pericardial effusion is rupture of a hepatic amoebic abscess into the pericardial space.[163] Mortality is high in these usually very sick patients despite aggressive treatment. In those who survive, constrictive pericarditis develops in a matter of weeks.[163]

Diseases of the Aorta

An important though uncommon group of diseases seen in this part of the world is comprised of the various types of nonspecific (Takayasu-type) aortitis.[67,112] No specific etiology or etiologic association has been established. Portions of the aorta involved show both aneurysmal sacculations (Fig. 12) and narrowing (Fig. 3). These patients present with hypertension, angina, myocardial infarction, or cerebrovascular symptoms. Kawasaki's disease has not so far been reported in Pakistan.

Even though hypertension is Pakistan's greatest cardiovascular problem, dissecting aneurysm of the aorta is a very rare problem. While a major reason may be underdiagnosis, this is not enough to explain the reporting of only 2 confirmed cases in the entire cardiologic literature despite the availability of angiography for over a decade. In these two patients, the dissection was of DeBakey's type II, i.e., localized to the ascending aorta.[164] If indeed this observation is correct, it would be a very worthwhile study to look at the aorta and the kind of changes or lack of changes that occur with hypertension and age in this population. Other documented causes of aortic aneurysm in Pakistan are atherosclerosis, syphilis,[113] and typhoid fever (Fig. 13).

Pulmonary Vascular Disease

Primary pulmonary hypertension is seen frequently and constitutes 8.3 percent of all cases of pulmonary hypertension due to various diseases other than rheumatic heart disease.[165] The disease is seen in all ages, and both sexes are involved. While a large number of traditional herbs and medicines are used by a large segment of the population, none has been incriminated in the causation of primary pulmonary hypertension.

An interesting fact is the complete absence of any data pertaining to pulmonary embolism. In this author's experience, even though the predisposing factors for the occurrence of pulmonary embolism are commonly present in our hospitalized patients, no case of pulmonary embolism or infarction has been documented. Cases of established pulmonary embolism and infarction treated by the author in Pakistan have been foreign nationals. There have been instances in which the terminal event in a long-standing or serious disease appeared clinically to be massive pulmonary embolism. However, in the absence of autopsy, this has never been confirmed. This problem remains another area in which anecdotal clinical experience shall have to be substantiated by large, well-planned scientific studies. Moreover, the reason for the low rate of pulmonary embolism should be studied if this is indeed true.

Cardiac Tumors

The only cardiac tumors reported in Pakistan are left and right atrial myxomas.[166–168] In one patient with a large right atrial myxoma almost filling the entire right ventricle and blocking the tricuspid valve (Fig. 14), the presenting complaints were "angina of effort," nonspecific ST and T wave changes on resting ECG, and a normal coronary arteriogram. The "angina" was relieved after successful surgery.

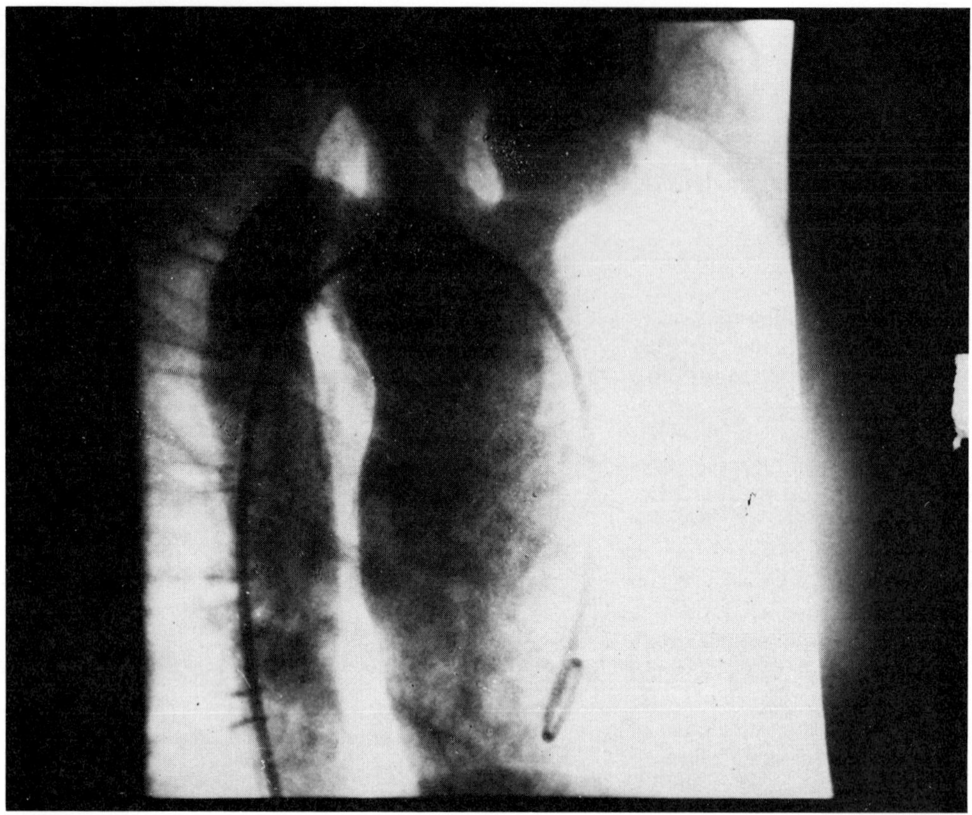

FIGURE 12 Aortogram in a patient with nonspecific (Takayasu-type) aortitis. Note the saccular appearance of the aorta.

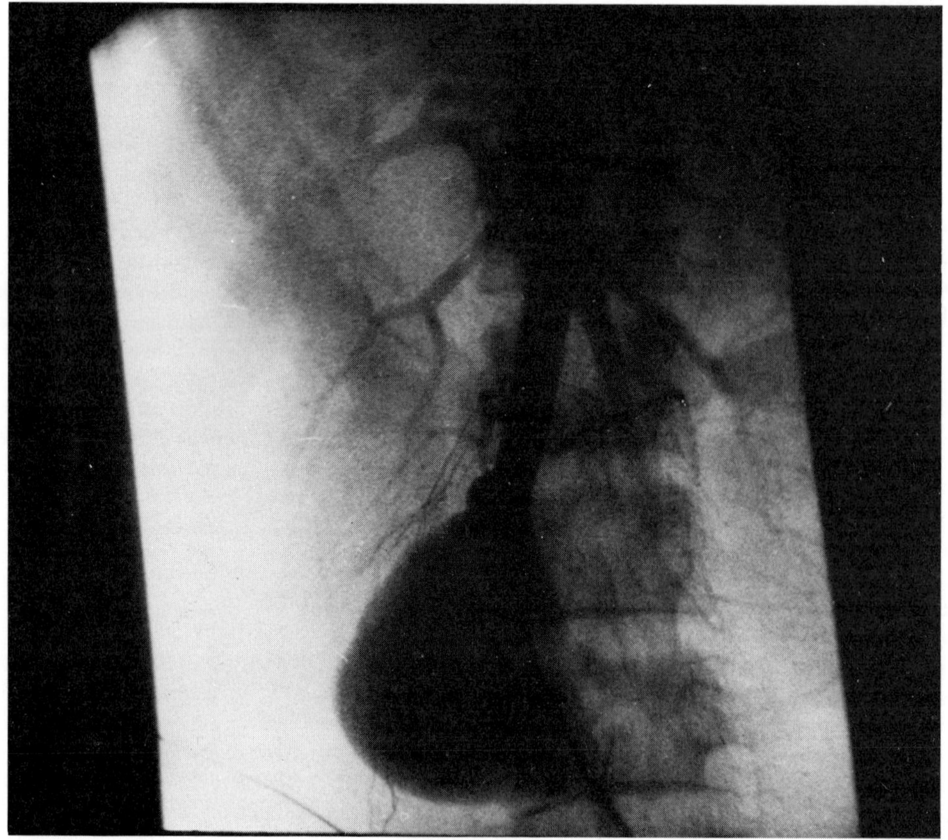

FIGURE 13 Abdominal aortogram showing a discrete abdominal aneurysm developing in the course of typhoid fever. (*Courtesy of Dr. A. Samad.*)

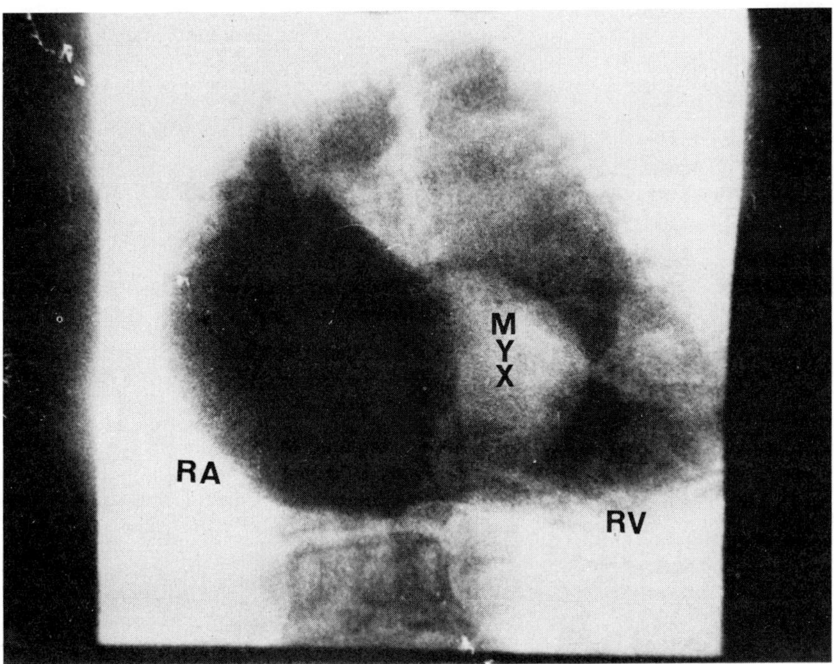

FIGURE 14 A right-sided angiogram showing a large egg-shaped and mobile right atrial myxoma (MYX) occupying the right atrium (RA) in systole and moving into the tricuspid valve and right ventricular inflow (RV) area in diastole.

TROPICAL CARDIOLOGY: A HYPOTHESIS

The term *tropical cardiology* stirs in the minds of many physicians the picture of unusual and bizarre diseases in people of a different genetic makeup. After having had the opportunity to study and practice cardiology in Western populations as well as in Pakistan, I have made a number of observations. The most impressive of these in the *similarity* of diseases that exist in apparently so dissimilar populations. The next impression is that the differences between the rural and urban populations in tropical countries are so much more marked than those in the developed Western countries. The pattern of cardiovascular diseases in the urban and affluent populations in the tropics resembles more and more that of Western populations. While differences in prevalence rates of various disorders do seem to exist between populations of the world, most of the major and outstanding differences are perhaps more due to differences in socioeconomic conditions and environmental factors than to predetermined genetic makeup. It seems quite probable that with time, the pattern of cardiovascular diseases may change in the tropics enough to render redundant the concept of tropical cardiology. However, before this happens, there seems to be a large natural experiment going on in the tropics and elsewhere for the world to study and document. It would be a pity if this opportunity were lost.

REFERENCES

1 "International Work in Cardiovascular Diseases," WHO, Geneva, 1969.

2 Shaper, A. G., Hutt, M. S. R., and Fejfar, Z.: Preface, in A. G. Shaper, M. S. R. Hutt, and Z. Fejfar (eds.), "Cardiovascular Disease in the Tropics," International Society of Cardiology, British Medical Association, London, 1974, p. v.

3 "Ischaemic Heart Disease Registers," Report of the Fifth Working Group, Copenhagen, 26–29 April, 1971, WHO Document EURO 8201(5).

4 Strasser, T., and Rotta, J.: The Control of Rheumatic Fever and Rheumatic Heart Disease: An Outline of WHO Activities, *WHO Chron.*, 27:49, 1973.

5 "Encyclopaedia Brittanica," vol.13, 15th ed. Encyclopaedia Brittanica, Inc., Chicago, 1980, pp. 892–905.

6 "Encyclopedia Americana," vol.21. Americana Corporation, New York, 1976, pp. 132–134L.

7 "Pakistan, Basic Facts 1980–1981," 19th ed. Government of Pakistan Finance Division, Economic Adviser's Wing, Islamabad, 1981.

8 "National Accounts of Pakistan. Product and Expenditure 1976 to 1980," Statistics Division, Government of Pakistan, Islamabad, 1980, p. 22

9 Faruqui, N.: "Abridged Life Table for Urban and Rural Areas in Pakistan," Pakistan Development Review no. 3, Pakistan Institute of Economics, Karachi, 1974.

10 Khan, M. K. H.: Abridged Life Tables for Males and Females, *Pak. J. Med. Res.,* 1:73, 1958.

11 Akhtar, R.: "Pakistan Year Book, 1980–1981," 8th ed., East and West Publishing Co., Pakistan, 1981, p. 327.

12 Kannel, W. B.: Incidence, Prevalence, and Mortality of Cardiovascular Disease, in J. W. Hurst et al. (eds.), "The Heart," McGraw-Hill Book Company, New York, 1982, p. 621.

13 Hashmi, J. A.: An Epidemiological Study of Heart Disease in Pakistan, *J.P.M.A.,* 15:439, 1965.

14 Raza, M., Hashmi, J. A., Abbasi, A. S., et al.: A Study of Blood Pressure of Pakistani School Children Age 5–14 Years, *Pak. Heart J.,* 4:47, 1971.

15 Abbasi, A. S., Hashmi, J. A. Robinson, R. D., Jr., et al.: Prevalence of Heart Disease in School Children of Karachi, *Am. J. Cardiol.,* 18:544, 1966.

16 Syed, S. A., Raza, M., Hashmi, J. A., et al.: "Establishment of Comprehensive Research and Rehabilitation Programme for Persons of Various Forms of Heart Disease," Project V.R.A. Pak-8-66, National Institute of Cardiovascular Diseases, Karachi, 1973.

17 Mirza, M. A.: Prevalence of Hypertension, *Pak. Armed Forces Med. J.,* 26:1, 1976.

18 Ilyas, M., Peracha, M. A., Ahmed, R., et al.: Prevalence and Pattern of Rheumatic Heart Disease in the Frontier Province of Pakistan, *J.P.M.A.,* 29:165, 1979.

19 Ahmed, I.: Hypertension among Shopkeepers and Clerks, *J.P.M.A.,* 26:180, 1976.

20 Ilyas, M., Sherazi, S. H., Shah, M., et al.: Peshawar Hypertension Study: Epidemiological Profile of Juvenile and In-Service Population, *J.P.M.A.,* 30:174, 1980.

21 Malik, S. M., Jaffery, S., Ahmed, S., and Khanum, Z.: Prevalence of Heart Disease in School Children of Islamabad, *Pak. Heart J.,* 14:2, 1981.

22 Rahimtoola, R. J., Majid, I., Ramzan, A., and Ahmed, Q.: Blood Pressure Study in Children: Preliminary Data, *Pak. Heart J.,* 14:8, 1981.

23 Usman, S., Bano, K. A., Haider, Z., et al.: Study of Blood Pressure Pattern and Screening for Glycosuria in Urban and Rural Population—A Pilot Study, *J.P.M.A.,* 31:138, 1981.

24 Hill, A. B.: "Principles of Medical Statistics," 7th ed., Oxford University Press, London, 1961, pp. 27 and 47.

25 Epidemiology of Cardiovascular Diseases (Princeton Conference Report), *Am. J. Public Health,* 50 (suppl.10):12, 1960.

26 Pirzada, M. A., and Khan, M. A.: Coronary Heart Disease in West Pakistan, *Pak.J.Med.Res.,* 2:9, 1962.

27 Ibrahim, M., and Ahmad, K. A.: A Preliminary Survey of Coronary Heart Disease, *Pak.J.Med.Res.,* 2:10, 1959.

28 Rab, S. M., Quaderi, M. A., and Choudhry, G. M.: A Study of Coronary Artery Disease in East Pakistan, *J.P.M.A.,* 16:227, 1967.

29 Khan, N., Ahmed, I., Ali, M. L., et al.: Study of Chronic Rheumatic Endocarditis in Multan, *Medicus,* 26:71, 1963.

30 Pervez, M. A., Ahmed, S., and Ahmed, S.: Hospital Morbidity Pattern in Jinnah Postgraduate Medical Centre, Karachi, *Pak. J. Med. Res.,* 10:308, 1969.

31 Abbasi, A. S., Hashmi, J. A., Robinson, R. D., Jr., et al.: Experience with Rheumatic Fever and Rheumatic Heart Disease in Karachi, *Medicus,* 31:245, 1966.

32 Rahimtoola, R. J., and Rehman, H.: Acute Rheumatic Fever in Children, *J.P.M.A.,* 22:185, 1972.

33 Khan, N. A., Shah, M. Z., and Roghani, M. T.: Epidemiology of Coronary Heart Disease in Peshawar, *Pak. Heart J.,* 6:64, 1973.

34 Beg, M. A., Siddiqui, M. K., Ahmed, N., Abbasi, A. S., and Syed, S. A.: Atherosclerosis in Karachi—A Retrospective Study of the Clinical Pattern of Coronary Heart Disease in Cardiac Admissions, *J.P.M.A.,* 18:412, 1968.

35 Rahimtoola, R. J., Majid, I., Shafqat, H., and Qureshi, A. F.: Congenital Heart Disease in Children visiting JPMC, *Pak. Heart J.,* 13:21, 1980.

36 Iftikhar, A. R.: Figures for Admission and Deaths January 1st, 1980 to December 31st, 1981 at the National Institute of Cardiovascular Diseases, unpublished data, Karachi.

37 Khan, A. R.: Disease Category in Patients Admitted May 1st to October 31, 1981, at the National Institute of Cardiovascular Diseases, unpublished data, Karachi.

38 Aziz, H., Beg, M. R., Ahmad, J., Hafeez, N., and Hasan, Z.: "Cerebrovascular Disease—An Interim Report," (proceedings 19th Annual Medical Symposium, Karachi, Pakistan, Dec. 19–24, 1981), JPMC Symposium Committee, Karachi, 1981.

39 Chaudhry, M. S.: Some Observations on the Coronary Artery Pattern and Intercoronary Anastomoses in Human Hearts, *Medicus,* 30:160, 1965.

40 Sattar, A. B. M. A., and Khan, B.: Atherosclerosis in Karachi. A Study of an Unselected Autopsy Series. Part 1, *J.P.M.A.,* 17:245, 1967.

41 Rashid, H., and Jafery, N. A.: Atherosclerosis in Karachi. A Study of an Unselected Autopsy Series. Part 2, *J.P.M.A.,* 17:252, 1967.

42 Ahmed, F. S.: Pathology of Hypertrophic Obstructive Cardiomyopathy, *Pak. Armed Forces Med. J.,* 23:61, 1972.

43 Khalil, K. A.: Statistics of the State Life Insurance Corporation of Pakistan, unpublished data, 1979–1981.

44 Rogers, L.: Life Insurance in the Tropics, *Br. Med.J.,* 1:219, 1928.

45 Clarke, J. T.: The Nature of the Rheumatic Poison, *J. Trop. Med.,* 35:55, 1932.

46 Scott, H.: The Incidence of Rheumatic Infection in India. *Indian Med. Gaz.,* 73:271, 1938.

47 *WHO* Prevention of Rheumatic Fever, 2d Report of Expert Committee on Rheumatic Diseases, *Tech. Rep. Ser.*, 126, 1957.

48 Shaper, A. G.: Coronary Heart Disease, in A. G. Shaper, M. S. R. Hutt, and Z. Fejfar (eds.), "Cardiovascular Disease in the Tropics," International Society of Cardiology, British Medical Association, London, 1974, p. 148.

49 Fejfar, Z.: Tropical Cardiology and the W.H.O., in A. G. Shaper, M. S. R. Hutt, and Z. Fejfar (eds.), "Cardiovascular Disease in the Tropics," International Society of Cardiology, British Medical Association, London, 1974, p. 1.

50 "Heart Disease in Adults, U.S., 1960–1962," U.S. Public Health Service publication 1,000, ser. 11, no. 6, September 1964.

51 Kannel, W. B., and Sorlie, P.: Hypertension in Framingham, in O. Paul (ed.), "Epidemiology and Control of Hypertension," Stratton Intercontinental Medical Book Corp., New York, 1975, p. 553.

52 Truswell, A. S., Kennelly, B. M., Hansen, J. D. L., and Lee, R. B.: Blood Pressure of Kung Bushmen in Northern Botswana, *Am. Heart J.*, 84:5, 1972.

53 Sehgal, A. K., Krishnan, I., Malhotra, R. P., and Gupta, H. D.; Observations on the Blood Pressure of Tibetans, *Circulation,* 37:36, 1968.

54 Shaper, A. G., Leonard, P. J., Jones, K. W., and Jones, M.: Environmental Effects on the Body Build, Blood Pressure and Blood Chemistry of Nomadic Warriors Serving in the Army in Kenya, *East African Med. J.,* 46:282, 1969.

55 Cruz-Coke, R., Etcheverry, R., and Negel, R.: Influence of Migration on Blood Pressure of Easter Islanders, *Lancet,* 1:697, 1964.

56 Syed, S. A., Beg, M. A., Bhimjee, S., et al.: Study of Blood Pressure in Urban and Rural Populations of Pakistan, *Pak. Heart J.,* 3:35, 1970.

57 Bano, K. A., Haider, Z., and Rana, I. A.: Study of Blood Pressure in Women Taking Oral Contraceptives, *J.P.M.A.,* 30:157, 1980.

58 Beg, M. A., Abbasi, A. S., Raza, M., Hashimi, J. A., Masood, A., and Syed, S. A.: Blood Pressure Findings in Relation to Hardness and Softness of Drinking Water in a Single Community in Pakistan, *Pak. Heart J.,* 3:33, 1970.

59 Haider, Z., Bano, K. A., Usman, S. Din, F. U., and Rana, I. A.: Blood Lipids in Non-Obese Patients with Newly Diagnosed Diabetes Mellitus and Untreated Hypertension, *J.P.M.A.,* 30:57, 1980.

60 Haider, Z., Usman, S., Jabeen., M., Bano, K. A., Obaidullah, S., and Fayyaz, A.: Profile of Hyperlipidemia in Various Patient Groups and Controls, *Pak. J. Med. Res.,* 20:63, 1981.

61 Haider, Z., Shahid, M., Jabeen, F., and Chowdhry, M. A. I.: Mild Hypertension, *J.P.M.A.,* 26:54, 1976.

62 Haider, Z., Bano, K. A., Zubair, M., and Shahid, M.: Diagnostic Evaluation of Hypertension, *J.P.M.A.,* 27:375, 1977.

63 Shareef, M., Bhimjee, S., Rehman, S., and Syed, S. A.: Hypertension under Forty, *Pak. Heart J.,* 2:49, 1969.

64 Yusuf, R.: Symposium on Hypertension, *J.P.M.A.,* 12:151, 1962.

65 Haider, Z., Bano, K. A., Zubair, M., and Shahid, M.: Hypertension Clinic in a General Hospital, *J.P.M.A.,* 27:410, 1977.

66 Hussain, A., and Siddiqi, B.: "Pheochromocytoma—A Surgically proven Case Report" (proceedings 19th Annual Medical Symposium, Karachi, Pakistan, Dec. 19–24, 1981), JPMC Symposium Committee, Karachi, 1981.

67 Ilyas, M., Peracha, M. A., and Ali, N.: Takayasu's Disease, *J.P.M.A.,* 25:81, 1975.

68 Kassim, A. M., and Sharif, M.: Treatment of Severe and Malignant Hypertension with Guanethidine, *J.P.M.A.,* 12:125, 1962.

69 Peracha, M. A., Ahmad, R., Saeed, M., and Ilyas, M.: Acute Effects of Clonidine on Blood Pressure in Normal Individuals and Patients with Hypertension, *J.P.M.A.,* 25:131, 1975.

70 Bano, K. A., Haider, Z., and Rana, I. A.: Comparative Study of Anti-Hypertensive Effect of a Thiazide Diuretic, Propranolol and Prazosin in Mild to Moderate Hypertension, *Pak. J. Med. Res.,* 20:102, 1981.

71 Siddiqui, M. A., and Sharif, M.: Propranolol in the Treatment of Hypertension, *Pak. Heart J.,* 11:32, 1978.

72 Muhammad, A.: Propranolol in the Treatment of Hypertension, *Pak. Heart J.,* 5:77, 1972.

73 Muhammad, A.: Acebutolol in Hypertension, *Pak. Heart J.,* 14:11, 1981.

74 Haider, Z., and Bano, K. A.: A Follow-Up Study of Patients with Mild and Moderate Hypertension, *J.P.M.A.,* 30:227, 1980.

75 Chohan, R. I., Din, F. U. Bano, K. A., and Haider Z.: Changes in Blood Lipids during Anti-Hypertensive Treatment, *J.P.M.A.,* 28:68, 1978.

76 Restrepo, C.: Atherosclerosis, in A. G. Shaper, M. S. R. Hutt, and Z. Fejfar (eds.), "Cardiovascular Disease in the Tropics," International Society of Cardiology, British Medical Association, London 1974, p. 125.

77 Galgav S., Rowly, D. A., and Kohut, R. I.: Atherosclerosis of Human Aorta and Its Coronary and Renal Arteries, *Arch. Pathol.,* 7:558, 1961.

78 Hill, H. R., Camps, F. E., Rigg, K., and McKinney, B. E. G.: Atherosclerosis: Results of a Pilot Survey in a North London Area. *Br. Med. J.,* 1:1190, 1961.

79 Enos, W. F., Holman, R. H., and Beyer, J.: Coronary Disease among United States Soldiers Killed in Action in Korea, *J.A.M.A.,* 152:1090, 1953.

80 McGee, D., and Gordon, T.: The Results of the Framingham Study Applied to Four Other U.S.-Based

Epidemiologic Studies of Cardiovascular Disease, in W. B. Kannel and T. Gordon (eds.), "The Framingham Study. An Epidemiologic Investigation of Cardiovascular Disease," DHEW Publication NIH-76-1083, Washington, 1976.

81 Salel, A. F., Fong, A., Zelis, R., Miller, R. R., Borhani, N. O., and Mason, D. T.: Accuracy of Numerical Coronary Profile. Correlation of Risk Factors with Arteriographically Documented Severity of Atherosclerosis, *N. Engl. J. Med.*, 296:1447, 1977.

82 "Multicentre Study of Risk Factors for Coronary Heart Disease," PMRC Monograph no. 3, Pakistan Medical Research Council, Karachi, Pakistan, 1980.

83 Jaffery, N. A., Mahmood, Z., and Zaidi, S. H. M.: Habits and Dietary Pattern of Cases (and Controls) of Carcinoma of the Oral Cavity and Oropharynx, *J.P.M.A.*, 27:340, 1977.

84 Mahmood, Z.: Smoking and Chewing Habits of People of Karachi, *J.P.M.A.*, 32:34, 1982.

85 Beg, M. A., Siddiqui, M. K., Abbasi, A. S., Raza, M., Masood, A., and Syed, S. A.: Coronary Heart Disease in Young Adults—A Comparative Study of Risk Factors between Pakistanis and Americans, *J.P.M.A.*, 20:251, 1970.

86 Usman, S., Haider, Z., Din, F. U., Zubair, M., and Khan, I. A.: Clinical and Biochemical Profile in 55 Male Patients of Coronary Heart Disease, *Pak. J. Med. Res.*, 18:9, 1979.

87 Ibrahim, S., Hashmi, J. A., and Syed, S. A.: Prevalence of Coronary Heart Disease in Patients Suffering from Diabetes Mellitus, *Pak. J. Med. Res.*, 14:45, 1975.

88 Haider, Z., and Obaidullah, S.: Clinical Diabetes Mellitus in Patients, *Pak. J. Med. Res.*, 20:1, 1981.

89 Abbasi, A. S., Raza, M., Beg. M. A., and Syed, S. A.: Coronary Heart Disease in Pakistan: Serum Cholesterol in Healthy Adults and Patients with Coronary Heart Disease, *J.P.M.A.*, 18:285, 1968.

90 Kannel, W. B., Castelli, W. P., and Gorden, T.: Cholesterol in the Prediction of Atherosclerotic Disease. New Perspectives Based on the Framingham Study, *Ann.Intern.Med.*, 90:85, 1979.

91 Rahman, M. A.: Lipoprotein Study in Pakistani Subjects by Paper Electrophoresis, *Pak.J.Med.Res.*, 5:335, 1966.

92 Knuiman, J. T., Hermus, J. J., Hautavast, J. G. A. J., and Ilyas, M.: International Collaborative Study on Total and HDL-Cholesterol In 7–9 Year Old School Boys, *Pak. Heart J.* 12:15, 1979.

93 Hashmi, J. A., Afroze, N., Bano, S., et al.: Pattern of Blood Lipids in Patients Suffering from Anemia, *J.P.M.A.*, 19:131, 1969.

94 Hashmi, J. A., Afroze, N., and Syed, S. A.: Blood Lipids in Anemia: An Experimental Study, *J.P.M.A.*, 20:293, 1970.

95 Shaper, A. G.: "Diet in the Epidemiology of Coronary Heart Disease," Proceedings of the Nutrition Society, vol. 31: 1972, p. 297.

96 "State Bank of Pakistan Annual Report," Karachi, Pakistan, 1980–1981.

97 Rahman, M. A., Khan, S. N., and Samad, A.: Serum Trace Elements in Patients with Ischemic Heart Disease, *Pak. Heart J.*, 12:21, 1979.

98 Beg, M. A., Siddiqui, M. K., Hashmi, J. A., et al.: Serum Uric Acid in Patients with Coronary Heart Disease, *J.P.M.A.*, 20:35, 1970.

99 Zafar, H. M., Ahmad, I., Mallick, G. Q., Chaudhry, M. A., and Khan, M. A.: The Incidence of Ischemic Heart Disease in Adults at Multan: A Comparative Study of Risk between Pakistanis and Americans, *Pak. Heart J.*, 8:4, 1975.

100 Ahmed, N.: Diagonal Earlobe Crease as a Coronary Risk Factor, *Pak. Heart J.*, 12:18, 1979.

101 Hashmi, J. A., Raza, M., Beg, M. A., Siddiqui, M. K., Afroze, N., and Syed, S. A.: Blood Coagulation Studies in Patients Suffering from Coronary Heart Diseases, *J.P.M.A.*, 19:8, 1969.

102 Hashmi, J. A., Afroze, N., Ibrahim, S., and Syed, S. A.: Blood Fibrinolytic Activity and Plasma Fibrinogen in Ischemic Heart Disease, *J.P.M.A.*, 20:135, 1971.

103 Khan, N., Wahidi, N., Aslam, S., Khan, A. H., Shareef, M., and Syed, S. A.: "Pattern of Admission in South Ward, NICVD" (proceedings 15th Annual Medical Symposium, Karachi, Pakistan, December 1977), JPMC Symposium Committee, Karachi, 1977.

104 Shareef, M., Zafar, S., Syed, S. A., Faruqui, A. M. A., and Wahidi, N.: "In-Hospital Complications of Acute Myocardial Infarction" (proceedings 16th Annual Medical Symposium, Karachi, Pakistan, 16–21 December 1978), JPMC Symposium Committee, Karachi, 1978.

105 Akhtar, A. H., Haque, M., Akhtar, S. A., Jaffery, S., and Mohydin, M. A. Z.: An Experience with 100 Cases of Coronary Heart Disease Treated in an Intensive Therapy Unit, *Pak. Heart J.*, 4:26, 1971.

106 Ilyas, M.: Use of Electroconvulsive Therapy Machine for Cardioversion, *J.P.M.A.*, 22:138, 1972.

107 Faruqui, A. M. A., Ahmed, A. S., and Syed, S. A.: "Treadmill Testing Two Weeks after Uncomplicated Myocardial Infarction" (proceedings of the 17th Annual Medical Symposium, Karachi, Pakistan, March 1980), JPMC Symposium Committee, Karachi, 1980.

108 Faruqui, A. M. A., Ahmed, I. S., and Syed, S. A.: Treadmill Testing Two Weeks after Myocardial Infarction: Comparison with Late Retesting, *Pak.Heart J.*, 13:3, 1980.

109 Faruqui, A. M. A., Ahmed, I. S., Shareef, M., and Syed, S. A.: "Serum Cholesterol Alterations in Acute Myocardial Infarction" (proceedings of the 4th All Pakistan Congress of Cardiology, Karachi, Pakistan, December 1979), Pakistan Cardiac Society, Karachi, 1979.

110 Haider, Z., and Zubair, M.: Variant Angina Pectoris (Prinzmetal Angina), *J.P.M.A.,* 25:308, 1975.

111 Faruqui, A. M. A.: "Acute Myocardial Infarction with Normal Coronary Arteries" (proceedings of the 17th Annual Medical Symposium, Karachi, Pakistan, March 1980), JPMC Symposium Committee, Karachi, 1980.

112 Shafqat, S. H., Haque, M., Rizwan, M., Sadiq, M., and Naheed, S.: Ischemic Heart Disease in Young Women, *Pak. Heart J.,* 12:26, 1979.

113 Hameedi, A. A., and Ali, S. M.: Cardiovascular Syphilis, *J.P.M.A.,* 15:499, 1964.

114 Rehman, S., and Ahmed, S.: Post Myocardial Infarction Syndrome, *Pak. Heart J.,* 1:80, 1968.

115 Qureshi, M. S.: Dressler's Syndrome, *Pak. Heart J.,* 5:24, 1972.

116 Shafqat, S. H., Hasan, I., and Samad, A.: "Systolic Murmur Following Acute Myocardial Infarction" (proceedings of the 15th Annual Medical Symposium, Karachi, Pakistan, December 1977), JPMC Symposium Committee, Karachi, 1977.

117 Raza, M., Ibrahim, S., and Syed, S. A.: "Pan" Angina, *J.P.M.A.,* 24:108, 1974.

118 Beg, M. A., Siddiqui, M. K., Abbasi, A. S., Ahmad, N., and Syed, S. A.: Atherosclerosis in Karachi. A Retrospective Study of Coronary Heart Disease in Cardiac Admissions, *J.P.M.A.,* 17:236, 1967.

119 Samad, A., Rehman, M., Kundi, A., and Syed, S. A.: "Early Onset Ischemic Heart Disease, Clinical and Angiographic Correlates" (proceedings of the 19th Annual Medical Symposium, Karachi, Pakistan, December 1981), JPMC Symposium Committee, Karachi, 1981.

120 Samad, A., Rehman, M., Kundi, A., Khakwani, A., and Syed, S. A.: Calcified Post Myocardial Infarction Left Ventricular Aneurysm in a Young Woman, *Pak.Heart J.,* 14:9, 1981.

121 Faruqui, A. M. A.: Coronary Arteriography and Coronary Artery Bypass Surgery, *Pak.Heart J.,* 13:31, 1980.

122 Hashmi, J. A.: Certain Anthropometic Features of Adult Pakistani Males, *J.P.M.A.,* 16:15, 1996.

123 Ahmed, N., Beg, M. A., Abbasi, A. S., and Syed, S. A.: Electrocardiogram in Healthy Individuals—A Study of 1832 Subjects, *J.P.M.A.,* 18:3, 1968.

124 Faruqui, A. M. A.: "Ventricular Tachycardia in 'Normal' Heart" (proceedings of the 5th All Pakistan Congress of Cardiology, Lahore, Pakistan, December 1981), Pakistan Cardiac Society, Lahore, 1981.

125 Samad, A., Hameedi, S. A., Shafqat, S. H., and Syed, S. A.: Isolated Idiopathic QT Interval Prolongation, *Pak. Heart J.,* 8:21, 1975.

126 Ilyas, M., Khan, S. M., Sherazi, S. M. H., Shah, M., and Hassan, A. U.: Cardio-Auditory Syndrome, *J.P.M.A.,* 30:159, 1980.

126a Samad, A., and Shareef, M.: "QT-Interval Prolongation and Ventricular Tachycardia with Prenylamine" (proceedings of the 14th Annual Medical Symposium, Karachi, Pakistan, December 1976), JPMC Symposium Committee, Karachi, 1976.

127 Robinson, R. D., Sultan, S., Abbasi, A. S., et al.: Acute Rheumatic Fever in Karachi, Pakistan, *Am.J.Cardiol.,* 18:548, 1966.

128 Rahimtoola, R. J., Shafqat, H., and Ramzan, A.: Acute Rheumatic Fever and Rheumatic Carditis in Children, *Pak.Heart J.,* 13:2, 1980.

129 DeSa, L. M., Abbasi, A. S., Billoo, A. G., Sultan, S., and Syed, S. A.: Streptococcal Throat Infection in Pediatrics Out-Patient Population, *Pak. J. Med. Res.,* 7:186, 1968.

130 Cherian, G., Krishnaswami, S., Sukumari, I. P., and John, S.: Variations in the Practice of Cardiology: Some Problems Encountered in India, in P. N. Yu and J. F. Goodwin (eds.), "Progress in Cardiology," Lea and Febiger, Philadelphia, 1980, p. 147.

131 Billoo, A. G., Abbasi, A. S., Sultana, S., DeSa, L., and Syed, S. A.: Prophylaxis against Recurrence of Rheumatic Fever, *Pak. Heart J.,* 1:8, 1968.

132 Bland, E. F.: Declining Severity of Rheumatic Fever, *N. Engl. J. Med.,* 262:598, 1960.

133 Samad, A.: Editorial, *Pak. Heart J.,* 12:1, 1979.

134 Syed, S. A., Abassi, A. S., Raza, M., et al.: "Studies in the Efficacy of Corrective Heart Surgery on Psychological, Social and Vocational Status of Patients with Rheumatic Heart Disease" (Project V.R.A. Pak 12-67), National Institute of Cardiovascular Diseases, Karachi, 1973.

135 Ahmad, F. S.: Pathology of Rheumatic Heart Disease, *Rawal Med. J.,* 6:713, 1975.

136 Samad, A., Rehman, M., Faruqui, A. M. A., and Syed, S. A.: "Pattern of Mitral Valve Leaflet Prolapse in Rheumatic Mitral Stenosis" (proceedings IX World Congress of Cardiology, Moscow, USSR, June 1982, abstract 475), International Society and Federation of Cardiology, Moscow, 1982.

137 Samad, A., Raja, K., Rehman, M., and Syed, S. A.: Effect of Sublingual Isordil on Hemodynamics of Rheumatic Valve Disease, *Pak. Heart J.,* 12:25, 1979.

138 Ilyas, M., and Haidry, J. G.: Juvenile Mitral Stenosis: A Pathogenic Puzzle, *J.P.M.A.,* 30:254, 1980.

139 Ansari, N. M.: Rheumatic Valvular Lesions in Children and Adolescents, *Pak. Heart J.,* 12:12, 1979.

140 Ahmad, M., Yusuf, A. R., and Khan, A. H.: Mitral Valvotomy, *Pak. J. Med. Res.,* 3:182, 1964.

141 Rehman, M., Samad, A., Mohsin, M., and Shareef, M.: Surgery for Rheumatic Heart Disease in Children and Adolescents, *Pak. Heart J.,* 12:24, 1979.

142 Kundi, A., Samad, A., and Shafqat, S. H.: "Mid-Systolic Click and Late Systolic Murmur (Barlow's) Syndrome" (proceedings of the 15th Annual Medical

Symposium, Karachi, Pakistan, December 1977), JPMC Symposium Committee, Karachi, 1977.

143 Faruqui, A. M. A., and Ahmad, I. S.: First Year of Echocardiography in Pakistan, *Pak. Heart J.*, 12:3, 1979.

144 Ahmed, I. S., Faruqui, A. M. A., and Syed, S. A.: Mitral Valve Prolapse Syndrome: Experience in Pakistan, *Pak. Heart J.*, 13:16, 1980.

145 Aziz, K. U.: Care of Heart Disease in Children, *Pak.J.Med. Res.*, 11:9, 1972.

146 Rahimtoola, R. J., Majid, I., Shafqat, H., and Gureshi, A. F.: Congenital Heart Disease in Children Visiting JPMC, *Pak. Heart J.*, 13:21, 1980.

147 Aziz, K. U.: Statistics of the Congenital Heart Disease Workup clinic at the National Institute of Cardiovascular Diseases, October 1980 to October 1981, unpublished data, Karachi.

148 Shafqat, S. H., and Tahira, I.: A Study of Congenital Heart Disease in Karachi, *Pak. Heart J.*, 11:7, 1978.

149 Kassim, A. M., Hameedi, A. A., Shareef, M., and Khan, A. H.: A Study of Congenital Heart Disease, *J.P.M.A.*, 19:695, 1964.

150 Samad, A., Rehman, M., and Syed, S. A.: Aneurysm of the Sinus of Valsalva, *Pak. Heart J.*, 13:3, 1980.

151 Sharma, S., Munsi, S. C., Katdare, A. D., Thawani, A., and Parulkar, G. B.: Isolated Critical Pulmonary Valve Stenosis—A Need for Further Classification, *Indian Heart J.*, 33:169, 1981.

152 Faruqui, A. M. A., Ahmed, I. S., and Syed, S. A.: "Apparent Aorto-Mitral Non-Continuity" (proceedings IX World Congress of Cardiology, Moscow, USSR, June 1982, abstract 0073), International Society and Federation of Cardiology, Moscow, 1982.

153 Malik, S. M.: "Peripartal Cardiomyopathy" (proceedings of the 19th Annual Medical Symposium, December 1981), JPMC Symposium Committee, Karachi, 1981.

154 Ahmed, I. S., Faruqui, A. M. A., and Syed, S. A.: Hypertrophic Cardiomyopathy: Experience in Pakistan, *Pak. Heart J.*, 13:30, 1980.

155 Waiz, A.: Tropical Eosinophilia, *Pak. Armed Forces Med. J.*, 17:22, 1967.

155a Khan, N.: Tropical Eosinophilia, *Pak.J.Med. Res.*, 1:30, 1958.

156 Ahmed, F. S.: Cardiopathies of Obscure Origin: A Necropsy Study, *Pak. Heart J.*, 4:5, 1971.

157 Yusuf, A. R., and Khan, A. H.: Constrictive Pericarditis, *Pak. J. Med. Res.*, 3:267, 1964.

158 Ansari, N. M. A.: Chronic Constrictive Pericarditis, *Pak. Heart J.*, 11:4, 1978.

159 Hassan, Z. U., Bowes, D. E., and Walford, R.: The Diagnosis and Management of Constrictive Pericarditis, *Pak. Heart J.*, 5:19, 1972.

160 Kaleta, J.: Tuberculosis in the World and in Pakistan, *Med. Gaz.*, April 15, 1982.

161 Samad, A., Jatoi, A. G., and Aleem, N.: Left Atrial Enlargement in Chronic Constrictive Pericarditis: Clinical Implications, *Pak. Heart J.*, 11:18, 1978.

162 Khan, Z. A.: "Constrictive Pericarditis" (proceedings of the 5th All Pakistan Congress of Cardiology, December 1981), Pakistan Cardiac Society, Karachi, 1981.

163 Rab, S. M., Noor, M., and Yee, A.: The Changing Etiology of Constrictive Pericarditis, *Pak.Heart J.*, 2:21, 1969.

164 Samad, A., Faruqui, A. M. A., Rehman, M., and Syed, S. A.: Aortic Dissection, *Pak. Heart J.*, 14:2, 1982.

165 Samad, A., and Rehman, M.: "Pulmonary Hypertension: Etiology and Clinical Implications" (proceedings of the 16th Annual Medical Symposium, December 1978), JPMC Symposium Committee, Karachi, 1978.

166 Ilyas, M., Peracha, M. A., Ahmad, R., Samad, A., Kabir, M., and Ahmed, F. S.: Left Atrial Myxoma—Case Report, *J.P.M.A.*, 24:206, 1974.

167 Faruqui, A. M. A., Syed, S. A., and Shareef, M.: Right Atrial Myxoma, *Pak. Heart J.*, 13:24, 1980.

168 Kiani, M. U. R.: "Atrial Myxomas" (proceedings of the 5th All Pakistan Congress of Cardiology, December 1981), Pakistan Cardiac Society, Karachi, 1981.

Clinical Essays on The Heart

Volume 2

Clinical Essays on The Heart

Volume 2

Edited by

J. Willis Hurst, M.D.

Candler Professor of Medicine (Cardiology)
Chairman, Department of Medicine
Emory University School of Medicine

Chief of Medicine, Emory University Hospital

Chief of Medicine, Grady Memorial Hospital

Head, Medical Section
Emory University Clinic
Atlanta, Georgia

McGraw-Hill Book Company

New York St. Louis San Francisco Auckland Bogotá Guatemala Hamburg
Johannesburg Lisbon London Madrid Mexico Montreal New Delhi
Panama Paris San Juan São Paulo Singapore Sydney Tokyo Toronto

NOTICE

Medicine is an ever-changing science. As new research and clinical experience broaden our knowledge, changes in treatment and drug therapy are required. The editors and the publisher of this work have made every effort to ensure that the drug dosage schedules herein are accurate and in accord with the standards accepted at the time of publication. Readers are advised, however, to check the product information sheet included in the package of each drug they plan to administer to be certain that changes have not been made in the recommended dose or in the contraindications for administration. This recommendation is of particular importance in regard to new or infrequently used drugs.

To N.W.H. with love

J.W.H.

Contents

List of Contributors

Ralph Berg, Jr., M.D.
Department of Cardiothoracic Surgery, Deaconess and Sacred Heart Medical Centers, Spokane, Washington

Eugene H. Blackstone, M.D.
Cardiovascular Research Professor of Surgery, University of Alabama in Birmingham, School of Medicine and Medical Center, Birmingham, Alabama

James H. Chesebro, M.D.
Associate Professor of Medicine, Consultant in Internal Medicine, Mayo Medical School, Rochester, Minnesota

Lawrence H. Cohn, M.D.
Professor of Surgery, Harvard Medical School; Division of Thoracic & Cardiovascular Surgery, Brigham and Women's Hospital, Boston, Massachusetts

John J. Collins, Jr., M.D.
Professor of Surgery, Harvard Medical School; Chief, Division of Thoracic & Cardiac Surgery, Brigham and Women's Hospital, Boston, Massachusetts

C. Richard Conti, M.D.
Professor of Medicine and Chief, Division of Cardiology, University of Florida, College of Medicine, Gainesville, Florida

Denton A. Cooley, M.D.
Surgeon-in-Chief, Clinical Assistant Professor of Surgery, Texas Heart Institute of St. Luke's Episcopal and Texas Children's Hospitals and The University of Texas Health Science Center, Houston, Texas

Delos M. Cosgrove, M.D.
Surgeon, Department of Thoracic and Cardiovascular Surgery, The Cleveland Clinic Foundation, Cleveland, Ohio

Joe M. Craver, M.D.
Associate Professor of Surgery (Cardiovascular and Thoracic), Department of Surgery, Emory University School of Medicine, Atlanta, Georgia

Gordon K. Danielson, M.D.
Professor of Surgery, Mayo Medical School, Rochester, Minnesota

Michael E. DeBakey, M.D.
Chancellor, Olga Keith Wiess Professor of Surgery and Chairman, Cora and Webb Mading Department of Surgery, Baylor College of Medicine, Houston, Texas

Giacomo A. DeLaria, M.D.
Assistant Professor of Surgery, Rush Medical College, Chicago, Illinois

Marcus A. DeWood, M.D.
Director, Cardiovascular Research, Deaconess and Sacred Heart Medical Centers, Spokane, Washington

John S. Douglas, Jr., M.D.
Associate Professor of Medicine (Cardiology), Assistant Professor of Radiology, Emory University School of Medicine, Atlanta, Georgia

J. Michael Duncan, M.D.
Associate Surgeon, Clinical Assistant Professor of Surgery, Texas Heart Institute of St. Luke's Episcopal and Texas Children's Hospitals and The University of Texas Health Science Center, Houston, Texas

Paul A. Ebert, M.D.
Professor of Surgery, Chairman, Department of Surgery, University of California, San Francisco, San Francisco, California

Gray Ellrodt, M.D.
Assistant Professor of Medicine, University of California at Los Angeles School of Medicine, Director of Medical Intensive Care Unit, Cedars-Sinai Medical Center, Los Angeles, California

René G. Favaloro, M.D.
Head, Institute of Cardiology and Cardiovascular Surgery at the Guemes Hospital; Professor of Cardiac Surgery at El Salvador University School of Medicine, Buenos Aires, Argentina

Robert L. Feldman, M.D.
Assistant Professor of Medicine, Division of Cardiology, University of Florida, College of Medicine, Gainesville, Florida

William H. Frishman, M.D.
Associate Professor of Medicine, Albert Einstein College of Medicine; Chief, Department of Medicine, Hospital of the Albert Einstein College of Medicine, Bronx, New York

Carl C. Gill, M.D.
Surgeon, Department of Thoracic and Cardiovascular Surgery, The Cleveland Clinic Foundation, Cleveland, Ohio

Leonard A. R. Golding, M.D.
Surgeon, Department of Thoracic and Cardiovascular Surgery, The Cleveland Clinic Foundation, Cleveland, Ohio

Andreas R. Gruentzig, M.D.
Professor of Medicine (Cardiology) and Radiology; Director, Interventional Medicine, Emory University School of Medicine and Emory University Hospital, Atlanta, Georgia

Charles R. Hatcher, Jr., M.D.
Professor of Surgery (Thoracic and Cardiovascular); Chief of Division of Thoracic and Cardiovascular Surgery, Emory University School of Medicine; Acting Director, Woodruff Medical Center; Director, Emory University Clinic, Atlanta, Georgia

Lloyd L. Hefner, M.D.
Professor of Medicine, Physiology and Biophysics, University of Alabama in Birmingham, School of Medicine and Medical Center, Birmingham, Alabama

Jay Hollman, M.D.
Former Fellow in Medicine (Cardiology), Department of Medicine, Emory University School of Medicine, Atlanta, Georgia, currently staff member, Cleveland Clinic Foundation, Cleveland, Ohio

J. Willis Hurst, M.D.
Candler Professor of Medicine (Cardiology), Chairman of the Department of Medicine, Emory University School of Medicine; Chief of Medicine and Cardiology, Emory University Hospital; Chief of Medicine Grady Memorial Hospital; Chief of the Medical Section Emory University Clinic, Atlanta, Georgia

Douglas D. Johnson, M.D.
Cardiac Surgeon, Northwest Cardiac Surgery Associates; Clinical Assistant Professor of Surgery, University of Washington, Seattle, Washington

Ellis L. Jones, M.D.
Associate Professor of Surgery (Cardiovascular and Thoracic), Department of Surgery, Emory University School of Medicine, Atlanta, Georgia

Robert B. Karp, M.D.
Professor of Surgery, University of Alabama in Birmingham, School of Medicine and Medical Center, Birmingham, Alabama

Siavosh Khonsari, M.B., B.Ch.
Associate Professor of Cardiopulmonary Surgery, Oregon Health Sciences University; Chief, Cardiopulmonary Surgery, Veterans Administration Hospital, Portland, Oregon

Spencer B. King, III, M.D.
Professor of Medicine (Cardiology) and Radiology, Emory University School of Medicine; Director, Cardiac Catheterization Laboratory, Emory University Hospital, Atlanta, Georgia

James K. Kirklin, M.D.
Assistant Professor of Surgery, University of Alabama in Birmingham, School of Medicine and Medical Center, Birmingham, Alabama

John W. Kirklin, M.D.
Fay Fletcher Kerner Professor of Surgery, Director, Division of Cardiothoracic Surgery, University of Alabama in Birmingham, School of Medicine, Birmingham, Alabama

Gerald M. Lawrie, M.D.
Associate Professor of Surgery, Cora and Webb Mading Department of Surgery, Baylor College of Medicine, Houston, Texas

William A. Lell, M.D.
Professor and Vice Chairman, Department of Anesthesiology; Director, Cardiovascular Anesthesia Division, University of Alabama in Birmingham, School of Medicine and Medical Center, Birmingham, Alabama

Floyd D. Loop, M.D.
Chairman, Department of Thoracic and Cardiovascular Surgery, The Cleveland Clinic Foundation, Cleveland, Ohio

Bruce W. Lytle, M.D.
Surgeon, Department of Thoracic and Cardiovascular Surgery, The Cleveland Clinic Foundation, Cleveland, Ohio

D. Craig Miller, M.D.
Assistant Professor of Cardiovascular Surgery, Stanford University School of Medicine, Stanford, California

Donald W. Miller, Jr., M.D.
Cardiac Surgeon, Northwest Cardiac Surgery Associates; Clinical Associate Professor of Surgery, University of Washington, Seattle, Washington

Koonlawee Nademanee, M.D.
Assistant Professor of Medicine, University of California at Los Angeles School of Medicine; Director of Coronary Care Unit, Wadsworth Veterans Administration Medical Center, Los Angeles, California

Hassan Najafi, M.D.
Professor and Chairman, Department of Cardiovascular-Thoracic Surgery, Rush Medical College, Chicago, Illinois

Thomas A. Orszulak, M.D.
Instructor in Surgery, Mayo Medical School, Rochester, Minnesota

Albert D. Pacifico, M.D.
Professor of Surgery, University of Alabama in Birmingham, School of Medicine and Medical Center, Birmingham, Alabama

Jeffrey M. Piehler, M.D.
Instructor in Surgery, Mayo Medical School, Rochester, Minnesota

James. R. Pluth, M.D.
Professor of Surgery, Mayo Medical School, Rochester, Minnesota

Francisco J. Puga, M.D.
Assistant Professor of Surgery, Mayo Medical School, Rochester, Minnesota

William J. Rogers, M.D.
Associate Professor of Medicine, University of Alabama in Birmingham, School of Medicine and Medical Center, Birmingham, Alabama

Hartzell V. Schaff, M.D.
Assistant Professor of Surgery, Mayo Medical School, Rochester, Minnesota

Richard J. Shemin, M.D.
Assistant Professor of Surgery, Harvard Medical School; Division of Thoracic and Cardiac Surgery, Brigham and Women's Hospital, Boston, Massachusetts

Norman E. Shumway, M.D.
Chairman and Frances and Charles Field Professor of Cardiovascular Surgery, Stanford University School of Medicine, Stanford, California

Bramah N. Singh, M.D., D. Phil.
Professor of Medicine, University of California at Los Angeles School of Medicine; Director of Cardiovascular Research Laboratory, Wadsworth Veterans Administration Medical Center, Los Angeles, California

Albert Starr, M.D.
Professor and Chief, Division of Cardiopulmonary Surgery, Oregon Health Sciences University, Portland, Oregon

Robert W. Stewart, M.D.
Surgeon, Department of Thoracic and Cardiovascular Surgery, The Cleveland Clinic Foundation, Cleveland, Ohio

Edward B. Stinson, M.D.
Thelma and Henry Doelger Professor of Cardiovascular Surgery, Stanford University School of Medicine, Stanford, California

Paul C. Taylor, M.D.
Surgeon, Department of Thoracic and Cardiovascular Surgery, The Cleveland Clinic Foundation, Cleveland, Ohio

Daniel J. Ullyot, M.D.
Professor of Surgery, Associate Director, Cardiothoracic Surgery, Department of Surgery, University of California, San Francisco, San Francisco, California

Nanette K. Wenger, M.D.
Professor of Medicine (Cardiology), Emory University School of Medicine; Director, Cardiac Clinics, Grady Memorial Hospital, Atlanta, Georgia

George L. Zorn, Jr., M.D.
Associate Professor of Surgery, University of Alabama in Birmingham, School of Medicine and Medical Center, Birmingham, Alabama

The theme of this issue of *Clinical Essays on The Heart* is "The Treatment of Atherosclerotic Coronary Heart Disease." Coronary disease continues to be the most common type of heart disease, and more people die of it than any other disease. We have made some progress in preventing it, but the disease continues to be a major health problem. The prevalence and seriousness of the disease justify a book on its treatment.

The book is divided into the following parts:
- New drugs used in the treatment of atherosclerotic coronary heart disease
- Coronary bypass surgery in the treatment of atherosclerotic coronary heart disease
- Coronary angioplasty in the treatment of atherosclerotic coronary heart disease
- Rehabilitation of patients with atherosclerotic coronary heart disease

I selected authors who are expert in their field and requested that they, whenever possible, describe their own experience in the treatment of atherosclerotic coronary heart disease.

The authors writing on the use of drugs reported their views—not as pharmacologists but as physicians who know the importance of drugs. The cardiac surgeons reported the results of their *total* experience.

It is unlikely that this bench mark (total experience) will be reported in a single book in this way again. Accordingly, I believe this issue of *Essays* will be used as a reference book for many years to come. I regret that several surgeons could not contribute because of other commitments.

Andreas Gruentzig joined the Department of Medicine of Emory University School of Medicine in 1980. He not only developed the technique of coronary angioplasty but has done more balloon dilatations than anyone. Accordingly, he, Jay Hollman, and other colleagues were asked to write a complete treatise on the subject of coronary angioplasty. This could not be published in a journal or a standard textbook and shows the value of the *essay* type of book. The article on angioplasty will become the source where others look for details that cannot be easily found elsewhere.

Although all patients with atherosclerotic coronary heart disease do not need a formal rehabilitation program, some patients do. Accordingly, the last part of this book deals with rehabilitation.

The title of this series of books, *Clinical Essays on The Heart*, was chosen after a great deal of thought and after discarding the title *Updates on The Heart*. An *essay* gives an author more freedom than is possible in a scientific journal or standard textbook. It is my hope that the essays in this issue of *Clinical Essays on The Heart* will be valuable to practicing physicians and surgeons.

I wish to thank Carol Miller who takes my scribbles and translates them into much prettier type. I thank Robert McGraw, Joseph Brehm, Donna McIvor, Paulette Williams, and Deborah Sheridan of McGraw-Hill publishers for their superb help and sustained interest.

I thank my wife Nelie. No Nelie—no book.

J. Willis Hurst, M.D.

PART I

New Drugs Used in the Treatment of Atherosclerotic Coronary Heart Disease

The Use of Nitrates in the Treatment of Ischemic Heart Disease[*]

C. RICHARD CONTI, M.D., and
ROBERT L. FELDMAN, M.D.

In the recent past, only glycerol trinitrate in its sublingual form was considered to be effective therapy for patients with myocardial ischemia. Subsequently the use of all forms of nitrates has increased tremendously.

The clinician has been overwhelmed by the increasing number of nitrate preparations as well as the expanded use of these preparations for prophylaxis and treatment of both myocardial ischemia and congestive heart failure.

The purpose of this chapter is to review extensively what is known about these widely used therapeutic substances in order to provide the practitioner with a thorough understanding of the uses and limitations of nitrates.

AVAILABLE PREPARATIONS, PHARMACOKINETICS, AND DOSES

T. Lauder Brunton appears to have been the first physician to use nitrates to relieve angina pain. In 1857, Brunton administered amyl nitrite to a patient with angina pectoris by inhalation; he noted a rapid relief of the patient's angina. In 1879, William Murrell noted that the physiological action on blood pressure and heart rate of amyl nitrite was mimicked by sublingual glycerol trinitrate. He was perhaps the first physician to establish the routine use of the drug for relief of angina and as a prophylactic agent to be taken prior to exercise. Since then several other organic nitrates have been found to be potent vasodilators. In common with one another they contain polyol esters of nitric acid. Except for amyl nitrite, which is a nitrite ester, the presently available compounds useful in clinical practice are organic nitrates. The use of the term *nitroglycerin* is incorrect in this context, since nitrates are not "nitro compounds." Nitro compounds are not vasodilators. However, glycerol trinitrate is so commonly referred to as nitroglycerin or trinitroglycerin that this name has become accepted over the years. In this chapter the abbreviation GTN will be used instead of glycerol trinitrate.

Amyl Nitrite

Amyl nitrite is available for administration by inhalation in two different doses. Although amyl nitrite has been found to relieve acute angina episodes, its duration of action is brief and side effects are common. Thus, it is rarely used at present in the treatment of angina. Its most frequent use is as a provocative agent to aid in the diagnosis of hypertrophic cardiomyopathy.

Nitrates

There are several different nitrate compounds available to practitioners in the United States for use in the treatment and prophylaxis of angina episodes. These nitrate compounds are available in numerous preparations for administration by different routes (Table 1). Glycerol trinitrate is available in several formulations.

Glycerol Trinitrate (GTN)

PARENTERAL GTN

Glycerol trinitrate for parenteral use has recently been approved by the Food and Drug Administration and is available from several manufacturers. It has become clear that the handling and storage of parenteral GTN is extremely important. In contrast to nitroprusside, GTN (parenteral) is not inactivated by room or fluorescent light.[1] Glycerol trinitrate stored in glass containers has been stable in normal saline or 5% dextrose solutions (D5W) for periods greater than 48 h at temperatures between 4 and 40°C.[1] When stored in plastic bags, however, the potency of a GTN solution decreases rapidly and is affected by temperature and by the bag volume.[1,2] Thus, if stored in a plastic bag at 4°C for 24 h, approximately 75 percent of the GTN remains in solution, and at 48 h 60 percent remains in solution. The remaining GTN has been absorbed by the plastic. At room temperature this absorption by plastic is enhanced so that at 24 h approximately 50 percent of the GTN has been absorbed, and only 40 percent remains in solution at 48 h. At higher temperatures the absorption is accelerated further as parti-

[*]From the Department of Medicine, Division of Cardiology, University of Florida College of Medicine, Gainesville, Florida.

TABLE 1
Organic nitrates available for clinical use

Generic name	Chemical structure	Preparation	Dose	Trade name	Dosing frequency
Amyl nitrite	H_3C—CHCH$_2$CH$_2$ONO / H_3C	Inhalation	0.18 or 0.3 mL	Vaporale	
Glycerol trinitrate	H_2C—O—NO_2 / HC—O—NO_2 / H_2C—O—NO_2	Parenteral	50–100 μg/mL	Nitro-bid IV, Nitroglycerin injection, Nitrostat IV, Tridil	2–4 min (half-life)
		Sublingual	0.15,0.3,0.4,0.6 mg	USP, Nitro-bid, Nitrol, Nitrostat	5–30 min
		Buccal	1,2,5 mg	Susadrin	4–6 h
		Oral	1.3,2.5,6.5,9.0 mg	Nitro-bid, Nitrong, Nitroglycerin Capsules, Nitrospan	4–8 h
		Topical	2% over 5,8,10,15,20 cm^2	Nitro-bid, Nitrol, and Nitrong ointment	4–5 h
				Nitro-disc, Nitro-dur, Transderm-nitro	24–48 h
Isosorbide dinitrate		Sublingual	2.5,5 mg	USP, Dilatrate, Iso-bid, Isordil, Laserdil, Sorbide, Sorbitrate	30–60 min
		Chewable	5,10 mg		30–180 min
		Oral	5,10,20,40 mg		2–6 h
Erythrityl tetranitrate	H_2C—O—NO_2 / HC—O—NO_2 / HC—O—NO_2 / H_2C—O—NO_2	Sublingual	5,10,15 mg	USP, Cardilate	30–60 min
		Oral	10 mg		2–6 h
Pentaerythritol tetranitrate		Oral	10,20,30,40,60 mg	USP, Duotrate, Pentritol, Peritrate	4–6 h

tioning between the plastic and the solution is faster. The rate of loss of GTN to plastic is greater when dissolved in D5W than in normal saline and is greater if the plastic bag volume is smaller rather than larger. This latter fact is due to the contact area per unit volume being much greater in small as compared to large plastic bags; therefore, a more rapid partitioning of GTN to the plastic occurs. Other important factors are the infusion set used between the intravenous container and the patient and the rate of infusion. Commercial infusion sets usually contain polyvinyl chloride, and GTN is lost into this tubing. Although for clinical purposes equilibrium between the solution and tubing probably occurs within several hours, the precise dosage administered to the patient may not be constant even after infusions as long as 24 h. The actual dose of GTN reaching the patient is not only related to the length of time the GTN solution has been exposed to the intravenous tubing but also related to the flow rate.[1] Unfortunately, the effect of flow rate on the amount of GTN delivered to the patient is not linear. At low flow rates, such as 0.5 mL/min, between 50 and 75 percent of the GTN in solution can be absorbed by the intravenous tubing. At slightly faster flow rates, such as 1 mL/min, between 25 and 50 percent of the GTN will be absorbed by the IV tubing, and at a faster rate, such as 2 mL/min, 25 to 30 percent of the administered GTN is absorbed. In addition to the type of tubing and the rate of administration, the length of the intravenous tubing between the glass bottle and the patient is also of importance. All these factors produce the potential for small changes in the concentration of GTN over time.

Before being mixed with either normal saline or D5W, GTN for parenteral use is stored in glass ampules. Depending on the manufacturer, the undiluted GTN also contains various solvents and diluents. These include propylene glycol, ethanol, lactose, and citrate in several concentrations and combinations. These additional substances do not appear to have any clinically important effect when GTN is administered intravenously. We have also not found any detrimental effects when administering parenteral GTN containing small quantities of ethanol and propylene glycol directly into a coronary artery.[3,4] When used intravenously the usual starting dose of nitroglycerin should be approximately 10 μg/min. However, as discussed above, the actual amount of GTN to reach the patient may differ depending on temperature, infusion rates, tubing, etc. This estimated dose of GTN can be increased by either doubling or increasing the dose by 10-μg increments, depending upon the physiological response in individual situations, until the desired effect is seen. The usual dosage of GTN necessary to produce a "clinical effect" varies between 10 and 200 μg/min. However, 20 to 30 percent of patients require much larger doses of GTN. One must remember, however, that because of absorption by the infusion apparatus, only a percentage of the calculated dose of GTN may actually reach the patient. This dose may change over time, and patients need to be monitored continuously.

Parenteral GTN has clinical applicability when given by the intracoronary route during diagnostic cardiac catheterization.[3,4] It can be used to diagnose and relieve coronary artery spasm and to prevent coronary spasm during intervention procedures such as intracoronary streptokinase infusion or percutaneous transluminal coronary angioplasty. It produces a slightly greater dilation of epicardial coronary arteries than does sublingual GTN.[4–7] When administered in this fashion, doses as small as 5 μg produce considerable coronary dilation (Fig. 1). The magnitude of dilation seen with this small dose is approximately 66 percent of maximal dilation. Doses of 50 μg or less administered into the coronary artery produce coronary dilation but no important systemic hemodynamic effects. Maximal coronary dilation occurs with doses between 100 and 200 μg administered directly into the coronary artery. To relieve coronary artery spasm, doses between 50 and 100 μg are sufficient in the usual case. The duration of the physiological effect of intracoronary GTN is unknown. In several cases of patients with coronary artery spasm given a single dose of intracoronary GTN, spasm has recurred 10 to 15 min later (Fig. 2). This may reflect the physiological half-life of the drug.

NONPARENTERAL GLYCEROL TRINITRATE

Sublingual GTN Nonparenteral nitrate administration has been the mainstay of antiangina treatment for years. For acute relief of an angina episode sublingual GTN has been the drug treatment of choice for over 100 years. Other nitrate preparations, such as isosorbide dinitrate and erythrityl tetranitrate, are also available for administration by the sublingual route. Their onset of action appears to be delayed in comparison with sublingual GTN, and it is not clear that their duration of action is longer. Thus, there is little reason to recommend their use for most patients. Sublingual GTN tablets are available in dosages from 0.15 to 0.6 mg. Once a bottle is opened, the potency of the tablet diminishes slowly over time. In order to ensure potency open bottles should be kept only 30 to 60 days. If no local burning or tingling sensation is noted under the tongue with administration of sublingual GTN, the potency of the tablets should be questioned. After administration of a sublingual GTN tablet (0.6 mg) investigators have found peak plasma levels averaging between 1.5 and 2.5 ng/mL.[8–10] With serial measurements of plasma GTN, levels are measurable by 30 s in many patients. Peak plasma levels occur between 2 and 5 min after GTN administration. The half-life of GTN after sublingual administration is approximately 5 min. By 20 to 30 min after sublingual administration of GTN very little of the drug can be measured in the plasma. These plasma level determinations correlate nicely with physiological changes in measurements of heart rate, blood pressure, and left ventricular dimension (echocardiography).[10] The effect of GTN on these physiological variables peaks between 2 and 5 min and then diminishes slowly over the next 5 to 10 min. By 20 to 30 min after GTN administration no important physiological effects can usually be detected.

The most commonly used sublingual GTN dose is 0.4 mg. This is appropriate for the majority of patients as important side effects or inability to abort an angina episode are uncommon with this dose. Lower dosages are useful in patients with side effects such as headache or hypotension after the 0.4-mg dose. Either 0.15 or 0.3 mg of GTN may be used in these patients and are usually effective in relieving angina episodes. Although these dosages are not usually used, it is possible that they could be effective in relieving angina in the vast majority of patients who are now routinely given 0.4-mg tablets. In occasional patients the 0.4-mg dosage does not seem to be sufficient to relieve angina, and multiple tablets are necessary. In these patients a

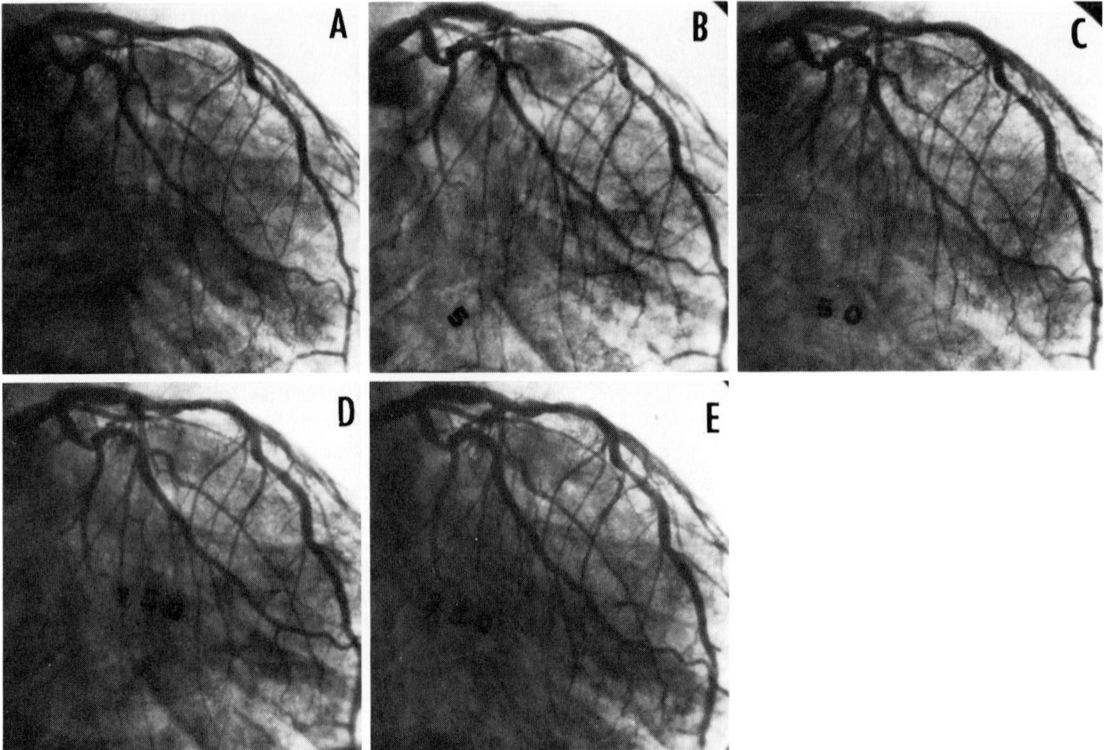

FIGURE 1 Angiographic sequence showing changes in coronary diameter after increasing doses of intracoronary nitroglycerin. Compared to the control angiogram *(A)* coronary artery dilation was apparent after 5 µg *(B)*. Further coronary artery dilation occurred after 50 µg *(C)*. After the 150- *(D)* and 250-µg *(E)* doses little further change in coronary diameters was apparent. *(From R. L. Feldman, J. D. Marx, C. J. Pepine, and R. C. Conti, Analysis of Coronary Responses to Various Doses of Intracoronary Nitroglycerin, Circulation, 66(suppl. 2):321, 1982. Used with permission.)*

0.6-mg tablet may be preferable. After sublingual GTN the interpatient variability of plasma nitroglycerin concentration is large. Whether patients who require different GTN dosages to relieve angina have similar plasma levels at the time angina is relieved is unclear.[8] It may be that some patients are able to achieve a peak GTN plasma level of approximately 2 ng/mL with low-dose GTN while others need a higher dose to achieve similar plasma concentrations. Any interpatient variability between changes in physiological parameters and plasma levels has not been studied in detail.

Buccal GTN   Recently, buccal lozenges of GTN have become available. GTN is stored in a matrix for sustained release, and physiological effects for up to 6 h have been documented.[11] They may also be used by many patients to abort acute angina episodes. Their precise role in antiangina therapy has yet to be determined. This mode of administration seems to be helpful in most patients who respond to other forms of long-acting nitrates. Most patients find the tablets unobtrusive, tasteless, and acceptable for either prophylactic

use before activity or continuous use throughout the day. Although eating with the lozenge in place is potentially a problem, patients have usually not complained of this. However, other patients with dentures often find the lozenge uncomfortable.

Oral nitrate preparations   Oral nitrates for long-term prophylaxis or continuous use are available with various preparations including GTN, isosorbide dinitrate, erythrityl tetranitrate, and pentaerythritol tetranitrate. Although for years there was controversy about the potential effectiveness of these compounds, the recent use of large doses has demonstrated beyond doubt clinical effectiveness.[12-20] Previously, when smaller doses of these compounds were used, physiological effects and blood levels of active drug could not be measured.[14-17] This led some physicians to question effectiveness of oral nitrates and their place in clinical practice. In the past several years multiple studies using larger dosages of each of these long-acting compounds have demonstrated persistent physiologic effects such as decreased blood pressure and left ven-

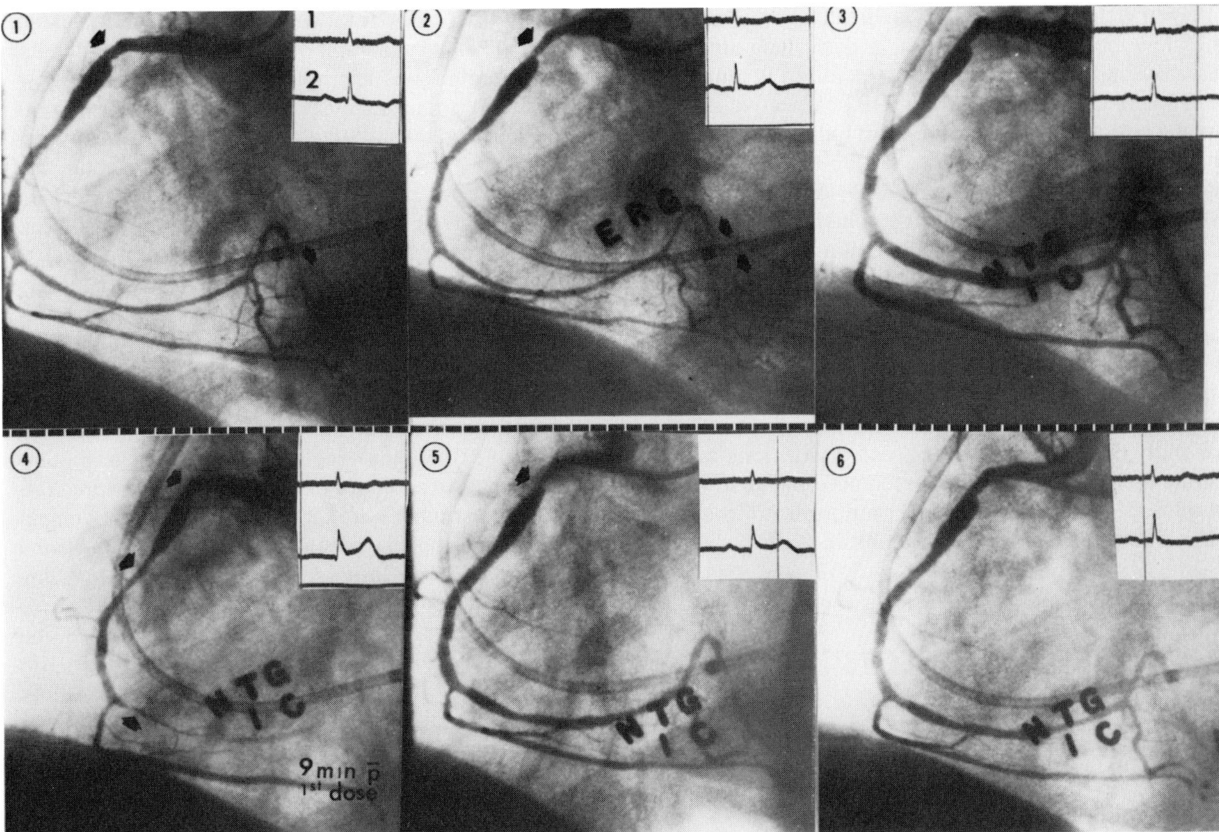

FIGURE 2 Angiographic and electrocardiographic sequence showing changes in coronary artery diameter during a sequence of spontaneous and ergonovine-induced episodes of angina and relief of angina after nitroglycerin and nifedipine. Panel 1 demonstrates the control right coronary artery angiogram showing stenoses in the proximal and distal portion of the right coronary artery (arrows) and electrocardiographic leads I and II. During ergonovine-induced chest discomfort (panel 2) further narrowing is noted in the proximal coronary stenosis and more severe narrowing in the distal coronary artery (arrows). Electrocardiographic lead II now shows mild ST-segment elevation. In panel 3, following the administration of 50 μg of intracoronary nitroglycerin, the electrocardiogram has returned toward base line, and coronary artery dilation is noticed both proximally and distally. Panel 4 was obtained 9 min after the first dose of intracoronary nitroglycerin; it shows severe narrowing in the proximal, mid, and distal portion of the right coronary artery with no contrast material filling the most distal portion (arrows). Marked ST-segment elevation is noted in electrocardiographic lead II. Panel 5 demonstrates some resolution of coronary spasm following further intracoronary GTN (100 μg) but persistent ST-segment elevation in lead II and severe stenosis in the proximal and distal portions of the right coronary artery. In panel 6 following further intracoronary GTN (100 μg) and buccal nifedipine (10 mg), the electrocardiogram and angiographic changes have returned toward the control.

tricular dimension by echocardiographic analysis and prolongation of exercise duration. Some studies have also documented persistence of the active drug in plasma for many hours.

Transdermal GTN   The transcutaneous administration of GTN has become popular in the past several years.[15,16,21–24] Only an occasional patient develops skin irritations to either the ointment, patch, or adhesive used to deliver the GTN through to the skin.[25] Plasma levels obtained with the 2% GTN ointment applied at doses from 1 to 3 in. several times daily have been shown to be comparable to those achieved after sub-lingual and intravenous GTN administration.[8] Plasma levels obtained after the new "patch" delivery systems appear to be lower than those obtained in most cases by ointment or sublingual administration. One problem many physicians and patients have had with GTN ointment has been its messy nature. This had made the product unacceptable for some patients and stimulated development of the new patches. To use GTN ointment appropriately the medication needs to be spread over a suitable area for absorption, as its physiologic effects are directly related to both the amount applied and the surface area to which it is applied. Carelessly applied GTN ointment is only poorly absorbed, and is less likely to yield acceptable clinical results. In this regard, the new patches are simpler and provide uniform interpatient dosing as patient cooperation is minimal.

Topical GTN has been found to be effective in producing effects in patients with heart failure, myocardial infarction, and chronic angina for up to 6 h when administered as an ointment and 24 to 48 h when administered through the new patch systems. Important clinical differences have not been demonstrated between the three different commercial brands of GTN patches.

A clinical comparison of long-acting buccal, oral, and topical nitrates has not been done. However, there is no reason to expect major differences between preparations as long as a sufficient dosage of each is administered to produce similar physiologic effects. Thus, for individual patients being treated with long-acting nitrate preparations, patient preference relative to route of administration and daily cost are probably the two most important variables to be considered.

PHYSIOLOGICAL EFFECTS OF NITRATES

Physiological responses to nitrates are multiple.[14–16,26] These physiological effects can be divided into direct coronary and noncoronary, or systemic, effects. The relative portion of coronary and noncoronary effects seen with the different nitrate preparations appears related both to the dose of drug and to the manner in which the drug is administered. These differential responses will be discussed in detail in the section dealing with potential mechanisms of action of the nitrates.

Coronary Effects of GTN

Glycerol trinitrate produces several direct coronary effects. Many of these effects, such as coronary artery dilation, have also been documented after sublingual or oral doses of other nitrates.[3–7,27–29] In response to GTN, dilation of large epicardial coronary arteries, smaller intramural coronary arteries, and some coronary artery stenoses occurs. The percentage of dilation differs for different coronary segments.[4,7] Smaller, more distally located segments dilate more than proximally located and larger coronary segments. The percentage of dilation of coronary artery stenoses is usually modest; however, some stenoses dilate considerably while others do not appear to dilate at all.[4–7,27–29] It is not appropriate to necessarily equate coronary artery dilation with an increase in coronary blood flow or an improvement in transmural myocardial perfusion. Coronary flow is controlled at the arteriolar level. Even in patients with severe coronary artery disease, the ability to increase "total coronary flow" above resting values appears preserved during stress. Present angiographic techniques are not capable of visualizing arterioles. In animals, nitrates have been shown to improve perfusion distal to totally or subtotally obstructed coronary arteries in some species. Either total flow and/or the endocardial/epicardial flow ratio usually improve in certain species such as the dog with well-developed collaterals.[30–36] However, in species such as the pig, which has only poorly developed collaterals, GTN is not uniformly able to improve perfusion.[37] In human beings, detailed studies on transmural flow distribution await technological advances to enable accurate measurements of endocardial-epicardial perfusion and metabolism. Present studies using inert gas radioactive isotopes, regional coronary thermodilution, or measurement of distal coronary pressure techniques to estimate coronary flow to large left ventricular regions suggest coronary flow increases in some patients but not in others.[38–43] It is probable that flow responses in patients will vary depending on the severity of coronary disease, contribution of reversible changes in coronary stenosis tone (i.e., coronary stenosis dilation) to the level of resting coronary flow, degree of reversible ischemia in the resting state, and the individual coronary collateral circulation of each patient. In patients with normal coronary arteries, coronary flow falls, and coronary resistance, calculated as the ratio of mean blood pressure to mean flow, increases. In patients with coronary artery disease, sublingual GTN appears to improve flow in some regions perfused by severely diseased arteries. However, this is not a universal response. Some patients with totally occluded vessels appear to increase flow to the region formerly perfused by the occluded artery after sublingual GTN.[38] However, this is not a consistent finding in all patients with totally occluded arteries. Why flow appears to increase in some patients and not to change or to decrease in others with similar anatomy is not clear. Intracoronary GTN transiently increases coronary artery flow in human beings.[44,45] This flow increase lasts less then 1 min even if intracoronary administration is continued. This increased flow does not appear to prevent or reverse ischemia as pacing- or exercise-induced angina is not relieved with intracoronary GTN administered by bolus injection.[44,45]

Systemic Effects of GTN

The noncoronary, or systemic, effects of nitrates include arterial and venodilation.[14–16] With systemic nitrate administration either by sublingual, buccal, or oral routes a larger decrease in right atrial and pulmonary artery pressures as compared to systemic arterial pressure is usually seen. These changes are usually accompanied by a decrease in stroke volume and baroreceptor-mediated reflex increases in heart rate. With intravenous administration of GTN similar changes in systemic hemodynamics are usually seen; however, if nitroglycerin is administered initially as a bolus, a transient increase in stroke volume and cardiac output may occur, as arteriolar dilation may be the initial predominant effect (Fig. 3).[46] Unfortunately the arteriolar dilation is transient, lasting less than 1 min. In patients with heart failure, the decrease in afterload produced by GTN may lead to a sustained improvement in cardiac output.[47] In these patients the magnitude of cardiac output change will vary widely between patients and probably could not be predicted beforehand. With intracoronary administration of GTN a separation of the systemic and coronary effects is possible. With

doses less than or equal to 50 μg no change in systemic hemodynamics occurs, while near-maximal coronary artery dilation is apparent. With larger doses changes in pressure and heart rate similar to those seen with intravenous GTN become apparent. We suspect this is related to the dose of GTN reaching the systemic circulation.

CELLULAR ACTION AND METABOLISM OF NITRATES

Nitrates produce relaxation of almost all smooth muscle cells. The specific nitrate receptor(s) and binding of nitrates to this receptor have not been well-

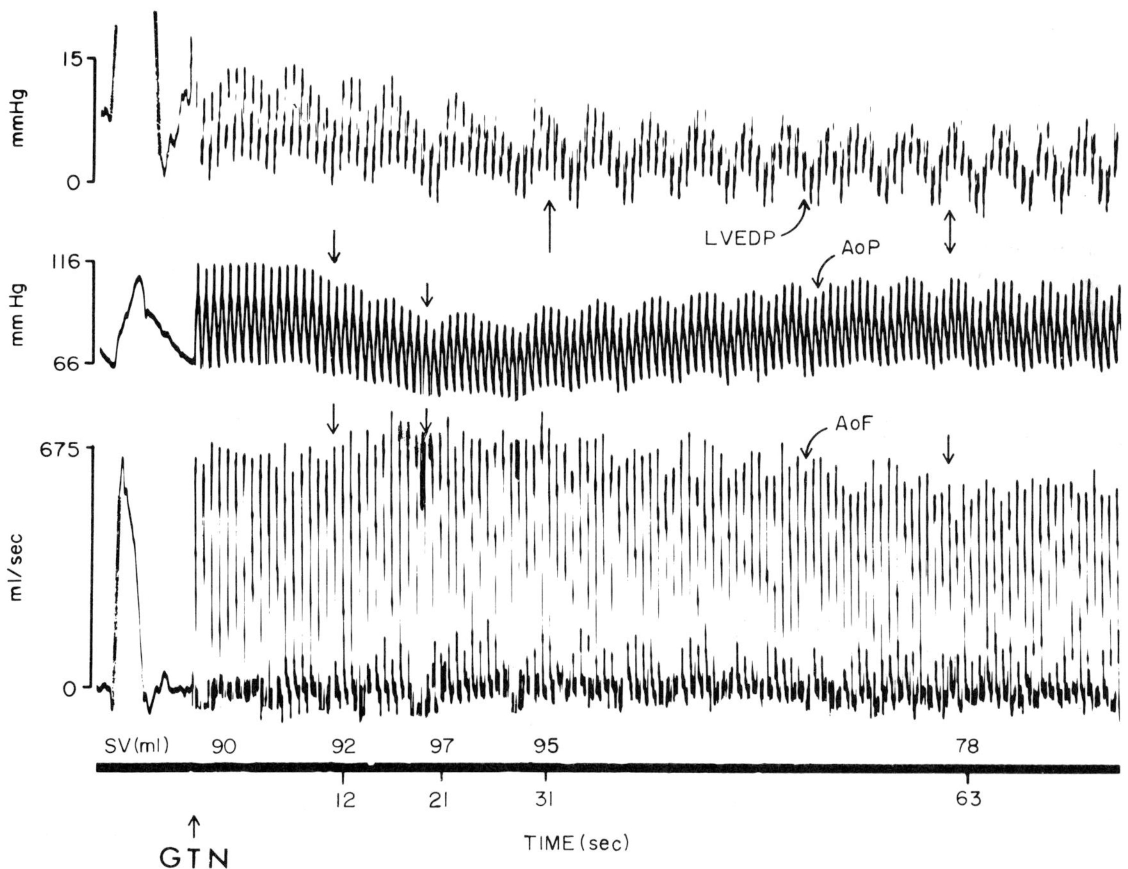

FIGURE 3 Simultaneous recording of high-gain left ventricular pressure (top panel), aortic pressure (mid panel), and aortic root blood velocity (lower panel) in a patient with angina. GTN indicates the point at which intravenous nitrates were administered (150 μg) into the right atrium. The first significant hemodynamic change was a fall in systolic pressure associated with an increase in stroke volume. This occurred 21 s after right atrial injection. At 31 s left ventricular end-diastolic pressure decreased without any noticeable effect on stroke volume. By 63 s arterial pressure rose and left ventricular end-diastolic pressure decreased further associated with a fall in stroke volume. *(From P.R. Lichtlem, H.G. Engel, A. Schrey, and H.J.C. Swan (eds.), Nitrates III, Cardiovascular Effects, Springer-Verlag, New York, 1981. Used with permission.)*

characterized. It is believed that nitrates bind with sulfhydryl groups on specific sites on the smooth muscle cell wall.[48,49] This interaction may lead to activation of guanylate cyclase.[50] Nitrates have also been shown to activate prostaglandin synthesis and release.[51,52] In particular, prostacyclin synthesis has been shown to be stimulated in human endothelial cell cultures.[51] Prostacyclin is a potent smooth muscle relaxant and inhibitor of platelet aggregation. Stimulation of prostacyclin synthesis by GTN may be an important mechanism through which GTN produces its effect.

The metabolism of all nitrates is by reductive hydrolysis of the nitrate moieties.[14,53] This hydrolysis occurs principally in the liver and is catalyzed by the enzyme glutathione–organic nitrate reductase. This enzyme catalyzes the conversion of organic nitrate esters into denitrated metabolites. The partially and fully denitrated metabolites are much less potent vasodilators than the parent compounds. In most cases they are physiologically inactive in the concentrations found after nitrate administration. A small amount of nitrate metabolism also appears to be handled by plasma proteins and red blood cells, but this has been studied less extensively.[54] The ability of the liver to reduce nitrates is the principal reason that large oral doses are necessary to achieve physiological responses. The enzyme system must be overwhelmed by large doses before any nitrate escapes "first-pass" metabolism.

CLINICAL PHARMACOLOGY AND ACTIONS OF NITRATES

The coronary and noncoronary effects of GTN and other nitrates are both potentially important mechanisms to relieve myocardial ischemia. Although the clinical effectiveness of nitrate compounds in relieving episodes of transient myocardial ischemia is unchallenged, the precise mechanism of this beneficial effect remains unclear.[26] Considerable investigation of this topic has been done, and conflicting opinions raised. More recently, as our knowledge of the many important different mechanisms which produce clinical symptoms of myocardial ischemia in patients has increased, our understanding of how nitrates are beneficial in different clinical circumstances has become clearer.

First, let us reconsider the physiological actions of GTN. The direct coronary effects of GTN include dilation of large coronary arteries, small intramural coronary arteries, and conduit vessels that carry collateral flow to severely narrowed or totally narrowed vessels.[4–7,26–29,33,34] The diameter of many coronary artery stenoses also increases. Measurements of coronary blood flow in patients with severe coronary artery disease have shown the potential for coronary blood flow to increase after GTN in some regions perfused by either collateral flow or severely stenosed arteries.[38–43] The noncoronary effects of nitroglycerin are those of arterial dilation and venodilation. Dilation of the systemic venous system will lower right-sided heart pressures and left ventricular filling pressures and volume. Systemic arterial dilation usually occurs to a lesser extent, but arterial pressure usually also decreases. These effects should decrease left ventricular oxygen demand. The decreased left ventricular volume and diastolic pressure could favor endocardial perfusion.

Next let us consider the wide spectrum of patients who have angina. At one extreme are those with only rest angina and in whom coronary artery spasm is the predominant mechanism responsible for transient myocardial ischemia. These patients may or may not have atherosclerotic coronary artery disease, but coronary disease does not necessarily play a principal role in the production of angina. On the other extreme are patients who have only exertional angina in whom severe atherosclerotic coronary narrowings are present and in whom myocardial oxygen supply is limited during stress. The majority of patients fit somewhere between these two extremes. Various degrees of atherosclerotic coronary stenosis are present in these patients, and changes in coronary tone may contribute to their clinical syndrome. Within this framework, some patients have only rest angina whereas others have only exertional angina. Other patients have predominantly exercise angina but appear to have a variable angina threshold; i.e., angina is more easily provoked early during the day than later and angina may occur with a specific activity on some days but not on others. Thus, the patient population with ischemic heart disease is not homogeneous.

If the various physiological effects of the nitrates are matched with the different groups of patients, one can conceptualize how GTN and other nitrates potentially relieve myocardial ischemia in each group. For instance, in a patient with rest angina due to coronary artery spasm, GTN will reverse or prevent coronary artery spasm (Fig. 4). Thus, coronary artery dilation is the primary physiological effect responsible for the relief of myocardial ischemia in this patient. In contrast is the patient with severe coronary artery stenosis and reproducible angina during exercise. In this patient GTN decreases venous return, left ventricular size, and aortic pressure, thus decreasing myocardial oxygen demand. Thus, the peripheral systemic effects of GTN are the principal mechanism by which myocardial ischemia is relieved in this patient. Obviously, in individual patients the coronary or the noncoronary effect of GTN may be of principal importance with variable contribution from the other effect of GTN. Additionally, the ability of GTN to redistribute blood flow and

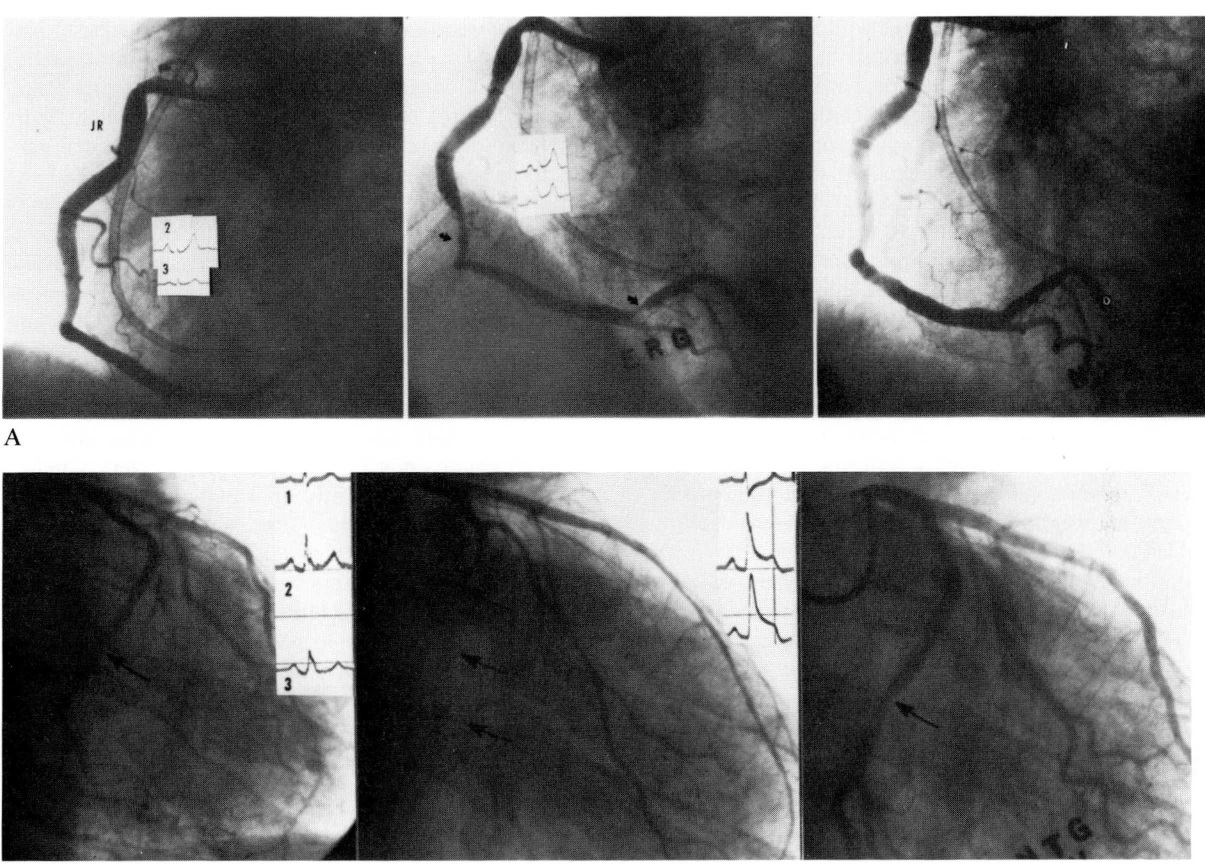

FIGURE 4 Angiographic and electrocardiographic sequences from two patients with coronary artery spasm reversed by GTN. The patient shown in (A) had coronary artery spasm involving the right coronary artery and the patient shown in (B), the circumflex coronary artery. In both patients the left panel shows control angiographic and electrocardiographic findings, the middle panel, findings during angina, and the right panel, findings after administration of GTN. In both patients coronary spasm and ST-segment elevation occurred during angina and were reversed by GTN.

to dilate certain coronary artery stenoses may be important in some individuals. In a few instances, patients with exercise-induced angina have been shown to have coronary spasm during exercise, accompanied by either ST-segment depression or elevation.[55–59] To evaluate the possibility that coronary spasm was the usual mechanism responsible for exercise-induced angina we performed coronary angiography before and during pacing- or exercise-induced angina in a small group of patients.[45] All patients had exercise-induced angina accompanied by ST-segment depression; none had rest angina. In these patients, angiography evidence for coronary artery spasm during exercise or pacing-induced angina was not apparent. In fact, there was either no change in coronary artery size or even mild dilation as the usual physiological response to pacing or exercise stimuli. This increase in coronary

artery size was apparent in both nonstenotic segments, some coronary artery stenoses, and in regions distal to coronary artery stenoses. In these patients, a bolus of intracoronary GTN (50 to 100 μg) during pacing- or exercise-induced angina did not relieve myocardial ischemia. However, there was a further increase in large-vessel coronary artery size and a transient further increase in coronary artery blood flow. Larger doses of intravenous nitroglycerin ($\geq$200 μg) were then administered and angina improved and the electrocardiogram normalized as blood pressure and coronary blood flow decreased. Thus, in patients with exercise-induced angina the role of the direct coronary effects of nitrates seems to be small. These studies support previous ones by Ganz and Marcus, who showed that pacing-induced angina was not relieved by small doses of intracoronary GTN but was relieved by larger doses of intravenous

GTN.[44] In an occasional patient with severe coronary artery disease GTN may favorably redistribute coronary blood flow to a large region perfused by either a severely stenosed or a totally occluded coronary artery. In this instance the direct coronary effect may be important. However, in the majority of patients with exercise-induced angina these direct coronary effects do not seem of principal importance.

In this regard there are important differences between various GTN preparations. Parenteral GTN, in particular intracoronary GTN, has the potential to produce maximal coronary artery dilation with only minimal systemic effects.[4] Intracoronary GTN also causes a transient increase in coronary flow; however, even if the intracoronary infusion is continued, coronary autoregulation rapidly adjusts flow to basal levels.[60] Several patients with either spontaneous or ergonovine-provoked coronary spasm in whom sublingual GTN did not promptly relieve an episode of myocardial ischemia have been reported.[3] These patients uniformly obtain relief from ischemia with small doses of GTN (50 to 200 μg) administered directly into the affected coronary artery. However, compared to sublingual GTN the physiological effect of intracoronary GTN is relatively short-lived. Several patients have experienced recurrent episodes of ischemia shortly after having an initial episode abolished by intracoronary GTN administration (Fig. 2). Perhaps the combination of intracoronary GTN followed by sublingual or oral GTN or another long-acting nitrate may be appropriate acute therapy to treat coronary spasm and prevent recurrence. Oral nitrates also have direct coronary effects.[27] Both transdermal preparations and oral nitrate preparations are effective therapy in managing many patients with coronary spasm.[61,62]

Since nitrates are often used in combination with beta-adrenergic blocking agents and calcium antagonists to treat patients with ischemic heart disease, a brief comparison of the mechanism(s) by which they produce a beneficial effect is of interest (Table 2). Beta blockers appear to be beneficial because of their direct cardiac and systemic effects of decreasing heart rate and blood pressure at rest and during exercise.[63–65]

TABLE 2
Mechanism of beneficial action in patients with ischemic heart disease

	Nitrates	Beta blockers	Calcium antagonists
Heart rate	↑	↓ ↓	↑↓
Blood pressure	↓	↓	↓ ↔
Cardiac output	↓ ↑	↓	↑
Coronary size	↑ ↑	? ↓ ↔	? ↑ ↔
Left ventricular:			
End-diastolic pressure	↓	? ↑ ↔	↔
End-diastolic volume	↓	↑	↔

Thus, myocardial oxygen demand is decreased at rest and during exercise in most patients. Additionally, myocardial contractility is decreased, thus producing further sparing of myocardial oxygen demands. However, there are several deleterious effects of beta blockers in patients with ischemic heart disease. In patients with compensated heart failure beta blockers, through the mechanisms discussed above, may rarely precipitate myocardial failure. By decreasing myocardial contractility beta blockers usually increase left ventricular chamber size, which increases wall stress and oxygen demand. Additionally, coronary vascular resistance is increased with beta blockade.[65] For this reason these drugs are considered to be coronary artery vasoconstrictors; however, the precise effect of beta blockade on large-vessel coronary artery size has not been measured. Thus, in a patient with predominantly exertional angina and preserved left ventricular function beta blockers usually produce a beneficial clinical effect. In patients with both rest and exercise-induced angina the role of beta blockers is undergoing reevaluation, and in other patients with predominantly rest angina and coronary artery spasm, beta blockers may not be helpful and may even exacerbate symptoms.[66]

The mechanism by which calcium antagonists alleviate myocardial ischemia have been less well studied.[67–69] These drugs are considered to be coronary artery vasodilators. Many investigators have found them to increase coronary artery blood flow in some patients and animal models with coronary artery obstruction.[70,71] However, others have not confirmed that observation.[72] The effects of the calcium antagonists on large-vessel coronary artery size and coronary artery stenosis diameter have only been recently studied. In preliminary reports Brown et al.[73] have suggested that intravenous verapamil produces minimal coronary artery dilation. Feldman et al. studied the effects of buccal nifedipine on coronary artery size and found no consistent increase in large-vessel coronary artery diameter or in coronary artery stenosis diameter.[74] In the same patients nifedipine plus intracoronary nitroglycerin produced coronary artery dilation similar to that in other patients who received intracoronary nitroglycerin alone (Fig. 5). The calcium antagonists do not seem to produce uniform effects on determinants of myocardial oxygen consumption. At rest diltiazem has little effect on heart rate and blood pressure but may blunt the tachycardia and hypertensive response to exercise.[75] Similarly, verapamil appears to have little effect on blood pressure and heart rate at rest but usually decreases blood pressure and heart rate during exercise.[76] Stroke volume is increased with both these drugs to a small degree at rest but whether changes in stroke volume and cardiac output occur during exercise or not is less clear. In general no major effect on left ventricular filling pressure or venous pressures is

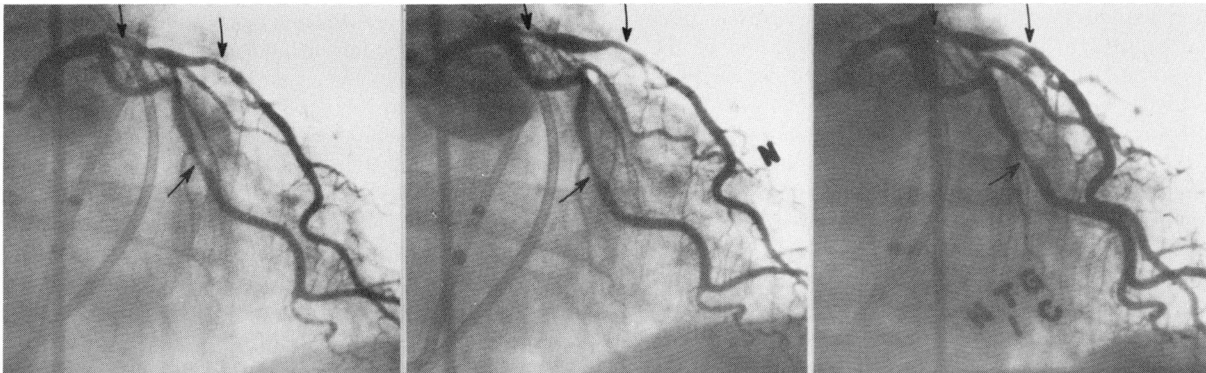

FIGURE 5 Angiographic sequence of left coronary artery angiograms from a patient with previously documented coronary artery spasm. The control angiogram is on the left, the angiogram following buccal nifedipine (10 mg) in the middle, and the angiogram following intracoronary GTN (200 μg) on the right. Several areas of stenosis are noted in the anterior descending and circumflex arteries (arrows). Following nifedipine, minimal coronary artery dilation is noted; however, following administration of intracoronary GTN, there is marked dilation when compared to responses after nifedipine alone.

seen with these two agents. By contrast, nifedipine usually produces a decrease in arterial pressure both at rest and during exercise. There is a reflexly mediated increase in heart rate with this drug. In general there is little venodilation, but left ventricular filling pressure may decrease in patients in whom it is raised initially. This may be because of the marked decrease in aortic pressure and unloading of the left ventricle. Stroke volume is consistently increased with this drug at rest, but its effect during exercise on stroke volume and cardiac output has not been studied in detail. Despite their inability to cause important dilation of epicardial coronary arteries in the resting state, an important property of calcium antagonists may be their ability to prevent coronary artery spasm.

In summary, patients with predominantly rest angina who likely have coronary artery spasm are best treated by various combinations of nitrates and calcium antagonists. On the other hand, patients with exercise angina are probably best initially treated with nitrates and beta blockers. In other patients in whom changes in coronary artery tone are perhaps important in addition to coronary atherosclerosis, combinations of all three types of antianginal agents may be useful.

GENERAL INDICATIONS AND CONTRAINDICATIONS TO THE USE OF NITRATES

Indications

The commonest general indication for use of nitrates has been for the treatment and prevention of myocardial ischemia. All forms of nitrates, i.e., sublingual, oral, transdermal, and parenteral, have been used to accomplish that goal. Thus, patients with exertional angina or rest angina fall into that category.

Nitrates have been used early in the course of an evolving myocardial infarction with the hope of diminishing peri-infarction ischemic zones and perhaps limiting infarction size.[77–86] In addition, in patients with myocardial infarction, nitrates provide relief of pulmonary congestion by lowering left ventricular end-diastolic pressure and thus diminishing pulmonary venous pressure.[81,85,87–90]

Nitrates have also been used in some patients as an adjunct to other therapy to produce controlled hypotension during surgical procedures.[90–92]

Although nitrates are not necessarily effective in all forms of left ventricular failure, the drugs do seem to have clinical effectiveness in patients whose congestive symptoms are related to a ''stiff'' left ventricle, specifically patients with recent acute myocardial infarction.[87–90] In addition, in this setting, nitrates reverse ischemia or limit the size of the ischemic myocardium and perhaps improve systolic function of the ventricle. Thus, paradoxically nitrates may raise systemic blood pressure and increase cardiac output in select cases. This is generally not the case in the patient with heart failure due to a dilated cardiomyopathy.

Another use of nitrates that is becoming increasingly popular is in the management of perioperative hypertension.[91–93] A common example is the patient in the immediate postsurgical period recovering from cardiopulmonary bypass procedures.

Contraindications

Patients who are known to have an exaggerated response to nitrates or an idiosyncratic reaction to nitrates should not be given these drugs. However, in some instances, patients who develop severe hypotension or severe headache after administration of the drugs can be given smaller doses and these reactions avoided.

Topical preparations, especially the ointment form of the drug, have produced skin irritations in some patients, requiring discontinuance of this therapy.[25] However, sometimes this can be avoided by altering the site of the application or changing the topical preparation.

Nitrates should not be given to patients who are obviously hypotensive for unknown reasons or who have uncorrected hypovolemia. The problem of hypovolemia is best illustrated in the patient with a recent myocardial infarction who has been sweating profusely for a prolonged period of time prior to admission to the hospital. In this particular patient, pooling of blood in the periphery after GTN administration may have disastrous effects. However, it can be corrected by raising the legs and infusing intravenous fluids. Another example of hypotension secondary to nitrate use is seen commonly in the catheterization laboratory, especially in patients who have had fluid restriction for 8 or 12 h. Of course these conditions can be promptly treated when recognized, but more importantly they should be avoided.

Patients with known increased intracranial pressure, e.g., secondary to head trauma or cerebral hemorrhage, may be at increased risk after nitrate administration because cerebral vascular dilation may further increase intracranial pressure.[94]

Patients with specific conditions such as constrictive pericarditis and pericardial tamponade should be given nitrates with caution because the fall in right- and left-sided filling pressures may further diminish cardiac output and produce significant hypotension.

In addition to the obvious contraindications to the use of the drug, one must be aware that prolonged periods of hypotension may have deleterious effects on the brain, heart, liver, and kidneys secondary to poor perfusion. Thus, for example in a patient who has known liver disease, there may be further alteration of function of this organ under conditions of poor perfusion. In addition, myocardial ischemia in a few instances has been aggravated because of GTN-induced hypotension.

ADVERSE REACTIONS, COMPLICATIONS, AND TOXICITY OF NITRATES

In spite of the widespread use of nitrates, no long-term studies in animals have been performed to evaluate their carcinogenic potential. It is also not known whether nitrates can cause fetal harm when administered to a pregnant woman or can affect reproduction capacity; nor is it known whether nitrates are excreted in human milk.

Nitrates should be used with caution in patients receiving pentobarbital anesthesia since they will prolong pentobarbital sleep time.[95] Nitrates also potentiate the hypotensive and anticholinergic effects of tricyclic antidepressants.[95] Thus, one must be aware of the concomitant administration of these agents. Nitrates also have an additive effect to many other hypotensive agents and may precipitate severe hypotension in patients receiving antihypertensive therapy.

Recently Gibson et al. reported the occurrence of methemoglobinemia in a patient receiving high doses of parenteral GTN [30 μg/(kg)(min)].[96] If this occurs, there is decreased oxygen delivery to the cell which may be deleterious in a patient with ischemic myocardium.

All things considered, however, nitrates have relatively few adverse reactions, the most frequent one being headache. This occurs in a significant, but small, percentage of patients. Sometimes the headache can be diminished or abolished by decreasing the dose. If this fails to alleviate the headache, when appropriate the concomitant use of mild analgesics such as aspirin or acetaminophen can sometimes allow continued use of nitrates.

Several patients receiving nitrates will note an increase of heart rate. This usually is a secondary phenomenon due to decreased venous return and activation of cardiac reflexes to maintain cardiac output at a normal level. A few patients are nauseated and vomit after the administration of the drug. Others report restlessness, apprehension, muscle twitching, palpitations, dizziness, and abdominal pain. The exact mechanism for these adverse reactions is not clear. When topical preparations are used, a few patients have reported drug rash or, in rare instances, an exfoliative dermatitis.[25]

Paradoxical bradycardia and increased angina pectoris may accompany nitrate-induced hypotension. The mechanism of bradycardia is not understood, but paradoxical narrowing of the coronary arteries occurring after the administration of nitrates has also been reported, and this may contribute to that problem.[97,98]

If nitrate preparations are administered to patients with either normal or low pulmonary capillary wedge pressures, they may be especially sensitive to the hypotensive effects of the drug.

PROBLEMS OF NITRATE TOLERANCE AND NITRATE DEPENDENCE

In 1888, Stuart was concerned that nitrate tolerance was a common problem in clinical practice.[99] This was based on his report of a case of a patient requiring 1,200 mg of nitrates to achieve the same hypotensive effect as the initial dose of 0.6 mg. This concern was further amplified in reports indicating withdrawal symptoms in workers exposed to nitrate compounds on a daily basis when taken away from their work environment.[48,100] It is probably true that chronic exposure to nitrates by munitions workers can result in tolerance since many workers report disappearance of headaches after several days of work. In addition, the rebound phenomenon, i.e., vasoconstriction, that has been reported in these individuals is likely to occur. What is not clear, however, is whether this type of exposure to nitrates has any relevance to the use of these compounds in clinical practice. In fact, experienced clinicians treating large numbers of patients with ischemic heart disease rarely, if ever, note patients who develop tolerance or a decreased effectiveness of the nitrates they have currently administered.

In clinical practice, the problem of nitrate tolerance and nitrate dependence does not seem to be an important one.[48] Perhaps this is in part related to the intermittent administration of the drug. Until recently, nitrates have been administered on a 4- to 8-hourly basis and, in many instances, are not administered throughout the night during sleep. Thus, it is unlikely that most patients who were receiving nitrates were developing constant blood levels. In these patients a steady-static nitrate blood level is unlikely, and it is more likely that a pulse dose of the drug is being administered. This would allow for the recovery from the initial dose. The next administration of the drug would begin with either a low or an absent blood level of nitrates.

One intriguing and not uncommon situation bears further comment. Patients with chronic angina treated with nitrates with a satisfactory result may develop increasing frequency or duration of angina attack despite continuance of nitrates. These patients, by current definition, have unstable angina. Since the pathophysiology of unstable angina is not clear, it is attractive to hypothesize that nitrate tolerance could be responsible. Unfortunately, there are insufficient data to verify this hypothesis.

Several authors have reported long-term decreases in angina frequency in patients taking oral nitrates.[11–22,101–103] It seems unlikely, based on these studies, that nitrate tolerance, as we understand it, was active.

It seems reasonable to conclude that at the present time the evidence for clinically important nitrate tolerance in patients with either ischemic heart disease or congestive heart failure is not strong.[104] However, there are no data testing the long-term effects in patients receiving newer transdermal preparation by which blood levels are maintained for a 24-h period. In all previous studies constant levels of nitrates probably have not been maintained.

Despite the lack of evidence for clinically important nitrate tolerance, it seems prudent to be cautious about the rapid and precipitious withdrawal of nitrate preparations, particularly in patients treated with high-dose nitrates. Clinicians have been concerned about the withdrawal of beta blocker therapy for angina pectoris, but have often ignored the problem of nitrate withdrawal in this patient population. When nitrates are discontinued, levels decline rapidly, and the pharmacological effect parallels this. In contrast the physiological effect of beta blockers is generally prolonged over several days even after discontinuance of the drug. Therefore, one should perhaps have more concern about nitrate withdrawal than beta blocker withdrawal.

CLINICAL USEFULNESS OF NITRATES
Stable Angina

The physiological effects of nitrates have been described previously, but it is worth reviewing what happens to systemic and coronary hemodynamics in patients with stable angina. Beneficial effects of nitrates are due to (1) reduction of systemic blood pressure, (2) reduction of left ventricular end-diastolic pressure, (3) reduction of left ventricular volume, and (4) dilation of epicardial coronary arteries and collateral channels. The above effects combine to decrease myocardial oxygen consumption and diminish any effect of coronary vasoconstriction on coronary blood flow. These effects occur in patients regardless of the type of nitrate preparation used or route of administration (except intracoronary). In a typical patient with stable angina pectoris, sublingual nitrates are commonly used to abort an attack of angina. In addition, sublingual nitrates can be used to prevent angina. For example, many patients learn to recognize situations which invariably provoke angina. In these instances, the use of sublingual nitrates prior to the anticipated provocative stimulus often will prevent angina from occurring and allow the patient to proceed without chest pain or symptoms usually experienced during an ischemic event.

Often it is necessary for physician and patient to experiment with dose titration for the prevention and treatment of attacks of angina pectoris. For example, if too large a dose is used, the patient may complain of a headache, become hypotensive, develop tachycardia, and lose interest in continuing the medication. Thus, the physician should try to establish a dose that is both effective in treating the ischemic event and have the least side effects. In the experience of many physicians, nitrate doses of 0.4 mg or less, given sublingually, are effective treatment for most attacks of angina in patients with stable symptoms. Physicians should instruct patients about the use of GTN. For example, patients should understand that the effectiveness of the drug is lost if the medication is not fresh. One can never be certain of the duration of the effectiveness of the drugs. As a general rule, if usual symptoms are not relieved promptly or if burning of the tongue or headache associated with the administration of sublingual GTN does not occur, the drug should be replaced.

In the usual circumstance, patients with angina who have taken sublingual GTN to relieve symptoms should sit or lie down. This accomplishes two goals. First, it decreases myocardial oxygen consumption, and second, it may prevent syncope due to postural hypotension.

Long-acting nitrate preparations should not be used to treat individual attacks but are effective in prevention of subsequent episodes of myocardial ischemia. Several preparations are available (Table 1). After a great deal of controversy over the last several years, it has finally been established that these drugs are effective for managing patients with angina pectoris.[11–22,101–103] Current evidence indicates the "long-acting preparations" produce an effect lasting several hours. This can be documented by showing alterations of blood pressure, left ventricular end-diastolic pressure, heart rate, left ventricular volume, and exercise tolerance.[21–24,101–105]

Topical nitrate preparations can be used in the same manner as the oral long-acting nitrates. The ointment form of the drug probably has a physiological effect lasting 3 to 4 h.[22,23,105] Some of the newer transdermal preparations may last 24 h or more (at least as determined by plasma levels of GTN). Reichek and colleagues have reported an increase in exercise capacity of patients for periods up to 3 h after GTN ointment treatment.[21] Minor and Conti have shown that the ointment reduces blood pressure and diastolic dimension (M-mode echo) and slightly increases heart rate beginning 15 to 20 min after application and lasting for up to 4 h.[105] In the same group of patients, sublingual GTN had an effect beginning in 5 to 10 min and lasting up to 1 h.

Unstable Angina

In the group of patients loosely defined as those with angina severe enough to require prompt admission to a coronary care unit for treatment and concern about the possibility of myocardial infarction, nitrates in all forms have been used liberally. Until recently the mainstay of therapy has been sublingual GTN to treat an individual attack and long-acting nitrate preparations and transdermal preparations to prevent subsequent attacks. In these patients it may be necessary to use high and frequent doses of long-acting or parenterally administered preparations.[61,62,106–108]

Patients with unstable angina seem ideally suited

for treatment with intravenous GTN, a preparation recently available for clinical use. Although clinical experience with the use of this drug in this situation is not vast, it is obvious that intravenous GTN can provide rapid and controlled alteration of the systemic hemodynamics and favorably alter the myocardial oxygen supply-and-demand equation. Several groups have reported a marked reduction in frequency of angina episodes in patients who were considered "refractory" to maximum standard medical therapy.[107,108] Nitroglycerin was infused at an average dose of approximately 50 µg/min for a period of several days. Our personal experience is similar to that reported in the literature.

When intravenous GTN is used in this situation, infusion rates should begin at a low dose.[107] One should begin with 5 to 10 µg/min, monitoring the effect on blood pressure and heart rate (if a balloon flotation catheter is used for measurement of pulmonary artery pressure and cardiac output, this will provide additional capability to adjust precisely the hemodynamic state of the patient). The drug can be increased by 5 to 10 µg/min every 5 min until symptom relief or hypotension occur. An alternative approach to continuous infusion is intermittent injection of an IV bolus dose of GTN in the 25- to 200-µg range. Bogoert and colleagues suggest that the intermittent use of GTN may be more effective in producing coronary vasodilation than steady state GTN levels.[109] No study has been published comparing effectiveness of the different modes of GTN therapy in this group of patients with rest angina.

Variant Angina

It is now generally accepted that the syndrome of variant angina, i.e., rest angina associated with transient ST-segment elevation on the electrocardiogram, is due to a drastic reduction in coronary blood flow secondary to a transient reduction in epicardial coronary lumen diameter. This being the case, it follows logically that any agent that dilates epicardial coronary arteries (or prevents constriction) will be effective as treatment for episodes of myocardial ischemia and also perhaps in preventing future episodes. In most instances, coronary spasm can be effectively reversed by sublingual or intravenous GTN. In a few instances, however, both spontaneous or provoked coronary artery spasm (with ergonovine) require the direct administration of GTN into the coronary circulation.[3,110] Recent experiences in the catheterization laboratory provoking coronary spasm with ergonovine prompted us to have parenteral GTN available for immediate use. In our experience, the intracoronary administration of this drug is the most effective way to reverse coronary spasm when provoked with ergonovine.

Myocardial Infarction

Until recently, textbooks of medicine and cardiology have recommended that nitrates be avoided in patients with acute myocardial infarction. The principal concern was that nitrate-induced hypotension reduced coronary perfusion pressure and perhaps extended the infarction. Some of this concern relates to the lack of hemodynamic monitoring capabilities in the past. Many patients who became hypotensive probably were hypovolemic. Hemodynamic monitoring might have shown a "normal" systemic blood pressure and a low or normal left ventricular filling pressure (i.e., ≤12 mmHg). A filling pressure of even 12 mmHg, which is "normal," should be considered abnormally low in patients with an evolving myocardial infarction since the effects of the infarction on diastolic compliance elevate the filling pressure. In this situation, nitrates would tend to precipitate hypotension more commonly than when the filling pressure is elevated. Obviously the clinician must individualize the use of nitrates in the early phases of acute myocardial infarction to avoid unwanted hemodynamic responses.

The use of nitrates in patients with acute myocardial infarction can be grouped into four major headings. First, the treatment of the symptoms of myocardial ischemia during the initial presentation; second, "limitation" of infarction size; third, treatment of pulmonary congestion; and fourth, treatment of recurrent ischemic cardiac pain.

When nitrates are used to treat the symptom of cardiac pain in the early stages of acute myocardial infarction, many patients will obtain relief or at least have their morphine requirements diminished.[107] If the decision to use nitrates is made, the intravenous form of the drug probably should be used. It does not make a great deal of sense to use sublingual, oral, or topical forms of the medication in this setting. If an unwanted side effect does occur, simply stopping the intravenous preparation usually rapidly reverses that effect. If pain is not completely relieved with nitrate preparations, then standard analgesic agents such as morphine sulfate should be used.

The use of nitrates to limit infarction size is attractive. Animal experiments have shown that this can occur.[36,83] Unfortunately, in human beings there is no good way to quantitate infarction size. Several studies using parameters such as CK and CK-MB isoenzymes to estimate infarction size have provided conflicting results.[84] Although it seems reasonable to expect that nitrates might limit infarction size, studies have not conclusively proved that hypothesis.

Glycerol trinitrate is effective treatment of pulmonary edema secondary to acute myocardial infarction. Intravenous GTN rapidly reduces left ventricular end-diastolic pressure, which in turn decreases pulmonary venous pressure and relieves pulmonary congestion. In addition, lowering left ventricular end-diastolic pressure allows better perfusion of subendocardium, probably decreases peri-infarction ischemic zones, and may improve systolic function of the ventricle, increasing cardiac output.

In patients recovering from acute myocardial infarction, chest pain occasionally occurs during hospitalization. In some instances this may be due to coronary artery spasm or extension of the myocardial infarction. In others it may occur as activity is increased. Often this is due to limitation of coronary flow in regions distant to the recent infarction. In these patients sublingual, oral, or topical nitrates may be effective. However if prolonged pain recurs, the patient should be considered as a complicated infarct, and intravenous GTN should be infused while awaiting further evaluation of the patient.

An important caution must be added to the above recommendations. Although it is clear that intravenous nitrates can have a beneficial effect in many patients with myocardial infarction, adverse effects can occur. Thus, the intravenous drug should be given only in patients continually monitored.

Patients Undergoing Coronary Artery Bypass

There are two major indications for the use of nitrates in this group of patients. First, the patients with postoperative hypertension and second, patients in whom there is a suspicion of postoperative coronary artery spasm.

It is relatively common for patients in the immediate postoperative stage to develop persistent arterial hypertension associated with an increase in peripheral vascular resistance and a decrease in cardiac output.

In a randomized study comparing intravenous GTN and nitroprusside, Flaherty and colleagues showed that both vasodilators at nearly equal infusion rates lowered arterial pressure and peripheral vascular resistance equally in the majority of patients.[91] They also found that intravenous GTN appeared to have more favorable effects on the pulmonary circulation with a greater lowering of mean pulmonary artery pressure. In addition, GTN seemed to decrease intrapulmonary shunting compared to nitroprusside; thus, arterial oxygen saturation was higher during GTN infusion.

Recently Buxton and colleagues reported coronary artery spasm occurring in six patients who had unexpected hemodynamic collapse within 2 hs after cardiopulmonary bypass for myocardial revascularization.[111] All six had profound hypotension and recurrent ST-segment elevation of ECG leads II, III, and aV_F. All had either normal or noncritical lumen irregularities

18

of the right coronary artery and more than 70 percent narrowing in the left coronary circulation. Coronary artery spasm which was reversed after intracoronary GTN was demonstrated angiographically in one patient. A patent right coronary artery was found at autopsy in another patient. Three patients died despite large intravenous doses of GTN. Two patients who were unresponsive to intravenous GTN recovered after direct GTN infusion into the right coronary artery. The authors conclude that although a history of variant angina may predispose the patient to perioperative coronary spasm, coronary spasm may occur in patients without prior evidence of variant angina.

Patients Undergoing Coronary Angiography

Glycerol trinitrate administered either sublingually, intravenously, or by the intracoronary route is a potent large-vessel coronary artery dilator. If the drug is given prior to performing coronary angiography, coronary spasm, either generalized or localized, will not be seen. Thus, if one's goal is to detect coronary artery spasm, then nitrates should not be given prior to angiography. Glycerol trinitrate given after "routine" angiography is performed provides important anatomic information about the presence or absence of fixed coronary stenoses.[5,7,29]

Another use of nitrates in the catheterization laboratory is to evaluate ventricular performance.[112,113] Often one finds areas of regional wall motion abnormalities in patients with obvious coronary artery stenoses. Although the patient may not have chest pain or ECG changes consistent with myocardial ischemia at the time of study, administration of GTN often will reverse these wall motion abnormalities, suggesting that reversible ischemia rather than irreversible injury or infarction was the cause.

Chronic Congestive Heart Failure

Balloon flotation catheters and thermodilution cardiac output measurements provide important information about the relationship of cardiac output to left ventricular pressure in acutely ill cardiac patients. Mehta and Mehta have reported the effect of intravenous GTN on this relationship in heart failure patients admitted to a cardiac care unit.[114] In their study continuous infusion of GTN was used in doses adjusted to produce optimal hemodynamics in each patient (20 to 70 μg/min, mean 55 $\pm$ 7 μg/min). Cardiac output was measured by the thermodilution technique at control and after 15 min of drug infusion. Under these conditions left ventricular filling pressure consistently fell, cardiac

output was not significantly altered, heart rate increased, and mean arterial pressure declined slightly. In this group of patients cardiac performance was improved because cardiac output was maintained despite a lower filling pressure. It is not known what would have happened had the dose of GTN been increased above 100 μg/min.[46]

Bassenge and colleagues have shown a differential effect of GTN on arteries and veins related to the dose of the drug.[115] They report the continuous infusion of low-dose GTN [0.5 μg/(kg)(min) to 2 μg/(kg)(min)] results in venous dilation as the dominant effect, whereas continuous infusion of high-dose GTN [greater than 2 μg/(kg)(min)] results in arterial dilation as the dominant effect. In addition, Flaherty et al. have shown a potent arterial dilator effect of high-dose GTN in human beings.[80] They demonstrated a striking decrease in arterial pressure in hypertensive patients following intravenous GTN infusion of an average dose of 111 ± 29 μg/min.

The clinical implications of these observations are that low-dose GTN may have a detrimental effect in some patients with heart failure who are dependent on high filling pressure (Frank-Starling mechanism) for maintaining or increasing stroke volume. However, in patients with heart failure due to myocardial ischemia, low-dose GTN may produce a beneficial effect, i.e., the decrease in left ventricular end-diastolic pressure and volume may increase subendocardial myocardial perfusion and thus improve systolic function of the ventricle. These data also suggest that if a decrease in systemic vascular resistance is necessary to increase cardiac output, high-dose GTN should be used. It is thus doubtful that topical or "routine dose" oral preparations will increase cardiac output.

COMPARISON OF THE EFFECTIVENESS OF ISOSORBIDE DINITRATE AND NIFEDIPINE IN PATIENTS WITH PROVEN CORONARY ARTERY SPASM

The recent availability of calcium antagonists has been enthusiastically welcomed by practicing physicians. Numerous uncontrolled trials using these agents have shown them to be efficacious in managing patients with ischemic heart disease. Encouraged by results of this nature, Hill and colleagues did a randomized double-blind trial to evaluate the clinical effectiveness of the calcium antagonist nifedipine compared to that of isosorbide dinitrate in patients with coronary artery spasm.[116] During each phase there was dose titration. Both nifedipine and isosorbide dinitrate could be increased from an initial dose of 40 mg/day to a maximum dose of 120 mg/day unless limited by undesirable side effects such as headache or hypotension. Results of this trial in 26 patients indicate that one patient died suddenly during nifedipine therapy and one died during isosorbide dinitrate therapy. One patient dropped out after initial double-blind nifedipine phase, and two could not tolerate isosorbide dinitrate therapy, one due to headache and one due to severe hypotension. In the other 21 patients who completed all phases of the study, angina frequency decreased during both the nifedipine and isosorbide dinitrate phases as compared to the lead-in phase. Glycerol trinitrate consumption decreased similarly. A greater than 50 percent decrease in angina frequency compared with lead-in occurred in 18 of 24 patients during nifedipine and 15 of 21 patients during isosorbide dinitrate (p = ns) therapy. Comparing nifedipine with isosorbide dinitrate phases, 11 patients were better during the nifedipine phase ($\geq$50 percent decrease in angina frequency), 7 were better during the isosorbide dinitrate phase, and 3 others were similar (<50 percent difference) during nifedipine and isosorbide dinitrate treatment. No difference occurred comparing responses to nifedipine and isosorbide dinitrate in patients with and without severe coronary artery disease.

It is clear from data of this type that both nifedipine and isosorbide dinitrate are effective therapy of angina in patients with coronary artery spasm. An important aspect of the therapy with isosorbide dinitrate was that frequently patients responded to higher doses of isosorbide dinitrate than otherwise may have been used. In addition, many patients had a significantly different response to one therapy compared to the other: frequently when one drug was not effective, the other was. In clinical practice it is highly likely that both nitrates and calcium antagonists will be used in combination rather than separately. The effectiveness of combination compared to single drug therapy has not been studied.

SUMMARY

Nitrates are available in many preparations. These include parenteral, sublingual, buccal, oral, and transdermal. The most common route of administration is sublingually, but the intravenous preparation is being used more frequently especially in the acute situation, i.e., following cardiac surgery and during acute myocardial infarction.

Nitrates have a direct effect on the coronary arteries as well as noncoronary, or systemic, effects. Coronary effects include dilation of epicardial coronary arteries and decrease of coronary vascular resistance in some patients. Systemic effects are primarily due to periph-

eral venous dilation, which results in decreased venous return, decreased filling pressure, and decreased diastolic volume of the ventricles.

Nitrates produce relaxation of almost all smooth muscle cells. This may come about by nitrates stimulating prostacyclin synthesis. Nitrates are metabolized in the liver by reductive hydrolysis, and this is the principal reason that large oral doses are necessary to achieve physiological responses.

The beneficial effects of nitrates probably are related to a combination of coronary and noncoronary effects of the drug. However, patients with different forms of ischemic heart disease may respond differently. For instance, in a patient with rest angina due to coronary artery spasm, nitrates will reverse or prevent coronary artery spasm. In contrast, the patient with severe coronary artery stenosis and reproducible angina during exercise may obtain relief because nitrates decrease venous return, left ventricular size, and left ventricular pressure, thus decreasing myocardial oxygen demands.

Nitrates can be combined with beta blockers and calcium antagonists. Each of these drugs when used in combination may increase the overall beneficial effects for patients with ischemic heart disease.

The commonest general indication for the use of nitrates has been for the treatment and prevention of myocardial ischemia. In patients with myocardial infarction, nitrates provide relief of pulmonary congestion by lowering left ventricular end-diastolic pressure. Nitrates can be used in patients as an adjunct to other therapy to produce controlled hypotension during surgical procedures or for the management of perioperative hypertension in patients recovering from cardiopulmonary bypass procedures.

Idiosyncratic reactions to nitrates are rare, but if they occur, administration of the drug should not be repeated. Unwanted side effects such as hypotension or severe headache can sometimes be controlled by administering smaller doses of the drug. If this fails, the concomitant use of mild analgesics can sometimes allow continued use of nitrates in appropriate patients.

Although nitrates are commonly used during the early phases of acute myocardial infarction, they should be avoided in the patient who is volume-depleted even though the blood pressure is in the normal range.

The problem of nitrate tolerance and nitrate dependence does not seem to be an important one in the clinical practice of cardiology. Perhaps this is in part related to the intermittent administration of the drug. Despite the lack of evidence for clinically important nitrate dependence, it seems prudent to be cautious about rapid and precipitous withdrawal of nitrate preparations, particularly in patients treated with high doses.

Nitrates have been shown to be clinically useful in patients with stable angina, unstable angina (particu-

20

larly in combination with beta blockers), variant angina, and myocardial infarction. Other patients who may benefit are those who are undergoing coronary artery bypass, i.e., for control of postoperative hypertension or in patients in whom there is a suspicion of postoperative coronary artery spasm. Nitrates are also used in the catheterization laboratory to evaluate or detect coronary artery spasm as well as to evaluate ventricular performance in patients with chronically ischemic left ventricles. Although nitrates are useful in patients with chronic congestive heart failure, they probably are not as effective when used alone as when combined with other agents that decrease peripheral vascular resistance. For example, the combination of nitrates and Apresoline has been found to be an effective way to manage chronic heart failure. When nitrates are used to manage heart failure, doses should be as high as tolerated since low-dose nitroglycerin probably is primarily a venodilator and has little effect on changing peripheral vascular resistance.

When used in appropriate patients, in appropriate doses, nitrates can be effective therapy of myocardial ischemia. However, in clinical practice it is highly likely that nitrates, calcium antagonists, and beta blockers will be used in combination rather than separately.

REFERENCES

1 Baaske, D. M., Amann, A. H., Wagenknecht, D. M., Mooers, M., Carter, J. E., Hoyt, H. J., and Stoll, R. G.: Nitroglycerin Compatibility with Intravenous Fluid Filters, Containers, and Administration Sets, *Am. J. Hosp. Pharmacol.*, 37:201, 1980.

2 McNiff, B. L., McNiff, E. F., and Fund, H. L.: Potency and Stability of Extemporaneous Nitroglycerin Infusions, *Am. J. Hosp. Pharmacol.*, 36:173, 1979.

3 Pepine, C. J., Feldman, R. L., and Conti, C. R.: Action of Intracoronary Nitroglycerin in Refractory Coronary Artery Spasm, *Circulation*, 65:411, 1982.

4 Feldman, R. L., Marx, J. D., Pepine, C. J., and Conti, C. R.: Analysis of Coronary Responses to Various Doses of Intracoronary Nitroglycerin, *Circulation*, 66:321, 1982.

5 Feldman, R. L., Pepine, C. J., Curry, R. C., Jr., and Conti, C. R.: Case against Routine Use of Glyceryl Trinitrate before Coronary Angiography, *Br. Heart J.*, 40:992, 1978.

6 Feldman, R. L., Pepine, C. J., Curry, R. C., Jr., and Conti, C. R.: Coronary Arterial Responses to graded doses of Nitroglycerin, *Am. J. Cardiol.*, 43:91, 1979.

7 Feldman, R. L., Pepine, C. J., and Conti, C. R.: Magnitude of Dilatation of Large and Small Coronary Arteries by Nitroglycerin, *Circulation*, 64:324, 1981.

8 Wei, J. Y., and Reid, P. R.: Quantitative Determination of Trinitroglycerin in Human Plasma, *Circulation*, 59:588, 1979.

9 Armstrong, P. W., Armstrong, J. A., and Marks, G. S.: Blood Levels after Sublingual Nitroglycerin, *Circulation*, 59:585, 1979.

10 Wei, J. Y., and Reid, P. R.: Relation of Time Course of Plasma Nitroglycerin levels to Echocardiographic, Arterial Pressure and Heart Rate Changes after Sublingual Administration of Nitroglycerin, *Am. J. Cardiol.*, 48:778, 1981.

11 Reicheck, N., Priest, C., Kienzle, M., Kleaveland, J. P., Bolton, S., and Sutton, M. S.: Angina Prophylaxis with Buccal Nitroglycerin: A Rapid Onset Long-acting Nitrate, *Adv. Pharmacother.*, 1, Karger, Basel, 1982, in press.

12 Markis, J. E., Gorlin, R., Mills, R. M., Williams, R. A., Schweitzer, P., and Ransil, B. J.: Sustained Effect of Orally Administered Isosorbide Dinitrate on Exercise Performance of Patients with Angina Pectoris, *Am. J. Cardiol.*, 43:265, 1979.

13 Danahy, D. T., Burwell, D. T., Aronow, W. S., and Prakash, R.: Sustained Hemodynamic and Antianginal Effect of High Dose Oral Isosorbide Dinitrate, *Circulation*, 55:381, 1976.

14 Needleman, P., and Johnson, E. M., Jr.: Vasodilators and the Treatment of Angina, in L. S. Goodman and A. Gilman (eds.), "The Pharmacological Basis of Therapeutics," Macmillan, New York, 1980.

15 Aronow, W. S.: Clinical Use of Nitrates. 1. Nitrates as Antianginal Drugs, *Mod. Concepts Cardiovasc. Dis.*, 48:31, 1979.

16 Abrams, J.: Nitroglycerin and Long-acting Nitrates. *N. Engl. J. Med.*, 302:1234, 1980.

17 Abrams, J.: Usefulness of Long-acting Nitrates in Cardiovascular Disease, *Am. J. Med.*, 64:183, 1978. (Editorial)

18 Rowe, G. G., Chelius, C. J., Afonso, S., Gurtner, H. P. and Crumpton, C. W.: Systemic and Coronary Hemodynamic Effects of Erythrityl Tetranitrate, *J. Clin. Invest.*, 40:1217, 1961.

19 Parker, J. C., DiCarlo, F. J. and Davidson I. W. F.: Comparative Vasodilator Effects of Nitroglycerin, Pentaerythritol Trinitrate and Biometabolites, and Other Organic Nitrates, *Eur. J. Pharmacol.*, 31:29, 1975.

20 Shane, S. J., Iazzetta, J. J., Chishold, A. W., Berka, J. F., and Leung D.: Plasma Concentrations of Isosorbide Dinitrate and Its Metabolites after Chronic High Oral Dosage in Man, *Br. J. Clin. Pharmacol.*, 6:37, 1978.

21 Reichek, N., Goldstein, R. E., Redwood, D. R., and Epstein, S. E.: Sustained Effects of Nitroglycerin Ointment in Patients with Angina Pectoris, *Circulation*, 50:348, 1974.

22 Awan, N. A., Miller, R. R., Maxwell, K. S., and Mason D. T.: Cardiocirculatory and Antianginal Actions of Nitroglycerin Ointment, *Chest*, 73:14, 1978.

23 Slutsky, R., Battler, A., Gerber, K., Gordon, D., Froelicher, V., Karliner, J., and Ashburn, W.: Effect of Nitrates on Left Ventricular Size and Function during Exercise: Comparison of Sublingual Nitroglycerin and Nitroglycerin Paste, *Am. J. Cardiol.*, 45:831, 1980.

24 Colfer, H., Stetson, P., Lucchesi, B. R., Wagner, J., and Pitt, B.: The Nitroglycerin Polymer Gel Matrix System: A New Method for Administering Nitroglycerin Evaluated with Plasma Nitroglycerin Levels, *J. Cardiovasc. Pharmacol.*, 4:521, 1982.

25 Hendricks, A. A. and Dec, G. W., Jr.: Contact Dermatitis Due to Nitroglycerin Ointment, *Arch. Dermatol.*, 115:853, 1979.

26 Feldman, R. L., and Conti, C. R.: Relief of Myocardial Ischemia with Nitroglycerin: What Is the Mechanism?, *Circulation*, 64:1098, 1981. (Editorial.)

27 Gensini, G. G., Kelly, A. E., DaCosta, B. C. B., and Huntington, P. P.: Quantitative Angiography: The Measurement of Coronary Vasomobility in the Intact Animal and Man, *Chest*, 60:522, 1971.

28 Rafflenbeul, W., Urthaler, F., Russell, R. O., Lichtlen, P., and James, R. N.: Dilatation of Coronary Artery Stenoses after Isosorbide Dinitrate in Man, *Br. Heart J.*, 43:546, 1980.

29 Brown, B. G., Bolson, E., Petersen, R. B., Pierce, C. D., and Dodge, H. T.: The Mechanisms of Nitroglycerin Action: Stenosis Vasodilatation as a Major Component of the Drug Response, *Circulation*, 64:1089,1981.

30 Cohen M. V., Downey, J. M., Sonnenblick, E. H., and Kirk, E. S.: The Effects of Nitroglycerin on Coronary Collaterals and Myocardial Contractility, *J. Clin. Invest.*, 52:2836, 1973.

31 Swain, J. L., Parker, J. P., McHale, P. A., and Greenfield, J. C., Jr.: Effects of Nitroglycerin and Propranolol on the Distribution of Transmural Myocardial Blood Flow during Ischemia in the Absence of Hemodynamic Changes in the Unanesthetized Dog, *J. Clin. Invest.*, 63:947, 1979.

32 Malindzak, G. S., Jr., Green, H. D., and Stagg, P. L.: Effects of Nitroglycerin on Flow after Partial Constriction of the Coronary Artery, *J. Appl. Physiol.*, 29:17, 1970.

33 Winbury, M. M.: Redistribution of Left Ventricular Blood Flow Produced by Nitroglycerin. An Example of Integration of the Macro- and Microcirculation, *Circ. Res.*, 27, 29(suppl. 1):140, 1971.

34 Fam, W. M., and McGregor, M.: Effect of Nitroglycerin and Dipyridamole on Regional Coronary Resistance, *Circ. Res.*, 22:649, 1968.

35 Becker, L. C., Fortuin, N. J., and Pitt, B.: Effect of Ischemia and Antianginal Drugs on the Distribution of Radioactive Microspheres in the Canine Left Ventricle, *Circ. Res.*, 28:263, 1971.

36 Jugdutt, B. I., Becker, L. C., Hutchins, G. M., Bulkley, B. H., Reid, P. R., and Kallman, C. H.: Effect of Intravenous Nitroglycerin on Collateral Blood Flow and Infarct Size in the Conscious Dog, *Circulation*, 63:17, 1981.

37 Most A. S., Williams, D. O., and Millard, R. W.: Acute Coronary Occlusion in the Pig: Effect of Nitroglycerin on Regional Myocardial Blood Flow, *Am. J. Cardiol.*, 42:947, 1978.

38 Mehta, J., and Pepine, C. J.: Effect of Sublingual Nitroglycerin on Regional Flow in Patients with and without Coronary Disease, *Circulation*, 58:803, 1978.

39 Horwitz, L. D., Gorlin, R., Taylor, W. J., and Kemp, H. G.: Effects of Nitroglycerin on Regional Myocardial Blood Flow in Coronary Artery Disease, *J. Clin. Invest.*, 50:1578, 1971.

40 Knoebel, S. B., McHenry, P. L., Bonner, A. J., and Phillips, J. F.: Myocardial Blood Flow in Coronary Artery Disease, *Circulation*, 47:690, 1973.

41 Parker, J. O., West, R. O., and DiGiorgi, S.: The Effect of Nitroglycerin on Coronary Blood Flow and the Hemodynamic Response to Exercise in Coronary Artery Disease, *Am. J. Cardiol.*, 27:59, 1971.

42 Horwitz, L. D., Gorlin, R., Taylor, W. J., and Kemp, H. G.: Effects of Nitroglycerin on Regional Myocardial Blood Flow in Coronary Artery Disease, *J. Clin. Invest.*, 50:1578,1971.

43 Goldstein, R. E., Stineon, E. B., Scherer, J. L., Seningen, R. P., Grehl, T. M., and Epstein, S. E.: Intraoperative Coronary Collateral Function in Patients with Coronary Occlusive Disease, *Circulation*, 49:298, 1974.

44 Ganz, W., and Marcus, H. S.: Failure of Intracoronary Nitroglycerin to Alleviate Pacing-induced Angina, *Circulation*, 46:880, 1972.

45 Pepine, C. J., Feldman, R. L., and Conti, C. R.: Observations on the Role of Coronary Artery Spasm in Stress-induced Angina. *Circulation*, 62(suppl. 2):312, 1980.

46 Conti, C. R., Christie, L. G., Nichols, W. W., Feldman, R. L., Pepine, C. J., and Mehta, J.: Early Hemodynamic Responses to Single Dose Intravenous Nitroglycerin Time Course Relationships, in Lichtlen, P. R., Engel, H. J., Schrey, A., and Swan, N. J. C. (eds.), "Nitrates III: Cardiovascular Effects," Springer-Verlag, Berlin, New York, 1981, p. 151.

47 Aronow, W. S.: Clinical Use of Nitrates. II. Nitrates in Congestive Heart Failure, *Mod. Concepts Cardiovasc. Dis.*, 48:37, 1979.

48 Needleman, P., and Johnson, E. M., Jr.: Mechanism of Tolerance Development to Organic Nitrates, *J. Pharmacol. Exp. Ther.*, 184:709, 1973.

49 Needleman, P., Jakschik, B., and Johnson, E. M., Jr.: Sulphydryl Requirement for Relaxation of Vascular Smooth Muscle, *J. Pharmacol. Exp. Ther.*, 187:324, 1973.

50 Gruetter, C. A., Kadowitz, P. J., and Ignarro, L. J.: Methylene Blue Inhibits Coronary Arterial Relaxation and Guanylate Cyclase Activation by Nitroglycerin, So-

dium Nitrite, and Amyl Nitrite, *Can. J. Physiol. Pharmacol.*, 59:150, 1981.

51 Morcillio, E., Reid, P. R., Dubin, N., Ghodagaonkar, R., and Pitt, B.: Myocardial Prostaglandin E Release by Nitroglycerin and Modification by Indomethacin, *Am. J. Cardiol.*, 45:53, 1980.

52 Levin, R. I., Jaffe, E. A., Weksler, B. B., and Tack-Goldman, K.: Nitroglycerin Stimulates Synthesis of Prostacyclin by Cultured Human Endothelial Cells, *J. Clin. Invest.*, 67:762, 1981.

53 Needleman, P., Blehm, D. J., and Rotskoff, K. S.: Relationship between Glutathione-Dependent Denitration and the Vasodilator Effectiveness of Organic Nitrates, *J. Pharmacol. Exp. Ther.*, 165:286, 1969.

54 DiCarlo, F. J. and Melgar, M. D.: Binding and Metabolism of Nitroglycerin by Rat Blood Plasma, *Proc. Soc. Exp. Biol. Med.*, 131:406, 1968.

55 Waters, D. D., Chaitman, B. R., Dupras, G., Theroux, P., and Mizgala, H. F.: Coronary Artery Spasm during Exercise in Patients with Variant Angina, *Circulation*, 59:580, 1979.

56 Fuller, C. M., Raizner, A. E., Chahine, R. A., Nahormek, P., Ishimori, T., Verani, M., Nitishin, A., Mokotoff, D., and Luchi, R. J.: Exercise-induced Coronary Artery Spasm: Angiographic Demonstration, Documentation of Ischemia by Myocardial Scintigraphy and Results of Pharmacologic Intervention, *Am. J. Cardiol.*, 46:500, 1980.

57 Specchia, G., de Servi, S., Falcone, C., Bramucci, E., Angoli, L., Mussini, A., Marinoni, G. P., Montemartini, C., and Bobba, P.: Coronary Arterial Spasm as a Cause of Exercise-induced ST-Segment Elevation in Patients with Variant Angina, *Circulation*, 59:948, 1979.

58 Boden, W. E., Bough, E. W., Korr, K. S., Benham, I., Gheorghiade, M., Caputi, A., and Shulman, R. S.: Exercise-induced Coronary Spasm with S-T Segment Depression and Normal Coronary Arteriography, *Am. J. Cardiol.*, 48:193, 1981.

59 Yasue, H., Omote, S., Takizawa, A., Nagao, M., Miwa, K., and Tanaka, S.: Exertional Angina Pectoris Caused by Coronary Arterial Spasm: Effects of Various Drugs, *Am. J. Cardiol.*, 43:647, 1979.

60 Schaper, W.: Effects of Drugs on Collateral Circulation, in W. Schaper (ed.), "The Pathophysiology of Myocardial Perfusion," Elsevier–North Holland, Amsterdam, 1979, p. 471.

61 Hill, J. A., Feldman, R. L., Pepine, C. J., and Conti, C. R.: Randomized Double-blind Comparison of Nifedipine and Isosorbide Dinitrate in Patients with Coronary Arterial Spasm, *Am. J. Cardiol.*, 49:431, 1982.

62 Salerno, J. A., Previtali, M., Medici, A., Chimienti, M., Bramucci, E., Lepore, R., Specchia, G., and Bobba, P.: Treatment of Vasospastic Angina Pectoris at Rest with Nitroglycerin Ointment: A Short-Term Controlled Study in the Coronary Care Unit, *Am. J. Cardiol.*, 47:1128, 1981.

63 Nies, A. S., and Shand, D. G.: Clinical Pharmacology of Propranolol, *Circulation*, 52:6, 1975.

64 Frishman, W., and Silverman, R.: Clinical Pharmacology of the New Beta-adrenergic Blocking Drugs. Part 2. Physiologic and Metabolic Effects, *Am. Heart J.*, 97:797, 1979.

65 Schang, S. J., Jr., and Pepine, C. J.: Effects of Propranolol on Coronary Hemodynamic and Metabolic Responses to Tachycardia Stress in Patients with and without Coronary Disease, *Cath. Cardiovasc. Diag.*, 3:47, 1977.

66 Robertson, R. M., Wood, A. J. J., Vaughn, W. K., and Robertson, D.: Exacerbation of Vasotonic Angina Pectoris by Propranolol, *Circulation*, 65:281, 1982.

67 Ellrodt, G., Chew, C. Y. C., and Singh, B. N.: Therapeutic Implications of Slow-Channel Blockade in Cardiocirculatory Disorders, *Circulation*, 62:669, 1980.

68 Pepine, C. J., and Conti, C. R.: Calcium Blocker in Coronary Heart Disease. Part II, *Mod. Concepts of Cardiovasc. Dis.*, 50:61, 1981.

69 Pepine, C. J., and Conti, C. R.: Calcium Blockers in Coronary Heart Disease, *Mod. Concepts Cardiovasc. Dis.*, 50:67, 1981.

70 Lichtlen, P. R., Engel, H.-J., and Hundeshagen, H.: Regional Myocardial Blood Flow in Normal and Poststenotic Areas after Nitroglycerin, Beta Blockade (Atenolol), Coronary Dilatation (Dipyridamole), and Calcium Antagonism (Nifedipine), *Herz*, 2:81, 1977.

71 Bourassa, M. G., Cote, P., Theroux, P., Tubau, J. F., Genain, C., and Waters, D. D.: Hemodynamics and Coronary Flow following Diltiazem Administration in Anesthetized Dogs and in Humans, *Chest*, 78:224, 1980.

72 Ferlinz, J., and Turbow, M. E.: Antianginal and Myocardial Metabolic Properties of Verapamil in Coronary Artery Disease, *Am. J. Cardiol.*, 46:1019, 1980.

73 Brown, B. G., Pierce, C. D., Petersen, R. B., Singh, B. N., Bolson, E. L., and Dodge, H. T.: Verapamil, A Mild Epicardial Coronary Dilator, Inhibits Sympathetic and Ergonovine-induced Coronary Constriction in Humans, *Circulation*, 64(suppl. 4):50, 1981.

74 Feldman, R. L., Hill, J. A., Conti, J. B., Conti, C. R., and Pepine, C. J.: Analysis of Coronary Responses to Nifedipine Alone and in Combination with Intracoronary Nitroglycerin, *Am. Heart J.*, 105:651, 1983.

75 Hossack, K. F., and Bruce, R. A.: Improved Exercise Performance in Persons with Stable Angina Pectoris Receiving Diltiazem, *Am. J. Cardiol.*, 47:95, 1981.

76 Frishman, W. H., Klein, N. A., Strom, J. A., Willens, H., LeJemtel, T. H., Jentzer, J., Siegel, L., Klein, P., Kirschen, N., Silverman, R., Pollack, S., Doyle, R., Kirsten, E., and Sonnenblick, E. H.: Superiority of Verapamil to Propranolol in Stable Angina Pectoris: A Double-blind, Randomized Crossover Trial, *Circulation*, 65(suppl. 1):51, 1982.

77 Epstein, S.E., Kenth, K. M., Goldstein, R. E., Borer,

J. S., and Redwood, D. R.: Reduction of Ischemic Injury by Nitroglycerin during Acute Myocardial Infarction, *N. Engl. J. Med.*, 292:29, 1974.

78 Kim, Y. I., and Williams, J. R., Jr.: Large Dose Sublingual Nitroglycerin in Acute Myocardial Infarction: Relief of Chest Pain and Reduction of Q Wave Evolution, *Am. J. Cardiol.*, 49:842, 1982.

79 Awan, N. A., Amsterdam, E. A., Vera, Z., DeMaria, A. N., Miller, R. R., and Mason, D. T.: Reduction of Ischemic Injury by Sublingual Nitroglycerin in Patients with Acute Myocardial Infarction, *Circulation*, 54:761, 1976.

80 Flaherty, J. T., Reid, P. R., Kelly, D. T., Taylor, D. R., Weisfeldt, M. L., and Pitt, B.: Intravenous Nitroglycerin in Acute Myocardial Infarction, *Circulation*, 51:132, 1975.

81 Bussmann, W. D., Lohner, J., and Kaltenbach, M.: Orally Administered Isosorbide Dinitrate in Patients with and without Left Ventricular Failure Due to Acute Myocardial Infarction, *Am. J. Cardiol.*, 39:91, 1977.

82 Tomoda, H., and Suzuki, Y.: Effect of Sublingually Administered Isosorbide Dinitrate on Ischemic Injury in Patients with Acute Myocardial Infarction, *Jap. J. Med.*, 19:192, 1980.

83 Epstein, S. E., Borer, J. S., Kent, K. M., Redwood, D. R., and Goldstein, R.: Protection of Ischemic Myocardium by Nitroglycerin: Experimental and Clinical Results, *Circulation*, 53:191, 1976.

84 Bussmann, W. D., Bartman, F., Berghoft, E., Wagner, P., and Kaltenbach, M.: Random Study on the Effect of Intravenous Nitroglycerin on CK and CK-MB Infarct Size, *Circulation*, 56:65, 1977.

85 Bussmann, W. D., Barthe, G., Klupzig, H., and Kaltenbach, M.: A Controlled Study of Intravenous Nitroglycerin Treatment for Two Days in Patients with Recent Myocardial Infarction, *Clin. Cardiol.*, 3:399, 1980.

86 Bussmann, W. D.: The Role of Nitroglycerin in Acute Myocardial Infarction, in Lichtlen, P. R., Engel, J. H., Schrey, A., and Swan, H. J. C., (eds.), "Nitrates III: Cardiovascular Effects," Springer-Verlag, Berlin, New York, 1981, p. 329.

87 Baxter, R. H., Tait, C. M., and McGuinness, J. B.: Vasodilator Therapy in Acute Myocardial Infarction. Use of Sublingual Isosorbide Dinitrate, *Br. Heart J.*, 39:1067, 1977.

88 Williams, D. O., Amsterdam, E. A., and Mason, D. T.: Hemodynamic Effects of Nitroglycerin in Acute Myocardial Infarction, *Circulation*, 51:421, 1975.

89 Mantle, J. A., Russell, R. O., Jr., Moraski, R. E., and Rackley, C. E.: Isosorbide Dinitrate for the Relief of Severe Heart Failure after Myocardial Infarction, *Am. J. Cardiol.*, 37:263, 1976.

90 Rabinowitz, B., Tamari, I., Elazar, E., and Neufeld, H. N.: Intravenous Isosorbide Dinitrate in Patients with Refractory Pump Failure and Acute Myocardial Infarction, *Circulation*, 65:771, 1982.

91 Flaherty, J. T., Magee, P. A., Gardner, T. L., Potter, A., and MacAllister, N. P.: Comparison of Intravenous Nitroglycerin and Sodium Nitroprusside for Treatment of Acute Hypertension Developing after Coronary Artery Bypass Surgery, *Circulation*, 65:1072, 1982.

92 Kaplan, J. A., Dunbar, R. W., and Jones, E. L.: Nitroglycerin Infusion during Coronary Artery Surgery, *Anesthesia*, 45:14, 1976.

93 Fahmy, N. R.: Nitroglycerin as a Hypotensive Drug during General Anesthesia, *Anesthesia*, 49:17, 1978.

94 Rodgers, M. C., Trayst, R., Man, R. J., and Epstein, M. H.: Nitroglycerin Effects on Intracranial Pressure, *Am. J. Cardiol.*, 43:342, 1979.

95 Dicarlo, R. J.: Nitroglycerin Revisited: Chemistry, Biochemistry, Interactions, *Drug Metabol. Rev.*, 4:1, 1975.

96 Gibson, G. R., Hunter, J. B., Raabe, D. S., Jr., Manjoney, D. L., and Ittleman, F. P.: Methemoglobinemia Produced by High-Dose Intravenous Nitroglycerin, *Ann. Intern. Med.*, 96:615, 1982.

97 Come, P. C., and Pitt, B.: Nitroglycerin-induced Severe Hypotension and Bradycardia in Patients with Acute Myocardial Infarction, *Circulation*, 54:624, 1976.

98 Feldman, R. L., Pepine, C. J., and Conti, C. R.: Unusual Vasomotor Coronary Arterial Responses after Nitroglycerin, *Am. J. Cardiol.*, 42:517, 1978.

99 Stewart, D. D.: Tolerance to Nitroglycerin, *J.A.M.A.*, 44:1678, 1905.

100 Lang, R. E., Reid, M., Tresch, D., Keelam, N., Bernhard, V., and Collidge, G.: Nonatheromatous Ischemic Heart Disease following Withdrawal from Chronic Industrial Nitroglycerin Exposure, *Circulation*, 46:666, 1972.

101 Windsor, W., and Berger, H. J.: Oral Nitroglycerin as a Prophylactic Antianginal Agent: Clinical, Physiologic, and Statistical Evidence of Efficacy Based on a Three Phase Experimental Design, *Am. Heart J.*, 90:611, 1975.

102 Cold, S. L., and Kaye, H.: Antianginal Effects of Oral Controlled Release Nitroglycerin in Patients with Coronary Artery Disease. Double Blind Randomized Multiple Cross-over Study, *Clin. Res.*, 23:177, 1975.

103 Davidoff, M. E., and Mroczek, W. J.: The Effect of Sustained Release Nitroglycerin Capsules on Anginal Frequency and Exercise Capacity, *Angiology*, 28:181, 1977.

104 Abrams, J.: Nitrate Tolerance and Dependence, *Am. Heart J.*, 99:113, 1980.

105 Minor, J.A., and Conti, C. R.: Topical Nitroglycerin for Ischemic Heart Disease, *J.A.M.A.*, 239:2166, 1978.

106 Distante, A., Maseri, A., Severi, S., Biagini, A., and Chierchia, S.: Management of Vasospastic Angina at Rest with Continuous Infusion of Isosorbide Dinitrate, *Am. J. Cardiol.*, 44:533, 1979.

107 Mikolich, J. R., Nicoloff, N. B., Robinson, P. H., and Logue, R. B.: Relief of Refractory Angina with Continuous Intravenous Infusion of Nitroglycerin, *Chest*, 77:375, 1980.

108 Dauwe, F., Affaki, G., Waters, D. D., Thero, X. P., and Mizdla, H. F.: Intravenous Nitroglycerin in Refractory Unstable Angina, *Am. J. Cardiol.*, 43:416, 1979.

109 Bogoert, M. G., Russell, M. T., and Shaepdryver, A. F.: The Metabolic Fate of Nitroglycerin in Relation to its Vascular Effects, *Eur. J. Phamacol.*, 12:224, 1970.

110 Buxton, A., Goldberg, S., Hirshfeld, J. W., Wilson, J., Mann, T.,Williams, D. O., Overlie, P., and Oliva, P.: Refractory Ergonovine-induced Coronary Vasospasm: Importance of Intracoronary Nitroglycerin, *Am. J. Cardiol.*, 46:329, 1980.

111 Buxton, A. E., Goldberg, S., Harken, A., Hershfield, J., and Kaster, J.: Coronary Artery Spasm Immediately after Myocardial Revascularization Recognition and Management, *N. Engl. J. Med.*, 304:1249, 1981.

112 McEwan, M. P., Berman, N. D., Morch, J. E., Feiglin, D. H., and McLaughlin, P. R.: Effect of Intravenous and Intracoronary Nitroglycerin on Left Ventricular Wall Motion and Perfusion in Patients with Coronary Artery Disease, *Am. J. Cardiol.*, 47:102, 1981.

113 Helfant, R. H., Pine, R., Meister, S. G., Feldman, M. S., Trout, R. G., and Banka, V. S.: Nitroglycerin to Unmask Reversible Asynergy. Correlation with Post Coronary Bypass Ventriculography, *Circulation*, 50:108, 1974.

114 Mehta, J., and Mehta, P.: Compared Effect of Nitroprusside and Nitroglycerin on Platelet Aggregation in Patients with Heart Failure, *J. Cardiovasc. Pharmacol.*, 2:25, 1980.

115 Bassenge, E., Holtz, J., Kinabeter, H., and Kolin, A.: Threshold Doses of Nitroglycerin for Coronary Artery Dilation, Afterload Reduction, and Venous Pooling in Conscious Dogs, in Lichtlen, P. R., Engel, H. J., Schrey, A., and Swan, H. J. C. (eds.), "Nitrates III: Cardiovascular Effects," Springer-Verlag, Berlin, New York, 1981. p. 238.

116 Hill, J. A., Feldman, R. L., Pepine, C. J., and Conti, C. R.: Randomized Double Blind Comparison of Nifedipine and Isosorbide Dinitrate in Patients with Coronary Arterial Spasm, *Am. J. Cardiol.*, 49:431, 1982.

Beta-Adrenergic Blockade in the Treatment of Coronary Artery Disease

WILLIAM H. FRISHMAN, M.D.

The introduction of beta-adrenoceptor blocking drugs in clinical medicine has provided one of the major pharmacotherapeutic advances in this century. Beta-blockers were initially conceived for the treatment of patients with angina pectoris and arrhythmias; however, it soon became clear that they had much to offer in a diversity of clinical disorders which includes systemic hypertension, hypertrophic cardiomyopathy, mitral valve prolapse, migraine, glaucoma, and thyrotoxicosis.[1,2] Recent clinical trials with 1 to 2 years of active treatment have demonstrated that some beta-blockers are effective in reducing the risk of cardiovascular death and reinfarction in patients who are recovering from an acute myocardial infarction.[3,4] Beta-blockers have also been suggested as a treatment modality for reducing the extent of myocardial injury and mortality during the acute phase of myocardial infarction,[5] but their role in this situation is unclear.

In this article the molecular and clinical pharmacology of beta-adrenergic blockade will be reviewed. Also, the effects of beta-adrenergic blockade in experimental and clinical myocardial ischemia will be discussed.

THE BETA-ADRENOCEPTOR: CHANGING CONCEPTS
Hormonal and Drug Receptors

The effects of an endogenous hormone or an exogenous drug depend ultimately on the physicochemical interactions between the hormone or drug and functionally important molecules in an organism. In most situations, these interactions initially involve the combination of the drug or hormone with macromolecular structures of cells called *receptors*. *Agonists* are agents that interact with a receptor and elicit a response; *antagonists* interact with receptors and prevent the action of agonists.

As shown by Sutherland et al., in many of these interactions the circulating hormone or drug is the first "messenger."[6] It interacts with its specific receptor located on the external surface of the target cells; the drug or hormone-receptor complex activates the enzyme adenyl cyclase, located on the internal surface of the plasma membrane of the target cell. The active adenyl cyclase accelerates the intracellular formation of cyclic adenosine monophosphate (cyclic AMP), the second "messenger," which then stimulates or inhibits various metabolic or physiological processes.[6,7]

Until recently most research on receptor action bypassed the initial binding step and the intermediate steps and examined either the accumulation of cyclic AMP or the end step, the physiological effect. In the past fews years, however, research techniques have become available to study the initial binding of the receptor. Many of these involve the use of radioactive agonists or antagonists (radioligands) that attach to and label the receptors.[7,8] A great deal of information about receptors has been obtained with these techniques, which have helped to explain the many drug and hormone actions.

The Beta-Adrenergic Receptor

The catecholamines norepinephrine and epinephrine are important regulators of many physiological and metabolic effects in human beings. Norepinephrine acts primarily as a neurotransmitter released from sympathetic nerve terminals, and epinephrine functions as a circulating hormone released from the adrenal medulla.[7] Ahlquist performed detailed studies 35 years ago in which he thought to characterize the receptors by which catecholamines such as epinephrine and norepinephrine exert their physiological effects.[9] His studies indicated that there were two major types of receptors: alpha- and beta-adrenoceptors. Adrenergic receptors have since been subclassified into discrete beta 1 and beta 2 as well as alpha 1 and alpha 2 subtypes. Later studies by other investigators emphasized the accompanying changes in the intracellular second "messengers." The recent development of radioligand labeling techniques have greatly aided the investigation of adrenoreceptors, their physiological regulation, and clinical alterations.[7,8]

The older classical concept of adrenoreceptors as static entities in cells which simply serve to initiate the chain of events that lead to hormone action is no longer tenable. The newer theory is that the adrenoceptors are subject to a wide variety of controlling influences. The result of these influences is to regulate dynamically the number of adrenoceptors in tissues. It is likely that the changes in tissue concentration of receptor sites help to mediate important fluctuations in tissue sensitivity to drug action.[9]

There are significant clinical and therapeutic implications in these new principles. An apparent increase in the number of beta-adrenoceptors, and thereby a supersensitivity to agonists, may be induced by chronic exposure to antagonists.[8] This up-regulation of beta-adrenoceptors was described by Glaubiger and Lefkowitz and may explain the "beta blocker withdrawal phenomenon," which occurs in patients with coronary artery disease upon sudden discontinuation of beta-adrenoceptor blocking therapy.[10] With prolonged beta-adrenoceptor blocker therapy, receptor occupancy by catecholamines would be diminished and the number of available receptors increased. With sudden withdrawal of the beta-adrenoceptor blocker, an increased pool of sensitive receptors would be open to endogenous catecholamine stimulation. The resultant adrenergic stimulation could precipitate angina pectoris or a myocardial infarction.[11]

The effects of thyroid hormone on adrenoceptor numbers in experimental studies may provide at least a partial explanation for the therapeutic efficacy of beta-adrenergic blockers in the treatment of patients with thyrotoxicosis.[12] The receptor-binding sites have been shown to be increased in hyperthyroidism and decreased in hypothyroidism.[8] The number of beta-adrenoceptors has also been shown to increase with acute alcohol withdrawal after chronic ingestion, which may explain the reported beneficial effects of propranolol in this situation.

The concentration of beta-adrenoceptors in the membrane of mononuclear cells significantly decreases with age.[7] This might explain the progressive resistance to beta-adrenoceptor blocker therapy reported with increasing age of the hypertensive population. As shown in a study of Buhler et al., a good response to beta-adrenoceptor blocker therapy occurred in 90 percent of hypertensive patients in their twenties, but the percentage of responders fell progressively with increasing age.[13]

Using radioligand techniques a decrease in beta-adrenoceptor sites in the myocardium has been demonstrated in patients with chronic congestive heart failure.[14,15] An apparent reduction in beta-adrenoceptors has also been associated with the development of refractoriness or desensitization to endogenous and exogenous catecholamines, a phenomenon caused by the prolonged exposure of these adrenoceptors to high levels of catecholamines.[14] This desensitization phenomenon is not caused by changes in receptor formation or degradation but rather by catecholamine-induced changes in the conformation of the receptor sites which render them ineffective.[8] These changes are reversible over a period of hours.[8]

Beta-adrenoceptor blocking drugs do not induce desensitization or changes in the conformation of receptors. They do, however, block the ability of catecholamines to desensitize receptors, and this may explain their suggested use in chronic congestive heart failure.[16]

The new information regarding adrenoreceptors has led to a better understanding of the physiological and pharmacologic mechanisms that regulate their function. These new concepts concerning adrenoreceptor function and regulation have also increased our understanding of adrenergic receptors and sympathoadrenal activity in disease states.

BETA-ADRENOCEPTOR BLOCKING DRUGS: BASIC PHARMACOLOGIC DIFFERENCES

As a class of drugs, the beta-adrenoceptor blockers have been so successful that many of them have been synthesized, and over 15 are available on the world market.[2] The application of these agents has been accelerated by the development of drugs possessing a degree of selectivity for two subgroups of the beta-adrenoceptor population: beta 1–receptors in the heart and beta 2–receptors in the peripheral circulation and bronchi.[1] More controversial has been the introduction of beta blocking drugs with alpha-adrenergic blocking actions, varying amounts of intrinsic sympathomimetic activity (partial agonist activity), and nonspecific membrane stabilizing effects.[2] There are also pharmacokinetic differences between beta blocking drugs which may be of clinical importance.[1,2]

Six beta-adrenoceptor blockers are now marketed in the United States: propranolol for angina pectoris, arrhythmias, systemic hypertension, migraine prophylaxis, hypertrophic cardiomyopathy, and soon to be marketed for reducing the risk of cardiovascular mortality and reinfarction in survivors of an acute myocardial infarction; nadolol for hypertension and angina pectoris; timolol for hypertension and for reducing the risk of cardiovascular mortality and reinfarction in survivors of myocardial infarction, and, in topical form, for glaucoma; atenolol, metoprolol, and pindolol are approved for hypertension.[1,17–20] Labetalol, oxprenolol, and acebutolol are in the process of being approved for clinical use.

Despite the extensive experience with beta blockers in clinical practice, there are no studies suggesting that one of these agents has major advantages or disadvantages in relation to another for treatment of cardiovascular diseases. When any available beta blocker is titrated to the proper dose, it can be effective in patients with arrhythmia, hypertension, or angina pectoris.[1,2,12,17–20] However, one agent may be more effective in reducing adverse reactions in certain patients and for specific clinical situations.

Potency

Beta-adrenoceptor blocking drugs are competitive inhibitors of catecholamine binding at beta-adrenoceptor sites. They reduce the effect of any concentration of catecholamine agonist on a sensitive tissue. The dose-response curve of the agonist is shifted to the right; a given tissue response requires a higher concentration of agonist in the presence of beta blocking drugs.[1] Beta 1 blocking potency can be assessed by the inhibition of tachycardia produced by isoproterenol or exercise; potency varies from compound to compound (Table 1). These differences in potency are of no therapeutic relevance; however, they do explain the different drug dosages needed to achieve effective beta-adrenergic blockade when initiating therapy in patients or when switching from one agent to another.[1,21]

Structure-Activity Relationships

The chemical structures of most beta-adrenergic blockers have features in common with the agonist isoproterenol (Fig. 1)—an aromatic ring with a substituted ethanolamine side chain linked to it by an —OCH_2 group.[1,22] The beta blocker timolol has a catecholamine-mimicking side chain, but it is attached to a five-membered heterocyclic ring containing nitrogen and sulfur (a thiadiazole) which is, in turn, attached to another heterocyclic ring containing nitrogen and oxygen (a morpholino compound). It is possible that the thiadiazole-morpholino structure may confer on timolol as yet unidentified unique properties compared to other beta blockers.

Most beta blocking drugs exist as pairs of optical isomers and are marketed as racemic mixtures. Almost all the beta blocking activity is found in the negative (−) levorotatory stereoisomer. The two stereoisomers of beta-adrenergic blockers are useful for differentiating between the pharmacologic effects of beta blockade and membrane stabilizing activity (possessed by both optical forms). The positive (+) dextrorotatory stereoisomers of beta blocking agents have no recognized clinical value.[1,21,22]

Membrane Stabilizing Activity

In high concentrations well above therapeutic levels, certain beta blockers have a quinidine-like, or "local anesthetic," membrane stabilizing effect on the cardiac action potential. This property is exhibited equally by the two stereoisomers of the drug and is unrelated to beta-adrenergic blockade and to any therapeutic antiarrhythmic effects. There is no evidence that membrane stabilizing activity is responsible for any direct negative inotropic effects of beta blocking drugs since drugs with and without this property equally depress left ventricular function.[1,23] Membrane stabilizing activity can manifest itself clinically during massive beta blocker intoxications.[24]

TABLE 1

Pharmacodynamic properties of the beta-adrenoceptor blocking drugs

Drug	Beta 1 blockade potency ratio (propranolol = 1.0)	Relative beta 1 selectivity	Intrinsic sympathomimetic activity	Membrane stabilizing activity
Acebutolol	0.3	+	+	+
Atenolol	1.0	+ +	0	0
Labetalol*	0.3	0	0	0
Metoprolol	1.0	+ +	0	0
Nadolol	1.0	0	0	0
Oxprenolol	0.5–1.0	0	+ +	+
Pindolol	6.0–8.0	0	+ + +	+
Practolol	0.3	+ +	+ +	0
Propranolol	1.0	0	0	+ +
Sotalol	0.3	0	0	0
Timolol	6.0–8.0	0	0	0
Isomer:				
D-propranolol				+ +

*Labetalol has additional alpha-adrenergic blocking activity and direct vasodilatory actions.

SOURCE: Frishman.[2]

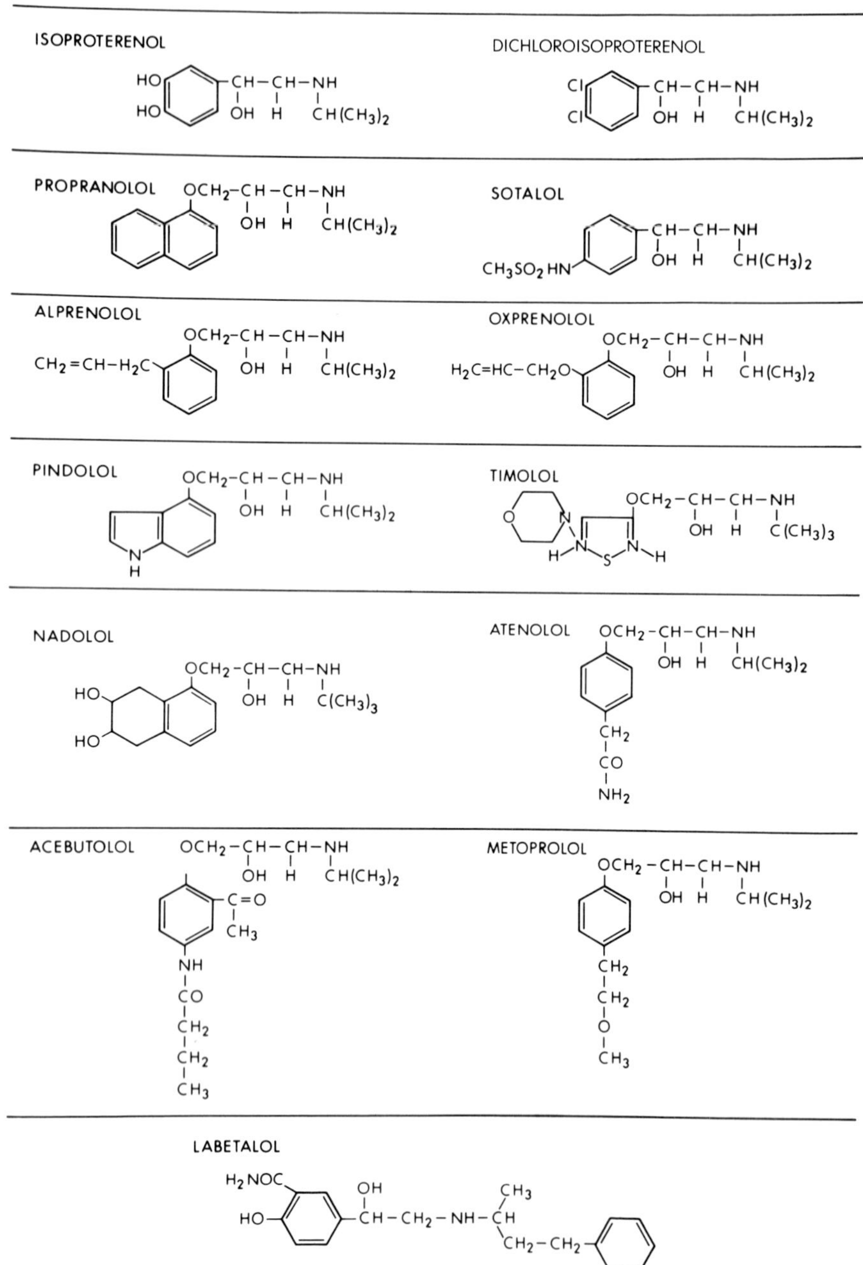

FIGURE 1 Molecular structures of isoproterenol and some beta-adrenergic blocking drugs.

Selectivity

Beta-adrenoceptor blockers may be classified as selective or nonselective according to their relative abilities to antagonize the actions of sympathomimetic amines in some tissues at lower doses than those required in other tissues.[1,17] When used in low doses, beta 1–selective blocking agents such as atenolol and metoprolol inhibit cardiac beta 2–receptors but have less influence on bronchial and vascular beta-adrenoceptors (beta 2). In higher doses, however, beta 1–selective blocking agents will also block beta 2–receptors. Because selective beta 1 blockers have less of an inhibitory effect on the beta 2–receptors, they have two theoretical advantages. The first is that beta 1–selective agents may be safer than nonselective ones in patients with obstructive pulmonary disease since beta 2–receptors remain available to mediate adrenergic bronchodilatation. In some clinical trials in patients with asthma, relatively low doses of beta 1–selective agents caused a lower incidence of side effects than did similar doses of propranolol. However, even selective beta blockers may aggravate bronchospasm in certain patients, so that these drugs should generally not be used in patients with bronchospastic disease. The second theoretical advantage is that unlike nonselective beta blockers, beta 1–selective blockers in low doses may not block the beta 2–receptors that mediate dilatation of arterioles. This property might be an advantage in treatment of hypertension with relatively low doses of beta 1–adrenergic drugs, but this possibility has not been demonstrated. During infusion of epinephrine, nonselective beta blockers can cause a pressor response by blocking beta 2–receptor–mediated vasodilatation, since alpha-adrenergic vasoconstrictor receptors are still operative. Selective beta 1–antagonists may not induce this pressor effect in the presence of epinephrine and may lessen the impairment of peripheral blood flow. It is possible that leaving the beta 2–receptors unblocked and responsive to epinephrine may be functionally important in some patients with asthma, hypoglycemia, hypertension, or peripheral vascular disease treated with beta-adrenergic blocking drugs.[1,17]

Intrinsic Sympathomimetic Activity (Partial Agonist Activity)

Certain beta-adrenoceptor blocking drugs have intrinsic sympathomimetic activity (partial agonist activity). In a beta blocker, this property is identified as a slight cardiac stimulation which can be blocked by propranolol.[1,20,21] The beta blocking drugs with this property slightly activate the beta receptor in addition to preventing the access of natural or synthetic catecholamines to the receptor. Dichloroisoprenaline, the first beta-adrenoceptor blocking drug synthesized, exerted such marked partial agonist activity that it was unsuitable for clinical use.[21] However, compounds with less partial agonist activity are effective beta blocking drugs. Partial agonist effects of beta-adrenoceptor blocking drugs such as pindolol and oxprenolol differ from those of the agonist epinephrine or isoproterenol in that the maximum pharmacologic response that can be obtained is less, although the affinity for the receptor is high. In the treatment of patients with arrhythmia, angina pectoris of effort, or hypertension, drugs with mild to moderate partial agonist activity appear to be as efficacious as beta blockers lacking this property.[12,20] It is still debated whether the presence of partial agonist activity in a beta blocker constitutes an overall advantage or disadvantage in cardiac therapy.[20] Drugs with partial agonist activity cause less slowing

of the heart rate at rest than propranolol or metoprolol, although the increments in heart rate with exercise are similarly blunted. They may reduce peripheral vascular resistance and may also depress atrioventricular conduction less than agents lacking this property.[20] It has been claimed by some investigators that partial agonist activity in a beta blocker protects against myocardial depression, bronchial asthma, and peripheral vascular complications.[20,25] The evidence supporting these claims is not definite, and more definitive clinical trials are necessary to resolve these questions.

Alpha-Adrenergic Blocking Activity

Labetalol is a beta blocker with antagonistic properties at both alpha- and beta-adrenoceptors.[26] Before labetalol, only antagonists acting at alpha- or beta-adrenoceptors, but not at both, were available. Labetalol has been shown to be 6 to 10 times less potent than phentolamine at alpha-adrenoceptors, 1.5 to 4 times less potent than propranolol at beta-adrenoceptors, and is itself 4 to 16 times less potent at alpha- than at beta-adrenoceptors.[26] Labetalol, like other beta blockers, has been shown to be a useful agent in the treatment of arrhythmias, hypertension, and angina pectoris.[27] However, unlike most beta blocking drugs, the additional alpha-adrenergic blocking actions of labetalol lead to a reduction in peripheral vascular resistance which may maintain cardiac output in patients.[26] Whether concomitant alpha-adrenergic blocking activity is actually advantageous in a beta blocker remains to be determined.

Pharmacokinetics

Although the beta-adrenergic blocking drugs as a group have similar pharmacologic effects in cardiovascular disease, their pharmacokinetics are markedly different (Tables 2 and 3).[1,2,21] Their varied aromatic ring structures lead to differences in completeness of gastrointestinal absorption, amount of first-pass hepatic metabolism, lipid solubility, protein binding, extent of distribution in the body, penetration into the brain, concentration in the heart, rate of hepatic biotransformation, pharmacologic activity of metabolites, and renal clearance of a drug and its metabolites which may influence the clinical usefulness of these drugs in some patients.[1,21] The desirable pharmacokinetic characteristics in this group of compounds are a lack of major individual differences in bioavailability and in metabolic clearance of the drug, and a rate of removal from the active tissue sites that is slow enough to allow longer dosing intervals.[1]

30

TABLE 2
Pharmacokinetic properties of beta-adrenoceptor blocking drugs

Drug	Extent of absorption (% of dose)	Extent of bioavailability (% of dose)	Dose-dependent bioavailability (major first-pass hepatic metabolism)	Interpatient variations in plasma levels	Beta blocking plasma concentrations	Protein binding (%)	Lipid solubility*
Acebutalol	≃70	≃ 50	No	7-fold	0.2–2.0 μg/mL	30–40	Weak
Atenolol	≃50	≃ 40	No	4-fold	0.2–5.0 μg/mL	<5	Weak
Labetalol	>90	≃ 33	Yes	10-fold	0.7–3.0 μg/mL	≃50	Weak
Metoprolol	>90	≃ 50	No	7-fold	50–100 ng/mL	12	Moderate
Nadolol	≃30	≃ 30	No	7-fold	50–100 ng/mL	≃30	Weak
Oxprenolol	≃90	≃ 40	No	5-fold	80–100 ng/mL	80	Moderate
Pindolol	>90	≃ 90	No	4-fold	5–15 ng/mL	57	Moderate
Practolol	>90	≃100	No	4- to 7-fold	1.5–5.0 μg/mL	≃40	Weak
Propranolol LA	>90	≃ 30	Yes	20-fold	20–100 ng/mL	93	High
Propranolol (Long-acting)	>90	≃ 20	Yes	10–20 fold	20–100 ng/mL	93	High
Sotalol	≃70	≃ 60	No	4-fold	0.5–4.0 μg/mL	0	Weak
Timolol	>90	≃ 75	No	7-fold	5–10 ng/mL	≃10	Weak

*Determined by the distribution ratio between octanol and water.

SOURCE: Frishman.[2]

TABLE 3
Elimination characteristics of orally active beta-adrenoceptor blocking drugs

Drug	Elimination half-life (N)	Total body clearance (mL/min)	Urinary recovery of unchanged drug (% of dose)	Total urinary recovery (% of dose)	Predominant route of elimination*	Active metabolites	Drug accumulation in renal disease
Acebutolol	3–4	6–15	≃40	>90	RE	Yes	No
Atenolol	6–9	130	≃40	>95	RE	No	Yes
Labetalol	3–4	2,700	<1	>90	HM	No	No
Metoprolol	3–4	1,100	≃3	>95	HM	No	No
Nadolol	14–24	200	70	70	RE	No	Yes
Oxprenolol	2–3	380	2–5	70–95	HM	No	No
Pindolol	3–4	400	≃40	>90	RE (≃40% unchanged & HM)		
Practolol	6–8	140	>90	>90	RE	No	Yes
Propranolol LA	3–4	1,000	<1	>90	HM	Yes	No
Propranolol (Long-acting)	10	1,000	<1	>90	HM	Yes	No
Sotalol	8–10	150	≃60	>90	RE	No	Yes
Timolol	4–5	660	≃20	65	RE (≃20% unchanged & HM)	No	No

*RE denotes renal excretion and HM hepatic metabolism.

SOURCE: Frishman.[2]

The beta-adrenergic blocking drugs can be divided by their pharmacokinetic properties into two broad categories: those eliminated by hepatic metabolism, which tend to have relatively short plasma half-lives, and those eliminated unchanged by the kidney, which tend to have longer half-lives.[1] Propranolol and metoprolol are both lipid-soluble, are almost completely absorbed from the small intestine, and are largely metabolized by the liver. They tend to have highly variable bioavailability and relatively short plasma half-lives.[1] A lack of correlation between the duration of clinical pharmacologic effect and plasma half-life may still allow these drugs to be administered once or twice daily.[1] In contrast, agents like atenolol and nadolol are more water-soluble, are incompletely absorbed through the gut, and are eliminated unchanged by the kidney.[18,19] They tend to have less variable bioavailability in patients with normal renal function, in addition to having longer half-lives, which permits one dose a day. This latter property may be useful in those patients who find compliance with beta blocker therapy a problem.

Recently, a long-acting preparation of propranolol was approved for marketing. The propranolol is part of a soluble matrix inside tiny spheroids made up of an insoluble membrane. Gastrointestinal fluid enters the spheroids and propranolol exits via a concentration gradient into the gut lumen and then the bloodstream. LA propranolol absorption is not dependent on gastric acidity or enzymatic action. Long-acting propranolol is metabolized by the liver in its first pass, an effect similar to conventional propranolol.

Specific pharmacokinetic properties of individual beta-adrenergic blockers (first-pass metabolism, active metabolites, lipid solubility, and protein binding) may be important to the clinician.[1,2,21] When drugs with extensive first-pass metabolism are taken by mouth, they undergo so much hepatic biotransformation that relatively little drug reaches the systemic circulation.[1,21] Depending on the extent of the first-pass effect, an oral dose of beta blocker must be larger than an intravenous dose to produce the same clinical effects. Some beta-adrenergic blockers are transformed into pharmacologically active compounds rather than inactive metabolites.[21] The total pharmacologic effect therefore depends on the amounts of both the drug administered and its active metabolites. Characteristics of lipid solubility in a beta blocker have been associated with the ability of the drug to concentrate in the brain. Many side effects of these drugs which have not been clearly related to beta blockade seem to result from their actions on the central nervous system (lethargy, mental depression, and hallucination). It is still not clear, however, whether drugs that are less lipid-soluble cause fewer of these adverse reactions.[18,19]

Clinical Implications

The beta-adrenoceptor blockers appear to have a similar spectrum of therapeutic cardiovascular effects despite the presence or absence of selectivity or partial agonist activity (Table 4).[1,2,12] Generally, if one agent in adequate doses does not work, neither will another; nor is it helpful to add one beta blocker to another in the hope of improving the therapeutic response. A similar profile of side effects is seen in about 5 to 10 pecent of patients receiving beta blocking drugs. Most of these effects are mild and transient; they include dizziness, fatigue, paresthesias, depression, and gastrointestinal disturbances.[1,28] When mild side effects are encountered, they can sometimes be counteracted by lowering the dose of beta blocker or by changing from one beta blocker to another. The most important cardiovascular side effects are rare in patients with normal left ventricular function.[28] These reactions, which include pulmonary edema, hypotension, and heart block, accompany the use of any beta blocker and appear most often in patients who are dependent on stimulation of the sympathetic nervous system for preservation of myocardial function.[1] In bronchospastic disease the beta blockers with beta 1 selectivity, alpha blocking actions, or partial agonist activity may be of use in some patients.[1] The value of peripheral vascular sparing effects with beta 1–selective agents or labetalol and of decreased brain uptake with hydrophilic beta blocking compounds is less well established.[1,26]

EFFECTS OF BETA-ADRENERGIC BLOCKADE IN ISCHEMIC HEART DISEASE

It is estimated that 4 million Americans have ischemic heart disease.[29] Beta-adrenergic blockers have potent anti-ischemic actions that enable them to be used in many patients with angina pectoris and myocardial infarction.[30] To understand the therapeutic effects of beta blockers, it is important to review briefly current thoughts regarding the pathophysiology of ischemic heart disease.

PATHOPHYSIOLOGY OF MYOCARDIAL ISCHEMIA

As our understanding of the coronary circulation has increased, it is clear that myocardial ischemia results from an imbalance in the supply of oxygen to the heart relative to myocardial demand (Fig. 2).[29–31] Myocardial

TABLE 4

Pharmacodynamic properties and cardiac effects of beta-adrenoceptor blocking drugs

Drug	Relative beta 1 selectivity	Intrinsic sympathomimetic activity	Membrane stabilizing activity	Resting heart rate‡	Exercise heart rate	Myocardial contractility	Resting blood pressure	Resting atrioventricular conduction	Anti-arrhythmic effect
Acebutolol	+	+	+	↓	↓	↓	↓	↓	+
Atenolol	+	0	0	↓	↓	↓	↓	↓	+
Labetalol*	0	0	0	↓ ↔	↓	↓	↓	↓ ↔	+
Metoprolol	+	0	0	↓	↓	↓	↓	↓	+
Nadolol	0	0	0	↓	↓	↓	↓	↓	+
Oxprenolol	0	+ +	+	↓ ↔	↓	↓ ↔	↓	↓ ↔	+
Pindolol	0	+ + +	+	↓ ↔	↓	↓ ↔	↓	↓ ↔	+
Practolol	+	+ +	0	↓ ↔	↓	↓ ↔	↓	↓ ↔	+
Propranolol	0	0	+ +	↓	↓	↓	↓	↓	+
Sotalol	0	0	0	↓	↓	↓	↓	↓	+
Timolol	0	0	0	↓	↓	↓	↓	↓	+
Isomer									
D-pro-pranolol†	0	0	+ +	↔	↔	↓ ↔	↔	↓ ↔	+

*Labetalol has additional alpha-adrenergic blocking properties and direct vasodilatory activity.

†Effects of D-propranolol occur with doses in human beings well above the therapeutic level. The isomer also lacks beta blocking activity.

‡↓ = reduction; ↑ = increase; ↔ = no change.

SOURCE: Frishman.[2]

oxygen requirements are determined by multiple factors. Oxygen supply, on the other hand, depends directly on the coronary blood flow since myocardial metabolism is almost totally aerobic and most of the oxygen in coronary arterial blood is taken up by the heart in a single passage.[31]

Determinants of Myocardial Oxygen Consumption

Myocardial oxygen consumption (MVO_2) is determined by several factors of varied importance. Of lesser quantitative importance are the basal metabolism of the myocardium, external contractile element work, and the activation energy required for depolarization and electromechanical coupling.[32,33] The major hemodynamic determinants of myocardial oxygen consumption are the contractile state of the heart, myocardial wall tension developed in systole, and heart rate (Fig. 3).[32,33] Myocardial oxygen consumption is also influenced by the metabolic substrate available to the heart for use in energy production, and by transmembrane calcium fluxes.[34]

Probably the most important hemodynamic factor determining myocardial oxygen consumption is the tension development, which is determined by the production of systolic pressure and ventricular volume (Laplace phenomenon).[30] Nearly as important is the heart rate, and because it also enters the supply part

of the equation by limiting the time for coronary flow to occur, heart rate has a critical role in the balance of supply and demand.[30] Contractility is of much less importance, and its role can be unpredictable when changes in heart size significantly alter wall tension.[30]

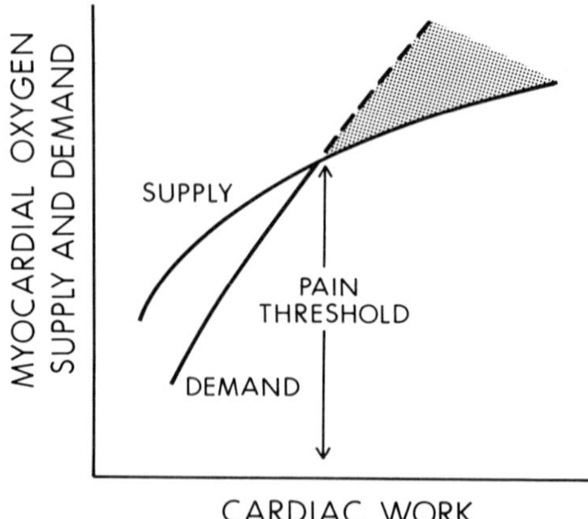

FIGURE 2 Oxygen supply and demand relationship in myocardial ischemia. As myocardial oxygen demand increases with cardiac work, a point is reached where oxygen demand exceeds supply, resulting in ischemia (gray zone) and clinical symptoms. (*From W. H. Frishman: Multifactorial Actions of β-Adrenergic Blocking Drugs in Ischemic Heart Disease. Circulation, 67(suppl. 1):11, 1983.*[31] *Used by permission of the American Heart Association, Inc.*

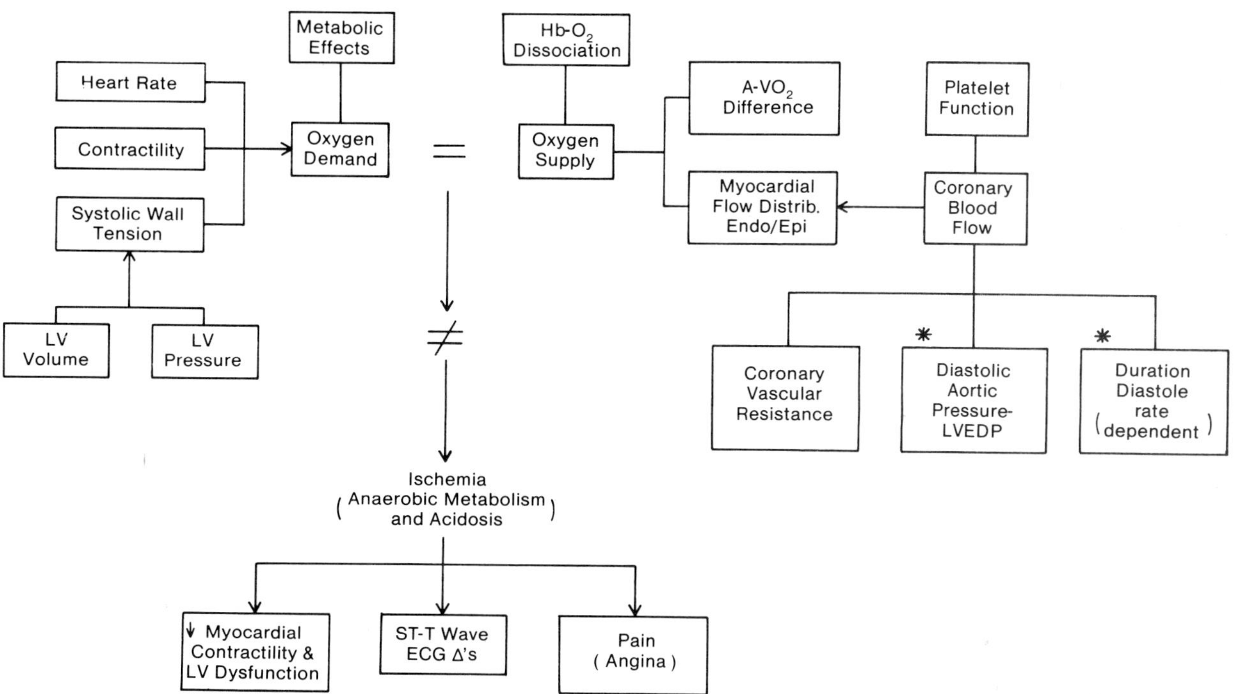

FIGURE 3 Factors in balance of oxygen demand and supply in the heart. Normally, diastolic pressure and heart rate do not limit coronary blood flow, and supply is autoregulated at the arteriolar level. When a coronary artery is largely obstructed or when flow is occurring via collaterals, the major determinants of flow become the diastolic perfusion pressure (aortic diastolic pressure less the diastolic filling pressure) and the heart rate, which determines the time spent by the heart in diastole. The consequences of an imbalance in demand and supply are depicted below. LVEDP = left ventricular end-diastolic pressure. *(From W. H. Frishman, Multifactorial Actions of β-Adrenergic Blocking Drugs in Ischemic Heart Disease. Circulation 67(suppl. 1):11, 1983.[31] Used by permission of the American Heart Association, Inc.)*

Determinants of Coronary Blood Flow in Normal Vessels

Coronary blood flow occurs primarily in diastole, when the heart is relaxed, and flow is distributed uniformly.[30] The aortic diastolic pressure represents the perfusion pressure of the myocardium in the normal heart; a coronary perfusion pressure of approximately 60 mmHg and above is required to maintain appropriate flow to meet myocardial oxygen needs.[35] As pressure falls below 60 mmHg, there is a linear decline in coronary blood flow.[36]

Under normal circumstances when myocardial oxygen demands increase, coronary blood flow can be augmented by local arteriolar vasodilatation.[30] The coronary circulation autoregulates its flow over a wide range in response to changes in myocardial oxygen demands. Adenosine is the primary substance identified as the mediator of this autoregulatory response;[35] other factors have also been suggested.

Superimposed on these autoregulatory factors is the sympathetic nervous system. The coronary vessels are richly supplied by adrenergic nerve endings. Norepinephrine stimulates the alpha-constrictor receptors and slightly modifies the normal autoregulatory capabilities of the vessels.[35] The precise importance of this superimposed adrenergic tone is uncertain but may be of significance in the presence of marked elevations in plasma catecholamines.

Determinants of Coronary Blood Flow in Obstructed Vessels

When there is substantial obstruction of a large coronary artery, the distal vessels become dilated and local autoregulation is lost.[30] At this point, mechanical factors become the dominant determinants of coronary blood flow to the affected region.[30] One of these mechanical factors is the pressure gradient forcing blood into the heart during diastole.[30] This pressure gradient is related to the difference between the diastolic aortic pressure and the filling pressure in the left ventricle.[30] Another physical factor that determines coronary flow is the time in diastole when blood flow can occur. This diastolic time for coronary blood flow is inversely related to the heart rate, and when tachycardia occurs, this diastolic time is seriously reduced.[30]

In addition to these physical factors, variable amounts of spasm of smooth muscle in the large arterial walls, especially in the areas of partial coronary obstruction, may be present and may further reduce coronary flow. On the other hand, coronary collateral vessels may contribute an increase in flow although they have limited ability to dilate (Fig. 3).

Independent of the cause, when oxygen supply does not rise to match oxygen requirements, the heart reverts to anaerobic metabolism and local ischemia ensues.[30,34] This is marked by metabolic acidosis that is accompanied by the rapid development of decreased ventricular wall motion, ST-segment alterations in the electrocardiogram, and chest pain that is interpreted by the patient as angina pectoris.[30,34] It should be noted that although pain might be quite variable, ventricular wall motion becomes seriously impaired as soon as ischemia ensues.

Angina pectoris results from the development of myocardial ischemia, which may be the result of either a decrease in coronary blood flow or an increase in oxygen need that is not met by an increase in coronary blood flow as shown in Fig. 3.[29] For example, with exercise, sympathetic tone is enhanced and leads to an increase in heart rate, contractility, and blood pressure. All these factors lead to an increase in the oxygen requirements of the heart. At the same time, the increase in heart rate leads to a reduction in the diastolic time for coronary blood flow to occur and therefore may lead to a decrease in coronary blood flow.[30] Thus, when heart rate increases, there is both a decrease in coronary flow and an increase in oxygen need. Spasm of vessels may also occur from augmented sympathetic tone, which may further reduce coronary blood flow. All of these factors combine to produce ischemia, which makes the anginal pain worse. In any particular case, the dominant factors may vary in importance, and indeed in the same patient they may change from time to time. Persistence of the ischemic state over a sustained period will ultimately lead to the development of myocardial infarction.

Other Factors Contributing to Myocardial Ischemia

PLATELET ACTIVITY

Heightened platelet activity has been described in patients with coronary and cerebral vascular diseases[37–39] and in conditions considered to be risk factors in the pathogenesis of cardiovascular disease such as diabetes mellitus,[40] hyperlipidemia,[41] cigarette smoking, and hypertension.[42] Therefore, platelets are postulated to have an important role in acute and chronic myocardial ischemia. Clinical events may result during the sequence of platelet activation, reactions of adhesion, aggregate formation, release of granular constituents, and thromboxane A_2 generation resulting in an ischemic ventricular arrhythmia induced by small-vessel platelet microembolization and local thromboxane A_2–induced vasoconstriction.[43–45] Whereas angina pectoris might be manifest if the microemboli disaggregated and vasospasm were transient, myocardial infarction would follow extensive permanent occlusion of small vessels or localized narrowing by vasospasm and extension of platelet thrombus formation at the site of intimal thickening.[43] Direct experimental and indirect clinical studies support the concept that platelets are important in ischemic cardiovascular events, but the relationship to spasm and to other possibly even more important mechanisms is unclear.[43,46] Acute myocardial infarction and mural thrombogenesis appear to have the greatest evidence of being platelet-related.[43] The hypothesized importance of platelets in the pathogenesis of many cardiovascular diseases has stimulated interest in drugs that modify platelet behavior.[47]

The Oxyhemoglobin Equilibrium Curve

Alterations in the oxyhemoglobin equilibrium curve may also influence oxygen supply to the myocardium. Decreased hemoglobin affinity for oxygen reflected in a rightward shift in the oxyhemoglobin equilibrium curve results in increased oxygen delivery to tissues.[48] Increased erythrocyte 2,3-diphosphoglycerate is one means by which the oxyhemoglobin equilibrium curve is shifted to the right.[48] Decreased hemoglobin affinity for oxygen would permit increased oxygen delivery to the myocardium compromised by inadequate coronary perfusion and improve the ischemic state.[48] On the other hand, those physiological variables which shift the oxyhemoglobin equilibrium curve to the left would increase the affinity of hemoglobin for oxygen, and reduce tissue oxygen delivery, thereby aggravating myocardial ischemia.[48]

BETA-ADRENERGIC BLOCKERS IN ISCHEMIC HEART DISEASE

Rational therapy in ischemic heart disease has been directed toward reversing the pathophysiological events discussed above.[49] Specific therapy for angina pectoris with pharmacologic agents was first undertaken over 100 years ago with amyl nitrite and nitroglycerin. Then 20 years ago Black searched for an antianginal drug which could improve myocardial ischemia by reducing the effects of sympathetic nervous stimulation on the heart. The discovery of beta-adrenergic antagonists by Black and others initiated one of the most important advances in the pharmacotherapy of ischemic heart disease.[1,29]

Effects of Beta Blockers on Myocardial Oxygen Demands

Beta blockers may be expected to protect the heart from the deleterious effects of physiological and psychological stresses. By reducing catecholamine-induced increments in heart rate, in velocity and extent of myocardial contraction, and in blood pressure, beta blockers reduce the oxygen requirements of the heart at any level of activity (Fig. 4).

The beta 1–receptors in the heart mediate increases in both heart rate and contractility and are blocked by both selective and nonselective beta blockers. Thus, beta blockers frequently cause reduction in heart rate at rest, although the most beneficial effect in reducing episodes of angina may be by blocking the heart rate

EFFECTS OF β- BLOCKERS

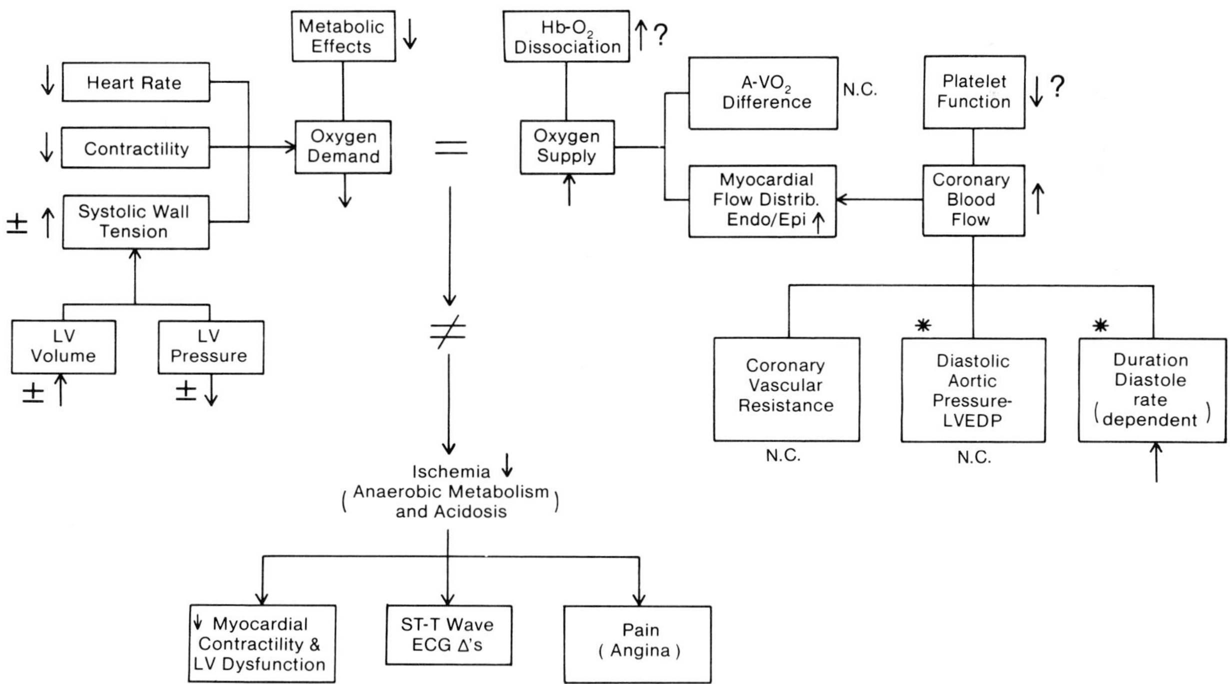

FIGURE 4 Effects of beta-adrenergic blockade on myocardial oxygen supply and demand. Beta-adrenergic blockers reduce overall myocardial oxygen requirements by their effects on heart rate, contractility, and blood pressure. At the same time, oxygen supply and coronary flow may be augmented by an increased diastolic perfusion time secondary to a reduction in heart rate. LVEDP = left ventricular end-diastolic pressure; NC = no change. (*From W. H. Frishman: Multifactorial Actions of β-Adrenergic Blocking Drugs in Ischemic Heart Disease. Circulation 67(suppl. 1):11, 1983.*[31] *Used by permission of the American Heart Association, Inc.*)

response to exercise. This fact is exemplified by beta blockers that have intrinsic sympathomimetic activity. Although they have little effect on heart rate at rest, and therefore would probably not be very beneficial in unstable angina, they do limit the heart rate response to exercise and therefore are efficacious in exercise-induced angina pectoris.[50]

The direct effects of beta blockers on contractile state are relatively minor. Since beta blockers block the effects of catecholamines, they will especially block the increased contractility associated with exercise. This effect on contractility will also tend to reduce myocardial oxygen demand and may be beneficial in patients with angina pectoris. One side effect of the reduction in heart rate and contractility, however, is reduction in cardiac output at rest and during exercise. These effects will reduce the maximum exercise tolerance in patients taking beta blockers.

Although beta blockers are an important class of drugs in the management of hypertension,[12] they tend to have variable effects on blood pressure in normotensive patients with ischemia. If they do produce a slight reduction in blood pressure, this will be helpful in reducing myocardial oxygen demands. Beta blockers have little effect on heart size in patients with normal left ventricular function.

There are, however, some inherent problems in beta blocker therapy in patients with ischemic heart disease. Beta blockers can increase myocardial oxygen requirements of the heart by increasing left ventricular fiber length and end-diastolic pressure, particularly in patients with overt heart failure. At the same time, by increasing left ventricular end-diastolic pressure, the drugs may limit an already compromised subendocardial blood flow. These factors could easily offset the beneficial reduction in heart rate and blood pressure with beta-adrenoceptor blockage. Also, in some patients cardiac impulse formation may be greatly impaired and atrioventricular conduction diminished to a degree that causes cardiac arrest.[51] It is for these reasons that beta blockers should be avoided in patients with myocardial failure and intrinsic sinus node and conduction disease who may be dependent on sympathetic tone to maintain their left ventricular integrity and heart rhythm.

Effects on Coronary Blood Flow

Beta blockers are very useful in the control of myocardial ischemia in patients because of their ability to decrease myocardial oxygen consumption at rest as well as to reduce the amount of oxygen required during exercise. A given state of exercise can be attained with a smaller increment in myocardial oxygen consump-

tion. This tends to abort or postpone the development of clinical ischemia.[52] In addition, the same level of exercise can be obtained at a slower heart rate, which allows more time in diastole for coronary blood flow to occur (Fig. 4).[30,53] It also has been hypothesized that beta-adrenergic blockers can improve myocardial oxygen supply by increasing coronary collateral flow.[54–56] In animal experiments using propranolol and pindolol, some investigators have demonstrated an improvement in collateral blood flow to the ischemic myocardium and a relative redistribution of blood flow favoring the ischemic subendocardium. Other investigators have not made this observation or have demonstrated an actual reduction in collateral coronary flow.[57] The actual effects of beta blockers on coronary collaterals and the relative distribution of myocardial flow in human beings has yet to be determined.

Beta-adrenoceptor blocking drugs do have the potential to decrease coronary blood flow in some patients.[58] The reduction of cardiac output with beta blockers leads to an increase in calculated systemic vascular resistance. The reduction in myocardial oxygen demand leads to an increase in cardiovascular resistance as mediated by the autoregulatory capabilities of the coronary system. It is not true, though, that this increase in cardiovascular resistance is necessarily a detrimental effect. Rather, it reflects the autoregulatory response of the coronary circulation to a reduction in oxygen demand.[59] Certainly, in some patients with coronary artery spasm, increased frequency of symptoms may occur when beta blockers are given.[60] This may relate to blockade of beta 2–vasodilating receptors in the coronary arteries so that unopposed alpha and other constrictive influences may lead to more severe spasm and symptoms. In this latter situation calcium-entry blockers and nitrates may have a therapeutic advantage over beta blockers.

Other Possible Anti-Ischemic Effects of Beta Blockers

EFFECTS ON PLATELETS

Propranolol, when added to normal platelets in vitro, has been demonstrated to inhibit platelet aggregation induced by ADP, epinephrine, collagen, thrombin, and the ionophore A23187.[61,62] The drug affects mainly the secondary phase of aggregation and serotonin release, while it has little effect on primary aggregation.[61,62] Platelet adhesion to collagen and the availability of platelet factor 3 are also inhibited by the drug. It has also been shown from in vitro measurements of platelet activity in peripheral venous and coronary sinus blood that therapeutic doses of propranolol can normalize the heightened platelet aggregability of patients with angina pectoris, and that platelets return to their hyperaggregable state after treatment withdrawal.[37,38,63] From in vivo experiments in rats, propranolol was also found to prevent isoproterenol- and stress-induced platelet aggregation in the microcirculation.[47]

Several lines of evidence suggest that propranolol alters platelet behavior through mechanisms other than beta-adrenergic blockade. First, only alpha-adrenergic receptors are found on platelet membranes.[64] Second, platelet aggregation in vitro can be inhibited to the same extent by both optical isomers of propranolol which have "local anesthetic" or membrane stabilizing activities;[61] the levorotatory stereoisomer has 100 times the beta blocking potency of the dextrorotatory isomer. Third, practolol, an alpha-adrenergic blocker which lacks both lipid solubility and membrane stabilizing activity, has no effects on platelet aggregation.[61,62] Thus, it appears that the membrane effect of propranolol, rather than its beta-adrenergic blocking property, is contributing to the drug's antiplatelet activity. Since other beta blockers lacking antiplatelet activity (e.g., practolol)[61] have been shown to be equally efficacious to propranolol in their anti-ischemic actions,[52] it is questionable whether altering platelet function contributes to the cardioprotective actions of this class of drugs in ischemic heart disease.

THE EFFECTS OF ERYTHROCYTES AND THE OXYHEMOGLOBIN EQUILIBRIUM CURVE

Propranolol, when added to a red blood cell suspension, has a direct effect on the cell membrane leading to an altered Gibbs-Donnan equilibrium and a decrease in intraerythrocyte pH.[65,66] By the classical Bohr effect, this could result in a shift of the oxyhemoglobin equilibrium to the right, and it appears to occur without a quantitative change in total 2,3-diphosphoglycerate. Oski et al. found that approximately 30 percent of 2,3-diphosphoglycerate may be normally found on red blood cell membranes, and therefore may be incapable of binding to deoxyhemoglobin.[67] They reported that propranolol administration in vitro released membrane-bound 2,3-diphosphoglycerate.[67] This, they postulated, then combined with deoxyhemoglobin and decreased the affinity of hemoglobin for oxygen.

Not all reported data confirm a shift to the right of the oxyhemoglobin dissocation curve with propranolol. Lichtman et al., on the basis of studies in six normal subjects and two patients with ischemic heart disease, concluded that propranolol had no significant effects on P_{50} (partial pressure of oxygen).[68] Frishman and associates, in a placebo-controlled double-blind study of 19 patients with angina pectoris, found no effects of propranolol on P_{50} or 2,3-diphosphoglycerate level when measured at rest or during exercise.[69] Therefore, it is still controversial whether the therapeutic effect of beta-adrenergic blockers in treatment of myocardial ischemia is accounted for in part by alterations in the oxyhemoglobin equilibrium curve.

ALTERATIONS IN MYOCARDIAL SUBSTRATE UTILIZATION

Beta blockers can also reduce myocardial oxygen demands by altering the metabolic substrate utilized by the heart and by inhibiting transmembrane calcium fluxes.[70] During myocardial infarction, adrenergic activity stimulates lipolysis, resulting in increased circulating free fatty acids. This, in turn, may augment free fatty acid uptake by the heart, which increases myocardial oxygen consumption and the risk of malignant arrhythmias.[29,34,71] During experimental myocardial infarction, beta blockers decrease lipolysis and myocardial free fatty acid uptake, thereby shifting the utilization of myocardial substrate from fatty acids to glucose.[70,71] Moreover, beta blockers may decrease glycogenolysis.[72] In patients with acute myocardial infarction, Mueller et al. found that propranolol shifted myocardial metabolism from free fatty acids to carbohydrates and decreased myocardial oxygen consumption, while causing lactate production to revert to extraction.[73] The degree to which alterations in myocardial metabolism are contributing to the beneficial effects of beta-adrenergic blocking drugs in human ischemic heart disease is not known at this time.

EFFECTS ON THE MICROVASCULATURE

Using colloidal carbon black as a marker, it was demonstrated that propranolol reduced ischemic microvascular damage during experimental myocardial infarction in dogs.[74] This marker, which identifies damage to vessels, was injected intravenously 5 min after release of a 1-h coronary occlusion in control and in propranolol-treated animals. The intravascular carbon was allowed to circulate for 2 h, during which time it is normally cleared by the reticuloendothelial system unless it is retained by damaged vessels. Significantly fewer vessels labeled by carbon black were found in propranolol-treated groups, suggesting decreased microvascular injury. However, since significant microvascular damage occurs only after myocardial cell injury, it appears unlikely that propranolol's primary action is through protection of the microvasculature.

Other Actions of Beta-Adrenergic Blockade

All beta blockers have been found to exert a powerful suppressive effect on plasma renin secretion both at rest and during stress activation. Owing to the attendant aldosterone-lowering effect, beta blockers slightly improve plasma potassium levels and may protect patients with myocardial ischemia from the dangers of hypokalemia.[75]

Welman and coworkers showed that low plasma concentrations for propranolol [0.1 mg/(mL)(L)] can stabilize cardiac lysosomal membranes in the presence of acute anoxia. In a subsequent study they found that patients on long-term propranolol therapy have a delayed release of plasma lysosomal and cytosolic enzymes after an acute myocardial infarction. These changes may lead to a reduction in electrical instability and myocardial injury.[76]

Finally, serious questions have been raised recently about whether long-term beta blocker use in ischemic heart disease might accelerate atherosclerosis by reducing plasma high-density lipoprotein levels and increasing triglyceride levels.[77] Although this issue needs further clarification, especially if beta blockers are to be considered for long-term use in patients with ischemic heart disease, recent data would suggest that these drugs have no detrimental effects on plasma lipid levels.[78]

Clinical Applications

The beneficial effects of beta blockers on the supply-and-demand equation have impacted greatly on the therapy of ischemic heart disease. First, 90 percent of patients who have angina pectoris on the basis of obstructive coronary artery disease will demonstrate an improvement in exercise tolerance and a reduction in chest pain with beta blocker therapy.[52] With increased exercise capabilities, the secondary benefit of training can be obtained in patients. This result may allow even greater increments in exercise performance for a given degree of ischemic heart disease. Second, because these agents favorably influence many of the determinants of myocardial oxygen consumption and supply, they have been considered for use in patients with "intermediate" ischemic syndromes and myocardial infarction to prevent the undesirable consequences of increased sympathoadrenal discharge.[51,52,74] The more left ventricular function is determined by the mechanical and contractile properties of ischemic areas, the more likely it is that beta blockers will have a beneficial effect in these situations.[51,78] The use of beta-adrenoceptor blockade in the "intermediate" syndrome and in the early stages of acute myocardial infarction may interrupt stepwise development of myocardial necrosis, salvage jeopardized tissue, and improve immediate mortality rate and long-term ventricular function.[79] Finally, the anti-ischemic effects of beta blockers may explain their beneficial effects in reducing the risks of cardiovascular mortality and nonfatal reinfarction in patients who have survived an acute myocardial infarction.[80] Whether or not beta blockers can protect patients with ischemic heart disease from their first myocardial infarction has yet to be determined.[51]

USE OF BETA BLOCKERS IN ANGINA PECTORIS

Angina pectoris is believed to occur when myocardial oxygen demand exceeds supply, i.e., when coronary blood flow is restricted by coronary atherosclerosis and spasm.[1,2] Since the conditions which precipitate anginal attacks (exercise, emotional stress, food, etc.) cause an increase in cardiac sympathetic activity, it might be expected that blockade of cardiac beta-adrenoceptors would relieve the symptoms of the anginal syndrome. It is on this basis that the initial clinical trials with beta blocking drugs in angina were initiated.[81] The findings of these and later studies led to the widespread clinical use of these drugs in patients with angina pectoris.[82–84]

Virtually all beta blockers, whether or not they have partial agonist activity, membrane-stabilizing activity, general or selective beta blocking properties, produce some degree of increased work capacity without pain.[12] Therefore, it must be concluded that it results from their common characteristic blockade of cardiac beta-receptors.[85] For example, both D- and L-propranolol have membrane stabilizing activity but only L-propranolol has significant beta blocking activity. The racemic mixture (D- and L-propranolol) causes a decrease in heart rate and force of contraction in dogs, while the D isomer has hardly any effect.[86] In human beings, D-propranolol, which has "membrane" but no beta blocking properties, has been found ineffective in angina pectoris using very high doses.

The effect of beta blocking drugs on acute exercise in patients with angina pectoris is of interest. Although exercise tolerance improves, the increment in heart rate and blood pressure with exercise is blunted, and the pressure-rate product (systolic blood pressure times heart rate) achieved when pain occurs is less than that reached during a control run.[87] This depressed pressure-rate product at the onset of pain (about 20 percent reduction from control) occurred with various intravenously administered beta blocking drugs that differed in certain properties: propranolol (membrane-stabilizing activity); oxprenolol (membrane-stabilizing and intrinsic sympathomimetic activity); and sotalol (minimal membrane-stabilizing activity).[88] Thus, although there is increased exercise tolerance with beta blockade, patients exercise less than might be expected. This probably represents the potentially adverse effect of beta blockers in increasing left ventricular size, causing increased left ventricular wall tension and an increase in oxygen consumption at a given blood pressure.[89]

All beta blockers will limit the heart rate increment with exercise; however, they cause differing effects on the resting heart rate (Table 4).[2] Propranolol and metoprolol slow the resting pulse more than do oxprenolol, pindolol, and practolol; D-propranolol had very little resting pulse–slowing activity. Morgan et al. also found differences in pulse-slowing activity among four beta blockers they tested: propranolol and timolol reduced pulse rate more than pindolol and alprenolol.[90] It would appear that beta blockers lacking partial agonist activity slow the resting pulse rate more than the beta blockers that have partial agonist activity.[2,50]

A possible explanation as to why drugs with intrinsic sympathomimetic activity do not affect the resting heart rate to the same degree that they affect the increment in heart rate with exercise is probably related to the increased sympathetic tone with exercise.[20] At rest, without a high degree of sympathetic activity, the intrinsic sympathomimetic effect will be more apparent than the beta blocking effect, the converse being true with exercise.[20]

The therapeutic benefit of beta blockade in angina pectoris is now established beyond question. There are many double-blind studies with various designs demonstrating a significant reduction in the frequency of anginal attacks and an improvement in exercise tolerance.[12] Observed improvement is dose-related, and dosage must be titrated for each individual patient. Although they were studied using different trial protocols, all the various beta blocker compounds, despite their differing pharmacologic characteristics and activities, appear to have similar effects in the relief of angina.[12,18,50]

Acebutolol

Acebutolol (Sectral) is a beta 1–selective blocker with weak intrinsic sympathomimetic activity and membrane stabilizing activity which is not approved for clinical use in the United States.

TRIALS VERSUS PLACEBO

Fiserova et al. demonstrated a considerable reduction in anginal attacks and increased exercise tolerance in a study involving 14 patients who received a fixed daily dose of acebutolol (600 mg daily) for a 6-week period.[91]

Twenty-three patients with documented coronary artery disease were placed in a double-blind study by Rod et al.[92] to assess the antianginal efficacy of acebutolol (200 mg three times daily and 400 mg three times daily). Both dosages were found to be therapeutically effective. With the larger daily dose (1,200 mg), heart rate decreased further compared to the lower dose, and there was a greater improvement in exercise tolerance.

Substantial support for the efficacy of acebutolol in angina pectoris is provided in a multicentric study by DiBianco et al:[93] 44 patients with chronic stable angina were entered in a double-blind, placebo-controlled, randomized, crossover trial. Compared to placebo, acebutolol was found to significantly reduce spontaneous anginal frequency, decrease nitroglycerin consumption, and increase exercise capacity.

Further support for the efficacy of acebutolol was provided in a double-blind crossover trial by Steele and Gold in which 20 men with angiographically documented coronary artery disease were treated with acebutolol (400 mg three times daily in 19 patients; 300 mg three times daily in 1 patient).[94] Their results suggest that acebutolol increases exercise performance and decreases the occurrence of angina symptoms compared to placebo in male patients with coronary artery disease.

COMPARATIVE STUDIES

A 28-week, multicenter, placebo-controlled, randomized, double-blind, crossover study comparing the antianginal efficacy of acebutolol versus propranolol in 46 male patients was conducted by DiBianco et al.[95] Dosages of acebutolol and propranolol were 1,650 ± 375 mg/day and 219 ± 50 mg/day, respectively. When compared to placebo, acebutolol produced a greater reduction in systolic, mean, and diastolic blood pressures and a smaller reduction in resting heart rate than propranolol. This difference may relate to the partial agonist property of acebutolol. Both agents produced a similar improvement in exercise duration and exercise work. Anginal frequency and nitroglycerin use were decreased significantly by both acebutolol and propranolol.

DePonti et al. investigated the comparative antianginal efficacy of nifedipine alone, acebutolol alone, and nifedipine plus acebutolol in a randomized, double-blind, placebo-controlled study of 16 patients with documented coronary artery disease.[96] Both agents, when used alone, improved exercise tolerance. At the doses used, nifedipine was found to be more efficacious than acebutolol. The drug combination was more effective than any of the single-drug treatments.

Atenolol

Atenolol (Tenormin) has relative beta 1 selectivity and no intrinsic sympathomimetic activity or membrane stabilizing activity. It is not approved for use in angina pectoris in the United States.

OPEN STUDIES

Daltro and Lion conducted an open study in which 10 chronic angina patients were treated with atenolol 100 mg in a single dose for a minimum period of 30 days.[97] Atenolol was effective in reducing anginal frequency, nitroglycerin consumption, heart rate, systolic blood pressure, and ECG ST-segment deviations. It also prolonged exercise time. Langbehn et al. treated 125 patients with coronary artery disease and previous myocardial infarction with 50 mg of atenolol twice daily for 4 weeks.[98] In their study, the number and severity of anginal attacks were reduced significantly.

The comparative efficacy of atenolol at three dose levels (100 mg once daily, 100 mg twice daily, and 200 mg once daily) was investigated by Backman et al.[99] Five patients were given atenolol at each dose level for a period of 4 weeks. The three doses were determined to be equally effective in reducing resting and exercise heart rates and in increasing maximum work time.

INVESTIGATIONS VERSUS PLACEBO

Roy et al. in a trial of 11 patients with severe angina, found that atenolol, in doses of 50, 100, and 200 mg administered twice daily, produced a significant reduction in anginal attacks and nitroglycerin consumption when compared to placebo.[100] A dose response relationship was also suggested by their results. There was some improvement in exercise tolerance with atenolol which was not statistically significant. The efficacy of atenolol as compared to placebo was further demonstrated in a randomized, double-blind investigation of 19 patients by Erikssen et al.[101] In this study, doses of 50 mg twice daily and 100 mg twice daily caused significant drops in resting heart rate, exercise heart rate, blood pressure, and double-product in all patients. A significant increase of 44 percent in bicycle exercise performance was observed at the different dose levels. van der Vijgh et al. evaluated the therapeutic effectiveness of a single daily oral dose of atenolol 100 mg and 200 mg in a double-blind, crossover, randomized study of 10 patients.[102] Compared to placebo, significant reductions in resting and exercising heart rates were observed with both doses. Maximal effects were obtained 3 to 6 h following the dose, with persistent effects throughout the 24-h post dose period.

Reductions in systolic and diastolic blood pressure, an attenuation of ST-segment changes, a decrease in anginal frequency, and an improvement in exercise tolerance were reported with both doses. Jackson et al. in a definitive, single-blind dose-ranging trial of 10 patients, reported that once-daily dosing with 25, 50, 100, and 200 mg of atenolol significantly decreased the frequency of anginal attacks and nitroglycerin consumption.[103] The best results were obtained with 100-mg and 200-mg doses. The 24-h ambulatory electrocardiographic recordings showed a decrease in mean hourly heart rate throughout the dosing period, with preservation of diurnal variation. Maximal, symptom-limited, treadmill exercise tests performed 3 h after drug ingestion showed significant increases in exercise time and a decrease in double-product and heart rate for all doses, especially with 100 mg and 200 mg. Exercise time 24 h after drug ingestion was still improved with a decrease in maximum heart rate and double-product, 100- and 200-mg doses again being the most effective. Atenolol serum levels correlated with the percent reduction in exercise heart rate and increased exercise time. These investigators concluded that the 100-mg once-daily dose of atenolol was preferable for relief of angina and for increasing exercise tolerance.

The long-term efficacy of once-daily atenolol was investigated by Schwartz et al. in a placebo-controlled, single-blind, dose-finding trial involving nine patients with chronic stable exercise-induced angina.[104] Two-week drug-dosing periods using 25, 50, 100, and 200 mg of oral atenolol were followed by daily treatments of 100 or 200 mg for a period of 1 year. Throughout the study, angina frequency and nitroglycerin use were decreased compared to placebo base line. The 24-h ambulatory electrocardiographic monitor studies and treadmill exercise tests demonstrated a sustained heart rate decrease. Exercise duration until angina onset was prolonged during all periods of atenolol administration. Maximal improvement in exercise tolerance and angina relief was not observed until after 3 months of atenolol therapy despite stable serum drug concentrations.

COMPARATIVE STUDIES

Jackson et al. demonstrated in a double-blind randomized comparison trial of oral atenolol and oral propranolol that twice-daily doses of 25, 50, and 100 mg of atenolol were as effective as propranolol 80 mg three times daily.[105] All dose levels were found to decrease anginal attacks, consumption of nitroglycerin, resting and exercise heart rate, and resting and exercise systolic blood pressure, and to prolong exercise time. Of the 14 patients, 9 continued in a trial comparing the effects of atenolol 200 mg once daily versus 100 mg twice daily. Both regimens were found to be equally effective in reducing anginal attacks, nitroglycerin consumption, systolic blood pressure, and heart rate. Ambulatory electrocardiographic monitoring demonstrated that atenolol consistently reduced heart rate throughout the 24-h period whether given once or twice daily.

Haghfelt et al. demonstrated in a double-blind crossover study that equipotent doses of atenolol and propranolol comparably decreased the frequency of anginal attacks and improved working capacity.[106] A greater reduction in the exercising double-product was noted with atenolol. The employment of a once-daily 100-mg dose of atenolol produced similar antianginal effects to propranolol use in doses up to 320 mg daily.

Metoprolol

Metoprolol (Betaloc, Lopressor) has relative beta 1 selectivity and no intrinsic sympathomimetic or membrane activity. It is not approved for clinical use in angina in the United States.

DOSE-FINDING TRIAL

Uusitalo et al. assessed the antianginal efficacy of metoprolol using single oral doses of 50, 100, and 200 mg in a dose-finding trial involving 23 patients.[107] The effects were assessed 1½ h following ingestion of the dose. Resting systolic blood pressures were similar with all three doses while resting heart rates were lower with 200 mg than with 50 mg. The mean exercise heart rate at the highest comparable work load was lowest with the 200-mg dose, followed by the 100-mg and 50-mg doses. Systolic blood pressure during exercise did not differ significantly. The total work capacity and the time until the onset of anginal pain was significantly greater with metoprolol 200 mg than with the other two dosage regimens.

COMPARATIVE STUDIES

Using equipotent doses of metoprolol and propranolol, Comerford and Besterman compared the antianginal effects of the drugs in a double-blind, crossover study in 14 patients, with long-term follow-up of 72 weeks.[108] Metoprolol was noted to cause a greater increase in total work and exercise tolerance to ST-segment depression than propranolol. Borer et al. performed a comparative, crossover, placebo-controlled study using equipotent doses of metoprolol (150 and 300 mg daily) and propranolol (120 and 240 mg daily) in 10 patients with angina pectoris.[109] A comparable reduction in anginal frequency and nitroglycerin consumption and an improvement in total work performed was

demonstrated with both agents. Resting and exercise heart rates were decreased by both metoprolol and propranolol. Conversely, arterial pressure was unchanged at rest but was decreased with exercise. The maximum dose of both medications was preferred by most patients. Finally, Frick and Luurila performed a double-blind investigation in 20 patients to compare equipotent doses of metoprolol (450 mg/day) and propranolol (360 mg/day) with respect to their antianginal effects.[110] Both agents were equally effective in improving exercise tolerance and relieving angina pectoris.

In a randomized, double-blind, crossover, placebo-controlled trial Thadani et al. compared propranolol, practolol, oxprenolol, metoprolol, and tolamolol with respect to their antianginal effects.[111] Sixteen patients participated in the investigation. All five agents caused a significant improvement in exercise tolerance, a reduction in ST-segment depression, resting heart rate, blood pressure, and double-product. The optimal dose for metoprolol was 200 mg/day.

Thadani et al. conducted a follow-up double-blind, placebo-controlled, randomized, crossover investigation to assess the comparative antianginal effect of these five agents on a long-term basis.[112] Twenty-three patients participated in this 6-month study. Equipotent doses of practolol (100 mg), oxprenolol (40 mg), propranolol (40 mg), metoprolol (50 mg), and tolamolol (50 mg) were provided for the patients on a twice-daily basis. Anginal frequency and nitroglycerin consumption were comparably reduced by all five drugs in comparison to placebo, and exercise tolerance was improved. In addition, significant reductions in ST-segment depression, exercising heart rate, systolic blood pressure, and double-product were noted with each of the five drugs—effects markedly different from those obtained with placebo. The investigators concluded that all five drugs were equally effective antianginal agents with sustained use.

Twenty patients participated in a placebo-controlled, double-blind, crossover study comparing the antianginal efficacy of the calcium-entry blocker verapamil (360 mg/day) and metoprolol (200 mg twice daily).[113] Subjective parameters (mean daily rate of anginal episodes and nitroglycerin consumption) decreased with both agents. Although both verapamil and metoprolol significantly increased exercise capacity, the former had a significantly greater effect. On the other hand, the rest and exercise double-products were reduced only by metoprolol.

Labetalol

Labetalol (Trandate, Normodyne) is a nonselective beta blocker with alpha-blocking and direct vasodilatory activities, and no membrane stabilizing or partial agonist activity. The drug is not approved for the treatment of angina in the United States.

TRIALS VERSUS PLACEBO

The antianginal effects of oral labetalol were demonstrated in a pilot single-blind placebo-controlled study of 10 patients with hypertension and stable angina pectoris.[27] Compared to placebo, labetalol significantly reduced blood pressure, heart rate, angina attacks, and nitroglycerin consumption, and improved exercise tolerance (Fig. 5).[27] Double-blind studies comparing labetalol to propranolol are now in progress.

Nadolol

Nadolol (Corgard) is a long-acting nonselective beta blocker which lacks intrinsic sympathomimetic activity and membrane stabilizing activity. It is approved for clinical use in angina pectoris in the United States.

TRIALS VERSUS PLACEBO

Multiple studies have been performed in patients with stable angina demonstrating the once-daily use of nadolol to be superior to placebo in reducing the fre-

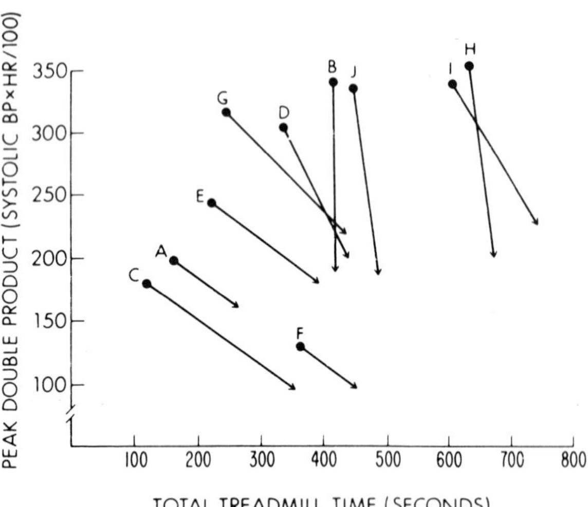

FIGURE 5 Effects of placebo and maximal labetalol dose on the duration of treadmill exercise and peak heart rate–blood pressure product at the end point of exercise. Compared with placebo baseline measurements (closed circles), exercise time increases and peak heart rate–blood pressure product decreases with labetalol (arrows). *(From W. H. Frishman, J. Strom, M. Kirschner, et al., Labetalol Therapy in Patients with Systemic Hypertension and Angina Pectoris: Effects of Combined Alpha and Beta-adrenoceptor Blockade, Am. J. Cardiol., 48:917, 1981.[27] Used with permission.)*

quency of anginal attacks, in decreasing nitroglycerin consumption, and in increasing the capability for exercise.[18,114] Shapiro et al. confirmed these results with nadolol in a double-blind, randomized, placebo-controlled study involving 37 patients.[115] Compared to placebo, the drug (in a fixed dose of 240 mg once daily) significantly decreased the number of angina attacks, nitroglycerin consumption, resting and peak heart rates, and peak rate-pressure products 24 h post dose; exercise time and work were significantly prolonged.

COMPARATIVE TRIALS

Studies have been conducted to assess the relative efficacy of nadolol once daily to propranolol four times a day.[18] Ling and Groel showed that nadolol given once daily is as effective an antianginal agent as propranolol four times a day.[116] Prager, in a trial involving 29 patients comparing nadolol once daily and propranolol four times daily, noted that both drugs had similar effects regarding the number of anginal attacks and nitroglycerin consumed.[117] Nadolol produced a better performance in exercise time. Conversely, Furberg et al. observed that optimal daily dosages of nadolol (100 mg) and propranolol (112 mg) were equally effective in prolonging exercise time in patients with angina.[118] These investigators also noted the continuing antianginal effectiveness of nadolol on a long-term basis (23 months).

In a more extensive study, Jones and Mir compared the antianginal efficacy of conventional propranolol, long-acting propranolol, sustained-release oxprenolol, and nadolol in a randomized, double-blind, crossover trial in 12 patients.[119] A fixed dose regimen of 160 mg once a day was used for all four medications. Observations were made 24 h following a single 160-mg dose. All the drugs were found to cause a reduction in anginal attack rate and nitroglycerin use. Exercise tolerance was prolonged more by propranolol, long-acting propranolol, and nadolol than with sustained-release oxprenolol. Subjectively, patients preferred nadolol and long-acting propranolol over the other two preparations.

Oxprenolol

Oxprenolol (Trasicor, Iset) is nonselective with membrane stabilizing activity and intrinsic sympathomimetic activity. It is not approved for clinical use in the United States.

OPEN TRIALS

In a simple, noncomparative study assessing the antianginal efficacy of oxprenolol in general practice, Watt found complete or substantial relief of symptoms in 80 percent of the patients studied.[120] Monitored release studies were performed in Great Britain by Burley to assess the antianginal efficacy of oxprenolol in 5,492 patients with angina of effort.[121] Of the patients, 5,238 were followed in general practice. Of these, 4,403 were treated with oxprenolol alone. Oxprenolol was added to long-acting nitrates in the remaining patients. The favorable response rate in all three groups was found to be 85 to 90 percent with the optimal oxprenolol dose being 120 to 200 mg/day.

STUDIES VERSUS PLACEBO

Using a fixed-dosage regimen (80 mg three times daily) of oxprenolol in 13 patients with angina, Sandler and Pistevos failed to show a significant beneficial effect of the drug on angina or exercise performance.[122] Bianchi et al., using a fixed dose of oxprenolol 40 mg four times per day in 62 patients, demonstrated a decrease in frequency of angina attacks and in nitroglycerin consumption.[123] Both these studies used 2-week assessment periods and lacked appropriate run-in periods (the run-in period prior to a trial provides an opportunity for patients to become familiar with the experimental protocol and for adjustment of drug dosage). Wilson et al., performing a 2-week trial using a variable dose schedule (60 to 400 mg oxprenolol per day) that was preceded by a run-in period, demonstrated a significant antianginal benefit with oxprenolol in 17 of 18 patients.[124] These results were confirmed in a double-blind, placebo-controlled study performed by Taylor and Thadani.[125] A single oral dose of 160 mg was effective in improving exercise tolerance, in attenuating exercise tachycardia and decreasing systolic blood pressure. Maximal effects were noted 1 h post dose and declined slowly over 8 h.

Forrest utilized a placebo-controlled, randomized, double-blind design to assess the comparative antianginal efficacies of oxprenolol (40 mg) and practolol (100 mg).[126] Both agents were equally effective in decreasing the frequency of anginal attacks and nitroglycerin consumption. Other studies comparing oxprenolol with other beta blockers were described earlier.[111,112]

TRIALS WITH SUSTAINED-RELEASE OXPRENOLOL

Forrest conducted a study in which 102 patients were treated in an open-protocol study with once-daily, sustained-release oxprenolol (160 mg per tablet).[127] Eighty-eight patients were successfully managed on once-daily oxprenolol, and 70 percent achieved significant benefit with a single morning dose of 160 mg. The mean number of anginal attacks and mean nitroglycerin consumption were both significantly reduced. Majid et al.

compared the antianginal efficacy of sustained-release oxprenolol (160 mg/day) and conventional propranolol (40 mg three times daily) in a double-blind, randomized, placebo-controlled, crossover study in 18 patients.[128] Relative to placebo values, both agents comparably reduced the frequency and severity of anginal attacks, prolonged exercise tolerance, and decreased exercise heart rate.

More recently Olowoyeye et al. compared sustained-release oxprenolol (160 mg/day) to propranolol (40 mg four times daily).[129] Twenty-three patients participated in this randomized, double-blind, crossover trial. The overall antianginal efficacy of the two drugs did not significantly differ. Resting heart rate was significantly higher 7½ and 24 h following a dose of oxprenolol than it was 4 and 12 h after a propranolol dose. Exercise tolerance 24 h post oxprenolol was significantly less than 7½ h after oxprenolol and less than 4 and 12 h post propranolol.

Pindolol

Pindolol (Visken) is a nonselective beta blocker with intrinsic sympathomimetic activity and no membrane stabilizing effect or beta 1 selectivity. Pindolol is not approved for clinical use in angina pectoris in the United States.

TRIALS VERSUS PLACEBO

Leary and Asmal assessed the antianginal efficacy of 15 to 25 mg of pindolol daily in 15 patients with chronic angina and coexistent moderate hypertension.[130] The investigators used a single-blind, randomized design. In this study, pindolol was found to be effective in decreasing supine and erect blood pressure, the frequency of anginal episodes, and nitroglycerin consumption.

In a randomized, double-blind, crossover study of 20 patients, Storstein investigated the effects of IV (0.4 mg) pindolol and oral pindolol (5 mg three times daily) on exercise tolerance and electrocardiographic ST-segment changes.[131] Pindolol significantly decreased heart rate at rest and during exercise. The time intervals before the appearance of ST-segment depression were significantly increased, and exercise tolerance was enhanced.

In two recent studies, pindolol was demonstrated to have, at best, a modest beneficial effect in patients with angina pectoris.[132,133] Each of these trials employed a double-blind, crossover protocol design and studied 12 patients with chronic stable angina and documented coronary artery disease. Dwyer et al. found that pindolol (15 mg/day and 30 mg/day) slightly decreased the number of anginal episodes and nitroglycerin tablets consumed while showing evidence of beta blockade during exercise.[132] However, they could not demonstrate any effect on exercise endurance with either dose. Harston and Friesinger demonstrated that a dosage of 5 mg four times daily of pindolol did not significantly reduce nitroglycerin consumption and anginal episodes.[133] Also treadmill exercise tolerance and ST-segment depression with exercise were not significantly altered. However, there was a statistically significant reduction in myocardial oxygen demand as measured by the double-product of blood pressure and pulse during exercise. The investigators concluded that pindolol significantly reduced myocardial oxygen demand, but clinical ischemia was not significantly reduced. They suggested possible mechanisms to explain the disparity between reduction in estimated myocardial oxygen demand (double-product) and objective improvement in ischemia.[134] These include coronary spasm and altered regional flow resulting from beta blockade. Alternative explanations proposed were the relatively small fixed dose of pindolol and the small number of patients studied in their trial.[133,134]

COMPARATIVE TRIALS

Frishman et al. in a large, placebo-controlled clinical study of 41 patients with classical angina pectoris observed that pindolol (10 to 40 mg/day in four divided doses) reduced angina attacks (Fig. 6) and nitroglycerin

consumption and increased exercise tolerance (Fig. 7) at least as effectively as propranolol (40 to 160 mg/day in four divided doses).[20,50] Both drugs effectively blunted increments in blood pressure and heart rate with exercise. However, unlike propranolol, pindolol with partial agonist activity did not affect the resting heart rate (Fig. 8). The investigators concluded that although beta blocking drugs are effective in patients with angina pectoris of effort, in patients with angina pectoris at rest or with low heart rates, propranolol and other beta blockers without partial agonist activity would probably have a distinct advantage over pindolol.

Cocco et al. assessed the comparative antianginal efficacy of pindolol (10 mg three times daily) and nifedipine (10 mg three times daily) in 42 patients with stable angina utilizing a single-blind, randomized, parallel study protocol.[135,136] Pindolol and nifedipine were found to cause equal reductions in angina attacks and nitroglycerin consumption while improving exercise tolerance. Exercise heart rate was slightly decreased with pindolol and slightly increased with nifedipine. Nifedipine was found to be more effective in relieving asymptomatic myocardial ischemia than pindolol.

Propranolol

Propranolol (Inderal, Inderal-LA) is nonselective with membrane stabilizing activity and no intrinsic sympathomimetic activity. There have been many trials of propranolol using different daily dosages that have demonstrated its clinical effectiveness in angina.[137,138] Propranolol is approved for clinical use in angina in the United States as a conventional tablet and as a long-acting sustained-release capsule.

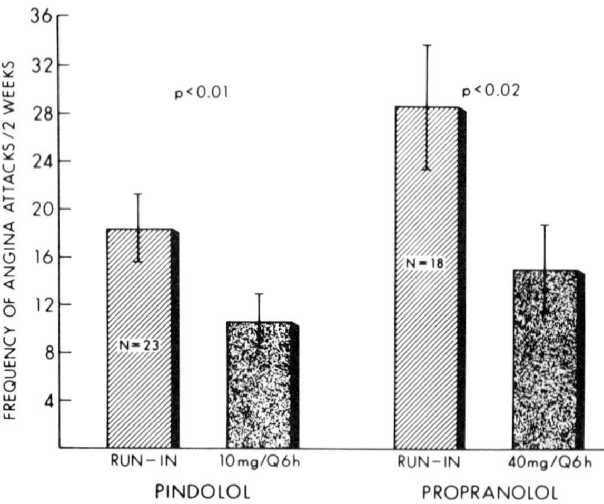

FIGURE 6 Effects of pindolol and propranolol on angina attack frequency. A significant decrease in the frequency of anginal attacks in 2 weeks is seen with both pindolol 40 mg/day and propranolol 160 mg/day compared to the run-in period. There was no significant difference in the effectiveness of the two drugs in reducing the frequency of angina attacks. *(From W. H. Frishman, J. Kostis, J. Strom, et al., A Comparison of Pindolol and Propranolol in Treatment of Patients with Angina Pectoris: The Role of Intrinsic Sympathomimetic Activity, Am. Heart J., 98:526, 1979.[50] Used with permission.)*

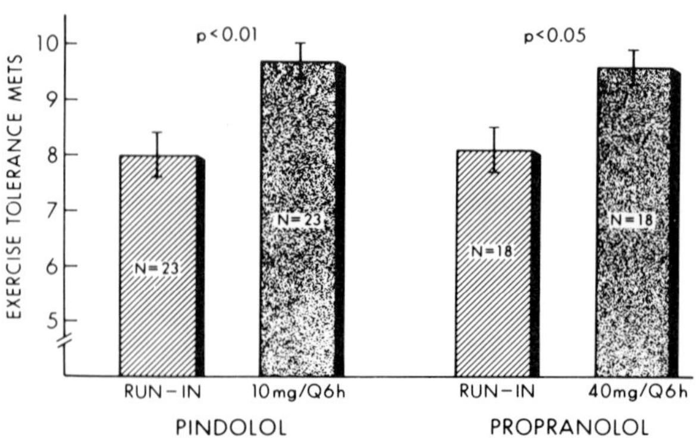

FIGURE 7 Effects of pindolol and propranolol on exercise tolerance in patients with angina pectoris. A significant improvement in mean total work performance occurs with both pindolol and propranolol compared to the run-in period. *(From W. H. Frishman, J. Kostis, J. Strom, et al., A Comparison of Pindolol and Propranolol in Treatment of Patients with Angina Pectoris. The Role of Intrinsic Sympathomimetic Activity, Am. Heart J., 98:526, 1979.[50] Used with permission.)*

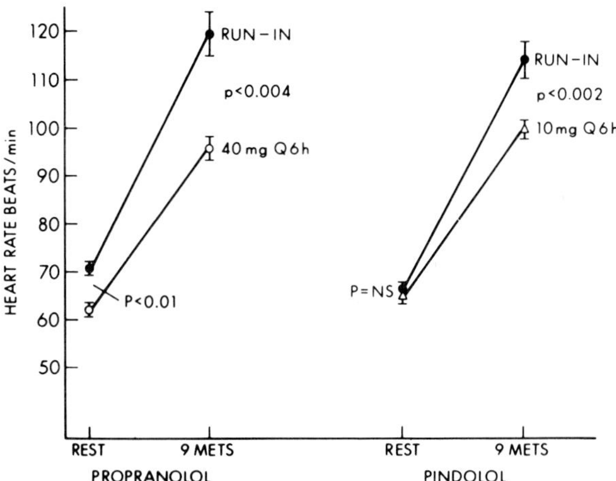

FIGURE 8 Effects of pindolol and propranolol on heart rate at rest and during exercise (9 mets). A significant decrease in the resting heart rate and the heart rate increment with exercise is seen with propranolol (160 mg/day) compared to the run-in period. There is no change in the resting heart rate in patients treated with pindolol (40 mg/day). However, the heart rate increment with exercise is significantly blunted. *(From W. H. Frishman, J. Kostis, J. Strom, et al., A Comparison of Pindolol and Propranolol in Treatment of Patients with Angina Pectoris. The Role of Intrinsic Sympathomimetic Activity, Am. Heart J., 98:526, 1979.[50] Used with permission.)*

A dose-dependent reduction of anginal attacks with propranolol was well demonstrated in an early study by Prichard and Gillam.[139] Sixteen patients were administered four different dose levels of propranolol and placebo in a double-blind fashion. The average doses ranged from 0 (placebo) to 417 mg/day. As the dosage increased, there was a progressive decrease in the number of anginal attacks and in the amount of nitroglycerin used, giving a linear dose-response curve, whose slope did not flatten even at the 417-mg dosage level (suggesting that maximum effect had not yet been obtained).

Alderman et al. conducted a double-blind, placebo-controlled, randomized, crossover study in 17 patients assessing the comparative efficacy of doses of 80, 160, and 320 mg of propranolol.[140] Significant decreases in the frequency of anginal episodes and nitroglycerin consumption were noted with 160 mg and 320 mg. A significant improvement in exercise tolerance was only achieved with 320 mg. Resting heart rate was significantly decreased by all three doses. While standing systolic blood pressure was significantly decreased by all three doses, standing diastolic blood pressure and supine diastolic and systolic blood pressures were not. The investigators also confirmed the prominent linear relationship between clinical response and the log of the propranolol dosage which was noted previously by Prichard and Gillam.[139]

Thadani and Parker assessed the comparative duration of effect of single oral doses of 80 and 160 mg of propranolol during acute and sustained therapy in nine patients.[141,142] Treadmill walking time to onset of angina, total duration of exercise, and total external work performed were significantly increased 1, 8, and 12 h post dose with both acute and sustained therapy. Similar effects were observed with 80 and 160 mg. The improvement in exercise tolerance was accompanied by a significant decrease in the magnitude of ST-segment depression. Rest and exercise heart rates, systolic blood pressure, and double-product were significantly reduced with propranolol. These effects were noted 12 and 24 h post dose.

In a more recent trial involving 25 patients, Thadani and Parker investigated the comparative efficacy of propranolol given twice a day or four times a day.[143] The same total daily dose of 160 or 320 mg was administered with each dosing regimen. A double-blind, crossover, randomized design was used in this trial. Similar results were obtained in the frequency of anginal episodes, prolongation of exercise time, reduction in ST-segment depression, and decrease in heart rate, systolic blood pressure, and double-product with both dosage regimens. The investigators concluded that in the treatment of stable angina, propranolol given twice daily is as effective as the same dose given four times daily.

TRIALS WITH SUSTAINED-RELEASE PROPRANOLOL

The comparative antianginal efficacy of standard formulation propranolol (40 mg four times daily) and sustained-release propranolol (160 mg once daily) was assessed in a double-blind, placebo-controlled, crossover, randomized trial in eight patients.[144] The frequencies of anginal episodes and nitroglycerin consumption were decreased by both formulations. The peak heart rate increment was reduced by both long-acting and standard propranolol, as was the maximal double-product and the degree of ST-segment depression.

The equivalent antianginal efficacy of long-acting propranolol (160 mg once daily) and standard propranolol (40 mg four times daily) was further supported in a trial by Parker et al.[145] Twenty patients participated in this double-blind, crossover, placebo-controlled, randomized study. A similar reduction in anginal episodes and nitroglycerin consumption was observed with both formulations. Resting values for heart rate, systolic blood pressure, and rate-pressure product were similar when determined 25.4 h after a dose of long-acting propranolol and 10.7 h after standard propranolol. When the patients exercised at these times, patients on long-acting propranolol and standard propranolol had similar walking times to the onset of angina and to the development of moderate angina. The values for heart rate, systolic blood pressure, and rate-pressure product were similar at rest and during exercise during these two treatment programs. Sustained-release propranolol has recently received FDA approval for once daily use in angina.

COMPARATIVE STUDIES

See above "Acebutolol," "Atenolol," "Metoprolol," "Nadolol," "Oxprenolol," and "Pindolol."

Eleven patients participated in a short-term, single-blind, randomized, crossover trial by Leon et al. to assess the comparative antianginal efficacy of propranolol (160 to 320 mg/day), verapamil (480 mg/day), and a combination of these two drugs (propranolol optimal dose, verapamil 160 to 480 mg).[146] Each of the regimens significantly increased exercise time, with propranolol having the least effect and the combination the greatest.

The comparative efficacy of propranolol and verapamil was further investigated by Johnson et al. in a double-blind, randomized, placebo-controlled, crossover study involving 18 patients.[147] Doses of propranolol, 40 mg and 80 mg every 6 h, and verapamil, 80 mg and 120 mg every 6 h, were administered to the participants. Low- and high-dose propranolol as well as high-dose verapamil significantly reduced the frequency of anginal episodes, while nitroglycerin consumption was only significantly reduced by high-dose verapamil. Episodes of ST-segment deviations noted on 24-h ambulatory ECG monitoring were decreased only with high-dose verapamil. Propranolol alone produced a significant reduction in resting heart rate. Peak heart rate was significantly decreased with both agents but significantly more with propranolol. Verapamil significantly decreased resting systolic blood pressure while propranolol significantly reduced exercise systolic blood pressure. Both agents produced a significant and comparable reduction in exercise-induced ST-segment deviation.

In addition, a study was conducted by Subramanian et al.[149] comparing the antianginal effects of propranolol and verapamil used alone and as combination therapy. Twenty-two patients participated in this double-blind, placebo-controlled, crossover study (verapamil 360 mg/day; propranolol 240 mg/day; verapamil 360 mg/day and propranolol 120 mg/day). A significant increase in exercise time was observed with all three regimens. The combination had a significantly greater effect than verapamil alone, which in turn was significantly better than propranolol.

In another double-blind, randomized, crossover trial, Frishman et al. further demonstrated the comparable effectiveness of verapamil and propranolol in patients with stable angina.[148]

Lynch et al. conducted a double-blind, placebo-controlled, randomized, crossover study to assess the comparative antianginal efficacy of propranolol (240 and 480 mg/day) and nifedipine (30 and 60 mg daily) and a combination of both drugs.[150] The incidence of anginal pain and nitroglycerin consumption were significantly decreased with both drugs when compared with placebo, but propranolol produced significantly greater reductions than nifedipine for both variables. While there was no significant difference between the propranolol doses, the higher dose of nifedipine produced a significantly greater reduction in these variables than the lower dose. When the higher doses of these two drugs were combined, an additional decrease in anginal frequency and nitroglycerin consumption was observed. Furthermore, the number of episodes of ST-segment depression observed on a Holter electrocardiogram significantly decreased from placebo base line with both agents used alone, and a significantly greater effect was noted with the combination.

In a double-blind, placebo-controlled, randomized, crossover trial Kenmure and Scruton further assessed the comparative efficacy of nifedipine (10 mg three times daily), propranolol (80 mg three times daily), and a combination (nifedipine 10 mg three times daily and propranolol 40 mg three times daily).[151] Twenty-one patients participated in the study. Both agents used alone significantly reduced the frequency of anginal episodes, with propranolol having a greater effect (not statistically significant) than nifedipine. The drug combination had the greatest effect. Comparable results were seen relating to nitroglycerin consumption. Nifedipine produced no change in heart rate but did cause a significant fall in systolic and diastolic blood pressures. Propranolol caused a significant decrease in both heart rate and blood pressure. The combination produced a lesser reduction in heart rate than with propranolol alone, but a greater fall in both systolic and diastolic blood pressures.

These results were supported by a double-blind, placebo-controlled, randomized, crossover trial conducted by Dargie et al.[152] Sixteen patients participated in this study, which utilized 30 and 60 mg/day of nifedipine and 240 and 280 mg/day of propranolol. The frequency of angina and consumption of nitroglycerin tablets were significantly decreased by all active treatments. The effect of propranolol was slightly greater than that of nifedipine. Although the high dose of propranolol provided no additional benefit, nifedipine at 60 mg/day was significantly more effective than nifedipine at 30 mg/day for both parameters. A further significant reduction in both variables occurred with the high-dose combination of propranolol and nifedipine. Both propranolol and nifedipine alone significantly reduced the area of exercise-induced ST-segment depression, with the combination producing an additional reduction. The combination and propranolol alone produced a significant and comparable reduction in double-product. All three dosage regimens significantly reduced the episodes of ST-segment depression seen on Holter ECG monitoring with a greater reduction with combination treatment. Resting systolic and diastolic blood pressures were decreased with the higher doses of nifedipine and propranolol alone and by both doses of the combination. Propranolol and combination therapy significantly decreased exercise systolic blood pressure and resting heart rate.

In two additional studies, the antianginal efficacy and safety of combined nifedipine-propranolol treatment was confirmed.[153,154]

Sotalol

Sotalol (Betacordone, Sotacor) has no intrinsic sympathomimetic activity, no membrane stabilizing activity, and no cardioselectivity. Sotalol is not available for clinical use in the United States.

TRIALS VERSUS PLACEBO

In a fixed, multidose level (80, 160, 320, 640, 1,280 mg sotalol per day) trial in nine patients, Toubes et al. demonstrated a significant decrease in the frequency and severity of anginal attacks and a reduction in nitroglycerin consumption at all dose levels.[155] Contrasting results were obtained in a double-blind crossover trial of 15 patients performed by Kentala et al.[156] A fixed daily dose of 160 mg was utilized in this study. Sotalol was observed to significantly decrease resting heart rate and systolic blood pressure with a significant increase in heart volume. The frequency of anginal attacks and nitroglycerin consumption were not significantly altered; however, a relatively low drug dose was utilized. Sotalol was found to decrease significantly the number and intensity of anginal attacks in a double-blind crossover study of 69 patients conducted by Milei and Fortunato.[157] The antianginal efficacy of sotalol was further supported by the results of a double-blind, crossover study of 17 patients conducted by Slome, who determined that 320 mg of sotalol (160 mg twice daily) was effective in significantly decreasing the mean number of angina attacks, nitroglycerin consumption, and heart rate at rest and during exercise.[158] This dosage regimen also significantly improved exercise tolerance.

Timolol

Timolol (Blocadren) is a drug which has no beta 1 selectivity, intrinsic sympathomimetic activity, or membrane stabilizing activity. This drug is not approved for clinical use in the United States for the treatment of angina pectoris.

TRIALS VERSUS PLACEBO

Brailovsky, using an average dose of 30 mg of timolol in a large multinational, multicenter trial in 390 patients, found a highly significant reduction in the frequency of anginal attacks and nitroglycerin consumption compared with placebo.[159]

In a 2-day double-blind, randomized, crossover investigation of 16 patients, Villa et al. showed that timolol, compared to placebo, significantly increased exercise duration, decreased resting and exercise double-product, and delayed the onset of ischemic ST-segment depression during exercise.[160]

The beneficial effects of timolol were also demonstrated by Aronow et al. in a double-blind, randomized, crossover study of 23 patients with chronic angina.[161] Utilizing the optimal timolol dose for each patient (10 to 30 mg twice daily) these investigators found that compared to placebo, timolol significantly reduced anginal frequency, nitroglycerin consumption, resting and exercise heart rate and blood pressure (systolic and diastolic), and double-product. Timolol also prolonged exercise duration and reduced electrocardiographic manifestations of myocardial ischemia.

DiSegni et al. in a single-blind, controlled study of 20 stable angina patients assessed the efficacy of timolol in doses of 10 to 30 mg/day.[162] They determined that timolol caused a significant decrease in the number of anginal attacks and nitroglycerin consumption. Significant reductions in resting heart rate and blood pressure and exercising blood pressure were also noted. Work capacity was found to improve significantly.

Aronow et al., in the most recent of these trials, investigated the effect of timolol on exercise duration 2 h and 12 h post ingestion.[163] Doses of 10 to 30 mg of timolol twice daily were used in this double-blind, randomized, crossover study of seven patients. Exercise duration to angina or marked fatigue was prolonged in 100 percent of patients 2 h after drug ingestion and in 43 percent of patients 12 h post dose. The mean exercise duration was significantly increased at both testing intervals.

COMBINED USE OF BETA BLOCKERS WITH OTHER ANTIANGINAL THERAPIES IN STABLE ANGINA
Nitrates

Combined therapy with nitrates and beta blockers may be more efficacious for treatment of angina pectoris than either drug alone (Table 5).[164] The primary effect of beta blockers is a reduction of resting heart rate and the heart rate response to exercise. Since nitrates produce a reflex increase in heart rate owing to a re-

48

TABLE 5

Hemodynamic effects of nitrates, beta blockers, and combination treatment

	Nitrates	Beta blockers	Combination
1 Heart rate	↑ (reflex)	↓	↓ ↔
2 Contractility	↑ (reflex)	↓	↔
3 Wall tension:	↓	↔	↓
a Systemic blood pressure	↓	↓	↓
b Left ventricular volume	↓	↑	↔ ↑
4 Coronary resistance	↓	↑ ↔	↓ ↔

TABLE 6

Hemodynamic effects of calcium-entry blockers, beta blockers, and combination treatment

	Ca^{2+} blockers	Beta blockers	Combination
1 Heart rate	↓ ↔ ↑ (reflex)	↓	↓ ↔
2 Contractility	↓ ↔ (reflex)	↓	↓ ↔
3 Wall tension:	↓	↔	↓
a Systolic blood pressure	↓	↓	↓
b Left ventricular volume	↓ ↔	↑	↑ ↔
4 Coronary resistance	↓	↑ ↔	↓ ↔

duction in arterial pressure, concomitant beta blocker therapy will be extremely effective because it will block this reflex increase in heart rate. Similarly, the preservation of diastolic coronary flow with a reduced heart rate will also be beneficial.[30] In patients with the potential for further heart failure who might have a slight increase in heart size with the beta blockers, the nitrates will counteract this tendency by reducing heart size due to peripheral venodilation. During the administration of nitrates, the reflex increase in contractility that is mediated through the sympathetic nervous system will be checked by the presence of beta blockers. Similarly, the increase in coronary resistance associated with beta blocker administration can be ameliorated by the administration of nitrates.[164]

Calcium-Entry Blockers

Calcium-entry blockers are a new group of antianginal drugs which block transmembrane calcium currents in vascular smooth muscle to cause vasodilation. Some calcium-entry blockers also will slow the heart rate and reduce atrioventricular conduction. Combined therapy of beta-adrenergic and calcium-entry blockers can provide substantial clinical benefits for patients with angina pectoris who remain symptomatic with either agent used alone (Table 6).[149,150–153] Because adverse effects can occur, however, patients being considered for such treatment need to be carefully selected and observed.[165]

ANGINA AT REST AND VASOSPASTIC ANGINA

Although beta blockers are effective in the treatment of patients with angina of effort, clinical studies in patients with angina at rest have largely been based on uncontrolled observations and have proved inconclusive. The rationale for therapy with beta blockers was based on an approach which considered the pathogenesis of chest pain at rest to be similar to that in patients with exertional symptoms. Recent studies, however, have emphasized that angina pectoris can be caused by multiple mechanisms and that coronary vasospasm is responsible for ischemia in a significant proportion of patients with angina at rest.[166,167] Therefore, drugs such as propranolol and other beta blockers that primarily reduce myocardial oxygen consumption but fail to exert vasodilating effects on the coronary vasculature may not be effective in patients in whom angina is caused by dynamic alterations in coronary luminal diameter rather than by an increase in myocardial metabolic demands.[168,169] Despite their theoretical dangers in rest and vasospastic angina, beta blockers have been successfully used alone and in combination with vasodilating agents.[170]

ADVERSE EFFECTS OF BETA BLOCKERS IN TREATMENT OF ANGINA PECTORIS

Any serious side effects of beta blockers are related to their beta-adrenergic blocking activity and are similar to those of propranolol.[1,2,28] It should be emphasized that the occurrence of unwanted depression of myocardial, electrical, and mechanical functions by beta-adrenergic blockers is related to the dependence of these functions in some patients on stimulation of the sympathetic nervous system rather than to the specific blocker or its dose within the therapeutic range.[28] Similarly, beta blockers will interfere with ventilatory function only in patients dependent on stimulation of beta 2–adrenoreceptors, i.e., patients with asthma or chronic obstructive pulmonary disease.

Other side effects of beta blockers have been rather uncommon and are generally mild and transient. Fatigue and dizziness have occurred in about 2 percent of patients. Nausea, diarrhea, abdominal discomfort, constipation, vomiting, indigestion, anorexia, bloating, and flatulence have been reported frequently, as have rashes, dry eyes, and dry mouth.[128] The oculomucocutaneous syndrome associated with the beta blocker practolol has not been reported with any other beta blocker.[28] Potential side effects of other beta blockers used in angina but not yet reported with nadolol include reversible mental depression and decreased performance on neuropsychometric tests.[19] Nadolol and atenolol with their low brain penetrations have been stated to cause fewer central nervous system side effects than the more lipophilic propranolol; however, further comparative studies need to be performed to substantiate this claim.[18,19]

BETA-ADRENOCEPTOR BLOCKER WITHDRAWAL

Following the abrupt cessation of beta blocker therapy after chronic administration, exacerbation of angina pectoris and, in some cases, acute myocardial infarction have been reported.[171,172] Two early double-blind randomized trials confirmed the reality of a propranolol withdrawal syndome.[173,174] The mechanism for the propranolol withdrawal effect is unclear and may be related to the multifactorial actions of the drug.[11] Reduced exercise tolerance following abrupt withdrawal of chronic propranolol therapy in patients with angina pectoris may be due to loss of sympathetic blockade of cardiovascular function resulting in an acute increase in myocardial oxygen demands. Our group demonstrated that abrupt propranolol withdrawal can possibly harm some patients with angina pectoris by causing rebound platelet hyperaggregability associated with increased anginal frequency, decreased exercise tolerance, and possible compromise of coronary blood flow.[175]

A "rebound" effect has not been well-defined with the other beta blocking agents. When necessary, it would appear prudent to discontinue beta blocker therapy gradually and cautiously in patients with ischemic heart disease.

BETA BLOCKER THERAPY IN MYOCARDIAL INFARCTION

Beta-Adrenoceptor Blockade as Protective Therapy in the Early Phase of Acute Myocardial Infarction and for Preinfarction Angina

In patients with acute myocardial infarction the presence of severe pain, tissue injury, and circulatory disturbances creates important physiological stresses which trigger an increased sympathoadrenal discharge.[51] This observation is based on evidence derived from several clinical studies in which measurements of urinary free catecholamine excretion and plasma catecholamine levels were elevated.[51]

An increase in sympathetic tone following myocardial infarction may have an important supportive role in maintaining contractile function in ischemic areas of the myocardium, as well as enhancing residual nonischemic areas.[51] However, there are two important and potentially deleterious consequences of an increase in sympathetic nervous activity. First, increased sympathoadrenal discharge may be the cause of serious cardiac arrhythmias after myocardial infarction. Second, the positive inotropic and chronotropic effects of catecholamines lead to an increase in total cardiac work and myocardial oxygen consumption by causing increments in heart rate, blood pressure, and contractility.[51] This may be critical in areas of the heart that may be receiving very limited blood flow and could extend necrosis.[51]

Beta-adrenergic blockers have been considered for use as standard therapy in patients with acute myocardial infarction to prevent the undesirable consequences of increased sympathoadrenal discharge: arrhythmogenesis and extension of myocardial injury.[5] These agents can reduce the determinants of increased myocardial oxygen consumption and may augment coronary blood flow by increasing diastolic perfusion time.[30] On the other hand, beta-adrenergic blockade can have unfavorable consequences in some cases of fresh infarction.[51] Cardiac impulse formation may be greatly impaired and conduction diminished to a degree that causes cardiac arrest. Furthermore, exacerbation of congestive heart failure in patients dependent on the positive inotropic effects of catecholamines is a well-recognized sequela of beta blockade.[51]

USE OF BETA BLOCKERS IN HEMODYNAMICALLY STABLE SURVIVORS OF MYOCARDIAL INFARCTION LATE IN THE HOSPITAL COURSE

Although beta blockers have been suggested for reducing the extent of myocardial injury and mortality during the acute phase of myocardial infarction, their role in this situation remains unclear.[176,177] Recent clinical trials of 1 to 2 years of treatment have demonstrated that some beta blockers are effective in reducing the risk of cardiovascular mortality and reinfarction in patients who are recovering from acute myocardial infarction.[3,4,176,178–189] The value of beta blockade in survivors of an acute myocardial infarction and the implications for clinical practice are described below.

The Clinical Problem

More than 500,000 patients are admitted to hospitals each year in the United States with a diagnosis of acute myocardial infarction.[190] For those with a first infarction there is a 12 to 18 percent hospital mortality rate, the figure being somewhat higher for those with recurrent infarction.[80] On discharge from the hospital, the patients remain at increased risk of cardiovascular morbidity and mortality. Patients under 70 years of age who survive a myocardial infarction have a 10 percent mortality rate during the first year, with a high proportion of the deaths occurring in the first 3 months.[80] Subsequent to the first year, there is a 4 to 6 percent annual mortality rate, which is four to eight times greater than that expected in an age-matched noncoronary population.[80] Approximately 85 percent of the deaths which occur after hospitalization for myocardial infarction are related to coronary artery disease, and almost half of them are sudden. Ventricular fibrillation is the primary mechanism for the sudden death.

A major goal of preventive treatment is to prolong life in the heterogeneous group of patients who are recovering from an acute myocardial infarction. A variety of therapeutic measures have been examined in an attempt to reach this goal, ranging from life-style measures (dietary modification, cessation of smoking, physical exercise), to specific drug treatments, to coronary reconstructive surgery.[80] Pharmacologic interventions have included anticoagulants,[191] drugs that inhibit platelet aggregation,[192] lipid-lowering agents,[193] calcium-entry blockers,[194] and antiarrhythmic drugs.[80] None of these interventions have been proved to be efficacious for reducing the risk of cardiovascular death in patients surviving the acute phase of myocardial infarction.[80] Of the multiple interventions evaluated, beta-adrenergic blockade is the only treatment modality clearly demonstrated to be effective.

Beta Blockade in the Postinfarction Period

For 20 years beta blockers have been used for the treatment of angina pectoris and arrhythmias. After the clinical introduction of propranolol in 1963, it was proposed that beta blocker administration might also offer the possibility of modifying the natural history of myocardial infarction by preventing the undesirable consequences of sympathoadrenal discharge.[195,196] However, since these drugs can depress left ventric-

ular function, beta blockers were initially avoided, or were used in dosages which today we would consider too small,[195–200] for fear of precipitating symptomatic heart failure in the already compromised myocardium. Only recently have long-term clinical trials provided evidence for the efficacy and safety of beta blocker therapy in prolonging life in patients surviving the acute phase of myocardial infarction.

THE LONG-TERM BETA BLOCKER POSTINFARCTION TRIALS
Trial Design

Since 1974, 11 major randomized controlled trials of beta blockers after myocardial infarction have been reported with treatment and mean patient follow-up extending from 9 to 48 months (Table 7).[3,4,178–189] Over 14,000 survivors of acute myocardial infarction were studied in attempts to document a reduction in total mortality rate, cardiovascular mortality rate, coronary mortality rate, sudden death, and nonfatal reinfarction. Six different beta blockers have been evaluated in these studies—alprenolol, oxprenolol, practolol, propranolol, sotalol, and timolol.[3,4,178–179] Long-term trials evaluating the beta blockers metoprolol and pindolol have been completed, but the findings are not yet available.

The size of each of the 11 trials, specification of the active intervention employed, the time between the infarct and the onset of treatment, and the duration of treatment are given in Table 7. In the presentation, all patients randomized have been included in the mortality rate estimates in order to maintain the randomization and reduce the potential bias induced by differential withdrawal of patients in the analysis.

Trial Results

The three trials from Scandinavia evaluating alprenolol (nonselective beta blocker with membrane stabilizing activity and intrinsic sympathomimetic activity) in the postinfarction population were the smallest of the 11 (Table 8).[178–182] Alprenolol is not available for clinical use in the United States. A statistically significant reduction in total mortality rate by the drug was not observed in any of these trials.[178–182] Wilhelmsson et al. and Ahlmark et al. reported a borderline significant effect on the incidence of sudden death, defined as death within 24 h from onset of symptoms.[180,181] In both trials, however, there were more nonsudden deaths in the alprenolol group than among the controls. The nonblinded study by Ahlmark et al. did report a significant reduction in the incidence of recurrent nonfatal myo-

TABLE 7
Design of long-term beta blocker trials

Trial	Patients randomized	Beta blocker	Daily dose (mg)	Mean entry time after MI	Mean length of follow-up (mo)
Wilhelmsson et al.[178,179]	230	Alprenolol	400	7–21 days after discharge	24
Ahlmark et al.[180,181]	393	Alprenolol	400	14 days after diagnosis	24
Barber et al.[183]	500	Practolol	600	< 1.0 days	24
Multicentre International Study[184,185]	3,053	Practolol	400	13.2 days	14
Andersen et al.[182]	480	Alprenolol	400	< 1.0 day	12
Baber et al.[186]	720	Propranolol	120	8.5 days	9
Norwegian Multicenter Study[3]	1,884	Timolol	20	11.5 days	17
BHAT[4]*	3,738	Propranolol	180–240	13.8 days	25
Hansteen et al.[187]	560	Propranolol	160	4–6 days	12
Julian et al.[188]	1,456	Sotalol	320	8.3 days	12
Taylor et al.[189]	1,103	Oxprenolol	80	14 mo†	48

*BHAT = Beta Blocker Heart Attack Trial.

†Time between infarction and entry into trial ranged from under 1 month to 7½ years.

cardial infarction, but design shortcomings limit the firm conclusions that can be drawn from this trial.[180,181]

Barber et al.[183] using the beta 1–selective blocker practolol (intrinsic sympathomimetic activity but no membrane activity) and initiating treatment upon hospital admission, did not observe any significant effect of treatment on survival. In contrast, the International Multicentre Study of practolol, a trial which was dis-continued earlier than scheduled because of the drug's toxicity, did note a 23 percent reduction in total mortality rate with the beta blocker, but this barely reached statistical significance.[184,185] Retrospective analysis, which must be interpreted cautiously, of the patient subgroup which remained in this trial suggested that any benefit of practolol on mortality rate was limited to patients with anterior wall infarcts. The oral prep-

TABLE 8
Results of long-term beta blocker trials

Trial	Patients randomized		Mortality rate (%)		
	Control	Intervention	Control	Intervention	*p* value*
Wilhelmsson et al.[178,179]	116	114	12.1	6.1	0.18
Ahlmark et al.[180,181]†	93	69	11.8	7.2	0.48
Barber et al.[183†‡]	147	151	31.3	27.2	0.51
Multicentre International[184,185]	1,520	1,533	8.2	6.3	0.051
Andersen et al.[182‡]	242	238	26.2	25.2	0.92
Baber et al.[186]	365	355	7.4	7.9	0.91
Norwegian Multicenter[3]	939	945	16.2	10.4	0.0003
BHAT[4§]	1,921	1,916	9.8	7.2	0.005
Hansteen et al.[187]	282	278	13.1	9.0	0.16
Julian et al.[188]	583	873	8.9	7.3	0.32
Taylor et al.[189]	471	632	10.2	9.5	0.78

*p values computed for chi-square test comparing the proportion of deaths in each group.

†Incomplete reporting.

‡Mortality rates include all inhospital deaths.

§BHAT = Beta Blocker Heart Attack Trial.

aration of practolol is no longer available for clinical use because of the oculomucocutaneous syndrome attributed to it.

The Norwegian Multicenter Group[3] demonstrated that timolol (nonselective beta blocker without membrane or intrinsic sympathomimetic activity), in a fixed dose of 20 mg/day in two divided doses, was of clear benefit in reducing total mortality rate by 36 percent and the rate of nonfatal reinfarction by 32 percent over an average follow-up period of 17 months. In contrast to the findings with alprenolol[182] and practolol,[184,185] the benefit of timolol was evident regardless of age and site of infarct.

The three trials of propranolol (nonselective beta blocker with membrane activity and no sympathomimetic activity) differ with regard to dosage schedule and patient population.[4,186,187] Baber et al.,[186] who restricted their trial to patients with anterior wall infarctions, used 120 mg daily. Hansteen et al. only studied high-risk survivors of a myocardial infarction and gave 160 mg in four divided doses.[187] The patients enrolled into the Beta Blocker Heart Attack Trial (BHAT) were predominately from the low- and intermediate-risk subsets of the postinfarction population.[4] The dose of propranolol was increased, based on serum drug levels, from 120 mg daily in the first month to 180 or 240 mg daily thereafter. Eighty-two percent of the patients were given 180 mg daily.[4]

The trial by Baber et al., the only study that observed a marginally higher mortality rate in the beta blocker group compared to the placebo group, experienced problems with drug compliance; moreover, the dosage could very well have been too small.[186] The equivalent beta blocking potency of 120 mg propranolol per day is lower than that used in all but one of the other 10 trials.

The Beta Blocker Heart Attack Study Group (BHAT) demonstrated that propranolol reduced mortality rate by 26 percent and the combined rate of coronary events (coronary deaths and nonfatal reinfarctions) by 23 percent over an average patient follow-up period of 25 months.[4,201] Benefit was also evident regardless of age and site of infarct. Similar to the findings of the Norwegian timolol study, the protective effect of propranolol was primarily seen in the first 12 to 18 months of intervention. The first-year placebo mortality rate of 11.3 percent in the timolol study[10] was about twice as high as that seen in BHAT (6 percent),[12] which suggests that a higher-risk population was studied in Norway. In spite of this difference in study populations, the treatment effect was similar with reductions in first-year mortality rate of approximately 33 percent with timolol and 39 percent in BHAT (in both trials patients were followed for a minimum of 1 year).

Survivors of an uncomplicated first infarct who made up over 60 percent of the BHAT population were ex-

cluded from enrollment in the propranolol trial by Hansteen et al.[187] That study reported a statistically significant reduction with propranolol in the incidence of sudden death, the primary end point of the trial. However, the difference of 32 percent in total mortality rate between propranolol and control did not reach statistical significance.

Sotalol (a nonselective beta blocker without membrane activity or intrinsic sympathomimetic activity which also possesses class III antiarrhythmic properties) was evaluted by Julian et al.[188] A statistically nonsignificant favorable trend (18 percent) for total mortality rate was reported. For the combined end point, fatal and nonfatal myocardial infarction, there was a significant difference of 41 percent between the sotalol and placebo groups.[188] Sotalol is not available for clinical use in the United States.

Oxprenolol (a nonselective beta blocker with membrane stabilizing activity and intrinsic sympathomimetic activity) was evaluated by Taylor et al. in low-risk male patients with uncomplicated myocardial infarction.[189] This trial entered patients from 1 month to 7½ years after infarction and provided the longest time for patient follow-up. Similarly to the trial of Baber et al. with propranolol,[186] a low beta blocking dose of oxprenolol (80 mg/day) was used in the study. Overall there was no significant difference in the mortality and nonfatal reinfarction rates between the placebo and oxprenolol treatment groups. Retrospective subgroup analyses suggested that the treatment effect was influenced by the time at which treatment was started after infarction. In patients in whom treatment was started within 4 months of infarction, total mortality rate was lower in the oxprenolol group compared to the placebo group. There was no apparent long-term benefit in mortality rate seen when treatment was started beyond 4 months. Oxprenolol is not available for clinical use in the United States.

INTERPRETATION OF TRIAL RESULTS

Overall, 10 of the 11 long-term trials showed a lower mortality rate in the beta blocker treatment group compared to placebo (Table 8). In three of the studies the difference in mortality rates was statistically significant;[3,4,184,185] in two, this decrease was highly significant;[3,4] and in the third, borderline (Table 8).[184,185]

A statistical test for homogeneity shows that the findings of all 11 trials are consistent with each other. However, this test is somewhat insensitive and does not prove equality. The pooled estimate of benefit for beta blockers is 23 percent. It should be pointed out that in pooling the results, one disregards trial differences in, for example, composition of patient population, type of dosage of intervention, and time of initiation and duration of treatment.

Eight of the nine trials reporting the incidence of nonfatal reinfarction found lower rates in the treatment group.[3,178,181,187–189,201] The most favorable effect was observed in the only nonblinded trial.[180,181] In only one of the trials did this lower incidence reach statistical significance.[3] However, a homogeneity test indicated that the results of each trial were consistent with those of the others.[202] When all the findings from the eight placebo-controlled double-blind trials are pooled, one finds a reduction in nonfatal reinfarction by 23 percent, a benefit identical to that for overall mortality rate.[3,178,187–189,201] Again, caution is advised when interpreting pooled results.

MECHANISM OF THE PROTECTIVE BENEFIT

When cause-specific death is analyzed in the beta blocker trials, it is seen that the reductions in total mortality rate were due to a reduction in cardiovascular and coronary mortality rates.[3,4,176,178–189] Although different definitions of sudden death were employed in the trials, the benefit from beta blocker treatment seems to stem particularly from the prevention of these deaths.[3,4,178,184,185,187,189] However, there is also evidence for a reduction in both nonsudden cardiac death and in nonfatal reinfarctions.[3,4,188,189,202] These findings raise the question of how beta blockers produce their protective actions.

Antiarrhythmic effects It has been shown in the long-term beta blocker postinfarction trials that the incidence of complex ventricular arrhythmias is reduced by these drugs.[188,203] Although they are not powerful antiarrhythmic agents, the beta blockers as a group can attenuate sympathetic cardiac stimulation and perhaps the potential for reentrant ventricular arrhythmias and sudden death.[52,204] The beta blockers can also inhibit lipolysis and reduce stress-induced increases in free fatty acids which can induce ventricular arrhythmias.[205,206]

Anti-ischemic effects Since nonsudden cardiovascular deaths and nonfatal reinfarctions are also reduced by beta blockade, protective mechanisms other than a primary antiarrhythmic effect must be considered. The anti-ischemic actions of the beta blockers may also play a major role in the beneficial effects of these drugs in the postinfarction period.[31]

CLINICAL USE

Although it has been clearly demonstrated that beta blocking drugs can prolong life in the postinfarction population, a number of important questions pertaining to their clinical use remain to be answered—who to treat, when to start and stop treatment, and which drug and dose regimen to use?

Who to treat? The long-term clinical trials have shown that 1 to 2 weeks after the acute event up to 20 percent of infarct survivors have absolute or relative contraindications to beta blockade, such as advanced congestive heart failure, Raynaud's phenomenon, a recent history of bronchial asthma, significant disorders of atrioventricular and sinus node function, and vasospastic angina.[28] This restricts the postinfarction population to whom beta blockade therapy can or should be administered. It appears from the results of the timolol and BHAT trials that the large majority of remaining patients stand to benefit from beta blocker treatment.[3,4] A large number of subgroup analyses conducted in the largest trials have failed to identify with certainty any subset of patients that does not benefit from beta blocker therapy.[3,4] Thus, a relative reduction of approximately 25 percent in total mortality rate in this population can be expected during the period of 1 to 2 years on such therapy. A trend towards an even greater relative benefit has been observed in patients 60 years of age or older and in those who suffered complications during their infarctions (ventricular tachyarrhythmias, mild left ventricular dysfunction).[3,4] Both these subgroups of patients have a fairly high expected mortality rate, making them prime targets for beta blocker treatment.

If the mortality risk of a population subgroup is high (e.g., 20 percent in the first year), treatment of 100 patients would prolong five lives assuming a 25 percent benefit from treatment. In the low-risk population (2 percent mortality in the first year), 1,000 patients would have to be treated to prolong five lives assuming the same relative benefit.

One may therefore question the wisdom of treating low-risk survivors of an acute myocardial infarction with beta blockers, as the hazards and costs of treatment may outweigh the potential benefit of protection from cardiovascular death. In this decision process, one must also consider that the risk of nonfatal reinfarction is favorably influenced by these drugs.[3,188,189,202]

A decision on starting beta blocker therapy in the postinfarction patient should probably be made irrespective of any consideration of performing coronary angiography or other studies to assess the patient's potential benefit from coronary reconstructive surgery. It is not known whether beta blockers are helpful as prophylactic therapy in patients who have undergone successful coronary bypass surgery after their infarction. Considering that the increased risk of morbidity and mortality in the postinfarction population appears to be multifactorial and is probably not totally elimi-

54

nated by coronary bypass surgery, it would seem prudent to administer beta blocker therapy to this population as well. Certainly, postinfarction patients with proven indications for beta blockade (angina pectoris, hypertension, supraventricular tachycardia) should be considered for treatment as these conditions arise.

When to start? The majority of the long-term trials initiated treatment 1 to 3 weeks after the acute event. By that time the patients had started their recovery and were in relatively stable condition. It was a clear advantage to start treatment while the patients were in the hospital. Two trials, the International Multicentre Study and BHAT, have compared the results in hospitalized patients recruited early versus late in the trial entry window.[207] In both it appears, although not definitively, that early initiation (6 to 9 days after the acute event) is advantageous compared to waiting for 2 to 3 weeks. Certainly from these studies there was no evidence of harm from starting treatment earlier.

It has been proposed that treatment be started upon hospital admission in order to reduce the high early inhospital mortality rate.[190] Recently the argument that treatment started within 6 to 12 h may limit infarct size and thereby subsequent mortality rate has been added.[177] A review of the reported acute phase beta blocker trials provides information on this matter.

Sixteen trials have evaluated the effects of acute intervention on early mortality rate, usually 4-week mortality rate.[187,188,196–200,208–217] In 10 of these trials, an oral treatment regimen was employed which was begun probably too late to favorably influence the size of or eventual development of an acute myocardial infarction.[183,196–200,209–213] In 7 of the 10, total mortality rate was higher in the beta blocker group than in the placebo group.[196–200,210,212,213]

In the other six trials, intravenous beta blocker therapy was started immediately (followed by oral treatment) to test whether the early intervention could influence mortality rate, presumably by limiting infarct size.[182,208,214–217] Three of these studies found a higher mortality rate in the beta blocker–treated group compared to a group given placebo therapy,[182,214,215] and three showed a lower mortality rate in the beta blocker group.[208,216,217] One of the latter studies using metoprolol showed a statistically significant reduction in mortality rate.[208] However, this trial had a longer treatment and patient follow-up period than most other acute intervention studies. Judged from the mortality curves, which did not start to diverge until after 5 to 7 days of treatment, the benefit seen with metoprolol may have been related to the 90-day oral maintenance regimen rather than the acute intravenous intervention. A second metoprolol trial which used the same dosage, enrolled all patients within 6 h from onset of symptoms, and also treated for 90 days did not show any benefit.[217]

The question of the value of early beta-adrenergic blocker therapy within 6 to 12 h of myocardial infarction in humans is now being readdressed in four cooperative acute phase trials being carried out in Europe and in the United States.[218] One of these studies using propranolol is the Multicentre Investigation of Limitation of Infarct Size trial (MILIS). Another is the International Study of Infarct Survival (ISIS) which will be testing atenolol eventually in 10,000 patients. At present, beta blockers have not received Federal Drug Administration approval for early intravenous use in patients with myocardial infarction except for the treatment of supraventricular tachyarrhythmias.

In summary, it seems prudent, based on the findings of the Norwegian timolol and BHAT studies, to start oral beta blocker therapy 6 to 9 days after the acute phase of myocardial infarction in hemodynamically stabilized patients who have no major contraindications to this treatment.

There are no conclusive data available regarding the benefit on long-term survival of beta blocker therapy begun months to years after an acute infarction. However, it seems reasonable to assume a beneficial effect on mortality and morbidity rates even if treatment is initiated within a few months after hospital discharge. This view is supported by the retrospective subgroup analyses from the trial of oxprenolol, which suggested benefit if treatment was started within 4 months, but a lack thereof if initiated more than 4 months after the acute infarction.[189]

When to stop? The results of the Norwegian timolol study and BHAT indicate a continuously increasing treatment benefit over approximately 18 months.[3,4] Beyond that point, the interpretation becomes less certain as there are fewer numbers of deaths and only BHAT continued to follow a substantial number of patients.[4]

At present, any decision to continue treatment beyond 18 months has to be based on clinical judgment rather than scientific data. The limited information available from the trials shows more deaths in the placebo group than in the beta blocker group out as far as 48 months.[3,4,189] This would indicate that perhaps there is some sustained benefit from continued treatment. If one is concerned with extended use of these drugs in the general postinfarction population, patients in the high-risk subset of infarct survivors who could potentially benefit the most from therapy with these drugs might nevertheless be a group considered for longer therapy.

Which drug and what dose? Each of the long-term postinfarction trials compared one beta blocking drug against placebo. Since no direct comparisons between drugs are available, it is not known whether any specific beta blocking compound has advantages over another when used as postinfarction therapy. Some investigators argue that the specific pharmacodynamic and pharmacokinetic differences which these drugs manifest (beta 1 selectivity, membrane stabilizing properties, intrinsic sympathomimetic activity, lipid solubility, protein binding) may be important so that the beta blockers are not interchangeable. Other investigators believe that the benefit of beta blocker therapy is conferred by the common class effect of beta 1–adrenergic blockade rather than by a specific compound. This is supported by the clinical trials, since six different beta blockers with varying pharmacologic properties demonstrated favorable trends on patient survival rate.[3,4,178–189]

The evidence at present is strongest for the use of oral timolol or propranolol, which have similar pharmacologic properties. Both drugs have been shown to reduce the risk of cardiovascular mortality in hemodynamically stabilized survivors of an acute myocardial infarction. In late 1981, timolol maleate became the first orally active beta blocker to be approved for this indication at a fixed daily dose of 20 mg to be used in two divided doses.[18] Propranolol will be approved, based primarily on the favorable findings from BHAT.[4] In this study, 180 to 240 mg of oral propranolol was employed in three divided doses and plasma drug levels utilized to monitor the drug regimen.[12] The 180-mg dose to which 82 percent of the patients were assigned is approximately equivalent in pharmacologic potency to 20 mg of timolol.[1,18]

Even though a thrice-daily regimen was tested in BHAT, there are findings that support a twice-daily dosing regimen for propranolol in survivors of myocardial infarction.[219] Both timolol and propranolol have similar plasma half-lives of 4 to 5 h but their pharmacodynamic half-lives are substantially longer, allowing the twice-daily dosing regimens for the treatment of patients with angina pectoris or systemic hypertension.[143,220,221] The pharmacodynamic studies in normal volunteers indicate that clinical beta blockade, as assessed by inhibition of exercise-induced tachycardia, is well-maintained over 24 h whether propranolol is given twice daily or thrice daily in doses of 160 to 240 mg/day.[219] The availability of a long-acting propranolol preparation may even allow once daily administration.

It is still not clear from the trials what the optimal dosage of beta blockers is, and whether a fixed dose beta blocker regimen is preferable for all postinfarction patients who are placed on treatment. Neither issue was carefully evaluated in the reported studies. In some acute and long-term trials of propranolol, there is evidence that with lower propranolol doses no clinical benefit was seen. In addition, high doses may be needed to treat coexisting disease states such as hypertension, arrhythmia, and angina pectoris. Following plasma drug levels is not helpful in determining clinical efficacy but may be used for monitoring patient compliance with the prescribed drug regimen.

Side effects—what are the risks? In making the decision whether or not to treat patients with beta blockers, the risk of treatment must be weighed against the benefit. Severe adverse reactions from beta-adrenoceptor antagonist were fairly infrequent in the long-term postinfarction trials. The proportion of patients taken off beta blockers for medical reasons in the 11 trials ranged from 5.7 to 20.7 percent.[3,4,178–189]

The composition of the patient population, the dosage, and the duration of treatment are factors that need to be considered in comparing these numbers. An enlightening finding in all trials was the high frequency of adverse effects reported by patients in the placebo groups.[3,4] It seems clear that many of the side effects seen with beta blockers are not directly drug-related in these patients with advanced coronary artery disease who are predominantly in the sixth and seventh decades of life, but rather indications of their underlying disease or changes in its course. Cardiovascular problems accounted for the greatest number of excess symptoms and signs in the beta blocker groups.[3,4,185,187–189] They included symptomatic congestive heart failure, hypotension with and without dizziness, bradycardia, and atrioventricular block. Heart failure was much less common than expected, perhaps because the studies excluded at entry patients with even moderate congestive heart failure.[222] Nonetheless, patients with a history of failure are more likely to develop problems. The high-risk patients assigned propranolol in the Norwegian study experienced a transient increase in heart failure within the first 2 weeks of treatment.[187]

Caution should be exercised when using beta blockers in the high-risk patients in whom myocardial and bronchial function may be dependent on stimulation from the sympathetic nervous system. Overall, the different beta blockers used in these trials were well-tolerated[3,4,178–183,186–189] and appeared to demonstrate similar safety profiles, except for practolol,[184,185] which caused a unique series of side effects.

Also detected in the trials was a high frequency of minor side effects which did not lead to treatment discontinuation.[3,4,178–189] These included mild cases of cold extremities, nausea, constipation, asthma, fatigue, mental depression, impotence, and dry eyes.

Clinical Impact

The reduction in cardiovascular mortality rate and recurrent myocardial infarction in infarct survivors given beta blockers represents an important breakthrough in the treatment of coronary artery disease. Beta blockers seem to act by delaying recurrent fatal and nonfatal coronary events. The long-term prognosis of those "saved" by beta blocker therapy remains uncertain since the underlying atherosclerotic heart disease is generally progressive, and most of these patients will ultimately die from it. Beta blockers appear to be only a partial and temporary answer for the prevention of the many deaths from coronary artery disease in Western societies.

REFERENCES

1 Frishman, W. H.: β-Adrenoceptor Antagonists New Drugs and New Indications, *N. Engl. J. Med.*, 305:500, 1981.

2 Frishman, W. H.: The Beta-Adrenoceptor Blocking Drugs, *Int. J. Cardiol.*, 2:165, 1982.

3 The Norwegian Multicenter Study Group: Timolol-Induced Reduction in Mortality and Reinfarction in Patients Surviving Acute Myocardial Infarction, *N. Engl. J. Med.*, 304:801, 1981.

4 Beta-Blocker Heart Attack Trial Research Group: A Randomized Trial of Propranolol in Patients with Acute Myocardial Infarction. I. Mortality Results, *J.A.M.A.*, 247:1707, 1982.

5 Braunwald, E.: Treatment of the Patient after Myocardial Infarction, *N. Engl. J. Med.*, 302:290, 1980.

6 Sutherland, E. W., Robinson, G. A., and Butcher, R. W.: Some Aspects of the Biological Role of Adenosine 3'5'-Monophosphate (Cyclic AMP), *Circulation*, 37:279, 1968.

7 Motulsky, H. J., and Insel, P. A.: Adrenergic Receptors in Man: Direct Identification, Physiologic Regulation, and Clinical Alterations, *N. Engl. J. Med.*, 307:18, 1982.

8 Lefkowitz, R.: Direct Binding Studies of Adrenergic Receptors: Biochemical, Physiologic, and Clinical Implications, *Ann Intern. Med.*, 91:450, 1979.

9 Ahlquist, R. P.: A Study of Adenotropic Receptors, *Am. J. Physiol.*, 53:586, 1948.

10 Glaubiger, G., and Lefkowitz, R. J.: Elevated Beta-Receptor Number after Chronic Propranolol Treatment, *Biochem. Biophys. Res. Commun.*, 78:720, 1977.

11 Shand, D. G., and Wood, A. J. J.: Propranolol Withdrawal Syndrome—Why?, *Circulation*, 58:202, 1978.

12 Frishman, W., and Silverman, R.: Clinical Pharmacology of the New Beta-adrenergic Blocking Drugs. Part 3. Comparative Clinical Experience and New Therapeutic Applications, *Am. Heart J.*, 98:119, 1979.

13 Buhler, F. R., Bukart, F., Benno, L. E., King, M., Marbet, G., and Pfisterer, M.: Antihypertensive Beta-blocking Action as Related to Renin and Age. A Pharmacological Tool to Identify Pathogenic Mechanisms in Essential Hypertension, *Am. J. Cardiol.*, 36:653, 1975.

14 Bristow M. R., Ginsberg, R., Minobe, W., et al.: Decreased Catecholamine Sensitivity and β-adrenergic-Receptor Density in Failing Human Hearts, *N. Engl. J. Med.*, 307:205, 1982.

15 Colucci, W. S., Alexander, R. W., Williams, G. H., et al.: Decreased Lymphocyte Beta-adrenergic-Receptor Density in Patients with Heart Failure and Tolerance to the Beta-adrenergic Agonist Parbuterol, *N. Engl. J. Med.*, 305:185, 1981.

16 Frishman, W. H.: Clinical Pharmacology of the New Beta-adrenergic Blocking Drugs. Part 13. The Beta-adrenergic Blocking Drugs: A Perspective, *Am. Heart J.*, 99:665, 1980.

17 Koch-Weser, J.: Metoprolol, *N. Engl. J. Med.*, 301:698, 1979.

18 Frishman, W. H.: Atenolol and Timolol, Two New Systemic β-Adrenoceptor Antagonists, *N. Engl. J. Med.*, 306:1456, 1982.

19 Frishman, W. H.: Nadolol: A New β-Adrenoceptor Antagonist, *N. Engl. J. Med.*, 305:678, 1981.

20 Frishman, W. H.: Pindolol: A New β-Adrenoceptor Antagonist with Partial Agonist Activity, *N. Engl. J. Med.*, 308:940, 1983.

21 Frishman, W.: Clinical Pharmacology of the New Beta-adrenergic Blocking Drugs. Part 1. Pharmacokinetic and Pharmacodynamic Properties, *Am. Heart J.*, 98:663, 1979.

22 Conolly, M. E., Kersting, F., and Dollery, C. T.: The Clinical Pharmacology of Beta-Adrenoceptor Blocking Drugs, *Prog. Cardiovasc. Dis.*, 19:203, 1976.

23 Opie, L. H.: Drugs and the Heart. 1. Beta-blocking Agents, *Lancet*, 1:693, 1980.

24 Frishman W., Jacob, H., Eisenberg, E., and Ribner, H.: Clinical Pharmacology of the New Beta-adrenergic Blocking Drugs. Part 8. Self-poisoning with Beta-Adrenoceptor Blocking Drugs: Recognition and Management, *Am. Heart J.*, 98:798, 1979.

25 Taylor S. H., Silke, B., and Lee, P. S.: Intravenous Beta-Blockade in Coronary Heart Disease: Is Cardioselectivity or Intrinsic Sympathomimetic Activity Hemodynamically Useful?, *N. Engl. J. Med.*, 306:631, 1982.

26 Frishman, W., and Halprin, S.: Clinical Pharmacology of the New Beta-adrenergic Blocking Drugs. Part 7. New Horizons in Beta-Adrenoceptor Blocking Therapy: Labetalol, *Am. Heart J.*, 98:660, 1979.

27 Frishman W. H., Strom, J., Kirschner, M., et al.: Labetalol Therapy in Patients with Systemic Hypertension and Angina Pectoris: Effects of Combined Alpha- and Beta-adrenergic Blockade, *Am. J. Cardiol.*, 48:917, 1981.

28 Frishman W., Silverman, R., Strom, J., Elkayam, U., and Sonnenblick, E.: Clinical Pharmacology of the New Beta-adrenergic Blocking Drugs. Part 4. Adverse Effects. Choosing a Beta-Adrenoceptor Blocker, *Am. Heart J.*, 98:256, 1979.

29 Hillis L. D., and Braunwald, E.: Myocardial Ischemia, *N. Engl. J. Med.*, 296:971, 1034, 1093, 1977.

30 Kirk, E. S., and Sonnenblick, E. H.: Newer Concepts in the Pathophysiology of Ischemic Heart Disease, *Am. Heart J.*, 103:756, 1982.

31 Frishman, W. H.: Multifactorial Actions of β-adrenergic Blocking Drugs in Ischemic Heart Disease: Current Concepts, *Circulation*, 67(suppl. 1):11, 1983.

32 Sonnenblick E. H., Ross, J., Jr., and Braunwald, E.: Oxygen Consumption of the Heart. Newer Aspects of Its Multifactorial Determination, *Am. J. Cardiol.*, 22:328, 1968.

33 Sonnenblick E. H., and Skelton, C. L.: Myocardial Energetics Basic Principles and Clinical Implications, *N. Eng. J. Med.*, 285:668, 1971.

34 Opie, L. H.: Myocardial Infarct Size. Part 1. Basic Considerations, *Am. Heart J.*, 100:355, 1980.

35 Berne R. M., and Rubio, R.: Coronary Circulation, in ''Handbook of Physiology. The Cardiovascular System,'' vol 1, ''The Heart,'' American Physiological Society, Bethesda, 1979, p. 873.

36 Stowe D. F., Mathey, D. G., Morres, W. Y., et al.: Segment Stroke Work and Metabolism Depend on Coronary Blood Flow in the Pig. *Am. J. Physiol.*, 234:H597, 1978.

37 Frishman W. H., Weksler, B., Christodoulou, J., Smithen, C., and Killip, T.: Reversal of Abnormal Platelet Aggregability and Change in Exercise Tolerance in Patients with Angina Pectoris following Oral Propranolol, *Circulation*, 50:887, 1974.

38 Mehta, J., Mehta, P., and Pepine, C.: Differences in Platelet Aggregation in Coronary Artery Sinus and Aortic Blood in Patients with Coronary Artery Disease: Effect of Propranolol, *Clin. Cardiol.*, 1:96, 1978.

39 Walsh P. N., Pareti, F. I., and Corbett, J. J.: Platelet Coagulant Activities and Serum Lipids in Transient Cerebral Ischemia, *N. Engl. J. Med.*, 295:854, 1976.

40 Kwaan H. C., Colwell, J. A., Cruz, S., Suwanwela, N., and Dobbie, J. G.: Increased Platelet Aggregation in Diabetes Mellitus, *J. Lab. Clin. Med.*, 80:236, 1972.

41 Carvalho A. C., Colman, R. W., and Lees, R.: Platelet Function in Hyperlipidemia, *N. Engl. J. Med.*, 290:434, 1974.

42 Poplawski A., Skorolska, M., and Niewiarowski, S.: Increased Platelet Adhesiveness in Hypertensive Cardiovascular Disease, *J. Atheroscler. Res.*, 8:721, 1968.

43 Harker L. A., and Ritchie, J. L.: The Role of Platelets in Acute Vascular Events, *Circulation*, 62 (suppl. 5):13, 1980.

44 Jorgensen L., Roswell, H. C., Hovig, T., Glynn, M. F., and Mustard, J. F.: Adenosine Diphosphate Induced Platelet Aggregation and Myocardial Infarction in Swine, *Lab. Invest.*, 17:616, 1967.

45 Haft J. I., Gershengorn, K., Kranz, P. D., and Oestreicher, R.: Protection against Epinephrine-induced Myocardial Necrosis by Drugs That Inhibit Platelet Aggregation, *Am. J. Cardiol.*, 30:838, 1972.

46 Folts J. D., Gallagher, K., and Rowe, G. G.: Blood Flow Reductions in Stenosed Canine Coronary Arteries: Vasospasm or Platelet Aggregation?, *Circulation*, 65:248, 1982.

47 Haft, J.: Role of Blood Platelets in Coronary Artery Disease, *Am. J. Cardiol.*, 43:1197, 1979.

48 Schrumph J., Sheps, D. S., Wolfson, S., Aronson, A., and Cohen, L. S.: Altered Hemoglobin-Oxygen Affinity with Long-term Propranolol Therapy in Patients with Coronary Artery Disease, *Am. J. Cardiol.*, 40:76, 1977.

49 Lesch, M., and Gorlin, R.: Pharmacological Therapy of Angina Pectoris, *Mod. Concepts Cardiovasc. Dis.*, 42:5, 1973.

50 Frishman W. H., Kostis, J., Strom, J., et al.: Clinical Pharmacology of the New Beta-Adrenoceptor Blocking Drugs. Part 6. A Comparison of Pindolol and Propranolol in Treatment of Patients with Angina Pectoris. The Role of Intrinsic Sympathomimetic Activity, *Am. Heart J.*, 98:526, 1979.

51 Frishman, W. H.: Clinical Pharmacology of the New Beta-Adrenoceptor Blocking Drugs. Part 12. Beta-Adrenoceptor Blockade in Myocardial Infarction: The Continuing Controversy, *Am. Heart J.*, 99:528, 1980.

52 Frishman, W. H., and Silverman, R.: Clinical Pharmacology of the New Beta-adrenergic Blocking Drugs. Part 2. Physiologic and Metabolic Effects, *Am. Heart J.*, 97:797, 1979.

53 Boudoulas H., Lewis, R. P., Rittgers, S. E., Leier, C. V., and Vasko, J. S.: Increased Diastolic Time: A Possible Important Factor in the Beneficial Effect of Propranolol in Patients with Coronary Artery Disease, *J. Cardiovasc. Pharmacol.*, 1:503, 1979.

54 Becker L. C., Fortuin, N. J., and Pitt, B.: Effect of Ischemia and Antianginal Drugs on the Distribution of Radioactive Microspheres in the Canine Left Ventricle, *Circ. Res.*, 28:263, 1971.

55 Vatner S. F., Baig, H., Manders, W. T., and Ochs, H.: Effects of Propranolol on Regional Myocardial Function, Electrograms, and Blood Flow in Conscious Dogs with Myocardial Ischemia, *J. Clin. Invest.*, 60:353, 1977.

56 Vatner S. F., Baig, H., Manders, W. T., and Murray, P. A.: Effects of a Cardiac Glycoside in Combination with Propranolol in the Ischemic Heart of Conscious Dogs, *Circulation*, 57:568, 1978.

57 Kloner R. A., Reimer, K., and Jennings, R.: Distribution of Coronary Collateral Flow in Acute Myocardial Ischemic Injury: Effect of Propranolol, *Cardiovasc. Res.*, 10:81, 1976.

58 Downey, J. M.: An Evaluation of the Coronary Constriction following Propranolol, *Eur. J. Pharmacol.*, 46:119, 1977.

59 Rubio R., and Berne, R.: Regulation of Coronary Blood Flow, *Prog. Cardiovasc. Dis.*, 18:105, 1975.

60 Gunther S., Muller, J., Mudge, G. H., and Grossman, W.: Therapy of Coronary Vasoconstriction in Patients

with Coronary Artery Disease, *Am. J. Cardiol.*, 47:157, 1981.

61 Weksler, B., Gillick, M., and Pink, J.: Effect of Propranolol on Platelet Function, *Blood*, 49:185, 1977.

62 Frishman, W. H., and Weksler, B. B.: Effects of β-Adrenoceptor Blocking Drugs on Platelet Function in Normal Subjects and Patients with Angina Pectoris, in H. Roskamm and K. H. Graefe (eds.), "Advances in β-Blocker Therapy: Proceedings of an International Symposium," Excerpta Medica, Amsterdam, 1980, p. 165.

63 Frishman W. H., Christodoulou, J., Weksler, B., Smithen, C., Killip, T., and Scheidt, S.: Abrupt Propranolol Withdrawal in Angina Pectoris: Effects on Platelet Aggregation and Exercise Tolerance, *Am. Heart J.*, 95:169, 1978.

64 Lefkowitz R.: Identification of α-adrenergic Receptors in Human Platelets by ³H Dihydroergocryptine Binding, *J. Clin. Invest.*, 61:395, 1978.

65 Pendleton R., Newman, D. J., Sherman, S. S., Brown, E. G., and Maya, W. E.: Effect of Propranolol upon the Hemoglobin-Oxygen Dissociation Curve, *J. Pharmacol. Exp. Ther.*, 180:647, 1972.

66 Manninen, B.: Movement of Sodium and Potassium and their Tracers in Propranolol-treated Red Cells and Diaphragm Muscle, *Acta Physiol. Scand. Suppl.*, 325:1, 1970.

67 Oski F., Miller, L., Delivoria-Papadopoulous, M., Manchester, J. H., and Shelburne, J. C.: Oxygen Affinity in Red Cells. Changes Induced In Vivo by Propranolol, *Science*, 175:1372, 1972.

68 Lichtman, M. A., Cohen, J., Murphy, M. S., Kearny, E. A., and Whitbeck, A.: Effect of Propranolol on Oxygen Binding to Hemoglobin In Vitro and In Vivo, *Circulation*, 49:881, 1974.

69 Frishman, W. H., Wilner, G., Smithen, C., Hayes, J., and Killip, T.: Effects of Exercise and Propranolol on Hemoglobin Oxygen Affinity in Patients with Angina Pectoris, *Clin. Res.*, 24:614, 1976.

70 Opie, L. H.: Myocardial Infarct Size. Part 2. Comparison of Anti-Infarct Effects of Beta-Blockade, Glucose-Insulin, Potassium, Nitrates and Hyaluronidase, *Am. Heart J.*, 100:531, 1980.

71 Kjekshus, J. K., and Mjos, O. D.: Effect of Inhibition of Lipolysis on Infarct Size after Experimental Coronary Occlusion. *J. Clin. Invest.*, 52:1770, 1973.

72 Marchetti, G. M., Merlo, L., and Nuseda, V.: Myocardial Uptake of Free Fatty Acids and Carbohydrates after Beta-adrenergic Blockade, *Am. J. Cardiol.*, 22:370, 1968.

73 Mueller, H. S., Ayres, S. M., Religa, A., and Evans, R. G.: Propranolol in the Treatment of Acute Myocardial Infarction: Effect on Myocardial Oxygenation and Hemodynamics, *Circulation*, 49:1078, 1974.

74 Kloner R. A., Rishbein, M. C., Cotran, R. S., Braunwald, E., and Maroko, P. R.: The Effect of Propranolol on Microvascular Injury in Acute Myocardial Ischemia, *Circulation*, 55:872, 1977.

75 Buhler, F. R., Laragh, J. H., Vaughan, E. D., Brunner, H. R., Gavras, H., and Baer, L.: Anti-hypertensive Action of Propranolol, *Am. J. Cardiol.*, 32:511, 1973.

76 Welman, E., Fox, K. M., Selwyn, A. P., and Carroll, B. J.: The Effect of Established β-Adrenoceptor Blocking Therapy on the Release of Cytosolic and Lysosomal Enzymes after Acute Myocardial Infarction in Man, *Clin. Sci. Mol. Med.*, 55:549, 1978.

77 Leren, P., Helgeland, A., Holme, I., Foss, P. O., Hjermann, I., and Lund-Larsen, P. G.: Effects of Propranolol and Prazosin on Blood Lipids. The Oslo Study, *Lancet*, 2:4, 1980.

78 Johnson, B.: The Emerging Problem of Plasma Lipid Changes during Anti-hypertensive Therapy, *J. Cardiovasc. Pharmacol.*, 4 (suppl.2):213, 1982.

79 Gold, H. K., Leinbach, R. C., and Maroko, P. R.: Propranolol-induced Reduction of Signs of Ischemic Injury during Acute Myocardial Infarction, *Am. J. Cardiol*, 38:689, 1976.

80 May, G. S., Eberlein, K. A., Furberg, C. D., Passamani, E. R., and DeMets, D. L.: Secondary Prevention after Myocardial Infarction: A Review of Long-term Trials, *Prog. Cardiovasc. Dis.*, 24:331, 1982.

81 Black J. W., and Stephenson, J. S.: Pharmacology of a New Adrenergic Beta-Receptor Blocking Compound (Nethalide), *Lancet*, 2:311, 1962.

82 Bjorntorp, P.: Treatment of Angina Pectoris with Beta-adrenergic Blockade, Mode of Action, *Acta Med. Scand.*, 184:259, 1968.

83 Prichard B. N. C., Aellig, W. H., and Richardson, G. A.: The Action of Intravenous Oxprenolol, Practolol, Propranolol, and Sotalol on Acute Exercise Tolerance in Angina Pectoris: The Effect on Heart Rate and the Electrocardiogram, *Postgrad. Med. J.*, 46:77, 1970.

84 Connolly M. E., Kersting, F., and Dollery, C. T.: The Clinical Pharmacology of Beta-Adrenoceptor Blocking Drugs, *Prog. Cardiovasc. Dis.*, 19:203, 1976.

85 Boakes, A. J., and Prichard, B. N. C.: The Effects of AH 5158, Pindolol, Propranolol, and *d*-Propranolol on Acute Exercise Tolerance in Angina Pectoris, *J. Pharm. Pharmacol.*, 47:673, 1973.

86 Barrett, A. M.: A Comparison of the Effect of (±) Propranolol and (+) Propranolol in Anesthetized Dogs; β-Receptor Blocking and Hemodynamic Action, *J. Pharm. Pharmacol.*, 21:241, 1969.

87 Gianelly, R. S., Goldman, R. H., Treister, B., and Harrison, D. C.: Propranolol in Patients with Angina Pectoris, *Ann. Intern. Med.*, 67:1216, 1967.

88 Prichard, B. N. C.: β-Receptor Antagonists in Angina Pectoris, *Ann. Clin. Res.*, 3:344, 1971.

89 Frishman, W., Smithen, C., Belfer, B., Kligfield, P., and

Killip, T.: Non-invasive Assessment of Clinical Response to Oral Propranolol, *Am. J. Cardiol.*, 35:635, 1975.

90 Morgan, T. O., Sabto, J., Anavekar, S. M., Louis, W. J., and Doyle, A. E.: A Comparison of Beta-adrenergic Blocking Drugs in the Treatment of Hypertension, *Postgrad. Med. J.*, 50:253, 1974.

91 Fiserova, J., Hlavecek, K., Vaura, M., Holik, F., and Munz, J.: Acebutolol (Sectral) in Angina Pectoris Treatment, *Acta Univ. Carol.*, 25:335, 1979.

92 Rod, J. L., Admon, D., Kimchi, A., Gotsman, M. S., and Lewis, B. S.: Evaluation of the Beta Blocking Drug Acebutolol in Angina Pectoris, *Am. Heart J.*, 98:604, 1979.

93 DiBianco R., Singh, S., Singh, J., et al.: Effects of Acebutolol on Chronic Stable Angina Pectoris—A Placebo-Controlled, Double-Blind, Randomized Crossover Study, *Circulation*, 62:1179, 1980.

94 Steele P., and Gold, F.: Favorable Effects of Acebutolol on Exercise Performance and Angina in Men with Coronary Artery Disease, *Chest*, 82:40, 1982.

95 DiBianco R., Singh, S., Shah, P., et al.: Comparison of the Antianginal Efficacy of Acebutalol and Propranolol. A Multicenter, Randomized, Double-Blind, Placebo-controlled Study, *Circulation*, 65:1119, 1982.

96 DePonti, C., DeBiase, A. M., Pirelli, S., et al.: Effects of Nifedipine, Acebutolol, and their Association on Exercise Tolerance in Patients with Effort Angina, *Cardiology*, 68 (suppl. 2):195, 1981.

97 Daltro, L. L., and Lion, M. F.: Treatment of Angina Pectoris with a New Beta Blocker Atenolol (Portuguese), *Rev. Bras. Med.*, 34 (suppl. 7):5, 1977.

98 Langbehn, A.F., Burmeister, G., Horst, H., Sonntag, F., and Klempein E. J.: Long-term Effects of the Beta-adrenergic Blocking Agent Atenolol (Tenormin) on Coronary Heart Disease, *Med. Klin.*, 73:101, 1978.

99 Backman H., Normi, H., and Sano, S.: Atenolol in Angina Pectoris—Preliminary Results of an Ergometric Dose Finding Study, *Acta Therapeutica*, 4:267, 1978.

100 Roy, P., Day, L., Sowton, E.: Effect of New Beta Adrenergic Blocking Agent, Atenolol (Tenormin), on Pain Frequency, Trinitrin Consumption and Exercise Ability, *Br. Med. J.*, 3:195, 1975.

101 Erikssen J., Osvik, K., and Dedichen, J.: Atenolol in the Treatment of Angina Pectoris, *Acta Med. Scand.*, 201:579, 1977.

102 van der Vijgh, W. J. F., Majid, P. A., deFeyter, P. J., Wardeh, R., and van der Wall, E. E.: Pharmacokinetics of Atenolol and Its Clinical Consequences in Patients with Angina Pectoris, *Int. J. Clin. Pharmacol.*, 18:375, 1980.

103 Jackson G., Schwartz, J., Kates, R. E., Winchester, M., and Harrison, D. C.: Atenolol: Once Daily Cardioselective Beta Blockade for Angina Pectoris, *Circulation*, 61:555, 1980.

104 Schwartz J., Jackson, G., Kates, R. E., and Harrison, D. C.: Long-term Benefit of Cardioselective Beta Blockade with Once-daily Atenolol Therapy in Angina Pectoris, *Am. Heart J.*, 101:380, 1981

105 Jackson, G., Harry, J. D., Robinson, C., Kitson, D., and Jewitt, D.: Comparison of Atenolol with Propranolol in the Treatment of Angina Pectoris with Special Reference to Once Daily Administration of Atenolol, *Br. Heart J.*, 40:998, 1978.

106 Haghfelt, T., Pindborg, T. and Thayssen, P.: Atenolol (Tenormin) in the Treatment of Angina Pectoris, *Ugeskr. Laeg.*, 142:2475, 1980.

107 Uusitalo, A., Keyrilainen, O., and Johnsson, G.: A Dose Response Study on Metoprolol in Angina Pectoris, *Ann. Clin. Res.*, 13 (suppl. 30):54, 1981.

108 Comerford, M. B., and Besterman, E. M. M.: An Eighteen Months' Study of the Clinical Response to Metroprolol, A Selective Beta 1–Receptor Blocking Agent, in Patients with Angina Pectoris, *Postgrad. Med. J.*, 52:481, 1976.

109 Borer, J. S., Comerford, M. B., and Sowton, E.: Assessment of Metoprolol, A Cardioselective Beta-blocking agent, during Chronic Therapy in Patients with Angina Pectoris, *J. Int. Med. Res.*, 4:15, 1976.

110 Frick, M. H., and Luurila, O.: Double-Blind Titrated-Dose Comparison of Metoprolol and Propranolol in the Treatment of Angina Pectoris, *Ann. Clin. Res.*, 8:385, 1976.

111 Thadani, U., Davidson, C., Chir, B., Singleton, W., and Taylor, S. H.: Comparison of the Immediate Effects of Five β-Adrenoreceptor Blocking Drugs with Different Ancillary Properties in Angina Pectoris, *N. Engl. J. Med.*, 300:750, 1979.

112 Thadani, U., Davidson, C., Singleton, W., and Taylor, S. H.: Comparison of Five Beta-Adrenoceptor Antagonists with Different Ancillary Properties during Sustained Twice Daily Therapy in Angina Pectoris, *Am. J. Cardiol.*, 68:243, 1980.

113 Arnman K., and Ryden, L.: Comparison of Metoprolol and Verapamil in the Treatment of Angina Pectoris, *Am. J. Cardiol.*, 49:821, 1982.

114 Heel R. C., Brogden, R. N., Pakes, G. E., Speight, J. M., and Avery, G. S.: Nadolol: A Review of Its Pharmacological Properties and Therapeutic Efficacy in Hypertension and Angina Pectoris, *Drugs*, 20:1, 1980.

115 Shapiro W., Park, J., DiBianco, R., Singh, S., Katz, R., and Fletcher, R.: Comparison of Nadolol, A New Long Acting Beta-Receptor Blocking Agent, and Placebo in the Treatment of Stable Angina Pectoris, *Chest*, 80:425, 1981.

116 Ling, A. S., and Groel, J. T.: Improved Physical Performance as a Therapeutic Objective in Patients with Angina, *Br. J. Clin. Pharmacol.*, 7 (suppl. 2): 1615, 1979.

117 Prager G.: Angina Pectoris: Effective Therapy Once Daily, *J. Int. Med. Res.*, 7:39, 1979.

118 Furberg B., Dahlqvist, A., Raak, A., and Wrege, U.: Comparison of the New Beta-Adrenoceptor Antagonist, Nadolol, and Propranolol in the Treatment of Angina Pectoris, *Curr. Med. Res. Opin.*, 5:388, 1978.

119 Jones, G. R., and Mir, M. A.: Comparison of Antianginal Efficacy of One Conventional and Three Long Acting Beta-Adrenoceptor Blocking Agents in Stable Angina Pectoris, *Br. Heart J.*, 46,503, 1981.

120 Watt, M.: Drug Surveillance in General Practice: A Study of Oxprenolol in the Treatment of Angina, *N.Z. Med. J.*, 81:200, 1975.

121 Burley, D. M.: Monitored Release Studies with Trasicor, in W. Schweizer (ed.), "Beta-Blockers—Present Status and Future Prospects," Hans Huber Publishers, Berne, 1974, p. 140.

122 Sandler, G., and Pistevos, A.: Clinical Evaluation of Oxprenolol in Angina Pectoris, *Br. Heart J.*, 34:847, 1972.

123 Bianchi, C., Lucchelli, P. E., and Starcich, R.: Beta-Blockade and Angina Pectoris. A Controlled Multicentre Clinical Trial, *Pharmacologica Clinica*, 1:161, 1969.

124 Wilson, D. F., Watson, O. F., Peel, J. S., and Turner, A. S.: Trasicor in Angina Pectoris: A Double-Blind Trial, *Br. Med. J.*, 2:155, 1969.

125 Taylor, S. H., and Thadani, U.: Oxprenolol in Angina Pectoris, *Br. J. Pharmacol.*, 58:412P, 1976.

126 Forrest, W. A.: A Double-Blind Clinical Trial in Angina Pectoris. A Comparison between Oxprenolol, Practolol and Placebo, *Br. J. Clin. Pract.*, 29:343, 1975.

127 Forrest, W. A.: Experience with a Sustained-release Formulation of Oxprenolol in the Management of Angina Pectoris in Hospital Out-patient Departments, *Curr. Med. Res. Opin.*, 5:669, 1978.

128 Majid, P. A., deFeijter, P. J., Wardeh, R., van der Wall E. E., and Roos, J.P.: Comparison of Clinical Effects of Propranolol (Inderal) with Once-daily Slow-release Oxprenolol (Slow Trasicor) in Angina Pectoris, *J. Int. Med. Res.*, 7:194, 1979.

129 Olowoyeye, J. O., Thadani, U., and Parker, J. O.: Slow Release Oxprenolol in Angina Pectoris: Study Comparing Oxprenolol, Once Daily, with Propranolol, Four Times Daily, *Am. J. Cardiol.*, 47:1123, 1981.

130 Leary, W. P., and Asmal, A. C.: Treatment of Coexistent Angina Pectoris and Hypertension with Pindolol, *S. Afr. Med. J.*, 49:11, 1975.

131 Storstein, L.: Effect of Intravenous and Oral Pindolol on Exercise Tolerance and Electrocardiographic Changes in Angina Pectoris, *J. Cardiovasc. Pharmacol.*, 2:739, 1980.

132 Dwyer, E. M., Jr., Pepe, A. J., and Pinkernell, B. H.: Effects of Beta-adrenergic Blockade with Pindolol Versus Placebo in Coronary Patients with Stable Angina Pectoris, *Am. Heart J.*, 103:830, 1982.

133 Harston, W. E., and Friesinger, G. C.: Randomized Double-Blind Study of Pindolol in Patients with Stable Angina Pectoris, *Am. Heart J.*, 104:504, 1982.

134 Harston, W. E., and Friesinger, G. C.: Variability of Response to Beta Receptor Blockade for Angina Pectoris in Clinical Trials: A Study of Pindolol, *Am. J. Cardiol.*, 50:722, 1982.

135 Cocco G., Strozzi, C., Chu, D., Amrein, R., and Castagnoli, E.: Therapeutic Effects of Pindolol and Nifedipine in Patients with Stable Angina Pectoris and Asymptomatic Resting Ischemia, *Eur. J. Cardiol.*, 10:59, 1979.

136 Cocco G., Strozzi, C., Chu, D., Amrein, R., and Castagnoli, E.: Therapeutic Effects of Pindolol and Nifedipine in Patients with Stable Angina Pectoris and Asymptomatic Resting Ischemia, *Br. J. Clin. Pract.*, 34 (suppl. 8):59, 1980.

137 Prichard, B. N. C.: β-Adrenoceptor Blocking Drugs in Angina Pectoris, in G. Avery (ed.), "β-Adrenoceptor Blocking Drugs," University Park Press, Baltimore, 1978, p. 85.

138 Prichard, B. N. C.: Propranolol in the Treatment of Angina: A Review, *Postgrad. Med. J.*, 52 (suppl. 4):35, 1976.

139 Prichard, B. N. C., and Gillam, D. M. S.: An assessment of Propranolol in Angina Pectoris. A Clinical Dose Response Curve and the Effect on the Electrocardiogram at Rest and on Exercise, *Br. Heart J.*, 33:473, 1971.

140 Alderman, E. L., Davies, R. O., Crowley, J. J. et al.: Dose Response Effectiveness of Propranolol for the Treatment of Angina Pectoris, *Circulation*, 51:964, 1975.

141 Thadani, U., and Parker, J. O.: Propranolol in Angina Pectoris: Duration of Improved Exercise Tolerance and Circulatory Effects after Acute Oral Administration, *Am. J. Cardiol.*, 44:119, 1979.

142 Thadani, U., and Parker, J. O.: Propranolol in the Treatment of Angina Pectoris—Comparison of Duration of Action in Acute and Sustained Oral Therapy, *Circulation*, 59:571, 1979.

143 Thadani, U., and Parker, J. O.: Propranolol in Angina Pectoris—Comparison of Therapy Given Two and Four Times Daily, *Am. J. Cardiol.*, 46:117, 1980.

144 Halkin, H., Vered, I., Saginer, A., and Rabinowitz, B.: Once Daily Administration of Sustained Release Propranolol Capsules in the Treatment of Angina Pectoris, *Eur. J. Clin. Pharmacol.*, 16:387, 1979.

145 Parker, J. O., Porter, A., and Parker, J. D.: Propranolol in Angina Pectoris—Comparison of Long-acting and Standard Formulation Propranolol, *Circulation*, 65:1351, 1982.

146 Leon, M. B., Rosing, D. R., Bonow, R. O., Lipson, L. C., and Epstein, S. E.: Clinical Efficacy of Verapamil Alone and Combined with Propranolol in Treating Patients with Chronic Stable Angina Pectoris, *Am. J. Cardiol.*, 48:131, 1981.

147 Johnson S. M., Mauritson, D. R., Corbett, J. R., Woodward, W., Willerson, J. T., and Hillis, L. D.: Double-Blind, Randomized, Placebo-controlled Comparison of

Propranolol and Verapamil in the Treatment of Patients with Stable Angina Pectoris, *Am. J. Med.*, 71:443, 1981.

148 Frishman, W. H., Klein, N. A., Strom, J. A., et al.: Superiority of Verapamil to Propranolol in Stable Angina Pectoris: A Double-Blind, Randomized Crossover Trial, *Circulation*, 65 (suppl. -l):51, 1982.

149 Subramanian B., Bowles, M. J., Davies, A. B., and Raftery, E. B.: Combined Therapy with Verapamil and Propranolol in Chronic Stable Angina, *Am. J. Cardiol.*, 49:125, 1982.

150 Lynch, P., Dargie, H., Krikler, S., and Krikler, D.: Objective Assessment of Antianginal Treatment: A Double-Blind Comparison of Propranolol, Nifedipine, and Their Combination, *Br. Med. J.*, 48:131, 1981.

151 Kenmure, A. C. F., and Scruton, J. H.: A Double-Blind Controlled Trial of the Anti-anginal Efficacy of Nifedipine Compared with Propranolol, *Br. J. Clin. Pract.*, 8:49, 1980.

152 Dargie, H. J., Lynch, P. G., Krikler, D. M., Harris, L., and Krikler, S.: Nifedipine and Propranolol: A Beneficial Drug Interaction, *Am. J. Med.*, 71:676, 1981.

153 Tweddel, A. C., Beattie, J. M., Murray, R. G., and Hutton I.: The Combination of Nifedipine and Propranolol in the Management of Patients with Angina Pectoris, *Br. J. Clin. Pharmacol.*, 12:229, 1981.

154 Fox, K. M., Jonathan, A., and Selwyn, A. P.: The Use of Propranolol and Nifedipine in the Medical Management of Angina Pectoris, *Clin. Cardiol.*, 4:125, 1981.

155 Toubes, D. B., Ferguson, R. K., Rice, A. J., Aoki, V. S., Funk, D. C., and Wilson, W. R.: β-Adrenergic Blockade Versus Placebo in Angina Pectoris, *Clin. Res.*, 18:345, 1970.

156 Kentala, E., Pyorala, K., and Frich, M. H.: Sotalol in the Treatment of Angina Pectoris—A Double-Blind, Crossover Study, *Ann. Clin. Res.*, 6:253, 1974.

157 Milei, J., and Fortunato, M. R.: A New Beta-adrenergic Blocking Agent, Sotalol, in the Treatment of Angina Pectoris. A Double Blind-crossed Treatment Study, *Rev. Bras. Pesqui. Med. Biol.*, 8:279, 1975.

158 Slome, R.: Sotalol in Angina Pectoris. A Double-Blind Study, *S. Afr. Med. J.*, 50:469, 1976.

159 Brailovsky, D.: Timolol Maleate (ML-950). A New Beta-blocking Agent for the Prophylactic Management of Angina Pectoris. A Multicentre, Multinational, Co-operative Trial, in B. Magnani (ed.), "Beta-adrenergic Blocking Agents in the Management of Hypertension and Angina Pectoris," Raven Press, New York, 1974, p. 117.

160 Villa, I., Dagenais, G. R., Dorian, W. D., and Burford, R. G.: Effects of Timolol on Exercise Tolerance in Patients with Angina Pectoris, in B. Magnani (ed.), "Beta-adrenergic Blocking Agents in the Management of Hypertension and Angina Pectoris," Raven Press, New York, 1974, p. 153.

161 Aronow, W. S., Turbow, M., Van Camp, S., Lurie, M., and Whittaker, K.: The Effect of Timolol vs. Placebo on Angina Pectoris, *Circulation*, 61:66, 1980.

162 DiSegni, E., Fidelman, E., David, D., Klein, H. O., and Kaplinsky, E.: The Beneficial Effect of the Beta Blocker Timolol in Stable Angina Pectoris, *Angiology*, 31:238, 1980.

163 Aronow W. S., Plasencia, G., Wong, R., and Landa, D.: Exercise Duration to Angina at Two and Twelve Hours After Timolol, *Clin. Pharmacol. Ther.*, 29:155, 1981.

164 Parmley, W. W.: The Combination of Beta-adrenergic-Blocking Agents and Nitrates in the Treatment of Stable Angina Pectoris, *Cardiol. Rev. Rep.*, 3:1425, 1982.

165 Packer, M., Leon, M. B., Bonow, R. O., Kieval, J., Rosing, D. R., and Bala Subramanian, V.: Hemodynamic and Clinical Effects of Combined Verapamil and Propranolol Therapy in Angina Pectoris, *Am. J. Cardiol.*, 50:903, 1982.

166 Maseri, A., L'Abbate, A., Ballestra, A. M., et al.: Coronary Vasospasm in Angina Pectoris, *Lancet*, 1:713, 1977.

167 Maseri, A.: Pathogenic Mechanisms of Angina Pectoris: Expanding Views, *Br. Heart J.*, 43:648, 1980.

168 Mehta, J., and Conti, C. R.: Verapamil Therapy for Unstable Angina Pectoris: Review of Double-Blind Placebo-Controlled Randomized Trials, *Am. J. Cardiol.*, 50:919, 1982.

169 Parodi, O., Simonetti, I., L'Abbate, A., and Maseri, A.: Verapamil Versus Propranolol for Angina at Rest, *Am. J. Cardiol.*, 50:923, 1982.

170 Conti, C. R.: Treatment of Unstable Angina: A Model for Step Care Therapy, *Cardiol. Rev. Rep.*, 3:1306, 1982.

171 Oka, Y., Frishman, W. H., Becker, R. M., et al.: Clinical Pharmacology of the New Beta-adrenergic Blocking Drugs. Part 10. Beta-adrenergic Receptor Blockade and Coronary Artery Surgery, *Am. Heart J.*, 99:255, 1980.

172 Frishman, W. H., Klein, N., Stom, J., et al.: Comparative Effects of Abrupt Withdrawal of Propranolol and Verapamil in Angina Pectoris, *Am. J. Cardiol.*, 50:1191, 1982.

173 Alderman, E. L., Coltart, J., Wettach, G. E., and Harrison, D. C.: Coronary Artery Syndrome after Abrupt Sudden Propranolol Withdrawal, *Ann. Intern. Med.*, 81:925, 1974.

174 Miller, R. R., Olson, H. G., Amsterdam, E. A., and Mason, D. T.: Propranolol Withdrawal Rebound Phenomenon. Exacerbation of Coronary Events after Abrupt Cessation of Anti-anginal Therapy, *N. Engl. J. Med.*, 293:416, 1975.

175 Frishman W. H., Christodoulou, J., Weksler, B., Smithen, C., Killip, T., and Scheidt, S.: Abrupt Propranolol Withdrawal in Angina Pectoris: Effects on Platelet Aggregation and Exercise Tolerance, *Am. Heart J.*, 95:169, 1978.

176 Turi, Z. G. and Braunwald, E.: The Use of Beta-Blockers after Myocardial Infarction, *J.A.M.A.*, 249:252, 1983.

177 Hampton, J. R.: Should Every Survivor of a Heart Attack Be Given a Beta Blocker?, *Br. Med. J.*, 285:33, 1982.

178 Wilhelmsson, C., Vedin, J. A., Wilhelmssen, L., Tibblin, G., and Werko, L.: Reduction of Sudden Deaths after Myocardial Infarction by Treatment with Alprenolol. Preliminary Results, *Lancet*, 2:1157, 1974.

179 Vedin A., Wilhelmsson, C., and Werko, L.: Chronic Alprenolol Treatment of Patients with Acute Myocardial Infarction after Discharge from Hospital. Effects on Mortality and Morbidity, *Acta Med. Scand. Suppl.*, 575:1, 1975.

180 Ahlmark G., Saetre, H., and Korsgren, M.: Reduction of Sudden Death after Myocardial Infarction, *Lancet*, 2:1563, 1974.

181 Ahlmark G., and Saetre, H.: Long-term Treatment with Beta-Blockers after Myocardial Infarction, *Eur. J. Clin. Pharmacol.*, 10:77, 1976.

182 Andersen, M. P., Bechsgaard, P., Frederiksen, J., et al.: Effect of Alprenolol on Mortality among Patients with Definite or Suspected Acute Myocardial Infarction, *Lancet*, 2:865, 1979.

183 Barber J. M., Boyle, D. McC., Chaturvedi, N. C., Singh, N., and Walsh, M. J.: Practolol in Acute Myocardial Infarction, *Acta Med. Scand. Suppl.*, 587:213, 1975.

184 Multicentre International Study: Improvement in Prognosis of Myocardial Infarction by Long-term Beta-Adrenoceptor Blockade Using Practolol, *B. Med. J.*, 3:735, 1975.

185 Multicentre International Study: Reduction in Mortality after Myocardial Infarction with Long-term Beta-Adrenoceptor Blockade. Supplementary Report, *Br. Med. J.*, 2:419, 1977.

186 Baber, N. S., Wainwright-Evans, D., Howitt, G., et al.: Multicentre Postinfarction Trial of Propranolol in 49 Hospitals in the United Kingdom, Italy, and Yugoslavia, *Br. Heart J.*, 44:96, 1980.

187 Hansteen V., Moinichen, E., Lorentsen, E., et al.: One Year's Treatment with Propranolol after Myocardial Infarction: Preliminary Report of Norwegian Multicentre Trial, *Br. Med. J.*, 284:155, 1982.

188 Julian D. G., Prescott, R. J., Jackson, F. S., and Szekely, P.: A Controlled Trial of Sotalol for One Year after Myocardial Infarction, *Lancet*, 1:1142, 1982.

189 Taylor, S. H., Silke, B., Ebbott, A., Sutton, G. C., Prout, B. J., and Burley, D. M.: A Long-term Prevention Study with Oxprenolol in Coronary Heart Disease, *N. Engl. J. Med.*, 307:1293, 1982.

190 May, G. S., Furberg, C. D., Eberlein, K. A., and Geraci, B. S.: Secondary Prevention Trials after Myocardial Infarction: A Review of Short-term Acute Phase Trials, *Prog. Cardiovasc. Dis.*, 25:335, 1983.

191 Frishman, W. H., and Ribner, H.: Anticoagulation in Myocardial Infarction. A Modern Approach to an Old Problem, *Am. J. Cardiol.*, 43:1207, 1979.

192 Persantine-Aspirin Reinfarction Study Research Group: Persantine and Aspirin in Coronary Artery Disease, *Circulation*, 62:449, 1980.

193 The Coronary Drug Project Research Group: Clofibrate and Niacin in Coronary Heart Disease, *J.A.M.A.* 231:360, 1975.

194 Myocardial Infarction Study Group: Secondary Prevention of Ischemic Heart Disease: A Long-term Controlled Lidoflazine Study, *Acta Cardiol.*, 34 (suppl. 24):7, 1979.

195 Snow, P. J. D.: Treatment of Acute Myocardial Infarction with Propranolol, *Am. J. Cardiol.*, 18:458, 1966.

196 Snow, P. J. D.: Effect of Propranolol in Myocardial Infarction, *Lancet*, 2:551, 1965.

197 Balcon R., Jewitt, D. E., Davies, J. P. H., and Oram, S.: A Controlled Trial of Propranolol in Acute Myocardial Infarction, *Lancet*, 2:919, 1966.

198 Clausen J., Felsby, M., Schonau Jordensen, F., Lyager Nielsen, B., Roin, J., and Strange, B.: Absence of Prophylactic Effect of Propranolol in Myocardial Infarction, *Lancet*, 2:920, 1966.

199 Multicentre Trial: Propranolol in Acute Myocardial Infarction, *Lancet*, 2:1435, 1966.

200 Norris, R. M., Caughey, D. E., and Scott, P. J.: Trial of Propranolol in Acute Myocardial Infarction, *Br. Med. J.*, 2:398, 1968.

201 Goldstein, S.: Propranolol in Patients with Acute Myocardial Infarction: The Beta-Blocker Heart Attack Trial, *Circulation*, 67 (suppl. 1):53, 1983.

202 Furberg, C. D., and Bell, R. L.: What Is the Effect of Beta-Blocker Therapy on Recurrent Myocardial Infarction?, *Circulation*, 67 (suppl. 1):83, 1983.

203 Morganroth, J., Lichstein, E., Hubble, E., and Harrist, R.: Effect of Propranolol in Ventricular Arrhythmias in the β-Blocker Heart Attack Trial, *Circulation*, 66 (suppl. 2):328, 1982. (Abstract.)

204 Koppes, G. M., Beckmann, C. H., and Jones, F. G.: Propranolol Therapy for Ventricular Arrhythmias 2 Months after Myocardial Infarction, *Am. J. Cardiol.*, 46:322, 1980.

205 Hjalmarson, A.: Myocardial Metabolic Changes Related to Ventricular Fibrillation, *Cardiology*, 65:226, 1980.

206 Opie, L. H.: Myocardial Infarct Size. Part 1. Basic Considerations, *Am. Heart J.*, 100:355, 1980.

207 Baber, N. S., and Lewis, J. A.: Beta-Adrenoceptor Blockade and Myocardial Infarction: When Should Treatment Start and for How Long Should It Continue?, *Circulation*, 67 (suppl. 1):71, 1983.

208 Hjalmarson, A., Elmfeldt, D., Herlitz, J., et al.: Effect on Mortality of Metoprolol in Acute Myocardial Infarction, *Lancet*, 2:823, 1981.

209 Barber, J. M., Murphy, F. M., and Merrett, J. D.: Clinical Trial of Propranolol in Acute Myocardial Infarction, *Ulster Med. J.*, 36:127, 1967.

210 Briant, R. B., and Norris, R. M.: Alprenolol in Acute Myocardial Infarction: Double-Blind Trial, *N.Z. Med. J.,* 71:135, 1970.

211 Wilcox, R. G., Roland, J. M., Banks, D. C., Hampton, J. R., and Mitchell, J. R. S.: Randomized Trial Comparing Propranolol with Atenolol in Immediate Treatment of Suspected Myocardial Infarction. *Br. Med. J.,* 280:885, 1980.

212 Wilcox, R. G., Rowley, J. M., Hampton, J. R., Mitchell, J. R. S., Roland, J. M., and Banks, D. C.: Randomized Placebo-controlled Trial Comparing Oxprenolol with Disopyramide Phosphate in Immediate Treatment of Suspected Myocardial Infarction, *Lancet,* 2:765, 1980.

213 Coronary Prevention Research Group: An Early Intervention Secondary Prevention Study with Oxprenolol following Myocardial Infarction, *Eur. Heart J.,* 2:389, 1981.

214 Evemy, K. L., and Pentecost, B. L.: Intravenous and Oral Practolol in the Acute Stages of Myocardial Infarction, *Eur. J. Cardiol.,* 7:391, 1978.

215 Johansson, B. W.: A Comparative Study of Cardioselective Beta-Blockade and Diazepam in Patients with Acute Myocardial Infarction and Tachycardia, *Acta Med. Scand.,* 207:47, 1980.

216 Yusuf S., Ramsdale, D., Peto, R., et al.: Early Intravenous Atenolol Treatment in Suspected Acute Myocardial Infarction, *Lancet,* 2:273, 1980.

217 McIlmoyle L., Evans, A., Boyle, D. McC., et al.: Early Intervention in Myocardial Ischemia. Proceedings of the British Cardiac Society, *Br. Heart J.,* 47:188, 1982. (Abstract.)

218 Cutler, J. A.: Ongoing Trials of Beta-Blockers in the Secondary Prevention of Coronary Heart Disease: A Review. *Circulation,* 67 (suppl. 1):62, 1983.

219 Mullane, J. F., Kaufman, J., Dvornik, D., and Coelho, J.: Propranolol Dosage, Plasma Concentration, and Beta-Blockade, *Clin. Pharmacol. Ther.,* 32:692, 1982.

220 Berglund G., Anderson, O., Hansson, R., and Olander, R.: Propranolol Given Twice Daily in Hypertension, *Acta Med. Scand.,* 94:513, 1973.

221 McLeod S. M., Harnet, P., Kaplan, H., et al.: Antihypertensive Efficacy of Propranolol Given Twice Daily, *Can. Med. Assoc. J.,* 121:737, 1979.

222 Julian, D.: Can Beta-Blockers Be Safely Used in Patients with Recent Acute Myocardial Infarction Who Also Have Congestive Heart Failure?, *Circulation,* 67 (suppl. 1):61, 1983.

Calcium Antagonists: Cardiocirculatory Effects and Therapeutic Applications

BRAMAH N. SINGH, M.D., GRAY ELLRODT, M.D., and KOONLAWEE NADEMANEE, M.D.

Over 10 years ago Fleckenstein[1] observed that changes in myocardial contractility and in the gross electrophysiologic properties of isolated cardiac muscle produced by calcium-free media could be mimicked closely not only by certain divalent cations but also by such compounds as verapamil and prenylamine. He designated such compounds as "specific calcium antagonists": they were thought to act by inhibiting calcium-mediated excitation-contraction coupling (EC) in cardiac muscle. This pharmacologic concept represented the culmination of a number of important advances which were made in the 1960s and early 1970s in our knowledge of cardiac electrophysiology. For example, it was demonstrated that in partially depolarized cardiac muscle, an inward calcium current was the main depolarizing current.[2,3] Perhaps more important, the voltage clamp technique[4] permitted the "separation" of depolarizing currents in normal cardiac muscle into two channels, "rapid" and "slow," each capable of being selectively blocked by certain pharmacologic interventions.[5] Finally, it was demonstrated that the flow of calcium current through the slow channel was augmented by epinephrine.[6] The group of compounds which Fleckenstein[1] called calcium antagonists has since been found to inhibit not only the slow channel in normal myocardial tissues and nodal fibers solely dependent on the slow channel for depolarization but also slow channel–dependent potentials arising pathologically.[2,3] These properties, most readily demonstrable in isolated tissues, have now become the basis for the delineation of a class of chemically heterogeneous compounds which also competitively block calcium influx in vascular smooth muscle. Various terms have recently been used to categorize these compounds: calcium antagonists, calcium entry blockers, slow-channel inhibitors, calcium channel blockers. It is now recognized that as a class they exhibit distinctive pharmacologic properties in common characterized by variable potencies for coronary and peripheral vasodilatation, negative inotropism, and depression of AV conduction, features which are of direct clinical relevance.[7] An increasing plethora of calcium antagonists is under investigation. The pharmacologic properties of these compounds, when considered together, clearly demonstrate the overall clinical utility of calcium antagonists in the treatment of numerous cardiocirculatory disorders.[8–10] Indeed, the therapeutic spectrum of calcium antagonists closely rivals that of beta-adrenoceptor blocking drugs. In this chapter, the expanding role of this "new" class of therapeutic agents is delineated in relation to their electrophysiological, hemodynamic, and pharmacokinetic properties with a particular reference to verapamil, nifedipine, and diltiazem.

ELECTROPHYSIOLOGICAL CONSIDERATIONS

An understanding of the pharmacologic properties of calcium antagonists presupposes some familiarity with the basic elements of cardiac and smooth muscle electrophysiology. This is briefly reviewed here relative to the significance of role of calcium and calcium channel activity in cardiac and smooth muscle cells.

Voltage clamp in heart muscle[4] permits the separation of the early inward currents into two discrete components, which allows the identification of two types of myocardial fibers. In the first ("fast-response"), the inward current is carried by sodium with rapid activation and inactivation kinetics and high conduction velocity. The threshold of activation is -60 to -70 mV, membrane potential being the primary determinant of the refractory period in such fibers. The fast response is selectively inhibited by tetrodotoxin and local anesthetic drugs. In such fibers, the depolarizing role of the slow inward current (carried essentially by calcium) can be demonstrated only after the fast response has been inactivated. Normally, when the membrane is depolarized (by the fast Na current) to -35 to -45 mV, the slow channel is activated. Its kinetics of activation and inactivation are sluggish. In fibers with fast-response characteristics, the slow inward current serves two main functions. First, it is responsible for excitation-contraction coupling. Second, because of its long time constant of inactivation, the slow channel contributes to the maintenance of the action potential plateau in fast-response fibers. Thus, the selective inhibition of the slow inward current in myocardial fibers which normally have fast-response characteristics will result in a marked reduction in contractility and in an acceleration of the action potential plateau.

The role of the slow inward current in excitation-contraction coupling and the generation of the plateau phase of the action potential in fast-response fibers must be distinguished from its dominant role as the main depolarizing current in certain normal myocardial cells. Such myocardial cells, termed "slow-response" fibers,[2,3] have been described in the mitral annulus and coronary sinus[3,11,12] but are of the greatest physiological importance in the sinoatrial and atrioventricular nodes. The overall similarities and differences between the fast and slow inward currents in cardiac muscle are summarized in Fig. 1. The cardiac electrophysiological effects of slow-channel inhibitors may be interpreted within the framework of the changes produced by this class of drugs on the two current systems.

In the case of vascular smooth muscle, their precise action is, however, less well understood, undoubtedly due to the fact that steps to excitation-contraction coupling in this tissue are still not clearly defined[13] and are more complex than those in cardiac muscle.[4] Furthermore, they may differ in various regional circulations. It is known, however, that contraction in vascular smooth muscle can be initiated by the activation of potential-dependent calcium channels or by the stimulation of receptor-operated channels.[14] The influx of calcium through such channels may trigger the release of sarcolemmal stores of calcium or of calcium from the sarcoplasmic reticulum. As the concentration of intracellular Ca^{2+} increases, the combination of the calcium modulator protein, calmodulin, and calcium leads to the activation of the myosin light chain kinase with the resultant phosphorylation of one of the myosin light chains. This allows the interaction of the actin and myosin, and contraction ensues. The initial rapid phasic contraction is dependent on the release of small amounts of calcium from the intracellular pools, but it is likely that the more sustained tonic contractions in vascular smooth muscle results from the transmembrane transfer of calcium through the potential-dependent or receptor-operated channels. The subsequent phosphatase-mediated dephosphorylation of myosin light chain P increases and predominates over the myosin light chain kinase-mediated phosphorylation reaction. The calmodulin-calcium light chain kinase complex then decreases in concentration as the intracellular calcium is either taken up into storage intracellular sites or leaves the cell.[14] At present, it is not known as to how various calcium antagonists precisely affect the trans-sarcolemmal passage of calcium or its intracellular movements in vascular smooth muscle. Nevertheless, it should be noted that transmembrane potentials which result from the superfusion of isolated strips of coronary artery in physiological media containing tetraethylammonium (TEA) are consistently depressed by calcium antagonists such as verapamil[15] with the consequent relaxation of the contraction. A similar action in other vascular tissues undoubtedly accounts for the

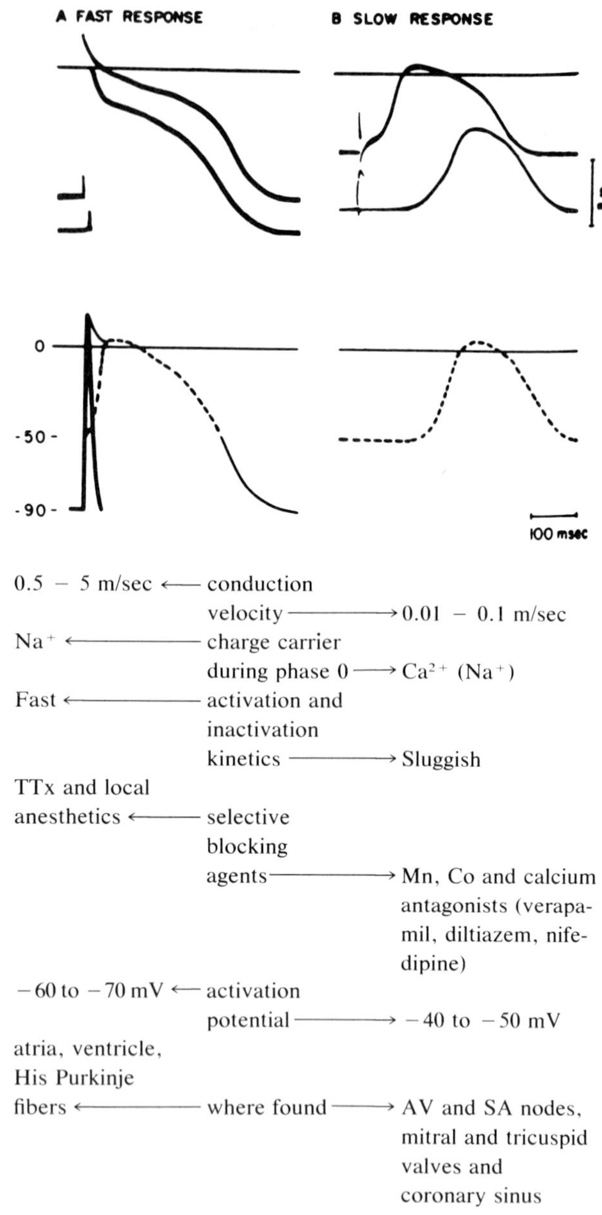

FIGURE 1 The configuration of the action potentials dependent on fast-channel ("fast response") and slow-channel ("slow response") activities for depolarization. In the upper panels two action potentials from each type of fiber are shown; in the lower panel, the time course of fast-channel (solid lines) and slow-channel (broken lines) activities is shown. Note the kinetic and other differences between slow- and fast-response fibers.

known propensity of slow-channel inhibitors to induce peripheral vasodilatation, a property which is of crucial importance in modulating the overall cardiocirculatory dynamics due to myocardial slow-channel blockade.[8,9]

The overall electrophysiological and hemodynamic effects of individual slow channel-blocking drugs are dependent on a number of factors. Perhaps the most significant is the relative blocking potencies with respect to the slow channel-dependent functions in cardiac and vascular smooth muscle. Since the inotropic, chronotropic as well as the dromotropic effects are also affected by the impulse traffic in the cholinergic and sympathetic terminals to the heart, the interaction of slow channel-blocking drugs with the autonomic nervous system is also significant. For example, verapamil and diltiazem (but not nifedipine and its derivatives) exert noncompetitive sympathetic antagonistic actions which may influence their overall cardiocirculatory effects (see below).

General Pharmacologic Properties of Slow Channel-Blocking Drugs

It is not the intent here to discuss at length the detailed general pharmacologic properties of calcium antagonists. Only those features which are essential to an appreciation of their electrophysiological and hemodynamic effects are emphasized. Figure 2 shows the chemical structures of the clinically most significant

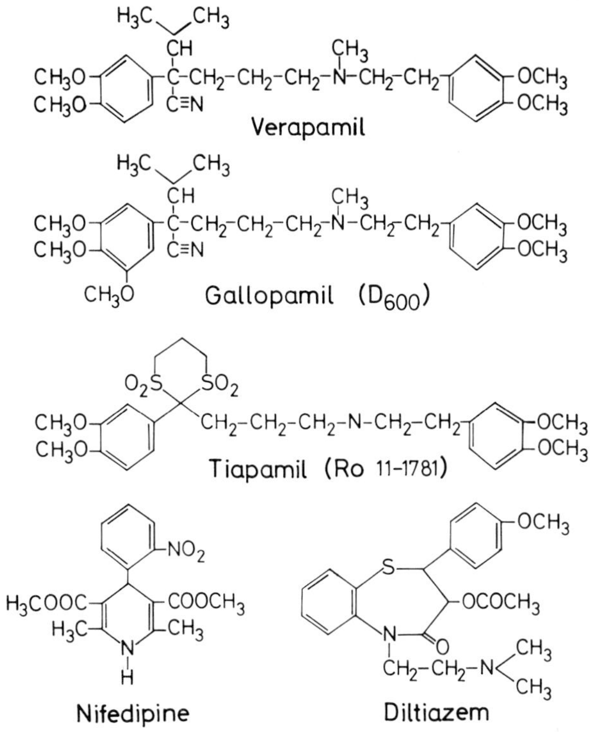

FIGURE 2 The chemical structures of some calcium antagonists. Verapamil is the prototype; gallopamil and tiapamil are congeners of verapamil. Nifedipine and diltiazem are structurally different from verapamil, but they share with it the common property of inhibiting the slow channel in the heart and of blocking calcium fluxes in vascular smooth muscle.

compounds. It will be evident that gallopamil (a methoxy derivative of verapamil) and tiapamil share close structural similarities with verapamil (a papaverine derivative), the prototype slow-channel inhibitor. In contrast, both nifedipine and diltiazem are structurally dissimilar; the former is a dihydropyridine derivative whereas the latter is a benzothiazepine derivative. In this chapter, neither perhexilene nor lidoflazine are considered. They are coronary and smooth muscle dilators,[7] but they both block the fast sodium current in relatively low concentrations.[16,17] For this reason, it is doubtful whether they can be considered ''selective'' slow-channel inhibitors although the concept of peripheral vascular tissue selectivity may be developed to account for the coronary and peripheral vasodilator actions of such compounds as lidoflazine.[18] Table 1 summarizes the salient features of the pharmacology of the ''conventional'' slow channel-blocking drugs. It should be emphasized that the known quantitative differences and similarities among the compounds are merely estimates from available experimental observations; they do, however, provide a framework for the interpretation of the known clinical cardiocirculatory actions of the compounds.[8,9] Particularly noteworthy is the fact that, in the case of some of the compounds, a striking difference may be found with respect to their in vitro and in vivo effects. For example, nifedipine in vitro is undoubtedly the most potent calcium antagonist. In conscious animals and in human beings with the autonomic nervous system intact, the drug's depressant effect on atrioventricular conduction either is absent or may even be reversed. In contrast to the effects of verapamil and diltiazem, nifedipine does not exhibit nonspecific sympathetic antagonism.[19] Thus, its overall chronotropic and dromotropic effect is a balance between its direct effect on slow-response fibers in the sinoatrial and atrioventricular nodes and that due to the reflex response to peripheral vasodilatation.

Specific Electrophysiological Actions

In concentrations which are therapeutically meaningful, all calcium antagonists inhibit the slow inward current in a dose-dependent manner in all normal myocardial tissues.[7] The result is excitation-contraction uncoupling with a variable acceleration of plateau phase of the action potential.[7] Except in high concentrations, none of the compounds has an effect on the upstroke velocity of phase 0 of the action potential; ''membrane responsiveness'' is unaltered, as is conduction velocity or the resting membrane potential. Thus, the effective refractory period (ERP) is not significantly affected by verapamil and other calcium antagonists in isolated atrial, ventricular, or His-Purkinje fibers.

The most striking effects of slow-channel inhibition by calcium antagonists in healthy tissues are predictably found in those structures which are normally slow channel-dependent for their excitation, namely the sinoatrial (SA) and atrioventricular (AV) nodes.[20–22] In isolated preparations, the sinus node frequency is markedly slowed,[23,24] with dose-depressant effect on the slow-channel fibers in the isolated AV node, especially in its upper and middle portions. Both in the SA and AV nodes, the rate of rise and overshoot of the action potentials are lowered and conduction velocity is decreased.

In general, there is an excellent concordance between the overall experimental and clinical electrophysiological effects of verapamil, diltiazem, and nifedipine (see Table 1). As might be expected, none of the compounds has an effect on the QRS duration or on the QTc interval of the 12-lead ECG. Similarly, neither the infranodal conduction (HV interval) nor the ERPs of the atria, ventricles, His-Purkinje system, or the anomalous pathways (presumably all fast channel-dependent) are significantly affected by slow-channel blockade.[7]

As indicated in Table 1, neither verapamil nor the other slow channel-blocking agents[25–27] induces clinically significant alterations in the maximum sinus node recovery time (SNRT) or in sinoatrial conduction time (SACT) in patients with normal sinus node. In contrast, in patients with abnormal sinus node function, a marked lengthening of the SNRT as well as sinus arrest may result,[28] although such an effect is less pronounced in the case of nifedipine.

Perhaps the most striking and significant electrophysiological effect of calcium antagonists is on AV conduction (Table 1). For example, both diltiazem and verapamil lengthen the intranodal (AH interval) conduction time during sinus rhythm and they slow AV conduction in the anterograde and retrograde directions.[25,29] In contrast, nifedipine either has no effect or may even facilitate AV conduction,[30] at least in part because the expected direct depressant effect of the drug is offset by the autonomic reflexes activated by

TABLE 1

Comparative experimental and clinical electrophysiological effects of verapamil, nifedipine, and diltiazem*

Effects	Verapamil	Nifedipine	Diltiazem
Inhibitory effect of cardiac slow channel:			
In vitro	+ + +	+ + + +	+ + +
Relaxation of smooth muscle:			
In vitro	+ + +	+ + + +	+ +
In vivo	+ + +	+ + + +	+ +
Nonspecific sympathetic antagonism	+	0	+
Effect on heart rate:			
Isolated atria	↓ + + +	↓ + + + +	↓ + + +
Intact organism and human beings	↑ ↓	↑	↓
Effect on AV conduction:			
In isolated heart	↓ + + +	↓ + + + +	↓ + + +
In intact organism and human beings	↓ + + + +	0 to ↑	↓ + + +
Clinical electrophysiological properties:			
R–R interval	↑ ↓	↓	↑ ↓
QRS	0	0	0
Q-Tc	0	0	0
PR	↑	0	↑
A–H	↑	0	↑
H–V	0	0	0
Atrial ERP	0	0	0
AV node ERP	↑ ↑	±	↑
AV node FRP	↑ ↑	±	↑
Ventricular ERP	0	0	0
His-Purkinje ERP	0	0	0
Bypass tract ERP	±	0	?
Sinus node recovery time	0†	0	0†
Ventricular automaticity	0	0	0

*↓ = decrease; ↑ = increase; ↑ ↓ = variable effect; ERP = effective refractory period; FRP = functional refractory period.
†Prolonged in sick sinus syndrome.

its potent hypotensive action.[7,8] It is of practical importance that most calcium antagonists (except for nifedipine) also influence AV nodal refractoriness,[7,8] an effect that correlates reasonably well with the drugs' salutary effects in supraventricular tachyarrhythmias.[7] Verapamil and diltiazem prolong the functional as well as the effective refractory periods (ERP) of the AV node, and they also prolong the AV node Wenckebach cycle length.[7,25] However, there is little quantitative data available on the relative potencies of these compounds in this regard. Nevertheless, it appears that, despite equivalent depression of AV nodal conduction, verapamil affects AV nodal refractoriness to a greater degree than diltiazem,[27] a difference that is of clinical significance.

As in the case of AV nodal conduction, the effects of nifedipine on the ERP of the AV node are opposite to those of the other calcium antagonists (see Table 1). It *reduces* the AV nodal ERP and the AV node Wenckebach cycle length.[25,30]

Systemic Hemodynamic Effects

The net hemodynamic effects of the various calcium antagonists result from a complex interplay of their direct actions on the myocardium and the coronary and peripheral circulations, on the one hand, and the relevant reflex sympathetic discharge and the presence of competitive sympathetic antagonistic activity that some of the compounds have, on the other.[7,8] As in the case of their electrophysiological actions, there are significant differences among the calcium antagonists relative to their negative inotropic propensity in vitro and their net cardiocirculatory effects in intact animals and human beings. The net hemodynamic effect that becomes apparent will thus be dependent on the agent used, on the cardiac condition and the level of ventricular function present, on the integrity of the autonomic nervous system, and on the dose and the route of drug administration. Again, there is a close correlation between the experimental and clinical hemodynamic effects for the individual agents.[7]

Most reported hemodynamic data have dealt with the resting state and the responses after a single intravenous dose of nifedipine, verapamil, and diltiazem. In general, the effects can be accounted for by the inhibitory potencies of these compounds as they act on the myocardium and peripheral vasculature,[8] combined with their propensities to stimulate sympathetic reflex mechanisms and the intrinsic noncompetitive sympathetic inhibitory effects present in some of the compounds. The net effects of intravenous or sublingual nifedipine are consistent with profound peripheral vasodilatation and reflex increases in contractility in both normal subjects and those with underlying cardiac disease.[31–33] In patients with coronary artery disease

increments in heart rate, cardiac output, and contractility have been observed with sublingual nifedipine.[32] The drug also induces increases in left ventricular ejection fraction and mean velocity of circumferential fiber shortening without significantly changing the left ventricular end-diastolic pressure (LVEDP) or end-diastolic volume.[33] Occasionally, in patients with coronary artery disease, the LVEDP may, however, fall.[34] In patients with impaired left ventricular function sublingual nifedipine (20 mg) reduces LV afterload and myocardial oxygen demand, enhances diastolic performance, and improves systemic and pulmonary hemodynamics, left ventricular ejection fraction, and cardiac output.[35] It must be emphasized nevertheless that in the case of nifedipine, if the reflex effects consequent upon peripheral vasodilatation are blocked by beta blockade, profound hypotension and cardiac failure may result, especially in patients with impaired ventricular function. During exercise the amelioration of ischemia may influence the observed hemodynamic changes. During bicycle exercise, orally administered nifedipine can reduce the mean pulmonary capillary wedge pressure and blunt the increases in systolic arterial pressure, while permitting a significant increase in work load.[35] In patients with coronary artery disease paced to anginal threshold, the drug also attenuates increases in LVEDP.[36] Although further study is required, it appears that in patients with coronary artery disease with normal or moderately impaired ventricular function hemodynamic changes are relatively consistent. Nifedipine causes significant peripheral vasodilatation provoking reflex increases in heart rate, contractility, atrioventricular conduction, and stroke-volume indexes. Overall, without concomitant beta-adrenergic blockade and in patients without cardiac failure, these changes may not always be clinically beneficial,[37] and acute ischemia and myocardial infarction may sometimes be precipitated.

Verapamil has also been studied extensively in healthy individuals and in patients with a variety of cardiac diseases. In healthy adults a trivial negative inotropic action, easily abolished with the increased sympathetic excitation of exercise, is found.[38] In patients with cardiac disease in sinus rhythm, mean arterial pressure is reduced slightly, with a slight increase in cardiac output but without a significant fall in stroke volume. In patients with atrial fibrillation stroke volume has been reported to fall.[39] Following intravenous verapamil (10 mg) in patients with coronary or rheumatic heart disease, peak hemodynamic effects are observed in between 3 and 5 min with return to base line by 10 min. A marked fall in systemic vascular resistance accompanied by a modest fall in LV dP/dt_{max} has been observed.[40] A modest increase in right ventricular end-diastolic pressure, mean right atrial pressure, and mean pulmonary artery pressure has been found.[41] The effect of verapamil on ventricular ejection fraction (VEF) is variable. For example, in one series of patients, verapamil was found to increase significantly left ventricular ejection fraction,[41] while it had little effect in another.[42] In another study, which utilized gated radionuclide angiography, in 13 of 16 patients who had normal LVEF at rest verapamil decreased resting left ventricular ejection fraction but did not affect LVEF during exercise.[43] However, left ventricular diastolic filling was enhanced by the drug at rest and during exercise.

Thus, although the ejection fraction data from different centers are somewhat in conflict, in general the expected myocardial depressant effects of verapamil are found to be offset by its vasodilator properties for most patients. In patients with left ventricular ejection fraction between 30 and 75 percent, despite slight increases in mean pulmonary capillary wedge pressure, stroke volume and cardiac index generally remain unchanged or actually increase.[40,41,44–47]

Although diltiazem has been studied less extensively, its cardiocirculatory effects are similar to those of verapamil. Intravenous diltiazem (10 mg) administered to patients with essential hypertension significantly reduces mean arterial pressure and systemic vascular resistance, while increasing cardiac index. This occurs without a significant alteration in heart rate, pulmonary capillary wedge pressure, mean right atrial, or pulmonary artery systolic or diastolic pressures.[48] In patients with coronary artery disease intravenous infusion of 15 to 30 μg/(kg)(min) of diltiazem did not alter left ventricular ejection fraction.[49] However, with various oral doses different effects have been noted. Doses of 60 mg significantly decrease systolic arterial pressure and stroke-volume index without corresponding alterations in cardiac index, stroke-work index, heart rate, or systemic vascular resistance. These alterations are abolished by exercise.[50] Higher doses (90 mg PO tid) administered chronically to patients with coronary artery disease significantly reduce cardiac output, stroke volume, and stroke-work index. These effects are consistent with diltiazem's antianginal effects.[49] Thus, although the action of nifedipine, verapamil, and diltiazem may be qualitatively similar, quantitative differences among the compounds become apparent in patients relative to the variable competing direct, reflex, and extracardiac effects of the three calcium channel blockers; such differences may also be apparent during oral administration of the drugs (Fig. 3).[51]

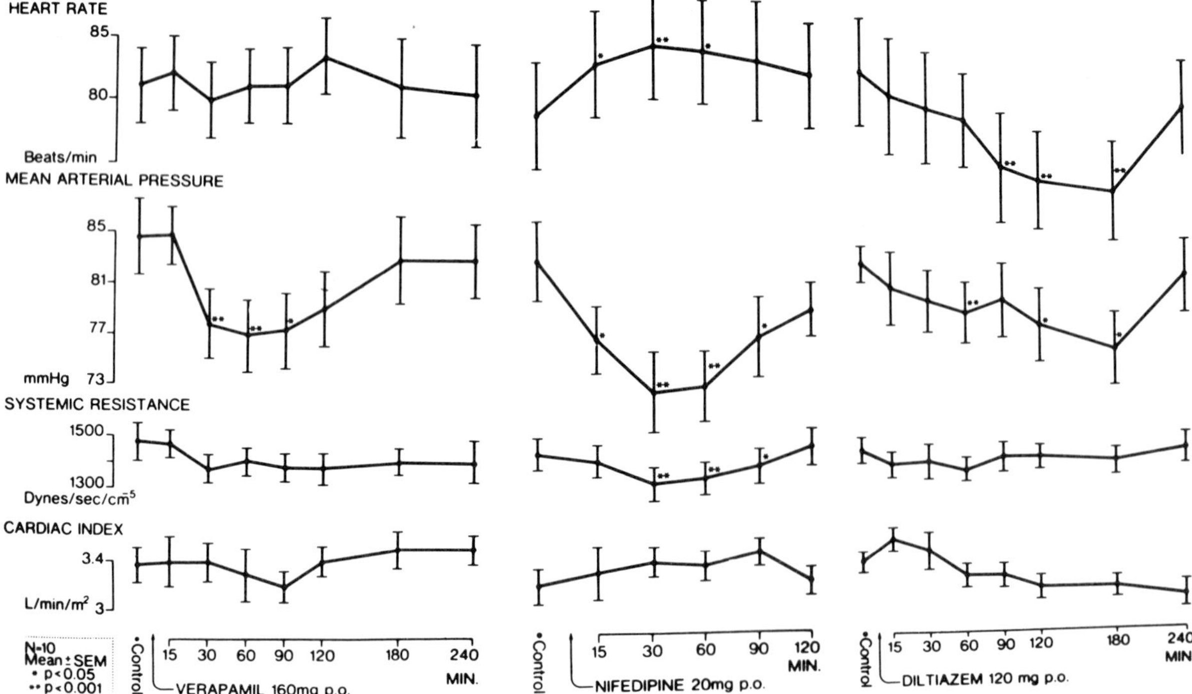

FIGURE 3 Hemodynamic effects of orally administered (single doses) calcium antagonists in patients with uncomplicated acute myocardial infarction. Measurements of the hemodynamic variables were made serially after the ingestion of the agent shown. Note that diltiazem produces a reduction in heart rate, verapamil a variable response, and nifedipine frank tachycardia, changes which are consistent with the known overall pharmacologic properties of the three compounds. (*Adapted from P. Theroux, D. D. Waters, J. C. Debaisieux, J. Szlachcic, H. F. Mizgala, Hemodynamic Effects of Calcium Ion Antagonists after Acute Myocardial Infarction, Clin. Invest. Med., 3:81, 1980. Reproduced with permission.*)[51]

Calcium Antagonists and the Coronary Circulation

The studies with parenterally administered drugs in experimental models of ischemia in the dog have yielded generally comparable findings,[52] emphasizing the essential pharmacologic similarities in the action of calcium antagonists with respect to the coronary circulation. The data suggest that these drugs dilate resistance as well as conductance coronary vessels; they reduce coronary vascular resistance, producing a variable change in coronary sinus flow and myocardial oxygen consumption. In experimental myocardial ischemia, a tendency for "coronary steal" is not induced by calcium antagonists but coronary collateral flow is augmented, a finding which is of clinical significance. There is a close concordance for the actions of diltiazem, nifedipine, and verapamil with respect to the coronary circulation in patients with ischemic heart disease. This is in line with the evolving knowledge that, as a class, these agents exert qualitatively similar therapeutic effects in various myocardial ischemic syndromes (see below).

Sublingual or intracoronary administration of nifedipine in patients with coronary artery disease has been shown to augment coronary flow by 100 percent in normal areas as well as in areas served by stenotic coronaries when flow is measured by the xenon-washout technique; the increases were relatively greater in poststenotic than in the normal areas and occurred under resting conditions as well as during continuous atrial pacing.[53,54] Sublingual nifedipine also significantly reduced the exercise-induced perfusion deficits as detected by thallium-201 myocardial imaging.[53,54] The drug had no effect on coronary sinus flow or myocardial oxygen consumption either at rest or during rapid atrial pacing; however, a decrease in myocardial oxygen extraction indicated coronary vasodilatation.[55,56] When administered intravenously, nifedipine induced an increase in the coronary sinus oxygen saturation[57] and an increase in coronary artery diameter in normal and poststenotic segments when injected by the intracoronary route.[34] Thus, the overall effects of nifedipine are consistent with a mild coronary vasodilatory action, reduced coronary arteriolar resistance, and increased myocardial blood flow without a significant reduction in myocardial oxygen consumption under resting conditions.[57,58] It is also known that coronary hemodynamic alterations induced by the cold pressor test or ergonovine are attenuated by nifedipine.[59] Although studies with diltiazem have been limited, its actions in this context are likely to be similar to those of nifedipine or verapamil. Studies with verapamil perhaps most clearly illustrate the overall effects of calcium antagonists on the coronary circulation in patients with coronary artery disease. From gross angiographic appearances, Mignault, in 1966,[60] concluded that IV verapamil did not alter the caliber of either normal or atherosclerotic vessels, whereas Luebs et al,[61] using myocardial clearance of rubidium as an index of coronary blood flow, found that IV verapamil increased coronary blood flow in patients without coronary artery disease while no such effect was apparent in patients with diseased vessels. Although a decrease in myocardial oxygen consumption and an increase in coronary arteriolar resistance has been suggested in one study[46] when verapamil is given intravenously, the bulk of the evidence suggests that, as in the case of the other calcium antagonists, verapamil *reduces* coronary arteriolar resistance without a significant effect on coronary sinus flow (measured by thermodilution) or myocardial oxygen consumption.[62-64] A computer-assisted quantitative angiographic technique has shown that the drug has the capability to dilate not only the normal but also stenotic coronary artery lesions by 10 to 20 percent[64] with comparable increases in the cross-sectional area and a significant decrease in estimated flow resistance. The quantitative angiographic technique has also demonstrated that intravenous verapamil has the potential to inhibit both sympathetic as well as ergonovine-induced coronary vasoconstriction in diseased human coronary arteries.[65] The overall findings on the effects of intravenously administered verapamil on coronary and systemic hemodynamics thus appear to illustrate a spectrum of action of calcium antagonists in general. These drugs produce a small but significant dilatation of not only normal but also the narrowed segments of the coronary arteries with a corresponding reduction in estimated flow resistance. Such vasodilatory response is accompanied by a fall in total coronary vascular resistance with the tendency for the coronary sinus blood flow to increase, suggesting that these drugs dilate both conductance and the resistance components of the coronary arteries. However, there is no change in myocardial oxygen consumption despite a significant reduction in the heart rate–blood pressure product under the influence of these drugs. During chronic oral therapy, the reduction in the heart rate–blood pressure product is considerably less than that after beta blockade[66] despite the use of dosage regimens producing identical effects on exercise-induced angina. Thus, it appears that, unlike the case with beta blocking drugs, the observed hemodynamic actions of calcium antagonists do not account for their potent documented antianginal effects in patients with coronary artery disease. The role of their vasodilator properties in this setting is nevertheless unclear, but the fact that they all tend to reverse the vasoconstriction induced by ergonovine and other provocative maneuvers provides the clear rationale for their therapeutic application in vasospastic ischemic myocardial syndromes.

THERAPEUTIC APPLICATIONS

The complete spectrum of the therapeutic utility of calcium antagonists is still not fully delineated. However, it appears to be at least as extensive as that for the beta-adrenoceptor blocking drugs. The cardiovascular conditions in which calcium channel-blocking drugs have either been found to be unequivocally effective or in which they appear to hold promise are listed in Table 2. It is emphasized that in certain clinical situations they may have advantages over beta blockers; in others they may be administered in combination with them to achieve optimum clinical results in certain major cardiovascular disorders.

Myocardial Ischemic Syndromes

The development of calcium antagonists as antianginal compounds in the 1970s has occurred simultaneously with the accumulation of evidence that a primary decrease in coronary blood flow may constitute an important and frequent mechanism that mediates the genesis of various myocardial syndromes in patients with an entire spectrum of coronary artery disease.[67–70] The compelling investigative results derived from hemodynamic and electrocardiographic monitoring,[69,71] angiographic studies,[69] and radioisotope perfusion imaging[67] have clearly documented that myocardial ischemia does not always result as a consequence of increased oxygen demand.[67–71] Thus, antianginal agents such as calcium antagonists which not only decrease myocardial demand but may also enhance coronary blood flow are of particular therapeutic interest since

TABLE 2
Therapeutic applications of calcium antagonists

1 Myocardial ischemic syndromes
  a Prinzmetal angina
  b Chronic stable angina
  c Unstable angina
  d Myocardial infarction
  e Myocardial preservation during open heart surgery
2 Cardiac arrhythmias
  a Supraventricular tachyarrhythmias
  b Ventricular arrhythmias
  c Prevention of sudden death in survivors of acute myocardial infarction
3 Systemic hypertension
  a Control of hypertensive emergencies
  b Chronic hypotensive therapy
4 Hypertrophic cardiomyopathies
5 Miscellaneous cardiovascular disorders
  a Pulmonary hypertension
  b Acute and chronic congestive heart failure
  c Cerebrovascular diseases
  d Raynaud's phenomenon
  e Inhibition of platelet aggregability

current evidence favors the concept that myocardial ischemia develops as a result of a complex interplay of structural coronary disease, normal vasomobility, and focal vascular hypersensitivity;[72] the relative significance of these features may vary with different ischemic myocardial syndromes.

PRINZMETAL VARIANT ANGINA

That coronary artery spasm is the underlying mechanism of variant angina is no longer in serious doubt.[69] Numerous controlled as well as uncontrolled studies have now attested to the value of calcium antagonists in controlling attacks of angina poorly responsive to conventional therapy.

Initial reports indicated that 40 to 80 mg of nifedipine daily dramatically reduced symptoms in such patients.[73–75] Experience in the United States with 127 patients with or without underlying fixed obstructive coronary lesions, most of whom had previously failed with conventional antianginal therapy, was striking even though the study was neither blinded nor statistically controlled. Nifedipine in doses of 40 to 160 mg/day completely eliminated spontaneous pain episodes in 63 percent of patients, and in 87 percent of patients decreased the frequency of attacks by at least 50 percent. Although side effects in this particular study occurred in 37 percent of patients, they were severe enough to require discontinuation of the drug in only 5 percent.[76] In a multicenter, randomized, double-blind withdrawal study comparing nifedipine to placebo the former was again demonstrated to be significantly more efficacious.[77] Nifedipine was also found to effectively block ergonovine-induced coronary spasm in patients with variant angina.[78] Furthermore, nifedipine has been shown to prevent malignant arrhythmias and conduction disturbances associated with variant angina attacks.[76,79,80]

Perhaps the most detailed and controlled study documenting the efficacy of a calcium antagonist in Prinzmetal angina, a double-blind placebo-controlled study utilizing objective end points (Fig. 4), has been with verapamil reported by Johnson et al.[81] The drug was found to reduce anginal frequency, nitroglycerin consumption, number of hospitalizations, and number of episodes of ST deviations apparent on ambulatory ECG readings over a 9-month period when compared to placebo; there were no side effects requiring reduction in dosage or discontinuation.[81] In another study with verapamil (120 to 320 mg daily for 8 months), it was found that 59 percent of patients became entirely asymptomatic, and an additional 29 percent had a reduction in pain episodes to less than two per month.[82] In a long-term follow-up study of verapamil, long-acting nitrates, or both in 138 patients with spontaneous angina associated with ST-segment elevation, results were also

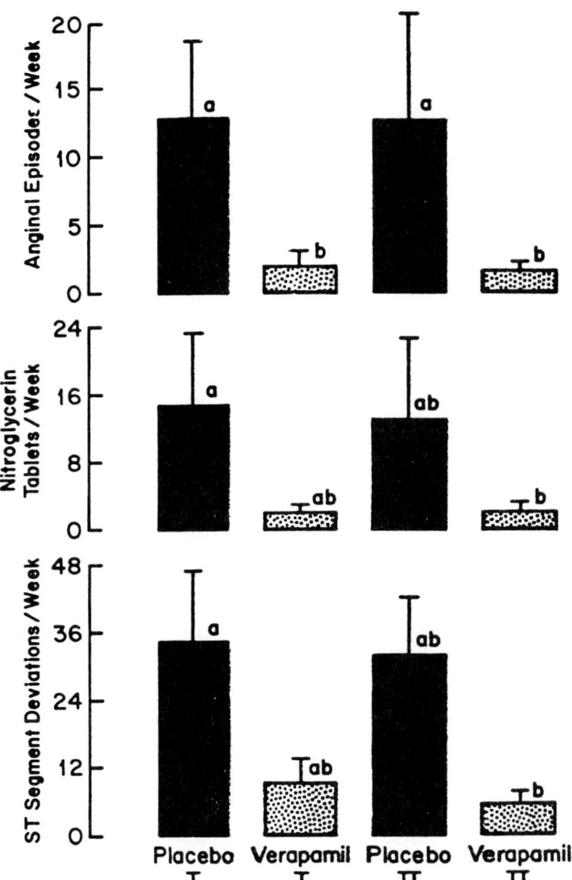

FIGURE 4 Double-blind placebo-controlled study of the effects of oral verapamil in Prinzmetal angina. Each phase shown contains the mean of weekly data over 2 months. Verapamil had a significant effect on ST-segment deviations recorded on 24-h Holter recordings, nitroglycerin consumption, and anginal episodes. *(From S. M. Johnson, D. R. Mauitson, J. T. Willerson, and L. D. Hillis, A Controlled Trial of Verapamil for Prinzmetal's Variant Angina, N. Engl. J. Med., 304(15):862, 1981. Reproduced with permission.)*

encouraging. By 1 year 20 percent, and by 4 years 50 percent of patients were asymptomatic, with remissions occurring more frequently in those with less severe underlying coronary artery disease.[83]

The experience with diltiazem, albeit less extensive, is comparable. For example, in a small double-blind crossover study, 240 mg daily of the drug significantly reduced the number of episodes of pain and the amount of nitroglycerin consumption while 120 mg/day was without effect.[84] A study of short- and long-term efficacy of diltiazem revealed that the short-term response, in which 7 of 12 patients had at least a 50 percent reduction in anginal frequency, was generally predictive of the long-term response at 16 months.[85] Finally, in a multicenter, randomized, controlled crossover study, 19 percent of patients on 120 mg of

diltiazem daily became pain-free while at 240 mg daily 30 percent became pain-free and experienced a 68 percent reduction in anginal frequency from study entry.[86]

Little is known about the relative efficacy of the various calcium antagonists in variant angina. In one direct comparison of verapamil, nifedipine, and placebo in 10 patients, most of whom were also taking isosorbide dinitrate, verapamil and nifedipine were equipotent in reducing the frequency of chest pain and ST-segment deviations and in reducing the number of nitroglycerin tablets consumed. Nifedipine, however, was associated with more frequent side effects.[87] In a large Japanese multicenter survey, both nifedipine and diltiazem completely eliminated evidence of ischemic syndromes in about 75 percent of patients, with clinical improvement in more than 90 percent, whereas verapamil eliminated variant anginal attacks in only 11 percent of cases but was effective in 86 percent,[88] but dose response comparisons were not made. In comparison of efficacy in preventing ergonovine-induced coronary vasospasm, although nifedipine, diltiazem, and verapamil all increased the spasm threshold, nifedipine was the most potent agent.[89] Although no systematic data are available, it is conceivable that calcium antagonists may be used in combination in resistant cases of Prinzmetal's angina since their mechanism of action in relaxing smooth muscle in the coronary circulation may differ. However, at present there is little systematic experience in this regard.

Although beta blockers may aggravate coronary vasospasm in patients with variant angina,[90] it is of interest that the combination of long-acting nitrates and calcium channel blockers may be more effective than either agent alone.[79,91] In patients with variant angina, withdrawal of nitrate preparations or calcium channel blockers is potentially dangerous and should therefore be done with caution.[77,79]

CHRONIC STABLE ANGINA

There is now an impressive body of evidence that when calcium antagonists are administered in optimal dosage regimens, they all reduce the frequency of angina and the extent of nitroglycerin consumption; they increase exercise duration on treadmill or on bicycle, and minimize the electrocardiographic, hemodynamic, metabolic, and functional abnormalities induced by exercise or atrial pacing.[92] There do not appear to be major differences in potency in this regard among various calcium antagonists. However, the precise mechanisms whereby these salutary effects are mediated are not fully elucidated but may result from net changes in oxygen demand as well as supply (Table 3). It is conceivable that a modulation of the normal coronary vasomobility with stenosis-dilatation may constitute a significant mechanism of the observed antianginal action of this class of compounds.[64]

TABLE 3

Potential mechanisms of action of calcium antagonists in chronic stable angina*

I Increased myocardial oxygen supply
   A Increased coronary blood flow (all agents)
      1 Coronary arterial dilatation
      2 Improved subendocardial perfusion
II Decreased myocardial oxygen demand
   A Decreased peripheral vascular resistance afterload (all agents)
   B Decreased myocardial contractility (verapamil)
   C Decreased heart rate (verapamil, diltiazem)

*Not all the postulated mechanisms have been verified in patients. They have been extrapolated from findings in experimental models of myocardial ischemia.

SOURCE: Adapted from Braunwald.[10]

Extensive studies with nifedipine have consistently shown efficacy of the drug in chronic stable angina. For example, a single sublingual dose of 10 or 20 mg of the drug has been found to reduce anginal frequency by 23 to 100 percent and increase exercise tolerance by 20 to 70 percent, as judged by graded stress testing against the background of placebo control.[93–95] The data from four double-blind-controlled studies, using a single dose of nifedipine, demonstrated an average reduction in exercise-induced ischemic ST depression of 32 percent.[9] The acute improvement in exercise-induced ST-segment deviations in patients with chronic stable angina appeared to persist for at least 6 weeks when therapy was continued with 20 mg of nifedipine three times daily. Qualitatively similar results have been obtained in over 4,000 patients treated from 2 weeks to 3 years.[93] Although the doses used in many of these early studies ranged from 10 to 60 mg daily, there was a suggestion that improvement in angina may be dose-dependent, and therefore 120 mg or more per day may be required for optimal therapy in some patients.[9]

Studies attempting to elucidate nifedipine's antianginal effects have shown a diminution in the rate-pressure product at any given work load.[96,97] Maximum systolic blood pressure was found to be decreased and the double-product at the onset of angina or at cessation of exercise was similar when compared with control, suggesting that the improved exercise capacity observed with nifedipine was due essentially to its ability to decrease afterload rather than to increase myocardial oxygen supply.[98,99] In a hemodynamic study in patients with coronary artery disease, 14 of 20 developed evidence of LV dysfunction and/or ischemia with exercise or pacing.[100] The sublingual administration of 20 mg of nifedipine shortened the duration of pain, reduced ST-segment depression, and reversed the hemodynamic abnormality. In a second group of patients with recent myocardial infarction, nifedipine re-duced left ventricular end-diastolic pressure and volume, and increased ejection fraction from 43 percent to 58 percent. In these patients with moderate left ventricular dysfunction, nifedipine appeared both safe and efficacious.[100]

It should be emphasized that in the case of nifedipine, reflex increases in heart rate almost invariably occur and may be dose-dependent. In general, however, such increases in heart rate do not appear to nullify or reverse the overall decreases in myocardial oxygen consumption resulting from alterations in the determinants of myocardial oxygen demand. Nevertheless, chest pain in patients with chronic stable angina treated with the drug may be aggravated in about 10 percent of patients.[9] At least the potentially deleterious effects of augmented heart rate and contractility induced by the drug can be obviated by the addition of various beta blockers to nifedipine in patients with chronic stable angina. Propranolol administered in combination with nifedipine not only abolishes the increase in resting heart rate but lowers heart rate, blood pressure, and hence the double-product at a given work load compared to either agent alone.[101] Clinically, the combination of nifedipine (10 mg tid) with propranolol (40 mg tid) or metoprolol leads to a greater decrease in anginal frequency and nitroglycerin consumption compared to that when either of the agents is used alone.[102,103]

Thus, the overall clinical experience suggests that nifedipine, used alone or in combination with beta blockers, is an effective and relatively safe drug for the treatment of patients with chronic stable angina. However, when combined with nitrates, side effects related to excessive peripheral vasodilatation may become troublesome.

In contrast, neither verapamil nor diltiazem has been found to exacerbate angina since reflex increases in heart rate and contractility are offset by their noncompetitive sympatholytic actions. Furthermore, their somewhat weaker peripheral vasodilator actions allow the concomitant use of long-acting nitrates, while their overall antianginal actions are comparable to those of nifedipine. It is further noteworthy that both agents can also be combined with beta antagonists although caution is warranted in patients with reduced ventricular function or with conduction system disease.[7]

A number of controlled double-blind clinical trials have demonstrated a significant reduction in frequency of anginal episodes and nitroglycerin consumption while improving exercise tolerance when verapamil was given at varying doses.[104–108] The precise mechanism by which the drug exerts its beneficial effect in chronic stable angina is, however, uncertain and appears multifactorial. The drug causes a 10 percent reduction in rate-pressure product at rest and a 12 percent reduction in rate-pressure product at submaximal exercise compared to over 30 percent reduction by beta blockers.[66]

In addition, at peak exercise and pressure-rate product, similar to that obtained on placebo, there appears to be less marked ST-segment depression, suggesting a favorable redistribution of coronary blood flow to ischemic zones.[109] The verapamil dose response relationship is of particular significance in patients with stable angina. At lower doses (e.g., 40 mg qid), the drug is essentially indistinguishable from a placebo,[106,110–111] with significant antianginal effects becoming evident at doses equal to or higher than 80 mg tid or qid. Doses higher than 480 mg daily are associated with significant side effects.[112]

Recent studies have also confirmed the efficacy of diltiazem in chronic stable angina, but the overall experiences are still limited compared to those with verapamil and nifedipine. Two recent multicenter, double-blind placebo-controlled trials have demonstrated that the drug significantly decreases anginal frequency and nitroglycerin consumption while increasing total exercise duration and the time to onset of angina.[113,114] In this setting, the drug appears safe with no effect on PR or QRS intervals. Side effects necessitating discontinuation of diltiazem have been very rare.[114] As with verapamil, the dose of diltiazem is an important determinant of the therapeutic response. In the earlier studies with the drug utilizing 30 to 60 mg tid signs or symptoms of myocardial ischemia were improved in about 55 percent of patients, but in 26 percent of patients placebo was more effective than diltiazem.[115,116] More recent studies have demonstrated that 240 mg of diltiazem daily is more efficacious than 180 mg daily, which is in turn more effective than 120 mg daily, emphasizing the dose-dependence of the beneficial effects.[113] It is possible that the major mechanism mediating the prolongation of duration of exercise by diltiazem in chronic stable angina is a reduction in the rate-pressure product.[113] As in the case of verapamil, the hemodynamic effects of diltiazem vary with the underlying hemodynamic status. For example, in a study in which patients were classified into two groups by resting pulmonary capillary wedge (PCW) pressure, those with a PCW less than 16 mmHg (group 1) or greater than 16 mmHg (group 2), 1 h following administration of 120 mg of diltiazem both groups experienced decreases in the frequency of anginal attacks, the mean systolic blood pressure, systemic vascular resistance, and the rate-pressure product. However, those patients with a PCW of greater than 16 had a significant increase in cardiac output and reduction of mean pulmonary artery pressure, mean PCW, and pulmonary vascular resistance at peak exercise, compared to placebo.[117] Thus, although experience is still limited, diltiazem appears efficacious and safe in chronic stable angina when used at an appropriate dose and may have therapeutically desirable effects in patients with disturbed left ventricular function, especially if the latter is due essentially to ischemia.

Comparison of calcium antagonists and other antianginal agents in chronic stable angina

As already noted, the antianginal efficacy of the calcium antagonists is dose-dependent. This is also true, of course, of other agents, and thus direct comparative studies are difficult to perform and evaluate. However, using the degree of ST-segment depression during an exercise tolerance test as a test criterion, single doses of several agents have been compared. Nifedipine (20 mg SL), propranolol (80 mg PO), pindolol (2.5 mg PO), and nitroglycerin (0.8 mg SL) appeared equally efficacious. Verapamil (5 mg IV) in this setting was somewhat less effective and isosorbide dinitrate (10 mg PO) and pentaerythrityl tetranitrate (150 mg PO) the least effective.[118] For the primary therapy of exertional angina, nifedipine appeared equal to isosorbide dinitrate in efficacy.[119] Nifedipine (10 mg tid) was approximately equipotent to propranolol (20 mg tid) but less effective when compared to higher beta blocking doses (40 or 80 mg tid) in reducing the frequency of anginal attacks.[102,119] Nifedipine (10 mg) appeared more effective than propranolol (20 mg) in reducing exercise-induced ST-segment depression, and more effective than metoprolol in enabling patients to tolerate greater work loads.[101,120]

Several recent studies comparing verapamil and propranolol have helped delineate approximate dose equivalence and further define differences. When reduction of anginal frequency, nitroglycerin consumption, and exercise-induced ST depression and prolongation of duration of treadmill exercise were used as test criteria, verapamil (120 mg tid) was found to be as effective as propranolol (100 mg tid).[106,111] In a double-blind randomized comparison of propranolol (80 mg qid) and verapamil (80 mg qid), both drugs improved exercise performance as judged by the prolongation of time to ST-segment depression, and there were comparable improvements in the ischemia-induced changes in ventricular ejection fractions. Neither drug, at these doses, reduced resting ejection fractions in this group, which had relatively well-preserved ventricular performance.[121] Another study using multiple-gated equilibrium blood pool imaging comparing oral verapamil (480 mg/day) to oral propranolol (320 mg/day) found comparable potency in reducing the ischemic consequences of exercise. It appeared that propranolol's beneficial effects were due essentially to its effects on myocardial oxygen demand, but verapamil's efficacy may have been due to additional mechanisms such as alteration of myocardial metabolism or primary changes in perfusion.[66] A comparison of two doses of propranolol (40 mg q6h and 80 mg q6h) to two of verapamil (80 mg q6h and 120 mg q6h) demonstrated that both propranolol and high-dose verapamil significantly reduced the need for nitroglycerin and decreased ST-segment deviations on ambulatory ECG recordings. Although neither drug had a deleterious effect on left ventricular volumes or left ventricular ejection fractions, propranolol worsened forced vital capacity and forced expiratory volume.[36] Finally, in a comparison of increasing doses of propranolol and verapamil, the latter produced greater improvement in exercise duration and in ischemic ST depression at the end of exercise. Of note was the observation that two patients experienced propranolol rebound while none had an exacerbation of angina during verapamil withdrawal.[122]

Little information is available comparing different calcium antagonists with one another. In one double-blind randomized trial of verapamil (120 mg tid) and nifedipine (20 mg tid), both drugs increased maximum work capacity, decreased anginal frequency, consumption of glyceryl trinitrate, and systolic blood pressure at rest and with exercise. The overall efficacy was felt to be equal, but side effects were more commonly encountered with nifedipine.[123]

UNSTABLE ANGINA PECTORIS

The role of calcium antagonists in this setting remains to be fully elucidated although the available experience and the known pharmacologic properties of this class of agents suggest an important alternative modality of therapy. At present it is uncertain whether they are superior to beta blockers, beta blockers plus nitrates, or high-dose long-acting nitrates.

Early results with nifedipine suggested that the addition of the drug (30 to 120 mg daily) to propranolol and long-acting nitrates could abolish rest pain in about 85 percent of patients acutely and during a 6-month follow-up.[124,125] In a large, double-blind randomized trial, the efficacy of adding nifedipine to propranolol and nitrates using failure of medical treatment (defined as sudden death, myocardial infarction, or bypass surgery within 4 months) as an end point, nifedipine was significantly more effective than placebo in the entire group. In the subset of patients with ST-segment elevation during attacks, the drug was particularly beneficial.[126]

In two controlled clinical trials, verapamil was also effective in reducing the number of ischemic episodes in patients with unstable angina.[127,128] Of particular interest is the recent demonstration that verapamil but not propranolol (given *without* nitrates) significantly reduced the frequency of myocardial ischemic episodes in such a subset of patients.[129] The precise significance of this observation merits further study. However, the overall experience indicates that calcium antagonists, either alone or with nitrates, provide an effective therapeutic modality for the initial medical control of unstable angina, particularly in the group of patients in whom coronary artery spasm may be involved in its pathogenesis.

MYOCARDIAL INFARCTION

Although coronary artery spasm has been implicated from time to time in the pathogenesis of acute myocardial infarction,[130] recent evidence from the use of coronary dilators during thrombolytic therapy has indicated that spasm is responsible for coronary occlusion in only a minority of patients.[131] Thus, the role of calcium antagonists in the early treatment of acute infarction is limited. However, experimental[132–134] and preliminary clinical[135] data suggest that as a class these agents have the potential to reduce infarct size, an effect that may be mediated by the inhibition of calcium entry into the myocardial cell, by augmentation of collateral perfusion,[133] and by the reduction in oxygen demand due to their hemodynamic effects. Whether such experimental observations will eventually be translated into a comparable clinical benefit in terms of a favorable effect on morbidity and mortality rates remains to be critically tested. On the other hand, a clear rationale exists for the role of these drugs in the control of recurrent myocardial ischemia in postinfarct patients and in the treatment of supraventricular tachycardias complicating the early phases of acute myocardial infarction.[136–139]

MYOCARDIAL PRESERVATION

It is known that following a period of coronary artery occlusion and subsequent reperfusion the accumulation of excess intracellular mitochondrial Ca^{2+} interferes with the cellular capacity to generate ATP and may contribute to cell necrosis in the ischemic myocardium.[140] The progressive ischemic contracture accompanied by abnormalities of systolic and diastolic ventricular function that supervene[141] is greatly minimized by pretreatment with calcium antagonists,[133] the beneficial effects being associated with a significant diminution in the accumulation of mitochondrial Ca^{2+}.[140] All three calcium antagonists, in a variety of experimental preparations,[132–134,140] have now been shown to reduce myocardial damage during coronary occlusion, especially during reperfusion,[142] and to preserve left ventricular function on cardiopulmonary bypass during protracted total ischemia,[143] while preliminary clinical experience indicates a reduction in myocardial enzyme release with a decreased incidence of myocardial injury as determined by technetium pyrophosphate scintigraphy.[144] Thus, it is clear that these preliminary experimental and clinical data on the use of various calcium antagonists are encouraging and suggest the potential utility of these agents in minimizing the severity of ischemic damage intraoperatively during open heart surgery. However, the relative potency of individual agents in this context is uncertain, and it is not clear whether as a class of agents they are superior to other cardioplegic regimens. It must nevertheless be emphasized that a great deal of the safety of these compounds intraoperatively and postoperatively may depend on their reflex actions induced by peripheral dilatation. If this were blocked by the concomitant therapy with beta antagonists (a regimen increasingly used), while ischemic injury might be reduced, severe hemodymanic depression might result from the negative inotropic actions of the compounds.

Cardiac Arrhythmias

For the most part, the antiarrhythmic effects of the slow-channel inhibitors are accountable in terms of their direct electrophysiological actions.[45] Since the AV node is slow channel-dependent and may become the site of either deranged impulse formation or con-

duction, calcium antagonists may be antiarrhythmic by either decreasing automaticity or preventing reentry in this region. These actions may be considered the "direct" antiarrhythmic properties of this class of drugs; they lead to termination of acute episodes of paroxysmal supraventricular tachycardia (PSVT), the slowing of the ventricular response in atrial fibrillation and atrial flutter, and the prevention of recurrent PSVT. As discussed earlier, calcium antagonists have little or no significant electrophysiological effect on ventricular muscle and are thus unlikely to be potent antiarrhythmic agents by "direct" action. However, by influencing the course of myocardial ischemia in patients with coronary artery disease, particularly vasospastic processes, the slow-channel blockers may exert significant "indirect" antiarrhythmic activity. The spectrum of the antiarrhythmic activities of calcium antagonists is summarized in Table 4. Most of the clinical

TABLE 4
Antiarrhythmic effects of calcium antagonists

Arrhythmia	Response to parenteral administration	Response during chronic prophylaxis
1 Sinus tachycardia	Variable	Of little value
2 Paroxysmal supraventricular tachycardia		
a AV nodal reentrant	90–100% conversion	Modest effect in preventing recurrence
b Circus movement (orthodromic) with bypass tract (overt or concealed)	80–90% conversion	Modest effect in preventing recurrence
c Circus movement (antidromic) with bypass tract	No effect	Of no value
d Sinus node or intraatrial reentrant	Probably effective	Effect unknown
e Ectopic atrial tachycardia	Produces AV block without conversion	Of little value
3 Paroxysmal atrial tachycardia with AV block (with or without digitalis toxicity)	May convert to sinus rhythm (? mechanism)	Effect unknown
4 Multifocal atrial tachycardia	Variable	Variable (more data needed)
5 Atrial fibrillation	Slows ventricular response (conversion to sinus rhythm rare)	Control of ventricular response at rest and with exercise excellent
6 Atrial flutter	Slows ventricular response (conversion to sinus rhythm rare)	Control of ventricular response at rest and with exercise good
7 Atrial flutter and fibrillation with W-P-W syndrome (wide QRS)	May accelerate ventricular response	Contraindicated
8 Ventricular tachyarrhythmias (including torsade de pointes)	Generally low rate of conversion except when due to coronary artery spasm	Rarely successful except secondarily by preventing myocardial ischemia

antiarrhythmic data on the calcium antagonists has been accumulated for verapamil. Preliminary studies with diltiazem are also encouraging. Nifedipine in vivo appears to have no "direct" antiarrhythmic properties but may have "indirect" antiarrhythmic activity in certain myocardial ischemic syndromes.

PAROXYSMAL SUPRAVENTRICULAR TACHYCARDIA—ACUTE TREATMENT

In most patients with paroxysmal supraventricular tachycardia (PSVT) the AV node constitutes the anterograde limb of the reentrant loop and the portion most susceptible to the depressant electrophysiological action of calcium antagonists (verapamil and diltiazem). This undoubtedly accounts for the consistent observation during a decade of clinical experience that intravenous verapamil promptly and predictably reverts 80 to 100 percent of cases of PSVT to sinus rhythm.[45,145–150] The usual dose of verapamil is 3 to 5 mg in children or 10 to 15 mg in adults. Recent studies have concentrated on mechanisms by which the drug exerts its salutary effects.[151,152] There is an increasing consensus that intravenous verapamil is now the drug of choice for the termination of PSVT due to reentry involving anterograde conduction through the AV node. Preliminary studies with other calcium antagonists (diltiazem, tiapamil, gallopamil) suggest that they may also be variably effective in the termination of narrow QRS complex PSVT.[153,154] A knowledge of diltiazem's electrophysiological effects, however, would suggest that the drug is likely to be less effective than verapamil in converting PSVT.[27,155]

In most cases of PSVT, verapamil induces reversion to sinus rhythm within 2 to 3 min although occasional cases convert within 10 min. The success rate can be further improved to nearly 100 percent by concomitant carotid sinus massage or the addition of 5 to 10 mg of edrophonium in rapid succession. Similar data exist for the therapeutic efficacy of verapamil in children and elderly persons. Several modes of conversion to sinus rhythm in PSVT have been reported with verapamil. The most common observation is an abrupt termination. In many cases the cycle length may prolong somewhat, followed by a brief pause before reversion to sinus rhythm. In other cases AV dissociation followed by junctional escape before restoration of sinus rhythm is observed, or rarely transient atrial fibrillation prior to reversion is seen.[145] Finally, the occurrence of premature ventricular contractions (without ventricular tachycardia) or the development of alternating cycle length before conversion have been reported.[146]

Limited information is available comparing "standard" therapy to verapamil or other calcium antagonists in PSVT. In one study using a crossover design, 5 mg of practolol converted 8 of 20 cases of PSVT,

whereas 5 mg of verapamil produced sinus rhythm in 19 of 20 cases. In 9 of the 12 cases in which the beta blocker had failed, verapamil was effective.[146a] Although insufficient systematic data exist comparing overall efficacy of slow-channel blockers to those of vagal maneuvers, intravenous tensilon, alpha agonists, or digoxin, alone or in combination, in certain instances verapamil offers distinct advantages. Where urgent termination is desirable, the delayed onset of action of digoxin (15 to 60 min or longer) may be unacceptable. Furthermore, with intravenous verapamil's short elimination half-life, dc electrocardioversion can be attempted reasonably promptly. In addition to verapamil's apparent higher conversion rate compared to beta blockers, the use of beta antagonists in bronchospastic syndromes, diabetes mellitus, and peripheral vascular disease is clearly less preferable to that of verapamil and diltiazem.

PAROXYSMAL SUPRAVENTRICULAR TACHYCARDIA—CHRONIC PROPHYLAXIS

Again, the most extensive experience has been obtained with verapamil, but diltiazem and other calcium antagonists which prolong AV conduction and refractoriness have potential applications. Because of the extremely variable pattern of recurrences of PSVT between patients and with the same patient, prophylactic efficacy is difficult to determine. Nevertheless, in patients with PSVT who initially responded to intravenous verapamil, long-term benefit has been observed.[156] In addition, in comparison with placebo the drug has been demonstrated to be both effective and well-tolerated.[157] It may be possible to predict long-term efficacy by response to intravenous verapamil studied by programmed electrical stimulation.[158,159] Although promising, more experience is needed in this regard.

Atrial fibrillation The administration of intravenous verapamil may produce three different responses in patients with atrial fibrillation. Perhaps the most common is temporary slowing of the ventricular response by inhibition of AV conduction.[160–162] However, unless an infusion is begun within 30 min, the ventricular response begins to accelerate almost immediately. In 25 percent or more of patients with atrial fibrillation verapamil, by an as yet unexplained mechanism, may lead to "regularization" of the ventricular response, without conversion.[145,163] Finally, an occasional patient may convert from atrial fibrillation to sinus rhythm,[146,153] especially those with recent onset of the arrhythmia and with relatively normal left atrial size. The administration of intravenous verapamil to already digitalized patients in atrial fibrillation can further decrease the ventricular response[164] by an additive depressant effect on the AV node.

Oral verapamil has been shown to be effective alone or in combination with digitalis in reducing resting ventricular response in atrial fibrillation, being especially effective in attenuating the exercise-induced increases in heart rate whereas digoxin's major effect is essentially on the resting ventricular response.[159,164–166] The potential summation of the effects of digoxin and verapamil in depressing AV node conduction, in addition to the significant interaction resulting in increased serum digoxin levels, should be emphasized in this setting.[164] Verapamil's efficacy in maintaining sinus rhythm after conversion from atrial fibrillation is unclear, but on electrophysiological grounds, the drug is unlikely to be particularly effective in this regard. In one recent controlled trial, quinidine was significantly more effective in producing cardioversion and maintaining it at 3 months.[167] Preliminary results with diltiazem reveal a slowed ventricular response and regularization.[154] As might be expected, nifedipine is without effect.

Atrial flutter The bulk of clinical experience in atrial flutter is again with verapamil. Here, the drug may be useful diagnostically and therapeutically. A single intravenous dose will generally increase the degree of AV block in atrial flutter with 2:1 block without converting the arrhythmia, thus distinguishing it from PSVT.[145,146] The slowing of ventricular response obviously may be therapeutically advantageous. Some patients for reasons that are not understood develop atrial fibrillation before reversion to sinus rhythm, while an occasional person is restored directly.[145] Consistent with the known electrophysiological effects of verapamil, however, the overall conversion rate is low. Limited data suggest that orally administered verapamil in combination with other antiarrhythmics may be of value in controlling the ventricular response in atrial flutter.[156] Other calcium antagonists with AV nodal inhibitory properties should also produce similar results.

Miscellaneous supraventricular tachyarrhythmias Although experience is limited, in a variety of supraventricular dysrhythmias other than those thus far discussed several potentially useful applications of verapamil are of interest. In one of two patients with sinus nodal tachycardia secondary to reentry within the SA node or its adjacent tissue, intravenous verapamil promptly terminated the tachycardia.[151] There are increasing data to suggest that intravenous verapamil is less effective in converting ectopic atrial tachycardia than paroxysmal supraventricular tachycardia of the reentrant type.[152] The efficacy of verapamil in patients with paroxysmal atrial tachycardia with block (not necessarily due to digitalis toxicity) has been evaluated. In 10 of 14 patients initial reversion of the arrhythmia to sinus rhythm was obtained, but subsequent relapse occurred in 4.[168] One study of supraventricular tachyarrhythmias associated with chronic pulmonary disease, including multifocal atrial tachycardia, suggests that verapamil may occasionally be beneficial.[169]

CALCIUM ANTAGONISTS IN PRE-EXCITATION SYNDROMES

The effects of the calcium antagonists, particularly verapamil, on arrhythmias complicating pre-excitation syndromes are predictable from their basic electrophysiological properties. Verapamil and diltiazem, but not nifedipine, depress AV nodal conduction in such patients. Verapamil generally appears to have minimal effect on the presumably fast channel-dependent bypass tracts. In one study the anterograde refractory period of the bypass tract was slightly shortened in most patients, unchanged in one, and minimally lengthened in several others. The shortening, however, was much less than that produced by digitalis.[170] In a second study verapamil shortened the anterograde effective refractory period of the accessory pathway in three of eight patients, and abbreviated the shortest cycle length with 1:1 conduction over the bypass tract in two patients.[171] From the known electrophysiological properties of the heart,[27,154] one may infer that diltiazem will have similar quantitative effects, but systematic data are not yet available. Thus, verapamil has been found to be effective in terminating the acute paroxysms of the narrow QRS (orthodromic) supraventricular tachycardia complicating the W-P-W (Wolff-Parkinson-White) syndrome.[172] The other calcium antagonists (except nifedipine) are likely to have variable potency in this regard, but their role in the chronic prophylaxis remain to be defined.

On the other hand, caution must be exercised in the use of calcium channel blockers in patients with pre-excitation syndromes complicated by atrial fibrillation or atrial flutter. Figure 5 illustrates the effects of intravenous verapamil in atrial fibrillation complicating the W-P-W syndrome. Agents which either shorten the effective refractory period of the bypass tracts (e.g., digitalis) or lengthen conduction over the AV node (digitalis, beta blockers, tensilon, and calcium antagonists) may augment the ventricular response rate and possibly precipitate ventricular fibrillation in such patients. In one electrophysiological study verapamil decreased the shortest R-R interval between pre-excited ventricular complexes during atrial fibrillation, and two patients demonstrated significant hemodynamic deterioration requiring cardioversion.[171] Thus, verapamil and other calcium antagonists are contraindicated in patients in whom atrial fibrillation or flutter complicate the W-P-W syndrome.

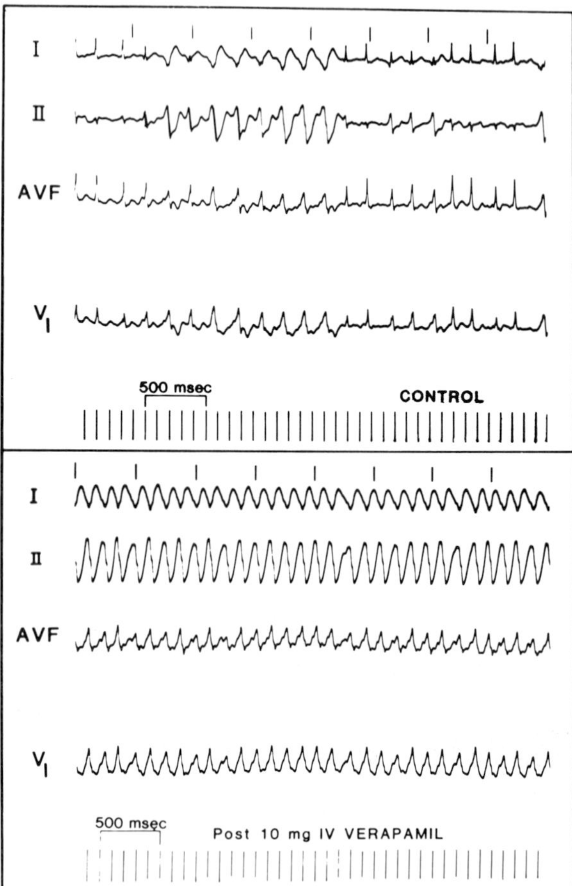

FIGURE 5 Effects of intravenous verapamil in atrial fibrillation complicating the W-P-W syndrome. *Upper panel:* Atrial fibrillation with fibrillatory impulses traversing the AV node (narrow QRS complexes) and the bypass tract (pre-excited impulses with wide QRS). *Lower panel:* Demonstrates changes after IV verapamil (10 mg). Note the marked increases in the ventricular responses over the bypass tract. (*From Johnson.*[81] *Reprinted by permission of the New England Journal of Medicine, 304(15):862, 1981. Reprinted with the permission of the author.*)

VENTRICULAR ARRHYTHMIAS

Despite promising theoretical and experimental considerations calcium antagonists appear to have a limited clinical role in ventricular arrhythmias. For example, there is a reasonable theoretical role for the slow channel in the genesis of the arrhythmias of obstructive cardiomyopathies[173] and those associated with mitral valve prolapse.[45] However, clinical experience to date, especially with hypertrophic cardiomyopathy, has not confirmed their efficacy.[174] Although a few controlled studies have demonstrated reduction in the number of PVCs complicating acute myocardial in-

farction,[175,176] the very limited experience in ventricular tachycardia associated with myocardial infarction or that occurring in the setting of chronic cardiac disease has been disappointing.[177]

Thus, preliminary evidence would suggest that calcium antagonists have little direct effect in ventricular arrhythmias.[178] Any apparent salutary effect may actually result from improved ischemia and therefore intramyocardial conduction through the drug's potent coronary vasodilatory properties.[179] Such an effect is likely to be most apparent in the setting of variant angina.[180] However, an occasional patient with recurrent ventricular arrhythmias resistant to the antiarrhythmic agents apparently responds to orally administered verapamil. The nature of such a beneficial response is unclear, and detailed studies of the patients who respond in this manner may reveal the underlying mechanisms involved.

Prevention of Sudden Death in Survivors of Acute Myocardial Infarction

An important question, as yet unanswered, is the role of calcium antagonists in the prevention of sudden cardiac death. The recent demonstration that beta blocking drugs can significantly reduce the risk of sudden death after myocardial infarction[181] and the presumption that this beneficial effect is due to decreased ischemia, not a primary antiarrhythmic effect, raises the possibility that the calcium antagonists may also be efficacious. Stringently controlled clinical trials will be needed to confirm or deny such a possibility, one that is likely to have an important impact on cardiovascular therapeutics if a favorable effect is demonstrated.

Systemic Hypertension

Calcium channel blockers are potent arterial dilators but their clinical utility in controlling systemic hypertension is essentially unexplored, and the definition of their value has lagged considerably behind those of their other clinical indications. A reassuring clinical observation is that the calcium antagonists nifedipine and verapamil appear to lower blood pressure to a degree directly related to pretreatment levels. For example, in normotensive patients with preserved ventricular function there is usually little or no reduction in blood pressure following administration of 10 mg of nifedipine orally or 5 mg of verapamil intravenously.[182,183] On the other hand, in patients with elevated blood pressures the degree of reduction is related directly to the basal levels of arterial pressure and systemic vascular resistance.[183,184] Thus, with doses of 10 mg of nifedipine orally or sublingually or 5 mg of intravenous verapamil the blood pressure reduction in severely hypertensive patients may be quite significant.[182,183] In the canine renovascular hypertension model nifedipine decreased systemic vascular resistance, lowered systolic and diastolic arterial pressure, induced tachycardia, and increased cardiac output. Unlike hydralazine, however, nifedipine reduced coronary vascular resistance and decreased myocardial oxygen consumption, thereby improving the myocardial supply-and-demand relationship.[185]

CALCIUM BLOCKERS AS ACUTE ANTIHYPERTENSIVE THERAPY

Several reports demonstrating the effectiveness of nifedipine in patients with hypertensive emergencies have been published.[186,187] In three patients in whom the average systemic arterial pressure was 307/164 mmHg, a 10-mg dose of nifedipine reduced the average blood pressure to 237/115 mmHg at 15 min. An additional 10 mg reduced the average systemic pressure to 176/89. In these same patients pulmonary arterial pressure fell progressively from 91/55 to 47/19 after the second dose of nifedipine. In a study of nifedipine in 43 patients in an emergency room nifedipine was also efficacious.[188] In those patients whose initial blood pressures were less than 110 mmHg diastolic, 10 mg of nifedipine administered sublingually decreased the average systolic pressure from 172 to 140 mmHg, and the average diastolic pressure from 109 to 88 mmHg. In that group of patients with more severe hypertension (diastolic pressure greater than 110 mmHg), the administration of 20 mg of nifedipine sublingually produced a decrease in average systolic pressure from 203 to 160 mmHg and in average diastolic pressure from 128 to 97 mmHg. The effect was seen within 1 to 5 min, and minimal adverse reactions were observed; these included facial flushing in three patients and symptomatic orthostatic hypotension in one. The antihypertensive effect of nifedipine in the acute situation generally persists for 3 to 5 h.[189–191]

CALCIUM CHANNEL BLOCKERS AS CHRONIC ANTIHYPERTENSIVE THERAPY

Data are still somewhat limited concerning the utility of the calcium antagonists as single agents in chronic antihypertensive therapy.[191,192] The efficacy of nifedipine in various studies appeared to be dose-related, with 10 mg three or four times daily producing a moderate decrease in arterial pressure,[191,193] and 30 mg orally producing more dramatic reductions in pressure.[194] The duration of antihypertensive action was also dose-related. At about 90 min after a 10-mg sublingual dose, blood pressure began to return toward base line, but

the hypertensive effect of a 20-mg dose was still present at 6 to 8 h.[195] During oral therapy over a 3-week period, 10 mg of nifedipine had an antihypertensive effect which lasted 8 to 12 h. Administration every 6 h significantly reduced blood pressure throughout the day without postural hypotension, development of drug resistance, sodium retention, plasma volume expansion, renin release, or production of angina pectoris. The average blood pressure fell from 198/122 to 165/97 mmHg. These preliminary results clearly indicate that nifedipine may be useful as a single agent in the control of hypertension.

The combination of nifedipine with either propranolol or methyldopa produces an additive hypotensive effect. Whereas 30 mg of nifedipine administered sublingually decreases systolic pressure by 27 percent and diastolic pressure by 28 percent, the addition of oral propranolol (0.2 mg/kg) was found to be mildly additive, with systolic pressure falling 32 percent, and diastolic pressure 30 percent from base line. In addition, the reflex increase in heart rate and plasma renin activity seen after a single dose of nifedipine was abolished, and its duration of antihypertensive action prolonged.[195] The addition of 250 mg of methyldopa every 6 h to nifedipine (10 mg every 6 h) produced a significant further reduction in arterial pressure (to 145/87 mmHg). This combination led to sustained efficacy over a 12-month follow-up.[188]

Experience with verapamil during prolonged trials has yielded conflicting results. The drug's hypotensive effect was not sustained in one trial of 320 to 640 mg daily over a 7-week period.[192] However, using a continuous intraarterial pressure monitoring system before and after 6 weeks of oral verapamil therapy (120 to 160 mg tid), the drug was demonstrated to produce a consistent reduction in arterial pressure. The effect was most prominent during the day and was accompanied by reduction in heart rate and no evidence of postural hypotension.[196] Preliminary studies with diltiazem (60 to 90 mg daily) demonstrated acute lowering of arterial pressure but gradual return to control values after several weeks of therapy.[197]

More information regarding the long-term efficacy of verapamil and diltiazem is needed before their role as single chronic antihypertensive agents is established. The delineation of dose-response characteristics and utility in hypertension of various etiologies is needed. In addition, the utility and safety of verapamil and diltiazem in combination with other antihypertensive drugs needs to be examined. Although experience remains limited, nifedipine, with its potent vasodilator properties, appears most promising in the acute and chronic treatment of hypertension. The combination of nifedipine and a beta blocker may prove of particular value in patients with combined hypertensive and coronary disease. It must be emphasized that while the reduction in arterial pressure by nifedipine and other calcium antagonists is likely to be confirmed by further studies, at present it is not certain whether the hypotensive actions will be accounted for solely by the peripheral dilator action of these drugs.

Hypertrophic Cardiomyopathy

Patients with hypertrophic cardiomyopathy have both systolic and diastolic abnormalities of ventricular function.[198] The degree of dynamic obstruction to left ventricular ejection is directly related to the inotropic state, and for this reason beta blockers have long been utilized in this context, albeit with a variable degree of success.[199] It is known, however, that propranolol reduces neither the incidence of serious ventricular arrhythmias nor the risk of sudden death.[173,174,200] The calcium channel blockers by their negative inotropic activity might be expected to exert a salutary effect in hypertrophic cardiomyopathy. It was found that calcium antagonists prevented the development of hereditary cardiomyopathy in hamsters, a disorder akin to hypertrophic obstructive cardiomyopathy and possibly related to abnormal calcium flux across myocardial cell membranes.[201] The most extensive data are available for verapamil. Early studies with the drug (480 mg daily) demonstrated significant improvement in symptoms compared to beta blockers. In uncontrolled clinical studies involving verapamil therapy, reductions in electrocardiographic signs of left ventricular hypertrophy and heart size assessed radiographically were observed.[202] Follow-up catheterization studies also demonstrated a decline in the resting outflow tract obstruction in 50 percent of patients, with decrease in left ventricular mass in 70 percent of patients.[203] Extensive studies by Rosing et al. have shown that an improvement in basal and provoked left ventricular outflow gradients is significant in most patients and is dependent on dose. Cardiac output remains unchanged or increases slightly, without significant increases in left ventricular end-diastolic pressure.[204]

A direct but uncontrolled comparison of verapamil and propranolol at varying doses has shown that both produce an increase in exercise tolerance of about 20 to 25 percent acutely. However, with long-term therapy exercise capacity deteriorates more frequently with propranolol and may actually increase with verapamil (120 mg qid). Patients symptomatically prefer verapamil. Unfortunately, a large number of patients develop significant side effects with long-term verapamil use including sinoatrial and atrioventricular node dysfunction, and occasionally severe myocardial dysfunction and heart failure.[205]

Abnormalities of diastolic function in patients with hypertrophic cardiomyopathy may also be improved with calcium antagonists. Verapamil has been shown to shorten the abnormally prolonged, isovolumic relaxation time in such patients.[206] Nifedipine has also been demonstrated to favorably modify abnormal left ventricular relaxation and diastolic filling rates in hypertrophic cardiomyopathy. This effect does not appear to be related to the depression of left ventricular systolic function. Administration of nifedipine alone could be deleterious through its potent abilities to stimulate reflex sympathetic discharge. The combined administration of nifedipine and propranolol has been demonstrated to be superior to the use of the calcium channel blocker alone.[207] The combination reduces left ventricular peak systolic pressure, total peripheral resistance, and resting left ventricular outflow gradient without altering cardiac index or pulmonary capillary wedge pressure, or inducing conduction defects.[207] A study of diltiazem in hypertrophic cardiomyopathy has demonstrated attenuation in exercise-induced elevation of pulmonary artery diastolic pressure, suggesting an improvement in left ventricular diastolic function.[208]

Thus, the calcium antagonists, alone or in combination with beta blockers, appear to improve both systolic and diastolic function in hypertrophic cardiomyopathy. Long-term follow-up studies and determination of comparative efficacy of the various calcium antagonists and combination regimens will be of great interest.

Miscellaneous Cardiovascular Disorders

The role of calcium antagonists is poorly defined in a number of cardiocirculatory disorders although the available data suggest promise (see Table 2). They will be discussed briefly in this chapter.

PULMONARY HYPERTENSION

Although promising from a theoretical and experimental standpoint, little controlled data are available concerning the efficacy of calcium channel blockers in the various forms of pulmonary hypertension. The effects of intravenous verapamil (mean dose 9.6 mg) have been reported in 12 patients with pulmonary hypertension.[209] The study group consisted of patients with a mean pulmonary artery pressure of 57 mmHg due to pulmonary fibrosis, congenital heart disease, or primary pulmonary hypertension. The drug caused a slight decrease in mean pulmonary artery pressure and right ventricular performance in several patients, while in others it had a marked negative inotropic effect with an increase in pulmonary arteriolar resistance. Overall, right atrial pressure, right ventricular end-diastolic pressure, pulmonary arteriolar resistance, and cardiac index were unchanged. Perhaps because of nifedipine's less inherent negative inotropic properties in human beings, very preliminary studies have suggested that it may be effective in some patients in specific clinical settings. In one case of primary pulmonary hypertension, nifedipine produced a 54 percent decrease in pulmonary vascular resistance, a 49 percent decrease in systemic vascular resistance, and a 90 percent increase in cardiac output. This improvement was maintained over a 3-month period.[210] In another study of patients with acute respiratory failure and chronic air flow obstruction, nifedipine dilated pulmonary vessels constricted by hypoxemia but had no further vasodilatory effect when hypoxemia was corrected. No adverse effects on arterial oxygenation were noted.[211]

Experience with diltiazem is limited. A case report demonstrating the drug's effectiveness in primary pulmonary hypertension has been published.[212] In one study of five patients with precapillary pulmonary hypertension, hemodynamic improvement occurred in four patients. The decline in pulmonary artery pressure and total pulmonary resistance at rest and during exercise was quite modest, however. No worsening of pulmonary gas exchange or ventilation-perfusion distribution was noted.[213]

It is thus apparent that although available data concerning calcium antagonists in pulmonary hypertensive states are encouraging, they are preliminary and essentially anecdotal. In addition, adverse effects have been noted probably due to inherent myocardial depressant properties and possibly due to differential vasodilatation of the pulmonary and systemic vascular beds. It is premature to conclude that calcium antagonists will make a major impact on the chronic prophylactic therapy of pulmonary hypertension.

ACUTE AND CHRONIC CONGESTIVE HEART FAILURE

While calcium antagonists are potent vasodilators and may function as agents to ameliorate heart failure by impedance reduction, it must be emphasized that as a class these compounds are unlikely to be the first-line therapy in this regard. Their greatest value may be in patients who have myocardial ischemia in the setting of cardiac decompensation. Available data suggest that nifedipine may be an effective preload- and afterload-reducing agent in the setting of acute pulmonary edema. The administration of 10 mg of nifedipine sublingually appeared to improve congestive heart failure secondary to hypertensive, rheumatic, or primary heart disease. The drug induced a sustained decrease in preload and afterload and appeared to enhance contractility.[214] Compared to nitrates, nifedipine had a greater tendency to increase cardiac output, without inducing venous pooling.[215] In patients with advanced chronic congestive heart failure the acute administration of nifedipine (20 mg sublingual) increased cardiac index and stroke-work index, while decreasing preload significantly. These changes appeared to be due to decreased systemic vascular resistance. However, sustained hemodynamic improvement has been noted in less than 50 percent of patients at 24 h with continuous therapy, suggesting tolerance or possible sodium retention.[217] The role of the other calcium antagonists in this setting is unexplored.

CEREBROVASCULAR DISEASE

Although information is tentative at present, nifedipine has been shown to prevent and reverse acute cerebral arterial spasm induced by injection of blood into the subarachnoid space.[216] In vitro nifedipine appears to exhibit a relatively selective activity preventing spasm induced particularly in the basilar artery when compared to that induced in the femoral arteries.[217] These experimental observations suggest potential applications in patients with subarachnoid hemorrhage, transient ischemic attacks, and perhaps migrainous syndromes.

RAYNAUD'S PHENOMENON

An open-label study of oral verapamil in patients with Raynaud's phenomenon associated with progressive systemic sclerosis demonstrated that 80 percent of patients had pronounced symptomatic improvement as judged by frequency and severity of attacks. In addition, there appeared to be a good correlation between symptomatic benefit and reappearance of digital pulse volume recordings after cold water immersion, and increased digital pulse pressures.[218] Clearly, further experience with calcium antagonists is needed in peripheral vasospastic syndromes.

INHIBITION OF PLATELET FUNCTION

Since platelet activation is in part a calcium-dependent process, the possibility that calcium antagonists may inhibit their function has been investigated in preliminary studies. In vitro, verapamil appears to reduce or prevent epinephrine-induced thromboxane-beta 2 release, platelet aggregation, and serotinin release and uptake. This has been observed in animals and healthy human volunteers.[219–221] The administration of verapamil to patients with coronary artery disease results in a rapid decrease in circulating platelet aggregates.[220]

Thus, in addition to the better studied application of calcium antagonists to supraventricular arrhythmias and ischemic syndromes, treatment of cerebral and peripheral vascular disorders appears promising. In addition, these drugs may exert "indirect" effects on cardiovascular function through mechanisms such as platelet inhibition; the clinical utility of such a potential therapeutic modality is essentially unexplored but merits further critical evaluation.

CLINICAL PHARMACOLOGY OF THE CALCIUM ANTAGONISTS

Table 5 summarizes the salient points on the pharmacokinetics and dosing schedules of nifedipine, verapamil, and diltiazem.

Ninety percent of orally or buccally administered nifedipine is absorbed.[222,223] The drug first appears in the plasma approximately 3 min after buccal administration and 20 min following oral administration, peak blood concentrations being reached 1 to 2 h after an oral dose. First-pass extraction by the liver is low, and systemic bioavailability is about 65 percent. Nifedipine is more than 90 percent protein-bound, and is completely metabolized to inactive polar forms. Approximately 80 percent of a given dose is excreted in the urine and 15 percent eliminated via the gastrointestinal

tract.[223] No accumulation of the drug or its metabolites has thus far been reported during chronic therapy. The plasma half-life is 4 to 5 h.[223]

The usual starting dose of nifedipine is 10 mg three times per day. The dose should be increased until relief of symptoms occurs, side effects develop, or the generally recommended maximal dose of 120 mg daily is reached. Adjustment of the dosing interval to every 4 h may be necessary if symptoms recur before the next scheduled dose.[9]

Diltiazem is rapidly and almost completely (90 percent) absorbed following oral administration. The drug first appears in plasma at 15 min with peak concentrations occurring after 30 min. The plasma half-life is about 4 to 5 h. A 50 percent first-pass effect has been observed with hepatic conversion to the active metabolite desacetyldiltiazem. Approximately 60 percent of the drug is hepatically metabolized with the remainder excreted by the kidneys. Diltiazem is about 80 percent protein-bound.[224–227] The usual oral dose of the drug is 30 to 60 mg every 8 h but doses up to 120 mg 8-hourly are well-tolerated.

Of all calcium antagonists, verapamil has been the most extensively studied from the pharmacokinetic and metabolic standpoint. The drug is well absorbed orally with measurable electrophysiological effects appearing

TABLE 5
Clinical pharmacokinetic parameters of three calcium antagonists

Parameter	Verapamil	Nifedipine	Diltiazem
Absorption:	79%	90%	90%
Bioavailability	10–20%	65–75%	45%
Onset of action	1–2 h (PO)	15 min (PO)	15 min (PO)
	½–1 min (IV)	2–3 min (SL)	2–3 min (IV)
Peak action	3–4 h (PO)	1–2 h (PO)	20 min
	2–5 min (IV)	20 min (SL)	———
Therapeutic plasma concentration	80–300 ng/mL	25–100 ng/mL	50–200 ng/mL
Elimination half-life	3–7 h (up to 26 h in hepatic cirrhosis)	4 h	4 h
Protein binding	87–93%	92–98%	80–86%
Metabolism:	Liver	Liver	Liver
Hepatic first pass	85%	20–30%	50%
Metabolites:			
Activity	20–25% (Nor-verapamil)	None	40–50% (Desacetyldiltiazem)
Accumulation	100%	None	10–30%
Excretion:			
Gastrointestinal	25%	15%	15%
Renal	75%	85%	85%
Dose	IV: 75–150 μg/kg	SL: 10–40 mg tid or qid PO: 10–40 mg tid or qid	IV: 75–150 μg/kg PO: 30–90 mg tid or bid
Interaction with other cardiovascular drugs	Digoxin	? Digoxin	———

at 2 h and peak action at 5 h following a single dose.[45,228] A disparity exists between verapamil's hemodynamic and electrophysiological effects. The hypotensive effect of the drug following intravenous administration is short-lived, with a peak effect of 5 min and dissipation of effect by 10 to 20 min.[40] The negative dromotropic effect is seen within 1 to 2 min, peak at 10 to 15 min, but may still be observed after 6 h. Preferential uptake and binding of verapamil by the atrioventricular node has been postulated to explain this observation.[45] Verapamil is about 90 percent protein-bound without significant clinical differences between normal subjects and patients with renal disease.[229] After either oral or intravenous administration the drug exhibits biexponential decay. An initial distribution phase of about 18 to 35 min is followed by an elimination phase of 3 to 7 h. Although verapamil is 90 percent absorbed by the oral route, a substantial first-pass effect in the liver reduces the overall bioavailability to about 10 to 20 percent.[230] Verapamil has been observed to accumulate to a greater extent than that predicted by its half-life secondary to decreased hepatic clearance. In addition, its active metabolite nor-verapamil accumulates 2.5-fold during attainment of steady state after oral dosing.[231] Variations in verapamil plasma concentrations may be explained by differences in hepatic blood flow.[232]

The clinical utility of following plasma levels of verapamil to guide therapy has been examined with conflicting results. Different patients demonstrate wide variations in serum levels on similar doses. Although plasma levels increased with increasing dose in patients with paroxysmal atrial tachycardia, they were not helpful in planning therapy in this study.[233] However, during chronic oral therapy for recurrent supraventricular tachycardias or vasospastic angina, although heart rate and P-R interval did not change significantly, plasma levels correlated with relief of symptoms.[234] In patients with hypertrophic cardiomyopathy, determination of plasma levels has been found to be of limited usefulness because of marked interpatient variation and the finding of similar serum levels in patients who responded to therapy and those who experienced serious side effects.[235] Thus, the role of plasma levels and the contribution of verapamil's metabolites need further study to clarify their role in the overall pharmacologic and therapeutic actions of this drug.

Although an initial dose of 5 mg administered intravenously over 60 s has been recommended for the termination of atrial arrhythmias, the most common dose is 10 mg (0.15 mg per kilogram of body weight). This should be given with electrocardiographic and blood pressure monitoring.[45] If the arrhythmia is not terminated by the initial injection, 10 mg may be administered within 30 min following the initial injection. If a continuous effect is desired, an infusion of 0.005 mg/(kg)/(min) may be administered. Dosage should be reduced in the presence of myocardial dysfunction. The usual initial dose of oral verapamil is approximately ten times the intravenous dose secondary to the extensive first-pass hepatic effect. Thus, a starting dose of 40 to 80 mg every 8 h is recommended. This may be rapidly increased over the next several days to the usual 240 to 360 mg/day. In patients without known contraindications doses as high as 720 mg daily have been suggested [45] and may be tolerated in a few patients.

SIDE EFFECTS

The major side effects of verapamil, nifedipine, and diltiazem are generally predictable from their inherent vasodilatory and relatively negative inotropic and chronotropic properties (see Table 6). Their side effects may also vary in relation to the route of administration.

Although the safety of nifedipine has not been thoroughly studied, a recent review of the records of over

TABLE 6
Adverse effects of calcium channel blockers

Nifedipine (17%)*	Verapamil (9%)*	Diltiazem (4%)*
Ankle edema	Constipation	Dizziness
Headache	Headache	Headache
Dizziness	Dizziness	Fatigue
Tinnitus	Nausea	Blurred vision
Flushing	Galactorrhea	Flushing
Hypotension	Hepatotoxicity	AV block
Aggravation of angina (occasionally)	AV block	
Nasal congestion	Congestive heart failure	

* Estimated overall incidence of side effects in therapeutic doses.

3,000 patients treated with the drug provides valuable basic information.[236] In this review of patients with various anginal syndromes, some complicated by congestive heart failure and many studied for longer than 6 months, about 60 percent of the patients reported no adverse side effects. Dizziness and light-headedness were reported in 12.1 percent of the total population but were more frequent in patients with congestive heart failure and in those on long-term therapy. Edema, swelling, and fluid retention occurred in 7.7 percent of the population and were also more common in patients with congestive heart failure and during long-term therapy. Disturbances of upper gastrointestinal tract function and headache occurred in about 7 percent of patients, while flushing or burning or a general or specific feeling of weakness were reported in 7.4 percent and 5.9 percent of cases, respectively. Less commonly reported side effects related to cardiovascular function included hypotension, precipitation of angina, preinfarction angina or myocardial infarction, and congestive heart failure in less than 4 percent of patients. The total percentage of patients in whom therapy was discontinued due to an adverse experience was 5 percent,[236] but the overall incidence of side effects may be considerably higher and has been estimated to be about 17 percent.

Following intravenous verapamil the adverse effects reported have been those expected from the drug's known pharmacologic properties. Perhaps the most common is a transient fall in blood pressure.[145,163] More serious side effects, including hypotension, bradycardia, and rarely ventricular asystole, have been observed, however.[237,238] In general, these latter occurred in patients receiving concomitant beta blocking drugs. Suicidal overdose with verapamil, manifested by unconsciousness, hypotension, anuria, and AV block has been reported.[239] These severe side effects of verapamil can be successfully treated with intravenous atropine (partially effective), catecholamine (particularly Isuprel), and intravenous calcium gluconate. Occasionally temporary transvenous ventricular pacing may be necessary.[240]

Overall, oral verapamil is well-tolerated. The most common side effects include constipation, dizziness, nausea, headache, and ankle edema. In general, these symptoms are relatively mild and can be managed symptomatically.[240] Less common side effects include galactorrhea [241] and reversible hepatic toxicity.[242] Prolongation of first-degree AV block occurs in a proportion of patients given chronic oral verapamil therapy, but in the absence of antecedent conduction system disease more advance grades of heart block are unusual. In patients with normal ventricular function the precipitation of clinically evident cardiac failure is very uncommon. The overall incidence of side effects following oral verapamil therapy is about 9 percent.

Experience with diltiazem is more limited in terms of side effects, and data are derived from studies in angina. Dizziness, headache, fatigue, blurred vision, flushing, and minor degrees of AV block have been reported when the drug is administered in daily doses of 240 to 360 mg. Overall, however, diltiazem appears to have the lowest incidence of side effects with estimates of about 4 percent.

CONTRAINDICATIONS AND PRECAUTIONS

The main contraindications to the use of calcium antagonists are dependent on the nature of the underlying disease and on the calcium antagonist being used.

Verapamil should be used with great caution in the presence of advanced heart failure, unstable AV block, disease of the conduction system including the sick sinus syndrome, and low blood pressure states such as cardiogenic shock. It must be emphasized, however, that in situations in which heart failure is related to persistence of a rapid atrial tachyarrhythmia, a prompt reversion to sinus rhythm by a calcium antagonist may lead to improvement in the clinical status. As already discussed under treatment of arrhythmias, verapamil and diltiazem are contraindicated in cases of atrial flutter or atrial fibrillation complicating the Wolff-Parkinson-White syndrome.[152,171]

Combination of Calcium Antagonists with Digitalis Glycosides

The two most important precautions in combining digitalis preparations and calcium channel blockers are the potential additive electrophysiological effects and the tendency for certain calcium antagonists to increase serum digoxin levels. Unless there is evidence of impaired AV conduction, prior digitalization is not a contraindication to the use of intravenous verapamil. In two studies of intravenous verapamil, 61 percent and 70 percent of patients were receiving maintenance oral digitalis at the time of administration of verapamil. In neither was a significant untoward reaction attributable to the combination.[145,163] The combination of intravenous diltiazem and digoxin in patients without SA or AV node disease appears to have an additive depressant effect with significant adverse effects.[27]

Verapamil has been shown to decrease renal clearance of digoxin and to increase its plasma concentration.[263] This effect appears to be dependent on the dose of verapamil used, and develops gradually over the first few days after addition of the calcium antagonist to a stable digoxin dose. In one study mean digoxin levels rose from 0.76 to 1.31 with 7 of 49 subjects developing signs and symptoms suggesting digitalis toxicity.[159] In a second study in patients with chronic atrial fibrillation, the mean serum digoxin levels rose from 1.6 to 2.7 mg/mL during addition of verapamil, but no patients developed evidence of digitalis intoxication.[164] Thus, caution and careful surveillance are advised in the concomitant administration of verapamil or diltiazem with digitalis preparations. Increases in serum levels of digoxin during nifedipine therapy have also been reported,[243] and its net hemodynamic effects appear to cause less myocardial depression. In properly selected patients, minimal side effects can be expected from the combination of beta-blockers and nifedipine. In a review of over 1,400 patients receiving this combination, the incidence of congestive heart failure and, indeed, all side effects was no greater with combined therapy than with nifedipine alone.[236]

A second study found no evidence that the incidence of side effects of combined therapy is any greater than with beta-blockers alone.[244]

Nevertheless, it must be emphasized that a major component of nifedipine's net hemodynamic effect is mediated through reflex adrenergic mechanisms and when these are not present, the drug may exert significant negative inotropic effect. Hemodynamic studies of the acute effects of nifedipine on left ventricular function in patients on beta-blockers reveal that the addition of the calcium channel blockers significantly depresses left ventricular dP/dt and systolic blood pressure.[245] The increase in cardiac output results from vasodilation compensating for the negative inotropic effect. Several anecdotal reports of heart failure associated with combined nifedipine and propranolol administration have already been published.[246,247] In addition, several reports of potentiation of nifedipine's hypotensive effects by beta-blockers have appeared.[183–248]

Combination of Calcium Antagonists with Beta-Blockers

The combination of a calcium antagonist and beta-blocker has been shown to be advantageous in a number of clinical settings. Care must be taken, however, in selecting patients to avoid untoward side effects.

The potentially deleterious effect of combining verapamil and beta-blockers has received the most attention. Persistent hypotension, bradycardia, high-grade AV block, and ventricular asystole have all been observed particularly with the intravenous administration of verapamil.[146,174,237,238,249] Of particular importance is to avoid the combined use of verapamil and its congeners in patients with overt or marginal hemodynamic

dysfunction. Whereas the administration of verapamil or practolol individually produces minor hemodynamic changes, the combined regimen produces a pronounced reduction in left ventricular contractility.[250] Caution must also be taken,[251,252] of course, in any patient with sick sinus syndrome and/or impaired AV conduction, where the additive effects of verapamil and beta-blockers may be disastrous. The combination of nifedipine with a beta-blocker theoretically poses less risk than does verapamil. Nifedipine has little effect on AV nodal function compared to verapamil.

Although diltiazem appears to have minimal intrinsic negative inotropic activity, its electrophysiological properties[25] would suggest similarity of action to that of verapamil during combined therapy with beta-blockers.

Thus, it appears that in selected patients with relatively normal ventricular function and intact impulse generation and conducting systems, the combination of a calcium channel antagonist and a beta-blocker is potentially advantageous. However, in patients with impaired hemodynamic performance or abnormalities of the SA or AV node, caution and extreme care must be exercised to obviate potentially life-threatening side effects during combination therapy, but careful selection of patients permits the combination therapy in many cases[43,253] despite the known electrophysiological interaction.[253,254]

THE RATIONAL CHOICE OF A CALCIUM ANTAGONIST IN CARDIOVASCULAR THERAPEUTICS

It will be evident that the overall spectrum of therapeutic activity of calcium antagonists rivals that of beta-adrenoceptor blocking drugs. However, unlike the case of beta-antagonists, calcium channel blockers differ often significantly with respect to their electrophysiological, pharmacologic, and hemodynamic actions. Their side-effect profile and pharmacokinetic characteristics also differ. These overall considerations therefore govern the choice of a particular calcium antagonist for a specific clinical indication. For example, in the case of supraventricular tachyarrhythmias, nifedipine is without effect and the most effective agent—both intravenously and orally—is verapamil. Its congeners may also be effective in this regard, as may be diltiazem, when their full spectrum of antiarrhythmic activity is elucidated. In the case of ventricular arrhythmias complicating coronary artery spasm, all calcium antagonists are likely to be effective, and the choice of an agent will be dictated by other clinical considerations. Similarly, for the control of nearly all myocardial ischemic syndromes (Prinzmetal's angina, unstable angina, chronic stable angina), verapamil, nifedipine, and diltiazem in appropriate dosage regimens are probably equi-effective. Which of the three agents the clinician might use will be dependent on one's familiarity with the agents and the presence of associated clinical features. For example, coexisting sick sinus diesase, AV conduction impairment, and moderate-to-greater degree of ventricular dysfunction will make nifedipine preferable to diltiazem or verapamil. For other cases of ischemic syndromes, one's choice will be dictated essentially by the frequency of side effects. The rational choice of various agents in other conditions (obstructive cardiomyopathies, myocardial preservation, hypertension, pulmonary hypertension, Raynaud's phenomenon, and other vasospastic syndromes) is at present limited by paucity of data relative to efficacy and side effects and must await further clinical evaluation.

CONCLUSIONS

The slow-channel blockers constitute a structurally diverse group of drugs with varying mechanism of action, predilections for site of greatest cardiovascular activity, and clinical efficacy, but they share the property of blocking the slow inward channel in heart muscle and of inhibiting calcium fluxes in smooth muscle. Their in vivo and in vitro actions must be distinguished. The overall in vivo actions represent a balance of the direct and sympathetically-mediated reflex activity interacting with varying degrees of intrinsic noncompetitive sympathetic antagonism present in some of the compounds. A knowledge of the pharmacodynamic and pharmacokinetic differences between the compounds allows one to select the most appropriate agent for a given clinical situation. The central role of calcium in the cellular processes in the heart and the vascular system forms the basis for the utility of this class of drugs in a wide variety of cardiovascular disorders. Their major clinical indications are various ischemic myocardial syndromes, certain cardiac arrhythmias, hypertension, and hypertrophic cardiomyopathies; their role in the prevention of sudden cardiac death, as in a miscellany of other cardiovascular disorders, remains to be determined. The development of the concept of calcium channel blockade and the synthesis and characterization of a plethora of specific antagonists such as verapamil, nifedipine, and diltiazem do nevertheless constitute a major advance in cardiovascular therapeutics. Further advances will depend on refinements in structure-activity relationships relative to tissue specificity of ionic channels as a basis for the development of more selective channel inhibitors.

REFERENCES

1 Fleckenstein, A.: Specific Inhibitors and Promoters of Calicum Action in the Excitation-Contraction Coupling of Heart Muscle and Their Role in the Prevention of Production of Myocardial Lesions, in P. Harris and L. Opie (eds.), "Calcium and the Heart," Academic Press, New York, 1971.

2 Cranefield, P. F.: "The Conduction of the Cardiac Impulse," Futura Publishing Company, New York, 1975.

3 Cranefield, P. F.: Action Potentials, Afterpotentials and Arrhythmias, Circ. Res., 41:415, 1977.

4 Hauswirth, O., and Singh, B. N.: Ionic Mechanisms in Heart Muscle in Relation to the Genesis and the Pharmacological Control of Cardiac arrhythmias, Pharmacol. Rev. 30:5, 1978.

5 Kohlhardt, M., Bauer, B., Krause, H., and Fleckenstein, A.: New Selective Inhibitors of the Transmembrane Ca Conductivity in Mammalian Myocardial Fibers. Studies with the Voltage Clamp Technique, Experiments, 28:288, 1972.

6 New, W., and Trautwein, W.: The Ionic Nature of Slow Inward Current and Its Relation to Contraction, Pflüegers Arch., 334:24, 1972.

7 Singh, B. N., Hecht, H. S., Nademanee, N., and Chew, C. Y. C.: Electrophysiologic and Hemodynamic Effects of Slow-Channel Blocking Drugs, Prog. Cardiovasc. Dis., 25:103, 1982.

8 Ellrodt, G., Chew, C. Y. C., and Singh, B. N.: Therapeutic Implications of Slow-Channel Blockade in Cardiocirculatory Disorders, Circulation, 62:669, 1980.

9 Stone, P. H., Antman, E. M., Muller, J. E., and Braunwald, E.: Calcium Channel Blocking Agents in the Treatment of Cardiovascular Disorders, Part II, Hemodynamic Effects and Clinical Applications, Ann. Intern. Med., 93:886, 904, 1980.

10 Braunwald, E.: Mechanism of Action of Calcium Channel Blocking Agents, N. Engl. J. Med., 307:1618, 1982.

11 Wit, A. L., and Cranefield, P. F.: Triggered Activity in Cardiac Muscle Fibers of the Simian Mitral Valve, Circ. Res., 38:85, 1976.

12 Wit, A. L., and Cranefield, P. F.: Triggered and Automatic Activity in the Canine Coronary Sinus, Circ. Res., 41:435, 1977.

13 Adelstein, R. S., and Hathaway, D. R.: Role of Calcium and Cyclic Adenosine 3', 5' Monophosphate in Regulating Smooth Muscle Contraction, Am. J. Cardiol., 44:783, 1979.

14 Triggle, D. J., and Swamy, V. C.: Pharmacology of Agents that Affect Calcium: Agonists and Antagonists, Chest, 78:174, 1980.

15 Harder, D. R., Belardinelli, L., Sperelakis, N., Rubio, R., and Berne, R. M.: Differential Effects of Adenorine and Nitroglycerin on the Action Potentials of Large and Small Coronary Arteries, Circ. Res., 44:176, 1979.

16 Einwachter, H. M., Keon, R., and Herb, J.: Effect of Lidoflazine on Membrane Currents and Contraction in Voltage-Clamped Frog Atrial Fibers, *Eur. J. Pharmacol.*, 55:225, 1979.

17 TenEick, R. E., and Singer, D. H.: Effects of Perhexiline on the Electrophysiologic Activity of the Mammalian Heart, *Postgrad. Med. J.*, 49(suppl. 3):32, 1973.

18 Zelis, R., and Flaim, S. F.: "Calcium Influx Blocker" and Vascular Smooth Muscle: Do We Really Understand the Mechanisms? *Ann. Intern. Med.*, 94:124, 1981.

19 Henry, P. D.: Comparative Pharmacology of Calcium Antagonists: Nifedipine, Verapamil, and Diltiazem, *Am. J. Cardiol.*, 46:1047, 1980.

20 Okada, R.: Effect of Verapamil on Electrical Activities of SA Node, Ventricular Muscle, and Purkinje Fibers in Isolated Rabbit Heart, *Jpn. Circ. J.*, 40:329, 1976.

21 Zipes, D. P., and Fischer, J. C.: Effects of Agents Which Inhibit the Slow-Channel on Sinus Node Automaticity and Atrioventricular Conduction in the Dog, *Circ. Res.*, 34:184, 1974.

22 Strauss, H. C., Prystowsky, E. N., and Scheinman, M. M.: Sinoatrial and Atrial Electrogenesis, *Prog. Cardiovasc. Dis.*, 19:385, 1977.

23 Singh, B. N.: "A Study of the Pharmacological Actions of Certain Drugs and Hormones with Particular Reference to Cardiac Muscle," Ph. D. Thesis, University of Oxford, England, 1971.

24 Refsum, H., and Landmark, K.: The Effect of Ca Antagonist Drug, Nifedipine, on the Mechanical and Electrical Activity of the Isolated Rat Atrium, *Acta Pharmacol. Toxicol.*, 37:369, 1975.

25 Kawai, C., Konishi, T., Matsuyama, E., and Okazaki, H.: Comparative Effects of Three Calcium Antagonists, Diltiazem, Verapamil, and Nifedipine, on the Sinoatrial and Atrioventricular Nodes—Experimental and Clinical Studies, *Circulation*, 63(suppl. 5):1035, 1981.

26 Sugimoto, T., Ishikawa, T., Kaseno, K., and Nakase, S.: Electrophysiologic Effects of Diltiazem, a Calcium Antagonist, in Patients with Impaired Sinus or AV Node Function, *Angiology*, 31:700, 1980.

27 Mitchell, L. B., Schroeder, J. S., and Mason, J. W.: Comparative Clinical Electrophysiologic Effect of Diltiazem, Verapamil, and Nifedipine—a Review, *Am. J. Cardiol.*, 49:629, 1982.

28 Carrasco, H. A., Fuenmayor, A., Barbosa, J. S., and Gonzalez, G.: Effect of Verapamil on Normal Sinoatrial Node Function and on Sick Sinus Syndrome, *Am. Heart J.*, 96:760, 1978.

29 Rizzon, P., Di Biase, M., Calabrese, P., Brindicci, G., and Chiddo, A.: Electrophysiologic Evaluation of Intravenous Verapamil in Man, *Eur. J. Cardiol.*, 6:179, 1977.

30 Rowland, E., Evans, T., and Krikler, D.: Effect of Nifedipine on Atrioventricular Conduction as Compared with Verapamil, *Br. Heart J.*, 42:124, 1979.

31 Debaisieux, J. C., Theroux, P., Waters, D. O., Mizgala, H. F., and Bourassa, M. G.: Hemodynamic Effects of Nifedipine and Diltiazem after an Acute Myocardial Infarction, *Circulation*, 82(suppl. 2):386, 1979.

32 Lydtin, H., Lohmoller, R., Lohmoller, G., Schmitz, H., and Walter, I.: Hemodynamic Studies on Adalat in Healthy Volunteers and Patients, in W. Lochner, W. Braasch, and G. Kroneberg (eds.), "2d International Adalat Symposium, New Therapy of Ischemic Heart Disease," Excerpta Medica, Berlin, 1975, p. 112.

33 Ludbrook P. A., Tiefenbrunn, A. J., Byrne, J. C., and Sobel, B. E.: Effects of Nifedipine on Left Ventricular Function—Their Dependence upon Reduced Impedance, *Circulation*, 62(suppl. 3):259, 1980.

34 Kober, G., Schulz, W, Bamberg, E, and Kaltenback, M.: Cardiac and Peripheral Effects of Nifedipine, in P. R. Lichtlen, E. Kimura, and N. Taira (eds.), "International Adalat Panel Discussion—New Experimental and Clinical Results," Excerpta Medica, Amsterdam, 1979, p. 86.

35 Grandjean, T., and Valenti, P.: Effects of Nifedipine on Effort-Tolerance and Left Ventricular Function during Exercise in Patients Suffering from Severe Angina Pectoris, in P. R. Lichtten, E., Kiumur, and N. Taira (eds.), "International Adalat Panel Discussion—New Experimental and Clinical Results," Excerpta Medica, Amsterdam, 1979, p. 118.

36 Johnson, S. M., Mauritson, D. R., Corbert, J. R., et al.: Double-Blind Randomized Placebo-Controlled Comparison of Propranolol and Verapamil in the Treatment of Patients with Stable Angina Pectoris, *Am. J. Med.*, 71:443, 1981.

37 Jariwalla, A. G., and Anderson, E. G.: Production of Ischemic Cardiac Pain by Nifedipine, *Br. Med. J.*, 1:1181, 1978.

38 Atterhog, J. H., and Ekelund, L. G.: Haemodynamic Effects of Intravenous Verapamil at Rest and during Exercise in Subjectively Healthy Middle-Aged Man, *Eur. J. Clin. Pharmacol.*, 8:317, 1975.

39 Ryden, L. S., and Slatre, R.: The Hemodynamic Effect of Verapamil, *Eur. J. Clin. Pharmacol.*, 3:153, 1971.

40 Singh, B. N., and Roche, A. H. G.: Effects of Intravenous Verapamil on Hemodynamics in Patients with Heart Disease, *Am. Heart J.*, 94:593, 1977.

41 Ferlinz, J., Easthope, J. L., and Aronow, W. S.: Effects of Verapamil on Myocardial Performance in Coronary Disease, *Circulation*, 59:313, 1979.

42 Chew, C. Y. C., Hecht, H. S. Collett, J. T., McAllister, F. G., and Singh, B. N.: Influence of the Severity of Ventricular Dysfunction on Hemodynamic Responses to Intravenously Administered Verapamil in Ischemic Heart Disease, *Am. J. Cardiol.*, 47:917, 1981.

43 Bonow, R. O., Leon, M. B., Rosing, D. R., et al.: Effects of Verapamil and Propranolol on Left Ventricular Systolic Function and Diastolic Filling in Patients with Coronary Artery Disease—Radionuclide Angiographic Studies at Rest and During Exercise, *Circulation*, 6 (suppl. 7):1337, 1982.

44 Ferlinz, J., Easthope, J. L., and Aronow, W. S.: Left Ventricular Function in Patients with Coronary Artery Disease after Verapamil Administration, *Clin. Invest. Med.*, 3:63, 1980.

45 Singh, B. N., Collett, J. T., and Chew, C. Y. C.: New Perspectives in the Pharmacologic Therapy of Cardiac Arrhythmias, *Prog. Cardiovasc. Dis.*, 22:243, 1980.

46 Ferlinz, J., and Turbow, M. E.: Antianginal and Myocardial Metabolic Properties of Verapamil in Coronary Artery Disease, *Am. J. Cardiol.*, 46:1019, 1980.

47 Vlieststra, R. E., Farias, M. A., Frye, R. L., Smith, H. C., and Ritman, E. L.: Effect of Verapamil on Left Ventricular Function—Randomized Placebo-Controlled Study, *Am. J. Cardiol.*, 47:406, 1981. (Abstract.)

48 Oyama, Y.: Hemodynamics and Electrophysiological Evaluations of Diltiazem Hydrochloride—A Clinical Study, in P. R. Lichtlen, E. Kimura, and N. Taira (eds.), "International Adalat Panel Discussion—New Experimental and Clinical Results," Excerpta Medica, Amsterdam, 1979, p. 169.

49 Bourrassa, M. A., Cote, P., Theroux, P., Tubau, J. F., Genain, C., and Waters, D. D.: Hemodynamics and Coronary Flow following Diltiazem Administration in Anesthetized Dogs and in Humans, *Chest*, 78:224, 1980.

50 Kinoshita, M., Motomura, M., Kusukawa, R., and Kawakita, S.: Comparison of Hemodynamic Effects between β-Blocking Agents and New Antianginal Agent, Diltiazem Hydrochloride, *Jpn. Circ. J.*, 43:587, 1979.

51 Theroux, P., Waters, D. D., Debaisieux, J. C., Szlachcic, J., and Migala, H. F.: Hemodynamic Effects of Calcium Ion Antagonists after Acute Myocardial Infarction, *Clin. Invest. Med.*, 3:81, 1980.

52 Osakada, G., Kumada, T., Gallagher K. P., Kemper, W. S., and Ross, J.: Effect of Verapamil on Exercise-Induced Regional Myocardial Dysfunction in Conscious Dogs, *Am. J. Cardiol.*, 47:416, 1981. (Abstract.)

53 Lichtlen, P. R., Engel, H. J., Wolf, R., and Hundeshagen, H.: Effect of Nifedipine on Regional Myocardial Blood Flow at Rest and in Pacing-Induced Ischemia, *Circulation*, 60 (suppl. 2):249, 1979. (Abstract.)

54 Lichtlen, P. R., Engel, J. G., Wolf, R., and Pretschner, P.: Regional Myocardial Blood Flow in Patients with Coronary Artery Disease after Nifedipine, in P. R. Lichtlen, E. Kimura, and N. Taira (eds.), "International Adalat Panel Discussion—New Experimental and Clinical Results," Excerpta Medica, Amsterdam, 1979, p. 69.

55 Stone, D. L., Stephens, J. D., and Banim, S. O.: Comparative Coronary Haemodynamic Effects of Nifedipine and Nitroglycerin, *Circulation*, 62 (suppl. 3):86, 1980.

56 Amende, I., Simon, R., and Lichtlen, P. R.: Early Effects of Nifedipine on Left Ventricular Diastolic Function in Man, *Circulation*, 62 (suppl. 3):259, 1980. (Abstract.)

57 Simonsen, S., and Nitter-Hauge, S.: Effect of Nifedipine (Adalat) on Coronary Hemodynamics in Patients with Coronary Arteriosclerotic Disease, *Acta Med. Scand.*, 204:179, 1978.

58 Hugenholtz, P. G., Michels, H. R., Serruys, P. W., and Brower, R. W.: Nifedipine in the Treatment of Unstable Angina, Coronary Spasm and Myocardial Ischemia, *Am. J. Cardiol.*, 47:163, 1981.

59 Gunther, S., Muller, J. E., Mudge, G. H., and Grossman, W.: Therapy of Coronary Vasoconstriction in Patients with Coronary Artery Disease, *Am. J. Cardiol.*, 47:157, 1981.

60 Mignault, S. H.: Coronary Cineangiographic Study of Intravenously Administered Isoptin, *Can. Med. Assoc. J.*, 95:1252, 1966.

61 Luebs, E. D., Cohen, A., Zaleski, E. J., and Bing, R. J.: Report on Therapy: Effect of Nitroglycerin, Intensain, Isoptin and Papaverine on Coronary Blood Flow in Man, *Am. J. Cardiol.*, 17:535, 1966.

62 Simonsen, S.: Effect of Verapamil on Coronary Hemodynamics in Patients with Coronary Heart Disease, *Eur. J. Cardiol.*, 8:9, 1978.

63 Simonsen, S.: Pharmacological Effects on Coronary Hemodynamics: A Comparative Study between Atenolol, Verapamil, Nifedipine, and Carbocromen, *Acta. Med. Scand.* (suppl.) 645:97, 1981.

64 Chew, C. Y. C., Brown, G. B., Singh, B. N., Wong, M., Pierce, C., and Petersen, R.: Effects of Verapamil on Coronary Hemodynamics and Vasomobility Relative to its Mechanism of Antianginal Action, *Am. J. Cardiol.*, 51:699, 1983.

65 Brown, B. G., Pierce, C. D., Petersen, R. B., Singh, B. N., Bolson, E. L., and Dodge, H. T.: Verapamil: A Mild Epicardial Coronary Dilator Inhibits Sympathetic and Ergonovine-Induced Coronary Constriction in Humans, *Circulation*, 64(suppl. 4):150, 1981.

66 Josephson, M. A., Hecht, H. S., Hopkins, J, Guerrero, J., and Singh, B. N.: Comparative Effects of Oral Verapamil and Propranolol on Exercise-Induced Myocardial Ischemia and Energetics in Patients with Coronary Artery Disease: Single-Blind Placebo Crossover Evaluation Using Radionuclide Ventriculography, *Am. Heart J.*, 103:978, 1982.

67 Maseri, A., Parodi, O., Severi, S., and Pesola, A.: Transient Transmural Reduction of Myocardial Blood Flow Demonstrated by Thallium-201 Scintigraphy as a Cause of Variant Angina, *Circulation*, 54:280, 1976.

68 Maseri, A., Pesola, A., Marzilli, M., et al.: Coronary Vasospasm in Angina Pectoris, *Lancet*, 1:713, 1977.

69 Maseri, A., Severi, S., et al.: 'Variant' Angina—One Aspect of a Continuous Spectrum of Vasospastic Myocardial Ischemia, *Am. J. Cardiol.*, 42:1019, 1978.

70 Maseri, A., L'Abbate, A., Chierchia, S., et al.: Significance of Spasm in the Pathogenesis of Ischemic Heart Disease, *Am. J. Cardiol.*, 44:788, 1979.

71 Figueras, J., Singh, B. N., Ganz, W., Charuzi, Y., and Swan, H. J. C.: Mechanism of Rest and Nocturnal Angina—Observations during Continuous Hemodynamic and Electrocardiographic Monitoring, *Circulation*, 59(suppl. 5):955, 1979.

72 Maseri, A., and Chierchia, S.: A New Rationale for the Clinical Approach to the Patient with Angina Pectoris, *Am. J. Med.,* 71:639, 1981.

73 Hosada, S., and Kimura, E.: Efficacy of Nifedipine in the Variant Form of Angina Pectoris, in A. D. Jatene and P. R. Lichtlen (eds.), "The Third International Adalat Symposium," Excerpta Medica, Amsterdam, 1976, p. 195.

74 Endo, M., Kanda, I., Hosada, S., Hayashi, H., Hirosawa, K., and Konno, S.: Prinzmetal's Variant Form of Angina Pectoris—Reevaluation of Mechanisms, *Circulation,* 52:33, 1975.

75 Muller, J. E., and Gunther, S. J.: Nifedipine Therapy for Prinzmetal's Angina, *Circulation,* 57:137, 1973.

76 Antman, E., Muller, J. E., and Goldberg, S.: Nifedipine Therapy for Coronary Artery Spasm Experience in 127 Patients, *N. Engl. J. Med.,* 302:1269, 1980.

77 Schick, E., et al.: Randomized Withdrawal from Nifedipine-Placebo Controlled Study in Patients with Coronary Artery Spasm, *Am. Heart J.,* 104:690, 1982.

78 Theroux, P., Waters, D. D. Affaki, G. S., Critten, J., Bonan, R., and Mizgala, H. F.: Provocative Testing with Ergonovine to Evaluate the Efficacy of Treatment with Calcium Antagonists in Variant Angina, *Circulation,* 60:504, 1979.

79 Heupler, R. A., Jr., and Proudfit, W. L.: Nifedipine Therapy for Refractory Coronary Arterial Spasm, *Am. J. Cardiol.,* 44:798, 1979.

80 Goldberg, S., Reichek, N., Wilson, J., Hirshfeld, J. W., Jr., Muller, J., and Kastor, J. A.: Nifedipine in the Treatment of Prinzmetal's (Variant) Angina, *Am. J. Cardiol.,* 44:804, 1979.

81 Johnson, S. M., Mauitson, D. R., Willerson, J. T., and Hillis, L. D.: A Controlled Trial of Verapamil for Prinzmetal's Variant Angina, *N. Engl. J. Med.,* 304(15):862, 1981.

82 Freedman, B., Dunn, R. F., Richmond, D. R., and Kelley, D. T.: Coronary Artery Spasm—Treatment with Verapamil, *Circulation,* 60 (suppl. 2):249, 1979. (Abstract.)

83 Severi, S., Davies, L., L'Abbate, A., and Maseri, A.: Long-term Prognosis of Variant Angina with Medical Management. *Circulation,* 60:(suppl. 2):250, 1979. (Abstract.)

84 Rosenthal, S. J., Ginsburg, R., Lamb, I., Baim, D. S., and Schroder, J. S.: Efficacy of Diltiazem for Control of Symptoms of Coronary Arterial Spasm, *Am. J. Cardiol.,* 46:1027, 1980.

85 Feldman, R. L., Pepine, C. J., Whittle, J., and Conti, C. R.: Short- and Long-term Responses to Diltiazem in Patients with Variant Angina, *Am. J. Cardiol.,* 49:554, 1982.

86 Schroeder, J. S., Feldman, R. L., Griles, T. D., et al.: Multiclinic Controlled Trial Diltiazem for Prinzmetal's Angina, *Am. J. Med.,* 72:227, 1982.

87 Johnson, S. M., Mauritson, D. R., Willerson, J. T., and Hillis, D. L.: Comparison of Verapamil and Nifedipine in the Treatment of Variant Angina Pectoris—Preliminary Observations in 10 Patients, *Am. J. Cardiol.,* 47:1295, 1981.

88 Kimura, E., and Kishida, H.: Treatment of Variant Angina with Drugs—A Survey of 11 Cardiology Institutes in Japan, *Circulation,* 63(suppl. 4):844, 1981.

89 Waters, D. D., Theroux, P., Dauwe, F., Critten, J., Affaki, G., and Mizgala, H. F.: Ergonovine Testing to Assess the Effects of Calcium Antagonist Drugs in Variant Angina, *Circulation,* 60(suppl. 2):248, 1979. (Abstract.)

90 Yasue, H., Omote, S., Takejawa, A., et al.: Pathogenesis and Treatment of Angina Pectoris at Rest as Seen from its Response to Various Drugs. *Jpn. Circ.,* 42:11, 1978.

91 Raizner, A. E., Gaston, W., Chahine, R. A., et al.: The Effectiveness of Combined Verapamil and Nitrate Therapy in Prinzmetal's Variant Angina, *Am. J. Cardiol.,* 45:439, 1980. (Abstract.)

92 Singh, B. N., Chew, C. Y. C., Josephson, M. A., and Packer, M.: Pharmacologic Mechanisms Underlying the Antianginal Actions of Verapamil, *Am. J. Cardiol.,* 50:886, 1982.

93 Ebner, F., and Dunschede, H. B.: Haemodynamics Therapeutic Mechanism of Action and Clinical Findings of Adalat Use Based on Worldwide Clinical Trials, in A. D. Jatene and P. R. Lichtlen (eds.), "The Third International Adalat Symposium," Excerpta Medica, Amsterdam, 1976.

94 Ekelund, L. G., and Atterhog, J. H.: Adalat and Beta Blockers—The Mechanism Studied with Two Series of Work Tests in Two Groups of Patients with Angina Pectoris, in W. Lochner, W. Braasch, and G. Kronenberg (eds.), "The Second International Adalat Symposium," Springer-Verlag, New York, 1975.

95 McIlwraith, G.: Adalat (Nifedipine) Under Loading Conditions, in W. Lochner, W. Braasch, and G. Kronenberg (eds.) "The Second International Adalat Symposium," Springer-Verlag, New York, 1975, p. 174.

96 Prempree, A., and Tabatznik, B.: Influence of Different Doses of Adalat on Angina Pectoris Induced by Exercise, in A. D. Jatene and P. R. Lichtlen (eds.), "The Third International Adalat Symposium," Excerpta Medica, Amsterdam, 1976, p. 113.

97 Stein, G.: Antianginal Efficacy of Different Doses of Adalat in Angina Pectoris Patients in a Double-Blind Trial, in A. D. Jatene and P. R. Lichtlen (eds.), "The Third International Adalat Symposium," Excerpta Medica, Amsterdam, 1980, p. 233.

98 Corbalan, R., Gonzalez, R., Chamorro, G., Munoz, M., Rodriquiz, J., and Casanegra, P.: Effect of a Calcium Inhibitor, Nifedipine, on Exercise Tolerance in Patients with Angina Pectoris, a Double-Blind Study, *Chest,* 79(3):302, 1981.

99 Moskowitz, R. M., Piccini, Nacarelli, G., and Zeliz, R.: Nifedipine Therapy for Stable Angina Pectoris—Preliminary Results of Effects on Angina Frequency and Treadmill Exercise Response, *Am. J. Cardiol.,* 44:811, 1979.

100 Majid, P. A., and DeJong, J.: Acute Hemodynamic Effects of Nifedipine in Patients with Ischemic Heart Disease, *Circulation,* 65(suppl. 6):1114, 1982.

101 Itoh, Y., Tamara, I., and Itoh, T.: Clinical Experience with Nifedipine, in K. Hashimoto, E. Kimura, and T. Kobayashi (eds.), ''The First Nifedipine Symposium,'' Tokyo Press, Tokyo, 1975, p. 251.

102 Kenmure, A. C. F., and Scruton, J. H.: Double-Blind Controlled Trial of the Antianginal Efficacy of Nifedipine Compared with Propranolol, *Br. J. Clin. Pract.,* 33:49, 1979.

103 Fox, K. M., Jonathan, S., and Selwyn, A. P.: The Use of Propranolol and Nifedipine in the Medical Management of Angina Pectoris, *Clin. Cardiol.,* 4:125, 1981.

104 Atterhog, J. H., and Porje, G.: Isoptin vid Angina Pectoris, *Lakartidningen,* 63:2071, 1966.

105 Neumann, M., and Luisada, A. A.: Double-Blind Evaluation of Orally Administered Iproveratril in Patients with Angina Pectoris, *Am. J. Med. Sci.,* 251:552, 1966.

106 Livesley, B., Catley, P. F., Campbell, R. C., and Oram, S.: Double-Blind Evaluation of Verapamil, Propranolol and Isosorbide Dinitrate against Placebo in the Treatment of Angina Pectoris, *Br. Med. J.,* 1:375, 1973.

107 Andreasen, F., Boye, E., Christoffersen, E., et al.: Assessment of Verapamil in the Treatment of Angina Pectoris, *Eur. J. Cardiol.* 2:443, 1975.

108 Bala-Subramanian, V., Parmasivan, R., Lahiri, A., and Raftery, E. B.: Verapamil in Chronic Stable Angina—A Controlled Study with Computerized Multistage Treadmill Exercise, *Lancet,* 1:841, 1980.

109 Brodsky, S. J., Cutler, S. S., Weiner, D. A., McCabe, C., Ryan, T., and Klein, M. D.: Treatment of Stable Angina of Effort with Verapamil—A Double-Blind Placebo Controlled Randomized Crossover Study, *Circulation,* 66(suppl. 3):569, 1982.

110 Phear, D. N.: Verapamil in Angina—A Double-Blind Trial, *Br. Med. J.,* 2:740, 1968.

111 Sandler, G., Clayton, G. A., and Thronicroft, S. G.: Clinical Evaluation of Verapamil in Angina Pectoris, *Br. Med. J.,* 3:224, 1968.

112 Pine, M. B., Citron, P. D., Bailly, D.J., et al.: Verapamil versus Placebo in Relieving Stable Angina Pectoris, *Circulation,* 65(suppl. 1):17, 1982.

113 Hossack, K. F., Pool, P. E., and Steele, P. Efficacy of Diltiazem in Angina on Effort—A Multicenter Trial, *Am. J. Cardiol.,* 49:567, 1982.

114 Strauss, W. E., McIntyre, K. M., Parisi, A. R., and Shapiro, W.: Safety and Efficacy of Diltiazem Hydrochloride for the Treatment of Stable Angina Pectoris—Report of a Cooperative Trial, *Am. J. Cardiol.,* 49:560, 1982.

115 Ono, K.: Clinical Effect of Herbesser on Ischemic Heart Disease—Double-Blind Studies with Inactive Placebo in Par, *Jpn. J. Clin. Exp. Med.,* 49:2304, 1972.

116 Mizuno, Y., Yasui, S., Tobata, I., et al.: Effect of CRD-401 on Ischemic Heart Disease, *Jpn. J. Clin. Exp. Med.,* 50:565, 1973.

117 Hossack, K. F., Pool, P. E., and Steele, P.: Efficacy of Diltiazem in Angina on Effort—A Multicenter Trial, *Am. J. Cardiol.,* 49:567, 1982.

118 Kalenbach, M.: Assessment of Antianginal Substances by Means of ST Depression in the Exercise EKG, in K. Hashimoto, E. Kimura, and T. Kobayashi (eds.), ''The First Nifedipine Symposium,'' Tokyo Press, Tokyo, 1975, p. 126.

119 Kimura, E., Mabuch, G., and Kikuchi, H.: Clinical Evaluation of the Effect of Nifedipine on Angina Pectoris by Sequential Analysis, in K. Hashimoto, E. Kimura, and T. Kobayashi (ed.), ''The First Nifedipine Symposium,'' Tokyo Press, Tokyo, 1975, p. 155.

120 Ekelund, L. G., and Ono, L.: Antianginal Efficacy of Nifedipine with and without a Beta-Blocker, Studied with Exercise Test—A Double-Blind, Randomized Subacute Study, *Clin. Cardiol.* 2:203, 1979.

121 Sadick, N., Tank, A. T. H., Fletcher, P. J., Morris, J., and Kelly, D.: A Double-Blind Randomized Trial of Propranolol and Verapamil in the Treatment of Effort Angina, *Circulation,* 66(suppl. 3):574, 1982.

122 Frishman, W. H., Klein, N. A., Strom, J. A., et al.: Superiority of Verapamil to Propranolol in Stable Angina Pectoris—a Double-Blind Randomized Crossover Trial, *Circulation,* 65(suppl. 1):51, 1982.

123 Dawson, J. R., Whitaker, N. H. G., and Sutton, G. C.: Calcium Antagonist Drugs in Chronic Stable Angina—Comparison of Verapamil and Nifedipine, *Br. Heart J.,* 46:508, 1980.

124 Moses, J., Feldman, M. S., and Helfant, R. H.: Efficacy of Nifedipine in the Intermediate Syndrome Refractory to Propranolol and Nitrate Therapy, *Am. J. Cardiol.,* 45:390, 1980. (Abstract.)

125 Previtali, M., Salerno, J. A., Tarazzi, L., et al.: Treatment of Angina at Rest with Nifedipine—A Short-Term Controlled Study, *Am. J. Cardiol.,* 45:825, 1980.

126 Gerstenblith, G., Ouyang, P., Achuff, S., et al.: Nifedipine in Unstable Angina—A Double-Blind, Randomized Trial, *N. Engl. J. Med.* 306(15):885, 1982.

127 Parodi, O., Maseri, A., and Simonetti, I.: Management of Unstable Angina at Rest by Verapamil—A Double-Blind Crossover Study in Coronary Care Unit, *Br. Heart J.,* 41:167, 1979.

128 Mehta, J., Pepine, C. J., Day, M., et al.: Short-Term Efficacy of Oral Verapamil in Rest Angina—A Double-Blind Placebo Controlled Trial in CCU Patients, *Am. J. Med.,* 71:977, 1981.

129 Parodi, O., Simonetti, I., L'Abbate, A., and Maseri, A.: Verapamil versus Propranolol for Angina at Rest, *Am. J. Cardiol.,* 50:923, 1982.

130 Oliva, P. D., and Breckenridge, J. C.: Arteriographic Evidence of Coronary Artery Spasm in Acute Myocardial Infarction, *Circulation,* 56:366, 1977.

131 Rentrop, P., Blanke, H., Korsch, K. R., Kaiser, H., Kostering, H., and Leitz, K.: Selective Intracoronary Thrombolysis in Acute Myocardial Infarction and Unstable Angina Pectoris, *Circulation*, 63:307, 1981.

132 Reimer, K. A., Lowe, J. E., and Jennings, R. B.: Effect of the Calcium Antagonist Verapamil on Necrosis following Temporary Artery Occlusion in Dogs, *Circulation*, 55:581, 1977.

133 Henry, P. D., Shuchleib, R., Clark, R. E., and Perez, J. E.: Effect of Nifedipine on Myocardial Ischemia—Analysis of Collateral Flow, Pulsatile Heat and Regional Muscle Shortening, *Am. J. Cardiol.*, 44:817, 1979.

134 Selwyn, A. P., Welman, E., Fox, K., Horlock, P., Pratt, T., and Klein, M.: The Effects of Nifedipine on Acute Experimental Myocardial Ischemia and Infarction in Dogs, *Circ. Res.*, 44:16, 1979.

135 Busman, W. D.: Use of Vasodilators in Acute Myocardial Infarction. Findings of the International Symposium on Limiting Infarct Size, *Tagung Dtsch. Gesellsch. Inves. Med.*, 129:1982. (Abstract.)

136 Hagemeier, F.: Verapamil in the Management of Supraventricular Tachyarrhythmias Occurring after Recent Myocardial Infarction, *Circulation*, 57:751, 1978.

137 Singh, B. N., Nademanee, K., and Feld, G.: Calcium Blockers in the Treatment of Cardiac Arrhythmias, in S. F. Flaim and R. Zelis (eds.), "Calcium Blockers: Mechanisms of Action and Clinical Applications," Urban and Schwarzenberg, Baltimore–Munich, 1982, pp. 245–264.

138 Singh, B. N., Nademanee, D., and Baky, S.: Calcium Antagonists: Uses in the Treatment of Cardiac Arrhythmias, *Drugs*, 25:125, 1983.

139 Sobel, B. E.: Calcium Antagonists in Cardiovascular Therapeutics, *Pract. Cardiol.*, 7:1, 1981.

140 Nayler, W. G., Ferrari, R., and Williams, A.: Protective Effect of Pretreatment with Verapamil, Nifedipine and Propranolol on Mitochondrial Function in the Ischemic and Reperfused Myocardium, *Am. J. Cardiol.*, 46:242, 1980.

141 Henry, P. D., Shuchleib, R., Davis, J., Weiss, E. S., and Sobel, B. E.: Myocardial Contracture and Accumulation of Mitochondrial Calcium in Ischemic Rabbit Heart, *Am. J. Physiol.*, 233:677, 1977.

142 Kloner, R. A., DeBoer, L. W. V., Carlson, N., and Braunwald, E.: The Effect of Verapamil on Myocardial Ultrastructure during and following Release of Coronary Artery Occlusion, *Exp. Mol. Pathol.*, 36:277, 1982.

143 Clark, R. E., Christlieb, I. Y., and Ferguson, T. B.: Laboratory and Initial Clinical Studies of Nifedipine, A Calcium Antagonist for Improved Myocardial Preservation, *Ann. Surg.*, 193:875, 1980.

144 Clark, R. E., Christlieb, I., Ferguson, T. B., et al.: Reduction of Consequences of Ischemia and Preservation of Myocardium with Nifedipine, *Am. J. Cardiol.*, 43:361, 1979b.

145 Heng, M. K., Singh, B. N., Roche, A. H. G., Norris, R. M., and Mercer, C. J.: Effects of Intravenous Verapamil on Cardiac Arrhythmias and on the Electrocardiogram, *Am. Heart J.*, 90:487, 1975.

146 Singh, B. N., Ellrodt, G., and Peter, C. T.: Verapamil—A Review of Its Pharmacological Properties and Therapeutic Uses, *Drugs*, 15:169, 1978.

146a Hartel, G., and Hartikainen, M.: Comparison of Verapamil and Practolol in Paroxysmal Supraventricular Tachycardia, *Eur. J. Cardiol.*, 4:87, 1976.

147 Kuhn, M.: Verapamil in the Treatment of PSVT, *Ann. Emer. Med.*, 10:538, 1981.

148 Anderson, C. J., and Reiser, J.: Calcium Antagonists and Cardiac Arrhythmias, *Am. Fam. Physician*, 23:214, 1981.

149 Krikler, D. M.: Calcium Ion Antagonists—Mechanisms of Action in Arrhythmias, *Clin. Invest. Med.* 3:29, 1980.

150 Dargie, H., Rowland, E., and Krinkler, D.: Role of Calcium Antagonists in Cardiovascular Disease, *Br. Heart J.*, 46:8, 1981.

151 Sung, R. J., Waxman, H. L., Elser, B., and Juma, Z.: Treatment of Paroxysmal Supraventricular Tachycardia and Atrial Flutter/Fibrillation with Intravenous Verapamil—Efficacy and Mechanism of Action, *Clin. Invest. Med.*, 3(1–2):41, 1980.

152 Rinkenberger, R. L., Prystowsky, E. N., Heger, J. J., Troup, P. J., Jackman, W. M., and Zipes, D. P.: Effects of Intravenous and Chronic Oral Verapamil Administration in Patients with Supraventricular Tachyarrhythmias, *Circulation*, 62:996, 1980.

153 Gmeiner, R., Ng, C. K., and Bstöttner, M.: Effect on Paroxysmal Reentrant Supraventricular Tachycardia of a Drug Affecting Calcium Transport (RO-11-1781), *Eur J. Clin. Pharmacol.*, 16:155, 1979.

154 Rozanski, J. J., Zaman, L., and Castellanos, A.: Electrophysiologic Effects of Diltiazem Hydrochloride on Supraventricular Tachycardia, *Am. J. Cardiol.*, 49:621, 1982.

155 Russell, D. C.: Electrophysiology and Antiarrhythmic Effects of Calcium Antagonists, *Scott. Med. J.*, 26(2):161, 1981.

156 Gonzalez, R., and Scheinmann, M. M.: Treatment of Supraventricular Arrhythmias with Intravenous and Oral Verapamil, *Chest*, 80(4):465, 1981.

157 Mauritson, D. R., Winniford, M. D., Walker, W. S., et al.: Oral Verapamil for Paroxysmal Supraventricular Tachycardia—A Long-term, Double-Blind Randomized Trial, *Ann. Intern. Med.*, 96(4):409, 1982.

158 Tonkin, A. M., Aylward, P. E., and Joel, S. E.: Verapamil in Prophylaxis of Paroxysmal Atrioventricular Nodal Reentrant Tachycardia, *J. Cardiovasc. Pharmocol.*, 2:473, 1980.

159 Klein, G. T., Gulamhussein, S., and Prystowsky, E. N.: Comparison of the Electrophysiologic Effects of

Intravenous and Oral Verapamil in Patients with Paroxysmal Supraventricular Tachycardia, *Am. J. Cardiol.*, 49:117, 1981.

160 Talano, J. V., and Feerst, D.: Verapamil—A New Class Antiarrhythmic Agent with a Variety of Beneficial Cardiovascular Effects, *Arch. Intern. Med.*, 140:314, 1980.

161 Aronow, W. S., Landa, D., and Plasencia, G.: Verapamil in Atrial Fibrillation and Atrial Flutter, *Clin. Pharmacol. Ther.*, 26:578, 1979.

162 Aronow, W. S., and Ferlinz, J.: Verapamil versus Placebo in Atrial Fibrillation and Flutter, *Clin. Invest. Med.*, 3(1–2):35, 1980.

163 Schamroth, L.: Immediate Effects of Intravenous Verapamil on Atrial Fibrillation, *Cardiovasc. Res.*, 5:419, 1971.

164 Schwartz, J., Keefe, D., Kates, R., Kirsten, E., and Harrison, D. C.: Acute and Chronic Pharmacodynamic Interaction of Verapamil and Digoxin in Atrial Fibrillation, *Circulation*, 65(6):1163, 1982.

165 Morganroth, J., Chen, C. C., Sturn, S., and Dreifus, L. S.: Oral Verapamil in the Treatment of Atrial Fibrillation/Flutter, *Am. J. Cardiol.*, 49:981, 1982.

166 Klein, H. O., Pauzner, H., Disengni, E., David, D., and Kaplinsky, E.: The Beneficial Effects of Verapamil in Chronic Atrial Fibrillation, *Ann. Intern. Med.*, 139:747, 1979.

167 Rasmussen, K., Wang, H., and Fausa, D.: Comparative Efficacy of Quinidine and Verapamil in the Maintenance of Sinus Rhythm after DC Conversion of Atrial Fibrillation, *Acta Med. Scand. (suppl.)*, 645:23, 1981.

168 Storstein, O., and Landmark, K. H.: Verapamil in the Treatment of Atrial Tachycardia with Block, *Acta Med. Scand.*, 198:483, 1975.

169 Rabkin, S. W. Tomlinson, C., Corbett, B. N., and Cuddy, T. E.: Verapamil and Supraventricular Tachyarrhythmias—Beneficial Effects in Patients with Chronic Pulmonary Disease, *Can. Med. Assoc. J.* 122:64, 1980.

170 Krikler, D. M., and Spurrel, R. A. J.: Verapamil in the Treatment of Paroxysmal Supraventricular Tachycardia, *Postgrad. Med. J.*, 50:447, 1974.

171 Gulamhusein, S., Ko, P., Carruther, S. G., and Klein, G. J.: Acceleration of the Ventricular Response during Atrial Fibrillation in the Wolff-Parkinson-White Syndrome after Verapamil, *Circulation*, 65(suppl. 2):348, 1982.

172 Hamer, A., Peter, T., Platt, M., and Mandel, W. J.: Effects of Verapamil on Supraventricular Tachycardia Patients with Overt and Concealed Wolff-Parkinson-White Syndrome, *Am. Heart J.*, 101:600, 1981.

173 Goodwin, J. F., and Krikler, D. M.: Arrhythmia as a Cause of Sudden Death in Hypertrophic Cardiomyopathy, *Lancet*, 2:937, 1976.

174 McKenna, W. J., Harris, L., and Perez, G.: Hypertrophic Cardiomyopathy—Comparison of Verapamil and Amiodarone in the Treatment of Arrhythmias, *Br. Heart J.*, 45:356, 1980.

175 Filias, N.: Verapamil—Behandlung Bei Herzrhythmusstörungen, *Scheveiz Rundschan Med.*, 3:66, 1974.

176 Fazzini, P. F., Marchi, F., and Pucci, P.: Effects of Verapamil on Ventricular Premature Beats of Acute Myocardial Infarction, *Acta Cardiol.*, 33:25, 1978.

177 Wellens, H. J. J., Bär, F. W., Lie, K. I., Düren, D. R., and Dohmen, H. J.: Effects of Procainamide, Propranolol and Verapamil on Mechanism of Tachycardia in Patients with Chronic Recurrent Ventricular Tachycardia, *Am. J. Cardiol.*, 40:579, 1977.

178 Wellens, H. J. J., Farre, J., and Bär, B. B.: The Role of the Slow Inward Current in the Genesis of Ventricular Tachyarrhythmias in Man, in D. P. Zipes, J. C. Bailey, and V. Elharrar (eds.), "The Slow Inward Current and Cardiac Arrhythmias," The Hague, Boston, 1980.

179 Elharrar, V., Gaum, W. E., and Zipes, D. P.: Effect of Drugs on Conduction Delay and Incidence of Ventricular Arrhythmias Induced by Acute Coronary Occlusion in Dogs, *Am. J. Cardiol.*, 39:544, 1977.

180 Kimura, E., Tanaka, K., Mizuno, K., Handa, Y., and Hashimoto, H.: Suppression of Repeatedly Occurring Ventricular Fibrillation with Nifedipine in Variant Form of Angina Pectoris, *Jpn. Heart J.*, 18:736, 1977.

181 The Norwegian Multicenter Study Group: Timolol-Induced Reduction in Mortality and Reinfarction in Patients Surviving Acute Myocardial Infarction, *N. Engl. J. Med.*, 304:801, 1981.

182 Aoki, K., Kondo, S., Moshizuk, A., et al.: Antihypertensive Effect of Cardiovascular Ca^{2+}-Antagonists in Hypertensive Patients in the Absence and Presence of Beta Adrenergic Blockade, *Am. Heart J.*, 96:218, 1978.

183 Brittinger, W. D., Schwarzbeck, A., Wittenmeier, K. W., et al.: Klinish-experimentelle Untersuchungen uber die blutdrucksenkende Wirkung von Verapamil, *Dtsch Med. Wochenschr.*, 95:1871, 1970.

184 Bartorelli, C., and Guazzi, M.: Cardiovascular Effects in Man of Nifedipine—Therapeutic Implications, in "Adalat. New Experimental and Clinical Results," Excerpta Medica, Amsterdam, 1979, p. 18.

185 Hiwatari, M., Satoh, K., and Taira, N.: Antihypertensive Effect of Nifedipine on Conscious Renal-Hypertensive Dogs, *Arzneim. Forsch.*, 29:256, 1979.

186 Kuwajiami, I., Veda, K., Kamata, C., et al.: A Study of the Effects of Nifedipine in Hypertensive Crises and Severe Hypertension, *Jpn. Heart J.*, 19:455, 1978.

187 Ueda, K., Kuwajima, I., Ito, H., Kuramoto, K., and Murakimi, M.: Nifedipine in the Management of Hypertension, in "Adalat—New Experimental and Clinical Results," Excerpta Medica, Amsterdam, 1979, p. 19.

188 Guazzi, M. D., Olivari, M. T., Polese, A., Fiorentini, C., Magrini, F., and Moruzzi, P.: Nifedipine, A New

Antihypertensive with Rapid Action, *Clin. Pharmacol. Ther.*, 22:528, 1977.

189 Olivari, M. T., Bartorelli, C., Polese, A., Fiorentini, C., Moruzzi, P., and Guazzi, M. D.: Treatment of Hypertension with Nifedipine, A Calcium Antagonist Drug, *Circulation*, 59:1066, 1979.

190 Beer, N., Gallegos, I., Cohen, A., Kline, N., Sonnenblick, E., and Frishman, W.: Efficacy of Sublingual Nifedipine in the Acute Treatment of Systemic Hypertension, *Chest*, 79(5):571, 1981.

191 Pederson, O. L.: Effects of Nifedipine on Blood Pressure, Regional Hemodynamics, Plasma Renin Activity and Plasma Catecholamines in Patients with Arterial Hypertension, *Acta. Med. Scand.*, 625:65, 1978.

192 Pederson, O. L.: Does Verapamil Have a Clinically Significant Antihypertensive Effect, *Eur. J. Clin. Pharmacol.*, 13:32, 1978.

193 Pederson, O. L.: Effect of Nifedipine on Plasma Renin, Aldosterone and Catecholamines in Arterial Hypertension, *Eur. J. Clin. Pharmacol.*, 15:235, 1979.

194 Aoko, K., Yoshida, T., Kato, S., et al.: Hypotensive Action and Increased Plasma Renin Activity by Ca^{2+}-Antagonist (Nifedipine) in Hypertensive Patients, *Jpn. Heart J.*, 17:479, 1976.

195 Pederson, O. L., and Mikkelsen, E.: Acute and Chronic Effects of Nifedipine in Arterial Hypertension, *Eur. J. Clin. Pharmacol.*, 14:375, 1978.

196 Gould B. A., Mann, S., Kieso, H., Subramanian, V. B., and Raftery, E. B.: The 24-hour Ambulatory Blood Pressure Profile with Verapamil, *Circulation*, (suppl, 1):22, 1982.

197 Sakuri, T., Kurita, T., Vagano, S., et al.: Antihypertensive Vasodilating and Sodium Diuretic Actions of D-*cis*-isomer of Benzothiazepine Derivative (CRD-401), *Acta Urol. Jpn.* 18:695, 1972.

198 Lorell, B. H., Paulus, W. J., Grossman, W., Wynne, J., and Cohn, P. F.: Modification of Abnormal Left Ventricular Diastolic Properties by Nifedipine in Patients with Hypertrophic Cardiomyopathy, *Circulation*, 65(suppl. 3):499, 1982.

199 Harrison, D. C., Braunwald, E., Glick, G., Mason, D. T., Chidsey, C. A., and Ross, J., Jr.: Effects of Beta Adrenergic Blockade on the Circulation with Particular Reference to Observations in Patients with Hypertrophic Subaortic Stenosis, *Circulation*, 29:84, 1964.

200 Hardarson, T., de la Calzada, C. S., Curiel, R., and Goodwin, J. F.: Prognosis and Mortality of Hypertrophic Obstructive Cardiomyopathy, *Lancet*, 2:1462, 1973.

201 Jasmin, G., and Proschek, L.: Prevention of Myocardial Degeneration in Hamsters with Hereditary Cardiomyopathy, in A. Fleckenstein and H. Roskamm (eds.), "Calcium Antagonismus," Springer-Verlag, Berlin, Heidelberg, and New York, 1980, p. 144.

202 Kaltenbach, M., Hopf, R., and Keller, M.: Treatment of Hypertrophic Obstructive Cardiomyopathy with Verapamil, a Calcium Antagonist, *Dtsch. Med. Wochenschr.*, 101:1284, 1976.

203 Kaltenbach, M., Hopf, R., Kober, G., Bussman, W. D., Keller, M., and Petersen, Y.: Treatment of Hypertrophic Obstructive Cardiomyopathy with Verapamil, *Br. Heart J.* 42:35, 1979.

204 Rosing, D. R., Kent, K. M., Maron, B. J., and Epstein, S. E.: Verapamil Therapy—A New Approach to the Pharmacologic Treatment of Hypertrophic Cardiomyopathy—II. Effects on Exercise Capacity and Symptomatic Status, *Circulation*, 60:1209, 1979.

205 Rosing, D. R., Kent, K. M., Borer, J. S., Seides, S. F., Maron, B. J., and Epstein, S. E.: Verapamil Therapy—A New Approach to the Pharmacologic Treatment of Hypertrophic Cardiomyopathy. I. Hemodynamic Effects, *Circulation*, 60:1201, 1979.

206 Hanrath, P., Mathey, D., Kremer, P., Sonntag, F., and Bleifeld, W.: Effect of Verapamil on Left Ventricular Relaxation and Filling in Hypertrophic Cardiomyopathy, *Am. J. Cardiol.*, 45:393, 1980. (Abstract.)

207 Landmark, K., Sire, S., Thaulow, E., Amlie, J., and Nitter-Hauge, S.: Haemodynamic Effects of Nifedipine and Propranolol in Patients with Hypertrophic Obstructive Cardiomyopathy, *Br. Heart J.*, 48:19, 1982.

208 Nagao, R., Omote, S., Hiromitsu, H., Horie, M., and Tanaka, S.: Diltiazem-Induced Decrease of Exercise Elevated Pulmonary Arterial Diastolic Pressure in Hypertrophic Cardiomyopathy Patients, *Am. Heart J.*, 102(4):789, 1981.

209 Landmark, K., Refsum, A. M., Simonsen, S., and Storstein, O.: Verapamil and Pulmonary Hypertension, *Acta Med. Scand.*, 204:299, 1978.

210 Camerini, F., Alberti, E., Klugmann, S., and Salvi, A.: Primary Pulmonary Hypertension—Effect of Nifedipine, *Br. Heart J.*, 44:352, 1980.

211 Simonneau, G., Escourrou, P., Deroux, P., and Lockhart, A.: Inhibition of Hypoxic Pulmonary Vasoconstriction by Nifedipine, *N. Engl. J. Med.* 304:1582, 1981.

212 Kambara, H., Fujimoto, K., Wahabayashi, A., and Kawai, C.: Primary Pulmonary Hypertension—Beneficial Therapy with Diltiazem, *Am. Heart J.*, 101(2):230, 1981.

213 Crevey, B. J., Dantzker, D. R., Bower, J. S., et al.: Hemodynamics and Gas Exchange Effects of Intravenous Diltiazem in Patients with Pulmonary Hypertension, *Am. J. Cardiol.*, 49:578, 1982.

214 Polese, A., Fiorentini, C., Olivari, M. T., and Guazzi, M. D.: Clinical Use of a Calcium Antagonist Agent (Nifedipine) in Acute Pulmonary Edema, *Am. J. Med.*, 66:825, 1979.

215 Henry, P. D.: Calcium Ion (Ca^{2+}) Antagonists—Mechanisms of Action and Clinical Applications, *Pract. Cardiol.*, 5:145, 1979.

216 Matsui, S., et al.: Hemodynamic Effects of Sublingual Nifedipine in Congestive Heart Failure, *Jpn. Circ. J.*, 43:1081, 1979.

217 Allen, G. S., and Bahr, A. L.: Cerebral Arterial Spasm (Pt 10) Reversal of Acute and Chronic Spasm in Dogs with Orally Administered Nifedipine, *Neurosurgery*, 4:43, 1979.

218 Kinney, E. L., Nicholas, G., Petrokuli, R., Zelis, R., and Pontoriero, C.: Verapamil in the Treatment of Raynaud's Phenomenon Due to Schleroderma, *Clin. Res.*, 28:351A, 1980.

219 Addonizio, V. P., Fisher, C. A., and Edmunds, L. H., Jr. Effects of Verapamil and Nifedipine on Platelet Activation, *Circulation*, 62(suppl. 3):326, 1980. (Abstract.)

220 Chierchia, S., Crea, F., Ber, W., et al. Antiplatelet Effects of Verapamil in Man, *Am. J. Cardiol.*, 47:399, 1981. (Abstract.)

221 Ribeiro, L. G. T., Brandon, T. A., Horak, J. K., Solis, T., and Miller, R. R.: Inhibition of Platelet Aggregation by Verapamil—Further Rationale for the Use of Calcium Antagonists in Coronary Artery Disease, *Circulation*, 62 (suppl. 3):293, 1980. (Abstract.)

222 Horster, F. A., Duhm, B., Maul, W., Medenwald, H., Patzschke, K., and Wegner, L. A.: Klinische Untersuchungen zur Pharmakokinetic von radioaktive markiertem (4-(2'-nitrophenyl)-2, 6 dimethyl-1, 4-dihydropyridin-305-dicarbonsauredimethylester). *Arzneim. Forsch.* 22:330, 1972.

223 Horster, F. A.: Pharmacokinetics of Nifedipine—^{14}C in Man, in W. Lochner, W. Braasch, and G. Kronenberg (eds.), ''The Second International Adalat Symposium,'' Springer-Verlag, New York, 1976, p. 124.

224 Piepho, R. W., Bloedow, D. C., Lacz, J. P., Runser, D. J., Dimmit, D. C., and Browne, D. K.: Pharmacokinetics of Diltiazem in Selected Animal Species and Human Beings, *Am. J. Cardiol.* 49:525, 1982.

225 Zelis, R. F., and Kinney, E. L.: The Pharmacokinetics of Diltiazem in Healthy American Men, *Am. J. Cardiol.* 49:529, 1981.

226 Kohno, K., Takenchi, Y., Etoh, A., and Noda, K.: Pharmacokinetics and Bioavailability of Diltiazem (CRD -401) in Dog, *Arzneim. Forsch.* 27:1424, 1977.

227 Meshi, T., Sugihara, J., and Sato, Y.: Metabolic Fate of CRD-401, *Chem. Pharm. Bull. (Tokyo)*, 19:1546, 1971.

228 Schlepper, M., Thormann, J., and Schwarz, F.: The Pharmacodynamics of Orally Taken Verapamil and Verapamil Retard as Judged by Their Negative Dromotropic Effects, *Arzneim. Forsch.*, 25:1452, 1975.

229 Keele, D. L., Yee, Y. G., and Kates, K. E.: Verapamil Protein Binding in Patients and in Normal Subjects, *Clin. Pharmacol. Ther.*, 29:21, 1981.

230 Schomerus, M., Spiegelhalder, B., Stieren, B., and Eichelbaum, M.: Physiological Disposition of Verapamil in Man, *Cardiovasc. Res.*, 10:605, 1976.

231 Shand, D. G., Hammill, S. C., and Aanonsen, L.: Reduced Verapamil Clearance during Long-term Oral Administration, *Clin. Pharmacol. Ther.*, 30:653, 1981.

232 Woodcock, B. L. G., Rietbrock, I., and Vohringer, H. F.: Verapamil Disposition in Liver Disease and Intensive Care Patients—Kinetics, Clearance and Apparent Blood Flow Relationships, *Clin. Pharmacol. Ther.*, 29:27, 1981.

233 Pritchett, E. L. C., Lee, K. L., and Hammill, S. C.: Efficacy of Oral Verapamil in Preventing Paroxysmal Atrial Tachycardia, *Circulation*, 64(suppl. 4):317, 1981. (Abstract.)

234 Reddy, C. P., McAllister, R. G., and Slack, J. C.: Absence of Specific Electrocardiographic End Points as Indicators of Drug Effect during Chronic Oral Verapamil Therapy, *Circulation*, 64(suppl. 4):138, 1981.

235 Leon, M. B., Rosing, D. R., and Jaoni, T. M.: Clinical Utility of Plasma Verapamil Levels in Patients with Hypertrophic Cardiomyopathy, *Am. J. Cardiol.*, 47:407, 1981.

236 Terry, R. W.: Nifedipine Therapy in Angina Pectoris: Evaluation of Safety and Side Effects, *Am. Heart J.*, 104 (3):681, 1982.

237 Benaim, M. E.: Asystole after Verapamil, *Br. Med. J.*, 2:169, 1972.

238 Boothby, C. B., Garrard, C. S., and Pickering, D.: Intravenous Verapamil in Cardiac Arrhythmias, *Br. Med. J.*, 2:348, 1972.

239 Immonen, P., Linkola, A., and Waris, E.: Three Cases of Severe Verapamil Poisoning, *Int. J. Cardiol.*, 1:101, 1981.

240 McGoon, M. D., Vlietstra, R. E., Holmes, D. R., and Osborn, J. E.: The Clinical Use of Verapamil, *Mayo Clin. Proc.*, 57:495, 1982.

241 Gluskin, L. E., Strasberg, B., and Shah, J. H.: Verapamil-Induced Hyperprolactinemia and Galactorrhea, *Ann. Intern. Med.*, 95:66, 1981.

242 Brodsky, S. J., Cutler, S. S., Weiner, D. A., and Klein, M. D.: Hepatotoxicity Due to Treatment with Verapamil, *Ann. Intern. Med.*, 94:490, 1981.

243 Belz, G. G., Doering, W., Munkes, R., Aust, P. E., and Belz, G.: Effects of Various Calcium Antagonists on Blood Level and Renal Clearance of Digoxin, *Circulation*, 64 (suppl. 4):24, 1981. (Abstract.)

244 Krikler, D. M., Harris, L., and Rowland, E.: Calcium Channel Blockers and Beta-Blockers—Advantages and Disadvantages of Combination Therapy in Chronic Stable Angina Pectoris, *Am. Heart J.*, 104:702, 1982.

245 Joshi, P. I., Dalab, J. J., Rutley, M. S., et al.: Nifedipine and Left Ventricular Function in Beta-Blocked Patients, *Br. Heart J.*, 45:457, 1981.

246 Nakamoto, K.: Nifedipine in the Management of Ischemic Heart Diseases, in K. Hashimoto, E. Kimura, and T. Kobayashi (eds.), ''Proceedings of the First International Nifedipin (Adalat) Symposium,'' Tokyo University Press, Tokyo, 1975, p. 279.

247 Anastassiades, C. J.: Nifedipine and Beta-Blocker Drugs, *Br. Med. J.*, 281:1251, 1980.

248 Opie, L. H., and White, D. A.: Adverse Interaction between Nifedipine and Beta-Blockade, *Br. Med. J.*, 281:1462, 1980.

249 Waxman, H. L., Myerburg, R. J., Appel, R., and Sung, R. J.: Verapamil for Control of Ventricular Rate in Paroxysmal Supraventricular Tachycardia and Atrial Fibrillation or Flutter—A Double-Blind Randomized Crossover Study, *Ann. Intern. Med.*, 94:1, 1981.

250 Seabra-Gomes, R., Richards, A., and Sutton, R.: Hemodynamic Effects of Verapamil and Practolol in Man, *Eur. J. Cardiol.*, 4:79, 1976.

251 Leon, M. B., Rosing, D. R., Bonow, R. O., Lipson, L. C., and Epstein, S. E.: Clinical Efficacy of Verapamil Alone and Combined with Propranolol in Treating Patients with Chronic Stable Angina Pectoris, *Am. J. Cardiol.*, 49:267, 1982.

252 Balasubramanian, V., Bowles, M. J., Daires, A. B., and Raftery, E. B.: Combined Therapy with Verapamil and Propranolol in Chronic Stable Angina, *Am. J. Cardiol*, 49:267, 1982.

253 Packer, M., Leon, M. R., Borow, R. O., Kieval, J., Rosing, D. R., and Balasubramanian, V.: Hemodynamic and Clinical Effects of Combined Verapamil and Propranolol Therapy in Angina Pectoris, *Am. J. Cardiol.*, 50:903, 1982.

254 Parker, M., Meller, J., and Medina, N.: Hemodynamic Consequences of Combined Beta-Adrenergic and Slow Channel Blockade in Man, *Circulation*, 65:660, 1982.

The Use of Streptokinase in the Early Stages of Myocardial Infarction[*]

JAY HOLLMAN, M.D., and
ANDREAS R. GRUENTZIG, M.D.

How much is a life worth? What price per gram of salvaged myocardium? What cost per met of increased exercise tolerance?

S. SCHEIDT, 1978[34]

The most effective treatment for acute myocardial infarction is not known. This is a curious statement when so many complex infectious and metabolic diseases have rather specific antimicrobial and hormonal antidotes. The disease, coronary atherosclerosis with its complications, inflicts some 1 million people annually and will kill more Americans than any other disease, and it has no fixed treatment.

The development of coronary care units, external defibrillators and temporary pacemakers in the 1960s permitted the more effective treatment of previously fatal arrhythmias. As a result hospital mortality rate for acute myocardial infarction was reduced from 30 to 40 percent to 11 to 21 percent.[1,2] The rhythm disturbances were often the consequences of myocardial infarction rather than the cause. But the new procedures were not able to alter the death of heart muscle.

Animal experiments showed that myocardial infarction is not a fixed process that is determined at the time of coronary occlusion but a process that evolves over several hours (Fig. 1).[3,4] The amount of myocardium lost could be altered during the peri-infarction period. Thus, the reduction of excess preload and afterload and the treatment of shock and heart failure were recognized as important measures to minimize the damage.[5]

Frustration still remains since infarctions still occur and left ventricular dysfunction with shock has replaced arrhythmias as the most common cause of death in the coronary care unit.

The best predictor of an unfavorable prognosis after an acute infarction is poor left ventricular function.[6] Accordingly, the best way to improve the rate of early and late mortality of myocardial infarction should be to salvage myocardium which is under jeopardy during the infarction. Thrombolytic therapy is a new promising means to accomplish this objective.

*From the Department of Medicine, Division of Cardiology, Emory University School of Medicine, Atlanta, Georgia.

OTHER METHODS FOR REDUCING INFARCT SIZE

In order to place streptokinase treatment for infarction in perspective, it is necessary to briefly review some of the other agents and methods that have been used to decrease infarct size. This is not intended to be a comprehensive review in order but rather a brief overview to understand other interventions and their efficacy compared to streptokinase.

Beta Blockers

Propranolol,[7] atenolol,[8] and alprenolol[9] when given acutely have been shown to decrease infarct size by enzyme assessment of infarction. Metoprolol[10] has also been shown to limit infarct size but only in anterior infarction or in patients treated less than 12 h after the onset of symptoms. Practolol,[11] metoprolol,[11] and propranolol[12] have been shown to limit the size of ischemic injury as assessed by precordial ST-segment mapping. Practolol, given acutely, has been shown to lower the mortality rate of patients with acute infarction who exhibit tachycardia.[13] Recent animal studies suggest that some beta blockers are more effective than others in myocardial preservation.[14]

Nitroglycerin

Flaherty et al.[15] first showed favorable effects with nitroglycerin on ST-segment elevation, and their observations were confirmed and expanded.[16] Using QRS precordial mapping, nitroglycerin has been shown to limit infarct size.[17] By treating patients with intravenous nitroglycerin within 8 h of symptoms, infarction size is limited as assessed by creatine kinase (CK) release curves.[18] Nitroglycerin, given intravenously, improves thallium perfusion defects[19,20] and improves ejection fraction, although the effect appears to be greatest in infarctions not complicated by left ventricular dysfunction.[19] Early wall motion improvement predicts late wall motion improvement.[21] Sublingual nitroglycerin has been shown to limit infarct size in normotensive patients as judged by precordial map-

"

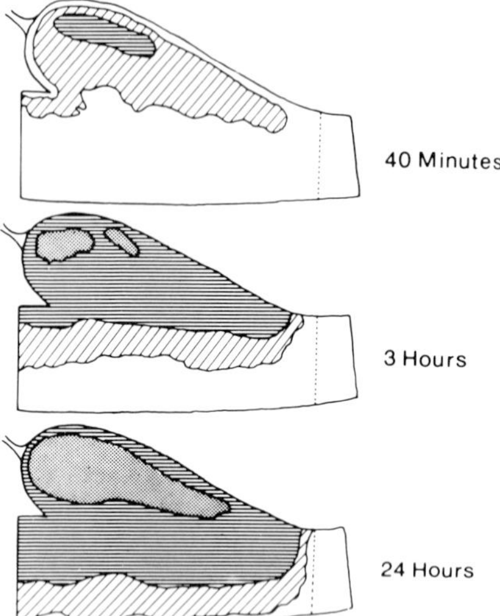

FIGURE 1 Diagrammatic summary of the progression of the wave front of ischemic cell death with respect to duration of coronary occlusion. Necrosis (all shaded areas) occurs first in the subendocardial myocardium and with longer durations of coronary occlusion involves progressively more of the transmural thickness of the ischemic zone. (Dashed line indicates the anatomic boundary between ischemic circumflex and nonischemic LAD coronary beds.)

Microvascular injury, evidenced by interstitial hemorrhage (horizontal cross-hatching), also progresses from subendocardial to subepicardial zones but the time scale is slower than that for myocyte necrosis. Complete cessation of microvascular perfusion may result in a central core (dotted areas) of necrotic muscle devoid of either hemorrhage or inflammatory response. Thus following either temporary or permanent coronary occlusions, the infarct may demonstrate, grossly and by light microscopy, a central core of relatively preserved necrotic muscle, a hemorrhagic midzone, and a peripheral zone of organizing necrosis. At 3 h after occlusion there is typically a significant amount of subepicardial myocardium which is viable and can be salvaged by reperfusion (*From K. A. Reimer, J. E. Lowe, M. M. Rasmussen, and R. B. Jennings; The Wavefront Phenomenon of Ischemic Cell Death. I. Myocardial Infarct Size vs. Duration of Coronary Occlusion in Dogs, Circulation, 56:786, 1977. Used with permission.*)

ping,[22,23] but no significant effect was seen on enzyme curves.[23] Intravenous nitroglycerin was reported to decrease the mortality rate of patients with heart failure,[17] and in another report it decreased the hospital mortality rate of patients with acute infarction.[24]

Hyaluronidase

Hyaluronidase has been shown to reduce myocardial infarction size as assessed by QRS precordial mapping studies.[25] Unlike beta blockade or nitroglycerin, hy-

aluronidase has no hemodynamic effect. This agent, along with propranolol, is currently being investigated in a multicenter investigation of the limitation of infarct size.

Glucose-Insulin-Potassium Infusion

Glucose, insulin, and potassium infusions require careful monitoring of blood chemistry. This therapy produces favorable effects on acute hemodynamics and improves ejection fraction.[26] Randomized trials have not shown a favorable effect on mortality rate or a reduction in infarct size as assessed by CK enzyme curves.[27]

Corticosteroid

Corticosteroid therapy was reported to decrease the hospital mortality rate of patients with acute infarction.[28] This effect could not be shown in a smaller randomized trial.[29] There is some evidence that corticosteroid therapy may be harmful,[30] particularly if it is used for a long period of time.[31]

Intraaortic Balloon Counterpulsation

Intraaortic balloon counterpulsation, while not strictly a medical therapy, offers an important theoretical advantage. Afterload reduction with nitroglycerin decreases myocardial work and oxygen consumption. But perfusion pressure of the coronary arteries and other vascular beds has to be maintained. Intraaortic balloon counterpulsation increases diastolic pressure in a short time interval without increasing end-diastolic aortic pressure. By increasing diastolic pressure it should increase antegrade flow to the infarct area if the vessel is severely stenosed without total occlusion. If total occlusion is present, increasing diastolic pressure may increase collateral flow to the border zones of the evolving infarction.

Despite these theoretical advantages, O'Rourke and associates were unable to show a decrease in infarction size in a randomized trial of patients with acute infarction heart failure.[32] Unfortunately, counterpulsation was not begun until a mean of 7.1 h following the onset of symptoms. In a small nonrandomized study, a favorable effect was observed on ST-segment elevation in anterior myocardial infarction if the left anterior descending artery was patent.[33] The known peripheral vascular complications associated with intraaortic balloon counterpulsation prohibits the widespread use of this technique.[34]

Other Agents

Oxygen has been shown to reduce precordial ST-segment elevation, but there are no data showing that this therapy can reduce infarct size in human beings.[35] Nonsteroidal anti-inflammatory agents, such as ibuprofen,[36] can reduce infarct size in animals as determined by postmortem studies, but no human data are available.

Other drugs, especially calcium-channel blockers[37–39] and prostaglandins,[40,41] are undergoing preliminary animal investigation. Human data are available on intravenous verapamil,[42] which has been shown to decrease ST-segment elevation in anterior infarction. In addition to a primary effect on infarct size, calcium antagonists may be useful in reducing any calcium injury associated with reperfusion. An encouraging preliminary report indicates that prostacyclin,[43] infused directly into the coronary artery, may open the vessel with or without prior urokinase.

Coronary sinus retroperfusion is an imaginative approach that has been shown to decrease infarct size in dogs with[44] or without[40] prostaglandin E_1 infusion. Retroperfusion with arterial blood in dogs can preserve myocardial contractility. Retroperfusion may be a more effective method of giving streptokinase since this method lysed coronary thrombi in dogs faster than the systemic infusion of the drug.[45]

Surgical Revascularization

Emergency surgical revascularization has been performed with an acceptable morbidity and mortality rate. Hospital mortality rate was less when the operation was performed soon after the onset of symptoms. Mortality rate was 3.1 percent in a group of patients operated on in less than 6 h, whereas those patients who were operated on after 6 h had a mortality rate of 7.7 percent.[46] The Spokane series showed favorable effects on mortality rate in surgically treated patients compared to medically treated controls, but patient selection is a problem since all patients did not undergo emergency surgery.[47] Phillips, in another uncontrolled study, showed emergency bypass surgery improved ejection fraction when the measurement made prebypass was compared to the measurement made at discharge.[48] This suggests that myocardial salvage occurred, since coronary bypass surgery usually has no effect on the ejection fraction at rest.[49] Favorable effect might be achieved, but it is extremely difficult to mobilize an entire catheterization and cardiac surgical team, perform the necessary procedures, and perform bypass surgery within 6 h. Early surgery may even reverse the infarction process completely if done within 2 h after the onset of the occlusion process as demonstrated by the favorable result of emergency coronary bypass surgery after coronary transluminal angioplasty. After 6 h the value of coronary artery bypass surgery is questionable.[50]

Conclusions

The purpose of this brief review of myocardial preservation data is to give the reader some insight concerning the various means of myocardial salvage. With these data in mind, it will be possible to review the published data on streptokinase. In summarizing the data on limitation of infarct size Rude, Muller, and Braunwald stated ''despite more than a decade of intense experimental and clinical research on interventions for limiting size of myocardial infarcts, no treatment was proven sufficiently efficacious that its routine use can be recommended.''[51]

THE PATHOPHYSIOLOGY OF MYOCARDIAL INFARCTION

Myocardial infarction is a dynamic event associated in many cases with coronary thrombosis. The thrombus is usually associated with severe underlying atherosclerosis but can also occur with trivial underlying disease. The atheromatous plaque associated with acute myocardial infarction is usually complicated by rupture, ulceration, or subintimal hemorrhage. The lumen of the coronary artery associated with such a lesion often shows a thrombus with varying degrees of recanalization.[52–55] Postmortem angiograms show these lesions to have irregular borders and intracoronary lucencies.[56] These complex lesions are the lesions most likely to be associated with a coronary thrombosis and acute myocardial infarction. Earlier investigators suggested that thrombosis was late and secondary to the infarction and decreased flow.[52,57] New cardiac catheterization data of acute infarction make such a hypothesis untenable. Coronary thrombosis is more likely secondary to acute or subacute changes in the lesion such as plaque rupture or coronary artery spasm.[58,59] The thrombus once formed initiates and/or perpetuates the ischemic injury until it undergoes lysis or is incorporated into the atherosclerotic process. If the clot lyses early, then an incomplete infarction occurs, but the artery is subject to rethrombosis with further ischemic injury.

The incidence of occlusion in the coronary artery supplying the infarcting area is higher early in the infarction than it is later.[60,61] This suggests that spontaneous lysis of clot or relief of coronary spasm may occur. When the arteriogram shows total occlusion, it is impossible to definitively distinguish coronary spasm, occluding plaque, and occluding thrombus. However, in many cases a filling defect that stains with dye suggests the presence of a thrombus. Thrombosis was identified by angiography in 70 percent of a series of 225 patients with acute infarction.[60] Coronary spasm with or without thrombosis may also be responsible for acute myocardial infarctions since intracoronary nitroglycerin relieves the total occlusion in some patients.[62]

While the role of thrombosis in the instigation of an infarction is not known, its role in the perpetuation of the infarction is clearer. The dissolution of the thrombus by intracoronary streptokinase is often associated with the dramatic relief of chest pain and restoration of hemodynamic stability.

THE HISTORICAL ASPECTS OF STREPTOKINASE THERAPY

Tillett and Garner discovered in 1933 that a filtrate of streptococci exhibited fibrinolytic activity.[63] The first human application of streptokinase was in 1949 when the investigators used it to liquefy a bloody pleural effusion, thus permitting proper drainage.[64] Johnson and McCarty performed the first intravascular thrombolysis by using the forearms of volunteers; they reported their results in 1959.[65]

Since coronary thrombosis is often associated with myocardial infarction, it seemed wise to investigate the use of thrombolytic therapy in such patients. Sherry and colleagues performed the first intravenous trial of streptokinase for acute infarction and published their results in 1958.[66] Even at that date it was realized that the technique might be beneficial if it could be applied early. The first intracoronary injection of streptokinase was reported in 1960.[67] The patient had an acute inferior infarction. Using a brachial approach the catheter was advanced to the right coronary cusp, and right cusp injections were performed. The results of these early studies are difficult to assess since the injection was performed before coronary angiography was available to the investigators.

American research then shifted from streptokinase to urokinase when the pharmaceutical house could not produce sufficiently pure compounds to meet our Federal Food and Drug Administration requirement. While American thrombolytic research shifted to pulmonary embolism, European drug companies produced enough purified streptokinase for several randomized trials [69–76] of streptokinase in acute myocardial infarc-

tion. Recent reanalysis of the data from these trials shows that intravenous streptokinase reduced the mortality of acute infarction by 20 percent.[77] Even though such a reduction is significant, it is hardly dramatic.

Galiano et al. were the first to do recanalization of a thrombus with a guide wire.[77a] Rentrop also used the guide wire to recanalize an acute occlusion occurring during streptokinase treatment.[79,80] Later, streptokinase following nitroglycerin was used for recanalization only.[81]

METHODS OF STREPTOKINASE THERAPY

Patient selection for streptokinase is as follows: Most investigators require the presence of chest pain associated with ST-segment elevation unrelieved by nitroglycerin as markers of early infarction. Some investigators[81,86] require that Q waves be absent in the leads with ST-segment elevations. Usual exclusion criteria are streptokinase allergy, recent cerebral vascular accident (because of the danger of changing a pale infarction into a hemorrhagic infarction), recent surgery, and abnormal coagulation. Patients are also excluded if they arrived at the hospital more than a certain period after the onset of chest pain. The period for exclusion ranges from 3 h[85] to 18 h.[84] Patients were excluded by some investigators if they were older than a certain arbitrary age such as 70 to 75 years.

Premedication is variable, but *most* workers give corticosteroids intravenously to avoid a pyrogenic reaction to streptokinase; 100 mg of hydrocortisone[83] or 1 g of methylprednisolone[84] may be used. If study purposes require assessment of LV function, ventriculography can be performed before initiation of therapy. However, some investigators[86] caution against ventriculography prior to arterial visualization and stabilization of the patient with successful thrombolysis because they experienced a death following initial ventriculography in a patient with severe three-vessel disease.[86] Certainly, injections of more than usual amounts of contrast material should be avoided if the patient is hemodynamically compromised.[87]

Several methods have been described for infusing streptokinase into the coronary artery. Ganz and colleagues[85] have advocated subselective infusion through a no. 2 French catheter just proximal to the total occlusion. Guide wire penetration of the clot has been initially used.[80] Others tried that and abandoned it.[88] Recently, balloon dilatation catheters are used for subselective streptokinase infusion, which permits the combination of both streptokinase infusion and angioplasty.[89] Others using this technique have increased their primary success rate with streptokinase from 68 percent to 89 percent,[90] but caution is advised, because introducing and using the dilatation catheter adds a certain risk, e.g., proximal dissection or penetration of the artery. The procedure might make the patient worse rather than better. The obstructed artery responsible for acute infarction is extremely reactive, and acute reclosure may happen even after successful angioplasty and thrombolysis.[91]

Nitroglycerin (100 to 450 μg) is usually given into the affected artery to make sure that spasm is not the cause for ongoing infarction. Remarkable enough, some artery will open up and the infarction reversed with this technique only. This occurs in less than 30 percent of the patients.[62] Others report only 7 percent of success with nitroglycerin.[92] After administration of nitroglycerin, a bolus infusion of approximately 10,000 to 50,000 U of streptokinase is given by most investigators[94] and then a continuous infusion of 2,000 to 4,000 U of streptokinase per minute is instituted.

Although most investigators use streptokinase, Ganz and colleagues[96] use thrombolysin (a combination of streptokinase and plasminogen). Mathey et al.[97] infuse 500 mg of plasminogen prior to streptokinase infusion.

The infusion is usually interrupted at 15-min intervals for repeat coronary arteriography to check on the success of the infusion. The coronary artery is also visualized if the patient's chest pain or electrocardiogram show sudden improvement. After 90 min to 2 h, if no reperfusion is obtained, the procedure is usually abandoned as a failure. In patients in whom the artery opens, the infusion is continued for an additional period, usually 30 min, at the same or reduced rate of infusion in order to decrease the chance of reocclusion. Occasionally further infusion will reduce the residual stenosis.[98]

After completion of the infusion, coronary angiogram and ventriculography are usually repeated.

When thrombolysis is successful, efforts are made to prevent reocclusion. For instance, aspirin (325 mg) is given orally,[86] or 1 g is given intravenously[88] by some groups prior to using streptokinase. In addition, heparin is given after the procedure, usually by intravenous infusion at 800 to 1,200 U/h. Most groups begin heparin after the partial thromboplastin time has fallen to less than twice normal and the arterial sheaths have been removed. Clinical follow-up data by Merx and colleagues suggest that early and full-dose heparin is the best mode of therapy to prevent reocclusion.[99] This is followed by oral anticoagulation or aspirin with or without dipyridamole.

After streptokinase therapy one must decide if the residual stenosis should be treated with dilatation or bypass surgery, or if medical therapy should be continued.

PHARMACOLOGY OF STREPTOKINASE

Streptokinase is derived from the purified filtrate of streptococcus cultures, and urokinase is derived from either human urine or from tissue cultures of human embryonic kidney cells.[100] Both act by activating the body's own lytic system. Urokinase directly activates plasminogen to plasmin while streptokinase must first form a complex with plasminogen. Plasmin will lyse fibrin and circulating fibrinogen. Fortunately, plasmin inhibitor concentration in the bloodstream is high, and plasmin inhibitor concentration in clots is low.[101]

As a foreign protein streptokinase is antigenic; therefore a loading dose may be useful to overcome antibodies.[95] Since neutralizing antibody titers are high and a pyrogenic reaction likely, streptokinase should be used no more often than once every 6 months.

EVIDENCE FOR EFFECTIVENESS
Mortality Rate

The most important variable, improved survival rate, is the easiest to measure. In the dog, if reperfusion occurs within 3 h, the 1-week survival is improved.[4]

In the Hoechst-Roussel registry of United States patients, where death was defined as any cardiac death up to day 28, 2.5 percent died in the group of patients who were successfully reperfused, and 18 percent died in the group in which reperfusion could not be achieved.[94] In another combined study of 204 patients from four West German centers, the cardiac death rate was 24 percent in the unsuccessful and 5.4 percent in the group of patients in whom successful recanalization occurred.[99] These differences were statistically significant in both the Hoechst-Roussel and the German registry. Both studies had a higher percentage of patients with major pump dysfunction and cardiac shock in the nonperfused group. Does the shock state and pump dysfunction interfere with the effectiveness of the streptokinase infusion, or does failure to open the artery prevent the myocardial salvage necessary to allow the patient to survive? Anecdotal evidence would suggest the latter, since establishment of reperfusion will often reverse the shock state.[97]

Although these studies may prove that patients whose arteries have been opened by streptokinase have a better rate of survival than those who do not, they do not prove that streptokinase is better than conventional therapy. Hopefully also, the patients who are streptokinase failures are not made worse by emergency catheterization and contrast agent infusions with their negative inotropic effects.

Comparison of mortality rates in these studies to routine medical therapy for myocardial infarction is difficult. Medically treated patients are stratified by a variety of prognostic variables: age of patient, location of infarction, blood pressure, and degree of heart failure, if present.[102,103] Mortality rate varies from 5 to 7 percent without heart failure to 60 to 80 percent with cardiogenic shock. DeWood[50] reported an inhospital mortality rate of 11.5 percent in 1978 using modern medical management. In a preliminary report, Weinstein et al.[104] compared the mortality rate of 23 successfully treated streptokinase patients with initial ejection fractions less than 35 percent with 28 coronary care unit patients with a similar low ejection fraction. While the difference in mortality rates was in favor of the successfully treated streptokinase patient, 4.3 percent versus 39.3 percent,[104] the study was not randomized and did not include the patients with low ejection fractions who failed with streptokinase. Nonetheless if one does open the artery of a patient with low ejection fraction, the prognosis may well be improved.

In a recent update of the data from the Intracoronary Streptokinase Registry of the European Society of Cardiology, the hospital mortality rate in streptokinase-treated patients was 11 percent. The mortality rate with a subtotal lesion was 9.6 percent, with a recanalized lesion, 7.6 percent, and when streptokinase failed to open the artery, 21 percent.[105] Therefore, although opening the artery appears to be associated with a better prognosis, the overall effect of this treatment on hospital mortality rate remains to be determined.

Ejection Fraction

Much of the published data on ejection fraction is summarized in Table 1.[84,86,97,105–109] Since the ejection fraction has been shown to be an important variable in determining the survival rate of patients following myocardial infarction,[6] it would logically follow that if the ejection fraction can be preserved, then long-term survival rate should be improved. But measuring the ejection fraction by invasive or noninvasive means requires time, which interferes with the treatment itself and with the final result. With acute interventions in myocardial infarction, an investigator cannot hope to simultaneously accurately measure the effect of what he or she is doing and still have time to do it. If one takes time to make the fine adjustments necessary to keep the method of measurement beyond criticism, one has probably spent too much time and the brief window of time during which any intervention would be of value has passed. Left ventricular ejection fraction is influenced by a variety of variables, including

the inotropic state, ventricular preload, and afterload. It is difficult to control these variables, making it difficult to compare the results of an acute study with the results of a chronic study. Since it is difficult to control these variables, there is a great variability in the results obtained in the acute state and chronic state. One study of conventionally treated infarctions showed that in about one-third of infarctions the ejection fraction improves, in one-third there is no change, and in one-third the ejection fraction deteriorates.[110] The ejection fraction fell as much as 14 percent and increased as much as 32 percent. Studying a group of first-time myocardial infarction patients treated in a conventional manner, Reduto et al. found that, on the average, left ventricular ejection fraction did not change from the acute study period to the chronic study period.[111]

The published data to date suggest the following conclusions: In large groups of patients, a small but significant improvement in ejection fraction will be detected when the measurement made during the acute study period is compared to the measurement made during the chronic study period. No significant improvement in overall ejection fraction can be expected if ejection fraction is greater than 50 percent; in groups of patients with ejection fraction less than 50 percent, successful lysis can be expected to improve overall ejection fraction, and improvement in regional myocardial wall motion is expected when comparing successful with unsuccessful thrombolysis.

The largest group of patients in whom acute and chronic ejection fractions have been measured is the 149 patients in the European Intracoronary Streptokinase Study. In the total group of patients the ejection fraction improved a modest but significant 2.3 percent after successful thrombolysis.[112] This study also showed significant inverse relationship between the initial ejection fraction and change in ejection fraction. Thus the most improvement occurs in the patients whose initial ejection fraction was poor; precisely the people who would need help the most. Twenty-three patients with ejection fractions less than 35 percent (mean 28.8 percent) had successful coronary thrombolysis. In the follow-up data, available in only 18, ejection fraction improved to 38 percent.[94]

Several investigators have demonstrated improvements in regional ejection fraction even when improvements in overall ejection fraction could not be demonstrated.[113–115] This effect might be due to the hyperkinesia of unaffected segments during the infarction prior to reperfusion. These hyperkinetic segments are able to compensate for the decrease in contractility in the ischemic and infarcting segment. Thus overall ejection fraction may be normal if the infarct is small while regional wall motion is severely hypokinetic. When the patients are studied at the time of discharge, if myocardial reperfusion has been successful, contrac-

TABLE 1
Ejection fraction studies comparing results of streptokinase infusion with controls*

Investigator	Number of patients reperfused	Ejection fraction pre	Ejection fraction post	Signifi-cance (p)	Type control	Number of patients in control	Control pre	Control post	Signifi-cance in control (p)	Significance comparing control to (p)	Time between deter-minations	EF Method
Mathey et al.[97]	11	37 ± 5†	47 ± 4†	<.0025	None	—	—	—	—	—	Late hosp.	Angiogram
Cowley et al.[105]	8	42 ± 5†	52 ± 5†	<.01	U	3	45 ± 8	30 ± 6	—	<.001	Late hosp.	Angiogram
Reduto[84]	18	45 ± 15‡	55 ± 7‡	<.007	CCU	10	47 ± 14	49 ± 16	ns	—	10 days	Radionuclide
					U	14	51 ± 15	52 ± 18	ns			
Smalling[86]	65	40 ± 14‡	48 ± 13‡	<.001	U	24	47 ± 17	47 ± 18	ns	—	10 days	Radionuclide
					CCU	30	41 ± 14	42 ± 14	ns			
Leiboff[106]	11	40 ± 9‡	58 ± 8‡	ns	U	8	41 ± 16	37 ± 11	ns	—	Study day	Unknown
Rentrop[107]	13	51 ± 10‡	57 ± 13‡	<.01	NA	18	52 ± 6	43 ± 8	<.02	<.05	25 ± 13	Angiogram
Shah[108]	13	47 ± 7‡	55 ± 14‡	<.05	CCU	12	39 ± 13	43 ± 19	—	—	96 ± 68 days	Angiogram
Walton[109]	12	50 ± 13‡	52 ± 13‡	ns	Placebo	18	49 ± 15	50 ± 13	ns	—	8–20 days	Radionuclide

*CCU = coronary care unit; U = unsuccessful; NA = nonattempted performed prior to use of SK; ns = not significant.

† ± Standard error of the mean.

‡ ± Standard deviation.

tility in the previously ischemic and infarcting segments may be improved, the stimulus to hyperkinesia in the nonischemic segments may be gone, and all segments may contract normally. Overall ejection fraction is still normal, but regional wall motion has changed. For this reason streptokinase infusion, even if successful, does not usually improve overall ejection fraction if the infarction is small. Thus, regional ejection fraction rather than overall ejection fraction appears to be the most sensitive index of reperfusion efficacy.

Rentrop et al.[116] reviewed their data and raised the possibility that there would be an interval of time during which reperfusion might be harmful. Patients who were reperfused at 3 to 6 h after onset of symptoms demonstrated no change in ejection fraction whereas patients reperfused before 3 h or after 6 h showed a rise in ejection fraction at the time of restudy. Although patients' demonstrating a fall in ejection fraction after successful streptokinase is disturbing, it must be remembered that the significance of a change in ejection fraction from the acute to the chronic study period after myocardial infarction is difficult to interpret. There is no good evidence that reperfusion increases infarct size (see below).

Three preliminary reports were recently published on randomized trials of streptokinase and its effect on the ejection fraction.[106,109,117] Two studies of 27 and 30 patients show no significant improvement in ejection fraction following the use of streptokinase. One study of 41 patients showed a significant rise in global ejection fraction compared to a conventionally treated control group.[118]

Although one randomized study did not show improved regional ejection fraction,[109] it showed a trend for improvement in streptokinase-treated patients. This group measured ejection fraction immediately following thrombolysis. A preliminary report by Gangadharan et al. showed left ventricular function requires 2 h for full recovery.[119]

One must conclude that the effect of streptokinase therapy on the ejection fraction has not been determined with absolute certainty.

Thallium

Thallium-201 scintigraphy has been used by several investigators to assess the efficacy of reperfusion.[84,120–125] All studies show an increase in thallium uptake in patients with successful reperfusion. Reduction in the thallium perfusion defect size immediately following reperfusion was predictive[121,125] of an improved late result, but failure to show a reduction of perfusion defect acutely did not exclude an improved late result.[121] Although thallium images can be difficult to quantify, particularly with intracoronary injections

where dosage is not proportional to flow, Schofer et al.[124] found that early thallium uptake predicted a good late functional result.

Combined intracoronary thallium-201 and technetium-99m pyrophosphate imaging[123,124] shows the complementary nature of these two techniques. Especially in subendocardial necrosis, thallium perfusion of the reperfused subepicardium may obscure the injury defect in the subendocardium. Schofer et al.[124] were able to show that the small thallium defects and small technetium pyrophosphate images correlated with the greatest improvement in regional ejection fraction.

A preliminary report of a randomized study[122] showed that reperfused patients showed a significant increase in the uptake of thallium compared to control patients treated conventionally. "Considerable overlap," however, existed. Interpretation of thallium data is complicated by the changing size of the defect in patients studied early after receiving conventional therapy.[126,127] Small infarctions are especially likely to show a reduction in defect size.[128] Intravenous nitroglycerin has also been shown to enhance the reduction of myocardial infarct size especially in small infarctions when assessed by thallium-201 imaging.[19,20]

Although the vast preponderance of thallium data suggests that infarct size can be reduced by successful early reperfusion, the variability of this method in assessing infarct size acutely makes randomized trials essential.

Relief of Chest Pain

Those involved with streptokinase therapy are impressed with the usual but not inevitable relief of chest pain that accompanies opening of the coronary obstruction. Some argue that this merely represents acceleration of the infarction.[129] This seems unlikely since the relief of chest pain is usually paralleled by sudden clinical improvement (e.g., reversal of shock, etc.) Chest pain relief has been documented by decreased morphine requirements in a randomized study where a streptokinase-treated group of patients was compared to a conventionally treated group of patients.[117]

ECG Evidence

Electrocardiographic precordial mapping using QRS voltage has been employed in studies to demonstrate the efficacy of hyaluronidase[25] and nitroglycerin[23] in limiting infarct size. Precordial ST-segment mapping has been used to show the efficacy of oxygen,[35] propranolol,[12] and nitroglycerin.[17] In none of these interventions, however, is the ST-segment shift as dramatic as it is with streptokinase therapy.[85] Reocclusion results in repeat ST-segment elevation. While the development of Q waves often accompanies the return of the ST segment to the isoelectric level, this probably does not mean an extension of injury but rather a more rapid progression in electrocardiographic infarct evolution. In a randomized trial using intracoronary streptokinase versus standard therapy, the streptokinase-treated group of patients had greater R wave loss at 6 h but less R wave loss at 10 days.[117] Other studies[99,130,131] also showed myocardial salvage by QRS mapping in anterior myocardial infarction, but another study did not show a similar benefit in inferior myocardial infarction.[99]

Creatine Kinase Curves

Creatine kinase (CK) curves have been used as evidence to support limitation of infarct size following the use of beta blockers[7–9] and nitroglycerin[18] trials. Most measurements of CK involve a measurement of enzyme activity in vitro. When a myocardial infarction exists without reperfusion, CK reaches the bloodstream via lymphatic channels. This delays the appearance of CK activity in the venous blood. Inactivation of CK in the lymph[132] results in a lower measurable CK activity in the venous blood. In reperfused infarcts, the CK appears earlier, and a higher percentage is in the active form (see Fig. 2).[133–135] This phenomenon is the so-called early washout of CK. Thus, traditional CK curves will overestimate a reperfused infarct size. The kinetics of CK disappearance after reperfusion are similar to the kinetics of an intravenous bolus injection of the enzyme.[136]

Blanke and colleagues[137] derived a linear relationship between CK curves and akinetic segments found at discharge by biplane ventriculography in 24 routinely treated patients with infarction. When they applied this relationship to 26 infarct patients who were successfully reperfused, the enzymatic prediction of infarct size exceeded the actual angiographic infarct size. However, when a new formula was derived, using only reperfused patients, a linear relationship could again be shown. Thus, while CK curves derived from nonperfused patients will not accurately estimate myocardial infarct size in reperfused patients, CK curves derived from reperfused patients will accurately estimate the infarct size of reperfused patients; the linear relationship is only shifted. Studies using such methods have not yet been reported.

Conclusions about Beneficial Effects of Intracoronary Streptokinase Infusions

No other method of limitation of infarct size has been as extensively evaluated as intracoronary streptokinase. Caution is justified since several methods have been claimed to limit the size of infarction, yet no method is uniformly used today to limit infarct size. Although a rather clear pattern of benefit is emerging for streptokinase infusion, the long-term outlook is not known.

HARMFUL EFFECTS OF STREPTOKINASE THERAPY

A method must show itself not only to be efficacious but also to have low side effects. Three areas of potential harm are associated with streptokinase therapy: (1) bleeding, (2) reperfusion arrhythmias, and (3) injury to viable myocardium. Of these, the first is due to the bleeding diathesis from the drug; the latter two are intrinsic to reperfusion.

Bleeding

Bleeding complications are not trivial. Since successful thrombolysis is followed by continuous heparin therapy (to prevent reocclusion), the cause of bleeding may be the lytic state from streptokinase or the anticoagulation effect from heparin.

By giving brief doses directly into the coronary artery it was hoped that the systemic lytic effect of strep-

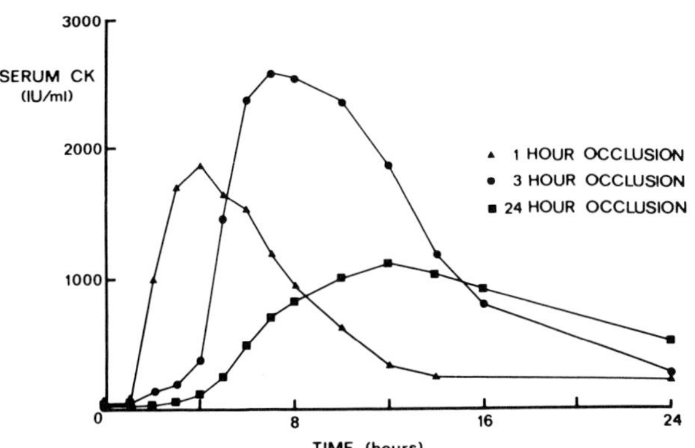

FIGURE 2 The different characteristic shapes of the serial blood CK curves for the three groups are shown by examples obtained from a dog with 24-h occlusion, a dog reperfused at 3 h, and a dog reperfused at 1 h. The rapid rise in CK level in blood is evident after reperfusion. (*From S. F. Vatner, H. Baig, W. T. Manders, and P. R. Maroko, Effects of Coronary Artery Reperfusion on Myocardial Infarct Size Calculated from Creatine Kinase, J. Clin. Invest., 61:1050, 1978. Used with permission.*)

tokinase would be eliminated. Three studies[99,138,139] have shown a significant depression of fibrinogen following usual doses of intracoronary streptokinase.[140] This depression of fibrinogen levels can last for 24 h. In one combined series of 204 patients,[99] bleeding occurred in 13 patients (6 percent). Six patients had groin site hematomas, one of which required surgical repair. Retroperitoneal hemorrhage occurred in two patients. Gastrointestinal bleeding requiring transfusion occurred in five patients, and one of these required surgery. Death from intracerebral hemorrhage is reported although the details are not published.[141] We have had one death from cerebral hemorrhage following combined coronary angioplasty and intracoronary streptokinase to a total dose of 240,000 IU. At this time the incidence of death from bleeding complications cannot be derived. In the most recently published trial of systemic (intravenous) streptokinase for acute infarction, the European Cooperative Study Group reported no deaths due to bleeding. Nonfatal intracerebral hemorrhage occurred in 2 of the 156 patients in the treatment group.[77] The fibrinogen level at its 24-h nadir following the use of intravenous streptokinase averaged 57 mg/dL;[77] in one trial using intracoronary streptokinase[139] the mean nadir of the fibrinogen level occurred at 6 h and was 54 mg/dL.[139] Significantly, in the trials with systemic streptokinase, anticoagulation was achieved with warfarin, which was given on admission and in the intracoronary streptokinase trials; heparin was given before and often within hours of the completion of successful lysis. Effective anticoagulation combined with low fibrinogen levels may increase the risk of serious hemorrhagic complications. Increased bleeding complications have been associated with the use of the Judkins technique, decline of fibrinogen level to less than 100 mg/dL, and streptokinase dosage greater than 200,000 IU.[99]

Because of these serious bleeding complications, the use of intracoronary streptokinase should be confined to randomized controlled clinical trials until definite proof of the effectiveness of the method has been shown.

Reperfusion Arrhythmias

In animals, ventricular fibrillation is most frequent when reperfusion occurs between 20 and 40 min after occlusion. Reperfusion after shorter or longer periods following coronary occlusion is not likely to induce ventricular fibrillation.[85] The most serious arrhythmia associated with reperfusion in human beings is bradycardia associated with inferior infarction reperfusion.[93] This idioventricular rhythm is often accompanied by hypotension.[86] Ventricular tachycardia or fibrillation occurred in 22 percent and some form of arrhythmia in 39 percent of one series of 72 reperfused patients.[83]

Increased automaticity and reentry may be important in the genesis of reperfusion arrhythmias.[142,143] Recent data suggest these arrhythmias may be due to increased alpha-adrenergic responsiveness[144] since in cats reperfusion arrhythmias can be prevented by high-dose alpha blockade.[145] More practically, it has recently been shown in dogs that reperfusion arrhythmias can be controlled with the local (intracoronary) infusion of phentolamine.[146] By using small local doses no systemic effects are seen. These new animal data need to be confirmed in humans.

Serious arrhythmias using the currently available methods of reperfusion do not appear to be an important problem. Infarct patients may be somewhat protected from the severe arrhythmias observed in animals because of the more gradual onset of reperfusion. Response to conventional therapy, except to pacing, is poor, but fortunately the duration of susceptibility to reperfusion arrhythmias is relatively short.[85]

Reperfusion Injury

The question of reperfusion injury has been under investigation since the early 1970s, when emergency bypass surgery was first being performed for acute myocardial infarction. Observations of deterioration in left ventricular function following bypass surgery lead to the postulation of hemorrhagic, postreperfusion injury. Montoya et al.[147] claimed that this would occur in patients with infarction who were operated on after 5 h. Balooki et al.[148] claimed that hemorrhagic infarction would occur in patients operated on 4 h after the onset of chest pain. Although hemorrhagic infarction was demonstrated in postmortem studies accompanying these surgical observations, no evidence was presented that hemorrhage itself was the cause of injury rather than the ischemic arrest of the heart during surgery.

Pathologists looking at patients dying following bypass surgery have observed subendocardial contraction band necrosis in areas supplied by patent bypass grafts.[149] Since contraction band necrosis is associated with reperfusion injury, the suggestion is that the reperfusion per se may have caused or aggravated the myocardial injury. Such injury is most likely due to ischemic injury during cardiac arrest or inadequate cardioplegia. Indeed widespread hemorrhagic subendocardial necrosis occurred in one-third of patients dying after valve surgery prior to the use of cardioplegia.[150]

It appears from rather extensive animal data that reperfusion injury is confined to areas where vascular injury has occurred and that the area of vascular injury is contained within a larger area of irreversible myocardial injury.

Experimental infarction in dogs proceeds in a wavefront manner from the subendocardium to the subepicardium. The longer the period of ischemia, the more likely that the infarction will be transmural. Reperfusion was associated with hemorrhage in this model, but the hemorrhagic zone was always contained in the zone of necrosis. Bresnahan et al. postulated that reperfusion in the close-chested dog model caused increased infarct size since 9 of 16 animals reperfused at 5 h had larger myocardial infarctions than were predicted from creatine kinase curves.[151] When myocardial biopsy showed increased hemoglobin content, it was presumed that reperfusion injury was responsible. Subsequent studies[133–135] have shown that conventional creatine kinase curves may overestimate infarct size by as much as two- to threefold when reperfusion occurs following coronary occlusion. The higher creatine kinase curve may be due to the washout phenomenon described earlier.

Several studies have failed to show a harmful effect of hemorrhagic infarction. Kloner and colleagues[152] have shown that damage to the ultrastructure of myocardial cells always precedes ultrastructure evidence of microvascular injury. The size of myocardial hemorrhage does not appear to be affected by giving intracoronary streptokinase following reperfusion,[154] further confirming that the hemorrhage is a consequence of microvascular injury and is not in itself harmful. Since myocardial injury antedates vascular injury, the only areas involved with hemorrhage are areas that are destined to die. Areas with intact vascular networks and ischemic but viable myocardium may be rescued by early reperfusion.[153] Hemorrhage, rather than being harmful, may actually benefit healing by accelerating the proliferation of granulation tissue[154a] and increasing the stiffness of the infarct region, leading to an early improvement in ejection fraction and decreasing the risk of subsequent aneurysm formation.[154a,155]

Thus, animal studies do not support the hypothesis that hemorrhagic infarction is harmful because the hemorrhage is always confined to areas of irreversibly damaged myocardial cells. But what about humans? One autopsy report on five patients who died from cardiac shock despite successful reperfusion showed hemorrhagic infarction in three patients. In each of these patients, the hemorrhage was confined to the area of necrosis.[156]

FACTORS WHICH INFLUENCE THE SUCCESS OF STREPTOKINASE THERAPY

The primary success rate using streptokinase infusion is about 75 percent. Unlike coronary angioplasty where primary success rate is clearly related to operator experience, there is not such a clear relationship with streptokinase (Table 2). This may in part be due to the fact that infusion from a coronary catheter does not require special skill beyond that needed for diagnostic studies. Therefore, unless one attempts mechanical recanalization or subselective infusion, the skills required are essentially the same as those for routine cardiac catheterization. If angioplasty and streptokinase infusion become a combined procedure, then operator skill will become more of a factor.

Although the loading dose of streptokinase and infusion rate vary (Table 1), no clear advantage is apparent for any infusion technique. The use of subselective infusion has not been shown to be clearly advantageous. One group which has used both methods saw no advantage to the subselective approach.[86]

Thrombolysin, a combination of streptokinase and plasminogen, is said by Ganz et al.[96] to be more effective, particularly in patients in whom arterial flow is slow. The investigators in Hamburg inject 500 U of human plasminogen prior to infusion of streptokinase.[97] The number of patients reported from individual centers is too small to evaluate the addition of plasminogen. Plasminogen level in the serum is usually elevated in acute myocardial infarction;[101] it is unlikely that the addition of plasminogen is of value.[68]

Urokinase[157] was shown to be equally effective as streptokinase in a double-blind randomized study at Vanderbilt; however, the primary success rate for streptokinase (47 percent) was rather low. Urokinase has the theoretical advantage of no antigenicity and thus no antibody inactivation and can be used frequently without pyrogenic reaction. Urokinase on a unit for unit basis cost (in 1982) more than six times as much as streptokinase.[101] Experience is still too limited to evaluate accurately the relative efficacy of urokinase and streptokinase in coronary thrombolysis. The two drugs are thought to be equally effective in treating peripheral artery thrombosis.[101]

Lee et al. related the duration of symptoms prior to streptokinase to the time required for successful lysis. In this study, the longer the duration of symptoms prior to the initiation of streptokinase, the longer the time required for successful lysis.[158] Data from a larger series do not confirm this observation.[86] In the pooled data from the Hoechst-Roussel registry, patients presenting less than 3 h following the onset of symptoms had a 85 percent chance of successful lysis, while patients presenting more than 9 h after the onset of symptoms had only a 70 percent chance of success.

A lower incidence of primary success occurs when the occlusion is in the circumflex artery (Table 3).[99] A combined study of four German centers attempted a guide wire recanalization of the circumflex artery but subselective infusion was not used.[159] The investigators considered their lack of success and increased incidence of reocclusion to be due to inability to deliver

TABLE 2
Table of primary success rate of streptokinase therapy

Medical center	Number of patients	Mean time to entry	Mean dosage (U)	Reperfused (%)	Reference
Medical College of Virginia	20	4.8	184,000	90	94
Boston Beth Israel Hospital	22	3.5	286,000	75	94
University of California, Davis	24	4.6	243,000	77	94
St. Louis University	12	3.1	195,000	42	94
University of Texas	65	7.1	104,000	66	94
Beaumont Hospital	66	2.6	211,000	88	94
Cedars-Sinai, Los Angeles	20	2.7	———	95	96
University Hospital Eppendorf, Hamburg	41	1.2	———	73	97
University Hospital Goettingen	29	———	———	76	88
Massachusetts General, Boston	25		———	76	187
Vanderbilt (streptokinase)	17	4.9	197,000	47	157
Vanderbilt (urokinase)	22	5.2	495,000	55	157
4 German centers*	204	———	———	63	99
European Cooperative Registry†	331	———	———	76	112

*Aachen, Goettingen, Hamburg, Berlin—note earlier separate reporting of Goettingen and Hamburg.

†Contains patients listed separately.

a sufficient quantity of streptokinase to the thrombus site since most of the streptokinase flowed down the patent left anterior descending artery. If subselective infusions are advantageous, it may be in such patients.

Merx et al.[160] report the difference a small amount of antegrade flow can make in success or failure with thrombolytic therapy. Of 18 patients with no antegrade flow, 5 were unresponsive to streptokinase infusion, whereas of the 15 patients with functionally occluded vessels but slight marginal antegrade flow there were no failures. Moreover, even the successful patients without antegrade flow required longer infusions of streptokinase.

TABLE 3
Primary success rates with different coronary arteries

Artery*	N	Success rate (%)	N	Reocclusion rate (%)
LAD	68	78	46	19
RCA	63	85	22	23
LCX	35	66	51	32

*LAD = left anterior descending; RCA = right coronary artery; LCX = left circumflex.

In summary, no agent or method of infusion has been shown to be superior to other agents or methods. There is not much evidence that operator experience improves the chances for success. Early presentation after the onset of chest pain may make success more likely. Streptokinase infusion into an occluded circumflex artery appears to have a lower success rate as compared to the streptokinase infusion of occlusion of the anterior descending artery and right coronary artery. The presence of even marginal antegrade flow improves primary success.

THERAPY AFTER SUCCESSFUL STREPTOKINASE THERAPY

Unfortunately initial success does not guarantee a good long-term result. The underlying arterial pathology is a ruptured plaque,[141] and there is usually some residual thrombus.[161] These lesions are "active" lesions and are subject to reocclusion with further loss of myocardium or death. Just as the prognosis is different for patients with stable and unstable angina, so the prognosis of patients who have had successful thombolysis will probably be different from that of other subgroups of patients.

Fioretti et al.[162] performed discharge exercise testing in patients who were discharged after successful streptokinase treatment. The findings were a higher incidence of chest pain (41 percent versus 16 percent) and ST-segment depression (61 percent versus 33 percent) in patients who had successful versus unsuccessful thrombolytic therapy. This may signify that heart muscle was salvaged, but it may also indicate that these patients are at greater risk for repeat infarction.

Merx et al.[99] studied 204 patients following streptokinase therapy. Of these patients 128 had occluded vessels and had successful thrombolysis. Twenty-six of these 128 went to bypass surgery, 9 within 1 day, and 17 during the hospitalization. Twenty-five patients reinfarcted; five of these patients died of heart failure in the coronary care unit. Of the 20 other cases of reinfarction, 15 had repeat angiography, and 14 showed reocclusion. While the incidence of reinfarction was not significantly higher in the occluded and recanalized group versus the group with initially occluded artery failing to respond to streptokinase (18.6 percent versus 8.1 percent), there was an alarming trend for patients who had had their vessels opened by streptokinase to reocclude and extend their infarction. This occurred despite anticoagulation with heparin. Two patients died from sudden death in the successfully recanalized group for a total hospital cardiac mortality rate of 5.4 percent. In a similar follow-up study of 34 patients, 4 of 21 patients treated medically suffered reinfarction or death.[163] Despite the difference in number of patients, the incidence of reinfarction is approximately 20 percent in both studies. Among the 32 successful patients reported from Society for Clinical Angiography Registry, 9 of 32 patients (28 percent) reoccluded by day 15.[92] Four out of five patients coming to autopsy had reocclusion at the site of thrombolysis[141]

Meyer et al.[91] studied the clinical course of 21 patients treated with streptokinase followed by percutaneous transluminal coronary angioplasty (PTCA). These 21 patients were compared to a control group of 18 patients suitable for PTCA but treated only with streptokinase. In the control group, 4 of 18 patients experienced reinfarction compared with 2 of 21 patients treated with streptokinase and PTCA. The mortality at 6 months was three deaths in 18 in the control group of 18 and one death in the streptokinase plus angioplasty group of 21. Those treated with combined modalities tended to be in a lower functional class than those treated with only streptokinase. In another group of 48 patients receiving combined treatment of streptokinase followed by coronary artery bypass grafting reinfarction was seen in only 2 of 48 patients (4 percent) although 2 additional patients died suddenly during hospitalization from arrhythmias. Bypass surgery improved left ventricular function as assessed by ventriculography.

In patients operated on less than 1 week after streptokinase therapy, graft occlusion rate to the artery supplying the infarct area was relatively high—17 percent (5 of 29 patients restudied). In patients operated on after 1 week, the graft to the infarct-related vessel was patent in all 13 patients restudied.[159]

Summary

Medical therapy with heparin infusion after successful streptokinase recanalization is associated with approximately 20 percent hospital reinfarction rate. About 25 percent of these reinfarctions will be fatal. Coronary angioplasty or coronary bypass surgery in appropriate patients appears to lower but does not eliminate the risk of reinfarction and death. Bypass graft patency in patients operated on in the first week following infarction and streptokinase therapy may be lower. It is clear that eliminating the thrombus does not eliminate the disease in the artery; these arteries may close from coronary artery spasm or rethrombosis since the nidus for thrombsis—ulcerated or ruptured atherosclerotic plaque—is not eliminated. The high reinfarction rate with its concomitant death rate makes aggressive therapy the best option for suitable patients.[164,165]

THE VALUE OF INTRACORONARY STREPTOKINASE COMPARED TO INTRAVENOUS STREPTOKINASE

Intravenous streptokinase holds two important advantages over intracoronary infusion: earlier application and less equipment and personnel required. Intravenous streptokinase can be given in the emergency room or by ambulance personnel.

The European experience with intravenous streptokinase has been reviewed[166] and analyzed.[77] The basic problem was that streptokinase was used hours after the diagnosis of myocardial infarction was established. Therefore, patients were entered in the study more than 6 h following the onset of chest pain. This delay may well have masked any benefit of the method. Despite this, reanalysis of the data combining several series[72–79] shows a reduction in mortality rate in the streptokinase group. From performing intracoronary streptokinase infusion and observing the effect of reperfusion in animals, it has been learned that the earlier reperfusion is instituted, the more likely successful myocardial salvage will result.

Spann et al.[167] studied 13 patients with angiographic evidence of coronary occlusion and electrocardiographic evidence of acute myocardial infarction. Clot lysis was achieved in six patients (46 percent) by the intravenous use of 850,000 U of streptokinase. Neuhaus[168] found angiographic evidence for arterial opening in 24 of 39 patients (62 percent) using an average intravenous infusion of 1,700,000 U of streptokinase over 60 min. The average time required to open the artery was 48 min.

In 59 patients not studied angiographically but treated within 6 h of the onset of symptoms, Schroeder[169] found 92 percent of these patients had early peaking of their CK curves—a sign of early reperfusion. Since early peaking of the CK enzyme curve has been correlated with decreased thallium defect and improved ejection fraction at discharge,[170] intravenous streptokinase may be even more successful than the angiographic studies indicate. Follow-up and correlative studies are indicated. The earlier intravenous streptokinase is started, the greater the probability of successful thrombolysis. Schroder et al.[169] observed that opening of the coronary artery was accomplished in six of eight patients receiving streptokinase less than 3 h after the onset of symptoms. Only 5 of 13 patients' arteries opened when they received intravenous streptokinase after 3 h.

Remarkably, despite larger total doses of streptokinase, no major bleeding complications were noted in these small series of patients or in a larger series of 85 patients.[169] Neuhaus reported on nine patients treated with an average dose of 1,550,000 U of streptokinase intravenously. Surprisingly, despite a 67 percent success rate, fibrinogen was only depressed to 0.181 ± 0.057 g/L.[171]

Accordingly, while intravenous therapy does not have the theoretical value of selective infusion, with its higher local concentration and possible combination with a mechanical procedure, it can open the artery in about 50 to 60 percent of patients within 1 h. Bleeding complications appear to be no more frequent despite larger doses of streptokinase, but the total number of patients treated is too small to give a final opinion regarding this complication. Despite the lower success rate with this technique, the cost is much less and the potential for widespread usage is much greater.

It would appear as though the primary success rate is lower with the use of intravenous streptokinase compared to the use of intracoronary streptokinase (Table 4). But if earlier application of intravenous streptokinase can improve primary success with the technique, then the difference between the two methods of streptokinase application may be small.

INDICATIONS FOR STREPTOKINASE
Acute Myocardial Infarction

Streptokinase therapy remains an investigational procedure, despite the Federal Food and Drug Administration's approval of streptokinase for intracoronary thrombolytic therapy.

The time that elapses from the onset of symptoms to reperfusion is clearly the important factor in myocardial salvage. Schwarz and colleagues showed that patients reperfused less than 4 h after the onset of symptoms had smaller infarctions as judged by peak creatine kinase and better global and regional wall motion when compared to a control group of patients reperfused after 4 h or to a control group of unreperfused patients. There was little difference between the two control groups.[172] Other groups have shown similar results.[173] If facilities and personnel are available so that there is a chance that reperfusion can be achieved in less than 4 h, then it is reasonable to attempt streptokinase infusion.

In patients who are seen later than 4 h after onset of chest pain, improvement in ejection fraction is dependent upon collateral flow or the presence of a marginal amount of antegrade flow. If either of these is present, the improvement in ejection fraction is more likely than if they are not.[173,174] In experimental infarction reperfusion of a pig after even 1 h of occlusion will not result in an improved ejection fraction or improvement in the electrocardiogram.[175]

In dogs improvement in mortality rate and myocardial salvage can be seen when reperfusion is initi-

TABLE 4
Efficacy of intravenous streptokinase

Institution	Number of patients	Dosage*	Success (%)	Reference
Temple University, Lancaster General	13	850,000 U	46	167
Klinikum der Universität Göttingen	39	1,700,000 U	62	168
Free University, Berlin	22	500,000 U	45	169

*Actual dosage or an average dose; in the Free University study either streptokinase or urokinase was given.

ated at 3 h.[3,4] Some decrease in infarct size may even be present with reperfusion at 6 h.[3] This difference between species is thought to be due to the presence of collateral vessels in the dog and their relative absence in the pig.[176]

Patients with severe underlying atherosclerotic lesions and good collateral vessels may have a longer period of time during which therapy may be successfully applied, but in both groups it is wise to intervene as quickly as possible.

But short of patients having a coronary angiogram within a few weeks prior to their infarction, are there any clinical markers in those patients presenting at 3 h or later that will distinguish a responder from a nonresponder to lytic therapy? Karsch and colleagues[177] found 76 percent of patients with acute infarction and antecedent chest pain within 1 month had collateral vessels, while only 33 percent of patients with infarction and no antecedent chest pain had collaterals. The overlap, however, is so great that this is little help for the clinician.

Randomized studies of patients presenting after 3 h are necessary in order to determine which patients presenting late can be helped.

Streptokinase for Bypass Graft Occlusion

Steptokinase therapy for bypass graft occlusion was first reported in 1980.[182] Subsequent reports[183,184] have shown pericardial hemorrhage and a cardiac tamponade can complicate infusion done within a week after surgery. Thrombolytic therapy within 1 week of surgery should be undertaken only if one is willing to tolerate a 33 percent incidence of pericardial hemorrhage requiring drainage and 10 to 15 percent incidence of tamponade requiring surgical rescue.

Streptokinase in Unstable Angina Pectoris

Unstable angina pectoris often precedes myocardial infarction. Since myocardial infarction is now clearly linked to coronary thrombosis, thrombosis may also be a part of the pathogenesis of unstable angina.[178] In one retrospective study of 129 patients undergoing coronary angiography less than 1 month after the onset of symptoms of unstable angina, 8 (6.2 percent) had angiographic evidence of coronary thrombosis.[179] Wolk et al. treated nine patients with either unstable angina or nontransmural myocardial infarction with intracoronary streptokinase; five of nine patients responded with either an increase of greater than 20 percent diameter or a shrinkage of greater than 2 mm of an in-

traluminal filling defect.[180] Vetrovec and colleagues reported their experience in 13 attempts at thrombolysis in patients with unstable or preinfarction angina.[181] Angiographic change consistent with thrombolysis occurred in 10 of their 13 attempts (77 percent); however, most changes were minor and the clinical importance of these results is yet to be determined.[181] Rentrop reported on six patients with unstable angina treated with intracoronary streptokinase; none showed angiographic evidence of improvement.[88] We have occasionally seen a residual filling defect consistent with the presence of a thrombus following coronary angioplasty. Although we have attempted intracoronary streptokinase infusion in these patients, none has shown any clear evidence of resolution. The thrombus of unstable angina is probably much older than the thrombus of acute myocardial infarction, and an old thrombus is less likely to respond to lytic therapy. Unless there is a recent onset of symptoms (<1 to 2 days), lytic therapy is probably not justified.

CONCLUSIONS AND PERSPECTIVE

Intracoronary streptokinase therapy has generated a great deal of excitement in both clinical and investigational cardiology.[182] Although investigations in human beings are still early and preliminary, lytic therapy seems to demonstrate myocardial salvage by more criteria than any other intervention.

It may be the quality of myocardium saved as well as the quantity. A rim of viable subepicardial muscle may be important in preventing rupture, expansion, aneurysm formation, and interventricular thrombus formation.[185] These complications are generally associated with transmural infarction. The nontransmural nature of infarctions associated with successful streptokinase therapy was documented by surgical observation in 10 patients and myocardial biopsy in 3 patients.[107] Although ischemic tissue immediately after reperfusion takes some time to recover full contractility, it can be made to contract earlier if inotropic drugs are given.[186] Such a combination of therapies may be useful in saving a patient's life in cardiogenic shock. Quality in addition to quantity of myocardium saved may be important and may contribute to the overall numbers of patients helped.

It is apparent that reperfusion must be done quickly and early after the onset of symptoms to be of maximal benefit. The primary success rate of intracoronary streptokinase therapy is about 60 to 80 percent.

Once the clot is lysed and (hopefully) myocardium is saved, the physician's responsibility has not ended. The underlying atherosclerotic disease must be treated to avoid repeat infarction, which occurs in about 20 percent of the patients. Angioplasty, bypass surgery, or vigorous medical therapy are indicated to preserve what has been gained.

REFERENCES

1 Lown, B., Falho, A. M., Hood, W. B., Jr., and Thorn, G. W.: The Coronary Care Unit: Perspectives and Directions, *J.A.M.A.,* 199:188, 1967.

2 DeWood, M. A., Berg, R., Jr., Spores, J., et al.: Medical and Surgical Management of Myocardial Infarction: A Retrospective Study, *Circulation,* 58(suppl. 2):17, 1978.

3 Reimer, K. A., Loew, J. E., Rasmussen, M. M., and Jennings, R. B.: The Wave Front Phenomenon of Ischemic Cell Death. I: Myocardial Infarct Size vs. Duration of Coronary Occlusion in Dogs, *Circulation,* 56:786, 1977.

4 Baughman, K. L., Maroko, P. R., and Vatner, S. F.: Effects of Coronary Artery Reperfusion on Myocardial Infarct Size and Survival in Dogs, *Circulation,* 63:317, 1982.

5 Hurst, J. W., King, S. B., III, Walter, P. F., Friesinger, G. C., and Edwards, J. E.: Atherosclerotic Coronary Artery Disease: Angina Pectoris, Myocardial Infarction and Other Manifestations of Myocardial Ischemia, in J. W. Hurst (editor-in-chief), "The Heart," 5th ed., McGraw-Hill Book Company, New York, 1982, p. 1009.

6 Taylor, G. J., Humphries, J. O., Mellitis, E. D., et al.: Predictors of Clinical Course, Coronary Anatomy and Left Ventricular Function after Recovery from Acute Myocardial Infarction, *Circulation,* 62:960, 1981.

7 Peter, T., Norris, R. M., Clarke, E. D., et al.: Reduction of Enzyme Levels with Propranolol after Acute Myocardial Infarction, *Circulation,* 57:1091, 1978.

8 Yusef, S., Ramsdale, D., Peto, R., et al.: Early Intravenous Atenolol in Suspected Acute Myocardial Infarction: Preliminary Report of a Randomized Trial, *Lancet,* 2:273, 1980.

9 Jurgensen, H. J., Frederiksen, J., Hansen, D. A., and Pedersen-Bjergaardo, O.: Limitation of Infarct Size in Patients Less than 66 Years Treated with Alprenolol, *Br. Heart J.,* 45:583, 1981.

10 Herlitz, J., Hjalmarson, A., Holmberg, S., et al.: Limitation of Infarct Size in Acute Myocardial Infarction with Metroprolol, *Am. J. Cardiol.,* 49:1004, 1982. (Abstract.)

11 Waagstein, F., and Hjalmarson, A. C.: Effect of Cardioselective Beta-Blockage of Heart Function and Chest Pain in Acute Myocardial Infarction, *Acta Med. Scand.* (suppl.), 587:201, 1975.

12 Gold, H. K., Leinbach, R. C., and Maroko, P. R.: Propranolol-induced Reduction of Signs of Ischemic Injury during Acute Myocardial Infarction, *Am. J. Cardiol.,* 38:689, 1976.

13 Barber, J. M., Boyle, D. M., Chaturvedi, N. C., Singh, N., and Walsh, M. J.: Practolol in Acute Myocardial Infarction, *Acta Med. Scand.* (Suppl.), 587:213, 1976.

14 Vik-Mo, H., Maroko, P. R., and Ribeiro, L. G. T.: Comparative Effects of Propranolol, Timolol and Metroprolol after Coronary Occlusion, *Circulation,* 66 (suppl. 2):85, 1982. (Abstract.)

15 Flaherty, J. T., Reid, P. R., Kelly, D. T. et al.: Intravenous Nitroglycerin in Acute Myocardial Infarction, *Circulation,* 51:132, 1975.

16 Bover, J. S., Redwood, D. R., Levitt, B., et al.: Reduction in Myocardial Ischemia with Nitroglycerin or Nitroglycerin plus Phenylephrine Administration during Acute Myocardial Infarction, *N. Engl. J. Med.,* 293:1008, 1975.

17 Chiche, P., Baligadoo, S. J., and Derrida, J. P.: A Randomized Trial of Prolonged Nitroglycerin Infusion in Acute Myocardial Infarction, *Circulation,* 60(suppl. 2):165, 1979. (Abstract.)

18 Bussman, W. D., Pasek, D. S., and Kaltenbach, M.: Reduction of CK and CK-MB Indexes of Infarct Size by Intravenous Nitroglycerin, *Circulation,* 63:615, 1981.

19 Flaherty, J. T., Weisfeldt, M. L., Bulkley, B. H., Kallman, C. H., and Becker, L. C.: Predictors of Patient Response to Intravenous Nitroglycerin Therapy, *Am. J. Cardiol.,* 49:1024, 1982. (Abstract.)

20 Becker, L. C., Bulkley, B. J., Pih, B., et al.: Enhanced Reduction of Thallium-201 Defects in Acute Myocardial Infarction by Nitroglycerin Treatment: Initial Results of a Prospective Randomized Trial, *Clin. Res.,* 26:219A, 1978. (Abstract.)

21 Durm, R. F., Botvinich, E. H., Benge, W., Chatterjee, K., and Parmley, W. W.: The Significance of Nitroglycerin-induced Changes in Ventricular Function after Acute Myocardial Infarction, *Am. J. Cardiol.,* 49:1719, 1982.

22 Awan, N. A., Amsterdam, E. A., Zakuddin, V., et al.: Reduction of Ischemic Injury by Sublingual Nitroglycerin in Patients with Acute Myocardial Infarction, *Circulation,* 54:761, 1976.

23 Kim, Y. I., and William, J. F.: Large Dose Sublingual Nitroglycerin in Acute Myocardial Infarction: Relief of Chest Pain and Reduction of Q Wave Evolution, *Am. J. Cardiol.,* 49:842, 1982.

24 Derrida, J. P., Sal, R., and Cliche, P.: Nitroglycerin Infusion in Acute Myocardial Infarction. Improved Mortality and EKG Criteria for Smaller Infarctions, *N. Engl. J. Med.,* 297:336, 1977.

25 Maroko, P. R., Hillis, L. D., Muller, J. E., et al.: Hyaluronidase Effect on ECG Evidence of Necrosis in Myocardial Infarction, *N. Engl. J. Med.,* 296:898, 1977.

26 Whitlow, P. L., Rogers, W. J., Smith, L. R., et al.:

Enhancement of Left Ventricular Function by Glucose-Insulin-Potassium in Acute Myocardial Infarction, *Am. J. Cardiol.*, 49:811, 1982.

27 Rogers, W. J., Segall, P. H., McDaniel, H. G., et al.: Prospective Randomized Trial of Glucose-Insulin-Potassium in Acute Myocardial Infarction, *Am. J. Cardiol.*, 43:801, 1979.

28 Barzilal, D., Plavnick, J., Hazani, A., et al.: Use of Hydrocortisone in the Treatment of Acute Myocardial Infarction, *Chest,* 61:488, 1972.

29 Madias, J. E., and Hood, W. B.: Effects of Methylprednisolone on the Ischemic Damage in Patients with Acute Myocardial Infarction, *Circulation,* 65:1106, 1982.

30 Roberts, R., deMello, V., and Sobel, B. E.: Deleterious Effects of Methylprednisolone in Patients with Myocardial Infarction, *Circulation,* 53(suppl. 1):204, 1976.

31 Bulkley, B. H., and Roberts, N. C.: Steroid Therapy during Acute Myocardial Infarction, *Am. J. Med.*, 56:244, 1974.

32 O'Rourke, M. F., Norris, R. M., Campbell, T. J., Chang, V. P., and Sammel, N. L.: Randomized Controlled Trial of Intraaortic Balloon Counterpulsation in Early Myocardial Infarction with Acute Heart Failure, *Am. J. Cardiol.*, 47:815, 1981.

33 Leinbach, R. C., Gold, H. K., Harper, R. W., Buckley, M. J., and Austen, W. G.: Early Intraaortic Balloon Pumping for Anterior Myocardial Infarction without Shock, *Circulation,* 58:204, 1978.

34 Scheidt, S.: Preservation of Ischemic Myocardium with Intraaortic Balloon Pumping: Modern Therapeutic Intervention or *primum non nocere?, Circulation,* 58:211, 1978. (Editorial.)

35 Madias, J. E., Madias, N. E., and Hood, W. B., Jr.: Precordial ST Segment Mapping. II. Effects of Oxygen Inhalation on Ischemic Injury in Patients with Acute Myocardial Infarction, *Circulation,* 53:411, 1976.

36 Jugjuh, B. I., Hutchins, G. M., Bulkley, B. H., and Becker, L. C.: Salvage of Ischemic Myocardium by Ibuprofen During Infarction in the Conscious Dog, *Am. J. Cardiol.*, 46:4, 1980.

37 Hamm, C. W., and Opie, L. H.: Protection of Infarcting Myocardium by Slow Channel Inhibitors (Calcium Antagonists), *Am. J. Cardiol.*, 49:942, 1982. (Abstract.)

38 Melin, J., Bulkley, B. H., Hutchins, G. M., and Becker, L. C.: Effectiveness of Delayed Treatment by Nifedipine in Reducing the Size of Experimental Myocardial Infarction in the Conscious Dog, *Circulation,* 66(suppl. 2):85, 1982.

39 Izquiedo, C., Roan, P., Buja, M., and Willerson, J. T.: Effects of Nifedipine and Verapamil during Acute Myocardial Infarction, *Am. J. Cardiol.*, 49:1005, 1982. (Abstract.)

40 Povzhitkov, M., Haendchen, R. V., Meerbaum, S., et al.: Protective Effect of Coronary Venous Prostaglan-din E, Retroperfusion during Acute Myocardial Ischemia, *Am. J. Cardiol.*, 49:1017, 1982. (Abstract.)

41 Lupinetti, F. M., Starnes, V. A., Law, K. H., Collins, J. C., and Hammon, J. W.: Prostacyclin Decreases Myocardial Infarct Size in Dogs Only in Doses that Cause Significant Vasodilation, *Am. J. Cardiol.*, 49:1005, 1982. (Abstract.)

42 Carvalho, M. A., Aloon, L., Mello, M. G., Jr., Carneiro, R. D., and Ribeiro, L. G. T.: Beneficial Effects of Verapamil on Myocardial Ischemic Injury: Evaluation by Precordial ST-Segment Mapping, *Clin. Res.*, 29:180A, 1981. (Abstract.)

43 Uchida, Y., Hanai, T., Hasegana, K., Kawamura, K., and Oshima, T.: Coronary Recanalization Induced by Intracoronary Administration of Prostacyclin in Patients with Acute Myocardial Infarction, *Circulation,* 66(suppl. 2):261, 1982. (Abstract.)

44 Glogar, D. H., Mohl, W., Mayr, H., et al.: Pressure-controlled Intermittent Coronary Sinus Occlusion Reduced Myocardial Necrosis, *Am. J. Cardiol.*, 49:1017, 1982. (Abstract.)

45 Meerbaum, S., Povzhitkor, M., Haendehen, R. V., et al.: Coronary Artery Thrombolysis by Streptokinase Coronary Venous Retroperfusion or Systemic Administration, *Am. J. Cardiol.*, 49:1046, 1982. (Abstract.)

46 DeWood, M. A., Spores, J., Shields, J. P., et al.: Acute Myocardial Infarction: A Decade of Experience with Reperfusion in 701 Patients, *Circulation,* 66(suppl. 2):93, 1982. (Abstract.)

47 Berg, R., Jr., Kendall, R. W., Duvoisin, G. E., et al.: Acute Myocardial Infarction, *J. Thorac. Cardiovasc. Surg.*, 70:432, 1975.

48 Phillips, S. J., Kongtahworn, C., Zeff, R. H., et al.: Emergency Coronary Artery Revascularization: A Possible Therapy for Acute Myocardial Infarction, *Circulation,* 60:241, 1979.

49 Kent, K. M., Bover, J. S., Grean, M. V., et al.: Effects of Coronary Artery Bypass on Global and Regional Left Ventricular Function during Exercise, *N. Engl. J. Med.*, 298:1434, 1978.

50 DeWood, M. A., Spores, J., Notske, R. N., et al.: Medical and Surgical Treatment of Myocardial Infarction, *Am. J. Cardiol.*, 44:1356, 1979.

51 Rude, R. E., Muller, J. E., and Braunwald, E.: Review: Efforts to Limit the Size of Myocardial Infarct, *Ann. Intern. Med.*, 95:736, 1981.

52 Roberts, W. C.: Coronary Arteries in Fatal Acute Myocardial Infarction, *Circulation,* 45:215, 1972.

53 Friedman, M., and Van den Borenkamp, G.: The Pathogenesis of Coronary Intramural Hemorrhages, *Br. J. Exp. Pathol.*, 47:347, 1966.

54 Ridolfi, R. L., and Hutchin, G. M.: Relationship between Coronary Artery Lesions and Myocardial Infarcts: Ulceration of Atherosclerotic Plaques Precipitating Coronary Thrombosis, *Am. Heart J.*, 93:468, 1977.

55 Horie, T., Sekiguchi, M., and Hirosawa, K.: Pathogenesis of Acute Myocardial Infarction: Histopathological Study of Coronary Arteries in 108 Necropsied Cases during Serial Section, *Br. Heart J.*, 40:153, 1978.

56 Levin, D. C., and Fallon, J. T.: Significance of the Angiographic Morphology of Localized Coronary Stenosis: Histopathologic Correlations, *Circulation*, 66:316, 1982.

57 Chandler, A. B., Chapman, I., Erhardt, L. R., et al.: Coronary Thrombosis in Myocardial Infarction. Report of a Workshop on the Role of Coronary Thrombosis in the Pathogenesis of Acute Myocardial Infarction, *Am. J. Cardiol.*, 34:823, 1974.

58 Dalen, J. E., Ockene, I. S., and Alpert, J. S.: Coronary Spasm, Coronary Thrombosis, and Myocardial Infarction: A hypothesis concerning the Pathophysiology of Acute Myocardial Infarction, *Am. Heart J.*, 104:1119, 1982.

59 Maseri, A., L'Abbate, A., Baroldi, G., et al.: Coronary Vasospasm as a Possible Cause of Myocardial Infarction: A Conclusion Derived from the Study of "Preinfarction" Angina, *N. Engl. J. Med.*, 299:1271, 1978.

60 DeWood, M. A., Spores, J., Notske, R., et al.: Prevalence of Total Coronary Occlusion during the Early Hours of Transmural Myocardial Infarction, *N. Engl. J. Med.*, 303:897, 1980.

61 Blanke, H., Rentrop, P., Karsch, K. R., and Kreuzer, H.: Coronary Angiographic and Ventriculographic Findings in the Acute and Chronic Stage of Myocardial Infarction, *Circulation*, 60(suppl. 2):69, 1979.

62 Oliva, P. B., and Breckinridge, I. C.: Arteriographic Evidence of Coronary Arterial Spasm in Acute Myocardial Infarction, *Circulation*, 56:366, 1977.

63 Tillett, W. S., and Garner, R. L.: The Fibrinolytic Activity of Hemolytic Streptococci, *J. Exp. Med.*, 58:485, 1933.

64 Tillett, W. S., and Sherry, S.: The Effect in Patients of Streptococcal Fibrinolysin (Streptokinase) and Streptococcal Deoxyribonuclease on Fibrinous, Purulent and Sanguinous Pleural Exudation, *J. Clin. Invest.*, 28:173, 1949.

65 Johnson, A. L., and McCarty, W. R.: The Lysis of Artificially Induced Intravascular Clots in Man by Intravenous Infusions of Streptokinase, *J. Clin. Invest.*, 39:426, 1959.

66 Fletcher, A. P., Alkjaersig, N., Synrniotis, F. E., and Sherry, S.: The Treatment of Patients Suffering from Early Myocardial Infarction with Massive and Prolonged Streptokinase Therapy, *Trans. Assoc. Am. Physicians*, 71:287, 1958.

67 Boucek, H. J., and Murphy, W. P.: Segmental Perfusion of the Coronary Arteries with Fibrinolysis in Man following a Myocardial Infarction, *Am. J. Cardiol.*, 6:525, 1960.

68 Sherry, S.: Personal Reflection on the Development of Thrombolytic Therapy and Its Application to Acute Coronary Thrombosis, *Am. Heart J.*, 102:1134, 1981.

69 Amery, A., Roeber, G., Vermeulen, H. J., and Verstraete, M.: Single-blind Randomized Multicentre Trial Comparing Heparin and Streptokinase Treatment in Recent Myocardial Infarction, *Acta Med. Scand.*, (*Suppl.*)505:5, 1969.

70 European Working Party: Streptokinase in Recent Myocardial Infarction: A controlled Multicentre Trial, *Br. Med. J.*, 3:325, 1971.

71 Heikinheimo, R., Ahrenberg, P., Honkapohja, H., et al.: Fibrinolytic Treatment in Acute Myocardial Infarction, *Acta Med. Scand.*, 189:7, 1971.

72 Dioguardi, N., Mannucci, P. M., Loho, A., et al.: Controlled Trial of Streptokinase and Heparin in Acute Myocardial Infarction, *Lancet*, 2:891, 1971.

73 Breddin, K., Ehrly, A. M., Fechler, L., et al.: Die Kurzzeitfibrinolyse beim akuten Myokardinfarkt, *Dtsch. Med. Wochenschr.*, 98:861, 1973.

74 Bett, J. H. N., Biggs, J. C., Castaldi, P. A., et al.: Australian Multicentre Trial of Streptokinase in Acute Myocardial Infarction, *Lancet*, 1:57, 1973.

75 Aber, C. P., Bass, N. M., Berry, C. L., et al.: Streptokinase in Acute Myocardial Infarction: A Controlled Multicentre Study in the United Kingdom, *Br. Med. J.*, 2:1100, 1976.

76 European Cooperative Study Group for Streptokinase: Treatment in Acute Myocardial Infarction. Streptokinase in Acute Myocardial Infarction, *N. Engl. J. Med.*, 301:797, 1979.

77 Stampfer, M. J., Goldhaber, S. Z., Yusuf, S., Peto, R., and Hennekens, C. H.: Effect of Intravenous Streptokinase on Acute Myocardial Infarction, *N. Engl. J. Med.*, 307:1180, 1982.

77a Galiano, N., Macruz, R., Arie, S., et al.: Enfarte Agudo Do Miocardio e Choque—Tratamento por Recanalizacao Arterial Atraves do Cateterisomo Cardiaco, *Arq. Bras. Cardiol.*, 25:197, 1972.

78 Rentrop, P., DeVivic, E. R., Karsch, K. R., and Kreuzer, H.: Acute Coronary Occlusion with Impending Infarction as an Angiographic Complication Relieved by Guidewire Recanalization, *Clin. Cardiol.*, 1:101, 1978.

79 Rentrop, P., Blanke, H., Wiegand, V., and Karsch, K. R.: Wiedereroffung verschlossener Kranzgefasse im akuten Infarkt mit hHlfe von Kathetern (transluminale Rekanalisation), *Dtsch. Med. Wochenschr.*, 104:1401, 1979.

80 Rentrop, P., Blanke, H., Karsch, K. R., and Kreuzer, H.: Initial Experience with Transluminal Recanalization of Recently Occluded Infarct-related Coronary Artery in Acute Myocardial Infarction. Comparison with Conventionally Treated Patients, *Clin. Cardiol.*, 2:92, 1979.

81 Rentrop, P., Blanke, H., Koestering, K., and Karsch,

K. R.: Acute Myocardial Infarction: Intracoronary Application of Nitroglycerin and Streptokinase in Combination with Transluminal Recanalization, *Clin. Cardiol.*, 5:354, 1979.

82 Kennedy, J. W., Fritz, J. K., and Ritchie, J. L.: Streptokinase in Acute Myocardial Infarction: Western Washington Randomized Trial—Protocol and Progress Report, *Am. Heart J.*, 104:899, 1982.

83 Timmis, G. C., Gangadhaven, V., Hauser, A. M., Ramos, R. G., Westveer, D. C., and Gordon, S.: Intracoronary Streptokinase in Clinical Practice, *Am. Heart J.*, 104:925, 1982.

84 Reduto, L. A., Freund, G. C., Gaeta, J. M., et al.: Coronary Artery Reperfusion in Acute Myocardial Infarction: Beneficial Effects of Intracoronary Streptokinase on Left Ventricular Salvage and Performance, *Am. Heart J.*, 102:1168, 1981.

85 Ganz, W., Ninomiya, K., Hashida, J., et al.: Intracoronary Thrombolysis in Acute Myocardial Infarction: Experimental Background and Clinical Experience, *Am. Heart J.*, 102:1145, 1981.

86 Smalling, R. W., Fuentes, F., Freund, G. C., Reduto, L. A., et al.: Beneficial Effects of Intracoronary Thrombolysis up to Eighteen Hours after Onset of Pain in Evolving Myocardial Infarction, *Am. Heart J.*, 104:912, 1982.

87 Popio, K. A., Ross, A. M., Oravec, J. M., and Ingram, J. T.: Identification and Description of Separate Mechanisms for Two Components of Renografin Cardiotoxicity, *Circulation*, 58:520, 1978.

88 Rentrop, P., Blanke, H., Karsch, K. R., et al.: Selective Intracoronary Thrombolysis in Acute Myocardial Infarction and Unstable Angina Pectoris, *Circulation*, 63:307, 1981.

89 Hartzler, G. O., Rutherford, B. D., and McConahay, D. R.: Percutaneous Coronary Angioplasty with and without Prior Streptokinase Infusion for the Treatment of Acute Myocardial Infarction, *Am. J. Cardiol.*, 49:1033, 1982. (Abstract.)

90 Cowley, M. J., Gold, H. K., Leinbach, R. C., et al.: Effect of Acute Coronary Angioplasty on Reperfusion Success Rates with Intracoronary Thrombolysis in Acute Myocardial Infarction, *Clin. Res.*, in press. (Abstract.)

91 Meyer, J., Merx, W., Schmitz, H., et al.: Percutaneous Transluminal Coronary Angioplasty Immediately after Intracoronary Streptolysis of Transmural Myocardial Infarction, *Circulation*, 66:905, 1982.

92 Schmitt, J. M., and Kennedy, J. W.: Preliminary Report of the Streptokinase Registry from the Society for Cardiac Angiography, *Am. J. Cardiol.*, 49:961, 1982. (Abstract.)

93 Van den Brand, M., Smissen, H. V. D., Serruyo, P. W., and Hooghoudt, T.: Potential Risks of Intracoronary Streptokinase during Acute Myocardial Infarction, *Circulation*, 64 (suppl. 4):246, 1981. (Abstract.)

94 Weinstein, J.: Treatment of Myocardial Infarction with Intracoronary Streptokinase: Efficacy and Safety Data from 209 United States Cases in the Hoechst-Roussel Registry, *Am. Heart J.*, 104:898, 1982.

95 Verstraete, M., Tytgat, G., Amery, A., and Vermylen, J.: Thrombolytic Therapy with Streptokinase Using a Standard Dosage, *Thromb. Diath. Haemorrh,* 16(suppl. 21):493, 1966.

96 Ganz, W., Buchbinder, N., Marcus, H., et al.: Intracoronary Thrombolysis in Evolving Myocardial Infarction, *Am. Heart J.*, 101:4, 1981.

97 Mathey, D. G., Juck, K.-H., and Tilsner, V.: Nonsurgical Coronary Artery Recanalization in Acute Transmural Myocardial Infarction, *Circulation*, 63:489, 1981.

98 Feldman, R. L., Crick, N. F., Pepine, C. J., and Conti, C. R.: Quantitative Coronary Angiography during Intracoronary Streptokinase in Acute Myocardial Infarction: How Long to Continue Thrombolytic Therapy, *Circulation*, 64 (suppl. 4):9, 1981. (Abstract.)

99 Merx, W., Dorr, R., Rentrop, P., et al.: Evaluation of the Effectiveness of Intracoronary Streptokinase Infusion in Acute Myocardial Infarction: Postprocedure Management and Hospital Course in 204 Patients, *Am. Heart J.*, 102:1181, 1981.

100 Bernik, M. B., and Kwaan, H. C.: Original of Fibrinolytic Activity in Cultures of the Human Kidney, *J. Lab. Clin. Med.*, 70:650, 1967.

101 Sharma, G. V. R. K., Cella, G., Parisi, A. F., and Sashara, A. A.: Thrombolytic Therapy, *N. Engl. J. Med.*, 306:1268, 1982.

102 Killip, T., III, and Kimball, J. T.: Treatment of Myocardial Infarction in a Coronary Care Unit, *Am. J. Cardiol.*, 20:457, 1967.

103 Norris, R. M., Brandt, P. W. T., Caughey, D. E., Lee, A. J., and Scott, P. J.: A New Coronary Prognostic Index, *Lancet*, 1:274, 1969.

104 Weinstein, J., Sonnenblick, E. H., Cowley, M. J., et al.: Improved Left Ventricular Function and Reduced Hospital Mortality Following Intracoronary Thrombolysis in Myocardial Infarction with Diminished Ejection Fraction, *Am. J. Cardiol.*, 49:961, 1982. (Abstract.)

105 Cowley, M. J., Hastillo, A., Betrovec, G. W., and Hess, M. L.: Effects of Intracoronary Streptokinase in Acute Myocardial Infarction, *Am. Heart J.*, 102:1149, 1981.

106 Roy, H., Leiboff, R. J., Wasserman, A. G., Bren, G. B., Varghese, P. J., and Ross, A. M.: A Randomized Controlled Trial of Intracoronary Streptokinase in Acute MI: Preliminary (Cautionary) Observations, *Circulation*, 66 (suppl. 2):334, 1982. (Abstract.)

107 Rentrop, K. P., Blanke, H., and Karsch, K. R.: Effects of Nonsurgical Coronary Reperfusion on the Left Ventricle in Human Subjects with Conventional Treatment, *Am. J. Cardiol.*, 49:1, 1982.

108 Shah, P. K., Ganz, W., Maddahi, J., Berman, D., Shellock, F., and Swan, H. J. C.: Intracoronary Thrombolysis in Early Acute Myocardial Infarction Improves Biventricular Function Compared to Conventional Therapy, *Circulation,* 64 (suppl. 4):194,1981. (Abstract.)

109 Walton, J., O'Neill, W., Colfer, H., et al.: Failure of Intracoronary Thrombolysis to Preserve Ventricular Function: Report of a Randomized Clinical Trial, *Circulation,* 66 (suppl. 2):1336, 1982. (Abstract.)

110 Wackers, F., Berger, H. J., and Zaret, B. L.: Spontaneous Changes of Global and Regional Left Ventricular Function during the First 24 Hours of Acute Myocardial Infarction. Implications for Evaluating Thrombolytic Therapy, *Circulation,* 64 (suppl. 4):196, 1981. (Abstract.)

111 Reduto, L. A., Berger, H. J., Cohen, L. S., Gottschak, A., and Zaret, B. L.: Sequential Radionuclide Assessment of Left and Right Ventricular Performance after Acute Transmural Myocardial Infarction, *Ann. Intern. Med.,* 89:441, 1978.

112 Rentrop, P., Chairman of the Intracoronary Streptokinase Registry of the European Society of Cardiology: Mortality and Functional Changes after Intracoronary Streptokinase Infusion, *Circulation,* 66 (suppl. 2):335, 1982.

113 Mathey, D., Sheehan, F. H., Schofer, J., Bleifeld, W., and Dodge, H. T.: LV Function following Intracoronary Thrombolysis in Acute Myocardial Infarction, *Circulation,* 66 (suppl. 2):335, 1982. (Abstract.)

114 Stack, R. S., Phillips, H. R., Grierson, D., Kong, Y., Peter, R. H., and Behar, V. S.: Changes in Segmental Function of Jeopardized Myocardium following Streptokinase Infusion, *Circulation,* 66 (suppl. 2):336, 1982. (Abstract.)

115 Sheehan, F. H., Mathey, D., Dodge, H. T., and Kuck, K. H.: Effect of Early Revascularization on Compensatory Hyperkinesis in Acute Infarction, *Circulation,* 66 (suppl. 2):336, 1982. (Abstract.)

116 Rentrop, K. P., Blanke, H., and Karsch, K. R.: Effects of Nonsurgical Coronary Reperfusion on the Left Ventricle in Human Subjects Compared with Conventional Treatment, *Am. J. Cardiol.,* 49:1, 1982.

117 Anderson, J. L., Marshall, H. W., Bray, B. E., Lutz, J. R., Frederick, P. R., Klausner, S. C., and Hagan, A. D.: A Randomized Trial of Intracoronary Streptokinase in Acute Myocardial Infarction, *Circulation,* 66 (suppl. 2):34, 1982. (Abstract.)

118 Freiman, J. A., Chalmero, T. C., Smith, H., and Kuebler, R. R.: The Importance of Beta, the Type II Error and Sample Size in the Design and Interpretation of the Randomized Control Trial. Survey of 71 ''Negative'' Trials, *N. Engl. J. Med.,* 299:690, 1978.

119 Gangadharan, V., Ramos, R. G., Hauser, A. M., et al.: Natural History of Left Ventricular Function following Intracoronary Thrombolysis, *Am. J. Cardiol.,* 49:962, 1982. (Abstract.)

120. Markis, J. E., Malagold, M., Parker, J. A., et al.: Myocardial Salvage after Intracoronary Thrombolysis with Streptokinase in Acute Myocardial Infarction, *N. Engl. J. Med.,* 305:777, 1981.

121 Maddahi, J., Ganz, W., Geft, I., et al.: Intracoronary Thrombolysis in Acute Myocardial Infarction: Assessment of Efficacy by Thallium 201 Scintigraphy, *Am. J. Cardiol.,* 49:973, 1982. (Abstract.)

122 Simoons, M. L., Serruys, P. W., Brand, V. D., et al.: Myocardial Salvage by Intracoronary Thrombolysis in Acute Infarcts, Documentation by Thallium Scintigraphy, *Am. J. Cardiol.,* 49:973, 1982. (Abstract.)

123 Maddahi, J., Geft, J., Hulse, S., Berman, D., Swan, H. J. C., and Ganz, W.: Intracoronary TC-99M-PYP Immediately Demonstrated Necrosis in Reperfused Myocardium and Complements Postreperfusion Intracoronary T1-1201 Imaging, *Circulation,* 66 (suppl. 2):342, 1982. (Abstract.)

124 Schofer, J., Stritzke, P., Kuck, K.-H., Bleifeld, W., Montz, R., and Mathey, D. G.: Dual Intracoronary Myocardial Scintigraphy with Thallium 201 and Technetium 99M Pyrophosphate Predicts Myocardial Salvage Immediately after Successful Intracoronary Thrombolysis, *Circulation,* 66 (suppl. 2):335, 1982. (Abstract.)

125 Schofer, J., Mathey, D., Kuck, K.-H., Montz, R., and Bleifeld, W.: Early Assessement of Salvaged Myocardium after Coronary Artery Recanalization by Sequential Intracoronary Thallium Scintigraphy, *Am. J. Cardiol.,* 49:962, 1982. (Abstract.)

126 Pohost, G. M., Zir, L. M., Moore, R. H., et al.: Differentiation of Transiently Ischemic from Infarcted Myocardium by Serial Imaging after a Single Dose of Thallium 201, *Circulation,* 55:294, 1977.

127 Smitherman, T. C., Osborn, R. C., Jr., and Nasahara, K. A.: Serial Myocardial Scintigraphy after Single Dose of Thallium-201 in Men after Acute Myocardial Infarction, *Am. J. Cardiol.,* 42:177, 1978.

128 Wackers, F. J. T., Sokole, E. B., Samson, G., et al.: Value and Limitations of Thallium-201 Scintigraphy in the Acute Phase of Myocardial Infarction, *N. Engl. J. Med.,* 295:1, 1976.

129 Sobel, B. E., and Bergmann, S. R.: Coronary Thrombolysis: Some Unresolved Issues, *Am. J. Med.,* 72 (suppl. 2):1, 1982.

130 Hollman, J., Gruentzig, A. R., King, S. B., III, and Douglas, J.: Acute Coronary Occlusion Immediately following Percutaneous Transluminal Coronary Angioplasty, *Circulation,* 66 (suppl. 2):4, 1982.

131 Blanke, H., Karsch, K. R., Schheeter, D., et al.: Preservation of R-Waves after Acute LAD Occlusion by Streptokinase Reperfusion, *Circulation,* 64(suppl. IV):9, 1981.

132 Robison, A. K., Grepp, D. R., and Sobel, B. E.: In activation of CPK in Lymph, *Circulation,* 52(suppl. 2):5, 1975. (Abstract.)

133 Vatner, S. F., Baig, H., Manders, W. T., and Maroko, P. R.: Effects of Coronary Artery Reperfusion on Myocardial Infarct Size Calculated from Creatine Kinase, *J. Clin. Invest.*, 61:1048, 1978.

134 Jarmakani, J. M., Limbird, L., Graham, T. C., and Marks, R. A.: Effect of Reperfusion on Myocardial Infarct, and the Accuracy of Estimating Infarct Size from Serum Creatine Phosphokinase in the Dog, *Cardiovasc. Res.*, 10:245, 1976.

135 Schuster, E. H., Kallman, C., and Bulkley, B. H.: Sizing Human Myocardial Infarcts from Creatine Kinase Curves: The Effects of Reperfusion, *Circulation*, 62(suppl. 3):216, 1980. (Abstract.)

136 Wei, J. Y., Markis, J. E., Malagold, M., and Blaustein, A.: Human Serum Creatine Kinase Kinetics following Reperfusion in Acute Myocardial Infarction, *Am. J. Cardiol.*, 49:1033, 1982. (Abastract.)

137 Blanke, H., Von Hardenberg, D., Karsch, K. R., et al.: Changes in Patients of CPK Kinetics following coronary Reperfusion, *Am. J. Cardiol.*, 49:1034, 1982. (Abstract.)

138 Cowley, M., Hastillo, A., Vectrovec, G., and Hess, M. L.: Fibrinolytic Effects of Low Dose Intracoronary Streptokinase Administration in Acute Myocardial Infarction, *Circulation,* 64(suppl. 4):10, 1981. (Abstract.)

139 Tabari, K. K., Rubinstein, M. D., Robinson, M. C., and Hanson, J. A.: Systemic Fibrinolysis Associated with Intracoronary Streptokinase Infusion, *Am. J. Cardiol.*, 49:974, 1982. (Abstract.)

140 Timmis, G. C., Hauser, A., Ramos, V., Gangadharan, D., and Westveer, G.: Regeneration of Fibrinogen after Intracoronary Streptokinase, *Circulation*, 66 (suppl. 2):262, 1982.

141 Fallon, J. T., Aretz, H. T., and Gold, H. K.: Coronary Arterial Pathology following Thrombolytic Therapy for Acute Myocardial Infarction, *Circulation,* 66:336, 1982.

142 Axelrod, P., Verier, R., and Lown, B.: Vulnerability to Ventricular Fibrillation during Acute Coronary Arterial Occlusion and Release, *Am. J. Cardiol.*, 36:776, 1975.

143 Penkoske, P. A., Sobel, B. E., and Cobb, P. B.: Disparate Electrophysiological Alterations Accompanying Dysrhythmia Due to Coronary Occlusion and Reperfusion in the cat, *Circulation*, 58:1023, 1978.

144 Corr, P. B., Shayman, J. A., Kramer, J. B., and Kipnis, R. J.: Increased Adrenergic Receptors in Ischemic Cat Myocardium, *J. Clin. Invest.*, 67:1232, 1981.

145 Sheridan, D. J., Penkoske, P. A., Sobel, B. E., and Cobb, P. B.: Alpha Adrenergic Contributions to Dysrhythmia during Myocardial Ischemia and Reperfusion in Cats, *J. Clin. Invest.*, 65:161, 1980.

146 Williams, L. T., Guewero, J. L., Leinback, R. C., and Gold, H. K.: Prevention of Reperfusion Dysrhythmias by Selective Coronary Alpha Adrenergic Blockage Intracoronary Infusion Phentolamine Block Reperfusion Arrhythmia in Dogs, *Am. J. Cardiol.*, 49:1046, 1982. (Abstract.)

147 Montoya, A., Mulet, J., Pifarre, R., et al.: Hemorrhagic Infarct following Myocardial Revascularization, *J. Thorac. Cardiovasc. Surg.*, 75:206, 1978.

148 Balooki, H., and Vargas, A.: Myocardial Revascularization after Acute Myocardial Infarction, *Arch. Surg.*, 111:1216, 1976.

149 Bulkley, B. H., and Hutchins, G. M.: Myocardial Consequences of Coronary Artery Bypass Surgery: The Paradox of Necrosis in Areas of Revascularization, *Circulation*, 56:906, 1977.

150 Najafi, H., Henson, D., Dye, W. S., et al.: Left Ventricular Hemorrhagic Necrosis, *Ann. Thorac. Surg.*, 7:550, 1969.

151 Bresnahan, G. F., Roberts, R., Shell, N. E., Ross, J., Jr., and Sobel, B. E.: Deleterious Effects Due to Hemorrhage after Myocardial Reperfusion, *Am. J. Cardiol.*, 33:82, 1974.

152 Kloner, R. A., Rude, R. E., and Carlson, N.: Ultrastructural Evidence of Microvascular Damage and Myocardial Cell Injury after Coronary Artery Occlusion: Which Comes First?, *Circulation,* 62:945, 1980.

153 Fishbein, M. C., Y-Rit, J., Lando, U., et al.: The relationship of vascular injury and myocardial hemorrhage to necrosis after reperfusion, *Circulation*, 62:1274, 1980.

154 Higginson, L. A. J., Sheldrick, K., Temple, V., and Beaulands, D. J.: Does Streptokinase Augment Reperfusion Hemorrhage?, *Circulation*, 66 (suppl. 2):86, 1982. (Abstract.)

154a Althaus, U., Gurtner, H. P., Baur, H., Hamburger, S., and Roos, B.: Consequences of Myocardial Reperfusion following Coronary Occlusion in Pigs: Effects on Morphologic, Biochemical and Hemodynamic Findings, *Eur. J. Clin. Invest.*, 7:437, 1977.

155 Pizada, F. A., Weiner, J. M., and Hood, W. B., Jr.: Experimental Myocardial Infarction. Accelerated Myocardial Stiffening Related to Coronary Reperfusion following Ischemia, *Chest*, 74:190, 1978.

156 Mathey, D. G., Klopell, G., and Kuch, K.-H.: Transmural Hemorrhagic Infarction following Intracoronary Streptokinase Clinical, Angiographic and Autopsy Findings, *Circulation*, 64(suppl. 4):194, 1981. (Abstract.)

157 Tennant, S., Campbell, W. B., Dixon, J., Page, H., Roach, A., and Kaiser, A.: Intracoronary Thrombolysis in Acute Myocardial Infarction: Comparison of Efficacy of Urokinase to Streptokinase, *Circulation*, 66 (suppl. 2):336, 1982.

158 Lee, G., Amsterdam, E. A., Low, R., Joye, J. A., et al.: Efficacy of Percutaneous Transluminal Coronary Recanalization utilizing Streptokinase Thrombolysis in Patients with Acute Myocardial Infarction, *Am. Heart J.*, 102:1159, 1981.

159 Mathey, D. G., Rodewald, G., Rentrop, P., et al.: Intracoronary Streptokinase Thrombolytic Recanalization and Subsequent Surgical Bypass of Remaining Atherosclerotic Stenosis in Acute Myocardial Infarction: Complementary Combined Approach Effecting Reduced Infarct Size, Preventing Reinfarction, and Improving Left Ventricular Function, *Am. Heart J.*, 102:1194, 1981.

160 Merx, W., Bethge, C. H., Effert, S., et al.: How Often Are "Occluding Thrombi" in Patients with Acute Myocardial Infarction Really Occluding?—Consequences for Selective Thrombolysis, *Circulation*, 64(suppl. 4):247, 1981.

161 Harrison, D. G., Ferguson, D. W., Kioschos, J. M., Marcus, M. L., and White, C. W.: Inapparent Persistent Thrombi following "Successful" Streptokinase Reperfusion during Acute Myocardial Infarction, *Circulation*, 66:335, 1982. (Abstract.)

162 Fioretti, P., Serruys, P. W., Rand, M., et al.: Incidence of Recurrent Myocardial Ischemia after Intracoronary Fibrinolysis in Acute Myocardial Infarction, *Am. J. Cardiol.*, 49:974, 1982.

163 Lee, G., Low, R. I., Takeda, P., et al.: Importance of Follow-up Medical and Surgical Approaches to Prevent Reinfarction, Reocclusion and Recurrent Angina following Intracoronary Thrombolysis with Streptokinase in Acute Myocardial Infarction, *Am. Heart J.*, 104:921, 1982.

164 Swan, H. J. C.: Thrombolysis in Acute Myocardial Infarction: Treatment of the Underlying Coronary Artery Disease, *Circulation*, 66:914, 1982. (Editorial.)

165 Kennedy, R. H., Kennedy, M. A., Frye, R. L., et al.: Cardiac Catheterization and Cardiac-Surgical Facilities: Use, Trends, and Future Requirements, *N. Engl. J. Med.*, 307:986, 1982.

166 Simon, T. L., Ware, J. H., and Stengle, J. M.: Clinical Trials of Thrombolytic Agents in Myocardial Infarction, *Ann. Intern. Med.*, 79:712, 1973.

167 Spann, J. F., Sherry, S., Carabello, B. A., et al.: High-dose, Brief Intravenous Streptokinase Early in Acute Myocardial Infarction, *Am. Heart J.*, 104:939, 1982.

168 Neuhaus, K. L., Tebbe, U., Sauer, G., Kstering, H., and Kreuzer, H.: Behandlung des Akuten Myokardinfarktes mit Streptase-Kurzinfusion. Kongress fur Thrombose and Blutgerinnung, unpublished data quoted in Spann et al.[167]

169 Schroeder, R., Biamino, G., Leitner, E. R., et al.: Intravenous Short-time Infusion of Streptokinase in Acute Myocardial Infarction, unpublished data quoted in Spann et al.[167]

170 Morrison, J., Ong, L., Reiser, P., Scherr, L.: Spontaneous Preservation of Left Ventricular Function during Myocardial Infarction, *Am. J. Cardiol.*, 49:1034, 1982. (Abstract.)

171 Neuhaus, K. L., Kostering, A., Tebbe, U., Sauer, G., and Kreuzer, H.: Intravenose kurzzeitstreptokinase—Therapie beim Frischen Myokardinfarkt, *2 Kardiol.*, 70:791, 1981.

172 Schwarz, F., Schuler, G., Katus, H., et al.: Intracoronary Thrombolysis in Acute Myocardial Infarction: Duration of Ischemia as a Major Determinant of Late Results after Recanalization, *Am. J. Cardiol.*, 50:933, 1982.

173 Rentrop, P., Blanke, H., Karsch, K. R., et al.: Changes in Left Ventricular Function after Intracoronary Streptokinase Infusion in Clinically Evolving Myocardial Infarction, *Am. Heart J.*, 102:1188, 1981.

174 Mehmel, H. C., Schwarz, F., Schuler, G., et al.: The Functional Result of Intracoronary Streptokinase Therapy after Myocardial Infarction May Be Determined by Collaterals, *Circulation*, 64 (suppl. 4):194, 1981. (Abstract.)

175 Capone, R. J., and Most, A. S.: Myocardial Hemorrhage after Coronary Reperfusion in Pig, *Am. J. Cardiol.*, 41:259, 1978.

176 Maroko, P.R., Kjekshus, J.K., Sobel, B.E., et al: Factors Influencing Infarct Size Following Experimental Coronary Artery Occlusion, *Circulation*, 43:67, 1971.

177 Karsch, K. R., Blanke, H., Schlueter, A., et al.: Relationship between Collaterals and History of Angina Pectoris in Acute Myocardial Infarction, *Circulation*, 64 (suppl. 4):107, 1981. (Abstract.)

178 Neill, W. A., Wharton, T. P., Fluri-Lundeen, J., and Cohen, I. S.: Acute Coronary Insufficency—Coronary Occlusion after Intermittent Ischemic Attacks, *N. Engl. J. Med.*, 302:1157, 1980.

179 Vetrovec, G. W., Cowley, W. J., Overton, H., and Richardson, D. W.: Intracoronary Thrombus in Syndromes of Unstable Myocardial Ischemia, *Am. Heart J.*, 102:1202, 1981.

180 Wolk, N. M., Mandelkorn, J., Singh, S., et al.: Evidence for Thrombosis in Acute Ischemic Syndromes Other than Transmural Infarction, *Circulation*, 64:197, 1981.

181 Vetrovec, G. W., Leinbach, R. C., Gold, H. K., and Cowley, M. J.: Intracoronary Thrombolysis in Syndromes of Unstable Ischemia: Angiographic and Clinical Results, *Am. Heart J.*, 104:946, 1982.

182 Rentrop, P., Blanke, H., Karsch, K. R., et al.: Recanalization of an Acutely Occluded Aortocoronary Bypass by Intragraft Fibrinolysis, *Circulation*, 62:1123, 1980.

183 Rentrop, P. K., Driesman, M., Blanke, H., Karsch, K., and Pichard, A.: Non-surgical Recanalization of Early and Late Bypass Occlusion, *Circulation*, 64 (suppl. 4):246, 1981. (Abstract.)

184 Holmes, D. R., Chesebro, J. H., Vlietstra, R. E., and

Orszulak, T. A.: Streptokinase for Vein Graft Thrombosis—A Caveat, *Circulation,* 63 (suppl. 4):729, 1981.

185 Bulkley, B.: Site and Sequelae of Myocardial Infarction, *N. Engl. J. Med.,* 305:337, 1981.

186 Mercier, J. C., Lando, U., Kanmatsuse, K., et al.: Divergent Effects of Inotropic Stimulation on the Mechanical Function of the Ischemic and the Severely Depressed Reperfused Myocardium, *Am. J. Cardiol.,* 47:442, 1981.

Coronary Bypass Surgery in the Treatment of Atherosclerotic Coronary Heart Disease

The Early and Late Results of Myocardial Revascularization: The Emory Experience*

CHARLES R. HATCHER, JR., M.D.,
JOE M. CRAVER, M.D., ELLIS L. JONES, M.D.,
SPENCER B. KING III, M.D., and
J. WILLIS HURST, M.D.

The major thrust of the development of coronary bypass surgery at Emory University began in the mid-1970s. It soon became apparent that coronary bypass surgery would relieve angina pectoris due to coronary atherosclerotic heart disease.[1-4] It also became apparent that the relief was not a placebo effect but was the result of improved coronary blood flow produced by the revascularization procedure.[5-8]

Since the procedure relieved angina pectoris due to the ischemia resulting from obstructive coronary disease, it seemed to us that it might prevent other clinical events due to myocardial ischemia secondary to coronary disease. We hoped it might prolong the lives of patients who suffered from this common and serious disease. Later the Veterans Administration randomized study proved that life could be prolonged in patients with angina pectoris due to left main coronary artery obstruction who had bypass surgery as compared to patients treated medically.[9] The Veterans Administration study also suggested but did not prove that the same was true for patients with triple-vessel disease who had less than normal ejection fraction.[10] Nonrandomized studies were available to show that symptomatic patients with triple-vessel disease and symptomatic patients with double-vessel disease lived longer with surgery than matched controlled patients treated medically.[11] There was no evidence that patients with single-vessel disease would live longer with bypass surgery when compared with medically treated controlled patients.[11] Patients with single-vessel disease were operated on to relieve angina. Since coronary bypass surgery relieved angina and since the procedure prolonged life in certain subsets of patients, we decided to make a major commitment of resources and personnel to develop the procedure at our institution. Accordingly, we added new faculty members to the cardiovascular laboratory, surgical staff, and cardiac anesthesia staff, and developed additional cardiac intensive care units and excellent cardiac nursing.[12] We also developed a computerized cardiac data bank to store and retrieve crucial data on all of our patients who had cardiac surgery.

We continued our work with coronary bypass surgery and have been pleased to attain an acceptable operative risk (under 1 percent) and a low perioperative infarction rate (4 to 6 percent) and an excellent graft patency rate.[13]

We began to use coronary angioplasty at Emory 3 years ago and shortly thereafter Dr. Andreas Gruentzig, who developed the technique, joined our staff.[14,15] This technique is used most often for patients with single-vessel disease who have evidence of myocardial ischemia. The initial success rate is now above 90 percent. Although approximately one-third of these patients have documented recurrence of the stenosis, redilatation is almost always possible. Patients who have unsuccessful coronary angioplasty have coronary bypass surgery and patients who have complications of angioplasty (approximately 4 percent) have emergency bypass surgery. His technique and the results of using it are discussed late in this book.

The following discussion outlines the details of the work at Emory University.

NUMBER OF PATIENTS OPERATED AT EMORY

By 1983, over 7,226 patients had coronary bypass surgery at Emory University Hospital. It is the most common surgical procedure performed at the Hospital. The analysis of results presented in this manuscript deals with the time 1973 to 1981.

THE PREOPERATIVE CLINICAL STATUS OF PATIENTS WHO HAVE HAD CORONARY BYPASS SURGERY

Between 1973 and 1981, 5,742 patients underwent myocardial revascularization at Emory University (Table 1). The preoperative cardiac status of these patients was as follows (Table 2): Almost all the patients had

*From the Departments of Surgery, Medicine, and Radiology, Emory University School of Medicine, Atlanta.

TABLE 1
Coronary revascularization Emory University Hospital, 1973–1981

Total cases		5,742
Series mortality	1.1%	65/5,742
Mortality 1976–1981	0.8%	44/5,357

TABLE 2
Preoperative clinical status

Prior MI	56%
Unstable angina	64%
Hypertension	39%
CHF by history	7%
Abnormal ST-T	15%

angina pectoris. Unstable angina pectoris, defined as initial onset angina, progressive angina, the occurrence of rest angina, or prolonged discomfort due to myocardial ischemia, was present in 64 percent of the patients. Previous myocardial infarction was noted in 56 percent of the patients. Other preoperative variables included hypertension in 39 percent, a history of congestive heart failure in 7 percent, and abnormal ST-T wave changes in 15 percent of the patients.

About 20 percent of the patients had single-vessel disease, 35 percent had double-vessel disease, 35 percent had triple-vessel disease, and 10 percent had left main coronary artery obstruction. Obstruction was considered to be significant when it occluded 75 percent of the cross-sectional area of an artery.

HOSPITAL MORTALITY RATE AND LONG-TERM SURVIVAL

Between 1973 and 1981, 5,742 patients had coronary bypass surgery at Emory University Hospital. The operative mortality rate was 1.1 percent for the entire series. The operative mortality rate from 1976 to 1981 was 0.8 percent (Table 1).

Hospital mortality and long-term survival rates have been related to the extent of vessel disease and status of ventricular contractility (Figs. 1 and 2). For statistical analysis patients are considered to have single-vessel disease when only one of the three arteries or its major branch has a lesion narrowing the cross-sectional area of the lumen by 75 percent or greater. Disease of a lesser degree may exist in the other vessels. Two- and three-vessel disease is identified using the same criteria but with the lesions being located in two or three of the arteries rather than in one.

Hospital mortality rate in patients with normal contractility (Fig. 2) varied from 0.1 percent in patients with single-vessel disease to 2.2 percent in patients

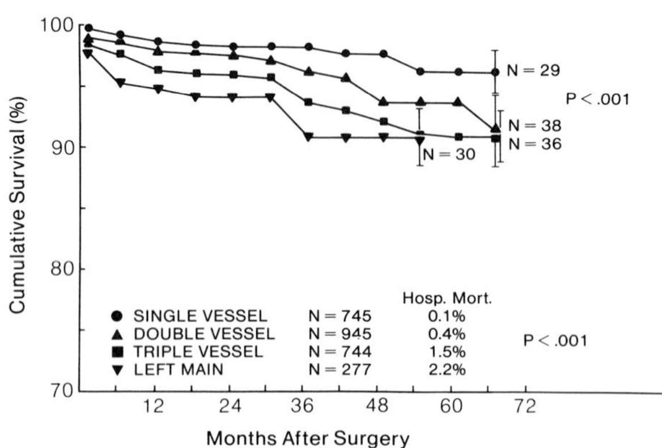

FIGURE 1 This figure shows the operative mortality and survival rates at 66 months of patients with *normal* ventricular contractility who had coronary bypass surgery at Emory University from 1973 through 1981. Note that the number of obstructed vessels influenced the operative mortality and survival rates.

with left main disease, and, correspondingly, the 66-month survival varied from 96 percent in patients with single-vessel disease to 91 percent in patients with left main and triple-vessel disease. The patients with double-vessel disease had a 66-month survival rate of 91 percent.

Patients with abnormal contractility (Fig. 2) had a hospital mortality rate that varied from 0.9 percent in patients with single-vessel disease to 1.8 percent in patients with left main coronary artery obstruction to 1.9 percent in patients with triple-vessel disease. The 42-month survival rate of patients who were operated

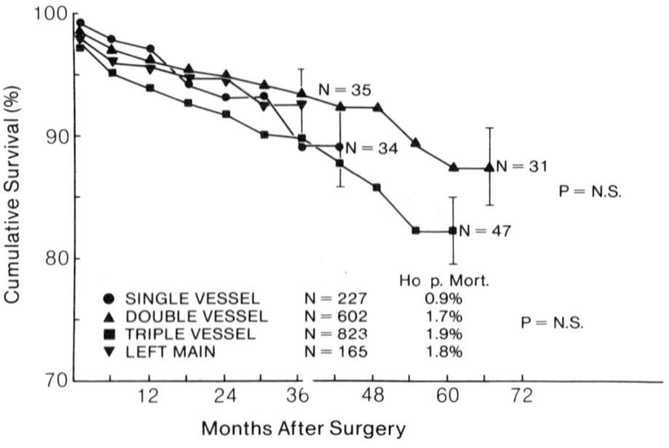

FIGURE 2 This figure shows the operative mortality and survival rates at 66 months of patients with abnormal contractility who had coronary bypass surgery at Emory University from 1973 through 1981. Note that the number of obstructed vessels influenced the operative mortality and survival rates. Note also that patients with abnormal ventricular contractility had a higher operative mortality rate and poorer survival rate than patients with normal ventricular contractility.

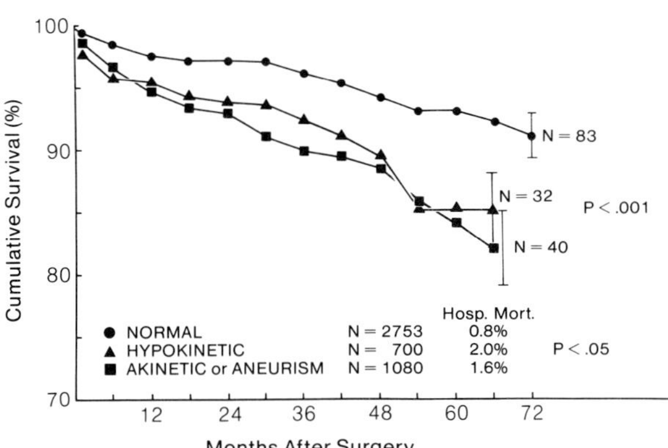

FIGURE 3 This figure indicates hospital mortality and survival rates at 66 months of patients with normal ventricular wall motion, patients with hypokinetic ventricles, and patients with ventricular aneurysms.

on with single-vessel disease was 89 percent. The 66-month survival rate of patients with double-vessel disease was 87 percent. The 60-month survival rate of patients with triple-vessel disease was 82 percent. The 36-month survival rate of patients with left main coronary artery obstruction was 93 percent.

Figure 3 illustrates the effect of abnormal ventricular wall motion on operative mortality and survival rates. Figure 4 illustrates the influence of an ejection fraction above and below 35 percent on the operative mortality rate and the long-term survival rate. Although the extent of vessel disease and the status of ventricular contractility are determinants of early and late mortality, the state of ventricular contractility at the time of surgery is the more significant of the two determinants of long-term survival.

Anginal status, hypertension, congestive heart failure, and the state of the preoperative electrocardiogram, are all determinants of patient survival (Figs. 5 to 8). One previous myocardial infarction did not influence patient survival rate significantly (Fig. 9). However, patients sustaining two or more prior infarctions showed decreased survival rates.

The data presented above indicate the appropriateness of performing myocardial revascularization before ventricular function is significantly compromised. Although patients with significant impairment of ventricular function may be operated upon with acceptable hospital mortality rate, the long-term results are significantly compromised by ventricular dysfunction.

Perioperative infarction, defined as the development of new Q waves in the electrocardiogram, occurs in 4.3 percent of patients. The influence of perioperative infarction on long-term survival of patients operated on between 1973 and 1981 is shown in Fig. 10.

Note that a perioperative infarction decreases the long-term survival rate slightly.

THE RELIEF OF ANGINA PECTORIS

The unique influence of myocardial revascularization on anginal relief postoperatively is apparent.[16] Our data indicate that there is significant relief of angina pectoris in about 90 percent of the patients regardless of clinical circumstances at the time of surgery, but this percentage decreases over time.

BYPASS SURGERY IN PATIENTS WITH RECENT INFARCTION

The role of myocardial revascularization immediately following myocardial infarction has yet to be determined.[17] It has been our policy to accept certain patients for surgery who have had a myocardial infarction and continue to have episodes of ischemic pain despite medical therapy. Between January 1976 and April 1980, 116 patients were operated upon within 1 month of the documented myocardial infarction.[18] These patients have been arbitrarially divided into those operated upon within 24 h of their infarction, those patients operated upon in 2 to 7 days after infarction, and those patients operated upon 1 week to 1 month after infarction. There was no hospital mortality in these patients. There has been no attempt at our institution to employ emergency bypass surgery as the primary treatment for acute myocardial infarction.

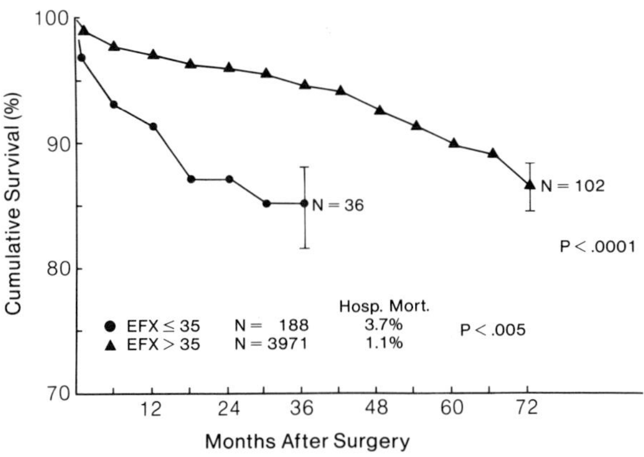

FIGURE 4 This figure shows the difference in hospital mortality and survival rates at 36 months of patients operated on at Emory University who had greater than 35 percent ejection fraction compared to patients who were operated on who had 35 percent or less ejection fraction.

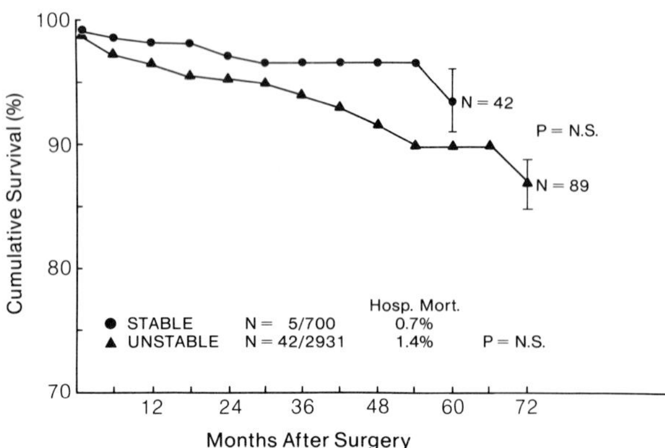

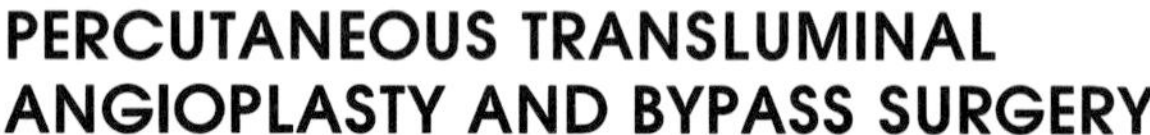

FIGURE 5 This figure compares the influence of stable angina and unstable angina on the operative risk and rate of survival at 60 months of patients who had coronary bypass surgery at Emory University.

PERCUTANEOUS TRANSLUMINAL ANGIOPLASTY AND BYPASS SURGERY

The ideal candidate for balloon angioplasty has proximal subtotal stenosis of a single coronary artery, exhibits proven myocardial ischemia, and is otherwise an acceptable candidate for bypass surgery. Expanding indications for coronary angioplasty have come to include some patients with multiple vessel disease, especially those in whom only one vessel would be bypassed surgically. Repeat percutaneous transluminal coronary angioplasty is indicated if angina recurs following initial dilatation. Coronary angioplasty has proved to be quite valuable in the management of selected patients who have recurrent angina following bypass

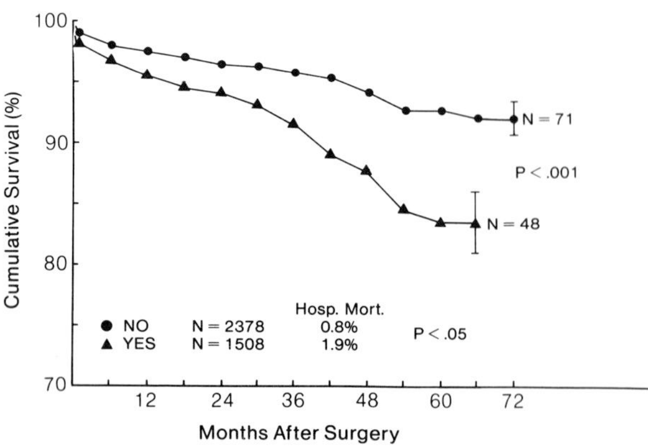

FIGURE 6 This figure compares the influence of hypertension on the operative mortality and survival rates at 66 months of patients who had coronary bypass surgery at Emory University.

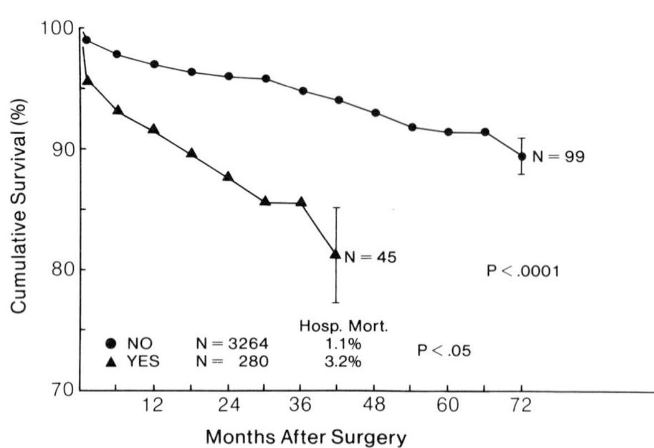

FIGURE 7 This figure shows the influence of congestive heart failure on the operative mortality and survival rates at 40 months of patients who had coronary bypass surgery at Emory University.

surgery due to either graft stenosis or additional disease of the native circulations.

To date, our group has performed over 2,000 coronary angioplasties. There has been 1 death in the series. The primary success rate has steadily increased to the level of 92 percent in 1982. Over 3 (3.7) percent of the patients have required emergency coronary artery bypass grafting, and 1.8 percent sustained myocardial infarction (new Q waves during or immediately following the procedure). Surgical support of the angioplasty effort has been designed to permit the institution of myocardial revascularization promptly following an angioplasty complication.[20]

Although approximately one-third of patients may have restenosis, it is possible to repeat the angioplasty.

NEW DATA: THE EUROPEAN COOPERATIVE STUDY

It appears that few people doubt the value of coronary bypass surgery in relieving angina pectoris due to coronary atherosclerotic heart disease. The European randomized study[19] makes it clear that symptomatic patients with left main coronary artery obstruction or triple-vessel coronary artery obstructions live longer when they have modern coronary artery surgery when compared to similar patients treated with modern drugs. The European study also supports the view that coronary bypass surgery will prolong the lives of patients with double-vessel disease when compared with medically treated patients when there is obstruction of the proximal portion of the left anterior descending coronary artery plus one additional vessel.[13,19] The European study showed that when the proximal portion of

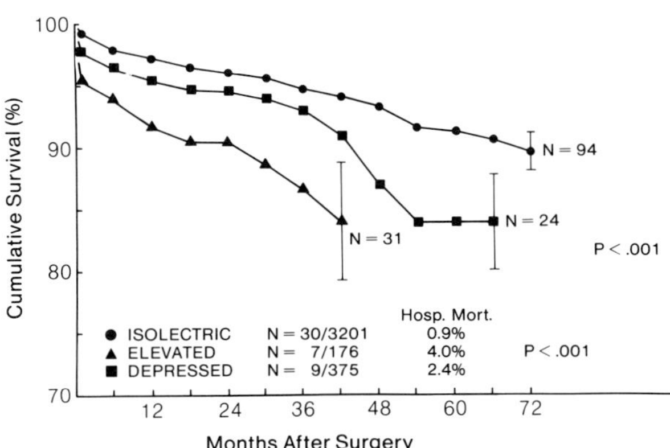

FIGURE 8 This figure shows the influence of perioperative ST-T wave change in the electrocardiogram on the operative mortality and survival rates at 40 months of patients who had coronary bypass surgery at Emory University.

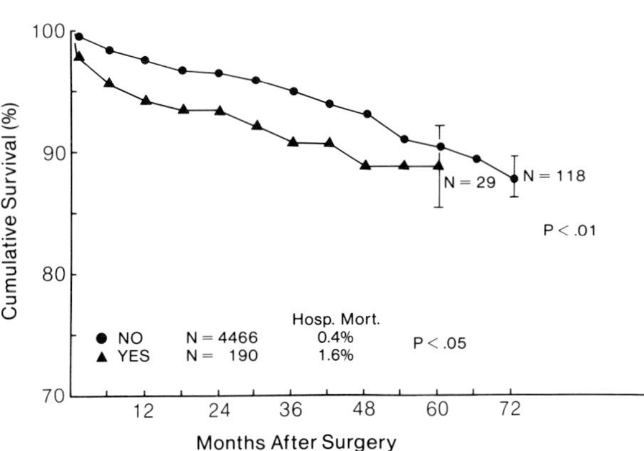

FIGURE 10 This figure shows the influence of perioperative infarction on the operative mortality and survival rates at 60 months of patients who had coronary bypass surgery at Emory University.

the left anterior descending artery was obstructed in patients with double-vessel disease who were treated medically, the 5-year survival rate was 82 percent.[19] When the left anterior descending artery was not obstructed, the 5-year survival rate for patients treated medically was 96 percent.[19]

THE FUTURE

The role of emergency surgery for evolving myocardial infarction must be addressed. The patients chosen for surgery are the same patients that are chosen for intracoronary streptokinase treatment. The debate regarding the use of these two approaches to reperfusion will continue for a few years until the indication for each is established.

It will be important to determine the proper approach to the asymptomatic patient with double-vessel disease or single-vessel disease who has objective evidence of ischemia but performs well on the treadmill despite ST-segment displacement.

It will be important to determine the long-term vessel patency after coronary angioplasty and which anatomic coronary lesions can be favorably altered with lasting benefit.

It will be necessary to determine the place of angioplasty in double- and triple-vessel disease and in patients with evidence of coronary artery obstruction but little evidence of ischemia.

The role of intraoperative coronary angioplasty must be carefully investigated.

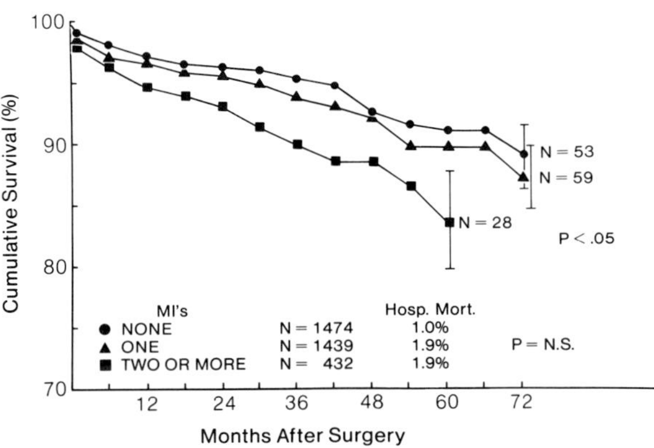

FIGURE 9 This figure shows the influence of no prior myocardial infarction, one prior infarction, and two or more infarctions on the operative mortality and survival rates at 60 months of patients who had coronary bypass surgery at Emory University.

SUMMARY

The results of coronary bypass surgery at Emory University have confirmed the studies done elsewhere.

We have found that angina pectoris is relieved in 90 percent of the patients who have the procedure; complete relief occurs in the majority of patients; bypass surgery can be performed with an overall operative risk of 1 percent; it is desirable to operate on patients before there is ventricular damage; patients have a 90 percent chance (or better) of living more than 5 years following coronary bypass surgery.

Coronary angioplasty is used primarily for patients with evidence of myocardial ischemia who have obstruction of a single coronary artery. Initial success occurs in about 90 percent of the patients and repeat angioplasty is possible in the 25 to 30 percent who have stenosis.

In practice we utilize medical treatment, surgical treatment, and coronary angioplasty. The three treatments are not viewed as competitive because there are rather specific indications for the use of each of the methods and medical therapy of some sort is almost always continued when either of the other methods is used.

Patients who were working at the time of bypass surgery return to work much more readily than patients who were not working when the procedure was done.[21]

REFERENCES

1 Sheldon, W C., Rincon, G., Pichard, A. D., Razavi, M., Cheanvechai, C., and Loop, F. D.: Surgical Treatment of Coronary Artery Disease: Pure Graft Operations, with a Study of 741 Patients Followed 3–7 Years, *Prog. Cardiovasc. Dis.*, 18(3):237, 1975.

2 Murphy, M. L., Hultgren, H. N., and Detre, K.: Treatment of Chronic Stable Angina: A Preliminary Report of Survival Data. The Randomized Veterans Administration Cooperative Study, *N. Engl. J. Med.*, 297:621, 1977.

3 Gott, V. L.: Outlook for Patients after Coronary Artery Revascularization, *Am. J. Cardiol.*, 33:431, 1974.

4 Ross, R. S.: Ischemic Heart Disease: An Overview, *Am. J. Cardiol.*, 40(5):665, 1977.

5 Lichtlen, P., Mocetti, T., Hlater, J., et al.: Postoperative Evaluation of Myocardial Blood Flow in Aorta-to-Coronary Artery Vein Bypass Grafting using Xenon-Residue Detection Technique, *Circulation*, 46:445, 1972.

6 Ormond, J., Platt, M., Mills, L., et al.: Thallium 201 Scintigraphy and Exercise Testing in Evaluating Patients Prior to and after Coronary Bypass Surgery, *Circulation*, 56(suppl. 3):131, 1977.

7 Marco, J. D.: Myocardial Perfusion following Bypass Surgery, in J. W. Hurst (ed.), "Update II:The Heart," McGraw-Hill Book Company, New York, 1980, p. 13.

8 Kent, K. M., Borer, J. S., Green, M. V., et al.: Effects of Coronary-Artery Bypass on Global and Regional Left Ventricular Function during Exercise, *N. Engl. J. Med.*, 298:1434, 1978.

9 Takaro, T., Hultgren, H. N., Lipton, M. J., et al.: The VA Cooperative Randomized Study of Surgery for Coronary Arterial Occlusive Disease. II. Subgroup with Significant Left Main Lesions, *Circulation*, 54(suppl. 3):107, 1975.

10 Read, R. C., Murphy, M. L., Hultgren, H. N., et al.: Survival of Men Treated for Chronic Stable Angina Pectoris: A Cooperative Randomized Study, *J. Thorac. Cardiovasc. Surg.*, 75:1, 1978.

11 Hurst, J. W., King, S. B., III, Logue, R. B., et al.: Value of Coronary Bypass Surgery: Controversies in Cardiology: Part I, *Am. J. Cardiol.*, 42:308, 1978.

12 Hatcher, C. R., Jr.: Coronary Bypass Surgery at Emory University Clinic: Service Organization, Surgical Technique, and Selected Surgical Results, in J.W. Hurst (ed.), "Update I:The Heart," McGraw-Hill Book Company, New York, 1979, p. 139.

13 Hurst, J. W., King, S. B., III, Walter, P. F., Friesinger, G. C., and Edwards, J. E.: Atherosclerotic Coronary Heart Disease: Angina Pectoris, Myocardial Infarction, and Other Manifestations of Myocardial Ischemia, in J. W. Hurst (ed.), "The Heart," 5th ed., McGraw-Hill Book Company, New York, 1982, p. 1091.

14 Gruentzig, A. R.: Technique of Percutaneous Transluminal Coronary Angioplasty, In J. W. Hurst (ed.), "The Heart," 5th ed., McGraw-Hill Book Company, New York, 1982, p. 1908.

15 Gruentzig, A. R.: Technique of Percutaneous Transluminal Coronary Angioplasty, in J. W. Hurst (ed.), "The Heart," 5th ed., McGraw-Hill Book Company, New York, 1982, p. 1904.

16 King, S. B., III, and Hurst, J. W.: The Relief of Angina Pectoris by Coronary Bypass Surgery, in J. W. Hurst (ed.), "Update II: The Heart," McGraw-Hill Book Company, New York, 1980.

17 Jones, E. L.: Use of the Coronary Bypass Operation in the Treatment of Selected Patients with Myocardial Infarction, in J. W. Hurst (ed.), "Update II:The Heart," McGraw-Hill Book Company, New York, 1980.

18 Jones, E. L., Waites, T. F., Craver, J. M., et al.: Coronary Bypass for Relief of Persistent Pain following Acute Myocardial Infarction, *Ann. Thorac. Surg.*, 32:33, 1981.

19 Second Interim Report by the European Coronary Surgery Study Group: Prospective Randomised Study of Coronary Artery Bypass Surgery in Stable Angina Pectoris, *Lancet*, 2:491, 1980.

20 Murphy, D. A., Craver, J. M., Jones, E. L., et al.: Surgical Revascularization following Unsuccessful Percutaneous Transluminal Coronary Angioplasty, *J. Thorac. Cardiovasc. Surg.*, 84:342, 1982.

21 Almeida, D., Bradford, J., Wenger, N. K., King, S. B., III, and Hurst, J. W.: Return to Work after Coronary Bypass Surgery, *Circulation*, 66(suppl. 2):220, 1982.

Coronary Bypass Surgery: The Total Experience at the Cleveland Clinic Foundation[*]

FLOYD D. LOOP, M.D.,
DELOS M. COSGROVE, M.D.,
PAUL C. TAYLOR, M.D.,
LEONARD A. R. GOLDING, M.D.,
BRUCE W. LYTLE, M.D., CARL C. GILL, M.D.,
and ROBERT W. STEWART, M.D.

These changes in the approach of treatment of patients with angina represent a complete turnaround of conventional teaching of ten years ago. Doctors need to recognize that the advice they used to give their patients is now outdated and that they have to learn how to take advantage of effective modern treatment for angina. Patients need no longer submit to the depressing deceleration of life that used to be their miserable medicine—the pill need not be bitter.

ANGINA: THE TREATMENT REVOLUTION[1]

Our experience in coronary artery surgery began on May 14, 1967. These early bypass operations were described by Favaloro.[2] Results from 1967 through 1970 have been reported periodically by Sheldon and colleagues and include a 10-year follow-up.[3] After 1970, all patients who underwent cardiac catheterization (or who were referred to us with films) and bypass surgery had clinical, angiographic, operative, and follow-up data coded into a cardiovascular information registry. All postoperative cardiac catheterization findings, cardiac events, including reoperation, and yearly follow-up are recorded in this data bank. After the initial 1967 to 1970 experience of 740 patients, we entered information from the first 1,000 patients who underwent isolated bypass procedures each year from 1971 through 1982. Thus, early results are available for all these years, 5-year results from 1973 through 1977 cohorts, and 10-year results from 1967 to 1970, 1971, and 1972.

INDICATIONS

There is considerable heterogeneity about referral to surgery, as shown in a Coronary Artery Surgery Study (CASS) report[4] of 11,352 patients referred for coronary artery surgery from geographically dispersed medical centers. In their survey, the relationship of severe proximal lesions to preserved wall motion in anterior and inferior left ventricular segments (defined as *myocardial jeopardy*) was the most frequent reason for surgical referral, followed by severity of angina, number of operable vessels, change in activity, unstable angina, and left main coronary artery disease. Between 1974 and 1979, the number of patients operated on for mild angina and for one-vessel disease decreased and the number of patients who underwent surgery for left main coronary artery disease increased. Assignment patterns among the 15 participating centers were diffuse; for example, the proportion of class IV angina patients referred to surgery varied from 28 percent in one hospital to 86 percent in another. These findings confirm that indications are still evolving and are based largely on results of surgery in the respective community. Although some serious differences remain in the optimal selection of patients for coronary bypass surgery, more than one therapeutic alternative is now available.

In the first 10 years of coronary artery surgery, relatively few of our patients were asymptomatic preoperatively (4 to 6 percent through 1976). In the past 5 years the percentage of patients without pain preoperatively has gradually increased to 14 percent in 1982. This selection of asymptomatic candidates is due to better pharmacologic management and represents more liberal indications. Today there is greater appreciation that the left anterior descending coronary artery is the most important of the three major vessels supplying the heart. Of all the lesions that may develop in the coronary arteries, the atherosclerotic plaque in the proximal portion of the anterior descending artery is most apt to cause a fatal infarct.[5] The final results of the prospective randomized study of patients with mild to moderate angina sponsored by the European Coronary Surgery Study Group[6] indicated that survival rate was improved significantly by surgery in patients

[*]From the Department of Thoracic and Cardiovascular Surgery, The Cleveland Clinic Foundation, Cleveland, Ohio.

with three-vessel disease and in patients with stenosis of the proximal third of the left anterior descending artery regardless of preoperative symptoms, "even when angina pectoris responds adequately to medical management."

Presently we recommend surgery for patients who have multivessel disease (ideally with focal proximal obstructions) regardless of symptom status. Surgery for one-vessel disease is based largely on an estimate of myocardial jeopardy. Anterior descending lesions are considered potentially the most dangerous. Balloon angioplasty may delay surgical intervention until multivessel disease develops, but the efficacy of this new therapy is not established. Single- or multivessel disease in asymptomatic patients with a positive submaximal exercise test has a higher priority for surgical treatment than in asymptomatic patients with negative exercise tests.[7]

Angina is a striking warning sign, but the absence of angina, especially in patients with multivessel disease, offers no long-term protection. The status of left ventricular function and extent of coronary atherosclerosis are the most important predictors of longevity, not severity of angina or any combination of risk factors.[8]

CLINICAL CHARACTERISTICS

Table 1 lists the pertinent clinical variables beginning with the initial experience of 1967 to 1970. Raw numbers may be obtained for any representative year by adding a zero to the percent (1,000 patients in each year). The median age has risen almost one decade in the 15 years surveyed. The number of female surgical candidates has increased (1967 to 1970 series excluded) to nearly 16 percent in 1982. Severe angina is defined as New York Heart Association class III or IV. From 22 to 31 percent of patients in all years had evidence of transmural infarction (new Q waves) on admission. However, approximately the same percentage of patients gave a history of myocardial infarction unconfirmed by Q waves. Diabetes is defined as clinical diabetes requiring insulin treatment. Hypertension means systolic pressure > 140 mmHg and diastolic pressure > 90 mmHg on admission to the hospital. A history of hypertension or use of diuretics was not considered sufficient information. Half the patients had a history of cigarette smoking. Hypercholesterolemia (>250 mg/dL) was found with increasing frequency in the later years.

Table 2 shows the prevalence of critical coronary atherosclerosis traditionally grouped into categories of one-, two-, and three-vessel disease. Left main coronary artery disease is listed independently. Patients with one-vessel disease have decreased in frequency to 8 percent of our practice in 1982. Patients with three-vessel disease make up two-thirds of surgical candidates, and the incidence of patients with left main disease has plateaued at 12 percent. The bottom line shows that abnormal left ventricular function has been found in more than one-half of our patients since 1979.

OPERATIVE RESULTS

Surgical trends Noteworthy surgical trends documented during the past 15 years include a doubling of mean grafts per patient from 1.5 in 1967 to 1970 to 2.9 in 1982. During the 1970s complete revascularization increased steadily. Complete revascularization is defined as grafts constructed to all arteries > 1 mm in diameter with lumen narrowing of 50 percent or more in diameter (nondominant right coronary artery excluded). Most frequently the reasons for incomplete revascularization are anatomic size of the vessel, dif-

TABLE 1
Preoperative clinical characteristics for representative years*

Clinical variable	1967–1970	1973	1976	1979	1982
Age (median)	50	53	55	56	59
Men	85%	89%	89%	88%	84%
Severe angina†	19%	47%	49%	45%	44%
Previous MI (Q wave)	22%	30%	25%	28%	31%
Diabetes	7%	7%	6%	7%	9%
Hypertension	10%	9%	7%	9%	8%
Cigarette smoking	58%	56%	53%	50%	46%
Cholesterol >250 mg/dL	35%	33%	47%	46%	50%
Triglycerides ≥140 mg/dL	60%	59%	70%	68%	62%

*Note rising median age which has increased nearly a decade when early years are compared with recent experience.

†Corresponds to New York Heart Association functional class III or IV.

TABLE 2
Prevalence of critical stenoses (≥50%) and left ventricular impairment for representative years*

Type	1967–1970(%)	1973(%)	1976(%)	1979(%)	1982(%)
One-vessel	56	17	15	10	8
Two-vessel	31	33	28	28	25
Three-vessel	13	50	57	62	67
Left main	9	8	12	12	12
LV asynergy	41	41	45	54	55

*One-vessel disease decreased in 1970 and accounts for only 8 percent of our surgical patients today. Three-vessel disease occurs in approximately two-thirds of patients and left main lesions have plateaued. Abnormal left ventricular contraction is documented in more than half of surgical patients in recent years.

fuse atherosclerosis, or presence of transmural scar tissue. In 1982, 82 percent of patients underwent complete revascularization according to these criteria. Aortic cross-clamp time per distal anastomosis has not changed appreciably over the years and has continued to average 10 min. Overall pump perfusion time has not increased significantly despite use of core cooling, cardioplegic solutions, and an increasing number of grafts per patient.

Operative mortality Operative mortality includes deaths in the operating room or during the hospital course. Operative mortality was highest in the 1967 to 1970 subset (3.0 percent). In the 1,000-patient cohorts from 1971 to 1982 mortality ranged from 0.4 to 1.8 percent, for an overall operative mortality of 1.0 percent. Interestingly, mortality in women was significantly higher (2.3 percent) than in men (0.9 percent) under age 60, but above age 60 the differences became insignificant as the mortality in men increased. Operative mortality increased sharply to 4.1 percent above age 70 in all 15 years surveyed.

Body surface area was a more significant operative risk predictor than gender. Men and women of the same size having the same status of other variables did not have significantly different risks of operative death.[9] Patients of smaller stature and less weight face a heightened risk of operative death probably because of smaller coronary vessel size, which implicates technical factors during graft construction.

Morbidity Table 3 shows morbidity for representative years. Except for neurologic deficit, all forms of major morbidity related to the bypass operation have decreased significantly when the early experience (1967 to 1970) is compared with that of later years. Perioperative myocardial infarction is defined as the appearance of new Q waves. We realize that this definition overlooks some intraoperative damage, but the definition is standardized for all years surveyed and documents a downward trend of operation-induced transmural myocardial infarction. Postoperative bleeding requiring reoperation for control declined after initiation of a blood conservation program in 1977.[10] Compared with 11 units of blood per patient per hospitalization in the early years, when blood was used to prime the oxygenator and administered liberally, blood transfusions today are infrequent. In 1982, 77 percent of patients who had isolated bypass grafts received no blood or blood products, and the number of units per patient per hospitalization decreased to 0.7 unit. Other complications such as respiratory insufficiency requiring prolonged intubation, stress gastrointestinal bleeding, and wound complications are significantly lower

TABLE 3
Morbidity rates after myocardial revascularization for representative years*

	1967–1970	1973	1976	1979	1982
Perioperative infarction	7.1%	3.9%	2.7%	1.6%	0.4%
Postoperative bleeding	10.0%	3.9%	7.3%	2.4%	1.8%
Blood units per case	11.0	6.4	5.7	1.3	0.7
Respiratory insufficiency	5.0%	1.6%	0.9%	0.6%	1.8%
Stroke	2.0%	1.9%	0.9%	2.0%	1.8%
GI bleeding	1.2%	1.4%	0.1%	0.2%	0.1%
Wound complication	2.0%	1.5%	0.6%	1.4%	1.1%

*Perioperative infarction has decreased consonant with use of cold chemical cardioplegia. The decrease in postoperative bleeding which requires reoperation is attributed to blood conservation techniques. Other major complications have decreased significantly when the first experience is compared with the most recent one. The exception is stroke, which is experienced by 1 to 2 percent of patients throughout all years.

TABLE 4
Saphenous vein graft patency in 1972–1982 patients*

Interval between surgery and catheterization (months)	Patients studied	Grafts studied	Number patent	Percent patent
Under 7	827	1,435	1,109	77.3
7–12	1,757	2,983	2,466	82.7
13–24	2,335	3,993	3,382	84.7
25–36	535	922	810	87.8
37–48	342	557	450	80.8
Over 48	1,172	1,775	1,325	74.6
Totals	6,968	11,665	9,542	81.8
Mean interval 26 months				

*The left-hand column indicates the interval in months between surgery and recatheterization, and the right-hand column shows patency for the respective interval. Overall saphenous vein patency at a mean interval of 26 months is 82 percent.

than in the early years of coronary artery surgery. Neurologic deficit persists at between 1 and 2 percent annually. Approximately half of these incidents result in little or no residual and half in major morbidity or death. Our patient population is older and manifests more multivessel disease and abnormal left ventricular function preoperatively, and yet the stroke rate has not increased. In patients above age 70, as mortality increases, the stroke rate also rises to 6 to 8 percent in all years.

LATE RESULTS
Graft Patency

Saphenous vein Saphenous vein graft patency is shown for varying intervals in Table 4. All patients who were restudied within the first 6 postoperative months had recurring angina which correlated with a lower graft patency rate. In the first 4 postoperative years vein graft patency remained in the 80th percentile, and overall for 7,000 recatheterized patients vein graft patency was 82 percent. Saphenous vein graft patency by vessel grafted was right coronary artery, 76.0 percent; left anterior descending, 83.3 percent; and circumflex, 77.8 percent.

Of 256 saphenous vein graft recipients undergoing recatheterization *serially,* first at 12 months or less (median 10 months) and then at 48 months or more (median 83 months), we found these results at the first catheterization: right coronary artery grafts, 127 of 151 (84 percent); anterior descending, 133 of 143 (93 percent); and circumflex, 85 of 100 (85 percent) patent. Of grafts patent at the first catheterization, the second catheterization yielded right coronary artery grafts, 94 of 127 (74 percent); anterior descending, 106 of 133 (80 percent); and circumflex, 60 of 85 (71 percent). Thus, after a median interval of 10 months, 88 percent of vein grafts were open, and of those that were open 75 percent remained open after a median interval of 83 months. Cumulative graft patency after a median interval of 83 months in these 256 patients was right coronary artery

TABLE 5
Internal mammary artery graft patency for patients 1972–1982*

Interval between surgery and catheterization (months)	Patients studied	Grafts studied	Number patent	Percent patent
Under 7	226	229	220	96.1
7–12	571	575	557	96.9
13–24	739	745	715	96.0
25–36	158	159	152	95.6
37–48	136	138	130	94.2
Over 48	280	281	268	95.4
Totals	2,110	2,127	2,042	96.0
Mean interval 19 months				

*The mammary artery graft patency for each interval is displayed in the right-hand column and overall patency is 96 percent after a mean interval of 18 months.

TABLE 6
Graft patency correlated with estimated severity of coronary artery narrowing

	Estimated reduction in lumen diameter*				
Graft†	0–49%	50–74%	75–99%	100%	Total grafts
IMA to anterior descending	10, 80%	154, 95%	665, 96%	304, 98%	1,133, 96%
Vein to anterior descending	34, 74%	245, 86%	1133, 85%	405, 90%	1,817, 86%
Vein to circumflex	40, 73%	315, 83%	992, 82%	397, 82%	1,744, 82%
Vein to right coronary	36, 92%	245, 79%	836, 81%	677, 77%	1,794, 79%

*The number of grafts studied is printed next to the patency.

†IMA = internal mammary artery. Both mammary artery and saphenous vein grafts show a satisfactory patency for preoperative "moderate" obstruction estimated at 40 to 50 percent.

grafts, 62 percent; anterior descending, 74 percent; and circumflex, 60 percent. The cumulative graft patency was 66 percent at 7 years.

Internal mammary artery Internal mammary artery graft patency is shown in the same format for varying intervals in Table 5. In contrast to the vein graft, the mammary artery has shown little attrition and the overall patency rate in 2,000 internal mammary artery grafts restudied is 96 percent. Nearly all of these grafts were constructed to the anterior descending artery. When vein graft patency was compared with internal mammary artery graft patency for the anterior descending alone, the mammary artery had a 96 percent patency in 1,557 arteries recatheterized as opposed to 83 percent for the saphenous vein in 2,999 restudies performed between 1974 and 1979.

Serial internal mammary artery graft studies at a mean interval of 14 months for 141 grafts studied initially showed a 98.5 percent patency. When these 139 open grafts were again restudied after a mean interval of 81 months, 134 (96.4 percent) were open. The overall internal mammary graft patency at 81 months was 134 of 141 (95.0 percent).

Mammary artery and vein graft patencies have been correlated with the severity of coronary artery obstruction (Table 6). Results in grafting the moderate obstruction (estimated 40 to 50 percent narrowing) support the extended grafting criteria that have evolved in the past 5 years.[11]

Angina Relief at 5 and 10 Years

Intermediate and late symptom status has been determined at 10 years for the 740 patients operated on from 1967 to 1970 and for the 1,000-patient cohorts operated

on in 1971 and 1972, and at 5 years for the 1,000-patient cohorts operated on each year from 1973 to 1977. Trained personnel in the cardiovascular registry elicited the follow-up information. Since angina cannot be accurately classified from telephone contact with patients, we recorded only complete angina relief at 5 and 10 years and correlated angina relief with extent of coronary atherosclerosis preoperatively, i.e., one-, two-, three-vessel, and left main artery disease (Table 7). We find no difference in postoperative angina status when comparing single to multivessel disease.

TABLE 7
Intermediate and late symptom status*

Cohort	1967–1970	1971–1972	1973–1977
Years of follow-up	10	10	5
Patients for whom angina status reported	442	1,545	4,474
Patients asymptomatic	287	976	3,100
Percent asymptomatic	64.9%	63.2%	69.3%
One-vessel	167 of 248 67.3%	220 of 300 73.3%	511 of 713 71.7%
Two-vessel	85 of 137 62.0%	427 of 700 61.0%	1,207 of 1,772 68.1%
Three-vessel	35 of 57 61.4%	329 of 545 60.4%	1,382 of 1,989 69.5%
Left main	27 of 46 58.7%	100 of 158 63.3%	303 of 433 70.0%

*Angina-free patients at 5 and 10 years are shown in percent and categorized according to one-, two-, three-vessel, and left main artery disease. No difference in angina relief is noted between one-vessel and multivessel disease patients.

Relief of angina Angina relief has been correlated with graft patency in patients who had a coronary arteriogram within the first 2 years postoperatively. At 5 years complete angina relief was reported in 431 of 613 (70 percent) patients who had all grafts patent. This figure was the same as 145 of 217 (67 percent) of patients who had at least one graft patent, but it was significantly better than the 30 percent (3 of 10) of patients who had all grafts occluded. At 10 years those with all grafts patent had a higher reported complete relief of angina, 217 of 330 (66 percent) than those who had at least one graft patent, 78 of 147 (53 percent), and those with all grafts occluded, 12 of 25 (48 percent).

In the 1967 to 1970 cohort, 42 (57.5 percent) of 73 surviving women and 320 (63.4 percent) of 505 surviving men were asymptomatic at *10 years*. For the 1971 and 1972 1,000-patient cohorts, 84 (56.0 percent) of 150 surviving women were angina-free in comparison with 944 (65.8 percent) of 1,435 surviving men at 10 years. All survivors among the first 1,000 surgical patients each year from 1973 to 1977 were contacted for a minimum follow-up of 5 years. At *5 years* 298 (60.6 percent) of 492 women were angina-free in comparison with 2,938 (71.4 percent) of 4,112 men. Thus, relief of angina 5 and 10 years postoperatively was less in women than in men.

Longevity

Ten-year survival rate Ten-year survival rate has been determined for three groups of patients: (1) 740 patients operated on in 1967 to 1970, (2) the first 1,000 patients in 1971, and (3) the first 1,000 patients in 1972. Survival curves include all early and late deaths and deaths from all causes. Ten-year survival rate for these three groups is shown in Fig. 1. The 1967 to 1970 patients had a 78 percent survival rate; however, more than half these patients had one-vessel disease preoperatively. The 1971 patients achieved a 76 percent 10-year survival rate and 1972 patients, 81 percent. The 5 percent higher survival rate in 1972 cannot be explained on the basis of preoperative clinical characteristics, operative mortality, or grafts per patient. The only significantly different variable was increased use of the internal mammary artery graft, which reached 26 percent in 1972 compared with minimal use in 1971. This finding bears watching in future years. For 342 single-vessel disease patients 10-year survival rate according to vessel grafted was left anterior descending, 90.2 percent, right coronary artery, 87.2 percent, and circumflex, 65.5 percent.

Five-year survival rate We assessed 5-year survival rate for 1,000-patient cohorts each year from 1973 through 1977. In Fig. 2 this 5-year follow-up for the

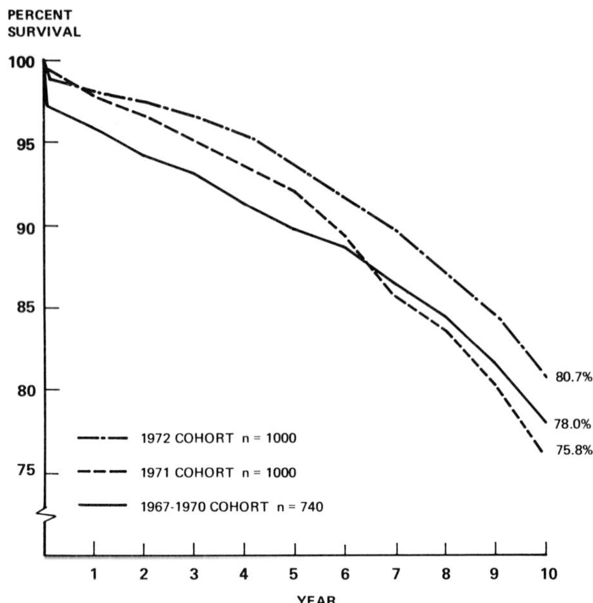

FIGURE 1 Ten-year survival rate for three cohorts of isolated myocardial revascularization patients. The 1967 to 1970 patients had a 78.0 percent 10-year survival rate; however, 56 percent of the patients in that cohort had one-vessel disease. In 1971 and 1972 the prevalence of one-vessel disease preoperatively was 18 percent. Survival rate of 1971 patients was 75.8 percent, and for 1972 10-year survival rate was 80.7 percent.

combined cohorts is divided into categories of one-, two-, three-vessel, and left main artery disease. In contrast to other reports we find a significant difference in 5- and 10-year longevity between single-vessel and multivessel disease patients. The overall 5-year survival is 93.6 percent for the 1973 to 1977 patients. In the single-vessel disease category, patients with left anterior descending lesions had a higher 5-year survival rate (96.6 percent) than patients with isolated circumflex (94.1 percent) or right coronary artery disease (95.5 percent). This finding is interesting because anterior descending obstruction is purportedly the most dangerous of serious obstructions in the three major arteries. We speculate that revascularization of the anterior descending artery offers more protection when the patient experiences progression in either the right or circumflex or both as opposed to patients who receive a bypass graft for either right or circumflex lesions and then later experience obstruction in the anterior descending artery.

For patients with normal or near-normal left ventricular function at operation 5-year survival rate is 94.0 percent, in contrast to 85.0 percent for the subset of patients with moderate or severe left ventricular dysfunction. Patients who underwent complete revas-

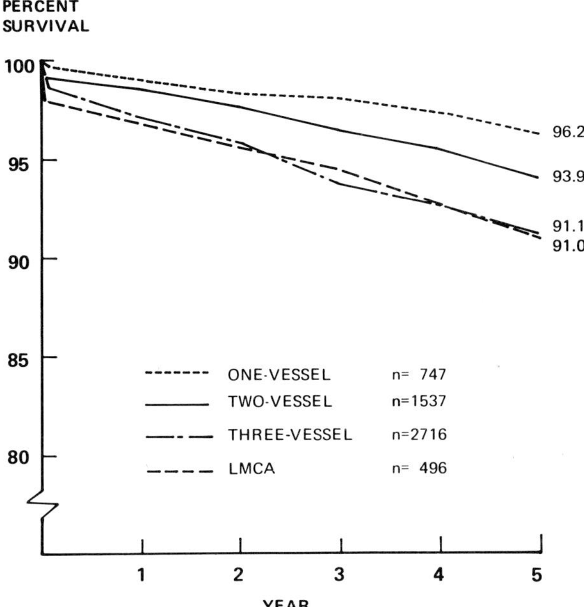

FIGURE 2 Five-year survival rate for 1973 to 1977 patients, who have been categorized according to the number of vessels involved (left main calculated independently). We find that one- and two-vessel patients have a higher survival rate than three-vessel or left main disease patients.

cularization (58 percent) achieved a 94.4 percent 5-year survival rate compared with 90.4 percent for those who underwent incomplete revascularization.

Fatal infarction   Late fatal myocardial infarction in the first 10 postoperative years was documented in 64 of 191 (34 percent) of 1967 to 1970 cohort late fatalities and in 148 of 392 (38 percent) late patient deaths in the 1971 to 1972 cohort. Of the 1973 to 1977 surgical patients followed for 5 years, 82 of 342 (24 percent) had documented fatal infarction. For these three groups, frequencies of late fatal myocardial infarction in patients who survived the operation were 8.9 percent, 7.5 percent, and 1.8 percent, respectively.

Nonfatal infarction   Nonfatal myocardial infarction was documented in 130 of 525 (25 percent) of the 1967 to 1970 surviving patients and in 268 of 1,585 (17 percent) of 1971 to 1972 surgical survivors during the first 10 postoperative years. In the first 5 years of follow-up for the 1973 to 1977 patients, 468 of 4,602 (10 percent) patients experienced nonfatal myocardial infarction. These data underestimate the true incidence of nonfatal myocardial infarction because an undetermined number were silent. Together the known fatal and nonfatal infarction rate annualized for 5-year follow-up is 3.2 percent per year (perioperative infarction included). For the 1971 to 1972 patients the annualized

rate per year over 10 years (perioperative infarctions included) is 2.8 percent. We have not calculated this figure for the 1967 to 1970 patients because the prevalence of single-vessel disease was unusually high.

REOPERATIONS

Coronary artery reoperations were performed in 17 percent of the 1967 to 1970 patients within the first 10 postoperative years. In the 1971 cohort, 10 percent were reoperated on in the next 10 years, but for 1972 patients, only 7 percent were reoperated on within 10 years. Our first coronary artery reoperation series of 1,000 patients (isolated bypass grafts only) was divided into four cohorts of 250 patients each.[12] Graft failure as a reoperative indication increased from 26 percent in the first cohort (1969 to 1976) to 40 percent in the last cohort (1981 to 1982), presumably due to more late graft closures 5 to 10 years postoperatively. Progressive atherosclerosis, most frequently in previously ungrafted vessels, has declined as an indication from 62 percent to 23 percent, which signifies more complete revascularization at the first operation. The prevalence of three-vessel disease among reoperation patients has increased to 73 percent and left main lesions to 18 percent; one-third of patients lose normal ventricular function in the interval between operations. This interval continues to lengthen and now averages 6½ years.

Table 8 lists mortality and major morbidity rates for

TABLE 8
Mortality and major morbidity rates*

	1967–1976	1976–1979	1979–1981	1981–1982
	12	8	6	5
Operative mortality	4.8%	3.2%	2.4%	2.0%
Perioperative	19	14	17	13
myocardial	7.6%	5.6%	6.8%	5.2%
infarction				
Bleeding requiring	22	29	19	11
reopening	8.8%	11.6%	7.6%	4.4%
Mean blood units	9.5	5.9	2.7	1.9
Neurologic deficit	5	3	6	6
	2.0%	1.2%	2.4%	2.4%
Respiratory	8	19	4	1
dysfunction	3.2%	7.6%	1.6%	0.4%
Wound	3	7	4	1
complication	1.2%	2.8%	1.6%	0.4%

*Our first 1,000 coronary artery reoperation patients have been divided into four 250-patient cohorts and the years of reoperation are shown above. Operative mortality has decreased from 5 percent to 2 percent, perioperative infarction rate declined slightly, and other complications have been significantly reduced with the exception of neurologic deficit. Blood conservation techniques have reduced blood usage from ten units per patient for each hospitalization to two units.

the time periods under consideration. Reoperative mortality rate has decreased from 5 to 2 percent, and every form of major morbidity except neurologic deficit has decreased when the incidence of complications in the early years is compared with the latest experience. The number of grafts per patient has increased from 1.4 to 2.3 in reoperations, and complete revascularization has increased from 65 to 76 percent. After a mean of 29 months, graft patency was 81 percent overall in 153 patients restudied after reoperation. Patency was similar for grafts to arteries previously involved with graft failure and for grafts to arteries not previously grafted. For patients in the first three cohorts (mean follow-up 57 months) 5-year actuarial survival was 89 percent. Survival rate was not significantly affected by the reason for reoperation, i.e., graft closure, progressive atherosclerosis, or combined indications.

REFERENCES

1 Angina: The Treatment Revolution, *Br. Med. J.*, 2:1167, 1979.

2 Favaloro, R. G.: Saphenous Vein Autograft Replacement of Severe Segmental Coronary Artery Occlusion. Operative Technique, *Ann. Thorac. Surg.*, 5:334, 1968.

3 Sheldon, W. C., Loop, F. D., and Proudfit, W.L.: Bypass Graft Surgery for Coronary Artery Disease. A 10–13 Year Follow-up Study of 741 Patients, *Am. J. Cardiol.*, 47:485, 1981. (Abstract.)

4 Alderman, E. L., Fisher, L, Maynard, C., et al: Determinants of Coronary Surgery in a Consecutive Patient Series from Geographically Dispersed Medical Centers. The Coronary Artery Surgery Study, *Circulation* 66(suppl. 1): i–6, 1982

5 Schuster, E. H., Griffith, L. S., and Bulkley, B. H. Preponderance of Acute Proximal Left Anterior Descending Coronary Arterial Lesions in Fatal Myocardial Infarction. A Clinicopathologic Study, *Am. J. Cardiol.*, 47:1189, 1981.

6 European Coronary Surgery Study Group: Long-term Results of Prospective Randomized Study of Coronary Artery Bypass Surgery in Stable Angina Pectoris, *Lancet*, 2:1173, 1982.

7 Epstein, S. E., Palmeri S. T., and R. E. Patterson: Evaluation of Patients after Acute Myocardial Infarction. Indications for Cardiac Catheterization and Surgical Intervention, *N. Engl. J. Med.*, 307:1487, 1982.

8 Proudfit, W. L., Bruschke, A. V. G., and Sones F. M. Jr.: Natural History of Obstructive Coronary Artery Disease. Ten-year Study of 601 Nonsurgical Cases, *Prog. Cardiovasc. Dis.*, 21:53, 1978.

9 Loop, F. D., Golding, L. R., MacMillan J. P., Cosgrove D. M., Lytle, B. W., and Sheldon, W. C.: Coronary Artery Surgery in Women Compared with Men: Analysis of Risks and Long-term Results, *J. Am. Coll. Cardiol.*, 1:383, 1983.

10 Cosgrove, D. M., Loop, F. D., and Lytle, B. W.: Blood Conservation in Cardiac Surgery, in A.N. Brest (ed.), "Cardiovascular Therapy," F. A. Davis Company, Philadelphia, 1982, 12:165-176.

11 Cosgrove, D. M., Loop, F. D., Saunders, C. R., Lytle, B. W., and Kramer, J. R.: Should Coronary Arteries with Less than 50% Stenosis Be Bypassed? *J. Thorac. Cardiovasc. Surg.*, 82:520, 1981.

12 Loop, F. D., Lytle, B. W., Gill, C. C., Golding, L. R., Cosgrove, D. M., and Taylor, P. C.: Trends in Selection and Results of Coronary Artery Reoperations, *Ann. Thorac. Surg.*, in press.

Coronary Bypass Surgery in the 1980s[*]

DONALD W. MILLER, JR., M.D., and
DOUGLAS D. JOHNSON, M.D.

> We may have heard a milestone in cardiac surgery today, because for years pathologists, cardiologists, and many surgeons have repeatedly stated that the pattern of coronary artery disease is so extensive that direct anastomosis can be done in only 5 to 7 percent of patients. If the exciting data by Dr. (W. Dudley) Johnson remain valid, and the grafts remain patent over a long period of time, a total revision of thinking will be required regarding the feasibility of direct arterial surgery for coronary artery disease.
>
> FRANK C. SPENCER, M.D., 1969[††]

We, the authors of this chapter, began our careers in cardiac surgery as thoracic surgery residents in 1972 and 1974, respectively, shortly after coronary bypass surgery began to be performed on a wide scale across the United States. In 1970, 2,000 bypass operations were performed nationwide. The number of bypass operations done rose to 50,000 per year by 1975, and by 1980 more than 100,000 bypass operations were being done each year in the United States.

The coronary bypass operation that we are now practicing in the 1980s, however, is considerably different from that which we were trained to do in the early 1970s. Over the last 10 years, important changes have occurred in the selection of patients for bypass surgery, in surgical techniques, and in the results of bypass surgery. An increasingly larger percentage of bypass operations are now being done in community hospital medical centers, and the composition of the cardiac surgical team now often includes a paraprofessional surgeons' or physicians' assistant in lieu of surgical residents. Also, a growing number of cardiac surgeons have established a computerized data registry in their practice for data storage and retrieval.

We propose to review these various developments in the practice of coronary bypass surgery. We will refer to our recent clinical experience, which illustrates well the current state of the art of this operation, and to several national surveys that we have conducted on techniques used for bypass surgery. The clinical experience presented in this chapter spans a period from July 1980, when we instituted a computerized data registry, through June 1982. During this 2-year interval, we carried out isolated coronary bypass surgery in 654 consecutive patients at the Swedish Hospital Medical Center in Seattle (Table 1). The surveys cited in this chapter were carried out in 1975 and 1980.

In 1975, we conducted a survey of techniques used for bypass surgery by 400 cardiac surgeons who collectively performed nearly 80 percent of the bypass operations done that year.[2] In 1980, we surveyed 677 cardiac surgeons who performed nearly 90 percent of the estimated 104,000 procedures done that year.[3] Also in 1980, we surveyed 811 cardiopulmonary perfusionists on their professional activities and the techniques they used for extracorporeal circulation for cardiac surgery.[4] These surveys provide a broad perspective on this operation and also document some of the important changes that have occurred on a nationwide scale in the techniques used for coronary bypass surgery since the early 1970s.

SELECTION OF PATIENTS FOR CORONARY BYPASS SURGERY

Two treatment goals can be defined for patients who have coronary heart disease: to improve quality of life and to extend survival.[5] Bypass surgery has been shown to achieve both of these goals in patients with coronary artery disease.[6,7]

Angina Pectoris

The primary indication for a bypass operation continues to be to relieve disabling symptoms of angina pectoris unresponsive to adequate treatment. In our last 654 patients who had isolated bypass surgery, 649 patients had symptoms of angina pectoris. Only 5 patients did not have angina. The definitions of "disabling" angina and "adequate" medical treatment, however, are quite subjective, and these criteria are interpreted in a variety of ways both by patients and their physicians. Furthermore, in recommending a bypass operation, the competence and record of the surgical team to which the patient would be referred for surgery must also be considered. A hypothetical retired male executive may feel that his quality of life is seriously impaired if he is unable to play golf without provoking anginal symptoms. He might want to undergo bypass surgery if the operative mortality risk is only 1 percent,

[*]From Northwest Cardiac Surgery Associates, Seattle, Washington

[†]Discussing one of the first papers that was presented on coronary bypass surgery by Dr. W. Dudley Johnson at the annual meeting of the American Surgical Association, April 30–May 3, 1969.

TABLE 1

Isolated coronary bypass surgery in 654 consecutive patients operated upon at the Swedish Hospital Medical Center, July 1980–June 1982

		Number of patients
Age (years) = mean (range)	60.7 (28–83)	
Patients ≥ 70 years old		115 (17.6%)
History of angina pectoris		649 (99.2%)
Preinfarction angina		27 (4.1%)
History of myocardial infarction		325 (49.7%)
Recent infarction (≤ 6 weeks)		81 (12.4%)
History of sudden death		27 (4.1%)
Number of diseased vessels (≥ 70% stenosis):		
One vessel		71 (10.8%)
Two vessels		158 (24.2%)
Three vessels		341 (52.2%)
Left main coronary stenosis (≥ 50% stenosis)		84 (12.8%)
Ejection fraction (629 patients) ≤ 40%		50 (7.9%)
Number of bypass grafts = mean (range)	3.2 (1–6)	
Time on cardiopulmonary bypass (min) = mean (range)	69.0 (19–160)	
Cardioplegic arrest time (min) = mean (range)	37.9 (7–86)	
Hospital stay postoperatively (days) = mean (range)	7.5 (4–114)	
Operative mortality:		12 (1.8%)
539 patients < 70 years		6 (1.1%)
115 patients ≥ 70 years		6 (5.2%)
Preoperative infarction (Q wave)		11 (1.7%)
Neurologic sequelae		9 (1.4%)
Bleeding requiring reoperation		7 (1.2%)
Sternal dehiscence		7 (1.2%)

but he might not feel sufficiently disabled to want to have surgery if the operative mortality risk is 5 percent.

It has now been established by randomized studies that a bypass operation improves survival in symptomatic patients with three-vessel coronary disease and in those with left main coronary artery stenosis.[7] A bypass operation is indicated, therefore, in patients with severe three-vessel disease or left main coronary artery stenosis even if their anginal symptoms are relatively mild. In our recent experience, 341 patient (52 percent) had three-vessel disease (greater than 70 percent arterial diameter narrowing) and 84 patients (12.8 percent) had left main coronary artery stenosis (greater than 50 percent narrowing). Of our patients 71 (10.8 percent) had single-vessel disease, and 158 patients (24.1 percent) had two-vessel disease.

Symptoms of angina pectoris are most disabling when they occur at rest. Anginal symptoms occurred at rest at some time in the course of their disease in 270 of our 654 patients (41 percent). Angina at rest could be controlled by hospitalization and medical treatment in all but 27 of these patients. Surgery was carried out on an elective basis during the same hospitalization after cardiac catheterization, or during a second hospitalization several days to several months after the arteriographic studies. Most patients who experience angina at rest (i.e., unstable angina) respond to medical management and do not require emergency coronary bypass surgery. Indeed, several studies have shown that emergency surgery for unstable angina carries a greater risk of myocardial infarction and operative mortality than does inhospital medical treatment followed by elective surgery when necessary.[8,9] The indications for a bypass operation in patients with unstable angina are essentially the same as those for patients who have only effort angina—to improve quality of life and, when severe multivessel disease is present, to extend length of life.

Only 27 of our patients (4.1 percent) had angina at rest that could not be controlled by inhospital bed rest, beta blocking agents, long-acting nitrates, and slow-channel calcium antagonists (i.e., had preinfarction angina). Continuous intravenous vasodilator therapy (22 patients) or intraaortic balloon pump support (5 patients) was necessary to stabilize these patients before coronary arteriography and bypass surgery were performed. Rest angina also occurred shortly after an acute myocardial infarction (i.e., postinfarct angina) in 8 patients.

In managing patients with medically refractory unstable angina, we first attempt to control their symptoms with an intravenous nitroglycerin drip while they are being monitored with continuously recorded pulmonary artery and radial artery pressures. If the patient's anginal symptoms still cannot be controlled, then intraaortic balloon pump support is established. This is usually done in the catheterization laboratory by the cardiologist with a percutaneously inserted intraaortic balloon. Hemodynamic support with an intraaortic balloon pump generally provides immediate relief of rest angina, as was the case in the five patients with preinfarction angina and in the four of our eight patients with postinfarct angina who required this treatment modality. Bypass surgery can then be carried out on a nonemergency basis in a hemodynamically stable patient.

Acute Myocardial Infarction

While some surgeons have advocated immediate bypass surgery for acute, uncomplicated myocardial infarction, this indication for a bypass operation remains controversial, particularly now in the 1980s following the introduction of streptokinase therapy for acute myocardial infarction.[10] Nevertheless, the experience of Berg and others has shown that bypass surgery can be carried out in the presence of an acute myocardial infarction with a very low operative mortality risk.[11] In our experience, 325 patients (50 percent) had a history of a previous myocardial infarction; 81 of these patients (25 percent) had a myocardial infarction within 6 weeks of surgery, and 29 patients were operated on within 2 weeks of their infarction (15 had a transmural infarction and 14 a nontransmural infarction). We carried out immediate bypass surgery for an acute, uncomplicated myocardial infarction in only 8 patients. Coronary arteriography had been done previously in all of these patients, and bypass surgery had been previously contemplated.

Cardiac surgeons have become more aggressive in performing bypass surgery shortly after a myocardial infarction, particularly in two types of patients: (1) those who continue to have angina at rest following an acute transmural or nontransmural myocardial infarction and (2) those who are found to have severe, multivessel coronary artery disease on arteriography which is done shortly after a nontransmural infarction. The risk of bypass surgery is not increased in patients who are operated upon early after a nontransmural

infarction.[6] Also, patients with postinfarct angina can be operated upon with a relatively low risk if they are first stabilized, with an intraaortic balloon pump if necessary. Immediate bypass surgery for an uncomplicated acute myocardial infarction, however, is not a widely accepted indication for a bypass operation.[6,10] At the present time, for many surgical teams the primary indication for immediate bypass surgery is failed coronary angioplasty.

Asymptomatic or Minimally Symptomatic Patients

Symptoms of angina pectoris develop in only approximately 30 to 40 percent of people who have coronary heart disease. The initial clinical event in the majority of people with coronary heart disease is either a myocardial infarction, sudden death, or the discovery of an abnormal electrocardiogram at rest or during exercise. Although they have no angina, some of these people will nevertheless have an impaired quality of life owing to their coronary disease. They "tire easily," or become short of breath with mild to moderate exertion from myocardial ischemia that occurs during exercise. Such patients are generally considered to be "asymptomatic" in the sense that they do not have symptoms of angina pectoris. Coronary arteriography is done usually because a treadmill test was found to be positive or because of a history of a myocardial infarction. If the physician can document exercise-induced myocardial ischemia by electrocardiographic or isotope studies, and if the patient is found on coronary arteriography to have advanced three-vessel disease (greater than 70 percent stenosis) or left main coronary artery stenosis, then a reasonable but as yet unproven argument can be made for recommending coronary bypass surgery.[5] If a minimally symptomatic patient with severe coronary artery disease tires easily or has dyspnea on exertion, a bypass operation can eliminate these symptoms. Also, since symptomatic patients who have severe multivessel coronary disease have improved survival with bypass surgery compared with medical treatment, it is reasonable to postulate that asymptomatic patients (i.e., those who do not have angina pectoris) with equally severe disease will also have an improved survival with surgery. Indeed, a variety of natural history studies of patients with angina pectoris have shown that the frequency and severity of anginal symptoms are unrelated to survival; other clinical findings such as hypertension, abnormalities on the resting electrocardiogram, and exercise-induced hypotension, along with the number of diseased coronary vessels found on arteriography, are much better predictors of survival.[6] Unfortunately, there are no studies that have been done that satisfactorily answer the question: Does bypass surgery improve survival in asymptomatic patients with coronary disease?[12]

In our practice, only 5 out of 654 patients, less than 1 percent, were asymptomatic. These patients had strongly positive ST-segment changes on treadmill test and were found to have severe multivessel coronary disease on arteriography.

Advanced Age

When we began our training in cardiac surgery in the early 1970s, bypass surgery was considered to be relatively contraindicated in people over the age of 70. But as the techniques of bypass surgery have improved, the operation has been extended to increasingly elderly patients. Most patients over the age of 70 can undergo coronary bypass surgery safely and enjoy a striking improvement in their quality of life. In the last 2 years, almost one out of every five of our patients having a bypass operation was over the age of 70 (115 of 654 patients). Indeed 11 of these patients were over the age of 80. Women constituted 30 percent of our patients over the age of 70, whereas only 15 percent of our patients less than 70 years old were women. The mean age of our patient population was 60.7 years, with age ranging from 28 to 83 years. Advanced age is no longer a contraindication for coronary bypass surgery.

SURGICAL TECHNIQUE

The surgical techniques used for coronary bypass surgery in the 1980s differ substantially from the surgical techniques that were used for this operation in the early 1970s. Simple bypass grafts and intermittent ischemic arrest characterized the coronary bypass operation done in 1975; sequential bypass grafts and continuous cold cardioplegic arrest are the hallmarks of the coronary bypass operation that is now practiced in the 1980s.[3,4]

Cardiopulmonary Bypass

As evidenced by both our 1975 and 1980 national surveys, the techniques used for cardiopulmonary bypass have become well-standardized.[2,4] We carry out cardiopulmonary bypass, as do most cardiac surgeons, with a disposable bubble oxygenator and a constant-output roller blood pump. The Silastic tubes through which blood flows through the extracorporeal circuit are connected to the patient with a cannula inserted into the ascending aorta and a cannula inserted into the right atrium. In the early 1970s, most surgeons also vented the left ventricle with a cannula inserted either through the apex of the left ventricle or through the right superior pulmonary vein, but in recent years an increasing number of surgeons, including us, no longer use a left ventricular vent for bypass surgery.[3] Before instituting cardiopulmonary bypass, adequacy of heparinization is confirmed by measuring the activated clotting time. Extracorporeal circulation is carried out with a flow rate of 2.4 L/(min)(m²), the blood pressure is maintained between 40 and 80 mmHg, and the patient is cooled to a systemic temperature of 30°C. Along with a growing number of cardiac surgeons,[4] we take special precautions to prevent air emboli by using a low-level photoelectric alarm on the bubble oxygenator and by using an air-bubble sensor that automatically shuts down the heart-lung machine when air bubbles are detected in the arterial line.

In our last 654 bypass operations, the average time on the heart-lung machine was 69 min, ranging from 19 to 160 min. During this time we placed an average of 3.2 bypass grafts per patient.

Cold Potassium Cardioplegia

Precise coronary artery bypass grafting requires a bloodless, motionless operative field, and in the early years of coronary bypass surgery, these necessary operating conditions were obtained by placement of a clamp across the ascending aorta to interrupt coronary blood flow and thereby produce ischemic cardiac arrest. In 1975, approximately 6 percent of cardiac surgeons had begun infusing a cold, potassium-enriched, physiological saline solution into the aortic root to achieve profound cardiac hypothermia and prompt electromechanical arrest.[2] The myocardial protection provided by cold cardioplegic arrest permitted the duration of aortic cross-clamping to be extended from 20 min, the upper limit for safely subjecting a heart to ischemic arrest during moderate systemic hypothermia (30°C), to 90 min or more when a cold potassium cardioplegic solution is infused intermittently through the aortic root.

By 1980, more than 90 percent of cardiac surgeons had adopted this technique of myocardial protection for coronary bypass surgery.[3] Sophisticated techniques have been devised to administer the cardioplegic solution and keep it cold. The system which we use is shown in Fig. 1. The cardioplegic solution consists of a Ringers lactate solution which is enriched with 15 mEq of KCl. It is continuously recirculated through an ice bucket using one of the secondary pump heads on the heart-lung machine in order to maintain the temperature of the solution at 4°C. When the aortic cross-clamp is applied, the cardioplegic solution is infused intermittently to maintain the intramyocardial temperature below 20°C, as measured by a thermistor probe placed into the interventricular septum.

In our 654 coronary bypass surgery patients, the

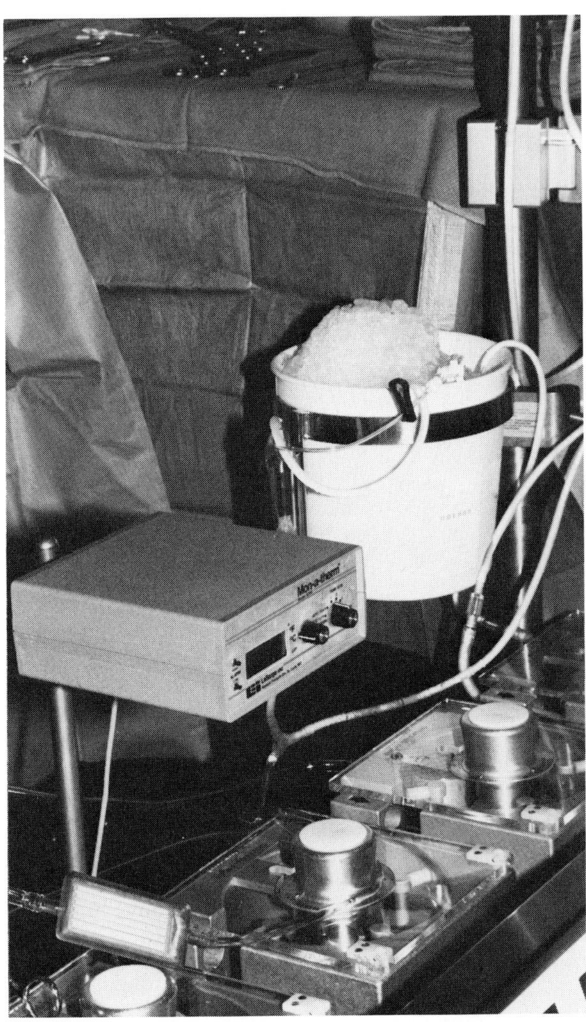

A

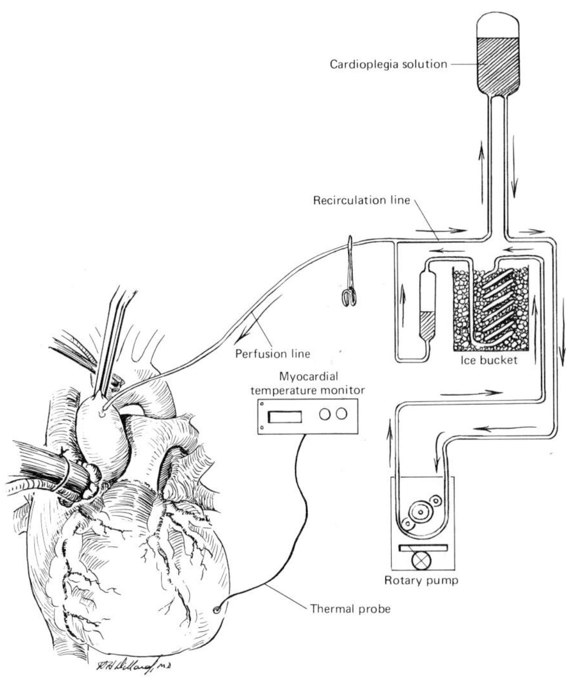

B

FIGURE 1 Delivery of cold potassium cardioplegic solution into the aortic root with the heart-lung machine. *(A)* An auxiliary pump head on the heart-lung machine is used to continuously recirculate the cardioplegic solution to maintain its temperature at 4°C. *(B)* The cardioplegic solution is intermittently infused into the aortic root after the aortic cross-clamp is applied, and the intramyocardial temperature is monitored with a thermistor probe, *(From D. H. Dillard and D. W. Miller, Jr., "Atlas of Cardiac Surgery," Macmillan Publishing Company, New York, 1983, plate XVIII. Reproduced with permission.)*

average cardioplegic arrest time was 37.9 min (range 7 to 86 min).

In 1980, 90 percent of cardiac surgeons surveyed used a crystalloid cardioplegic solution, and 10 percent used cold blood.[3] Other agents which are often added to the cardioplegic solution, in addition to potassium, include sodium bicarbonate, mannitol, glucose, insulin, magnesium, steroids, and, recently, nifedipine.[3,10] No one type of cardioplegic solution has been shown to be superior to another. Cold cardioplegic arrest is an important innovation which has substantially reduced the risk of coronary bypass surgery.

Sequential Bypass Grafts

This technique of bypass grafting (Fig. 2) is another important advance that has occurred in coronary bypass surgery.[10,13,14] Sequential grafts were used in 72 percent of our patients operated on over the last 2 years. Anterior sequential grafts employing two to four distal anastomoses were used in 308 patients to revascularize the left anterior descending coronary artery and its diagonal branches. Right- or left-sided posterior sequential grafts with two to five distal anastomoses were used in 399 patients to revascularize circumflex marginal branches and posterior descending branches of the right coronary artery. A single circular sequential graft with four to six distal anastomoses was employed in 42 patients.

In 1975, approximately 50 percent of surgeons surveyed reported that they had had some experience using sequential grafts.[2] In our second national survey in 1980, however, more than 90 percent of surgeons stated that they routinely used sequential grafts in their bypass operations.[3] A side-to-side saphenous vein–coronary artery anastomosis is more difficult to con-

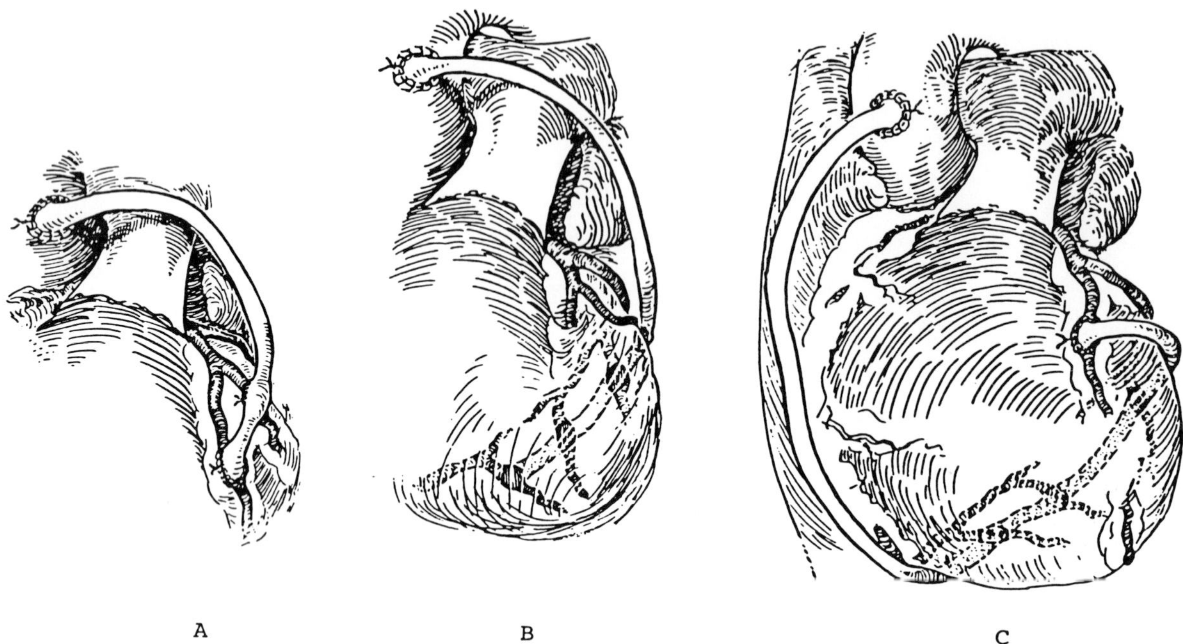

FIGURE 2 Types of sequential bypass grafts. *(A)* Anterior sequential graft with a side-to-side anastomosis to the diagonal artery and an end-to-side anastomosis to the left anterior descending coronary artery. *(B)* A left-sided posterior sequential graft. *(C)* A circular sequential graft. *(From D. H. Dillard and D. W. Miller, Jr., "Atlas of Cardiac Surgery," Macmillan Publishing Company, New York, 1983, plate XXIX. Reproduced with permission.)*

struct than an end-to-side anastomosis, but when expertly performed, sequential bypass grafts have been shown to have higher patency rates and more favorable hemodynamic characteristics than simple bypass grafts.[13,14] Sequential bypass grafts permit the surgeon to graft small, 1-mm coronary arteries that are not large enough to be revascularized with a simple bypass graft because the blood flow through the saphenous vein graft to that vessel alone might not be sufficient to maintain long-term graft patency. By reducing the number of proximal anastomoses that have to be performed, sequential grafts have the added advantage that manipulation of the ascending aorta is minimized. Minimizing manipulation of the ascending aorta will further decrease the rare but catastrophic complication of aortic dissection and will also shorten cardiopulmonary bypass time. We rarely construct more than two proximal anastomoses; one vein conduit is used for sequential anastomoses to coronary arteries on the anterior surface of the heart, and another vein conduit, directed either around the left or right side of the heart, is used to revascularize vessels on the posterior and lateral surface of the heart.

The saphenous vein remains the conduit of choice for coronary bypass grafting. The internal mammary artery is used routinely by only a very small percentage of surgeons,[2,3] and the cephalic vein is used for bypass grafting only when necessary.

RESULTS

The results of coronary bypass surgery have improved over the last 10 years, primarily, we believe, due to four important medical advances: (1) better stabilization of patients preoperatively with invasive hemodynamic monitoring and intravenously administered pharmacologic agents or intraaortic balloon pump support when necessary, (2) improved techniques of cardiac anesthesia, (3) the use of cold potassium cardioplegia for myocardial protection during construction of distal bypass graft anastomoses, and (4) the use of sequential grafts to achieve complete revascularization and minimize manipulation of the ascending aorta.

Operative Mortality Rate

The Collaborative Study on Coronary Artery Surgery (CASS), a large, multi-institutional study for the treatment of coronary artery disease begun in 1975, has provided a wealth of information on the clinical and angiographic predictors of operative mortality for bypass surgery.[15–17]

Within 3 years, more than 6,000 patients were entered into this registry. The overall operative mortality rate was 2.3 percent, ranging from 0.3 to 6.6 percent among the 15 participating institutions. Variables associated with an increased operative mortality rate were advanced age, female sex, left main coronary artery stenosis, left ventricular wall motion abnormalities, and emergency surgery.[16,17]

Our operative results are comparable to those of the CASS study. We had 12 inhospital deaths in our 654 patients (an operative mortality rate of 1.8 percent). Six deaths occurred in 539 patients under the age of 70 (1.1 percent). Six deaths occurred in 115 patients over the age of 70; 2 of 80 men died (2.5 percent), and four deaths occurred in 35 women over the age of 70 (11.4 percent) who underwent surgery. No deaths, however, occurred in the 11 patients over the age of 80 who underwent bypass surgery. In the CASS registry, 256 of 6,630 patients undergoing bypass surgery were greater than 70 years of age (3.9 percent), compared with 17.6 percent of our patients (115 of 654). The operative mortality rate for women over the age of 70 in the CASS registry was 16 percent (13 out of 81), and the operative mortality rate for men over the age of 70 was 7.4 percent (13 out of 175).

Unpredictable, nearly random, catastrophic events accounted for 5 of the 12 deaths in our 654 patients—an aortic dissection in one patient; a massive pulmonary embolism following a sternal dehiscence in another patient; a fatal transfusion reaction in one patient; a fatal cardiac tamponade following removal of the ventricular pacemaker wire in one elderly woman; and another fatal cardiac tamponade following heparin anticoagulation for a suspected pulmonary embolism in another elderly woman (no embolism was found at autopsy). The other seven deaths occurred in patients who had either preinfarction angina or an acute myocardial infarction preoperatively (three patients), very poor left ventricular function (one patient with an ejection fraction of 20 percent), poor renal function (one patient), or a perioperative myocardial infarction (two patients). The rare death that now occurs after coronary bypass surgery is increasingly due to essentially unpredictable, nearly random, catastrophic events such as those that occurred in 5 of our 12 patients who died.

Morbidity rate after coronary bypass surgery is quite low, as is reflected by our clinical experience. The average hospital stay after surgery for our 654 patients was 7.5 days. Less than 10 percent of patients stayed in the hospital longer than 10 days postoperatively. The most common complication was atrial flutter fibrillation, which occurred in 89 patients (14 percent). Premature ventricular beats requiring treatment occurred in 67 patients (10 percent), ventricular tachycardia occurred in 12 patients, and ventricular fibrillation in 6 patients (4 died). In this series 11 patients (1.7 percent) had one or more new Q waves $\geq$.04 s, evidencing a perioperative myocardial infarction. Inotropic drug support was necessary in 57 patients postoperatively (9 percent). Neurologic sequelae occurred in nine pa-

tients (1.4 percent). Seven patients underwent reoperation for bleeding, and seven patients sustained a sternal wound dehiscence. Only two patients developed renal insufficiency of sufficient severity that postoperative hemodialysis was required.

Effect of Bypass Surgery on Ventricular Function

Resting ventricular function is usually not improved by bypass surgery.[6] Many patients with chronic angina have normal resting ventricular function before surgery, so the surgeon cannot expect to "improve" with bypass grafts that which is already normal. Indeed, in 63 percent of our patients, ventricular function was either normal or borderline normal preoperatively. Also, other patients have segments of myocardium that are replaced by noncontractile scar tissue resulting from a previous myocardial infarction, and increased blood flow through bypass grafts will not make scar tissue contract.

In patients with coronary artery disease, ventricular performance can be normal at rest but will be impaired during exercise. Resting coronary blood flow is usually not impaired in people with coronary artery disease, but coronary blood flow during exercise (i.e., coronary flow reserve) will be reduced in patients with proximal stenoses in their coronary arteries that are greater than 50 percent arterial diameter narrowing. Coronary bypass grafts increase coronary flow reserve, and thereby improve ventricular performance during exercise, a benefit that has been well-demonstrated by hemodynamic studies and radionuclide ventriculography performed during exercise.[18] Improved cardiac output (mediated primarily by an improved heart rate response), an improved ejection fraction and wall motion score, and a decrease in end-systolic volume during exercise are commonly seen after myocardial revascularization with bypass grafts. These beneficial physiological effects also produce relief of anginal symptoms. Approximately 60 to 95 percent of the patients experience complete relief of anginal symptoms after bypass surgery.[19] On a 13.9-month mean follow-up of our 642 patients who survived bypass surgery, 532 patients (82.9 percent) have experienced complete relief of anginal symptoms.

Survival Rate

Randomized studies have shown that bypass surgery improves rate of survival in symptomatic patients with multivessel coronary artery disease, i.e., three-vessel disease and left main coronary artery stenosis. Nonrandomized studies indicate that bypass surgery improves survival rate in patients with two-vessel disease.[7] The survival rate of a patient with single-vessel disease is excellent with either medical or surgical treatment. Of our patients 96 percent were alive at a mean follow-up of 13.9 months.

The beneficial effects of bypass surgery on rate of survival are predicated on continued patency of the bypass grafts. Currently, in the community hospital setting only a small number of patients undergo repeat cardiac catheterization after bypass surgery, mainly patients with recurrent anginal symptoms. A large body of data has been collected, however, that indicates that 85 to 95 percent of saphenous vein bypass grafts are patent after the first year, and that the annual attrition rate for bypass grafts, during the first 5 to 7 years postoperatively, is approximately 1 percent per year.[6,13,14]

PRACTICE PATTERNS

Highly expert cardiac surgical teams now perform coronary bypass surgery in more than 600 hospitals throughout the United States. In our 1980 survey of 677 cardiac surgeons who performed 90 percent of the coronary bypass operations that year, only 138 surgeons (21 percent) performed bypass surgery in a university hospital.[3] Coronary bypass surgery in the United States is now largely carried out in community hospitals by surgeons who engage in a single-specialty group practice.

The cardiac surgical team now generally consists of a board-certified thoracic surgeon, an anesthesiologist who specializes in cardiac anesthesia, a board-certified cardiopulmonary perfusionist, a board-certified surgeons' or physicians' assistant or surgical resident, and specially trained operating room nurses; board-certified critical care nurses now provide care for these patients postoperatively.[3,4]

The results of cardiac surgery in community hospitals are comparable to those that are achieved in major university hospitals.[10] More than 50 percent of cardiac surgeons now engage in a single-specialty group practice; 13 percent are in solo private practice; 10 percent are in a multispecialty group practice; and 24 percent are staff surgeons at a university or federal hospital.[3] As is typical of many cardiac surgeons, we practice coronary bypass surgery at a community hospital medical center and work together in a single-specialty group practice.

COMPUTERIZED RECORD KEEPING

Computers are now widely used in medical practices for patient billing, accounting, appointment scheduling, and word processing. A number of cardiac surgical teams have established a computerized data registry that serves as a repository for a large body of clinical information of each of their patients that can be readily accessed and analyzed. Necessary demographic data, preoperative clinical information that prognostically stratifies each patient, relevant intraoperative data, information on surgical outcome and postoperative morbidity, and periodically updated follow-up information are entered into a computer.[20]

We began a computerized medical record-keeping system in our practice in 1980 (Fig. 3). Some cardiac surgical data registries, such as the CASS registry, are very extensive and require the services of one or more full-time data technicians for collecting and entering the information into the computer. A valuable data registry for cardiac surgical patients, however, can be obtained by collecting only approximately 100 items of information on each patient. We collect 106 items of information, 101 that can be expressed by an integer, and 5 items of information that require a text response (e.g., patient and physician names). One of our cardiopulmonary perfusionists collects this information, the data entry forms are reviewed by one of us, and a member of our office staff enters the data into the computer. A computerized medical record-keeping system such as the one we use permits surgeons to easily analyze their cardiac surgical experience and, when requested, to readily submit their results for peer review.

NEW DIRECTIONS

A synthetic or bioprosthetic conduit capable of maintaining a patency rate equal to that achieved with saphenous veins has yet to be developed. Such a prosthesis would eliminate the discomfort and potential morbidity which frequently attend harvesting the saphenous vein. Also, the best solution to use for cold cardioplegic arrest has yet to be defined. There is general agreement that the addition of potassium is an important adjunct, but opinion remains divided on the relative merits of using cold blood or a physiological saline solution and on the value of adding other pharmacologic agents. The addition of calcium antagonists to the cardioplegic solution offers an intriguing new approach to myocardial protection in cardiac surgery which is currently being investigated.

Intraoperative Coronary Angioplasty

This technique may open up a new dimension in coronary bypass surgery.[21] Some surgeons are beginning

Northwest Cardiac Surgery Associates
ADULT OPEN HEART SURGERY DATA REGISTRY

IDENTIFYING DATA

1. Patient Name _______________________________

2. Hospital Number _______________________________

3. Birthdate __________/__________________/______________

4. Sex: 1-Male   2-Female

5. Race: 1-White   2-Black   3-Oriental   4-Indian

6. Surgeon _______________________________

7. Referring Cardiologist _______________________________

8. Referring Physician _______________________________

DIAGNOSIS

9. Coronary Heart Disease Code _______________________________
   CODES =   0 = none
             1 = asymptomatic
             2 = effort angina
             3 = rest angina
             4 = preinfarction angina
             5 = acute myocardial infarction
             12 = postinfarct angina

10. Acquired Valve Disease Code _______________________________
    CODES =   none
              1 = mitral stenosis
              2 = mitral stenosis and regurgitation
              3 = mitral regurgitation
              4 = aortic stenosis
              5 = aortic insufficiency
              6 = mitral and aortic valve disease
              12 = mitral and tricuspid valve disease
              13 = aortic, mitral and tricuspid valve

11. Other Heart Disease Code _______________________________
    CODES =   0 = none
              1 = ventricular aneurysm
              3 = hypertrophic cardiomyopathy
              4 = atrial septal defect
              5 = other congenital heart disease
              6 = aortic dissection
              7 = ascending aortic aneurysm
              8 = bacterial endocarditis
              9 = tumor (myxoma)
              12 = other or more than one

OPERATION

12. Operation Date __________/__________________/______________

13. Bypass Surgery Code _______________________________
    CODES =   1 = none
              2 = isolated
              3 = reoperation
              4 = combined with valve surgery
              5 = with ventricular aneurysm
              6 = with other prodedures

14. Conduits Used Code _______________________________
    CODES =   1 = saphenous vein only
              12 = if cephalic vein used
              13 = if internal mammary artery used

15. Valve Surgery Code _______________________________
    CODES =   1 = none
              2 = isolated
              3 = reoperation
              4 = with bypass grafting
              5 = with other procedures

16. Valve Surgery Type Code _______________________________
    CODES =   0 = none
              1 = aortic valve replacement
              2 = aortic commissurotomy
              3 = mitral valve replacement
              4 = mitral commissurotomy
              5 = mitral reconstruction
              6 = tricuspid valve surgery
              12 = aortic and mitral valve
              13 = mitral and tricuspid valve
              14 = triple valve procedure

17. Valve Prosthesis Used _______________________________
    CODES =   1 = Carpentier-Edwards
              2 = Hancock
              3 = Bjork-Shiley
              4 = Ionescu-Shiley
              5 = Other or more than one

18. Valve Prosthesis Size _______________________________ mm

19. Other Cardiac Surgery Code _______________________________
    CODES =   1 = Patch closure aortic ring abscess
              2 = Ventricular aneurysmectomy
              4 = Septal myectomy
              5 = Closure atrial septal defect
              6 = Closure ventricular septal defect
              8 = Excision cardiac tumor
              9 = Resection ascending aorta
              11 = Other procedures

20. Other Noncardiac Procedures Code _______________________________
    CODES =   1 = Carotid endarterectomy
              3 = Other
              12 = Hemodialysis during cardiopulmonary bypass

CLINICAL FINDINGS

21. Angina   1-No   2-Yes

22. Myocardial Infarction   1-No   2-Yes

23. Time Since Infarct Code _______________________________
    CODES =   1 = less than 24 hours
              2 = 1-3 days
              3 = 4-7 days
              4 = 7-14 days
              5 = 15-21 days
              6 = 22-28 days
              7 = 4-6 weeks
              8 = 1½-6 months
              9 = more than 6 months

24. Congestive Heart Failure   1-No   2-Yes

25. NYHA Class (1-4) _______________________________

26. Sudden Death Code _______________________________
    CODES =   0 = none
              3 = out of hospital
              4 = in hospital

27. Previous Cardiac Surgery Code _______________________________
    CODES =   0 = none
              1 = coronary bypass surgery
              2 = aortic valve replacement
              3 = mitral commissurotomy
              4 = mitral valve replacement
              5 = other

FIGURE 3   One of the four pages from our Heart Surgery Data Registry form. Integer responses are entered for all medical attributes except for the patients' and referring doctors' names.

to use a balloon angioplasty catheter intraoperatively as an adjunct to bypass grafting. The balloon catheter is inserted through the coronary arteriotomy into the lumen of the artery to dilate secondary and tertiary obstructions. In the patient with diffuse coronary dis-ease a saphenous vein graft can be used to bypass a severe proximal obstruction while secondary, more distal obstructions are dilated with the angioplasty catheter. Clinical evaluation of this technique is now underway. Optimal utilization of intraoperative transluminal coronary angioplasty will probably require the performance of intraoperative coronary arteriography as well.[22]

Extended Endarterectomy

Coronary endarterectomy has long been performed in conjunction with bypass grafting in selected patients, particularly those with appropriate lesions involving the right coronary artery. Dr. W. Dudley Johnson has recently advocated extended endarterectomy in conjunction with bypass surgery for patients who have diffuse, essentially inoperable coronary disease.[23] Through a long arteriotomy incision (up to 8 cm in length) extensive endarterectomies are performed in the left anterior decending, diagonal, and circumflex marginal arteries. An onlay vein bypass graft is anastomosed along the entire length of the arteriotomy while the heart is being protected for an extended duration by cold cardioplegic arrest. The safety and efficacy of this technique has yet to be documented on a large scale, but it holds promise in patients with diffuse disease who might otherwise be declared inoperable.

Coronary bypass surgery has undergone considerable changes since we began our training in this field over a decade ago and will, undoubtedly, undergo further evolution in the years ahead. This expertly done, high-technology operation will continue to benefit many thousands of patients with advanced coronary artery disease until such a time as this disease can be prevented or successfully managed by nonoperative techniques.

REFERENCES

1 Spencer, F. C.: Discussion of a Paper by W. D. Johnson, R. F. Flemma, D. Lepley, Jr., and E. H. Ellison, Extended Treatment of Severe Coronary Artery Disease: A Total Surgical Approach, *Ann. Surg.*, 169:470, 1969.

2 Miller, D. W., Jr., Hessel, E. A., II, Wintersheid, L. C., et al.: Current Practice of Coronary Artery Bypass Surgery: Results of a National Survey, *J. Thorac. Cardiovasc. Surg.*, 73:75, 1977.

3 Miller, D. W., Jr., Ivey T. D., Bailey W. W., et al.: The Practice of Coronary Bypass Surgery in 1980, *J. Thorac. Cardiovasc. Surg.*, 81:423, 1981.

4 Miller, D. W., Jr., Binford, J. M., and Hessel, E. A.: Results of a Survey of the Professional Activities of 811 Cardiopulmonary Perfusionists, *J. Thorac. Cardiovasc. Surg.*, 83:385, 1982.

5 Miller, D. W., Jr., and Ivey, T. D.: Selection of Patients for Coronary Bypass Operations, *West. J. Med.*, 133:210, 1980.

6 Miller, D. W., Jr.: "The Practice of Coronary Artery Bypass Surgery," Plenum Medical Book Company, New York, 1977.

7 Hurst, J. W., King, S. B., III, Logue, R. B., et al.: Value of Coronary Bypass Surgery, *Am. J. Cardiol.*, 42:308, 1978.

8 Hutter, A. M., Jr., Russell, R. O., Jr., Resnekow, L., et al.: Unstable Angina Pectoris—National Randomized Study of Surgical vs. Medical Therapy: Results in 1, 2, and 3 Vessel Disease, *Circulation,* 55(suppl. 3):60, 1977.

9 Neill, W. A., Ritzman, L. W., Okies, J. E., et al.: Medical vs. Urgent Surgical Therapy for Acute Coronary Insufficiency: A Randomized Study, in S. H. Rahimtoola (ed.), Coronary Bypass Surgery, "Cardiovascular Clinics," vol. 8, no. 2, F.A. Davis Company, Philadelphia, 1977, pp. 179.

10 Dillard, D. H., and Miller, D. W., Jr.: "Atlas of Cardiac Surgery," Macmillan Publishing Company, New York, 1983.

11 Dewood, M. A., and Berg, R., Jr.: Coronary Artery Bypass Surgery: 13 Years' Experience with Chronic Stable Angina Pectoris, Unstable Angina Pectoris, and Acute Myocardial Infarction, in J.W. Hurst (ed.), "Clinical Essays on The Heart," vol. 2, McGraw-Hill Book Company, New York, 1983, p. 159.

12 Cohn, P. F.: Asymptomatic Coronary Artery Disease: Pathophysiology, Diagnosis, Management, *Mod. Concepts Cardiovas. Dis.*, 50:55, 1981.

13 Campeau, L., Crochet, D., Lesperance, J., Bourassa, M.G., and Grondin, C. M.: Postoperative Change in Aortocoronary Saphenous Vein Grafts Revisited: Angiographic Studies at Two Weeks and at One Year in Two Series of Consecutive Patients, *Circulation*, 52:369, 1975.

14 O'Neill, M. J., Wolf, P. D., O'Neill, T. K., et al.: A Rationale for the Use of Sequential Coronary Artery Bypass Grafts, *J. Thorac. Cardiovasc. Surg.*, 81:686, 1981.

15 Principal Investigators of CASS et al.: National Heart, Lung, and Blood Institute Coronary Artery Surgery Study, *Circulation,* 63(suppl. 2):1, 1981.

16 Kennedy, J. W., Kaiser, G. C., Fisher, L. D., et al.: Multivariant Discriminant Analysis of the Clinical and Angiographic Predictors of Operative Mortality, The Collaborative Study and Coronary Artery Surgery (CASS), *J.Thorac. Cardiovasc. Surg.*, 80:876, 1980.

17 Kennedy, J. W., et al.: Clinical and Angiographic Predictors of Operative Mortality from the Collaborative Study in Coronary Artery Surgery (CASS), *Circulation*, 63:793, 1981.

18 Newman, G. E., Rerych, S. K., Jones, R. H., and Sabiston, D. C., Jr.: Assessment of the Effects of the Aortocoronary Bypass Graft on Ventricular Function during Rest and Exercise, *J. Thorac. Cardiovasc. Surg.*, 79:617, 1980.

19 Miller, D. W., Jr., and Dodge, H. T.: Benefits of Coronary Artery Bypass Surgery, *Arch. Intern. Med.*, 137:1439, 1977.

20 Day, S. B., and Brandejo, J. F., (eds.): "Computers for Medical Office and Patient Management," Van Nostrand Reinhold Company, New York, 1982.

21 Walsh, E., Franzone, A. F., Weinstein, G. S., et al.: Use of Operative Transluminal Coronary Angioplasty as an Adjunct to Coronary Artery Bypass, *J. Thorac. Cardiovasc. Surg.*, 84:843, 1982.

22 Rainier, W. G., Sadler, T. R., Hilgenberg, A. D., et al.: Technique and Value of Operative Arteriography in Coronary Bypass Operations, *J. Thorac. Cardiovasc. Surg.*, 83:358, 1982.

23 Johnson, W.D.: Personal communication.

Coronary Artery Bypass Surgery: University of California, San Francisco Experience, 1969–1982[*]

DANIEL J. ULLYOT, M.D., and PAUL A. EBERT, M.D.

Our experience with coronary artery bypass at the University of California, San Francisco (U.C.S.F.) extends over a 13-year period from 1969 to 1982 inclusive. The experience was accumulated in three hospitals, each of which has a unique emphasis based on individual institutional referral patterns: Moffitt Hospital, a large university teaching hospital, the San Francisco Veterans Administration Hospital, a federal hospital with affiliations with the U.S. Public Health system and several military centers, and Peninsula Hospital, a private, community medical center.

From a historical perspective the experience can be classified into three reasonably distinct periods: a developmental phase (1969–1973), a mature phase in which most of the technical problems were solved (1973–1977), and an advanced phase during which the technology was extended (1978–1982).

DEVELOPMENTAL PHASE

Our initial experience was based on emulation of techniques originated at the Cleveland Clinic and St. Luke's Hospital in Milwaukee. Coronary arteriography was most advanced at the San Francisco Veterans Administration (VA) Hospital, where there had been an early interest in the VA study of the Vineburg procedure. As was true in numerous institutions across the country, there was a reluctance to study many patients with ischemic heart disease because of the deeply entrenched skepticism about the physiological efficacy of any surgical approach to the relief of angina. The anesthetic management of patients with myocardial ischemia was unsophisticated and was based on an extrapolation of experience in patients with valvular heart disease. The early emphasis was on prevention and treatment of low-output syndrome rather than on the regional myocardial supply-demand relationships in the presence of by-and-large good ventricular function. Up to that time emphasis had been on the evaluation of global function rather than on segmental or regional function.

There was uncertainty about the best way to achieve a dry field for distal anastomoses—whether to occlude the coronary arteries with slings, intracoronary occluders, or local pressure or to cross-clamp the aorta. We were, for a time, willing to accept a warm, fibrillating heart as theoretically preferable to risking infarction by cross-clamping the aorta. We were aware of the hazards of subendocardial ischemia and necrosis and made a point of venting the left ventricle to prevent distension, providing moderate systemic hypothermia (28°C) to maintain fibrillation, and keeping the mean systemic pressure at or above 70 mmHg while working on the fibrillating heart. Our early anastomotic technique was with interrupted silk without use of optical magnification.

Very early in our experience we opted to perform coronary anastomosis during aortic occlusion because of the superior exposure provided and because of the observation that few patients were harmed by this maneuver. Cross-clamping was intermittent and the proximal anastomosis was made during the period of reperfusion after each distal anastomosis. The heart was not defibrillated between periods of aortic occlusion.

We settled on a suture technique early in our experience which we have continued to use to the present: continuous technique using polypropylene suture with irrigation through the graft while tying to prevent purse-stringing the anastomosis. Most fortunate, we believe, was our early decision to employ optical magnification (4½-power loupes) which allowed improved accuracy in suture placement that was not required in most other types of cardiac surgery. This anastomotic technique using a single double-armed suture was technically simple and allowed deliberate placement of individual bites within an 8- to 10-min period for each distal anastomosis.

We had an early interest in coronary endarterectomy. Based on Sawyer's work we performed right coronary endarterectomy using carbon dioxide gas, although it soon became obvious that a similarly satisfactory endarterectomy could be accomplished using mechanical endarterectomy.

Surgical results during this period were remarkably good considering the relatively primitive and evolutionary nature of the technology. Coronary arteriography failed to adequately delineate surgical anatomy in many patients, and crises in the catheterization laboratory occurred not infrequently in elective studies. The patient risk seemed to be in phase with the technology of the period, however, at least in terms of

*From the Department of Surgery, University of California, San Francisco.

operative mortality rate, which remained in the 1 to 2 percent range and contrasted favorably with that seen in other types of cardiac surgery during the same period.

Few patients had more than three grafts placed, and many had one or two grafts. Patients with single- or double-vessel disease were considered ideal surgical candidates and uniformly did well from the standpoint of operative mortality rate and relief of symptoms. There was a reluctance to study patients with acute coronary syndromes, and patients with preinfarction angina who responded to medical treatment in the hospital were allowed to "cool off" over a 4- to 6-week interval or longer before elective study. Some of the higher-risk patients in this subgroup suffered infarction, thereby selecting a more favorable group for subsequent surgical treatment.

Recent myocardial infarction was considered a strong contraindication to surgical intervention, and a notion existed that failure to discover a recent, clinically silent myocardial infarction in a patient admitted for elective surgery often led to the dreaded phenomenon of "stone heart" following cardiopulmonary bypass.

Despite the low operative mortality rate, surgical results were marred by a disconcertingly high perioperative myocardial infarction rate, which was in the 10 to 20 percent range as measured by the incidence of new Q waves and possibly higher by other techniques. Most of these were clinically silent, and the long-term significance was unknown. Quantitation of infarct size was unavailable. Most patients did not undergo postoperative ventriculography. In the absence of late survival rate data and of symptoms of congestive heart failure in most patients sustaining perioperative infarction, this incidence of myocardial injury was accepted as a sequela of surgical management, perhaps clinically benign, in most patients. It was argued by some that this was an electrocardiographic phenomenon in which electrical forces developed by revascularization became evident when viewed electrocardiographically through an area of scar opposite the revascularized segment. Others argued that some of the symptomatic relief following surgical management was due to infarction of ischemic regions of myocardium.

MATURE PHASE

The next stage in coronary bypass surgery at U.C.S.F. was characterized by a substantial increase in the volume of patients studied and operated upon as the initial skepticism regarding the physiological benefit of surgical management gave way to cautious acceptance among the medical community. There were two developments which stimulated this quantum jump in the acceptance of surgical management.

The first of these was the discovery that patients with medically intractable coronary insufficiency syndromes could be safely and effectively managed surgically. Patients continuing to experience episodes of rest angina in the coronary care unit despite maximal medical management were studied and operated on urgently and were discharged pain-free 1 week later. This experience provided powerful evidence for the safety and efficacy of surgical intervention to even the most skeptical physicians. This advance was due in large part to improved management in the catheterization laboratory and to better anesthetic management. It was clear that catheterization laboratory mortality and morbidity rates were inversely related to patient volume. A sufficient experience had become concentrated in the hands of a few cardiologists at U.C.S.F. to allow high-quality studies to be obtained safely in most patients, including those with acute coronary syndromes. There was also a vigorous use of beta blocking agents to stabilize patients rapidly before they underwent catheterization and surgery. The use of heparin during study obviated some of the thrombotic complications occasioned by the change of catheters using the Judkins technique.

Cardiac anesthesiologists became much more sophisticated about the determinants of myocardial ischemia during induction and maintenance of cardiac anesthesia. Diversity of opinion among our anesthesiologists made us realize that the choice of anesthetic agent was unimportant, and the increased experience and understanding of those administering anesthesia were the important components of anesthesia's contribution to good surgical outcomes. Patients with severe ventricular dysfunction are regularly anesthetized with the so-called myocardial depressants, and patients with severe coronary artery disease are successfully anesthetized using nitrous narcotic techniques. Presurgical management improved as well. The practice of discontinuing beta blocking agents in apprehensive patients admitted for elective surgery because of the fear of low-output syndrome postoperatively led to emergency surgery in some patients for threatened myocardial infarction. This practice gave way to continuing propranolol in full therapeutic dosage and even to increasing the agent preoperatively and during anesthetic induction in many patients.

Operative technique advanced *pari passu* with increasing experience. Difficulty in finding the left anterior descending (LAD) artery or intramyocardial branches of the circumflex system and wasting time bypassing tiny filamentous branches which should not have been opened in the first place became a thing of the past. It was found that the posterior descending branch of the right coronary artery was often a superior site for anastomoses than the densely atherosclerotic main trunk at the crux. More grafts were placed, including those to major diagonal branches of the LAD and multiple branches of the circumflex system. All grafts were individually placed during this period, and a patient with five grafts, for example, would have five proximal anastomoses. The internal mammary artery was used selectively for LAD bypass, especially in young patients.

The second major factor leading to increased surgical volume was the recognition that patient survival rate appeared to be favorably influenced. As we followed our patients, it became evident that late mortality was a rare event. We were among the first to present evidence for improved survival rate with surgical management.[1] Lacking a control group, we used the scoring system of Friesinger, Page, and Ross and showed that patients with scores of 10 or greater (i.e., patients with triple-vessel disease) enjoyed a statistically significant expectation of improved rate of survival compared with historical controls, i.e., patients with similar extent of coronary atherosclerosis managed medically in the 1960s prior to the introduction of coronary bypass. In our published work we were careful to point out the methodological problems with this sort of comparison and showed that in our retrospective analysis our surgically managed patients were, if anything, higher-risk than the medically managed patients in that they were older, had worse ventricular function, and included patients (28 percent) with preinfarction angina by strict criteria (Fig. 1).

The Veterans Administration Combined Study published 3 years later suggested that with the exception of the subgroup of patients with left main stenosis, there was no difference in survival rate between patients managed medically or surgically when studied prospectively. Specifically, patients with triple-vessel disease exclusive of left main stem stenosis did not enjoy prolongation of life at a level of statistical significance compared with the medical cohorts in the VA study. These findings seemed to refute our earlier studies and stimulated one of the authors of the VA study to object strenuously to our work.[2]

This discrepancy prompted us to look more closely at the two studies. An important conclusion emerged: surgical quality is in itself a determinant of survival. No difference could be found between our veteran patients managed surgically during the 1972–1974 period of the VA Cooperative Study and either the medical or surgical cohorts in their study with respect to age, extent of coronary atherosclerosis, ventricular function, or other preoperative descriptors, and yet survival rate in our series was statistically better (Fig. 2).[3] What was different between our patients and those of the surgically managed patients in the VA Cooperative Studies were three factors related to surgical quality: operative mortality rate (0 versus 5.6 percent, $p < .05$), perioperative myocardial infarction rate (6 versus 18

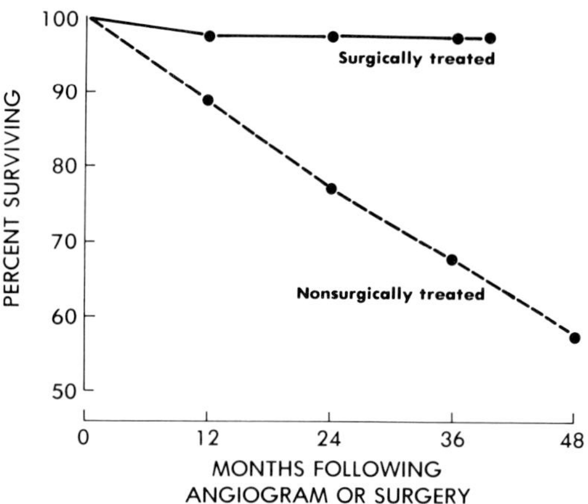

FIGURE 1 Cumulative survival rate at 1, 2, and 3 years among surgically treated patients (U.C.S.F. series of 149 consecutive patients) compared to published series of medically managed patients. Patients in both groups had scores of 10 or greater (Friesinger, Page, and Ross) equivalent to triple-vessel coronary artery disease. (*From D. J. Ullyot, J. Wisneski, R. W. Sullivan, and E. W. Gertz, Improved Survival after Coronary Artery Surgery in Patients with Extensive Coronary Artery Disease, J. Thorac. Cardiovasc. Surg., 70:405, 1975. Used with permission of the publisher.*)

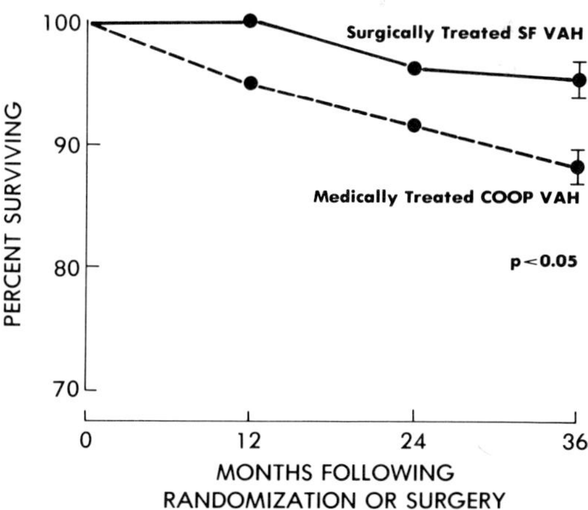

FIGURE 2 Cumulative survival rate at 1, 2, and 3 years comparing veteran patients with chronic, stable angina exclusive of those with left main stenosis at U.C.S.F. ($n = 88$) with those in VA Cooperative Study. The only discernible differences between the two groups were as follows:

	U.C.S.F.	VA Cooperative Study	Significance
Operative mortality rate	0%	5.6%	$p < .05$
Perioperative infarction rate	6%	18.0%	$p < .01$
Graft patency	86%	69.0%	$p < .001$

percent, $p < .01$), and graft patency rate (85 vs. 69 percent, $p < .001$). This work, part of a loud chorus of criticism of the VA Cooperative Study, attacked the quality of surgical management that led to doubtful conclusions.

A corollary of the assertion that coronary artery bypass confers improved survival on subgroups of patients with ischemic heart disease is the notion that late myocardial infarction rate must also be favorably reduced in surgically managed patients. In a longitudinal study of 200 consecutive, surgically managed patients followed as long as 53 months postoperatively (mean 27 months) only four late transmural infarctions (one fatal and three nonfatal) were found (Fig. 3).[4] A total of 2,304 electrocardiographic studies were examined for a total follow-up of 3,629 patient-months. Although the data were retrospective, compared with epidemiologic data such as those available in the Framingham Study they suggest a favorable impact of surgical management on late myocardial infarction rate even when all late deaths are taken as instances of myocardial infarction.

One caveat regarding the beneficial impact of surgical management was highlighted by this study: there remained a significant incidence of perioperative, transmural myocardial infarction, 8.5 percent in our study. An earlier study from our institution showed that one could no longer regard perioperative infarction as a benign event.[5] Using ventriculographic studies we showed that a new Q wave occurring in association with myocardial revascularization was invariably associated with a demonstrable impairment of wall motion corresponding to the electrocardiographic localization of the infarction. Although the incidence of perioperative, transmural infarction had fallen to the 5 to 10 percent range during this period, one could no longer rationalize this as a clinically insignificant event.

Postoperative hypertension was encountered in one-third to one-half of patients following coronary bypass. This phenomenon contrasted sharply with the hypotension and low-output syndrome often seen during the postoperative period in other types of cardiac surgery. Hypertension in the postoperative period was of concern because of increased bleeding and the potential for ischemia and infarction in patients who could not be completely revascularized. In a clinical study looking at hemodynamic variables we showed that postoperative hypertension following myocardial revascularization was due to increased systemic vascular resistance rather than to increased cardiac output attendant on improved myocardial blood flow.[6]

Our mature phase of coronary bypass at U.C.S.F. was characterized by a substantial increase in surgical volume, providing an experience no longer derivative of the institutions that pioneered coronary bypass in this country. Based on this experience we were able to make independent contributions to the evolving technology and to the understanding of the impact of surgery on survival rate, late myocardial infarction rate, the significance of perioperative myocardial infarction, and the mechanism of postoperative hypertension.

Patient selection was broadened during this period to include patients with acute coronary syndromes and poor left ventricular function. There was still reluctance to tackle patients in the throes of acute myocardial infarction and those with extensive distal disease. More grafts were placed in these seemingly higher-risk patients with a diminution in perioperative myocardial infarction rate and with a continued low mortality rate in the 1 to 2 percent range.

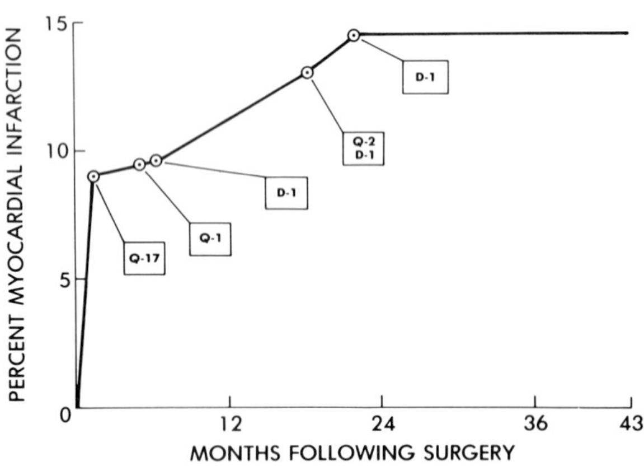

FIGURE 3 The cumulative myocardial infarction rate in 200 consecutive patients managed surgically at U.C.S.F. for a 43-month follow-up period. This represents a "maximal" rate and includes all perioperatively acquired new Q waves, late new Q waves, and *all* deaths (D) from cardiac disease. There were only five late myocardial events in this study in which 2,304 ECGs were examined for a total follow-up of 3,629 patient-months. (*From D. J. Ullyot, J. Wisneski, R. W. Sullivan, E. W. Gertz, and C. Ryan, The Impact of Coronary Artery Bypass on Late Myocardial Infarction, J. Thorac. Cardiovasc. Surg., 73:165, 1977. Used with permission.*)

ADVANCED STAGE

The advanced stage of coronary artery bypass at U.C.S.F. is characterized by the extension of operative indications to include patients with persistent angina complicating acute myocardial infarction and those with extensive distal atherosclerosis. Two technical changes occurred during this period: the routine use of cold crystalloid cardioplegia for myocardial protection during aortic cross-clamping and the use of sequential grafting.[7]

There was a further, substantial increase in surgical volume during this period due in large part to the general acceptance by the medical community of our earlier suggestion that survival is improved with surgical management in patients with extensive coronary atherosclerosis, i.e., significant obstruction of all three major coronary arteries. Also contributing to increased surgical volume are several interesting subgroups including patients with medically intractable ventricular tachyarrhythmias, those with previous myocardial revascularization and evidence of graft stenosis or progression of disease in native coronary vessels, and patients with acute coronary occlusion during or failing to benefit from percutaneous transluminal coronary angioplasty.

Based on our favorable experience in the surgical management of patients with coronary insufficiency, we extended our indications to include patients having rest angina refractory to medical therapy following acute myocardial infarction.[8] Our study was based on an experience of 30 consecutive patients who developed angina within 21 days of myocardial infarction, 22 of whom underwent surgical therapy, with only 2 (9 percent) operative deaths. We found that patients could be managed with a low operative mortality rate and that intraaortic balloon support was not required in the great majority.

Perhaps a word should be said about our use of the intraaortic balloon at our institution. We find that intraaortic balloon pumping is rarely necessary in our experience. When used, it is employed mainly in patients who cannot be weaned from cardiopulmonary bypass, which is approximately 3 percent of all patients undergoing coronary bypass with and without other cardiac repair. It is used rarely preoperatively and then just prior to cardiac catheterization and surgery in patients with hemodynamic instability. We have not found the device necessary for the management of angina or for improved safety in the management of patients with left main stem stenosis. We believe that this type of mechanical assistance belongs in the arsenal of all surgeons performing coronary bypass, but its frequent use is obviated by high-quality anesthetic and surgical management including careful postoperative care.

Surgical intervention during and within the early postinfarction period is stimulated by minitreadmill studies in patients following myocardial infarction prior to hospital discharge in whom ischemia is demonstrated at low levels of exercise. Patients treated in the early hours of myocardial infarction with intracoronary clot lysis may, on anatomic grounds or because of hemodynamic instability during treatment, be referred for urgent surgical revascularization. Our results with respect to operative mortality rate have been favorable in these subgroups, and we have not encountered hemorrhagic extension of infarction or uncontrollable bleeding related to the use of streptokinase.

We have not recommended direct surgical intervention in the early hours of uncomplicated myocardial infarction. We believe that from a logistical standpoint, clot lysis with or without balloon angioplasty makes more sense as an acute intervention for potential myocardial salvage and that surgery has a backup role should complications ensue.

Patients who in earlier years might have been refused surgery because of extensive distal coronary atherosclerosis are rarely turned down today. The use of sequential grafting and coronary endarterectomy including LAD and circumflex endarterectomy has extended surgical indications considerably. With increasing surgical experience one can usually find suitable segments for grafting in vessels considered not bypassable angiographically by earlier criteria.

In the mid-1970s we began to use cold crystalloid cardioplegia for valve replacement and for selected patients undergoing coronary bypass.[9] In a study of 204 patients in whom cold crystalloid cardioplegia was employed, only 9 patients underwent coronary bypass alone. Most of the patients in this study had valve replacement. At that time our results with intermittent aortic occlusion for distal coronary anastomoses were excellent, particularly when we practiced intermittent defibrillation during periods of reperfusion while the aortic anastomoses were performed. We converted to the exclusive use of cardioplegia for coronary bypass largely for technical reasons. It seemed easier to do all the small-vessel anastomoses at one time rather than shifting back and forth between coronary and aortic anastomoses. We also speculated that a single reperfusion period was preferable to multiple reperfusion periods. With the increasing use of sequential grafts one did not have an aortic anastomoses to do during periods of reperfusion corresponding to each distal anastomosis. We favor doing all distal anastomoses first during a single period of aortic occlusion followed by the aortic anastomoses, which are done during the rewarming period on total cardiopulmonary bypass while the heart is allowed to beat and recover from the effects of aortic occlusion.

We believe several points in the use of cardioplegia for coronary bypass grafting are worthy of emphasis. As soon as cardiopulmonary bypass is established, the heart is stopped by the infusion of cold cardioplegic solution into the aortic root. With experience one need not identify the sites for coronary anastomosis prior to the administration of cardioplegia. The delivery of cold solution to the myocardium is of paramount importance, outweighing, in our opinion, that of any constituent, additive, or combination of these in the solution itself. Myocardial temperature measurement using a needle thermistor is important to ensure adequate cooling, usually to the 8 to 10°C range. Frequently there are relatively warm regions of myocardium corresponding to poorly perfused myocardial segments. Grafts are placed to these regions first, and local cooling is accomplished by the infusion of cold (4°C) Ringers lactate solution through the graft using a hand-held syringe. The mean systemic pressure is kept at 50 mmHg or below during aortic occlusion to minimize tendency to myocardial rewarming through noncoronary collateral flow. Systemic hypothermia (28°C) should be used, particularly when multiple grafts or complex procedures are done. This is important for preservation of right atrial and right ventricular function and for preservation of sinoatrial conduction when relatively long (> 1 h) ischemic periods are contemplated. In such cases hypothermia to 21 to 23°C may be employed. We find that five or six distal anastomoses can be accomplished in 60 min or less of aortic occlusion. This requires an initial infusion of cardioplegic solution and one reinfusion at 20- to 30-min cross-clamp time in most cases. We believe that the left ventricle should be vented to facilitate exposure and to retard the rate of left ventricular rewarming. The heart should be allowed to beat on full bypass (not having to support the systemic circulation) for approximately one-half the aortic cross-clamp time while recovery takes place and the patient is rewarmed. The proximal anastomoses are performed during this reperfusion period. The mean aortic pressure is allowed to rise during the reperfusion period, since reperfusion is by way of the native coronary circulation while the aortic anastomoses are completed. Applying these principles we have found no evidence of deterioration in left ventricular function. Perioperative myocardial infarction rates decreased further to the 2 to 5 percent range during this period when cold cardioplegia was used exclusively.

We have had an interesting experience in the surgical management of patients with ischemic heart disease and ventricular tachyarrhythmia refractory to medical therapy.[10] Intraoperative ventricular mapping followed by subendocardial resection, encircling ventriculotomy, coronary artery bypass, and left ventricular aneurysm resection when appropriate has been employed in 14 patients with some good long-term results. These techniques appear to add benefit over coronary bypass and standard left ventricular aneurysmectomy. However, surgical management in these patients is still in a developmental phase and requires further long-term studies for validation.

We have extended our studies in the pathogenesis of perioperative myocardial infarction during this period. We developed a "relatively noninvasive" technique of assessing graft patency using contrast-enhanced computed tomography. We found a 94 percent sensitivity and a 92 percent specificity with this method compared to conventional graft arteriography.[11] In a random series an early graft patency rate of 94 percent was recorded.[12]

Applying this technique to 18 patients who sustained perioperative infarction by enzyme, electrocardiographic, and pyrophosphate scan criteria, we found that 14 of 18 grafts perfusing the region of infarction were patent.[13] Furthermore, in reviewing preoperative angiograms in these patients the segments of myocardium sustaining perioperative infarction were supplied by vessels with high-grade (> 90 percent) stenosis and with poor collateral flow.

Two important conclusions are drawn from these studies. Graft occlusion is an infrequent cause of perioperative myocardial infarction. Regions of myocardium at high risk for perioperative infarction can be identified preoperatively, and special attention is paid to their protection during aortic cross-clamping as described above.

Important advances in blood conservation have been made during this phase of our experience. Stimulated by favorable experience in managing Jehovah's Witness patients we developed strategies for limiting blood usage. We remove 800 to 1,000 mL of the patient's own blood from the side port in the venous line prior to instituting cardiopulmonary bypass. Blood volume is maintained during this maneuver by the simultaneous infusion of crystalloid prime from the arterial line. The blood is stored in the operating room at room temperature and reinfused after the administration of protamine. All blood remaining in the pump is collected and returned to the patient postoperatively. The "cell saver" is used in all patients undergoing second or third cardiac procedure.* Meticulous hemostasis is achieved prior to decannulation. Shed blood is collected in sterile bags in the chest tube drainage system and returned to the patient.† Using these techniques our current average blood utilization is less than 2 U per patient.

Importantly, anesthetic management has achieved a high level of sophistication. The anesthesiologists at U.C.S.F. deserve much credit for improved surgical results. We are uncertain as to the role of invasive monitoring in our results. With the advent of pulmonary artery catheters, we followed a national trend and used these extensively. For several years, however, we have used them less frequently, perhaps in 15 to 20 percent of cases.

In summary, the advanced period of coronary bypass at U.C.S.F. is characterized by an extension of indications to include patients considered high-risk by previous standards, including those with acute myocardial infarction and those with extensive distal coro-

*Haemonetics.

†Sorensen.

nary atherosclerosis. More grafts are placed, currently averaging four per patient. Complex cases are commonly performed, including frequent operations in patients who have had previous cardiac surgery, myocardial revascularization combined with valve replacement, left ventricular aneurysm resection, ventricular mapping, and resection or exclusion of arrhythmogenic foci, and carotid endarterectomy.

Despite greater extent of revascularization in higher-risk patients, including a higher frequency of complex, combined procedures, operative mortality rate has remained low. The majority of operative deaths are still due to cardiac causes. However, approximately one-third occur in "good-risk" patients, for example, those with stroke related to intracranial vascular disease. Perioperative myocardial infarction rate has declined further during this period, related, we believe, to the routine use of cold crystalloid cardioplegia and careful attention to myocardial cooling verified by regional myocardial temperature measurement. With the exception of a few cases associated with coronary angioplasty or intracoronary clot lysis, true emergency revascularization is a rarity. Catheterization laboratory misadventures are extremely rare even in a teaching environment. Urgency in coronary bypass has come to mean early surgical intervention at the first available elective opportunity on the regular operating room schedule.

PRESENT SURGICAL INDICATIONS

The major change in indications for coronary bypass surgery that has taken place at our institution during the past 5 years is the result of redefining the meaning of failure of medical therapy. Previously, medical therapy has been judged by its effect on symptoms, in particular angina pectoris. We reasoned that angina is a symptomatic manifestation of ischemia, and our primary therapeutic goal is to relieve ischemia. We recognized that some patients manifest ischemia without symptoms. Consequently we have systematically evaluated the effect of medical treatment with exercise stress testing, often in conjunction with thallium-201 myocardial scintigraphy. Patients who exhibit significant myocardial ischemia at low levels of exercise while receiving medical therapy are considered to be medical failures in addition to patients who continue to have angina.

With this redefinition of medical failure, the major clinical indication for coronary bypass surgery at our institution continues to be ischemia uncontrolled by medical therapy. In addition to patients with chronic stable angina, this approach also applies to patients with unstable or postinfarction angina, and to a smaller group of asymptomatic patients who undergo exercise

testing because of, for example, a history of myocardial infarction (especially young patients) or a strong presumption of important coronary artery disease.

Although our indications for coronary bypass are based primarily on physiological considerations, with objective testing for the documentation of ischemia in most cases, we recognize certain, primary *anatomic* indications for surgery based solely on angiographic data. Left main coronary artery stenosis greater than 50 percent still is the primary anatomic indication for surgery. However, the amount of myocardium at risk for infarction is taken into account and some patients with two- or three-vessel disease are also referred for surgery primarily because of anatomic considerations.

We are currently exploring the role of coronary bypass in the management of patients with acute infarction syndromes, in particular those who have been treated with streptokinase and continue to manifest ongoing ischemia.

The indications for coronary artery bypass have undergone continual evolution at our institution. We expect this evolutionary process to continue in step with improved diagnostic modalities, medical therapy, and surgical management.

REFERENCES

1 Ullyot, D. J., Wisneski, J., Sullivan, R. W., and Gertz, E. W.: Improved Survival after Coronary Artery Surgery in Patients with Extensive Coronary Artery Disease, *J. Thorac. Cardiovasc. Surg.*, 70(3):405, 1975.

2 Ullyot, D. J., Wisneski, J., Sullivan, R. W., and Gertz, E. W.: The Controversy over Coronary Arterial Surgery, *J. Thorac. Cardiovasc. Surg.*, 72(6):945, 1976. (Letters to the editor.)

3 Ullyot, D. J., Wisneski, J., Sullivan, R. W., and Gertz, E. W.: Improved Survival with Surgical Management in Patients with Chronic Stable Angina, *Am. J. Cardiol.*, 43:382, 1979. (Abstract.)

4 Ullyot, D. J., Wisneski, J., Sullivan, R. W., Gertz, E. W., and Ryan, C.: The Impact of Coronary Artery Bypass on Late Myocardial Infarction, *J. Thorac. Cardiovasc. Surg.*, 73(2):165, 1977.

5 Sternberg, L., Wisneski, J. A., Ullyot, D. J., and Gertz, E. W.: Significance of New Q Waves after Aortocoronary Bypass Surgery: Correlation with Changes in Ventricular Wall Motion, *Circulation*, 52:1037, 1975.

6 Hoar, P. F., Hickey, R. F., and Ullyot, D. J.: Systemic Hypertension following Myocardial Revascularization: A Method of Treatment using Epidural Anesthesia, *J. Thorac. Cardiovasc. Surg.*, 71(6):859, 1976.

7 Ullyot, D. J.: Current Controversies in the Conduct of the Coronary Bypass Operation, *Ann. Thorac. Surg.*, 30(2):192, 1980.

8 Brundage, B. H., Ullyot, D. J., Winokur, S., Chatterjee, K., Ports, T. A., and Turley, K.: The Role of Aortic Balloon Pumping in Post Infarction Angina: A Different Perspective, *Circulation,* 62(suppl. 1):119, 1980.

9 Roe, B. B., Hutchinson, J. C., Fishman, N. H., Ullyot, D. J., and Smith, D. L.: Myocardial Protection with Cold Ischemic Potassium Cardioplegia, *J. Thorac. Cardiovasc. Surg.,* 73(3):366, 1977.

10 Ullyot, D. J.: Discussion of Paper by A. H. Harken, L. N. Horowitz, and M. E. Josephson, Comparison of Standard Aneurysmectomy and Aneurysmectomy with Directed Endocardial Resection for the Treatment of Recurrent Sustained Ventricular Tachycardia, *J. Thorac. Cardiovasc. Surg.,* 80(4):532, 1980.

11 Brundage, B. H., Lipton, M. J., Herfkens, R. J., Berninger, W. H., Redington, R. W., Chatterjee, K., and Carlsson, E.: Detection of Patent Coronary Bypass Grafts by Computed Tomography: A Preliminary Report, *Circulation,* 61(4):826, 1980.

12 Ullyot, D. J., Turley, K., McKay, C. R., Brundage, B. H., Lipton, M. J., and Ebert, P. A.: Assessment of Saphenous Vein Graft Patency by Computed Tomography, *J. Thorac. Cardiovasc. Surg.,* 83(4):512, 1982.

13 Brindis, R., Lipton, M., McKay, C., and Brundage, B.: Graft Patency in Patients with Coronary Artery Bypass Operation Complicated by Perioperative Myocardial Infarction, *Am. J. Cardiol.,* 49:908, 1982. (Abstract.)

Coronary Artery Bypass Surgery: 13 Years' Experience with Chronic Stable Angina Pectoris, Unstable Angina Pectoris, and Acute Myocardial Infarction[*]

MARCUS A. DeWOOD, M.D., and
RALPH BERG, JR., M.D.

The general goal of coronary artery bypass graft surgery is to restore adequate blood flow distal to the point of a stenosed or occluded coronary artery. In selected patients, the effects of properly performed coronary bypass surgery may include prolongation of life by protection of myocardium at risk for dysfunction, reduction in risk of sudden cardiac death, prevention of myocardial infarction, relief of anginal symptoms, as well as attainment of normal or near-normal functional class.

When approaching the results of coronary artery bypass surgery, most essays include multiple operators, and oftentimes, multicentered results. When requested to provide the present paper, we decided that a personal experience by a single surgeon, although this involved fewer examples than would be the case with the results presented by many who have developed surgical treatment of coronary artery disease, could be valuable by offering a relatively uniform approach to therapy.

We approached this project aggressively. We found that comparing early coronary artery bypass without cardioplegia to modern bypass surgery with myocardial preservation techniques (i.e., cardioplegia plus hypothermia) offers some difficulties. Furthermore, when reviewing many years' experience with this form of therapy, the long-term results are increasingly difficult to evaluate because many patients eventually will suffer mortality or some morbidity. Distant events therefore may have less relation to the surgical procedure itself when taken in balance.

Because most patient classifications are matters of convenience and occasionally are artificially created, they can generate some illusion. For example, many patients with chronic stable angina pectoris come to the attention of the physician only because there has been some change in clinical status that prompts the patient to seek therapy. Yet these patients are not usu-ally placed in groups with unstable angina pectoris or acute myocardial infarction. Furthermore, although there are many technical factors involved in coronary bypass surgery, oftentimes these factors are difficult to measure or interpret but are taken for granted and perceived as uniform from operator to operator. Accordingly, subtle differences in technique receive little attention and yet may significantly alter the results. Assuming a relatively uniform case load, an adequate preoperative evaluation, as well as postoperative patient care, in the last analysis operative mortality and morbidity may be a reflection of the surgeon's value. Nevertheless, our survival data following coronary bypass surgery supports the concept that coronary anatomy and especially ventricular function at the time the patient enters the health care system are major determinants of the patient's future well-being.

In our hospitals, frequently the indication for coronary artery bypass is the presence of coronary lesions producing or threatening substantial myocardial damage. Because significant coronary lesions behave unpredictably and many offer the potential for creating major damage, patients scheduled for surgery are operated on with a minimum of procrastination. Change in the clinical state of the patient frequently prompts a more aggressive approach to therapy. This is especially so because we have found that the effectiveness of therapy wanes with the passage of time in many instances. For example, patients with acute evolving myocardial infarction appear to be best served if treatment begins within 6 h from symptom onset.

Medical and surgical management of coronary artery disease should be complementary and supportive. This has been achieved to the great benefit of patients in this community. While many of the patients involved in this report were managed jointly in the postoperative state by the authors, this paper reviews the 13-year experience of a single operator (R. Berg, Jr.) and reflects a relatively uniform surgical approach to the three major disease states associated with coronary artery disease—chronic stable angina, unstable angina pectoris, and acute myocardial infarction.

*From the Departments of Medicine and Surgery, Deaconess and Sacred Heart Medical Centers, Spokane, Washington.

INDICATIONS FOR CORONARY BYPASS SURGERY

Although chest pain is the generally accepted indication for coronary bypass surgery, it is recognized that the clinical expression of major coronary artery disease may range from no symptoms to incapacitating, resistant angina pectoris and in selected cases progression to acute myocardial necrosis. Alternatively, it is also well known that severe symptoms may occur in the presence of small-vessel or single-vessel disease. It cannot be uniformly stated, therefore, that chest pain should be the sole indication for coronary bypass. Many institutions now extend the indication for operation to multiple clinical situations that are usually based on an individual patient's needs.[1-8] These include a history of chronic stable angina pectoris with multivessel involvement, chronic stable angina pectoris with proximal left anterior descending coronary stenosis, worsening angina pectoris, ischemia-related rhythm disturbances, and, almost uniformly, significant left main coronary obstruction with or without symptoms. In our community, occasionally a patient presents with obstructive coronary disease in whom valvular heart disease is the primary indication for surgery. Usually these patients will undergo coronary bypass procedures. Furthermore, unstable angina pectoris and acute myocardial infarction are often treated surgically. Patients who have sustained previous myocardial infarction in whom a recurrent bout of necrosis might be fatal because of cumulative myocardial damage may also undergo coronary bypass surgery. Rarely, a patient undergoes surgical revascularization of the heart in the absence of symptoms, but usually this is because of multivessel disease in a young patient who demonstrates abnormal perfusion scintigraphy indicating inadequate perfusion. Over the past several years the procedure itself has gone from incomplete to complete revascularization, with complete revascularization being defined as insertion of a bypass graft into all vessels demonstrating 50 percent or more stenosis.

The goals in our coronary bypass surgery program are very basic. Although initially relief of pain was the sole indication for revascularization surgery, more physiological end points have been pursued. The first is to preserve myocardial function as it is encountered during evaluation of the patient. The second is protection of the patient from major clinical problems that might be based on ischemia-related events.

METHODS

Between 1969 and October of 1982 we analyzed the short-term (30-day) and the long-term mortality rates of 1,369 patients who underwent coronary bypass surgery at the Deaconess and Sacred Heart Medical Centers. For convenience, the patients were classified according to three standard clinical situations. Chronic stable angina included 920 patients, while surgical revascularization was performed on 274 patients with unstable angina pectoris; 175 patients were suffering acute myocardial infarction of both the transmural and subendocardial varieties. Eighty percent of the patient population was male. The age range was 28 to 81 years.

The patients who survived over the period of 13 years were contacted by patient questionnaire. This was followed by personal telephone conversation to explain any questions the patient might have had regarding the questionnaire or reasons for the study.

Each clinical classification was analyzed in relation to the presence of one-, two-, or three-vessel disease and was defined according to left ventricular function reflected by ejection fractions greater than or less than 50 percent. After analyzing each clinical state according to the number of vessels involved as well as left ventricular function, selected topics were examined. These selected topics of clinical importance included evaluation of sudden cardiac death, the possible prevention of myocardial infarction by coronary bypass surgery, and the functional class of each patient as well as the anginal status of the patient.

SURVIVAL WITH CHRONIC STABLE ANGINA PECTORIS

Table 1 demonstrates patient flow during the 13-year surgical experience described herein. Fifty-eight patients were lost to follow-up and were not included in subsequent analysis. The mean follow-up period was 6 years. The hospital mortality and the long-term mortality rates are demonstrated in the table on a year-by-year basis. As is demonstrated, the short-term hospital mortality rate for the period was 2.2 percent and, as expected, was highest in the early years and lowest with increasing experience. Overall, the 1-year survival rate was 96 percent. This is in keeping with the data described by Kouchoukos et al.,[9] who compared the 30-day hospital mortality rate of coronary bypass surgery in patients treated in 1970 to 1973 and in the period 1974–1977. The mortality rate in the earlier study period was 2.7 percent, while the mortality rate of the patients who underwent the procedure between 1974 and 1977 fell to 1.2 percent.

In our series the total mortality rate in the 13-year follow-up period rose to 14.8 percent. This data is similar to the results with surgical treatment of chronic stable angina pectoris reported by Greene et al.,[10] Lawrie and coworkers,[8] as well as Hurst et al.[7]

TABLE 1
Surgical experience with chronic stable angina

Year	Number of cases	30-day mortality		Additional deaths, first year	1-year survival rate (%)
		No.	Percent		
1969–1970	11	0	———	2	82
1970–1971	17	1	5.9	0	94
1971–1972	26	1	3.8	1	92
1972–1973	61	1	1.6	0	98
1973–1974	60	1	1.6	0	98
1974–1975	74	1	1.3	2	96
1975–1976	80	2	2.5	1	96
1976–1977	142	5	3.5	1	96
1977–1978	107	3	2.8	1	96
1978–1979	64	2	3.1	1	95
1979–1980	94	1	1.1	1	98
1980–1981	93	2	2.2	3	95
1981–1982	64	0	———	0	100
Oct. 1982	27	0	———	0	100
Totals	920	20	2.2	13	96

Influence of Multivessel Coronary Disease

SURVIVAL WITH SINGLE-VESSEL CORONARY ARTERY DISEASE

The effect of multivessel coronary disease on survival is described in Fig. 1. As is demonstrated, the short-term mortality rate for single-vessel disease was 2.8 percent and in the follow-up period rose to 14.4 percent over the 13-year study. These findings are similar to series describing results with conventional medical therapy for single-vessel coronary artery disease.[11–15] For example, age-, sex-, and race-matched survival

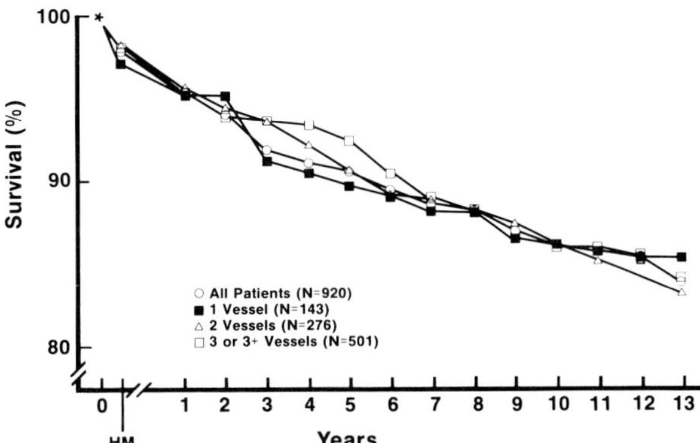

FIGURE 1 Survival curves of patients treated for chronic stable angina pectoris and classified by one- two- or three-vessel disease. As is shown, one vessel, two vessels, or three or more vessels were diseased in 143, 276, and 501 patients, respectively. The inhospital and long-term mortality rates were not significantly different in any of the groups.

curves generated by the Department of Health, Education and Welfare[16] suggest that survival data for patients with single-vessel disease undergoing coronary bypass and surviving hospitalization demonstrate a *5-year* life expectancy which is similar to conventional therapy.[16] It should be remembered, however, that during the period under study the modality employed for single-vessel disease associated with chest pain was coronary bypass surgery *after* a trial of conventional therapy. Therefore, the group described herein may not be completely comparable to those reports of results with conventional therapy. It is anticipated that with recent advances in the role of percutaneous transluminal coronary angioplasty for proximal discrete single-vessel stenosis, we may see an attractive alternative to bypass surgery, especially in single-vessel disease.

SURVIVAL WITH TWO-VESSEL CORONARY ARTERY DISEASE

The short-term mortality rate for two-vessel disease was 1.7 percent and rose to 17.1 percent over the 13-year follow-up period. This is comparable to the data described by Kouchoukos et al.,[17] who demonstrated a 93 percent survival rate in patients followed for 24 months and further revealed a significantly lower survival rate in the nonoperated surgical candidate group as compared to the operated patients.[17] Furthermore, the data of Greene and coworkers[18] show survival characteristics similar to those of the present study when two-vessel disease was treated surgically.

Conventional therapy for double-vessel coronary disease has proved to be similarly effective in two studies involving shorter periods of time (4 years) than the present study.[15,19] By contrast, the data supplied by the Cleveland Clinic,[14] which come from an angiographically documented study of the natural history of obstructive coronary disease, suggest that in longer follow-up the survival rate of patients demonstrating two-vessel coronary disease falls to 60 percent. Although there are obvious dangers in comparing results of different therapies between centers, it would therefore appear superficially that surgical management may offer some long-term protection in patients with two-vessel coronary disease. This will require further follow-up of conventionally managed patients in further trials, however.

SURVIVAL WITH THREE-VESSEL CORONARY ARTERY DISEASE

As is demonstrated in Fig. 1, the inhospital mortality rate for triple-vessel coronary artery disease in chronic stable angina pectoris was 2.0 percent and rose to 16.1 percent over the 13-year follow-up period. Other surgical series[17,18] support the concept that three-vessel coronary artery disease can be managed safely in the hospital. Furthermore, survival rate is improved over conventional therapy in patients with angiographically diagnosed three-vessel coronary artery disease.[11–14,19–21]

The data in the present study, as well as in other reports,[7,8,10,14,15,17,18,20,21] suggest that one of the primary determinants of survival in either conventionally or surgically treated triple-vessel coronary disease is the number of vessels involved and, therefore, compromise of coronary blood flow. These findings from multiple studies invoke a powerful argument in favor of coronary bypass surgery in patients with symptomatic triple-vessel disease.

Nevertheless, the value of coronary bypass surgery with three-vessel involvement in patients without symptoms is virtually unknown. Should the clinician wait for the patient who demonstrates triple-vessel coronary artery disease to develop symptoms before beginning therapy? Will the patient with three-vessel disease develop symptoms? These are open questions, but a powerful inferential argument can be made for prophylactic bypass by review of the series mentioned above as well as the results derived from the present study.

Influence of Left Ventricular Performance on Survival

With recent advances in operative techniques in conjunction with modern cardioplegia, increasing numbers of patients with impaired left ventricular function and multivessel involvement are being safely treated with coronary bypass surgery. As is shown in Fig. 2, we dichotomized the 920 patients with chronic stable angina pectoris according to ejection fraction greater or less than 50 percent. As is demonstrated, there were important differences in outcome between the two groups when viewed in this manner. The short-term mortality rate of the group with ejection fraction greater than 50 percent was 1.1 percent, but the short-term mortality rate of the group with significantly impaired left ventricular function reflected by ejection fraction less than 50 percent was 3.8 percent. Over the 13-year follow-up period the group with relatively normal left ventricular function sustained a total mortality rate of 11.7 percent, while the group with impaired left ventricular function demonstrated a total mortality rate of 22 percent. This confirms the experience reported by Kouchoukos and coworkers,[9] who reported on a similar group of patients and showed a 24-month survival rate of 85 percent for the 59 surgical patients.

As is shown by our data as well as by Vliestra,[22] Murphy and coworkers,[23] and Hammermeister et al.,[24] increased rate of survival in patient groups with relatively normal left ventricular performance can be anticipated. Some studies[22,24] have demonstrated that left ventricular performance is the variable most predictive of survival. Further supporting this view are data reported by Greene and coworkers,[18] who have shown that patients with an ejection fraction of 50 percent or more demonstrate survival curves that are only slightly less than that of the general public.

Further confirming the importance of left ventric-

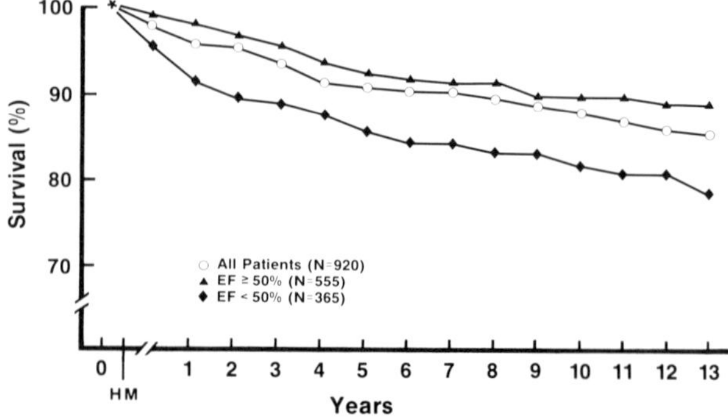

FIGURE 2 Survival curves in patients dichotomized by ejection fraction. Triangles (N = 555) indicate the group with ejection fractions greater than 50 percent prior to operation while the diamonds indicate patients whose ejection fraction was less than 50 percent. While there were minor inhospital differences in mortality rate (see text) there were significant differences ($p < .05$) at the end of 13 years between the groups.

ular performance as a major determinant of survival is the Coronary Artery Surgery Study (CASS) that recently described survival of medically treated patient groups sorted by various levels of ejection fraction.[15] This study clearly demonstrated that depression of left ventricular performance was associated with high mortality rate over a 4-year follow-up period. The reported mortality rate was somewhat higher than for our patients who had depression of ejection fraction but were treated with surgical revascularization. Likewise, Kouchoukos[9] and colleagues demonstrated only 67 percent survival rate in 89 patients managed with conventional therapy but with severe depression of left ventricular function. Importantly, of the 59 patients with similar left ventricular function who were treated surgically and followed longer than 2 years, there was no mortality. A total mortality rate of 22 percent over a 13-year period therefore appears to be acceptable in such patients.

In the present study there was a significantly different outcome depending on left ventricular function. Patients with normal left ventricular function frequently demonstrated flat survival curves, indicating that the process of left ventricular deterioration reflected by advancing mortality had been arrested. Furthermore, these data suggest that therapy aimed at preservation of left ventricular function and increased survival should begin before substantial damage occurs to the left ventricle whether due to acute or chronic necrosis. Surgical revascularization generally does not improve resting left ventricular function in patients with chronic stable angina.[25] Nevertheless, patients with both left ventricular dysfunction and disabling angina may benefit from surgical therapy.

SURVIVAL IN UNSTABLE ANGINA PECTORIS

Table 2 demonstrates patient flow during the 13-year experience described in this paper. Twenty-four patients were lost to follow-up and were not included in subsequent analysis. The mean follow-up period was 6 years. The short- and long-term mortality rates are demonstrated on an annual bases as well. Overall, the short-term mortality rate for the period under study was 1.8 percent, which was not significantly different from the overall figures for patients with chronic stable angina pectoris. The 1-year survival rate for the entire period under study was 96 percent, and the cumulative mortality rate in the 13-year follow-up period rose to 13.6 percent. This was also insignificantly different from the data for patients with chronic stable angina pectoris. The mortality rate overall of the group treated surgically for unstable angina pectoris is somewhat less than that reported at an earlier period (1972) after the unstable angina pectoris trial sponsored by the National Institutes of Health,[26] but is similar to the mortality sustained in the surgical group of the last 4 years (1973 to 1976) of the study.[26]

It is exceptionally difficult to compare results of the present study with the effects of medical or surgical therapy in the National Institutes of Health study[26] because 36 percent of the medical group underwent surgery for relief of continued angina. Furthermore, many patients considered to be too sick to be included in the medical series were operated on between coronary angiography and randomization. Therefore the medical and surgical results are difficult to interpret.

When reviewing overall results of other series that

TABLE 2
Surgical experience with unstable angina

| Year | Number of cases | 30-day mortality rate | | Additional deaths, first year | 1-year survival rate (%) |
		No.	Percent		
1969–1970	2	0	———	0	100
1970–1971	6	0	———	1	83
1971–1972	14	1	7.1	0	93
1972–1973	31	0	———	1	97
1973–1974	34	0	———	0	100
1974–1975	24	0	———	1	96
1975–1976	24	1	4.1	0	96
1976–1977	24	1	4.1	0	96
1977–1978	35	1	2.9	2	91
1978–1979	18	1	5.5	0	94
1979–1980	23	0	———	0	100
1980–1981	21	0	———	0	100
1981–1982	8	0	———	0	100
Oct. 1982	10	0	———	0	100
Totals	274	5	1.8	5	96

might shed value on the surgical therapy in unstable angina pectoris, it is clear that there are few medically treated series that have demonstrated similar long-term survival rates. The only long-term series given conventional therapy is that of Gazes.[27] Angiographic definition of the extent of disease in these patients is not known. One of the most unfavorable findings in their 10-year follow-up of patients with unstable angina was persistent angina in the hospital, which was associated with high mortality rate. It must be recognized, however, that the bulk of the data of the study group was generated during the 1960s and medical therapy was restricted mostly to short-acting oral nitrates. Nevertheless, in the National Institutes of Health study[26] continued medical therapy without later surgery (presumably in patients who had good results with initial medical therapy) still demonstrated more than 10 percent mortality in the follow-up period, which averaged 30 months.

Influence of Multivessel Coronary Disease

SURVIVAL WITH SINGLE-VESSEL CORONARY ARTERY DISEASE

The effect of multivessel coronary disease on survival in patients with unstable angina pectoris is depicted in Fig. 3. As is demonstrated, the mortality rate for single-vessel disease was 0 percent and rose to 8.7 percent in the follow-up period. These results with *single-vessel coronary disease* are precisely in concert with the

inhospital mortality rate for the National Institutes of Health (NIH) study of unstable angina treated surgically.[26]

SURVIVAL WITH TWO-VESSEL CORONARY ARTERY DISEASE

Where two-vessel coronary disease was discovered in the present study, the short-term mortality rate was 4.6 percent and rose to 16 percent in the follow-up period. This is demonstrated in Fig. 3. These short-term mortality rate figures are similar to the NIH's inhospital mortality rates with medical (4 percent) therapy, but slightly higher than the surgical (2 percent) results. Nevertheless, as the higher frequency of two- and three-vessel disease occurred in the NIH's study, more patients experienced significant angina pectoris and presumably crossed over to surgical therapy in the follow-up period.

SURVIVAL WITH THREE-VESSEL CORONARY ARTERY DISEASE

Triple-vessel disease was associated with a short-term mortality rate of 1 percent. This rose to 15 percent in the 13-year follow-up as is shown in Fig. 3. This inhospital mortality rate is much less than the 10 percent figure quoted in the NIH study for surgically treated unstable angina with triple-vessel disease.[26] Likewise, the long-term mortality rate in the present study appears to be somewhat more favorable than that in other reported series of patients given conventional therapy and having angiographic diagnosis.[28–30]

In our community we attempt to arrange surgery promptly for patients who have demonstrated failure of modern medical therapy. With this approach, the mortality rate has remained low with both conventional and surgical therapy.

It is important to recognize (Fig. 3) that the majority of patients in the present series demonstrate multivessel disease with a preponderance of three or more vessels being involved. Therefore the wisdom of waiting in this subgroup may be suspect. Frequently it is this group that is the most severely symptomatic, undergoes angiography, and is treated by surgical therapy. Perhaps an advantage to early angiography is that patients with chest pain but without multivessel disease or life-threatening lesions such as left main disease can be identified and usually be safely treated with medical therapy. Likewise, patients with normal coronary arteries but with a similar clinical presentation can be identified.

After reviewing the previously mentioned studies as well as our results, we conclude that unstable angina

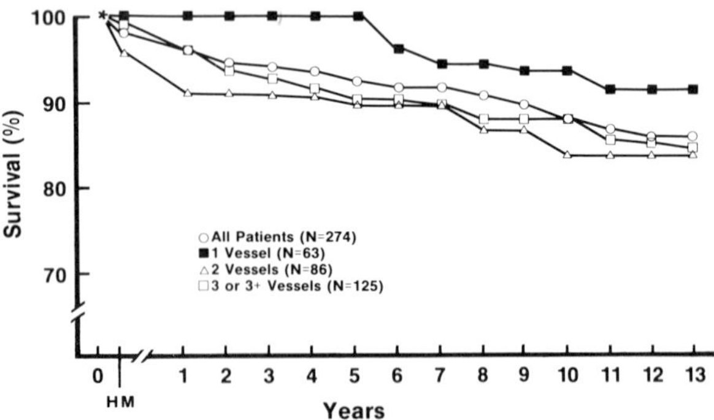

FIGURE 3 Survival curves in patients with unstable angina pectoris by one, two and three or more vessels diseased. As is shown the groups with two- and three-vessel disease behaved in a very similar manner after 3 years while the group with one-vessel disease demonstrated significantly ($p < .05$) better survival rates than two- or three-vessel disease patients. Mortality rates for all three groups were relatively low throughout the study. In many areas, the survival curves are flat, indicating that ischemic process was arrested.

can be treated with conventional therapy with a satisfactory outcome. However, if angiography demonstrates triple-vessel disease or left main disease, it appears there is no particular advantage in delaying surgery.

Influence of Left Ventricular Performance on Survival

Few studies have examined the influence of left ventricular performance on short- or long-term mortality rates. We therefore dichotomized our population at the 50 percent level. As is shown in Fig. 4, the short-term mortality rate in patients exhibiting an ejection fraction of 50 percent or more was 1.6 percent and rose to 11.3 percent in the long-term follow-up. By contrast, patients exhibiting an ejection fraction less than 50 percent experienced a short-term mortality rate of 3.8 percent, which rose to 18 percent in the follow-up period. Thus, left ventricular performance appeared to be a major determinant of short- and long-term mortality rates as was demonstrated in patients with chronic stable angina.

RESULTS WITH ACUTE MYOCARDIAL INFARCTION

Table 3 demonstrates patient flow during the 12-year experience with surgical reperfusion for acute evolving myocardial infarction. Eight patients were lost to follow-up and were not included in subsequent analysis. The mean follow-up period was 6 years. The data presented encompasses overall results with transmural and nontransmural infarctions. As with Tables 1 and 2, the inhospital mortality and long-term mortality rates are demonstrated in the table on an annual basis. As is shown, the hospital mortality rate for the period was 2.3 percent. Overall, the 1-year survival rate was 95 percent. This is in keeping with previous descriptions of surgical management of acute myocardial infarction,[31,32] and the work of Phillips and coworkers[33] has confirmed our findings.

The rationale for surgical reperfusion during early-evolving infarction is to reperfuse marginally ischemic areas and to protect myocardium that would otherwise progress to frank infarction. In transmural infarction, an especially important finding is the relatively high frequency of total coronary occlusion, which has been described recently[34] and confirmed by others.[35] Because success with reperfusion in preservation of function appears to vary inversely with the time interval from occlusion to reperfusion,[36] we have attempted to restore blood flow as early as possible following symptom onset.

By contrast, because nontransmural myocardial infarction is associated with much less frequency of total coronary occlusion,[37] there may be a longer period of time to protect ischemic myocardium or muscle distal to the point of insufficient blood flow. It should be noted, however, that total coronary occlusion appears to progress in subendocardial infarction. Therefore, timely restoration of blood flow in selected cases might offer protection of left ventricular function on a long-term basis.

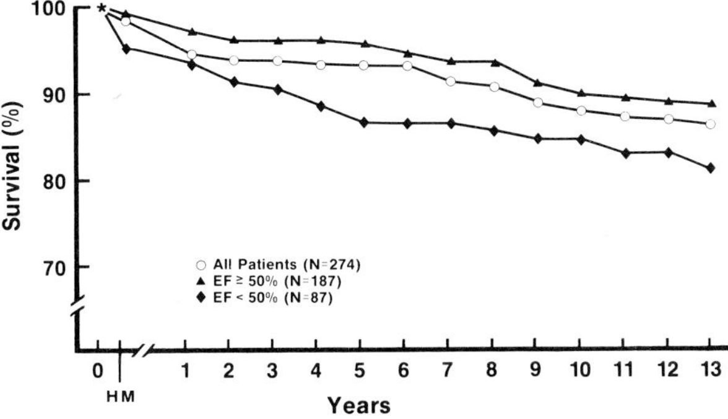

FIGURE 4 Survival curves in unstable angina pectoris patients when dichotomized by ejection fraction greater than or less than 50 percent. As is shown, there were significant differences both in hospital mortality rate as well as in long-term outcome when these patients were analyzed in terms of ejection fraction.

Survival with Multivessel Disease in Myocardial Infarction

The effect of multivessel coronary disease on survival in patients undergoing surgical reperfusion for acute myocardial infarction is demonstrated in Fig. 5. The short-term mortality rate with single-vessel disease was 1.8 percent and rose to 6.4 percent in the long term, while two-vessel disease was associated with 2.0 percent short-term mortality rate that rose to 15.4 percent in the follow-up period. There was a slightly higher mortality rate if three or more vessels were associated with the group suffering acute myocardial infarction. The mortality rate was 2.8 percent and rose to 17.0 percent over the study period. The low mortality rate associated with surgical reperfusion for the series is consistent with figures generated by Phillips et al.[33] and others[38–41] provided coronary bypass was performed during the early stages of myocardial necrosis.

The mortality rate progressively rose with two- or three-vessel disease as shown in Fig. 5. Nevertheless, there were multiple areas on each curve that were flat,

TABLE 3
Surgical experience with acute myocardial infarction

Year	Number of cases	30-day mortality rate		Additional deaths, first year	1-year survival rate (%)
		No.	Percent		
1971–1972	8	0	———	1	87
1972–1973	6	0	———	0	100
1973–1974	2	0	———	0	100
1974–1975	8	0	———	0	100
1975–1976	13	0	———	1	92
1976–1977	30	0	———	1	97
1977–1978	29	1	3.4	0	96
1978–1979	20	1	5.0	0	95
1979–1980	18	0	———	0	100
1980–1981	26	1	3.8	0	96
1981–1982	9	1	11.1	1	78
Oct. 1982	6	0	———	0	100
Totals	175	4	2.3	4	95

suggesting that the ischemic process had been effectively arrested. Since there are no controlled randomized trials that have angiographically investigated patients suffering acute myocardial infarction and then randomized these patients to conventional or surgical therapy, no comment can be made regarding comparisons with one-, two-, or three-vessel disease. However, the data of Proudfit and coworkers[14] does suggest that coronary artery disease in and of itself does carry progressive mortality whether due to one-, two-, or three-vessel disease. It might be expected, therefore, that patients suffering acute infarction with one-, two-, or three-vessel disease should demonstrate progressive mortality as do patients with chronic stable angina pectoris. This was not the case in all situations as can be seen in Fig. 5.

The inhospital and long-term mortality rates compare favorably with those of the previously published series from this community.[32] However, it should be noted that these patients have gone through a selection process involving several steps. For example, patients must survive long enough to be hospitalized. Oftentimes the patient is young and without debilitating diseases. Furthermore, the patient must present early to the hospital (within 6 h from symptom onset) and survive cardiac catheterization. It is then determined whether or not the patient is a surgical candidate. Therefore, an ''all comers'' is not practiced in this community. Instead, usually patients with anterior infarction are referred for surgical consideration as well as patients with multivessel involvement.

Influence of Left Ventricular Performance on Survival

As is shown in Fig. 6, left ventricular performance was a major predictor of outcome. As is shown, when left ventricular ejection fraction was greater than 50 percent, the short-term mortality rate was 1.1 percent, whereas if left ventricular ejection fraction was less than 50 percent, the mortality rate rose to 3.5 percent (difference nonsignificant). By contrast, differences in mortality rates became more marked in follow-up. The patient group with an ejection fraction greater than 50 percent experienced an 8.6 percent total mortality rate, whereas patients with depression of left ventricular ejection fraction experienced a 17.0 percent total mortality rate. Therefore, left ventricular function at the time of cardiac catheterization played a significant role in predicting the long-term mortality rate, but was less indicative of the short-term result.

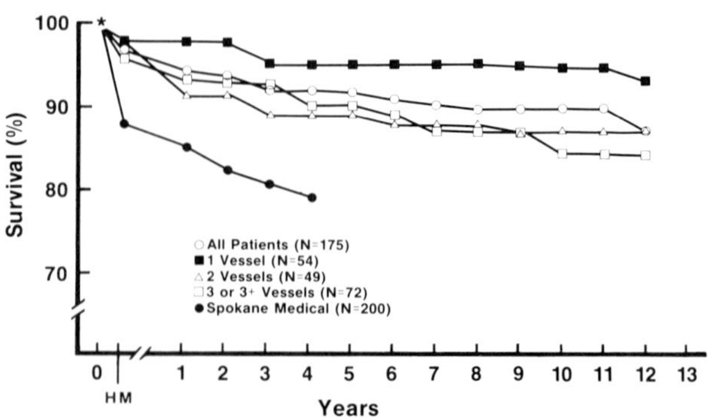

FIGURE 5 Survival curves of patients suffering acute myocardial infarction classified by one, two, and three or more vessels involved. As is shown, the inhospital mortality rates were similar between the three groups. However, in the long term the patient group with one-vessel disease demonstrated better survival rates than patients with two- and three-vessel disease.

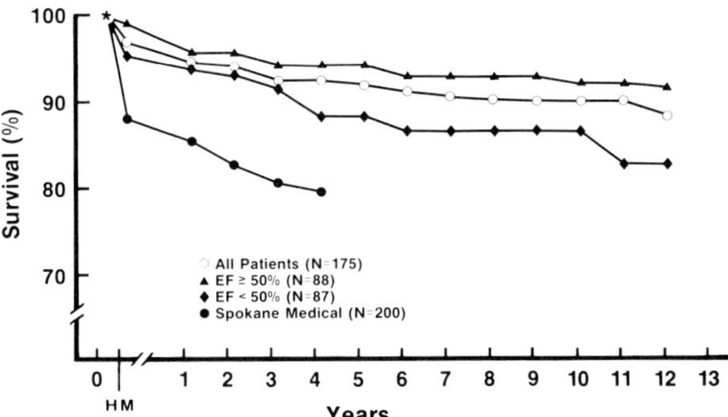

FIGURE 6 Survival curves in patients receiving surgical reperfusion for acute evolving myocardial infarction when dichotomized by ejection fraction greater than 50 percent (N = 88) or less than 50 percent (N = 87). As is shown, the inhospital and long-term mortality rates of the two groups are different at every point in the survival curves. This is especially marked at the end of the study. Other abbreviations as in Fig. 5.

EVALUATION OF SUDDEN DEATH FOLLOWING CORONARY BYPASS SURGERY

Sudden death related to coronary atherosclerosis is an important problem and is responsible for approximately 50 percent of coronary-related mortalities.[42] Unfortunately, patients who survive a bout of acute myocardial infarction remain at risk for major rhythm disturbances that lead to sudden unexpected mortality.[43] Autopsy studies[44] indicate that the majority of patients dying suddenly demonstrate severe coronary atherosclerosis with or without healed myocardial infarction, but oftentimes sudden death is without evidence of new necrosis or coronary thrombus.

The absence of acute myocardial infarction or coronary thrombosis suggests that ventricular rhythm disturbances triggered by unknown mechanisms cause the majority of sudden cardiac deaths. Canine studies suggest that deterioration of myocardial metabolism in ischemic areas of myocardium precedes deterioration in rhythm.[45]

If inadequate coronary blood flow is responsible for deterioration in metabolism and leads to ventricular dysrhythmias, an inferential argument could be made in favor of coronary bypass to prevent sudden cardiac death. Vismara and coworkers[43] at the University of California–Davis Medical Center analyzed 247 patients, 135 of whom had undergone coronary bypass grafting. The remainder of the group (N = 112) was given conventional medical therapy. Analysis of the data suggested severalfold reduction in sudden cardiac death in patients treated with coronary bypass surgery. Likewise, Hammermeister and coworkers[47] evaluated sudden death prospectively for 4 years in medically

and surgically treated patients matched for coronary atherosclerosis and ventricular function. For each subgroup analyzed, the incidence of sudden death was much lower in selected surgical cohorts. These data indicate that revascularization by coronary bypass surgery may reduce such fatalities in patients with multivessel disease.

As is shown in Fig. 7, our data indicate that whether patients had undergone revascularization surgery for chronic stable angina pectoris, unstable angina pectoris, or acute evolving infarction, there was similar reduction in sudden death relative to the group described by Vismara and coworkers[46] who were given conventional medical therapy. As is shown, the group with chronic stable angina pectoris demonstrated less than 5 percent incidence of sudden death in long-term follow-up. Likewise, the group with unstable angina demonstrated major reductions in the incidence of sudden death as did the group with acute myocardial infarction who had undergone surgical reperfusion. We conclude from the above series[43,46,47] as well as our own experience that sudden death may be avoided in selected surgically treated patients. However, there are no controlled randomized trials that evaluate sudden death in medically and surgically treated groups.

MYOCARDIAL INFARCTION FOLLOWING SURGICAL TREATMENT OF CORONARY ATHEROSCLEROSIS

Although the indications for surgical revascularization of the heart have expanded over the past several years, one of the areas of increasing interest is the possible prevention of myocardial infarction by prophylactic coronary bypass surgery. Although the location and extent of coronary obstruction obviously leaves variable degrees of myocardium at risk for future ischemic events, little is known regarding the incidence of myocardial infarction in patients with angiographically evaluated chronic stable angina pectoris. In this regard, probably an attitude of aggressive surgical management to prevent myocardial infarction *without careful case selection* is difficult to justify.

Although the expected mortality in chronic stable angina pectoris has been examined in multiple trials and publications, there is a surprising lack of data concerning the prevalence of acute myocardial infarction in chronic stable angina pectoris. Thus, it is difficult to know whether or not revascularization surgery protects the patients from subsequent coronary events recognized as myocardial infarction.

Although perioperative myocardial infarction may be a problem complicating evaluation of the efficacy of bypass surgery in prevention of future myocardial infarction, we could not demonstrate an adverse effect

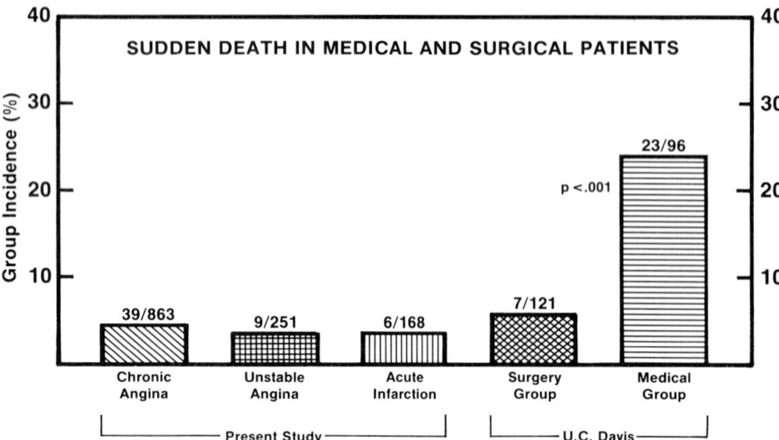

FIGURE 7 Sudden death in patients with chronic angina, unstable angina, and acute infarction in the present study compared to the group treated surgically or medically from the University of California at Davis. As is shown, there is a significant reduction in the incidence of sudden death in all treated groups. As is shown, the incidence of subsequent sudden death in the surgically treated patients is 5 percent or less in the present study. (*From Vismara et al., Improved Longevity due to Reduction of Sudden Death by Aortal Coronary Bypass in Coronary Atherosclerosis. Prospective Evaluation of Medical Versus Surgical Therapy in Matched Patients with Multivessel Disease, Am. J. Cardiol., 39:919, 1977. Reproduced with permission.*)

of the longevity of patients followed 5 or more years after the bypass procedure.[48]

We evaluated the subsequent myocardial infarction rate in all three groups described in the present paper. As is shown in Fig. 8, the group with chronic stable angina pectoris demonstrated a 10 percent incidence of subsequent myocardial infarction over the 13-year follow-up period, while the group with unstable angina pectoris had subsequent myocardial infarction in 12.4 percent of the population. As is shown in Fig. 8 of the survivors of infarction treated with reperfusion, there was a 16 percent incidence of subsequent myocardial infarction over the 12-year follow-up period. Thus, in all groups there is the potential for subsequent myocardial infarction, but as is shown in Figs. 1 to 6, the subsequent myocardial infarctions do not appear to account for major mortality in any of the groups. This may suggest that coronary bypass surgery offered effective treatment and possibly protection from future ischemic events of major consequence. Hammermeister et al.[47] found there was a reduction in the incidence of subsequent myocardial infarction in single-vessel coronary obstruction. Likewise, the frequency of unstable angina pectoris was significantly reduced by coronary bypass surgery in patients with two-vessel obstruction with depression of left ventricular function.

Prevention of myocardial infarction by coronary bypass surgery is difficult to evaluate in the absence of a randomized trial. It is recognized that this complication will occur in a relatively small percentage of patients on an annual basis. Unfortunately, in our experience recurrence of myocardial infarction most often involves progressive disease in the native circulation or problems with graft occlusion due to recurrent atherosclerosis in the bypass graft itself with or without coronary thrombosis.

EVALUATION OF FUNCTIONAL CLASS FOLLOWING CORONARY BYPASS SURGERY

The functional class of patients in this report was determined. Of the patients with chronic stable angina, unstable angina pectoris, and myocardial infarction, questionnaires were adequately answered in 735, 217, and 151 patients, respectively. Functional class was established by the following criteria: (1) no shortness of breath and no limitation of activity, (2) minor shortness of breath and limitation of activity with maximal exertion, (3) shortness of breath and limitation of exercise capacity with less than maximal exertion, and (4) severe restrictions in the ability to function normally based on cardiac disability.

As is shown in Fig. 9, of the patients treated for chronic stable angina 46 percent, 29.4 percent, 22 percent, and 2 percent were class I, II, III, or IV, respectively. In the unstable angina group 46 percent

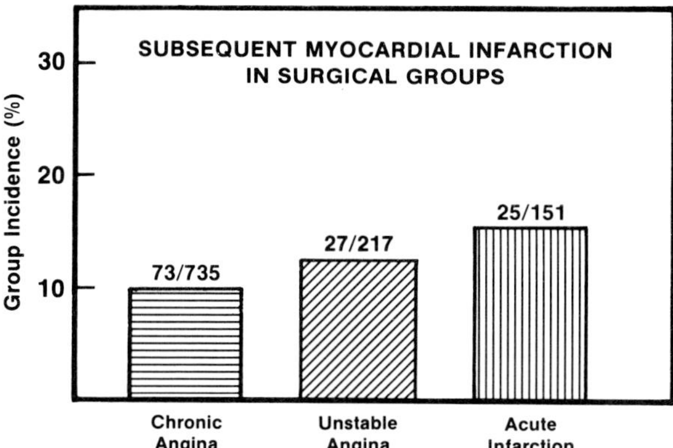

FIGURE 8 This figure indicates the incidence of subsequent myocardial infarction in the present study. As is shown, the patient group with chronic stable angina pectoris experienced a 10 percent myocardial infarction rate over the 13-year follow-up period while the group with unstable pectoris evidenced a 12.5 percent myocardial infarction rate. The group treated surgically for myocardial infarction experienced a 16.5 percent reinfarction rate in the 13-year follow-up. These subsequent myocardial infarctions were frequently due to advancing disease in the native circulation in an ungrafted vessel, atherosclerosis in a vessel distal to the insertion point of the bypass graft, and recurrent atherosclerosis in the bypass graft itself.

were completely without functional restrictions; 48 percent were in class II; while 30 percent were in class III; 4 percent classified themselves as class IV. In patients with acute myocardial infarction, classes I, II, III, and IV were present in 45 percent, 26 percent, 22 percent, and 6.5 percent, respectively. Overall, therefore, the majority of patient in this series were not limited in functional capacity or were limited only with maximum exercise. By contrast, very few patients classified themselves as having disabling symptoms due to heart disease.

RELIEF OF ANGINA PECTORIS

As is shown in Fig. 10, the anginal class of each group of patients was determined. The anginal class was divided into four types based on the occurrence of chest pain with activity. Clinical classification I was defined as no angina, II was defined as chest pain with maximal exertion, III included chest pain with less than maximal exertion. Clinical classification IV included chest pain with minor activity. As is shown in the figure, approximately 70 percent of each group was angina-free while approximately 25 percent of each group had angina only with maximum exercise. Five percent or less stated that they experienced angina pectoris with minor activity. Since these patients were followed for an average of 6 years, the question as to

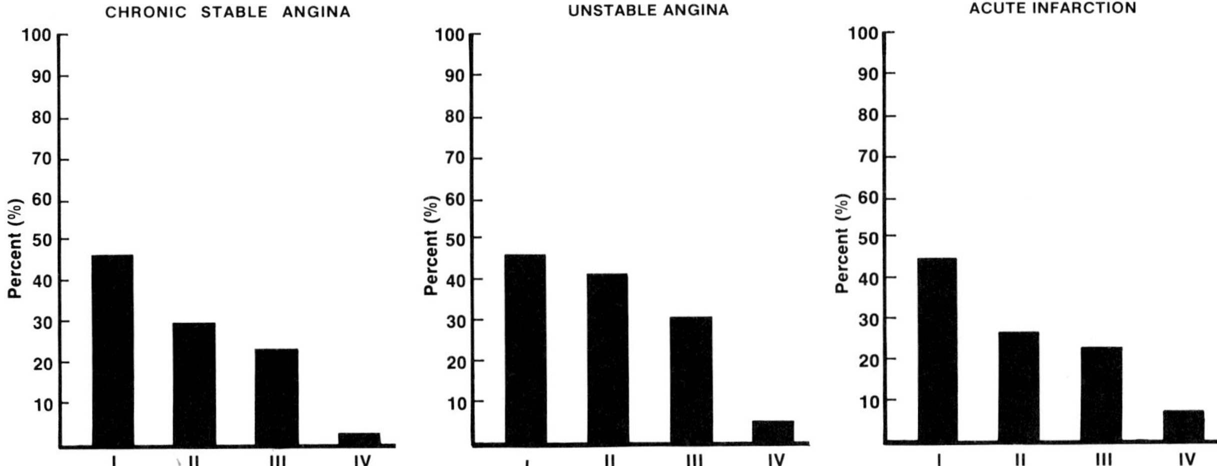

FIGURE 9 Figure 9 demonstrates results regarding functional class in chronic stable angina, unstable angina pectoris, and acute myocardial infarction. Class I was defined as no shortness of breath or limitation of movement with maximum exercise, class II was defined as shortness of breath with maximal exertion, while class III was defined as shortness of breath and limitation of exercise ability with less than maximal exertion, while class IV is defined as symptoms at rest. In the chronic stable angina group the incidence of classes I, II, III, and IV was 45.8 percent, 29.4 percent, 22.7 percent, and 2.1 percent, respectively. In the unstable angina group the incidence of each classification was 45.6 percent, 41.0 percent, 30.4 percent, and 4.6 percent, respectively. In the acute myocardial infarction patients the incidence of each classification was 44.4 percent, 26.5 percent, 22.5 percent, and 6.6 percent, respectively.

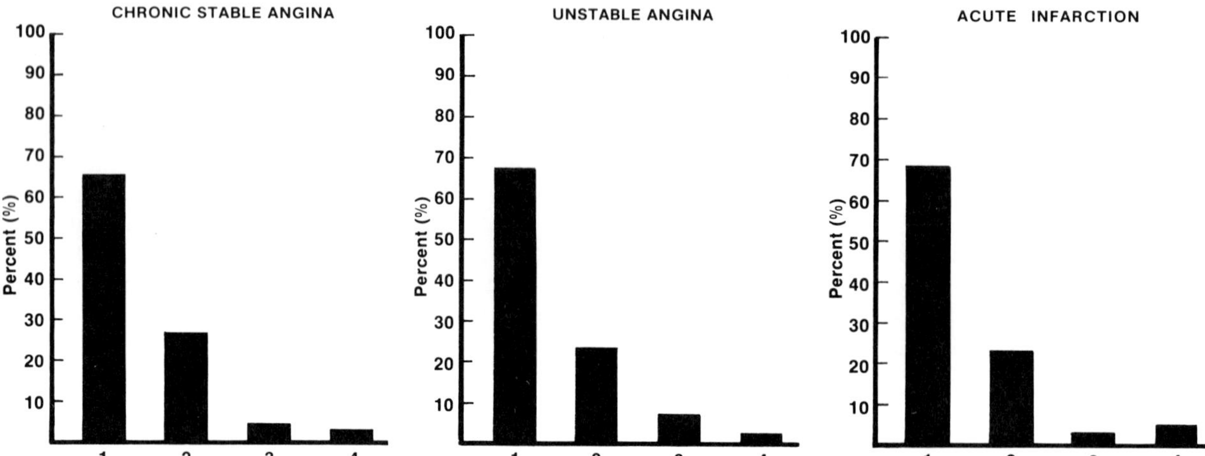

FIGURE 10 This figure demonstrates results regarding angina pectoris following coronary bypass surgery in chronic stable angina, unstable angina pectoris, and acute myocardial infarction. Angina was graded as 1 (no chest pain whatsoever), 2 (chest pain with maximal exertion), 3 (chest pain with submaximal exertion), or 4 (chest pain even with minor exertion). The incidence of each classification in the chronic stable angina group was 65.9 percent, 26.4 percent, 4.6 percent, and 3.0 percent, respectively. Similar results were obtained with the unstable angina group as well as the group having suffered acute myocardial infarction and treated with surgical reperfusion.

whether or not coronary bypass surgery results in sustained relief of exertional angina appears to be a settled issue. These data *cannot settle the questions surrounding the mechanisms of relief.* One must assume, however, that angina relief with low long-term mortality rate supports the concept that adequate myocardial perfusion of previously ischemic myocardium is likely the mechanism.

CONCLUSIONS

Although coronary artery bypass surgery has been shown to be associated with an acceptable mortality rate, morbidity rate, and favorable results in terms of the functional class and the prevalence of postoperative angina pectoris, many questions remain unanswered. Our data suggest that the recurrence of myocardial infarction is acceptably low, as is the incidence of sudden death relative to conventional therapy.

Careful examination of the literature concerning the benefit of coronary bypass surgery is helpful. Although there was some initial disappointment involving both the VA Cooperative Study on chronic stable angina and the National Institutes of Health study on unstable angina, the majority of firm conclusions showing the benefits of coronary bypass surgery that were addressed by each trial have now been satisfactorily answered. Skepticism generated by major trials (especially when the results published are premature) is justified. Acrimony regarding those results is not. In our community, treatment of coronary artery disease is viewed as complementary management.

It is likely the controversy will continue over the next several years regarding the most beneficial therapy for acute myocardial infarction. Even though the data cited in the present study appear favorable, we firmly believe that prospective controlled randomized trials are necessary to put the issue of reperfusion firmly in proper perspective. Finally, the value and limitations of coronary bypass surgery will probably require continued clinical research and further understanding of the basic mechanisms causative of coronary heart disease.

REFERENCES

1 Collins, J. J., Jr.: Indications for Coronary Bypass Surgery, *Am. J. Cardiol.*, 43:129, 1979.

2 Sheldon, W. C., Rincon, G., Pichard, A. D., Razavi, M., Cheanvechai, C., and Loop, F. D.: Surgical Treatment of Coronary Artery Disease: Pure Graft Operations, with a Study of 741 Patients Followed 3–7 Years, *Prog. Cardiovasc. Dis.*, 18:237, 1975.

3 Favaloro, R. G.: Direct Myocardial Revascularization: A Ten-Year Journey, *Am. J. Cardiol.*, 43:109, 1979.

4 Mundth, E. D., and Austen, G. W.: Surgical Measures for Coronary Heart Disease, *N. Engl. J. Med.*, 293:13,75,124, 1975.

5 Johnson, W. D., and Shores, R.: Coronary Bypass Surgery: Early and Long-term Results, in J. I. Haft and C.

P. Bailey (eds.), ''Advances in Management of Clinical Heart Disease,'' Futura Publishing Company, Mount Kisco, N.Y., 1978, p. 265.

6 Hall, R. J., Garcia, E., Mathur, V. S., Busch, U., Cooley, D. A., Gold, K. A., and Gray, A. G.: Longterm Follow-up after Coronary Artery Bypass, *Cleve. Clin. Q.*, 162, 1978.

7 Hurst, J. W., King, S. B., III, Logue, R. W., et al.: Value of Coronary Bypass Surgery, *Am. J. Cardiol.*, 42:308, 1978.

8 Lawrie, G. M., Morris, G. C., Jr., Howell, J. F., Tredici, T. D., and Chapman, D. W.: Improved Survival after 5 Years in 1,144 Patients after Coronary Bypass Surgery, *Am. J. Cardiol.*, 42:709, 1978.

9 Kouchoukos, N. T., and Oberman, A.: Coronary Artery Bypass Grafting, in C. E. Rackley and R. O. Russell, Jr. (eds.), ''Coronary Artery Disease: Recognition and Management,'' Futura Publishing Company, Mount Kisco, N.Y., 1979, p. 299.

10 Greene, D. G., Bunnell, I. L., Arani, D. T., et al.: Actuarial Analysis of Survival of 875 Cases of Coronary Bypass Surgery, in ''Proceedings of the VIII World Congress of Cardiology,'' 1978, p. 210, abstract 0487.

11 Bruschke, A. V. G., Proudfit, W. L., and Sones, F. M., Jr.: Progress Study of 590 Consecutive Nonsurgical Cases of Coronary Disease Followed 5–9 Years. I. Arteriographic Correlations, *Circulation*, 47:1147, 1973.

12 Burggraf, G. W., and Parker, J. O.: Prognosis in Coronary Artery Disease. Angiographic, Hemodynamic and Clinical Factors, *Circulation*, 51:146, 1975.

13 Brymer, J. F., Buter, T. H., Walton, J. A., Jr., and Willis, P. W., III.: A Natural History Study of the Prognostic Role of Coronary Arteriography, *Am. Heart J.*, 88:139, 1974.

14 Proudfit, W. L., Bruschke, A. V. G., and Sones, F. M., Jr.: Natural History of Obstructive Coronary Artery Disease: Ten Year Study of 601 Nonsurgical Cases, *Prog. Cardiovasc. Dis.*, 21:53, 1978.

15 Mock, M. B., Ringquist, I., Fisher, L., et al.: Survival of Medically Treated Patients in the Coronary Artery Surgery Study (CASS) Registry, *Circulation*, 66:562, 1982.

16 Department of Health, Education and Welfare: ''Life Tables,'' Vital Statistics of the United States, vol. 11, sec. 5, 1976.

17 Kouchoukos, N. T., Oberman, A., and Karp, T. B.: Results of Surgery for Disabling Angina Pectoris, in A. N. Brest and S. H. Rahimtoola (eds.), ''Cardiovascular Clinics (Coronary Bypass Surgery),'' F. A. Davis Company, Philadelphia, 1977, p. 157.

18 Greene, D. G., Bunnell, I. L., Arani, D. T., et al.: Preservation of the Myocardium by Coronary Bypass Surgery: The Effect on Survival, in J. W. Hurst (ed.), ''Update II. The Heart,'' McGraw-Hill Book Company, New York, 1980, p. 159.

19 Read, R. C., Murphy, M. L., Hultgren, H. N., and Takaro, T.: Survival of Men Treated for Chronic Stable Angina Pectoris. A Cooperative Randomized Study, *Thorac. Cardiovasc. Surg.*, 75:1, 1978.

20 Oberman, A., Kouchoukos, N. T., Harrell, R. R., et al.: Surgical Versus Medical Treatment in Disease of the Left Main Coronary Artery, *Lancet*, 2:591, 1976.

21 Webster, J. S., Moberg, C., and Rincon, G.: Natural History of Severe Proximal Coronary Artery Disease as Documented by Coronary Cineangiography, *Am. J. Cardiol.*, 33:195, 1974.

22 Vliestra, R. E., Assad-Morell, J. L., Frye, R. L., et al.: Survival Predictors in Coronary Artery Disease. Medical and Surgical Comparison, *Mayo Clin. Proc.*, 52:85, 1977.

23 Murphy, M. L., Hultgran, H. N., Detre, K., Thomsen, J., Takaro, T., and Participants of the Veterans Administration Cooperative Study: Treatment of Chronic Stable Angina. A Preliminary Report of Survival Data of the Randomized Veterans Administration Cooperative Study. *N. Engl. J. Med.*, 297:621, 1977.

24 Hammermeister, K. E., DeRouen, T. A., and Dodge, H. T.: Variables Predictive of Survival in Patients with Coronary Disease. Selection by Univariate and Multivariate Analyses from the Clinical, Electrocardiographic, Exercise, Arteriographic, and Quantitative Angiographic Evaluations, *Circulation*, 59:421, 1979.

25 Hammermeister, K. E., Kennedy, J. W., Hamilton, G. W., et al.: Aortocoronary Saphenous Vein Bypass. Failure of Successful Grafting to Improve Resting Left Ventricular Function in Chronic Angina, *N. Engl. J. Med.*, 290:186, 1974.

26 Russel, R. O., Jr., Moraski, R. E., Kouchoukos, N., Karp R., et al.: Unstable Angina Pectoris: National Cooperative Study Group to Compare Surgical and Medical Therapy. II. In-hospital Experience with Initial Follow-up Results in Patients with One, Two and Three Vessel Disease, *Am. J. Cardiol.*, 42:839, 1978.

27 Gazes, P. C., Mobley, E. M., Jr., Fanis, H. M., Jr., Duncan, R. C., and Humphries, G. B.: Preinfarction (Unstable) Angina—A Prospective Study—Ten Year Follow-up, *Circulation*, 48:331, 1973.

28 Scanlon, P. S., Nemickas, R., Moran, J. F., Talano, J. V., Amirparviz, F., and Pifarre, R.: Accelerated Angina Pectoris. Clinical, Hemodymanic, Arteriographic and Therapeutic Experience in 85 Patients, *Circulation*, 47:19, 1973.

29 Hultgren, H. N.: Medical Versus Surgical Treatment of Unstable Angina, *Am. J. Cardiol.*, 38:479, 1976.

30 Bertolasi, C. A., Trongé, J. E., Careeño, C. A., Jalon, J., and Vega, M. R.: Unstable Angina—Prospective and Randomized Study of Its Evolution, with and without Surgery, *Am. J. Cardiol.*, 33:201, 1974.

31 Berg, R., Selinger, S., Leonard, J., Grunwald, R. P., and O'Grady, W. P.: Immediate Coronary Artery Bypass for Acute Evolving Myocardial Infarction (AEMI), *J. Thorac. Cardiovasc. Surg.*, 81:493:, 1981.

32 DeWood, M. A., Spores, J., Notske, R. N., et al.: Medical

and Surgical Management of Myocardial Infarction, *Am. J. Cardiol.*, 44:1356, 1979.

33 Phillips, S., Kungtahworn, C., Zeff, R., et al.: Emergency Coronary Artery Revascularization: A Possible Therapy for Acute Myocardial Infarction, *Circulation* 60:241, 1979.

34 DeWood, M. A., Spores, J., Notske, R. N., et al.: Prevalence of Total Coronary Occlusion during the Early Hours of Transmural Myocardial Infarction, *N. Engl. J. Med.*, 303:897, 1980.

35 Mathey, D. G., Kuck, K. H., Tilsner, V., Krebber, H. J. and Bleifeld, W.: Nonsurgical Coronary Artery Recanalization in Acute Transmural Myocardial Infarction *Circulation*, 63:489, 1981.

36 Reimer, K. A., Lowe, J. E., Rasmussen, M. M. and Kennings, R. B.: The Wavefront Phenomenon of Ischemic Cell Death, *Circulation*, 56:786, 1977.

37 DeWood, M. A., Spores, J., Notske, R. N., et al.: Nontransmural (Subendocardial) Myocardial Infarction in Man. The Prevalence of Total Coronary Occlusion, *Am. J. Cardiol.*, 47:459, 1981.

38 Sustaita, H., Chatterjee, K., Matloff, J. M., Marty, A. T., Swan, H. J. C. and Fields, J.: Emergency Bypass Surgery in Impending and Complicated Acute Myocardial Infarction, *Arch. Surg.*, 105:30, 1972.

39 Cheanvechai, C., Effler, D. B., Loop, F. D., et al.: Emergency Myocardial Revascularization, *Am. J. Cardiol.*, 32:901, 1973.

40 Keon, W. J., Bedard, P., Shankar, K. R., Akyurekli, Y., Nino, A., and Berkman, F.: Experience with Emergency Aortocoronary Bypass Grafts in the Presence of Acute Myocardial Infarction, *Circulation*, 47(suppl. 3):151, 1973.

41 Scanlon, P. J., Nemickas, R., Tobin, J. R., Jr., Anderson, W., Montoya, A., and Pifarre, R.: Myocardial Revascularization during Acute Phase of Myocardial Infarction *JAMA*, 218:207, 1971.

42 Lown, B.: Sudden Cardiac Death: The Major Challenge Confronting Contemporary Cardiology, *Am. J. Cardiol.*, 43:313, 1979.

43 Vismara, L. A., Amsterdam, E. A., and Mason, D. T.: Relation of Ventricular Arrhythmias in the Late Hospital Phase of Acute Myocardial Infarction to Sudden Death after Hospital Discharge, *Am. J. Med.*, 59:6, 1975.

44 Reichenbach, D. D., Moss, N. S., and Meyer, E.: Pathology of the Heart in Sudden Cardiac Death, *Am. J. Cardiol.*, 39:865, 1977.

45 Corday, E., Heng, M. K., Meerbaum, S., Lang, T., Farcot, J., Osher, J., and Hashimoto, K.: Derangements of Myocardial Metabolism Preceding Onset of Ventricular Fibrillation after Coronary Occlusion, *Am. J. Cardiol.*, 39:880, 1977.

46 Vismara, L. A., Miller, R. R., Price, J. E., Karem, R., DeMaria, A. N., and Mason, D. T.: Improved Longevity due to Reduction of Sudden Death by Aortocoronary Bypass in Coronary Atherosclerosis: Prospective Evaluation of Medical Versus Surgical Therapy in Matched Patients with Multivessel Disease, *Am. J. Cardiol.*, 39:919, 1977.

47 Hammermeister, K. E., DeRouen, T. A., Murray, J. A., and Dodge, H. T.: Effect of Aortocoronary Saphenous Vein Bypass Grafting on Death and Sudden Death: Comparison of Nonrandomized Medically and Surgically Treated Cohorts with Comparable Coronary Disease and Left Ventricular Function, *Am. J. Cardiol.*, 39:925, 1977.

48 DeWood, M. A., Shields, J. P., Coulston, D. R., Rudy, L. W., O'Grady, W. P. and Grunwald, R. P.: Myocardial Necrosis during Coronary Bypass Surgery: Analysis of Markers of Cell Death and Relationship to Short- and Long-term Mortality, *Clin. Res.*, 31:179, 1983.

Coronary Artery Bypass Surgery: The Total Experience at the Oregon Health Sciences University[*]

SIAVOSH KHONSARI, M.B., and
ALBERT STARR, M.D.

I can promise to be sincere but not to be impartial.

GOETHE, 1907[1]

HISTORY

Coronary artery bypass graft surgery was first performed at The Oregon Health Sciences University hospitals in 1968 shortly after its introduction by Favaloro.[1a] Its role in the management of patients with coronary artery disease is now well-established, and the indications for its utilization continue to expand.

From 1968 through June 1982, 4,080 patients underwent coronary artery bypass graft surgery for angina, the major manifestation of ischemic heart disease. Four hundred and six additional patients who were operated on for a complication of coronary artery disease such as left ventricular aneurysm, ventricular septal defect, or mitral valve dysfunction, but who did not undergo concomitant coronary bypass grafting, are excluded from this report. There was a male/female predominance of 4:1 with a mean age of 58.3 years for the entire population. Follow-up has been accomplished by a full-time data management group[†] through office visits, questionnaires, and telephone contact with patients and referring physicians. The follow-up includes 15,149 patient-years with a mean of 3.7 years and maximum of 13.1 years.

Time Frame Influence

Review of our data reveals a continuous decrease in operative mortality from 7 percent during the first years of experience to 2 percent or less during the past 8 years (Table 1).

Actuarial long-term survival rate of all patients was 97($\pm$0.2) percent at 1 month, 89($\pm$0.6) percent at 5 years, 75($\pm$1.6) percent at 10 years, and 65($\pm$3.4) percent at 12 years (Fig. 1).

Previous reports from our institution by Anderson[2] and Rahimtoola[3] have referred to the influence of "time frame" on the results of coronary artery bypass graft surgery. In the present study, again, we find an important qualitative improvement in the group of patients operated on since 1974 as compared to the group operated on prior to 1974. The 8-year survival rate is 76($\pm$2.0) percent for the group operated upon between 1968 and 1973, and 83($\pm$1.3) percent in the group operated upon since 1974 (Fig. 2).

Factors Responsible for Improved Results

Many important factors have been responsible for this dramatic improvement. Certainly the frequency with which coronary artery bypass graft surgery was performed increased enormously, giving rise to greater surgical expertise and the attainment of superior operative techniques. At the same time, the introduction of Prolene as a refined suture material also improved the quality of anastomoses. The advanced monitoring of physiological parameters such as blood pressure, pulmonary artery wedge pressure, and cardiac output pre-, intra-, and postoperatively has contributed to continuous uninterrupted observation and evaluation of patients and, thus, to the safety of the operation.

Pharmacologic agents such as intravenous forms of nitroglycerin, nitroprusside, beta blockers, and, most recently, calcium antagonists have been most effective in ensuring a smooth induction of anesthesia and a satisfactory control of cardiac afterload and other hemodynamic parameters. The intraaortic balloon counterpulsation has been most helpful in augmenting cardiac performance in selected groups of patients with poor left ventricular function, particularly in the immediate postoperative period. To achieve maximum revascularization, the number of coronary arteries grafted per patient has increased substantially since 1974. Analyzing our data, we have noted that in terms of age, number of diseased vessels, incidence of wall

*From the Division of Cardiopulmonary Surgery, Oregon Health Sciences University, Portland, Oregon.

†Medical Data Research Center, Portland, Oregon.

TABLE 1
Operative mortality by year of operation*

Year of operation	Number of patients	Mean age (years)	Operative mortality rate (%)
1968–70	89	52	6.7
1971–72	199	53	5.0
1973–74	568	55	2.5
1975–76	782	57	1.5
1977–78	760	58	1.8
1979–80	794	59	1.5
1981–82	888	61	2.1
Overall	4,080	58.3	2.1

*p value $= .000$.

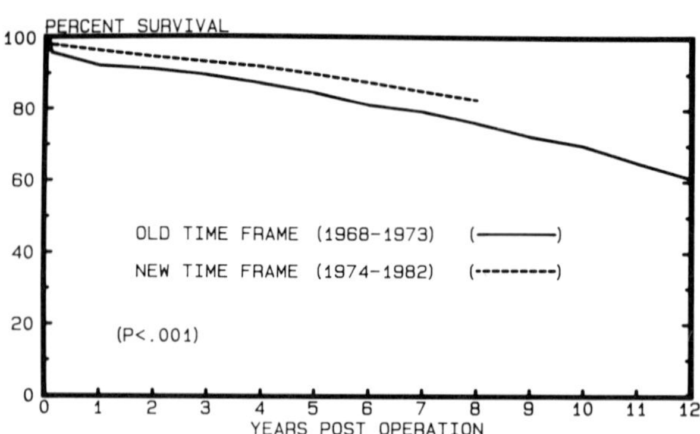

FIGURE 2 Actuarial survival rate for old and new time frames.

motion abnormalities, and prior infarctions, patients in the current time frame, if anything, are at higher risk than those in the previous time frame. From the foregoing data we can surmise that coronary artery bypass graft surgery in the current time frame has become an entity quite different from the operation performed prior to 1974. Therefore, a review and analysis of results obtained from only those patients operated on during the current time frame will reflect our true experience and current philosophy as to the management of patients with ischemic heart disease.

CURRENT TIME FRAME EXPERIENCE

From January 1974 through June 1982, 3,575 patients underwent coronary artery bypass graft surgery at the Oregon Health Sciences University and St. Vincent Hospital and Medical Center for angina. There was a male/female ratio of 4:1, and ages ranged from 24 to 84, with a mean of 59 years.

Indications for Surgery

Presence of angina pectoris without relief through adequate medical therapy has been the main indication for the performance of coronary artery bypass graft surgery in most instances (Fig. 3). However, we have been aggressive in recommending surgery for patients with unstable angina or those who continue to experience ischemic pain after a myocardial infarction, indicative of threatened extension of the infarction. High-grade obstruction of a coronary artery signifying ''critical'' anatomic lesions in the left anterior descending artery or left main coronary artery dictates surgical treatment even though a patient may be otherwise in a stable condition with mild symptoms. Selected patients with stable angina who seek a more active lifestyle are also occasional candidates for coronary surgery. The indications for coronary artery bypass graft surgery are continually expanding. Although we are currently operating on some patients with acute myocardial infarction and impending infarction who are temporarily stabilized by streptokinase, these patients are not included in the present review.

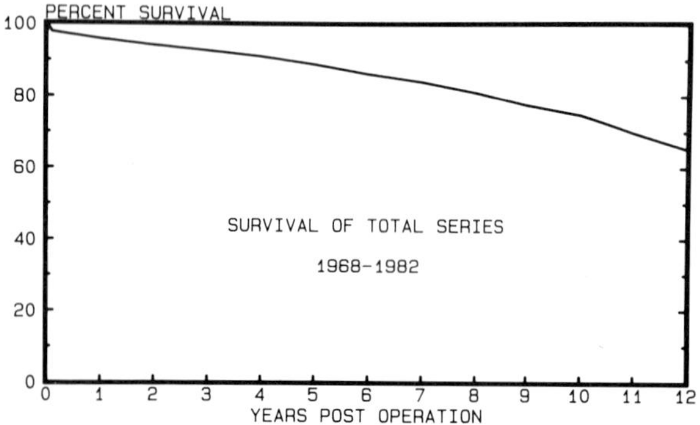

FIGURE 1 Actuarial survival rate for total series 1968–1982.

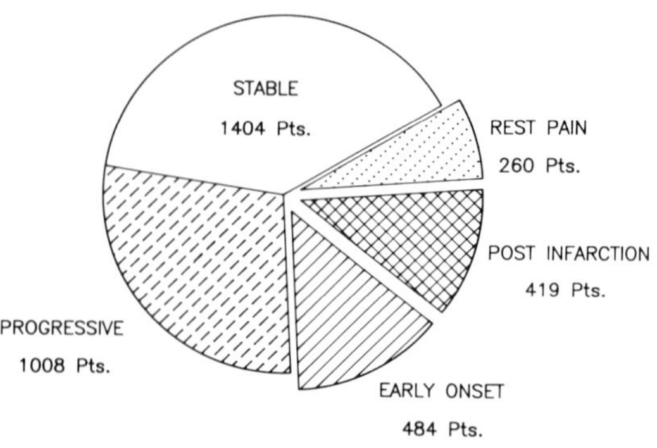

FIGURE 3 Major indications for coronary artery bypass graft surgery.

Surgical Technique

Our operative technique and postoperative management has remained essentially unchanged during the entire current time frame. The operations considered here were performed at the same hospital by the same surgical team. The heart is exposed through a median sternotomy incision, and the aorta and right atrial appendage are directly cannulated. The patient's temperature is lowered to 30°C during cardiopulmonary bypass. The left ventricle is rarely vented. Each distal anastomosis is performed during a short period of ventricular fibrillation and aortic cross-clamping, 5 to 15 min. At least 5 min of coronary flow is permitted between each distal anastomosis, during which time the proximal anastomosis is completed with the heart beating. A continuous suture technique with Prolene is used for all anastomoses. In recent years, cardioplegic arrest has been preferred in a select group of patients having associated procedures such as valve replacement. The saphenous vein has remained our preferred conduit for coronary artery bypass grafting. In some instances, we have selected internal mammary arteries, and, on rare occasions, the cephalic vein has been utilized when the saphenous vein was unavailable. The mean number of vessels diseased per patient was 2.7, and a mean of 2.5 vessels were grafted per patient.

RESULTS
Survival Rate

The actuarial survival curve for the 3,575 patients operated on during the current time frame is depicted in Fig. 4. After an initial operative mortality rate of 1.8 percent (63 patients), the long-term survival rate is

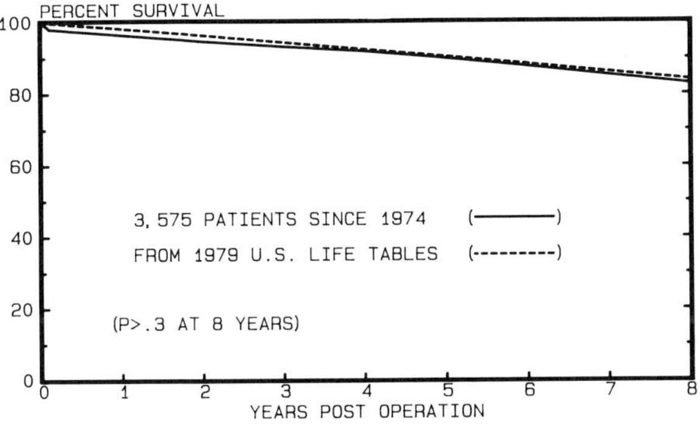

FIGURE 4 Actuarial survival rate for patients operated on during the current time frame compared to expected survival of the 1979 U.S. population matched for age, sex, and time at risk.

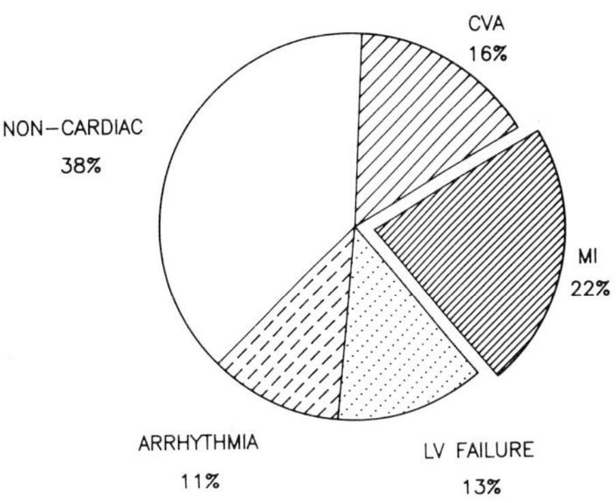

FIGURE 5 Causes of death during the first 30 days following surgery.

98(± 0.2) percent at 1 year, 90(± 0.7) percent at 5 years, and 83(± 1.3) percent at 8 years. The curve parallels closely the expected survival rate (84 percent at 8 years) taken from the 1979 U.S. Life Tables* of a population matched for sex, age, and time at risk.

The causes of death in the 63 patients dying in the first 30 days after surgery were myocardial infarction (22 percent), cerebrovascular accident (16 percent), left ventricular failure (13 percent), arrhythmia (11 percent), and non-cardiac-related (38 percent) (Fig. 5).

A total of 220 patients died during the follow-up period, with an attrition rate of 1.9 percent per year. Of late deaths 34 percent were non-cardiac-related. Sudden death (17 percent) and myocardial infarction (9 percent) were the leading causes of late death (Fig. 6). Perioperative infarction as diagnosed by elevation of cardiac enzyme levels and the appearance of new but permanent Q waves in the immediate postoperative

*U.S. Department of Health and Human Services. Provisional Data from the National Center for Health Statistics, vol. 31, no 6, Supplement, Sept. 30, 1982.

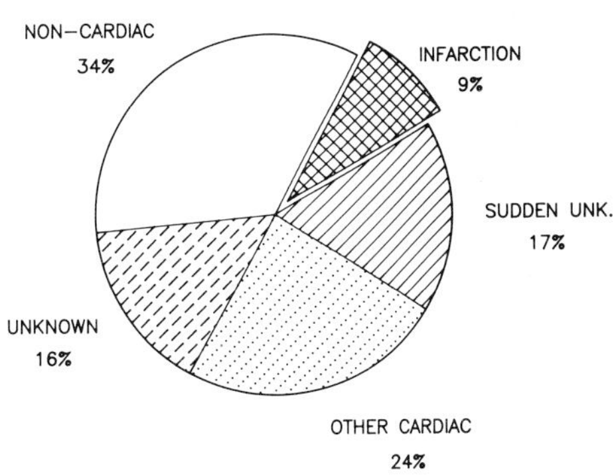

FIGURE 6 Causes of late death.

period was 3($\pm$0.3) percent. The development of late postoperative infarction during the follow-up period was 1.1($\pm$0.1) percent per patient-year.

Relief of Angina

It is now generally accepted that restoration of normal perfusion to previously ischemic myocardium is largely responsible for relief of angina.[4] Similarly, a decline in symptomatic improvement is highly suggestive of vein-graft occlusion.[5] For this reason, complete relief of symptoms is quite common early after surgery in most series, but angina tends to reappear in varying degrees of severity as the follow-up is extended.[6-11] This can be due to changes in the vein graft itself or as a result of atherosclerotic progression in the native circulation.[12] There were 2,358 patients available for functional class evaluation; of these, 59 percent have remained completely free of angina during an 8-year follow-up. Twenty-one percent, or 493 patients, developed angina only on severe exertion, 14 percent had pain with ordinary activity, and 6 percent developed angina with slightest exertion (Table 2).

As the length of follow-up increases, the need for reoperation requires careful consideration. Currently the reoperation rate at our institution is 0.9($\pm$0.1) percent per patient-year, but we anticipate a significant increase with the passage of time as these patients enter into the second decade of follow-up.

Multivariate Analysis

Meaningful analysis of survival rate in patients with coronary artery disease is a highly complex problem since there are many factors that can significantly influence the outcome. A multiple regression (Cox proportional hazard) survival rate analysis was obtained for 2,657 patients for whom cardiac catheterization, left ventricular angiography, and selected coronary arteriography were available. Sixteen variables which were expected to have an effect on survival were entered into the regression model.* However, only eight

*Computer program obtained from the Fred Hutchinson Cancer Research Center, Seattle, Washington.

TABLE 3
Results of multiple regression survival analysis

Variable	p value
1 Hypertension	<.001
2 Left-sided heart failure	<.001
3 Age	<.01
4 Poor left ventricular function	<.01
5 Cardiomegaly	<.01
6 Mitral regurgitation	<.05
7 Stable progressive angina	<.05
8 Number of diseased vessels	<.05

of these risk factors were noted to affect the long-term survival rate to a statistically significant degree. They are left-sided heart failure, hypertension, age, poor left-sided heart function, cardiomegaly, mitral regurgitation, stable-progressive angina, and number of diseased vessels (Table 3). Sex, year of operation, previous infarction, left main disease, acute myocardial infarction, arrhythmia, cardiomegaly, and number of graft placed did not have a significant effect on survival rate.

HYPERTENSION

Association of hypertension and coronary artery disease has been identified as affecting the long-term survival rate to a great degree. In our series, 2,223 patients were normotensive and their 8-year long-term survival rate was 87($\pm$1.4) percent. Similarly, long-term survival rate for 1,351 patients having hypertension in additional to coronary artery disease was reduced to 74($\pm$3.0) percent.

VENTRICULAR FUNCTION

Ventricular function is a significant risk factor affecting survival of patients with coronary artery disease. Poor ventricular function is manifested by an increase in left ventricular end-diastolic pressure, wall motion abnormalities with or without mitral valve regurgitation, or

TABLE 2
Percentage of patients per functional class

	Functional class I	Functional class II	Functional class III	Functional class IV
Stable (N = 930)	59	21	13	7
Progressive (N = 676)	56	22	15	7
Unstable (N = 752)	62	19	15	4

left-sided heart failure. We studied the isolated effects of each of these left ventricular (LV) abnormalities on the long-term survival rate in a group of 2,632 patients.

Left-sided heart failure   The presence of left-sided heart failure is highly significant and affects survival in a very profound way. One hundred eighty-eight patients had left-sided heart failure as part of their symptom complex. The 8-year long-term survival rate was 61($\pm$7.0) percent, compared to 84($\pm$1.3) percent for 3,386 patients who did not have left-sided heart failure.

Left ventricular end-diastolic pressure (LVEDP)   Measurement of left ventricular end-diastolic pressure is a very reliable index of ventricular function. In 626 patients, LVEDP was increased to greater than 15 mmHg, and the 8-year long-term survival rate was 80($\pm$1.9) percent as compared to 84($\pm$1.6) percent for the 2,030 patients with left ventricular end-diastolic pressure of less than 15 mmHg.

Cardiomegaly   Cardiomegaly also diminished survival rate considerably. Four hundred sixty-eight patients who had evidence of cardiomegaly on preoperative chest x-rays had an 8-year long-term survival rate of 72($\pm$3.1) percent as compared to 85($\pm$1.4) percent for 3,106 patients without cardiomegaly.

Mitral regurgitation   Only 94 patients showed evidence of mitral regurgitation on LV angiography. Presence of mitral regurgitation reduces the 8-year survival rate from 83($\pm$1.4) percent for the 2,563 patients with normal mitral valve function to 76($\pm$6.6) percent.

SUBSET ANALYSIS OF VARIOUS FORMS OF ANGINA AND LEFT VENTRICULAR FUNCTION ON SURVIVAL RATE

Evaluation of surgical results in patients with coronary artery disease should emphasize significant subsets identifiable with clinical symptoms which can significantly affect long-term survival rate.

The effect on survival rate of two variables, the urgency of clinical presentation and ventricular function, were studied. Figure 7 reveals a survival rate of 98($\pm$0.4) percent at 1 month, 88($\pm$1.2) percent at 5 years, and 79($\pm$2.7) percent at 8 years for the group of patients who had chronic stable angina as a presenting symptom and indication for coronary bypass surgery. Patients with progressive angina had a survival rate of 98($\pm$0.5) percent at 1 month, 90($\pm$1.1) percent at 5 years, and 80($\pm$2.5) percent at 8 years. Similarly, patients with unstable angina had a survival rate of 98($\pm$0.4) percent at 1 month, 92($\pm$1.1) percent at 5 years, and 89($\pm$1.5) percent at 8 years. Consid-

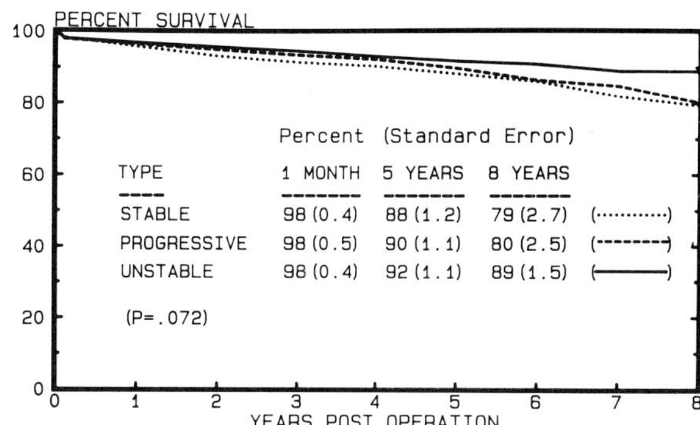

FIGURE 7 Actuarial survival rate by type of angina.

eration of ventricular function as an additive factor in this subset analysis reveals patients with stable angina and good left ventricular (LV) function had a survival rate of 99($\pm$0.3) percent at 1 month, 92($\pm$1.6) percent at 5 years, and 86($\pm$3.6) percent at 8 years (Fig. 8). Patients with stable angina and poor LV function, however, had survival of 96($\pm$1.0) percent at 1 month, 84($\pm$2.5) percent at 5 years, and 71($\pm$3.5) percent at 8 years (Figure 8). Patients with progressive angina and good LV function had a survival rate of 99($\pm$0.5) percent at 1 month, 94($\pm$1.4) percent at 5 years, and 83($\pm$3.4) percent at 8 years. Poor LV function in the same group of patients revealed a survival of 96($\pm$1.0) percent at 1 month, 85($\pm$2.2) percent at 5 years and 76($\pm$5.5) percent in 8 years (Fig. 9). Finally, patients with unstable angina and good LV function had a survival of 98($\pm$0.9) percent at 1 month, 92($\pm$1.6) percent at 5 years, and 89($\pm$2.2) percent at 8 years. Those patients with poor LV function had a survival of 98($\pm$0.7) percent at 1 month, 91($\pm$1.7) percent at 5 years, and 88($\pm$2.5) percent at 8 years (Fig. 10). This analysis clearly demonstrated that long-term survival rate was significantly superior in patients with unstable angina.

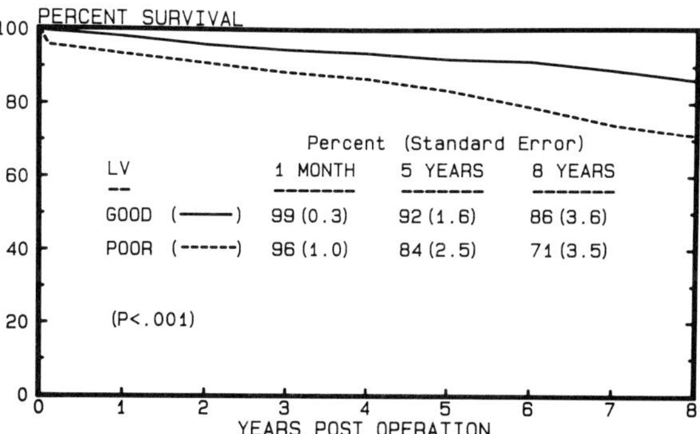

FIGURE 8 Actuarial survival rate showing influence of LV function in patients with stable angina.

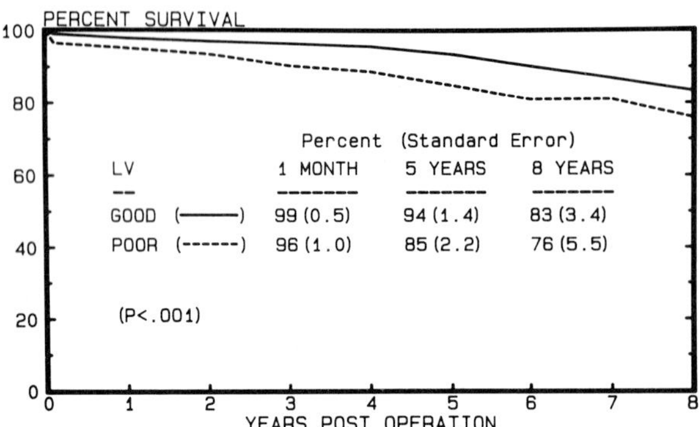

FIGURE 9 Actuarial survival rate showing influence of LV function in patients with progressive angina.

In addition, late survival is not compromised by poor LV function in the unstable angina group, suggesting a greater reversibility of ventricular function in this subset of patients.[13]

SUBSET ANALYSIS OF CORONARY ARTERY SURGERY ON CONCOMITANT AORTIC VALVE REPLACEMENT

From 1969 to 1981, 197 patients underwent aortic valve replacement and concomitant coronary artery bypass graft surgery. During the same period, 595 patients underwent isolated aortic valve replacement. Five-year relative survival rate* of patients with aortic valve replacement alone is 80 percent as compared to 82 percent for those patient who had coronary artery bypass surgery as well.[14] The 10-year relative survival rates are 73 and 80 percent, respectively. As the difference

*Relative survival rate equals actual observed survival rate divided by the expected survival rate computed from life tables.

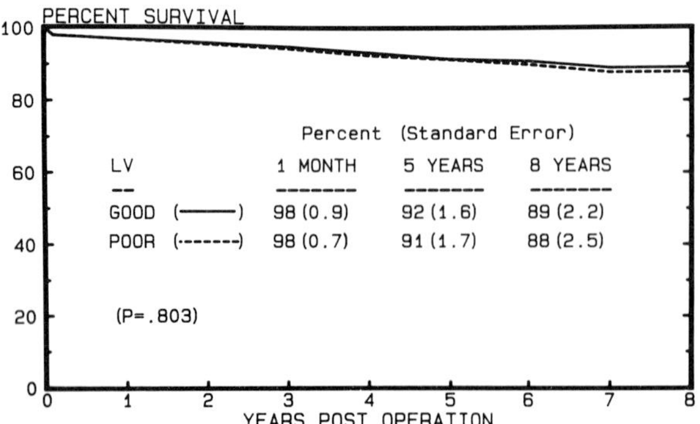

FIGURE 10 Actuarial survival rate showing influence of LV function in patients with unstable angina.

in long-term survival rate is not statistically significant, it can be surmised that concomitant coronary artery bypass graft with aortic valve replacement is not a risk factor and that the long-term survival rate parallels the prognostic curve as determined by aortic valve replacement alone.

CONCLUSION

On the basis of review of our total experience with coronary artery bypass graft surgery in 4,080 patients during the last 14 years, we are led to the following conclusions:

1 Time frame effect is an important factor. We have witnessed not only a distinct lowering in operative mortality rate and rate of perioperative infarction but also an improvement in late mortality rate for patients operated upon during the current time frame (1974 to 1982).

2 There have been at least 80 percent good clinical results and improvements in functional class of patients with angina over an 8-year period with only 1.1 percent per year risk of late infarction.

3 Some important survival determinants have been identified. They are left-sided heart failure, hypertension, age, poor left ventricular function, cardiomegaly, mitral regurgitation, stable/progressive angina, and number of diseased vessels. The overall attrition rate is 1.9 percent per year, of which two-thirds is cardiac-related.

4 Poor left ventricular function does not act as a negative survival determinant in patients with unstable angina, indicating the possible reversibility of left ventricular function in this subgroup of patients.

Of course, we cannot know for certain the future effect of coronary artery bypass graft surgery in patients with ischemic heart disease. Although some important determinants have been identified, we are still ignorant of all the factors that can influence coronary artery disease. Nevertheless, it is tempting to consider the relevance of past results for future risks. Such statistical techniques cannot at this time project the future accurately; however, it can be helpful in anticipating survival rate in a special group of patients from our past experience.

REFERENCES

1 Goethe: Spruche in Prosa, in "*Maximen und Reflexionen,*" Goethe-gesellschaft, Weimar, 1907, p. 33.

1a Favaloro, R. C.: Saphenous Vein Graft in the Surgical Treatment of Coronary Artery Disease: Operative Technique, *J. Thorac. Cardiovasc. Surg.*, 58:178, 1969.

2 Anderson, R. P., Rahimtoola, S. H., Bonchek, L. I., and Starr, A.: The Prognosis of Patients with Coronary Artery Disease after Coronary Bypass Operations. Time-related Progress of 532 Patients with Disabling Angina Pectoris, *Circulation*, 50:274, 1974.

3 Rahimtoola, S. H., Nunley, D., Grunkemeier, G., Teply, J., Lambert, L., and Starr, A.: Ten Year Survival after Coronary Bypass Surgery for Unstable Angina, *N. Engl. J. Med.*, 308:676, 1983.

4 McIntosh, H. D., et al.: Indications for Saphenous Vein Aortocoronary Bypass Surgery, in R. Paoletti and A. M. Gotto, Jr. (eds), "Atherosclerosis Reviews," vol. 1, Raven Press, New York, 1976, p. 185.

5 Campeau, L., Hermann, J., Lesperance, J., Grondin, C. M., Bourassa, M. G., Conti, R., et al.: Loss of Improvement of AP between One and Six Years after Aorta-Coronary Bypass Surgery: Correlations with Changes in Vein Grafts and in Coronary Arteries, *Circulation*, 58(suppl. 2):16, 1978.

6 Griffith, L. S. C., Achuff, S. C., Conti, R., et al.: Changes in Intrinsic Coronary Circulation and Segmental Ventricular Motion after Saphenous Vein Coronary Bypass Graft Surgery, *N. Engl. J. Med.*, 288:589, 1973.

7 Glassman, E., Spencer, F. C., Krauss, K. R., Weisinger, B., and Isom, O. W.: Changes in Grafted and Nongrafted Coronary Arteries following Saphenous Vein Bypass Grafting, *Circulation*, 49–50(suppl. 2):80, 1974.

8 Maurer, B. J., Oberman, A., Holt, J. H., Jr., et al.: Changes in Grafted and Nongrafted Coronary Arteries following Saphenous Vein Bypass Grafting, *Circulation*, 50:293, 1974.

9 Grondin, C. M., Lesperance, J., Bourassa, M. G., Pasternac, A., Campeau, L., and Grondin, P. Serial Angiographic Evaluation in 60 Consecutive Patients with Aortocoronary Artery Vein Grafts 2 Weeks, 1 Year, and 3 Years after Operation, *J. Thorac. Cardiovasc. Surg.*, 67:1, 1974.

10 Walker, J. A., Freidberg, H. D., et al.: Determinants of Angiographic Patency of Aortocoronary Vein Bypass Grafts, *Circulation*, 45,46(suppl. 1):86, 1972.

11 Sheldon, W. C., Loop, F. D., Flema, R. J., and Johnson, D. W.: Direct Myocardial Revascularization—1976. Progress Report on the Cleveland Clinic Experience, *Cleve. Clin. Q.*, 43(3):Fall, 1976, pp. 97.

12 Bourassa, M. G., Lesperance, J., Corbara, F., Saltiel, J., and Campeau, L.: Progression of Obstructive Coronary Artery Disease 5 to 7 Years after Aortocoronary Bypass Surgery, *Circulation*, 58(suppl.1)(3):100, 1978.

13 Cobanoglu, A., Freimanis, I., Grunkemeier, G. L., et al.: Enhanced Late Survival following Coronary Artery Bypass Surgery for Unstable Versus Chronic Angina, *Ann. Thorac. Surg.*, in press.

14 Nunley, D. L., Grunkemeier, G. L., Starr, A.: Aortic Valve Replacement with Coronary Bypass Surgery: Significant Determinants of Ten-Year Survival, *J. Thorac. Cardiovasc. Surg.*, 85:705, 1983.

Early Results of Coronary Artery Bypass Grafting in the Current Era[*]

JOHN W. KIRKLIN, M.D.,
EUGENE H. BLACKSTONE, M.D.,
ROBERT B. KARP, M.D., ALBERT D. PACIFICO, M.D.,
GEORGE L. ZORN, JR., M.D.,
JAMES K. KIRKLIN, M.D., WILLIAM A. LELL, M.D.,
WILLIAM J. ROGERS, M.D., and
LLOYD L. HEFNER, M.D.

Coronary artery bypass graft (CABPG) operations have been demonstrated to relieve angina pectoris, improve left ventricular function, and improve survival rate out to 10 years, in at least some subsets of patients.[1] The suggestion is strong that the long-term benefits of surgery are greatest when all the stenotic coronary artery narrowings are bypassed, so-called complete revascularization.[2] Available information indicates that the prognosis without surgery worsens, and the need for surgery, in theory at least, is greater as the coronary artery disease becomes more extensive and the left ventricular dysfunction more marked.[3] Recently, invasive forms of treatment, including the CABPG operation, have been extended to patients suffering acute myocardial infarction to reduce mortality and left ventricular damage.[4] This is because of the known mortality rate of 5 to 30 percent in acute myocardial infarction treated noninvasively, and the increased risk of late morbidity and mortality in patients with extensive postinfarction scarring.

The CABPG operation has evolved over the past 15 years, but only since the general adoption of complete revascularization and myocardial protection by cold cardioplegia has it approached its full potential value. In most institutions, this means that operations prior to about 1977 may not have produced early or late results comparable to those possible in the current era.[5]

Although the late results of the CABPG operation as it has been done in the current era are only beginning to be available, early results are now ready for study. It is the purpose of this report to describe these early results from our institution (University of Alabama in Birmingham, UAB). They indicate that the offering of operation to those in greatest need of myocardial revascularization has been accomplished with low hospital morbidity and mortality rates.

MATERIAL

At UAB 3,937 patients underwent the CABPG operation between January 1, 1977 and January 1, 1981. Among these, 3,851 underwent a primary CABPG operation, with or without another procedure,[†] and these are considered in detail (Table 1). Included are 153 patients who also underwent resection or plication of a large, full-thickness left ventricular scar (or aneurysm). In all, 210 patients underwent aneurysm resection with or without the CABPG operation (Table 2). Patients undergoing the CABPG operation within 1 month of the onset of an acute myocardial infarction in 1981 and 1982 are also reviewed.

EARLY RESULTS

Among the 3,851 CABPG patients, 38 died in (0.99 percent; CL[‡] 0.82 to 1.18 percent) the hospital after operation (Table 1). Among the total of 210 patients undergoing resection or plication of full-thickness left ventricular scars (aneurysms) with or without CABPG operation, 11 (5.2 percent; CL 3.7 to 7.3 percent) died.

INCREMENTAL RISK FACTORS FOR EARLY (INHOSPITAL) DEATH
Left Ventricular Dysfunction

Patients with severe left ventricular dysfunction (resting ejection fraction ≤ 0.30, or its equivalent cineangiographic appearance) had a higher hospital mortality rate (5 percent; CL 2 to 12 percent) than did those with

---

*From the University of Alabama in Birmingham, School of Medicine and Medical Center.

†This does not include patients whose primary procedure was for the aortic or mitral valve disease, isolated or in combination, who also underwent the CABPG operation.

‡CL = 70 percent confidence limits.

TABLE 1
Primary coronary artery bypass graft operation, UAB 1977–1981*

		Hospital deaths		
Category of CABPG	N	No.	%	CL (%)
Primary isolated	3,608	26	0.72	0.58–0.90
With simultaneous carotid endarterectomy	56	4	7	4–13
With other simultaneous vascular operations	4	0	0	0–38
With LV resection or plication (6 patients had plication)	153	7	4.6	2.9–7.0
With direct ventricular procedure for intractable VT	15	1	7	1–21
Other	15	0	0	0–12
Total	3,851†	38	0.99	0.82–1.18

*CL = 70% confidence limits; LV = left ventricular; VT = ventricular tachycardia; VSD = ventricular septal defect; p for table chi-square < .0001.

†18 patients (0 deaths) with ischemic heart disease whose *primary* procedure was not CABPG (e.g., mitral valve replacement, repair postinfarction VSD) are not included, and are tabulated under the primary procedure.

lesser degrees of dysfunction in the year 1977 (Table 3; data not yet analyzed for the entire current era). (*Moderate dysfunction* indicates ejection fraction ≤ 0.40 but > 0.30, or its equivalent appearance; *mild* ≤ 0.50 but > 0.40; *none* ≥ 0.5.) This information must be interpreted with the knowledge that patients with severe left ventricular dysfunction were operated upon only if evidences of right-sided heart failure (right atrial pressure greater than 15 mmHg, hepatomegaly, and fluid retention) were absent. The mortality rate for patients with severe dysfunction is the same as that for patients with left ventricular aneurysms, and emphasizes the unfavorable effect of extensive left ventricular scarring and poor function upon early results. However, patients with something less than severe left ventricular dysfunction did not have an increased risk of hospital death.

Extent of the Coronary Artery Disease

The extent of the coronary artery disease itself has no effect on hospital mortality rate in the current era (Table 4). This is particularly evident in the experience with left main coronary artery disease (Table 5). In spite of the fact that patients with this lesion had a mean age 2 years older than that of other patients ($p < .0001$), and that all but 16 had associated stenoses of other major coronary arteries (Table 6), the hospital

TABLE 2
Hospital deaths after isolated CABPG operation and after left ventricular aneurysm*

		Hospital deaths		
Category	N	No.	%	CL (%)
Primary isolated CABPG	3,608	26	0.72	0.58–0.90
"LV aneurysmectomy":	210	12	5.7	4.1–7.9
Isolated with or without CABPG	175	8	4.6	3.0–6.8
With MVR or MVA	8	1	12	2–36
With surgical treatment of ventricular tachycardia	13	1	8	1–24
With surgical treatment of VSD	6	1	17	2–46
Other	8	1	12	2–36

*CABPG = coronary artery bypass grafting; CL = 70 percent confidence limits; LV = left ventricular; MVR = mitral valve replacement; MVA = mitral valve annuloplasty; VSD = ventricular septal defect.

TABLE 3
Left ventricular dysfunction in relation to hospital mortality rate in primary CABPG at UAB (1977).*

LV dysfunction†	No.		Hospital mortality rate		
			No.	%	70% CL† (%)
None	286	5 of 704,	2	0.7	0.2–1.7
Mild	271	0.7%‡	——	0	0–0.7
Moderate	147	0.3–1.2%	3	2	0.9–4
Severe	39		2	5*	2–12
Total	743		7	0.9	0.6–1.5

*N = 757; no left ventriculogram data available in 14 patients (0 deaths); p chi-square for table = .007.

†LV = left ventricular; CL = confidence limits.

‡p chi-square for difference = .005.

mortality rate was no different than that for the remainder of the patients of this experience (Table 5). Special intraoperative measures for this group, such as preoperative intraaortic balloon pumping and the Swan-Ganz catheter, were not used.

This supports the idea that the CABPG operation provides good myocardial perfusion, even in patients with extensive coronary artery disease. A similar conclusion was reached by an earlier study, which showed no difference in 5-year survival after the CABPG operation between patients with two-vessel, three-vessel, and left main disease (Table 7).

Extensiveness of the Operation

The performing of extensive revascularizations does not increase the early risks of the operation in the current era, there being no relation between the number of distal anastomoses performed and the hospital mortality rate (Table 8). In the majority of patients, two-vein segments with multiple sequential grafts were used (Table 9).

Age of Patient

The age of the patient at the time of operation has an effect, although a small one, on hospital mortality rate (Table 10). It is not evident until age exceeds 60 years. Thus, the hospital mortality rate in the current era (1977–81) has been 0.3 percent (CL 0.2 to 0.8 percent) among the 2,362 patients less than 60 years old, and has been 1.4 percent (CL 1.1 to 1.9 percent) among those 60 years of age or older (p chi-square for this difference = .0002).

Recent Acute Myocardial Infarction

An experience is accumulating with the CABPG operation early after acute myocardial infarction (Table 11). Although the confidence limits around the proportions are still wide (0.6 to 15 percent), the CABPG operation within 24 h of the acute myocardial infarction has been surprisingly safe. The mortality rate in the patients operated upon more than 48 h after the infarction is related largely to the fact that these are patients who were doing poorly with medical management of their acute infarction.

COMMENT

In spite of earlier criticisms of the CABPG operation, it is now an accepted form of treatment for some subsets of patients with ischemic heart disease, and it may prove to be particularly effective in individuals with extensive or complicated chronic or acute disease. This review indicates that in the current era the hospital mortality rate of the isolated CABPG operation approaches zero (lower 70 percent confidence limit less than 1 percent, upper less than 5 percent) for most subsets of patients, even when extensive and complicated coronary artery disease is present. CABPG operations have been relatively safe even in patients who

TABLE 4
The relation of the extent of the coronary artery disease to hospital mortality rate after primary CABPG, UAB (1977)*

Major coronary arteries diseased (≥ 50% narrowing)	No.†	Hospital mortality rate		
		No.	%	70% CL‡ (%)
One	33	——	0	0–6
Two	162	2	1.2	0.4–2.9
Three	447	5	1.1	0.6–1.9
Left main	111	——	0	0–1.7
Total	753	7	0.9	0.6–1.4

*N = 757; these data for the entire current era are not yet available; p chi-square = .6.

†Data not available on 4 patients.

‡CL = confidence limits.

TABLE 5
CABPG operation for left main coronary artery disease ($\geq$ 50% stenosis), compared with the operation for patients without this, UAB (1977–1981)

		Left main experience: hospital deaths				Remaining experience: hospital deaths		
Major category	No.	N	%	CL* (%)	No.	N	%	CL* (%)
Primary isolated	519	5	1.0	0.5–1.6	3,089	21	0.68	0.53–0.87 (p = .5)
With simultaneous carotid endarterectomy	20	2	10	3–22	36	2	6	2–13 (p = .4)
With other simultaneous vascular operations	0	——	——	——	4	0	0	0–38
With LV* resection or plication	10	1	10	1–30	143	6	4.2	2.5–6.7
With direct ventricular procedure for intractable ventricular tachycardia	0	——	——	——	15	1	7	1–21
Other	1	0	0	0–85	14	0	0	0–13
Total	550	8	1.5	0.9–2.2	3,301	30	0.91	0.74–1.11 (p = .4)

*CL = 70% confidence limits; LV = left ventricular.

TABLE 6
(Associated coronary artery disease ($\geq$ 70% stenosis) in patients undergoing coronary artery bypass grafting for left main coronary artery disease ($\geq$ 50% stenosis), UAB (1977–1981)*

Lesions* (beside left main)	No.	Hospital deaths				
		No.	%	CL (%)		
Isolated	16	0	0	0–11		
RCA	30	0	0	0–6	0 of 87	
LCA	26	0	0	0–7	0% (CL 0–2.2%)	
CCA	15	0	0	0–12		
RCA + LCA	89	2	2.2	0.7–5.3†		p = .25
LCA + CCA	52	1	1.9	0.2–6.4	8 of 462	
RCA + CCA	40	1	2	0.3–8.3	1.7% (CL 1.1–2.6%)	
LCA + RCA + CCA	281	4	1.4	0.7–2.6		

*$\geq$ 70% luminal diameter stenosis; CL = 70% confidence limits; RCA = right coronary artery; LCA = left coronary artery; CCA = circumflex coronary artery; p chi-square for table = .96.

†In one additional patient LCA + CCA and no data regarding RCA survived.

TABLE 7
Actuarial 5-year survival rate of hospital survivors after the CABPG operation UAB (all operations prior to 1977)

	Survival at 5 years (%)		
Category	Surgical treatment (±SD)	Matched population	Significance level of difference
1-vessel	94.8 ± 2.63	94.9	p = .7
2-vessel	88.5 ± 2.47*	95.0	p = .003
3-vessel	89.8 ± 1.89*	95.0	p = .001
Left main	87.6 ± 3.90*	94.4	p = .05

*p for differences between these categories > .6. SD = standard deviation.

SOURCE: Reproduced with slight modifications from Kirklin et al., *Circulation*, 60:1613, 1979. Used with permission.

TABLE 8
Relation of hospital death (26 events) to number of distal anastomoses performed at primary CABPG operation without associated procedures (N = 3,608), UAB, 1977–1981*

Number of distal anastomoses	No.	Hospital deaths		
		N	%	CL (%)
1	115	0	0	0–1.7
2	460	3	0.7	0.3–1.3
3	906	3	0.33	0.14–0.67
4	1,087	9	0.8	0.5–1.2
5	672	6	0.9	0.5–1.4
6	265	4	1.5	0.8–2.7
7	77	1	1.3	0.2–4.4
8	22	0	0	0–8
9	3	0	0	0–47
10	1	0	0	0–85

*p for table chi-square = .7; CL = 70% confidence limits.

TABLE 9
Number of vein segments used during CABPG operation, UAB, 1977–1981*

Number of vein segments used	Left main experience			Remaining experience		
	No.	% of 550	CL* (%)	No.	% of 3,301	CL (%)
1	16	2.9	2.2–3.9	427	12.9	12.3–13.6
2	405	73.6	71.6–75.6	2169	65.7	64.8–66.6
3	129	23.5	21.5–25.5	702	21.3	20.5–22.0
4	0	0	0–0.4	3	0.09	0.04–0.18

*CL = 70% confidence limits.

TABLE 10
Age at operation in patients undergoing primary isolated CABPG operations, UAB, 1977–1981*

Age (yrs) at operation	N	Hospital deaths			
		N		%	CL (%)
20–30	8	0		0	0–21
30–40	124	1	8 of 2,362 =	0.8	0.1–2.7
40–50	659	2	0.3% (CL 0.2–0.5%)	0.3	0.1–0.7
50–60	1,571	5		0.32	0.18–0.54
60–70	1,063	12		1.1	0.8–1.6
70–80	182	6	18 of 1,246 =	3.3	2.0–5.3
80–90	1	0	1.4% (CL 1.1–1.9%)	0	0–85
Total	3,608	26		0.72	0.58–0.90

*p (logistic) = .0004; CL = 70% confidence limits.

have very recently sustained an acute myocardial infarction.

Other invasive methods, such as percutaneous transluminal coronary artery dilation, and in acute myocardial infarction intracoronary streptokinase, are also being used in many institutions including UAB. It remains to be seen whether their use can reduce the early (inhospital) mortality rate below that of the CABPG operation. Late follow-up studies out to 5 or more years after the intervention will determine their relative efficacies in prolonging life, protecting left ventricular myocardium, and relieving symptoms.

TABLE 11
CABPG operations within 1 month of acute myocardial infarction in patients without acute ventricular rupture or mitral incompetence, UAB (1981–1983)*

Interval since acute infarction	N	Hospital deaths		
		No.	%	CL† (%)
< 24 h	21‡	1	5	0.6–15
24 h < 48 h	1	——	0	0–85
48 h < 7 days	11	0	0	0–16
7 days < 1 month	28	3	11	5–20
Interval uncertain	16	1	6	0.8–20
Total	77	5	6	4–11

*p chi-square for table = .7.
†CL = 70% confidence limits.
‡3 were within 6 h of infarction.

REFERENCES

1 Mathur V. S., and Guinn, G. A.: Prospective Randomized Study to Evaluate Coronary Bypass Surgery: 10-Year (yr) Follow-up, *Circulation,* 66(suppl. 2):219, 1982. (Abstract.)

2 Loop, F. D., Cosgrove, D. M., Lytle, B. W., Thurer, R. L., Simpfendorfer, C., Taylor, P. C., and Proudfit, W. L.: An 11-Year Evolution of Coronary Artery Surgery (1967–1978), *Ann. Surg.,* 190:444, 1979.

3 Takaro, T., Peduzzi, P., Detre, K. M., Hultgren, H. N., Murphy, M. L., Bel-Kahn, J., Thomsen, J., and Meadows, W. R.: Survival in Subgroups of Patients with Left Main Coronary Artery Disease, *Circulation,* 66:14, 1982.

4 Selinger, S. L., Berg, R., Jr., Leonard, J. J., Grunwald, R. P., and O'Grady, W. P.: Surgical Treatment of Acute Evolving Anterior Myocardial Infarction, *Circulation,* 64(suppl. 2):28, 1981.

5 Miller, D. C., Stinson, E. B, Oyer, P. E., Jamieson, S. W., Mitchell, R. S., Reitz, B. A., Baumgartner, W. A., and Shumway, N. E.: Discriminant Analysis of the Changing Risks of Coronary Artery Operations: 1971–1979, *J. Thorac. Cardiovasc. Surg.,* 85:197, 1983.

Evolution of Coronary Bypass Surgery at Stanford University: The First 15 Years[*]

D. CRAIG MILLER, M.D.,
EDWARD B. STINSON, M.D., and
NORMAN E. SHUMWAY, M.D.

HISTORICAL OVERVIEW: EXPLORATORY ATTEMPTS, RESULTS, AND LESSONS LEARNED

The era of direct myocardial revascularization started at Stanford on October 23, 1968 when a 58-year-old lady[†] with a 16-year history of chest pain received a single saphenous vein graft to the distal left main coronary artery. The left main ostial stenosis was a congenital fibrous diaphragm, and not an atherosclerotic lesion. To accomplish this procedure, the heart was kept fibrillating continuously at normothermia, the main pulmonary artery was completely divided to facilitate the exposure, and the graft was sutured end-to-side to the distal left main coronary artery with interrupted no. 6-0 silk sutures. Cardiopulmonary bypass time totaled 107 min. Despite the primitive nature of these techniques, this patient remained asymptomatic until 1982; repeat arteriography at that time revealed a patent graft but a new important stenosis in the proximal left anterior descending (LAD) coronary artery. Parenthetically, this was the first, and the last, bypass graft placed directly into the left main coronary artery.

Following this first attempt 15 years ago, coronary artery bypass grafting (CABG) was cautiously applied to increasingly larger numbers of patients with various manifestations of ischemic heart disease.

Unstable Angina

In the early years (1969 to 1971) many patients with "preinfarction angina" or "impending myocardial infarction" were rushed to the operating room after emergency coronary angiography;[1–3] operative morbidity and mortality rates were relatively high.[3] Longer-term follow-up revealed generally excellent pain relief but no real improvement in terms of treadmill exercise testing or the occurrence of late myocardial infarction.[4]

Repeated assessment (at an average of 19 months postoperatively) showed that angina recurrence and other cardiac events were common after 36 months, although the 5-year actuarial survival rate was 86 percent.[5] An increased understanding of the pathophysiology of severe chest pain in these patients with unstable angina and the availability of beta blocking agents and vasodilators later ushered in a more "enlightened" approach. Such patients were stabilized or "cooled off" initially with intensive medical therapy, studied with coronary angiography semiurgently (usually within 1 week), and CABG was offered to selected patients on a semielective basis. Such a therapeutic strategy yielded more favorable early and late results.[6] Parenthetically, intraaortic balloon pump (IABP) counterpulsation has been employed only exceedingly rarely at Stanford to stabilize these patients.

A nonrandomized, prospective data bank study of 228 comparable patients (104 treated surgically and 124 treated medically) later showed convincingly that intensive initial medical therapy followed by semielective CABG was associated with superior survival and symptom relief compared to medical treatment alone over an 8-year interval.[6] The incidence of myocardial infarction (MI), however, was not significantly lower in the surgical cohort. This finding was related in part to a 13 percent incidence of perioperative MI (PMI) in this study (1970 to 1977), a complication which currently occurs (see below) in less than 3 percent of patients with unstable angina undergoing CABG.[6]

Revascularization for Life-Threatening Tachyarrhythmias

Another of our early attempts to broaden the indications for CABG proved to be less than completely successful. In 1973, we reported promising early results using CABG (with or without concomitant myocardial resection) to treat patients with refractory life-threatening ventricular tachycardia.[7] The introduction of clinical cardiac electrophysiology and the advent of activation sequence-guided electrophysiological surgery improved the outlook for these very ill patients.[8]

[*]From the Department of Cardiovascular Surgery, Stanford University School of Medicine, Stanford, California.

[†]Diagnosed and referred by Dr. Charles D. Miller, Redding, California.

Unfortunately, this new and promising therapeutic realm continues to be hampered by deficiencies in our fundamental knowledge of the pathogenesis and electrical mechanisms of these tachyarrhythmias.[9] Today it is clear in retrospect, however, that "blind" CABG with or without left ventricular aneurysmectomy offers little real hope of arrhythmia control and/or prolonged clinical benefit for this subset of patients with ischemic heart disease.

Chronic Stable Angina Pectoris

Chronic stable angina refractory to maximal medical therapy represented the most common indication for elective CABG in our early experience.[10,11] This subgroup of patients had the lowest operative risk in this early era (operative mortality rate of 0.8 percent between 1968 and 1972)[10] and appeared to benefit substantially in terms of angina relief.[11] In 1973, we reported 1-year results derived from a selected group of 102 patients with stable angina who underwent CABG between 1969 and 1971.[11] The operative mortality (OM) rate was 3.9 percent and the 1-year survival rate was 91 percent (including operative fatalities). The PMI rate (by ECG criteria) was 7 percent. The vast majority (85 percent) of patients had marked symptomatic improvement. The graft patency rate was 75 percent, but 95 percent of patients studied had at least one patent graft. The graft patency rate in patients operated upon after the institution of minor technical changes in 1970 was 82 percent. It is interesting to note that the average number of grafts constructed in this early era was only 1.7 per patient.

In 1974, we published a critical analysis of the results obtained in the first 400 consecutive patients undergoing CABG (with or without other concomitant procedures) over a follow-up interval ranging from 2 to 40 months [mean 10 ± 6 (SD) months].[10] Of surviving patients 88 percent were improved symptomatically, and 79 percent were completely free of angina. Stepwise regression analysis was employed to identify and rank preoperative variables that were independent predictors of overall outcome. The probability of a successful "late" result for patients undergoing isolated CABG was shown to be a function of only three variables: congestive heart failure (CHF), ECG abnormalities, and mitral regurgitation (MR). Thus, even at this early stage, the relatively limited efficacy of CABG for patients with advanced CHF and left ventricular (LV) dysfunction was apparent.

This early cohort of patients was later reevaluated when the follow-up period averaged 30 months[12] and 46 months.[13] Our 1975 article reported the 4-year overall actuarial survival rate to be 80 percent, although patients with severe CHF fared much worse.[12] The adverse influence of multivessel coronary artery dis-

ease (CAD) on survival in medically treated patients was well-appreciated at that time.[14] This was not the case in these surgically treated patients. In contrast to the earlier-reported[10] symptomatic status of these patients at an average follow-up time of 10 months, 13 percent showed further clinical improvement while 40 percent reported clinical deterioration with respect to chest pain 4 years following surgery. This longitudinal assessment signaled to us that the dramatic early postoperative angina relief in the vast majority of patients operated upon early in our experience might not be maintained over late follow-up periods due to progression of the underlying CAD in the native circulation, graft occlusion, or both.

These conclusions were corroborated by our 1977 report when this same patient cohort had been followed for an average of 46 months.[13] Over 75 percent of surviving patients, however, still exhibited some degree of functional benefit 4 years postoperatively in terms of angina or CHF, or both.

In 1978, we published our first analysis examining the question of whether or not these patients operated upon at the beginning (1968 to 1972) of our experience derived less satisfactory operative benefit than did patients operated upon subsequently.[15] The OM rate for the years 1972–1973 was 2.1 percent, compared to 4.9 percent earlier. More importantly, a trend was present showing superior medium-term (3 years) survival rates for patients operated upon after 1971. Moreover, 6 years postoperatively, 90 percent of the early (1968–1972) patients continued to have either no angina or only mild (NYHA class I-II) angina.

These longitudinal and sequential studies were informative, despite the inherent limitations of retrospective analyses. They formed the background for two later investigations which examined the long-term expectations of contemporary coronary artery surgery at Stanford and analyzed the ongoing dynamic interactions between changing indications for surgery and early operative risk (see below).

Bypass Grafting as a Concomitant Procedure

The controversy surrounding the efficacy of CABG in terms of prolonging life expectancy continued to be debated vigorously during the 1970s. Given this perspective and the markedly suboptimal early results of combined valve replacement and CABG, we carried out two parallel analyses to assess the surgical implications and results of such combined procedures.[16,17]

Coronary angiography was performed more frequently as a part of the cardiac catheterization evaluation of older patients with aortic or mitral valvular disease when the limited predictive value of the patient's symptoms, i.e., chest pain, became appreciated.

This was particularly germane in our specific patient population, where the average age of patients undergoing valve replacement was high; 61 years for aortic valve replacement (AVR)[16] and 59 years for mitral valve replacement (MVR).[17] In these studies the presence or absence of preoperative angina pectoris was of little value in predicting the coronary artery anatomy; we recommended that coronary angiography be performed routinely in all patients with valve disease undergoing catheterization who were older than 35 years of age. If important coronary stenoses (greater than 50 percent diameter narrowing) were present in vessels supplying substantial portions of left ventricular (LV) mass, we felt it prudent to bypass these vessels at the time of valve replacement. This philosophy was tempered in individual cases by the magnitude of the proposed operative procedure, the type, severity, and etiology of the underlying valvular lesions, and the patient's symptoms.[16,17] In general, diseased *nondominant* or *small* circumflex or right coronary arteries (and their branches) were ignored during concomitant valve replacement and CABG.

Assessment of the efficacy of such an aggressive policy was more difficult, and has been debated subsequently.[18,19] Our retrospective study of 111 patients with documented CAD undergoing AVR + CABG showed that although the operative risk was higher than that for patients *without* CAD undergoing isolated AVR (8 versus 2 percent), the medium-term survival rates were statistically indistinguishable.[16] For 97 patients undergoing combined MVR + CABG the operative risk was the same as that for patients without CAD;[17] medium-term survival was a function of the hemodynamic lesion (stenosis versus regurgitation) and the etiology of the mitral valvular disease (rheumatic versus degenerative versus ischemic), and was essentially independent of the presence or absence of CAD.

We inferred from these results that in the presence of coexistent *important* multivessel coronary disease, concomitant CABG did not add to the operative risk (and, in fact, might reduce this risk) and probably was responsible for neutralizing the expected adverse effect of CAD on postoperative survival. Hence, we continue to advocate an aggressive approach for such patients, who are being seen with increasing frequency as more and more elderly patients are considered for valve replacement.

Ischemic Cardiomyopathy

As mentioned previously, our early investigations showed that patients with advanced CHF and severe LV dysfunction undergoing CABG had lower postoperative survival rates than did patients with well-preserved LV function.[10,12,13,15] Despite these findings, a sizable number of patients with ischemic cardio-

myopathy (many who were referred to Stanford as possible cardiac transplantation candidates) underwent CABG. We attempted to ascertain in 1980 whether or not myocardial revascularization offered any real benefit to these desperately ill patients in terms of life expectancy or functional improvement. This was accomplished by comparing a concurrent, nonrandomized cohort of 55 patients with ischemic cardiomyopathy treated with CABG with 48 patients treated medically.[20,21] Multivariate logistic regression analysis was employed to normalize the two cohorts with respect to dissimilar entry characteristics. This adjustment had not been considered in previous studies,[22] rendering retrolective comparative differences in survival somewhat specious. Considering that these patients all had ejection fractions less than 0.35, most were operated upon in the early and mid-1970s, and a substantial number did not have angina, the operative mortality rate was not inordinately high (9 percent). The 5-year actuarial survival rate was markedly superior ($p = .0006$) for the surgical cohort [66 ± 7 percent (SEM)] compared to the medical cohort (18 ± 9 percent), as shown in Fig. 1. The proportion of deaths due to fatal myocardial infarction was also distinctly different: 11 versus 32 percent; respectively.[20] Excellent symptomatic improvement was seen after CABG for patients who presented with angina (59 percent of patients were without limiting symptoms 4 years postoperatively), but this figure was only 29 percent for 21 surgically treated patients who presented with CHF.

When the two patient populations were normalized using the multivariate logistic regression techniques, however, the treatment mode (CABG versus medical therapy) had only a weak ($p = .055$) predictive influence on survival. Treatment mode was overshadowed by the clinical severity of congestive heart failure and a refined measurement of ejection fraction.[20]

This investigation prompted us to reassess critically the risk-benefit guidelines surrounding CABG for patients who presented with ischemic cardiomyopathy and severe CHF but *without* exertional or rest angina. The dismal natural history of this subset of patients with end-stage ischemic heart disease is well-documented; furthermore, in our opinion, this poor prognosis justifies continued cautious attempts to help selected individuals by considering them to be candidates for bypass grafting (if they are not judged to be suitable transplant candidates).

RENAISSANCE: PARTICIPATION IN COOPERATIVE TRIALS

The prime importance of obtaining controlled prospective data regarding the clinical usefulness of coro-

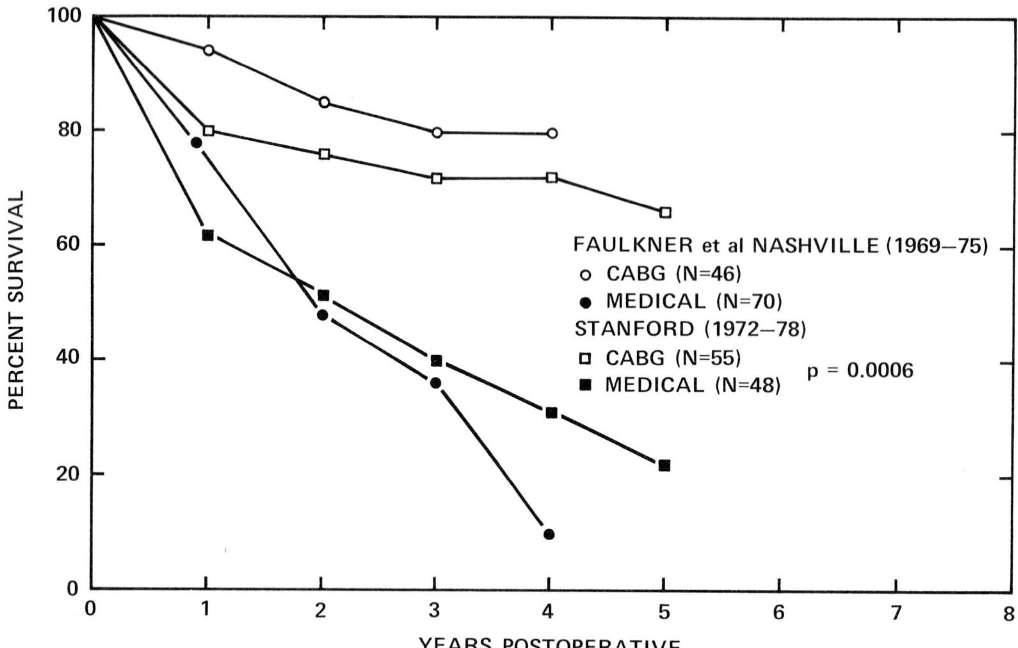

FIGURE 1 Actuarial survival rates in two retrospective comparative investigations of medical versus surgical treatment of patients with ischemic cardiomyopathy.[21,22] Despite the apparent marked enhancement of life expectancy with CABG, mode of treatment had only a marginal influence on survival rate in the multivariate logistic regression analysis, which normalized the Stanford medical and surgical cohorts for differences in entry characteristics (see text). (*From D. C. Miller, E. B. Stinson, and E. L Alderman, Surgical Treatment of Ischemic Cardiomyopathy: Is It Ever Too Late? Am J. Surg. 141:688, 1981. Used with permission of the authors and publisher.*)

nary bypass surgery was apparent shortly following the advent of direct myocardial revascularization at Stanford in 1968. The cardiology and cardiovascular surgery units at Stanford University Medical Center and the Palo Alto VA Medical Center are completely integrated, which led to participation in four major multicenter collaborative trials.

The NHLBI-sponsored Cooperative Unstable Angina Study Group randomly assigned patients with unstable angina to either medical or surgical therapy at nine centers. Stanford contributed 49 of the total of 288 randomized patients in this study (1972 to 1976). The results of this prospective trial are reported elsewhere in detail. This study was hampered by a high (36 percent) crossover rate (medical to surgical) within an average follow-up interval of 30 months and a relatively short period of follow-up, which made meaningful statistical conclusions difficult. Briefly, coronary bypass surgery proffered superior symptomatic benefit, but there was no statistically significant difference in survival or incidence of MI.

Our local prospective, nonrandomized data bank study, on the other hand, concluded that CABG did enhance life expectancy as well as provide more ef-

fective amelioration of symptoms.[6] This difference in survival rates retained its statistical significance whether the data were analyzed according to treatment assigned or by the crossover method. In our study, only 22 percent of patients initially treated with medical therapy required later CABG over a follow-up period extending to 10 years maximum.

The Collaborative Study in Coronary Artery Surgery (CASS) contained a randomized subprotocol as well as a substantially larger data registry. Fifteen major institutions in the United States and Canada prospectively registered and followed 24,959 patients who underwent coronary angiography. Of these, 6,176 were operated upon. Even though the randomized portion of this study is still unfinished, the data bank registry has already generated many valuable and important contributions,[23–28] including what is likely to be the most comprehensive assessment of the operative risk of CABG that will ever be published.[24] Interestingly, the most powerful predictors of operative mortality were (1) in which hospital the surgery was performed and (2) the need to proceed with CABG on an emergency or urgent basis.[24] In addition, many patient- and disease-related variables are found to be independent determinants of operative mortality.[24,25] The enormous data base generated by the CASS study promises to yield many additional important contributions in the future.

The Palo Alto VA Medical Center participated in both the Chronic Stable Angina and the Unstable Angina VA Cooperative Studies.[29–32] Although the *preliminary* results of the stable angina study spawned widespread debate and controversy,[29] longer-term follow-up has recently yielded new and valuable data confirming the capability of CABG to enhance life expectancy in certain subsets of patients.[30–32] Furthermore, important and novel prognostic information based on simple clinical characteristics have been derived from this study.[30,31]

The VA Unstable Angina Cooperative Study completed patient entry in 1982; follow-up will be extended beyond 5 years. It is hoped that a lower crossover rate, larger numbers of randomized patients, and a longer follow-up span in this study will answer some of the questions left unanswered by the NHLBI Cooperative Study.

Participation in these collaborative trials was well worth the time and effort extended. They provided rigorous scientific information pertaining to many unanswered questions and allowed us to compare our CABG results (confidentially) with those of the country as a whole.[24] We are currently planning to participate in a proposed NHLBI-sponsored prospective trial comparing the long-term efficacy of percutaneous transluminal coronary angioplasty (PTCA) versus CABG in patients with two-vessel coronary disease.

OPERATIVE FEATURES AND PERIOPERATIVE MANAGEMENT PHILOSOPHY

A brief summary of our technical approach should be included in this essay because our techniques differ substantially from those commonly used elsewhere.

Surgical and Technical Highlights

The cardinal feature of our operative management of patients undergoing CABG is *simplicity*. We use low-flow [30 to 40 mL/(kg)(min)], low-pressure [3.99 to 6.65 kPa mean arterial pressure (MAP)], nonpulsatile cardiopulmonary bypass (CPB), a bubble oxygenator, and only modest (29 to 30°C) systemic hypothermia. Two caval cannulas are used for more optimal venous drainage, and the venae cavae are not snared. Left ventricular venting is not employed, but frequently the left side of the heart is decompressed during the single period of ischemic arrest using either a small (no. 14 French) pulmonary artery sump vent connected to a coronary suction line or the cardioplegia tubing draining the ascending aorta by gravity into the oxygenator.

Our myocardial protection technique is also very simple: the heart is arrested and cooled rapidly by infusion of 500 mL of cold, hyperkalemic, asanguineous cardioplegic solution into the aortic root as profound topical hypothermia is started. Topical hypothermia is afforded by means of a *rapid* (200 mL/min) *continuous* drip of 4°C saline into the pericardial well coupled with continuous aspiration of this fluid. The left ventricle is kept constantly immersed under the cold saline; during the construction of grafts to obtuse marginal branches of the circumflex coronary artery, the cold saline is infused directly over the apex of the heart. This combination of low-flow, low-pressure CPB, two (unsnared) caval cannulas, continuous profound topical hypothermia, and single-dose cardioplegia ensures homogeneous cooling of the heart in the face of critical coronary stenoses and prevents rewarming of the heart during the cross-clamp interval without resorting to the additional complexity of profound *systemic* hypothermia or multidose cardioplegia.[33] The critical importance of assiduous attention to the topical hypothermia technique can not be overemphasized.

We essentially have used only autologous vein for the bypass graft conduits. The greater saphenous vein is preferred, but when this is unsuitable or not available, the lesser saphenous, cephalic, or basilic veins are used. Internal mammary artery grafts have been used only rarely, usually in the setting of either reoperation, when adequate autologous vein is not available, or when the patient has a small and/or diffusely diseased LAD. Adjunctive coronary endarterectomy has been used relatively often in carefully selected circumstances when diffuse distal CAD is encountered.[34]

All distal anastomoses are constructed first, using running Prolene sutures and a single period of uninterrupted ischemic arrest. Side-to-side anastomoses or "jump" grafts are reserved principally for LAD-diagonal or posterior descending artery (PDA)–distal right coronary artery combinations. We subscribe to a policy of "complete *regional* revascularization"; this implies placement of grafts to all regions of the LV which are jeopardized by proximal coronary stenoses. This philosophy does not imply, however, bypass grafting of *all* diseased vessels. Diseased coronary artery branches less than 1 mm in diameter are usually ignored or revascularized by means of a proximal (adjunctive) coronary endarterectomy when necessary.[34] In patients with critical (>60 percent diameter narrowing) stenoses of one or more coronary arteries, all other vessels with "marginal" lesions (35 to 49 percent narrowing) are also bypassed if they supply major regions of LV mass. After release of the aortic cross-clamp, the heart is resuscitated on CPB in the empty, beating state, the patient is rewarmed, and the proximal anastomoses are performed using a partial-occluding vascular clamp on the ascending aorta.

Parenthetically, the vast majority of cases are performed by the chief resident with the faculty member functioning in the role of the first assistant.

Postoperative Care

The vast majority of CABG patients are weaned off CPB using a sodium nitroprusside drip to keep the patient's mean arterial pressure (MAP) below 9.97 kPa. This allows transfusion of the blood volume remaining in the oxygenator back into the patient, minimizes myocardial oxygen demand, and may reduce hemorrhagic problems relating to anastomotic disruption or bleeding from friable tissues.[35] The synergistic effects of very low dose dopamine and nitroprusside in CABG patients with LV dysfunction have been documented by our group,[36] and this strategy is used frequently.

Postoperative invasive monitoring is also relatively simple. Left atrial lines are eschewed, and the use of flow-directed pulmonary artery catheterization is not routine. Customary invasive monitoring in uncomplicated cases includes urine output, MAP, ECG, and CVP. All patients are mechanically ventilated for at least 8 to 12 h postoperatively. This provides for optimal controllability of the patient's cardiodynamic subsystem during this critical period. Temporary atrial or atrioventricular sequential pacing has been helpful in selected patients, and is used on an individualized basis.

All postoperative management is carried out exclusively by the cardiovascular surgical housestaff in conjunction with the faculty and the intensive care unit (ICU) nursing staff. Appropriate subspecialty consultations are obtained when necessary. We believe this philosophy provides the most optimal postoperative care for the patient. As a corollary, we feel that teaching the nuances of postoperative care in terms of pharmacology and pathophysiology constitutes a critically important dimension of our resident training program. In patients with end-stage ischemic heart disease and advanced LV dysfunction, the caliber and intensity of postoperative care is probably as important as the intraoperative technical aspects of the case, if not more so.

One of our most valuable assets at Stanford is the expertise and dedication of the cardiovascular ICU nursing staff. The efforts of these talented individuals are commonly overlooked, but their crucial importance to the overall success of an open heart surgery program cannot be overemphasized. At Stanford these nurses function as integrated members of the cardiovascular surgical team with respect to ongoing patient assessment and decision-making.

Cardiac Anesthesia Management

Another invaluable asset at Stanford University Medical School is a dedicated, experienced cardiac anesthesia group,[37] which is organized as a separate division of the department of anesthesia. The members of this group are largely responsible for our overall results (see below). Key or unusual features of a particular patient's clinical or pathoanatomical situation are communicated to the cardiac anesthesiologist preoperatively. He or she, working with the anesthesia resident, is then solely responsible for the care of the patient during the induction phase. No input from the surgeon is necessary, barring any unforeseen major complication. Our cardiac anesthetic techniques are based on a slow narcotic (fentanyl is currently the preferred drug) and diazepam induction, and diazepam with supplemental narcotic maintenance thereafter. Volatile anesthetic agents are used only sparingly for control of blood pressure, optimizing the myocardial oxygen supply and demand ratio, or for the treatment of bronchospasm. During CPB, the MAP is kept in the targeted range (3.99 to 6.65 kPa) using a nitroprusside drip. Pharmacologic support during the period of weaning from CPB is a collaborative decision between the surgeon and the anesthesiologist. As described above, nitroprusside and low-dose [2 to 3 μg/(kg)(min)] dopamine are used liberally in our CABG patients.

CONTEMPORARY RESULTS AND EXPECTATIONS OF CORONARY BYPASS SURGERY
Early Operative Risk

Due to the dynamic and complex interactions between changing indications for CABG, criteria for patient selection, management methods, and early mortality and morbidity rates, it has been difficult to assess why the early risk of coronary surgery has declined. For example, the operative mortality (OM) rate was 0.7 ± 0.4 percent (70 percent confidence level) among 438 patients undergoing isolated CABG at Stanford in calendar year 1979; the perioperative myocardial infarction (PMI) rate was 2.8 ± 0.8 percent. On the other hand, the characteristics of the patients undergoing operation late in the 1970s indicated that they should be higher-risk CABG candidates compared to patients operated upon earlier in the decade,[38] according to previously reported criteria (Fig. 2).

We recently addressed this question using discrim-

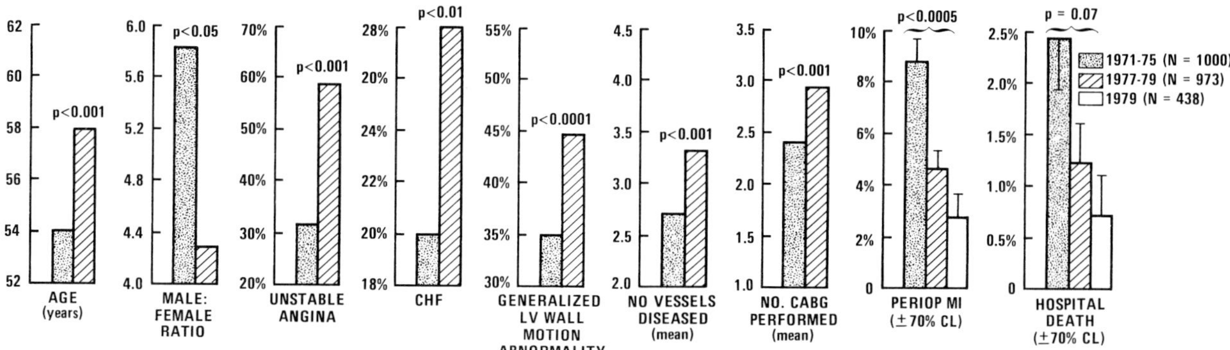

FIGURE 2 Graphic representation of the changing characteristic of patients undergoing CABG during the 1970s. Shown on the far right are the declining perioperative (PERIOP) MI and hospital death rates ± 70 percent confidence levels (CL), which would not have been expected given the simultaneous changes in patient-related and disease-related variables. Thus, more stringent patient selection criteria were *not* responsible for the superior results attained between 1977 and 1979. (*From D. C. Miller, E. B. Stinson, P. E. Oyer, et al., Discriminate Analysis of the Changing Risks of Coronary Artery Operations: 1971–1979, J. Thorac. Cardiovasc. Surg., 85:197, 1983. Used with permission of the authors and publisher.*)

inant analysis.[38] Two large cohorts of patients were studied. Group A included 1,000 consecutive patients operated upon between November 1971 and December 1975 and group B included 973 consecutive patients operated upon between July 1977 and December 1979. According to known criteria, the patients in group B were potentially a higher-risk cohort compared to group A in terms of OM and PMI (Tables 1 and 2). For example the proportion of patients undergoing single-vessel CABG fell from 18.5 percent (1971 to 1975) to 5 percent (1977 to 1979). Nevertheless, the OM rate declined from 2.4 ± 0.5 percent in group A to 1.2 ± 0.4 percent in group B ($p = .07$). Similarly, the PMI rate fell from 8.7 ± 0.9 percent to 4.6 ± 0.7 percent ($p = .0005$), as shown in Fig. 2.

Univariate and multivariate logistic regression analyses were used to identify preoperative variables for both cohorts that were *independent* significant determinants of OM and PMI. In the earlier era, a host of patient-related and disease-related characteristics were significant predictors of PMI (including age, acute preoperative MI, left main CAD, and mode of myocardial protection) (Table 3) and OM (emergency operation, left main CAD, severity of CHF, hypertension, and degree of MR) (Table 4). The findings were strikingly dissimilar for group B: only gender and coronary endarterectomy were significant independent determinants of PMI (Table 5). The only remaining (1977–79) independent predictors of OM were emergency operation and CHF,[38] as shown in Table 6. Thus, it was clear that the adverse impact of multiple patient-related and disease-related determinants of early postoperative risk had been neutralized over this decade by real improvements in patient management (Figs. 3 and 4).

Unfortunately, this type of analysis cannot ascertain which specific factors and management concepts were responsible for the superior results; moreover, it is likely that certain imponderable and/or unrecognized factors had some degree of influence on these improvements. In general terms, however, it can be inferred that more sophisticated medical, anesthetic, and nursing management and more refined surgical expertise were responsible for these improved results. We con-

TABLE 1

Clinical characteristics of the two patient cohorts*

Variable	Group A (1971–1975)	Group B (1977–1979)	p
Age:			
Years	54 ± 9	58 ± 10	<.001
Range	27–78	30–86	——
Male/female ratio	5.8:1	4.3:1	<.05
Hypertension	34%	41%	<.01
Diabetes mellitus	11%	16%	<.01
Hyperlipidemia	50%	62%	<.01
Renal insufficiency	2%	2%	ns
Carotid artery disease	2%	4%	<.02
Remote MI	54%	53%	ns
Acute MI	4%	4%	ns
Congestive heart failure	20%	28%	<.01
CHF code (1,2)†	1.96 ± 0.2	1.95 ± 0.2	ns
Severity of CHF (0–4)	0.53 ± 0.8	0.48 ± 0.9	ns
NYHA functional class IV	18%	26%	<.01
Severity of angina (1–4)	2.9 ± 0.7	3.1 ± 0.7	.005
Unstable angina	32%	58%	<.001

*ns = $p > .05$; MI = myocardial infarction; CHF = congestive heart failure; NYHA = New York Heart Association; continuous data represented as x̄ ± SD.

†1 = severe; 2 = none or mild.

SOURCE: From Miller, Stinson, Oyer, et al., Discriminate Analysis of the Changing Risks of Coronary Artery Operations: 1971–1979, *J. Thorac. Cardiovasc. Surg.*, 85:197, 1983. Used with permission of the author and publisher.

TABLE 2
Catheterization characteristics of the two patient cohorts*

Variable	Group A (1971–1975)	Group B (1977–1979)	p
Left main CAD (> 60%)	11%	14%	ns
No. vessels diseased (> 60%) (0–7)	2.7 ± 1.3	3.3 ± 1.2	<.001
CAD score (0–5)	2.6 ± 1.2	2.9 ± 1.2	<.001
Extent of CAD (1–4)	2.4 ± 0.9	2.7 ± 0.8	<.001
LV wall motion:	(N = 968)	(N = 960)	——
Normal left ventriculogram	32%	36%	
Segmental wall motion abnormality	33%	20% }	<.0001
Generalized wall motion abnormality	35%	44%	
LV wall motion score (1–3)	2.0 ± 0.8	2.1 ± .9	ns
Ejection fraction	61 ± 17% (N = 254)	58 ± 17% (N = 371)	.04
Range	3–94%	10–97%	——
Mitral regurgitation	9%	11%	ns
Degree of MR (0–4)	0.12 ± 0.4	0.14 ± 0.4	ns
LVEDP (kPa)	1.54 ± .09 (N = 654)	1.9 ± .09 (N = 873)	<.001
$\overline{PCW}$ (kPa)	1.09 ± .08 (N = 309)	1.4 ± .08 (N = 407)	<.001
$\overline{RA}$ (kPa)	.47 ± .04 (N = 348)	.63 ± .04 (N = 598)	<.001
Cardiac index [1/(m)(M²)]	.35 ± .08 (N = 359)	.37 ± .08 (N = 600)	ns

*ns = p > .05; N = number in sample; CAD = coronary artery disease; LV = left ventricular; MR = mitral regurgitation; LVEDP = LV end-diastolic pressure; $\overline{PCW}$ = mean pulmonary capillary wedge pressure; $\overline{RA}$ = mean right atrial pressure; continuous data presented as x̄ ± SD.
SOURCE: From Miller, Stinson, Oyer, et al., Discriminate Analysis of the Changing Risks of Coronary Artery Operations: 1971–1979, *J. Thorac. Cardiovasc. Surg.*, 85:197, 1983. Used with permission of the author and publisher.

TABLE 3
List of variables significantly related to PMI by univariate and multivariate analysis for group A (1971–1975)*

Variable†	Univariate analysis t	Univariate analysis p	Multivariate analysis F	Multivariate analysis p
Left main CAD	−3.2	.0012	9.24	.0024
Age	2.6	.0079	6.99	.0083
Acute preoperative MI	−2.3	.0196	6.43	.0114
Mode of myocardial protection	−2.4	.0151	5.82	.0160
CAD score	2.5	.0137	ns‡	ns
Coronary endarterectomy	−2.2	.0316	ns	ns
Extent of CAD	2.1	.0381	ns	ns
No. CABG	2.0	.0468	ns	ns
Unstable angina	−1.8	.0742	ns	ns
Remote MI	1.8	.0772	ns	ns
CABG score	1.8	.0661	ns	ns
No. vessels diseased	1.7	.0851	ns	ns
Congestive heart failure	−1.7	.0842	ns	ns
Severity of CHF	1.7	.0836	ns	ns

*Fourteen covariates were entered into the multivariate regression analysis, which yielded four determinants of PMI for this group.

†CAD = coronary artery disease; MI = myocardial infarction; CABG = coronary artery bypass graft; CHF = congestive heart failure.

‡ns = not significant.
SOURCE: From Miller, Stinson, Oyer, et al., Discriminate Analysis of the Changing Risks of Coronary Artery Operations: 1971–1979, *J. Thorac. Cardiovasc. Surg.*, 85:197, 1983. Used with permission of the author and publisher.

cluded that these advances had essentially nullified the concept that one can reliably identify high-risk CABG candidates. This is not to say, however, that these advances were capable of neutralizing the adverse *long-term* consequences of many of these preoperative characteristics, e.g., left ventricular dysfunction. The fact that emergency operation was the only strong independent determinant of OM in group B corroborated the findings of the CASS study[24] and confirmed our belief that coronary patients should be stabilized using intensive medical therapy before being taken to the operating room. The only other predictive variable for OM was CHF, which exerted in group B only a weak influence. Unfortunately, objective catheterization indexes of LV systolic pump function were not available in enough patients to allow them to be entered into the multivariate regression analyses; but this probably was not a major loss, because these parameters (e.g., ejection fraction) failed to attain important degrees of significance in the univariate analyses.

Late Results

The assessment of the long-term results of coronary bypass surgery at Stanford is confined to our experience with 1,000 consecutive patients undergoing isolated CABG between November 1971 and December

TABLE 4
Univariate and multivariate determinants of POM for group A (1971–1975)*

Variable†	Univariate analysis		Multivariate analysis	
	t	p	F	p
Emergency operation	−5.1	.0000	14.36	.0002
Left main CAD	−4.4	.0000	12.33	.0005
Severity of CHF (0–4)	4.0	.0001	8.93	.0029
Hypertension	−1.7	.0910	5.17	.0232
Degree of MR (0–4)	2.9	.0041	4.53	.0336
Acute preoperative MI	−3.5	.0005	ns	ns
Extent of CAD	3.0	.0028	ns	ns
LV wall motion score	2.8	.0059	ns	ns
CAD score	2.8	.0053	ns	ns
Age	2.6	.0086	ns	ns
CHF score	2.1	.0400	ns	ns
NYHA functional class	2.1	.0387	ns	ns
Gender	2.0	.0518	ns	ns
No. vessels diseased	1.7	.0996	ns	ns
$\overline{PCW}$ (N = 309)	1.8	.0728	——	——
LVEDP (N = 654)	2.3	.0189	——	——

*Sixteen variables were related to OM in a univariate sense, and 14 covariates were entered into the multivariate logistic regression. This yielded five important determinants of POM for this group.

†CAD = coronary artery disease; CHF = congestive heart failure; MR = mitral regurgitation; MI = myocardial infarction; LV = left ventricular; NYHA = New York Heart Association; $\overline{PCW}$ = mean pulmonary capillary wedge pressure; LVEDP = left ventricular end-diastolic pressure.

SOURCE: From Miller, Stinson, Oyer, et al., Discriminate Analysis of the Changing Risks of Coronary Artery Operations: 1971–1979, *J. Thorac. Cardiovasc. Surg.*, 85:197, 1983. Used with permission of the author and publisher.

1975. Follow-up for patients operated upon more recently (see above, "Early Operative Risk") remains too limited to reflect truly long-term outcome. Selected preoperative clinical and catheterization characteristics of this remote patient population are summarized in Tables 1 and 2, labeled as group A. Follow-up averaged 4.8 ± 1.2 years, extended to 7.3 years maximum, and was 98 percent complete. Some 424 patients were followed for greater than 5 years, and a cumulative total of 4,505 patient-years of follow-up was generated for analysis.

As a function of the remote time period when these patients underwent CABG, the OM and PMI rates were relatively high (2.4 and 8.7 percent, respectively) compared to today's standards. Also note that in this older era the average number of diseased major vessels per patient was only 2.1 and only an average of 2.4 grafts per patient were constructed. These and other disparities preclude direct extrapolation of the long-term results reported herein to patients undergoing CABG today.

TABLE 5
List of variables predictive of PMI for Group B (1977–1979)*

Variable†	Univariate analysis		Multivariate analysis	
	t	p	F	p
Gender	2.9	.0041	9.39	.0022
Coronary endarterectomy	−1.8	.0780	4.27	.0391
Year of operation	−2.3	.0237	ns‡	ns
Unstable angina	−2.0	.0480	ns	ns
Emergency operation	−1.9	.0661	ns	ns
$\overline{RA}$ (N = 598)	−2.1	.0398	——	——
Ejection fraction (N = 369)	2.1	.0380	——	——
LVEDP (N = 871)	−1.9	.0639	——	——

*Eight variables were related to PMI by univariate testing, but incomplete data prevented entry of the catheterization parameters into the multivariate logistic regression.

†$\overline{RA}$ = mean right atrial pressure; LVEDP = left ventricular end-diastolic pressure.

‡ns = not significant.

SOURCE: From Miller, Stinson, Oyer, et al., Discriminate Analysis of the Changing Risks of Coronary Artery Operations: 1971–1979, *J. Thorac. Cardiovasc. Surg.*, 85:197, 1983. Used with permission of the author and publisher.

SURVIVAL

As illustrated in Fig. 5, long-term survival rates for these 1,000 patients was highly satisfactory, especially when stratified according to number of vessels diseased. Cautious comparison of these survival rates with existing historical figures for medically treated patients[14] is very favorable, but not undertaken without considerable hazard.

TABLE 6
List of variables predictive of OM for group B (1977–1979)*

Variable	Univariate analysis		Multivariate analysis	
	t	p	F	p
Emergency operation	−3.8	.0002	14.68	.0001
Congestive heart failure	−2.2	.0292	4.76	.0294
Carotid disease	−2.0	.0425	ns†	ns
NYHA functional class‡	1.9	.0629	ns	ns

*For group B (1977–1979), only four variables were related to OM when tested singly. Multivariate analysis eliminated two of these: carotid disease and NYHA functional class.

†ns = not significant.

‡NYHA = New York Heart Association.

SOURCE: From Miller, Stinson, Oyer, et al., Discriminate Analysis of the Changing Risks of Coronary Artery Operations: 1971–1979, *J. Thorac. Cardiovasc. Surg.*, 85:197, 1983. Used with permission of the author and publisher.

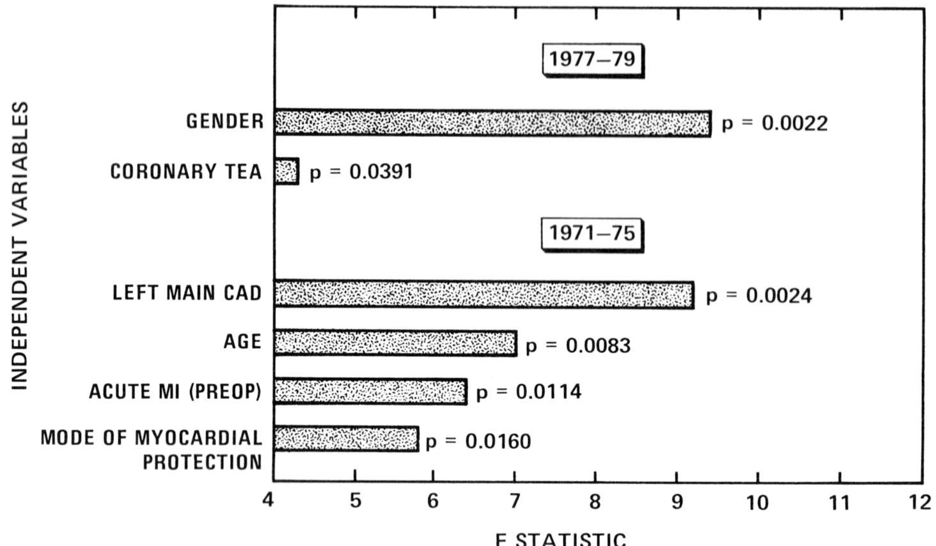

FIGURE 3 Relative discriminate influence of the independent predictors of PMI, subdivided according to era of operation. In the earlier group (1971–1975) left main disease had the strongest predictive influence of PMI, but no significant predictive value in the later (1977–1979) experience, where sex subsumed predominance. See text for additional details. TEA = endarterectomy; CAD = coronary artery disease; MI = myocardial infarction; Pre-op = preoperative. (*From D. C. Miller, E. B. Stinson, P. E. Oyer, et al., Discriminate Analysis of the Changing Risks of Coronary Artery Operations: 1971–1979. J. Thorac. Cardiovasc. Surg., 85:197, 1983. Used with permission of the authors and publisher.*)

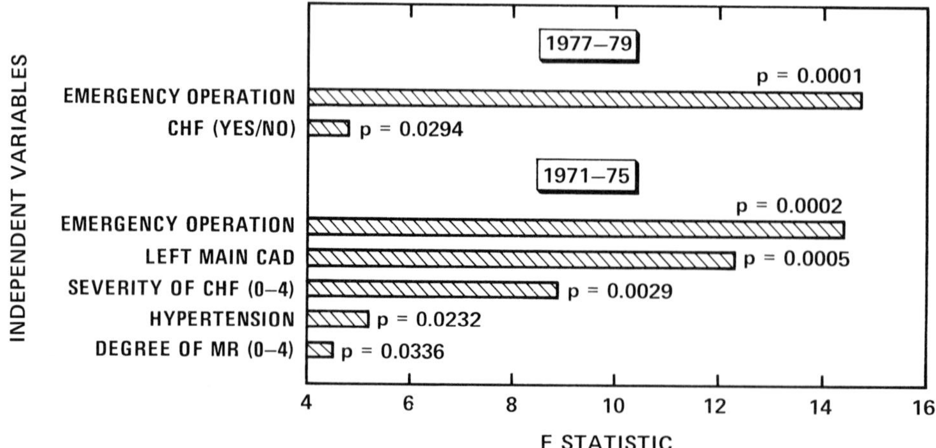

FIGURE 4 Relative predictive power of the independent determinants of operative mortality (OM) rate. The predictive influence of emergency operation was predominant in both groups. For the 1977–1979 cohort, the only other independent determinant of OM was congestive heart failure (yes/no), but its influence was quite weak, albeit significant. Abbreviations: CHF = congestive heart failure; CAD = coronary artery disease; MR = mitral regurgitation. (*From D. C. Miller, E. B. Stinson, P. E. Oyer, et al., Discriminate Analysis of the Changing Risks of Coronary Artery Operations: 1971–1979, J. Thorac. Cardiovasc. Surg., 85:197, 1983. Used with permission of the authors and publisher.*)

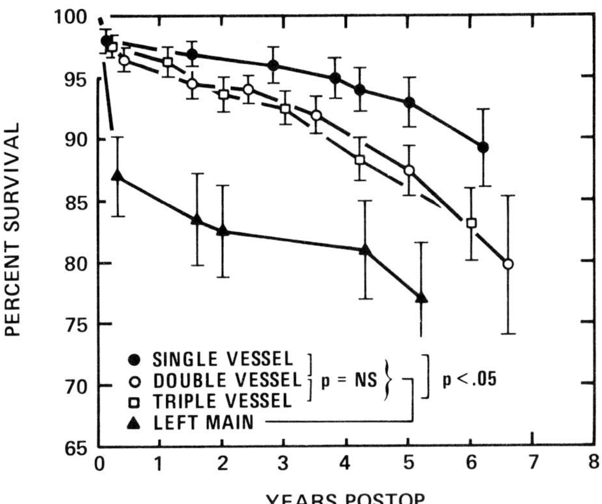

FIGURE 5 Actuarial survival rates (including operative deaths) of 1,000 patients undergoing isolated CABG between 1971 and 1975. The survival rates are stratified according to number of vessels diseased. The relatively lower survival rate for CABG patients with left main disease was due to a higher operative mortality rate during this era. This difference in operative mortality risk no longer exists, as outlined in the text and shown in Fig. 4.

It is more informative, but still imperfect, to compare the survival rates of these patients following CABG with the expected survivorship of the general population matched for age and sex. This was accomplished using a computerized simulation program and standard U.S. Census Bureau fiduciary tables. The results are shown in Figs. 6 and 7. Figure 6A illustrates the actuarial survival rate for these 1,000 CABG patients compared to the age- and sex-matched U.S. population. Due to the relatively high OM rate during this remote era, there was a statistically significant difference in survival out to 8 years. When the operative fatalities are excluded (Fig. 6B), there was no distinguishable difference in survival rate between the patients undergoing CABG and the "control" matched population. The actuarial 5-year survival rate for discharged CABG patients was 91 ± 0.5 percent. Inspection of Figs. 7A and B shows that the 183 discharged patients undergoing single CABG actually had a slight, but insignificant, advantage in survival rate over the control group, while the opposite trend (albeit also being statistically insignificant) was observed for the 794 discharged multivessel CABG patients. This is not surprising since the prognosis of medically treated patients with single-vessel CAD is extremely good for

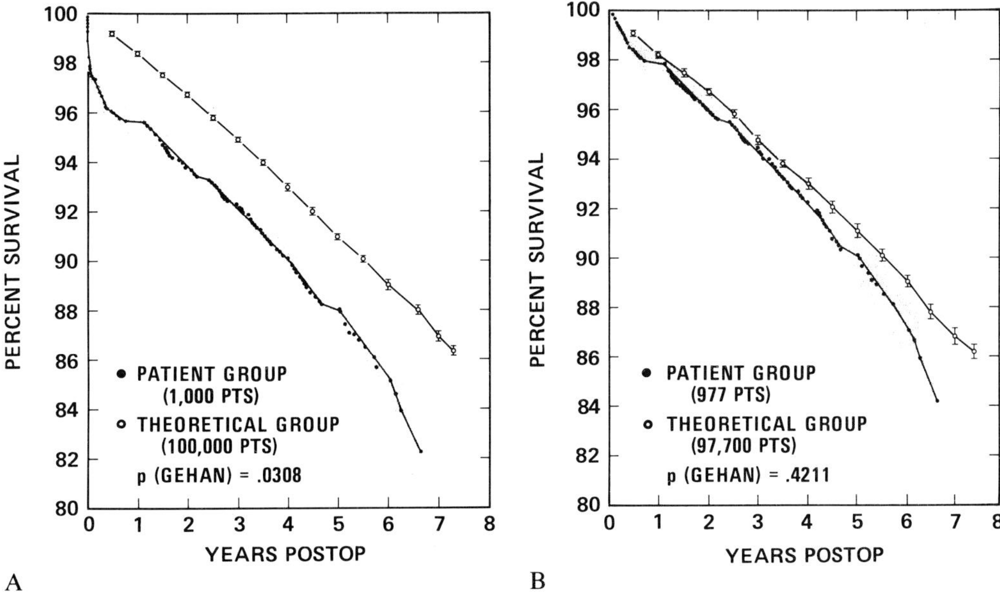

FIGURE 6 (A) Overall actuarial survival rate of 1,000 CABG patients (1971–1975) compared with a computer-simulated theoretical group matched for age and sex. Due to the higher operative mortality rate in this remote era (2.4 percent), there was a statistically significant difference in survival. (B) Similar actuarial survival rates comparing the 977 CABG patients who were discharged from the hospital against the same matched general population. The survival rate out to 8 years postoperatively is indistinguishable between the operated patients with coronary artery disease and the simulated control group. Given the current operative mortality rate of CABG at Stanford (less than 1 percent), it is expected, but not proven, that the long-term prognosis for all patients (not just discharged patients) undergoing CABG today would not be any different than that for an age- and sex-matched control group.

198

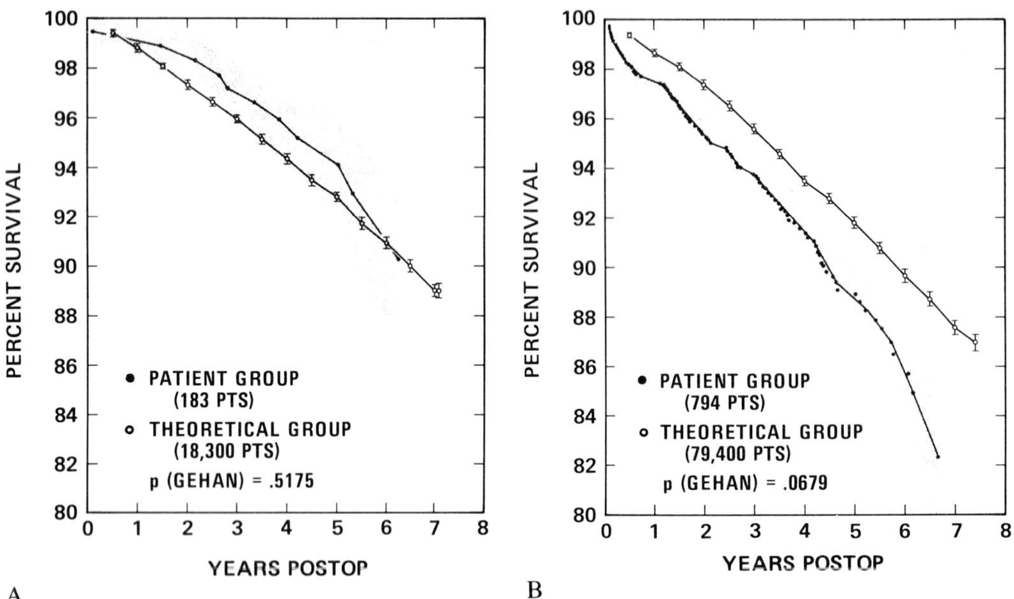

A   B

FIGURE 7 (*A*) A similar actuarial curve showing the survival of *discharged* CABG patients with single-vessel disease. (*B*) Comparison of the long-term actuarial survival rate for 794 patients with multivessel coronary artery disease who survived CABG between 1971 and 1975 compared to an age- and sex-matched control population. (See text for details.)

6 or 7 years;[32] it is only after this time threshold that one might expect to see differences in survival rates between patients with single-vessel CAD treated medically or surgically.

As shown above, the early operative risk of CABG

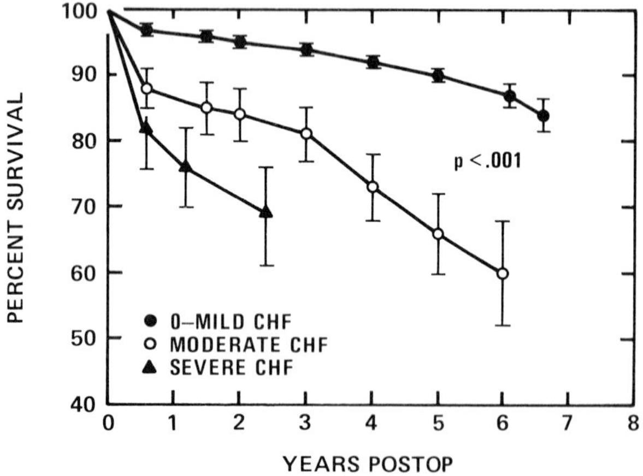

FIGURE 8 Long-term actuarial survival rates for 1,000 CABG patients (1971–1975) segregated according to degree of preoperative CHF. As described in the text, preoperative CHF no longer portends an inordinately high operative mortality rate, but the adverse impact of left ventricular dysfunction as manifested by congestive heart failure on long-term survival is readily apparent in this graph.

surgery is no longer a function of LV function, and even clinical CHF exerts only a weak, albeit significant, independent influence on OM (Table 6 and Fig. 4). Importantly, this was not the case in terms of long-term survival among these patients operated upon between 1971 and 1975. The adverse effect of preoperative clinical CHF on survival is shown in Fig. 8. Since the operative mortality and morbidity (PMI) rates surrounding coronary surgery are so low today, one message is clear: only earlier referral for surgery (prior to the irretrievable loss of viable myocardium) will favorably modify the postoperative prognosis of patients with moderate-to-severe CHF or LV dysfunction who undergo CABG.

SUDDEN DEATH

The incidence of late sudden death, a common manifestation of ischemic heart disease, was extremely low in these surgically treated patients. As shown in Fig. 9, the actuarial rate of late sudden death was only 4 ± 1 percent at 6 years. These 26 deaths occurred at a constant rate; thus, the linearized incidence of late sudden death (0.6 percent per patient-year) is a meaningful statistic. It is hazardous to compare these rates directly with similar figures for medically treated patients;[14] nevertheless, the exceedingly low incidence of sudden death seen in this study may well represent

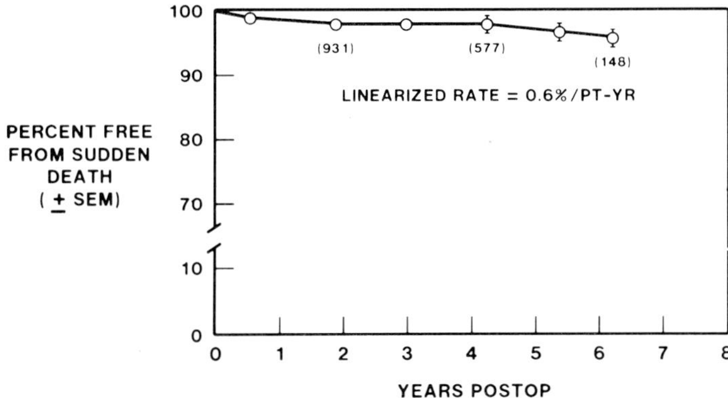

FIGURE 9 Actuarial rate of late sudden and/or unexplained death among 976 discharged CABG patients (1971–1975). Five years postoperatively, the actuarial rate of late sudden death was 3 ± 0.5 percent (± SEM). The linearized rate (precisely interpretable due to the constant occurrence rate of these events) was 0.6 percent per patient-year.

one of the key benefits of CABG surgery in terms of enhanced life expectancy.

Inspection of the causes of the 95 late deaths is also illuminating. As already noted, 27 percent (26 of 95) were sudden and unexplained; 14 percent (13 of 95) were caused by fatal MI, 4 percent were due to documented ventricular arrhythmias, and 19 percent (18 of 95) were associated with chronic, progressive CHF. Noncardiac causes included neoplasm (13 percent), suicide or accidental death (7 percent), and a variety of other miscellaneous diseases (14 percent).

MYOCARDIAL INFARCTION

Prospective, controlled studies have shown that the risk of myocardial infarction is not significantly reduced by CABG surgery. This, in our view, has been a disappointment; perhaps longer follow-up in the more recent randomized trials[25,39] will confirm our aspiration that successful CABG should be associated with a decreased incidence of MI.

Figure 10 illustrates in actuarial terms the MI rate in this older cohort (1971 to 1975) of patients undergo-

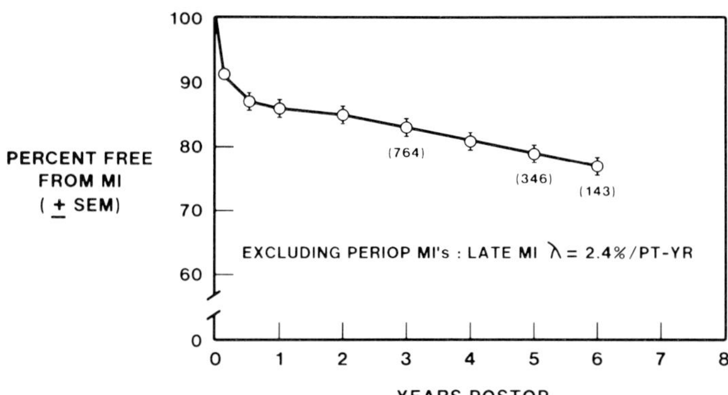

FIGURE 10 Actuarial rate of MI in patients undergoing CABG between 1971 and 1975. Of the 1,000 patients, 5 are excluded, as these patients died in the operating room. During this early era the perioperative MI rate was relatively high (8.7 percent), as reflected in the graph; currently the perioperative MI rate is 2.4 percent. After the early postoperative months, the rate of late MI occurred at a constant, linearized rate of 2.4 percent per patient-year. Excluding patients sustaining a perioperative MI, 88 ± 1 percent of patients were free of late MI 5 years postoperatively.

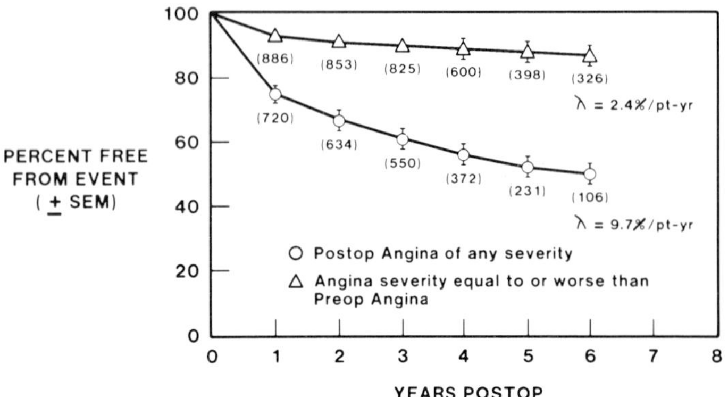

FIGURE 11 The recurrence of angina pectoris postoperatively depicted in actuarial format. The upper curve reflects recurrent angina which in terms of severity was equal to or worse than the preoperative angina status; the lower curve represents angina of any severity. Six years postoperatively 87 ± 1 percent of patients were improved compared to their preoperative angina status, but only 50 ± 2 percent were completely free of angina pectoris.

ing CABG, including patients who sustained a perioperative MI (8.7 percent). (As shown above, the current risk of PMI is in the range of 2.8 percent.[38]) Six years postoperatively, 77 ± 2 percent of patients were free from an MI. If one excludes the perioperative MIs, the linearized incidence of late MI was 2.4 percent per patient-year (Fig. 10). Of the 108 late MIs 13 (12 percent) were fatal, representing a linearized rate of late fatal MI of 0.3 percent per patient-year. Furthermore, the overall proportion of late deaths attributable to fatal infarction was 14 percent.

RECURRENCE OF ANGINA PECTORIS

As initially documented in our early investigations,[10,12,13] recrudescence of angina did occur as a function of time postoperatively. Our 1977 report included an average of 46 months of follow-up for the first 341 patients undergoing isolated CABG at Stanford; over 75 percent of surviving patients still reported some clinical benefit compared with their preoperative status 4 years postoperatively.[15]

Follow-up for the 1971 to 1975 cohort of 1,000 patients extended to 7.3 years and totalled 4,505 patient-years. Figure 11 depicts the functional status of these patients with respect to angina. At 6 years, 87 ± 1 percent of patients were free of angina pectoris considered to be worse or equivalent to their preoperative chest pain status. Only 50 ± 2 percent, however, remained completely angina-free at this same time. Linearized rates of angina recurrence are somewhat misleading because this phenomenon did not occur at a constant rate. As shown in Fig. 11, a large minority of patients redeveloped angina in the first postoperative

CONGESTIVE HEART FAILURE:

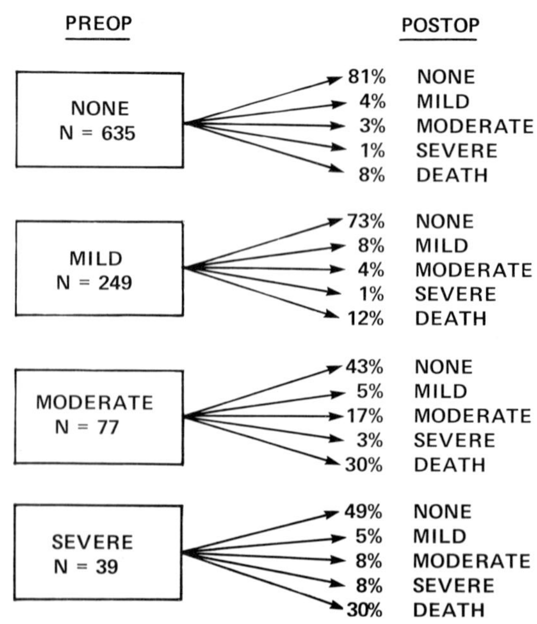

FIGURE 12 Functional improvement with respect to congestive heart failure following coronary artery bypass grafting (1971–1975). This assessment represents an average of 4.8 years of postoperative follow-up. While patients with moderate or severe preoperative CHF had relatively higher late fatality rates (Fig. 8), the majority of surviving patients experienced functional benefit in terms of heart failure.

year; thereafter, the likelihood of angina recrudescence over any given annual interval was much lower. Similar angina recurrence rates have been observed by other centers.[40]

Despite the fact that one-half of the patient population had recurrence of angina of some degree by 6 years, it is noteworthy that the severity of the chest pain and its attendant disability were equivalent to or worse than the preoperative status in only 13 ± 1 percent of patients. As a corollary, only a relatively small number of these patients with recurrent angina required late reoperation (see below).

CONGESTIVE HEART FAILURE

Irrespective of the deleterious impact of congestive heart failure on long-term survival (Fig. 8), the majority of surviving patients experienced some degree of improvement with regard to CHF. This is outlined in Fig. 12 stratified according to preoperative CHF status: 62 percent of the 39 patients with severe CHF, 48 percent of those with moderate CHF, and 73 percent of the 249 patients with mild CHF had improvement in their failure symptoms at an average of 4.8 years postoperatively. Unfortunately, objective ventriculographic data (basal and exercise) confirming improvement in LV systolic performance were not available in these patients, but have been reported by others.[41]

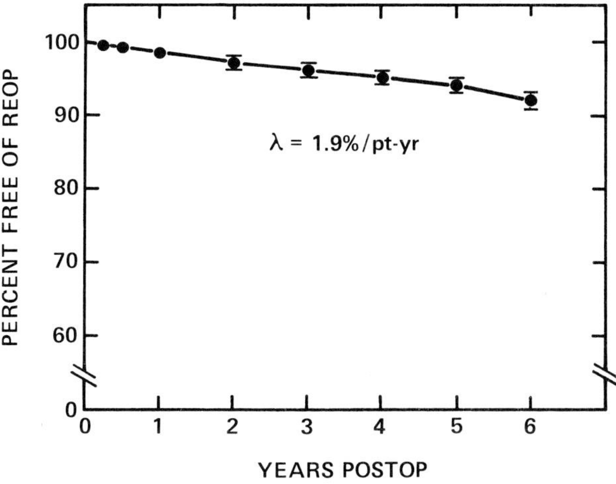

FIGURE 13 Actuarial incidence of first CABG *reoperation* in 1,000 patients undergoing initial CABG between 1971 and 1975. The linearized rate was 1.9 percent per patient-year, being significantly lower than the rate of overall angina recrudescence (Fig. 11). Over 94 percent of patients were free of reoperation 5 years postoperatively.

REOPERATION

As CABG surgery evolved, increasing numbers of patients redeveloped severe angina which mandated consideration of "redo" coronary bypass grafting.[42,43] This phenomenon had been seen earlier in patients undergoing peripheral arterial reconstruction for generalized atherosclerotic disease; as an example, less than ideal 5- to 10-year graft patency rates (50 percent or less) had prompted critical reassessment of the indications for femoropopliteal bypass grafting. Claudication due to simple superficial femoral artery occlusion or stenosis was shown to portend a relatively benign prognosis, and the claudication usually responded to conservative measures, e.g., cessation of smoking and a progressive exercise program. Given these facts, the indications for femoropopliteal bypass grafting thereafter became more stringent, generally being limited to cases of limb jeopardy or advanced symptoms which had caused vocational disability.

Such a large-scale reassessment of the indications for surgical intervention did not occur in the realm of CABG, probably because most of these patients had been initially referred only for incapacitating angina which was truly refractory to maximal medical therapy.

It was mentioned in the preceding section that only a minority of patients with postoperative angina pectoris had severe symptoms (Fig. 11). This correlated with the relatively low incidence of CABG reoperation in this series of 1,000 patients, as shown in Fig. 13. Six years postoperatively, 91 ± 1 percent of patients were free from reoperation. Reoperation occurred at a constant, linearized rate of 1.9 percent per patient-year. The need for reoperation beyond 6 years still remains poorly characterized, but it would not be unexpected, in our opinion, to see more CABG patients requiring reoperation between 7 and 10 years postoperatively due to accelerated graft atherosclerosis and the inexorable progression of disease in the native coronary arteries.

In our experience, *first* CABG reoperation was associated with a low risk of mortality and morbidity, essentially identical to that of the initial operation.[43] The likelihood of clinical benefit with respect to angina pectoris after first reoperation was similar to that obtained after the initial operation (Fig. 14). Although many patients again redeveloped angina following *reoperation,* the severity of the recurrent chest pain was usually less than that which prompted reoperation, as also shown in Fig. 14.

The survival rate after *first* CABG reoperation was almost identical to that following initial CABG (Fig. 15), but our data in this subset were limited to only 59 reoperation patients and a maximum follow-up span of 5 years. Repeated assessment of this issue focusing on the pathoanatomical conditions prompting reoperation as a function of time after initial CABG will be enlight-

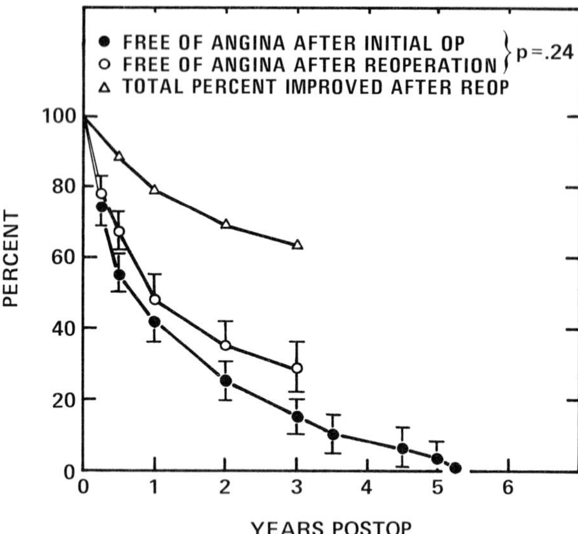

FIGURE 14 Actuarial graph describing the recurrence of angina following initial CABG (OP) and also following first CABG reoperation (REOP). The proportion of patients at various times completely free of angina following either the first or second CABG procedure is almost identical. The fraction of patients sustaining improvement in their anginal status after REOP CABG (triangles) is somewhat less than that following initial CABG operation (Fig. 11).

ening. Furthermore, additional information is necessary before the risk-benefit guidelines surrounding third and fourth CABG procedures in individual patients can be ascertained.

CURRENT INDICATIONS FOR CORONARY BYPASS SURGERY

As described above the indications for myocardial revascularization have changed substantially at Stanford over the first 15 years. In general, the indications for surgery have become liberalized as our experience has grown, the early operative risk has been reduced to nominal levels,[38] and the conclusive results from controlled collaborative trials documenting enhanced life expectancy in selected subsets of patients have been published;[30–32,39] however, patients with certain conditions judged in the past to represent reasonable indications for CABG (e.g., refractory ventricular tachycardia) are not currently considered to be candidates for isolated bypass grafting. Furthermore, the last decade has reflected an increasingly aggressive approach by our cardiologists to identify "high-risk" candidates with ischemic heart disease (with or without disabling symptoms), who are then referred for CABG.

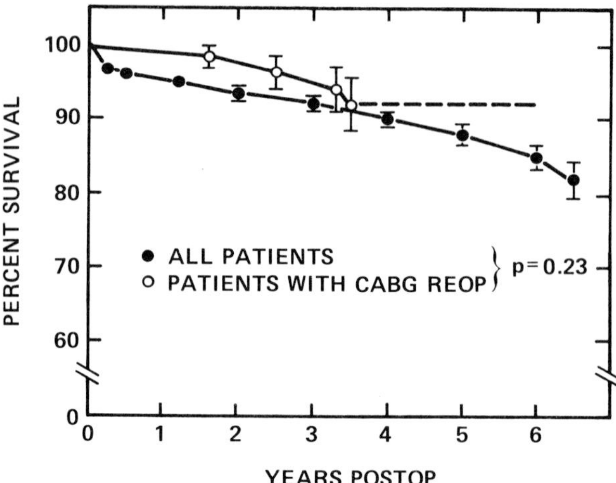

FIGURE 15 Actuarial survival rates following initial CABG and following first CABG reoperation (REOP). There was no statistical significant difference in survival out to 5 years, but long-term follow-up and number of REOP patients were limited.

The least arguable indication for CABG remains patients with chronic stable angina pectoris which has proven to be refractory to maximal medical therapy. Due to more effective medical therapy (principally the introduction of beta blocking drugs and calcium antagonists), poorly understood secular changes in the American population,[44] and the vast numbers of such patients who have already undergone CABG over the last 15 years, less than 50 percent of patients being referred for CABG today fall into this category at Stanford. The emergence of alternative revascularization procedures [namely, percutaneous transluminal coronary angioplasty (PTCA)] may also have had a recent impact on this issue, but this is unlikely due to the extremely small number of patients (< 3 percent) operated upon at Stanford currently who have single-vessel disease.

The most common current indication for CABG at Stanford is unstable angina. As mentioned previously, these patients are now managed with intensive medical therapy and then studied by coronary angiography during the same hospital admission. Rarely, IABP support is necessary. Selected patients are then referred for CABG based on pathological anatomy of the coronary arteries, LV function, and clinical considerations. It is too early to conclude whether the recent use of calcium antagonists has modified the clinical management of patients with unstable angina at Stanford vis-à-vis CABG, but these agents clearly have been helpful in the initial phase of medical stabilization. Given our recently published prospective, nonrandomized study (which provided compelling evidence that CABG significantly enhanced life expectancy in patients with unstable angina[6]), it is improbable that new advances in the medical therapy of these patients will alter our therapeutic philosophy.

Determination of "inoperability" has never been based on poor left ventricular function at Stanford. Indeed, our early attempts to revascularize patients with ischemic cardiomyopathy (defined as an ejection fraction of <0.35) with or *without* angina pectoris provided valuable information concerning the natural and surgical history of this end-stage disease.[20,21] Additionally, the *presence* of LV dysfunction (in conjunction with two- or three-vessel CAD or left main disease) has been shown by the VA Cooperative Study to be representative of patient subsets that benefit from CABG in terms of life expectancy.[30,31] We continue to be aggressive advocates of CABG for patients with angina pectoris (and/or dyspnea on exertion due to exercise-induced myocardial ischemia) who also have advanced LV dysfunction or CHF; on the other hand, revascularization probably offers little benefit to patients with ischemic cardiomyopathy who do not have anginal or "angina-equivalent" symptoms.

Similarly, diffuse CAD involving the distal vessels has not constituted a contraindication to CABG at Stanford. When necessary, adjunctive coronary endarterectomy is used in these circumstances, but represents an incremental risk factor for PMI.[34,38] In patients undergoing repeat CABG surgery, on the other hand, favorable coronary anatomy in the target vessels does correlate with clinical benefit.[43]

Clinical and angiographic recognition of coronary spasm has not had a large effect on our surgical practice. This is an area of intense investigation by our cardiologists, and most of these patients respond favorably to appropriate medical therapy. When a patient with coronary spasm superimposed upon fixed organic lesions in two or more vessels does not respond satisfactorily to medical management, CABG is considered. In this context it is important to optimize (using parenteral drugs) the patient's antispasm medication regimen throughout the entire perioperative period.

A growing proportion of patients being referred for CABG at Stanford represent "high-risk subsets." These patients are being operated upon principally for prolongation of life expectancy; amelioration of disabling symptoms is a secondary goal in these cases. Although the specific criteria used to identify such patients vary according to differences in individual and institutional judgment, certain generalizations can be made. Based on data derived from the VA Cooperative Stable Angina Pectoris Study[29,31,32] and the European Coronary Artery Surgery Group,[39] most patients with 50 percent or greater stenosis of the left main coronary artery are referred for CABG, irrespective of current symptomatic status. It must be emphasized, however, that low-risk subgroups of patients with left main disease do exist, are identifiable using clinical criteria alone, and may not benefit in terms of increased life expectancy after CABG.[31] Second, and again based on data derived from the VA Cooperative Study, "high-risk" patients characterized by either noninvasive criteria[30] or catheterization findings[32] are considered to be candidates for CABG in order to enhance survival. Using four simple clinical features (history of MI, history of hypertension, severe angina pectoris, and ST-segment depression on resting ECG) patients can be stratified into "high-, middle-, or low-risk" terciles.[30,31] Those patients in the high-risk tercile are referred for CABG. Anatomically, patients with multivessel CAD and LV dysfunction are also considered to be operative candidates with the goal of augmentation of life expectancy.[32] Patients who have two-vessel disease and normal LV function, regardless of symptoms, are also urged to consider CABG to enhance life expectancy if one of the lesions is a high-grade proximal LAD stenosis.[39]

Another subgroup that has tentatively emerged into an operative category consists of MI patients who thereafter are deemed "high-risk" on the basis of submaximal treadmill testing, radionuclide ventriculography, or ambulatory ECG monitoring.[45,46] If coronary angiography confirms that substantial volumes of viable LV mass are in jeopardy, CABG is recommended irrespective of angina status.

Early postinfarction angina is also being recognized more frequently as an indication for semiurgent coronary angiography and possible CABG. The risk of operation in these patients is low today,[47] but just because CABG can be performed safely in this setting does not mean it should be done routinely. Specifically, patients with early postinfarction angina who have "ischemia at a distance" and those who have "ischemia in the infarct zone" after a subendocardial MI probably will benefit from urgent CABG in terms of life expectancy.[48] This also is likely to be the case for patients in the immediate post-MI period who have echocardiographically documented "infarct expansion," since an alarming high fraction of these patients die in hospital of LV rupture with resultant pericardial tamponade.[49]

Cardiogenic shock due to an acute myocardial infarction is not an indication for emergency coronary angiography or CABG at Stanford unless postinfarction angina or certain electrophysiological abnormalities accompany and/or precipitate the low-output state.

We have not routinely operated upon patients in the very early hours of an acute, uncomplicated myocardial infarction because of logistical obstacles and scientific reservations. In this regard we look forward to evaluating the results of the prospective, randomized trial of emergency CABG versus medical therapy for patients with acute MI which is planned to be carried out in Spokane, Washington.

The use of intracoronary or intravenous streptokinase (SK) at Stanford has recently prompted surgical intervention within 1 week of an acute infarction. In our preliminary experience, a sizable minority of patients redeveloped severe chest pain 3 to 5 days after successful coronary thrombolysis, and many were then operated upon under emergency circumstances. This led to a more aggressive screening policy after successful SK therapy. If severe multivessel disease is documented, CABG is considered early (1 to 2 days) after successful coronary thrombolysis; if single-vessel CAD is present, then early PTCA is recommended. Only additional experience with various management sequences will identify the most judicious and prudent course of action.

Another small group of patients currently undergoing CABG at Stanford represents technical complications at PTCA. Our cardiology group (initially under the aegis of Dr. John Simpson) has been active in coronary angioplasty since 1979 and is a participant in the NHLBI PTCA registry. Approximately 8 percent of patients undergoing PTCA had a complication which led to emergency CABG. This has been performed to date without any operative deaths, and the number of patients requiring emergency CABG has declined with increased PTCA experience.

Concomitant CABG for patients undergoing valve replacement, LV aneurysmectomy, and other intracardiac procedure continues to be employed frequently at Stanford as dictated by individual judgment. Since the publication of our previous experience,[16,17] the operative risk of combined valve replacement and CABG has continued to fall, and we believe that revascularization of large amounts of jeopardized, viable LV mass in such patients with severe multivessel CAD is the most prudent approach.

SUMMARY

In conclusion, we have learned many lessons during our first 15-year experience with coronary bypass grafting; undoubtedly, more lessons remain to be learned as the clinical role of CABG continues to evolve. A major clinical shift over the last decade has been to deemphasize amelioration of symptoms in favor of prolonging life expectancy; the ultimate "efficacy" of this philosophy in terms of the overall net cost to society remains a debated, but probably moot, point. In an era of increasing cost-awareness and limited resources, many difficult social, economic, and philosophical issues remain to be addressed.

REFERENCES

1 Cohn, L. H., Fogarty, T. J., Daily, P. O., and Shumway, N. E.: Emergency Coronary Artery Bypass, *Surgery*, 10:821, 1971.

2 Pfeifer, J., Hultgren, H., Alderman, E., et al.: Surgical Intervention in Impending Myocardial Infarction, *Circulation* (suppl. 2):211, 1971.

3 Miller, D. C., Cannom, D. S., Fogarty, T. J., et al.: Saphenous Vein Coronary Artery Bypass in Patients with "Preinfarction Angina," *Circulation*, 47:234, 1973.

4 Berndt, T. B., Miller, D. C., Silverman, J. F., et al.: Coronary Bypass Surgery for Unstable Angina Pectoris, *Am. J. Med.*, 58:171, 1975.

5 Davidson, D. M., Lamb, I., and Schroeder, J. S.: Long-term Results of Coronary Artery Bypass Surgery for Unstable Angina: Incidence of Mortality, Myocardial Infarction, and Angina Resumption, *Clin. Cardiol.*, 3:297, 1980.

6 Hultgren, H. N., Shettigar, U. R., and Miller, D. C.: Medical vs. Surgical Treatment of Unstable Angina, *Am. J. Cardiol.*, 50:663, 1982.

7 Graham, A. F., Miller, D. C., Stinson, E. B., et al.: Surgical Treatment of Refractory Life-Threatening Ventricular Tachycardia, *Am. J. Cardiol.*, 32:909, 1973.

8 Mason, J. W., Stinson, E. B., Winkle, R. A., et al.: Surgery for Ventricular Tachycardia: Efficacy of Left Ventricular Aneurysm Resection Compared with Operation Guided by Electrical Activation Mapping, *Circulation*, 65:1148, 1982.

9 Mason, J. W., Stinson, E. B., Winkle, R. A., and Oyer, P. E.: Mechanisms of Ventricular Tachycardia: Wide, Complex Ignorance, *Am. Heart J.*, 102:1083, 1981.

10 Cannom, D. S., Miller, D. C., Shumway, N. E., et al.: The Long-term Follow-up of Patients Undergoing Saphenous Vein Bypass Surgery, *Circulation*, 49:77, 1974.

11 Alderman, E. L., Matlof, H. J., Wexler, L., et al.: Results of Direct Coronary-Artery Surgery for the Treatment of Angina Pectoris, *N. Engl. J. Med.*, 288:535, 1973.

12 Tecklenberg, P. L., Alderman, E. L., Miller, D. C., et al.: Changes in Survival and Symptom Relief in a Longitudinal Study of Patients after Bypass Surgery, *Circulation*, 51,52:98, 1975.

13 Alderman, E. L., Harrison, D. C., and Shumway, N. E.: Longevity and Symptom Relief in a Four-Year Follow-up of Coronary Surgery Patients, in J. C. Davila (ed.), "2d Henry Ford Hospital International Symposium on Cardiac Surgery," Appleton-Century-Crofts, Inc., New York, 1975, p. 605.

14 Oberman, A., Jones, W. B., Riley, A. P., et al.: Natural History of Coronary Artery Disease, *Bull. N.Y. Acad. Med.*, 48:1109, 1972.

15 Alderman, E. L., Brown, C. R., Sanders, G. R., and Stinson, E. B.: Survival following Bypass Graft Surgery, *Clev. Clin. Q.*, 45:157, 1978.

16 Miller, D. C., Stinson, E. B., Oyer, P. E., et al.: Surgical Implications and Results of Combined Aortic Valve Replacement and Myocardial Revascularization, *Am. J. Cardiol.*, 43:494, 1979.

17 Miller, D. C., Stinson, E. B., Rossiter, S. J., et al.: Impact of Simultaneous Myocardial Revascularization on Operative Risk Functional Result, and Survival following Mitral Valve Replacement, *Surgery*, 84:848, 1978.

18 Bonow, R. O., Kent, K. M., Rosing, D. R., et al.: Aortic Valve Replacement without Myocardial Revascularization in Patients with Combined Aortic Valvular and Coronary Artery Disease, *Circulation*, 63:243, 1981.

19 Kirklin, J. W., and Kouchoukos, N. T.: Aortic Valve Replacement without Myocardial Revascularization, *Circulation*, 63:252, 1981.

20 Miller, D. C., Stinson, E. B., and Alderman, E. L.: Surgical Treatment of Ischemic Cardiomyopathy: Is It Ever Too Late? *Am. J. Surg.*, 141:688, 1980.

21 Alderman, E. L., Miller, D. C., Stinson, E. B., et al.: Retrospective Comparison of Medical vs. Surgical Treatment of Coronary Disease in Patients with Severe Left Ventricular Dysfunction, *Circulation*, 62(suppl. 3):94, 1980. (Abstract.)

22 Faulkner, S. L., Stoney, W. S., Alford, W. C., et al.: Ischemic Cardiomyopathy: Medical vs. Surgical Treatment, *J. Thorac. Cardiovasc. Surg.*, 74:77, 1977.

23 Unstable Angina Pectoris: National Cooperative Study Group to Compare Surgical and Medical Therapy. II. In-Hospital Experience and Initial Follow-up Results in Patients with One, Two, and Three Vessel Disease, *Am. J. Cardiol.*, 42:839, 1978.

24 Kennedy, J. W., Kaiser, G. C., Fisher, L. D., et al.: Multivariate Discriminant Analysis of the Clinical and Angiographic Predictors of Operative Mortality from the Collaborative Study in Coronary Artery Surgery (CASS), *J. Thorac. Cardiovasc. Surg.*, 80:876, 1980.

25 Kennedy, J. W., Kaiser, G. C., Fisher, L. D., et al.: Clinical and Angiographic Predictors of Operative Mortality from the Collaborative Study in Coronary Artery Surgery (CASS), *Circulation*, 63:793, 1981.

26 Chaitman, B. R., Rogers, W. J., Davis, K., et al.: Operative Risk Factors in Patients with Left Main Coronary-Artery Disease (CASS), *N. Engl. J. Med.*, 303:953, 1980.

27 Chaitman, B. R., Bourassa, M. G., Davis, K., et al.: Angiographic Prevalence of High-Risk Coronary Artery Disease in Patient Subsets (CASS), *Circulation*, 64:360, 1981.

28 Chaitman, B. R., Fisher, L. D., Bourassa, M. G., et al.: Effect of Coronary Bypass Surgery on Survival Patterns in Subsets of Patients with Left Main Coronary Artery Disease (CASS), *Am. J. Cardiol.*, 48:765, 1981.

29 Murphy, M. L., Hultgren, H. N., Detre, K., et al.: Treatment of Chronic Stable Angina: A Preliminary Report of Survival Data of the Randomized VA Cooperative Study, *N. Engl. J. Med.*, 297:621, 1977.

30 Detre, K., Peduzzi, P., Murphy, M., et al.: Effect of Bypass Surgery on Survival in Patients in Low- and High-Risk Subgroups Delineated by the Use of Simple Clinical Variables, *Circulation*, 63:1329, 1981.

31 Takaro, T., Peduzzi, P., Detre, K., et al.: Survival in Subgroups of Patients with Left Main Coronary Artery Disease, *Circulation*, 66:14, 1982.

32 Takaro, T., Hultgren, H. N., Detre, K., Peduzzi, P.: The Veterans Administration Cooperative Study of Stable Angina: Current Status, *Circulation*, 65(suppl. 2):60, 1982.

33 Baumgartner, W. A., Miller, D. C., Stinson, E. B., et al.: Simple Adjuncts Which Maintain Septal Temperature Below 20°C without Multidose Cardioplegia or Deep Systemic Hypothermia, *Am. Heart J.*, 105:440, 1983.

34 Miller, D. C., Stinson, E. B., Oyer, P. E., et al.: Long-term Clinical Assessment of the Efficacy of Adjunctive Coronary Endarterectomy, *J. Thorac. Cardiovasc. Surg.*, 81:21, 1981.

35 Stinson, E. B., Holloway, E. L., Derby, G. C., et al.: Control of Myocardial Performance Early after Open-Heart Operation by Vasodilator Treatment, *J. Thorac. Cardiovasc. Surg.*, 73:523, 1977.

36 Miller, D. C., Stinson, E. B., Oyer, P. E., et al.: Postoperative Enhancement of Left Ventricular Performance by Combined Inotropic-Vasodilator Therapy with Preload Control, *Surgery*, 88:108, 1980.

37 Ream, A. K., and Fogdall, R. P.: "Acute Cardiovascular Management—Anesthesia and Intensive Care," J. B. Lippincott Company, Philadelphia, 1982.

38 Miller, D. C., Stinson, E. B., Oyer, P. E., et al.: Discriminant Analysis of the Changing Risks of Coronary Artery Operations, *J. Thorac. Cardiovasc. Surg.*, 85:197, 1983.

39 European Coronary Surgery Study Group: Long-term Results of Prospective Randomized Study of Coronary Artery Bypass Surgery in Stable Angina Pectoris, *Lancet*, 2:1173, 1982.

40 Campeau, L., Lesperance, J., Hermann, J., et al.: Loss of the Improvement of Angina between 1 and 7 Years After Aortocoronary Bypass Surgery, *Circulation*, (suppl. 1):1, 1979.

41 Hellman, C., Schmidt, D. H., Kamath, L., et al.: Bypass Graft Surgery in Severe Left Ventricular Dysfunction, *Circulation*, 62(suppl. 1):103, 1980.

42 Winkle, R. A., Alderman, E. L., Shumway, N. E., and Harrison, D. C.: Results of Reoperation for Unsuccessful Coronary Artery Bypass Surgery, *Circulation*, 51,52(suppl. 1):61, 1975.

43 Allen, R. H., Stinson, E. B., and Oyer, P. E.: Predictive Variables in Reoperation for Coronary Artery Disease, *J. Thorac. Cardiovasc. Surg.*, 75:186, 1978.

44 Kennedy, R. H., Kennedy, M. A., Frye, R. L., et al.: Cardiac Catheterization and Cardiac Surgical Facilities: Use, Trends and Future Requirements, *N. Engl. J. Med.*, 307:986, 1982.

45 Epstein, S. E., Palmeri, S. T., and Patterson, R. E.: Evaluation of Patients after Acute Myocardial Infarction, *N. Engl. J. Med.,* 307:1487, 1982.

46 Theroux, P., Waters, D. D., Halpern, C., et al.: Prognostic Value of Exercise Testing Soon after Myocardial Infarction, *N. Engl. J. Med.,* 301:341, 1979.

47 Jones, E. L., Waites, T. F., Craver, J. M., et al.: Coronary Bypass for Relief of Persistent Pain Following Acute Myocardial Infarction, *Ann. Thorac. Surg.,* 32:33, 1981.

48 Schuster, E. H., and Bulkley, B. H.: Early Post-infarction Angina: Ischemia at a Distance and Ischemia in the Infarct Zone, *N. Engl. J. Med.,* 305:1101, 1981.

49 Schuster, E. H., and Bulkley, B. H.: Expansion of Transmural Myocardial Infarction: A Pathophysiologic Factor in Cardiac Rupture, *Circulation,* 60:1532, 1979.

Coronary Bypass Surgery: The Total Experience at the Texas Heart Institute[*]

DENTON A. COOLEY, M.D., and J. MICHAEL DUNCAN, M.D.

> The philosophies of one age have become the absurdities of the next, and the foolishness of yesterday has become the wisdom of tomorrow.
>
> SIR WILLIAM OSLER, 1849–1919[1]

The surgical treatment of coronary artery occlusive disease by direct myocardial revascularization is now into its second decade. Few physicians in the early seventies could have accurately predicted the magnitude of the role that coronary bypass surgery (CBS) would play today in the treatment of ischemic heart disease. Numerous reports have documented the efficacy of the operation in relieving angina and improving the quality of life,[1a–6] and there is also substantial evidence which suggests that CBS prolongs life.[3,4,7–10] During a 12-year period at our institution, 22,284 patients underwent coronary bypass surgery. An analysis of this large group of patients forms the basis of this chapter.

CLINICAL MATERIAL

Between January 1970 and December 1981, a total of 22,284 patients underwent isolated coronary bypass surgery at the Texas Heart Institute (THI). An additional 2,828 patients had CBS combined with other cardiac procedures, but are not included in this analysis. There were 19,175 men (86 percent) and 3,109 women (14 percent) in the total series. Women were more prone to develop surgical disease later in life than men, and the percentage of female patients operated upon increased from the fourth through ninth decades of life (Table 1). The age of the patients ranged from the second to tenth decade, with the majority of patients operated upon in the fourth through seventh decades (Table 1). Atherosclerosis was the etiology of the coronary occlusive disease in the vast majority of patients. We classified 35 percent of the patients in New York Heart Association functional class IV, and 45 percent in class III. The number of patients undergoing CBS increased annually during the first 10 years of the

*Texas Heart Institute, Houston, Texas.

series, but remained relatively constant the last 2 years (Fig. 1). The percentage of patients 70 years of age and older increased annually (Table 2).

For the purpose of comparing the results of operations from the earlier years to the results in more recent years, the total 12-year experience was divided into two groups. Group I consisted of 5,829 patients (26 percent) operated upon from 1970 to 1975, and group II consisted of 16,455 patients (74 percent) operated upon from 1976 to 1981. Follow-up information, which was obtained from questionnaires sent directly to patients or referring physicians or from patient visits to the outpatient clinic, was in excess of 75 percent.

Operations were performed with standard extracorporeal circuits and bubble oxygenators. For patients in group I, the distal coronary anastomoses were performed during a single period of normothermic ischemic arrest. The distal coronary anastomoses were performed for most of the patients in group II after cardiac arrest was initiated with a single bolus (500 mL) of cold cardioplegic solution.[†]

Perioperative Mortality

Perioperative mortality rate refers to all deaths, regardless of cause, occurring within 30 days of operation. Mortality rate for the total series was 2.9 percent. The mortality rate for patients in group I was 4.9 percent, but decreased to 2.3 percent for patients in group II. In 1980 and 1981, mortality rate was 2.0 percent. Women had a perioperative mortality rate which was twice that of men during both periods of the study (Table 3). We attribute the progressive decline in perioperative mortality rate to a number of factors. During the earlier years of the study, greater surgical experience was probably most important; however, during the last 6 years of the series the most significant factor in reducing operative mortality rate was the use of cold chemical cardioplegic solution for myocardial protection. We began using cold cardioplegia routinely for

†THI cardioplegic solution: 500 mL 5% dextrose and 0.45% NaCl containing potassium chloride, 20 mM (20 mE) [1,492 mg]; magnesium chloride, 7.5 mM (15 mE) [1,527.03 mg]; sodium bicarbonate, 2.5 mM (2.5 mE) [210.0 mg]; calcium chloride, 1.0 mM (2.0 mE) [147.14 mg].

TABLE 1
Comparison of age and sex of coronary bypass patients at the Texas Heart Institute (January 1970 to December 1981)

Age (yr)	Patients	Men	%	Women	%
10–19	5	5	100.0	—	—
20–29	40	32	90.0	8	20.0
30–39	838	776	92.6	62	7.4
40–49	4,757	4,333	91.1	424	8.9
50–59	9,130	8.036	88.0	1,094	12.0
60–69	6,239	5,059	81.1	1,180	18.9
70–79	1,246	916	73.5	330	26.5
80–89	28	17	60.7	11	39.3
90–99	1	1	100.0	—	—
Total	22,284	19,175	86.1	3,109	13.9

SOURCE: R. J. Hall, M. A. Elayda, A. Gray, et al. Coronary Artery Bypass: Long-term Follow-up of 22,284 Consecutive Patients. *Circulation* 68 (suppl. 2), 1983, in press. Reproduced with permission of the American Heart Association.

all cardiac procedures in early 1977. Also of significance was the sharp decline in the incidence of perioperative myocardial infarctions from 10.2 percent prior to 1977 to 3.2 percent at present, better anesthetic and hemodynamic management, and more complete revascularization (Fig. 2).

Perioperative mortality rate was also related to the age of the patient at the time of surgery and progressively increased in men from the third through eighth decades (Table 4). Mortality rate in women was higher than in men for each decade, an observation reported previously.[11,12] We believe this higher mortality is related to the fact that women often have smaller coronary arteries and less satisfactory veins for bypass conduits, have more diffuse disease, and more frequently have intramyocardial coronary vessels.

INDICATIONS FOR OPERATION

Indications for myocardial revascularization in patients with coronary artery disease have been gradually expanded during the past 10 years as refinements in surgical techniques and improved methods of myocardial protection have resulted in a low operative mortality rate and improved survival rates in the majority of patients. Specific subsets of patients who were once denied operation because of an unacceptably high mortality rate, including those with coronary artery disease and left ventricular dysfunction or elderly patients with refractory angina, are now undergoing surgery with minimal risk and the expectation of a favorable functional result.

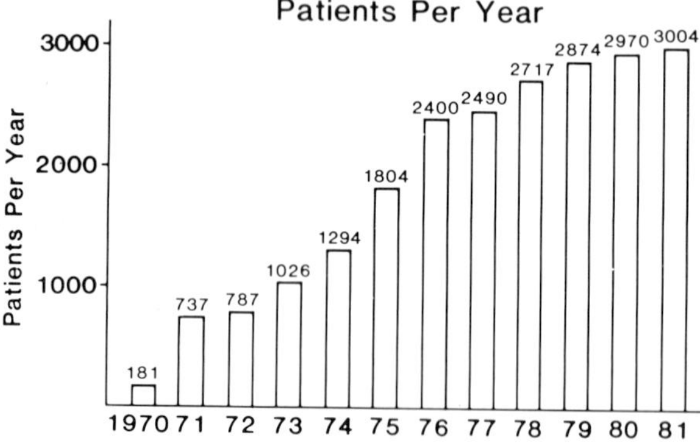

FIGURE 1 Number of patients who underwent isolated coronary artery bypass, including all reoperations during each year from 1970 through 1981. (*From R. J. Hall, M. A. Elayda, A. Gray, et al. Coronary Artery Bypass: Long-term Follow-up of 22,284 Consecutive Patients. Circulation 68 (suppl. 2), 1983, in press. Reproduced with permission of the American Heart Association.*)

TABLE 2
Coronary artery bypass surgery in patients 70 years and older at the Texas Heart Institute

Year	Total patients	Patients 70 yr & older	%
1970	181	—	—
1971	737	15	2.0
1972	787	14	1.8
1973	1,026	23	2.2
1974	1,294	44	3.4
1975	1,804	62	3.4
1976	2,400	113	4.7
1977	2,490	132	5.3
1978	2,717	171	6.3
1979	2,874	198	6.9
1980	2,970	258	8.7
1981	3,004	245	8.2
Total	22,284	1,275	5.7

SOURCE: R. J. Hall, M. A. Elayda, A. Gray, et al. Coronary Artery Bypass: Long-term Follow-up of 22,284 Consecutive Patients. *Circulation* 68 (suppl. 2), 1983, in press. Reproduced with permission of the American Heart Association.

TABLE 3
Early mortality rate related to sex

	Patients	Early mortality rate (%)
Total 1970–1981:	22,284	2.9
Men	19,175	2.6
Women	3,109	5.3
Group I 1970–1975:	5,829	4.9
Men	5,041	4.2
Women	788	9.1
Group II 1976–1981:	16,455	2.3
Men	14,134	2.0
Women	2,321	4.0

SOURCE: R. J. Hall, M. A. Elayda, A. Gray, et al. Coronary Artery Bypass: Long-term Follow-up of 22,284 Consecutive Patients. *Circulation* 68 (suppl. 2), 1983, in press. Reproduced with permission of the American Heart Association.

Angina Refractory to Medical Treatment

Patients with angina refractory to medical treatment constitute the majority of patients undergoing surgery at our institution (80 percent). If coronary angiography demonstrates double- or triple-vessel disease and the vessels are suitable for bypassing, surgery is recommended. In this large group of patients, 85 to 90 percent will be asymptomatic or significantly improved following complete revascularization. In a previous report, we noted that relief of angina was directly related to graft patency and completeness of revascularization.[3] Graft patency rates of 80 percent or greater for the first

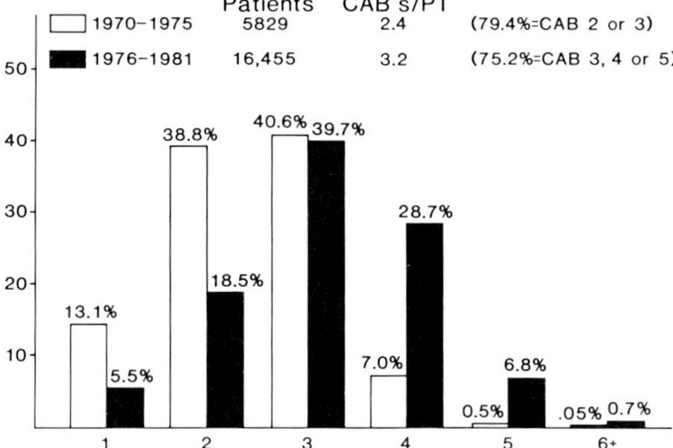

FIGURE 2 Number of coronary bypass grafts per patient during the years 1970 to 1975 (group I) and during 1976 to 1981 (group II). (*From R. J. Hall, M. A. Elayda, A. Gray, et al. Coronary Artery Bypass: Long-term Follow-up of 22,284 Consecutive Patients. Circulation 68 (suppl. 2), 1983, in press. Reproduced with permission of the American Heart Association.*)

TABLE 4
Comparison of early mortality rate related to age and sex

Age (yr)	Patients (men)	%	Patients (women)	%
10–19	5	20.0	——	——
20–29	32	——	8	12.5
30–39	776	1.2	62	6.5
40–49	4,333	1.5	424	5.7
50–59	8,036	2.1	1,094	4.8
60–69	5,059	3.8	1,180	5.0
70–79	916	5.3	330	7.0
80–89	17	5.9	11	9.1
90–99	1	——	——	——
Total	19,175	2.6	3,109	5.3

SOURCE: R. J. Hall, M. A. Elayda, A. Gray, et al. Coronary Artery Bypass: Long-term Follow-up of 22,284 Consecutive Patients. *Circulation* 68 (suppl. 2), 1983, in press. Reproduced with permission of the American Heart Association.

year with a 2 to 3 percent attrition rate thereafter are now being reported.[13,14]

Unstable Angina

Patients manifesting any of the clinical syndromes of unstable angina constitute approximately 5 to 10 percent of our surgical population. Once it is established either by electrocardiographic changes or with nuclear myocardial imaging that the patient's symptoms are a result of myocardial ischemia, aggressive medical treatment is initiated. If symptoms are relieved, the patient is monitored in the coronary care unit, and cardiac catheterization is performed within 24 h. For patients in whom symptoms persist despite maximal medical treatment including intravenous nitroglycerin, urgent coronary angiography is performed. Depending upon the clinical picture, an intraaortic balloon pump may be necessary for support in some patients.

Subsequent treatment for each patient depends on the extent and severity of the coronary pathology identified at catheterization. Patients who require intraaortic balloon support to control symptoms or those who remain unstable and have operable disease should undergo surgery at this time. Patients who remain stable on medical therapy undergo elective operation during the initial hospitalization, usually within 48 h. Patients with left main, triple-vessel, or double-vessel disease with suitable distal arteries are generally considered surgical candidates. Patients with single-vessel disease are candidates for percutaneous transluminal coronary angioplasty (PTCA) if the anatomy is favorable. If PTCA is not feasible or is unsuccessful, and the diseased artery supplies a large area of myocardium, surgery should be performed. The urgency for operation in all patients should depend primarily on the severity of the coronary pathology and the extent of myocardium at risk and not on the patient's symptoms.

Stable Angina

When evaluating the role of surgery in patients with stable angina, emphasis should be placed on the improved survival found in the surgical group compared to the survival of patients maintained on medical therapy. A decision for surgical treatment is made in patients who have documented myocardial ischemia, either on exercise testing or nuclear myocardial scans, and who have favorable anatomy for bypass grafting based on cineangiograms. We have reported previously that surgery increases survival rate in patients with left main, triple-vessel and probably double-vessel disease.[3] Mathur and associates[15] reported a series of 304 patients with triple-vessel disease who were followed for 5 years after operation. Survival rate in this group was 93.4 percent with an annual attrition rate of 1.3 percent. This survival rate is approximately the same as that expected for the "normal" U.S. population. Lawrie[16] and Kirklin[17] have reported similar findings.

Single-Vessel Disease

The treatment of patients with angina and single-vessel disease has changed at our institution in recent years with the success of percutaneous transluminal coronary angioplasty (PTCA). Most patients with high-grade stenosis of the anterior descending coronary artery proximal to the orgin of the first diagonal or septal branch are considered candidates for balloon dilatation. Success in relieving the obstruction has been achieved in 75 to 80 percent of the patients in this group.

Patients with isolated stenosis of the proximal right or circumflex coronary arteries are candidates for balloon dilatation if documented myocardial ischemia is present, and the diseased vessel supplies a large area of myocardium. Successful dilatations have been achieved in 65 to 75 percent of patients in this group. All patients having attempted PTCA must also be surgical candidates, and if the dilatation is unsuccessful or if complications occur during the procedure, surgical revascularization is performed.

Left Main Coronary Disease

All patients with left main coronary disease are considered candidates for surgery regardless of their symptomatic status. Numerous reports have documented that survival rate in this group of patients is uniformly poor with medical treatment alone. Tolano[18] reported a 1-year mortality rate of 39 percent, and Lim and associates[19] reported a mortality rate of 21.9 percent at 1 year, 34.7 percent at 2 years, and 51 percent at 5 years in medically treated patients. The Veterans Administration Study[20] and the European Cooperative Study[8] both demonstrated improved survival curves in surgically treated patients. In the VA study, patients treated medically had a cumulative survival rate of 68 percent at 1 year and 61 percent at 3 years, compared with 88 percent and 83 percent, respectively, in the surgical group. In a previous report from our institution, patients with left main disease (>70 percent stenosis) and an ejection fraction of 0.45 or greater had a cumulative 6-year survival rate of 90.2 percent.[3] The current perioperative mortality rate for all patients with left main disease (>50 percent stenosis) undergoing surgery at our institution is 2.5 percent.

Congestive Heart Failure with Coronary Disease

Congestive heart failure in patients with coronary disease was once considered a contraindication for coronary bypass surgery because of a high rate of operative mortality. Mortality rates greater than 30 percent were reported in the earlier years of myocardial revascularization. In recent years, however, the rate of operative mortality has declined, and rate of survival has improved as a result of more careful patient selection and better methods of myocardial protection during surgery.[3,21,22] We now believe that many patients with congestive heart failure who have angina can benefit from surgery both in symptomatic relief and improved survival rate.

Brockman et al.[23] reported an operative mortality rate of 2.0 percent in 51 patients with ejection fractions less than 0.35. All had angina preoperatively, and relief of angina was achieved in over 90 percent of the patients. A significant improvement in symptoms of congestive heart failure following surgery was also noted. Other reports have documented similar findings.[24–26] In a previously published series from our institute, Hall and associates reported an operative mortality rate of 2.03 percent in 148 patients with an ejection fraction of less than 0.45.[3] The 5-year survival rate in patients with abnormal ventricular function was 93.1 percent, which was not significantly different than the survival rate of patients operated upon with normal ventricles (94.3 percent). Patients with congestive failure who do not have angina but in whom reversible myocardial ischemia can be demonstrated might also be expected to improve following revascularization; however, surgery in this group is still controversial.

Patients who develop congestive heart failure as a

result of a mechanical defect following myocardial infarction, i.e., left ventricular aneurysm, ventricular septal defect, or mitral insufficiency, are also candidates for surgery. Surgical correction of the defect combined with myocardial revascularization in patients with coexisting coronary obstructions will result in improved survival and relief of symptoms in many patients. The prognosis in patients developing left ventricular aneurysms and congestive heart failure is poor, with late mortality rates at 3 and 10 years of 73 and 88 percent, respectively, having been reported.[27] We recently reported a perioperative mortality rate of 8.7 percent and a cumulative survival rate of 80 percent at 5 years and 65 percent at 7 years in 421 patients who underwent resection of left ventricular aneurysm combined with coronary bypass and ventricular septoplasty.[28] Following surgery 92 percent were asymptomatic or improved. Similar results have been reported by others.[29,30]

Acute Myocardial Infarction

Early coronary surgery in patients with acute evolving myocardial infarctions remains controversial. Our experience with surgical treatment in this group of patients is small, but reports from other centers have revealed encouraging results. Berg and associates reported a hospital mortality rate of 5.2 percent in 96 patients undergoing coronary bypass surgery for acute evolving myocardial infarction.[31] Phillips et al. reported similar findings.[32] The most favorable results occur in those patients who undergo surgery within 6 h of their infarction.

Other Indications for Coronary Bypass Surgery

Patients undergoing valvular heart surgery who also have coexisting coronary artery disease should have bypass grafting at the same operation. The mortality rate in these patients is high if the coronary disease is left untreated.

Patients with Prinzmetal's angina in whom significant, fixed coronary obstructions can be demonstrated should be considered for surgery.

Congenital coronary anomalies resulting in myocardial ischemia should be corrected at the time diagnosis is made. While different techniques have been utilized in treating these anomalies, bypass grafting is the technique used most commonly.

Patients with recurrent angina following coronary bypass surgery should be considered candidates for reoperation if their symptoms cannot be controlled medically, if they have unstable angina, or if left main coronary disease is present.

LONG-TERM SURVIVAL RATE

The overall survival rate for our entire series of 22,284 patients at 5 and 10 years was 89.6 percent and 70.2 percent, respectively (Fig. 3). The 5-year survival rate was better in group II patients than in group I, primarily due to the lower perioperative mortality rate in group II (Fig. 4). Average late attrition rates for the entire series of patients was 1.5 percent per year from 30 days to 5 years. This increased to 3.8 percent per year from 5 years to 10 years.

The 5-year survival rate was lower for women than men (87.2 percent versus 90 percent), the result of a higher perioperative mortality rate. However at 10 years the survival rate was almost identical (69.2 percent versus 70.4 percent) (Fig. 5).

The survival rate in patients with coronary artery disease has been shown to depend most consistently on the extent of disease, i.e., the number of diseased coronary vessels involved and ventricular function.[33,34] Natural history studies have concluded that the greater the number of diseased vessels or the more ventricular function is impaired, the worse the prognosis for survival.

Assuming the number of bypass grafts per patient correlates with the extent of coronary disease, survival curves were created for all patients receiving one to six or more grafts (Fig. 6). The 5-year survival rate ranged from 88.4 to 91.8 percent. The number of vessels bypassed did not significantly change the 5-year survival rate. The average late annual attrition rate from 30 days to 5 years was 1.2 to 1.6 deaths per hundred patients per year. The 10-year survival rate of 66.4 percent or better indicates an average overall attrition rate of 3.4 percent per year or less for the total series.

The age of the patient at the time of operation was also a determining factor in survival. There was a progressive decline in 10-year survival rate for patients in the fifth through eighth decades (Fig. 7).

As long-term results following coronary bypass surgery are now being reported by a number of centers, data are accumulating which support the belief that surgical treatment improves survival rate in at least some subsets of patients with coronary disease.

The prognosis for patients with left main disease treated medically is extremely poor. In one series, survival rate at 3 years was only 50 percent.[35] A 5-year survival rate of 88.2 percent in surgical patients with left main coronary artery disease has been reported from the Cleveland Clinic,[36] and the European Cooperative Surgery Study reported a 5-year survival rate of 93 percent in patients treated surgically.[8] We have previously reported a 4-year survival rate of 88.1 percent.[3] Clearly patients with left main coronary disease have a significantly improved survival rate with surgical treatment rather than with medical therapy.

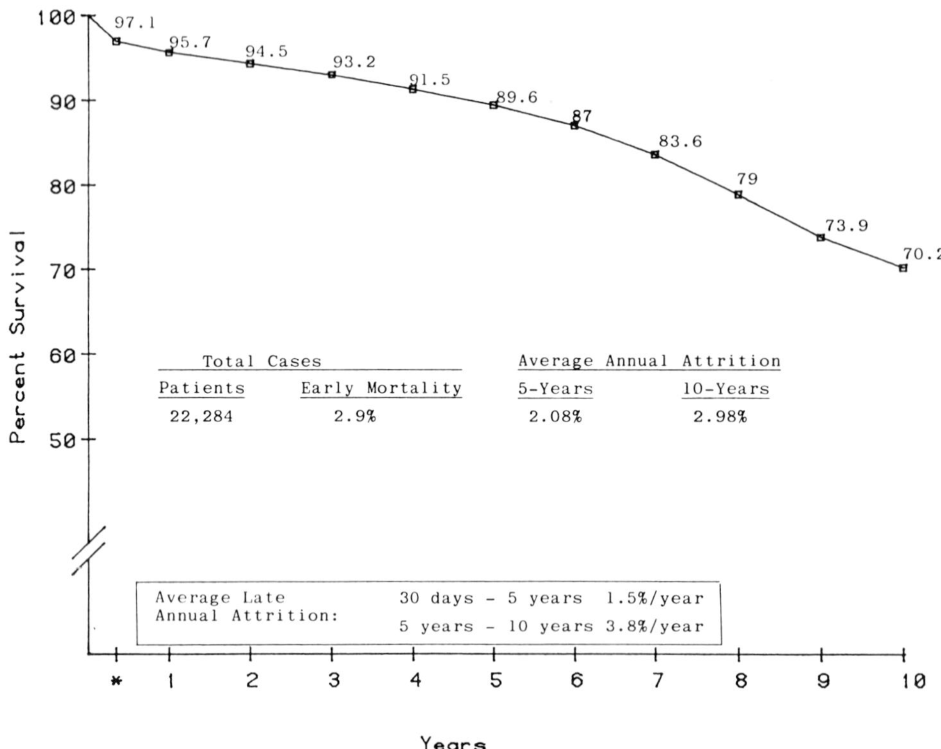

FIGURE 3 Life survival curve for all 22,284 patients in this series. The symbol (*) identifies the 30-day survival point on this and all subsequent figures. Average annual attrition = (100% − percent survival at x years) ÷ x years: This value includes both early and late mortality. Average late annual attrition expresses late attrition only and = (percent survivors at time x − percent survivors at time y) ÷ (x − y) years. (*From R. J. Hall, M. A. Elayda, A. Gray, et al. Coronary Artery Bypass: Long-term Follow-up of 22,284 Consecutive Patients. Circulation 68 (suppl. 2), 1983, in press. Reproduced with permission of the American Heart Association.*)

The prognosis of patients with triple-vessel disease treated nonsurgically is also poor. Numerous reports have documented the 4- and 5-year survival rates to be near 50 percent.[37,38] The overall 5-year survival rate in our series was 90 percent. The Cleveland Clinic reported a 5-year survival rate of 89.8 percent for patients with triple-vessel disease treated surgically.[39] Similar surgical results have been reported.[40,41] Mathur and associates also demonstrated that survival rate was significantly improved in patients with triple-vessel disease who uniformly did poorly on medical therapy, i.e., those with left ventricular dysfunction, severe symptoms, or severe disease (total or subtotal occlusion of all three major coronary arteries).[15] We believe these data lend strong support to the belief that coronary bypass surgery prolongs life in patients with triple-vessel disease.

Survival statistics on patients with single- or double-vessel disease treated nonsurgically are good. In patients with double-vessel disease treated medically 4- and 5-year survival rates have ranged from 69 to 85 percent.[37,38] The 5-year survival rate in our series for patients receiving two bypasses was 91.5 percent, which compares favorably to the nonsurgical group (Table 5). Similar favorable surgical results have also been reported.[39,42]

RELIEF OF ANGINA

The relief of angina in most patients following coronary bypass surgery is dramatic. Several prospective randomized studies have shown that following coronary bypass, 70 to 90 percent of patients will be asymptomatic or have significant improvement in their symptoms.[43–45] In contrast, fewer than 10 percent of patients treated medically become asymptomatic, and 50 percent continue to have angina which severely limits their activities.

The mechanism of action for relief of angina following surgery appears to be improved myocardial per-

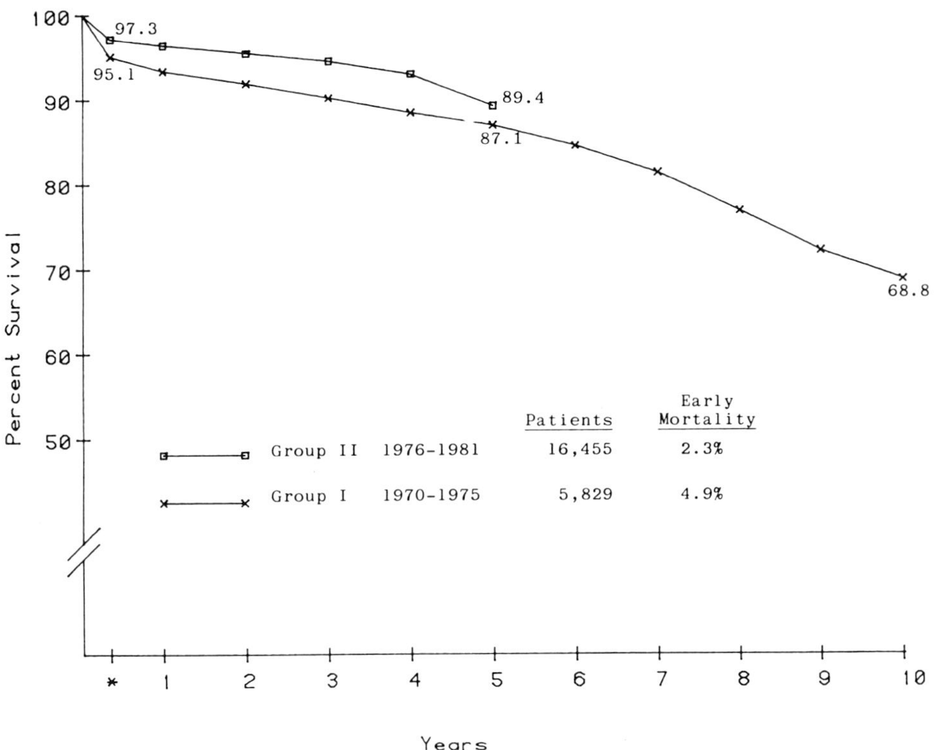

FIGURE 4 Life survival curves for patients in group II compared to patients in group I. (*From R. J. Hall, M. A. Elayda, A. Gray, et al. Coronary Artery Bypass: Long-term Follow-up of 22,284 Consecutive Patients. Circulation 68 (suppl. 2), 1983, in press. Reproduced with permission of the American Heart Association.*)

fusion. Completeness of revascularization and graft patency correlate well with symptomatic improvement.[3]

Of our patients 70 percent reported no angina from 1 to 10 years postoperatively; 16 percent reported angina was present but significantly improved. Angina was more frequent or more severe in 2.2 percent and was the same as preoperatively in 1.6 percent. Ten percent of our patients reported that angina was absent for some time before recurring later.

PREVENTION OF MYOCARDIAL INFARCTION AND SUDDEN DEATH

Myocardial infarction and lethal arrhythmias are the two major causes of cardiac mortality in patients with coronary artery disease. While many of the factors responsible for these terminal events in patients with coronary disease remain speculative, certain risk factors have been identified as predisposing to sudden death, including myocardial ischemia, premature ventricular arrhythmias, cardiac hypertrophy, and ventricular dysfunction.[46,47] Myocardial ischemia has been implicated as a cause of lethal arrhythmias,[48] and CBS has been reported to be effective in terminating refractory ventricular arrhythmias.[49]

In a prospective evaluation of medical versus surgical therapy in patients with multivessel disease, Vismara found a low incidence of sudden death in the surgical group (7 of 121, 6 percent) compared with a high incidence in the medical group (23 of 96, 24 percent).[50] The mean period of follow-up was 39 months. Myocardial ischemia has been shown to be a stimulus for the initiation and perpetuation of ventricular arrhythmias. The authors concluded that coronary bypass surgery had reduced the amount of ischemic myocardium at risk to developing arrhythmias and accounted for the lower incidence of sudden death in the surgical group.

In a nonrandomized study, Hammermeister et al. reported sudden death rates to be 1.8 to 10.9 times higher in medically treated patients than in patients treated surgically.[51] The most significant differences were in those patients with double-vessel disease with normal or moderately reduced ventricular function.

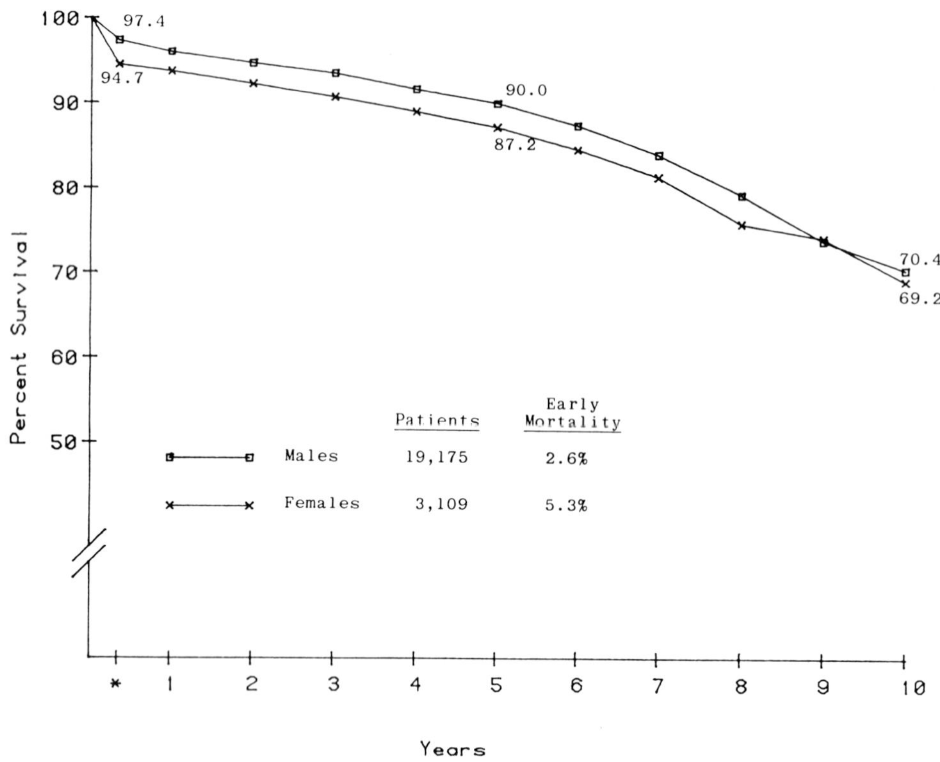

FIGURE 5 Life survival curves for female patients compared to male patients in the total series. *(From R. J. Hall, M. A. Elayda, A. Gray, et al. Coronary Artery Bypass: Long-term Follow-up of 22,284 Consecutive Patients. Circulation 68 (suppl. 2), 1983, in press. Reproduced with permission of the American Heart Association.)*

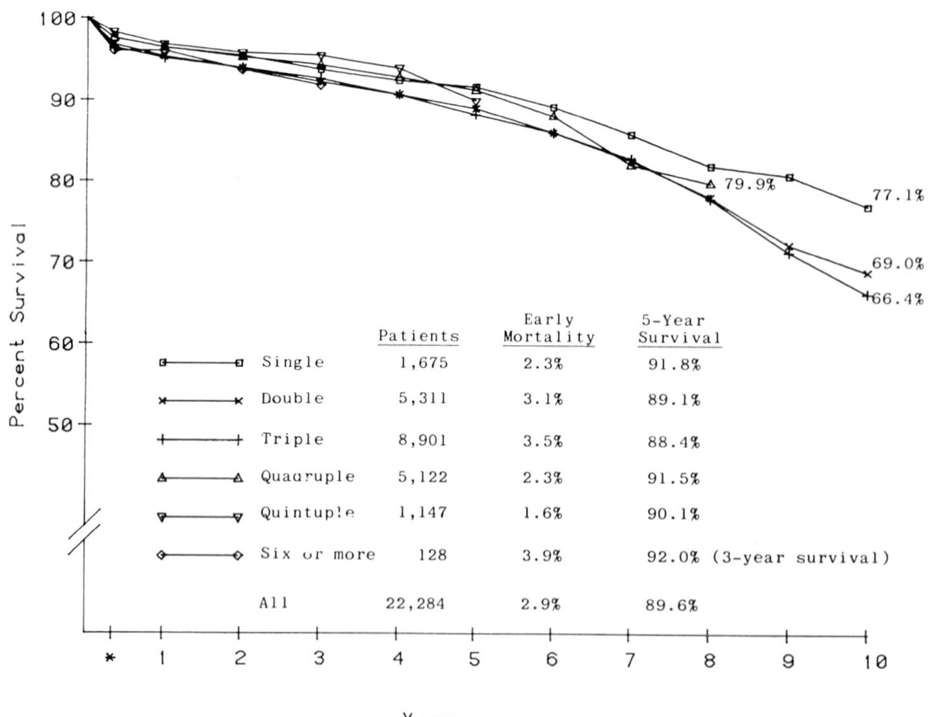

FIGURE 6 Life survival curves of all patients based upon the number of coronary arteries bypassed. *(From R. J. Hall, M. A. Elayda, A. Gray, et al. Coronary Artery Bypass: Long-term Follow-up of 22,284 Consecutive Patients. Circulation 68 (suppl. 2), 1983, in press. Reproduced with permission of the American Heart Association.)*

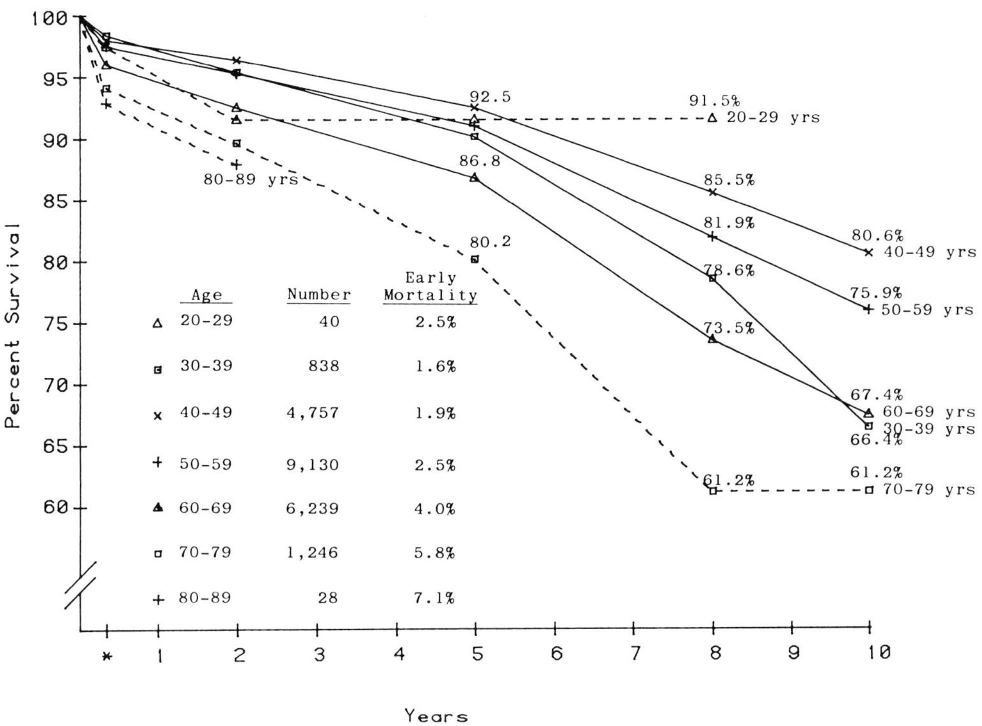

FIGURE 7 Life survival curves of all patients according to age at the time of coronary artery bypass. *(From R. J. Hall, M. A. Elayda, A. Gray, et al. Coronary Artery Bypass: Long-term Follow-up of 22,284 Consecutive Patients. Circulation 68 (suppl. 2), 1983, in press. Reproduced with permission of the American Heart Association.)*

Data from our series indicate that patients with left main, double- and triple-vessel disease have an improved survival over medically treated cohorts. This improved survival in surgically treated patients implies, but does not prove, that the incidence of fatal myocardial infarction and sudden death is less than in patients treated medically.

SUMMARY

From this brief analysis of a large series of patients, it can be seen that coronary bypass surgery can now be safely performed in all types of patients, even the high-risk group, with minimal mortality rate. The simple technique of bypassing an area of obstruction with a

TABLE 5

Five-year survival rate and average attrition rate per year for all patients in group II based upon the number of coronary arteries bypassed

Bypasses	Patients	Early mortality rate (%)	5-year survival rate (%)	Average attrition rate/yr (%)
Single	918	1.2	89.9	2.0
Double	3,048	1.9	91.5	1.7
Triple	6,536	2.7	87.6	2.5
Quadruple	4,716	2.2	90.3	1.9
Quintuple	1,118	1.4	93.1 (4-yr)	1.7
Six or more	125	4.0	92.0 (3-yr)	2.7
Total	16,455	2.3	89.4	2.1

new conduit is the only way that a significantly greater amount of blood can be brought to an ischemic area of the myocardium. The actual relief of symptoms and prolongation of life results only with increased blood flow to the myocardium.

In the final analysis, long-term survival, no late complications, and relief of symptoms are essential features in documenting the efficacy of the procedure. Based on our experience, coronary artery bypass improves both the quality and length of life in patients with severe coronary artery occlusive disease.

REFERENCES

1 Osler, W.: Chauzinism in Medicine, *Montreal Med. J.* 31:684, 1902.

1a Carey, J. S., and Cukingnam, R. A: Subjective Multivariate Analysis by Computer for Evaluation for Coronary Artery Bypass, *Arch. Surg.*, 111:769, 1976.

2 Guiney, T. E., Gubenstein, J. J., and Sanders C. A., et al.: Functional Evaluation of Coronary Bypass Surgery by Exercise Testing and Oxygen Consumption, *Circulation*, 48(suppl. 3):141, 1973.

3 Hall, R. J., Mathur, V. S., Garcia, E. G., and deCastro, C. M.: The Prolongation of Life by Coronary Bypass Surgery, in J. W. Hurst (ed.), "Update II: The Heart," McGraw-Hill Book Company, New York, 1980, p. 175.

4 Wukasch, D. C., Cooley, D. A., Hall, R. J., Reul, G. J., Sandiford, F. M. and Zillgitt, S. L.: Surgical Versus Medical Treatment of Coronary Artery Disease: Nine Year Follow-up of 9,061 Patients, *Am. J. Surg.*, 137:201, 1979.

5 McIntosh, H. D., and Garcia, J. A.: The First Decade of Aortocoronary Bypass Grafting, 1967–1977: A Review, *Circulation*, 57:405, 1978.

6 Favaloro, R. G.: Direct Myocardial Revascularization: A Ten-Year Journey, Myths, and Realities, *Am. J. Cardiol.*, 43:109, 1979.

7 Hultgren, H. N., Takaro, T., Iletre, K. M. and Murphy, M. L.: Aortocoronary Artery Bypass Assessment after 13 Years, *J.A.M.A.*, 240:1353, 1978.

8 European Coronary Surgery Study Group: Prospective Randomized Study of Coronary Bypass Surgery in Stable Angina Pectoris: Second Interim Report by the European Coronary Surgery Study Group, *Lancet*, 2:492, 1980.

9 Rahimtoola, S. H., Greenkemeier, G., Tepley, S., et al.: Changes in Coronary Bypass Surgery Leading to Improved Survival, *J.A.M.A.*, 246:1912, 1981.

10 Greene, D. G., Bunnel, I. L., Arnai, D. R., et al.: Long-term Survival after Coronary Bypass Surgery: Comparisons of Various Subsets of Patients with General Populations, *Br. Heart J.*, 45:417, 1981.

11 Hall, R. J., Dawson, J. J, Cooley, D. A., et al.: Coronary Artery Bypass, *Circulation*, 48(suppl. 3):146, 1973.

12 Bolooki, H., Vargas, A., and Green R.: Results of Direct Coronary Artery Surgery in Women, *J. Thorac. Cardiovasc. Surg.*, 69:271, 1975.

13 Lawrie, G. M., Morris, G. C., Chapman, D. W., et al.: Patterns of Patency of 596 Vein Grafts up to Seven Years after Aortocoronary Bypass, *J. Thorac. Cardiovasc. Surg.*, 73:443, 1977.

14 Kouchoukos, N. T., Karp, R. B., Oberman, A., et al.: Long-term patency of Saphenous Vein Grafts for Coronary Bypass Grafting, *Circulation*, 58(suppl. 1):96, 1978.

15 Mathur, V. S., Hall, R. J., Garcia, E., DeCastro, C. M., and Cooley, D. A.: Prolonging Life with Coronary Bypass Surgery in Patients with Three-Vessel Disease, *Circulation*, 62(suppl 1):90, 1980.

16 Lawrie, G. M., Morris, G. L., Howell, J. F., Tredici, T. D., and Chapman, D. W.: Improved Survival after 5 Years in 1,144 Patients after Coronary Bypass Surgery, *Am. J. Cardiol.*, 42:709, 1978.

17 Kirklin, J. W., quoted by Hurst, J. W., King, S. B., Logue, R. B., et al.: Value of Coronary Bypass Surgery: Controversies in Cardiology, Part I, *Am. J. Cardiol.*, 42:308, 1978.

18 Tolano, J. V., Scanlon, P. J., Meadows, W. R., et al.: Influence of Surgery on Survival in 145 Patients with Left Main Coronary Artery Disease, *Circulation*, 52(suppl. 1):105, 1975.

19 Lim, J. S., Proudfit, W. L., and Sones, F. M.: Left Main Coronary Arterial Obstruction: Long-term Follow-up of 141 Nonsurgical Cases, *Am. J. Cardiol.*, 36:131, 1975.

20 Takaro, T., Hultgren, H. N., Lipton, M. J., et al.: The VA Cooperative Randomized Study of Surgery for Coronary Arterial Occlusive Disease: II, Subgroup with Significant Left Main Lesions, *Circulation*, 54(suppl. 3):107, 1976.

21 Kay, J. H., Redington, J. V., Mendez, A. M., et al.: Coronary Artery Surgery for the Patient with Impaired Left Ventricular Function, *Circulation*, 46(suppl. 2):49, 1972. (Abstract.)

22 Faulkner, S. L., Stoney, W. S., Alford, W. C., et al.: Ischemic Cardiomyopathy: Medical vs. Surgical Treatment, *J. Thorac. Cardiovasc. Surg.*, 74:77, 1977.

23 Brockman, S. K., Cobanoglu, M. A., and Brest, A. N.: The Surgical Management of Coronary Artery Disease with Myocardial Dysfunction, in D. C. McGoon (ed.), "Cardiac Surgery," F. A. Davis Company, Philadelphia, 1982, p. 93.

24 Mitchel, B. F., Alivizatos, P. A., Adam, M., et al.: Myocardial Revascularization in Patients with Poor Left Ventricular Function, *J. Thorac. Cardiovasc. Surg.*, 69:52, 1975.

25 Isom, W. W., Spencer, F. C., Glassman, E., et al.: Long-term Survival following Coronary Bypass Surgery in Patients with Significant Impairment of Left Ventricular Function, *Circulation,* 51,52(suppl. 1):141, 1975.

26 Hellman, C., Schmidt, D. H., Kamath, M. L., et al.: Bypass Graft Surgery in Severe Left Ventricular Dysfunction, *Circulation,* 62(suppl. 1):103, 1980.

27 Schlicter, J., Hellerstein, H. K., and Katz, L. N.: Aneurysm of the Heart: A Correlative Study of One Hundred and Two Proved Cases, *Medicine (Baltimore),* 33:43, 1954.

28 Reddy, S. B., Cooley, D. A., Duncan, J. M., et al.: Left Ventricular Aneurysm: Twenty-Year Surgical Experience with 1572 Patients at the Texas Heart Institute, *Cardiovasc. Dis., Bull. Texas Heart Institute,* 8:165, 1981.

29 Cosgrove, D. M., Loop, F. D., Irarrazaval, M. J., et al.: Determinants of Long-term Survival after Ventricular Aneurysmectomy, *Ann. Thorac. Surg.,* 26:357, 1978.

30 Shaw, R. C., Ferguson, T. B., Weldon, C. S., et al.: Left Ventricular Aneurysm Resection: Indications and Long-term Follow-up, *Ann. Thorac. Surg.,* 25:336, 1978.

31 Berg, R., Kendall, R. V., Duvoisin, G. F., et al.: Acute Myocardial Infarction: A Surgical Emergency, *J. Thorac. Cardiovasc. Surg.,* 70:432, 1975.

32 Phillips, S. J., Kongtahworn, C., Zeff, R. H., et al.: Emergency Coronary Artery Revascularization: A Possible Therapy for Acute Myocardial Infarction, *Circulation,* 60:241, 1979.

33 Friesinger, G. C., Page, E. E., and Ross, R. S.: Prognostic Significance of Coronary Arteriography, *Trans. Assoc. Am. Physicians,* 83:70, 1970.

34 Humphries, J. O., Kuller, L., Ross, R. S., et al.: Natural History of Ischemic Heart Disease in Relation to Arteriographic Findings: 12-Year Study of 224 Patients, *Circulation,* 49:489, 1974.

35 Cohen, M. V., and Gorlin, R.: Main Left Coronary Artery Disease: Clinical Experience from 1964–1974, *Circulation,* 52:275, 1975.

36 Loop, F. D., Lytle, B. W., Cosgrove, D. M., et al.: Atherosclerosis of the Left Main Coronary Artery: Five Year Results of Surgical Treatment, *Am. J. Cardiol.,* 44:195, 1979.

37 Proudfit, W. L., Bruschke, A. V., and Sones, F. M.: Natural History of Obstructive Coronary Artery Disease: Ten-Year Study of 601 Nonsurgical Cases, *Prog. Cardiovasc. Dis.,* 21:53, 1978.

38 Harris, P. J., Harrell, F. E., Lee, K. L., et al.: Survival in Medically Treated Coronary Artery Disease, *Circulation,* 60:1259, 1979.

39 Loop, F. D., Cosgrove, D. M., Lytle, B. W., et al.: An 11-Year Evaluation of Coronary Arterial Surgery (1967–1978), *Ann. Surg.,* 190:444, 1979.

40 Fowler, B. M., Jacobs, M. L., Zir, L., et al.: Late Graft Patency and Symptom Relief after Aorta-Coronary Bypass, *J. Thorac. Cardiovasc. Surg.,* 79:288, 1980.

41 Cameron, A., Kemp, H. G., Shimomura, S., et al: Aortocoronary Bypass Surgery: A 7-Year Follow-up, *Circulation,* 60(suppl. 1):9, 1979.

42 Hammermeister, D. E., DeRouen, T. A., and Dodge, H. T.: Evidence from a Nonrandomized Study that Coronary Surgery Prolongs Survival in Patients with Two-Vessel Coronary Disease, *Circulation,* 59:430, 1979.

43 Mathur, V. S., Guinn, G. A., Anastassiades, L. C., et al.: Surgical Treatment for Stable Angina Pectoris: Prospective Randomized Study, *N. Engl. J. Med.,* 292:709, 1975.

44 Sheldon, W. C., Rincon, G., Pichard, A. D., et al.: Surgical Treatment of Coronary Artery Disease: Pure Graft Operations, with a Study of 741 Patients Followed 3 to 7 Years, *Prog. Cardiovasc. Dis.,* 18:237, 1975.

45 Kouchoukos, N. T., Oberman, A., and Karp, R. B.: Results of Surgery for Disabling Angina Pectoris, *Cardiovasc. Clin.,* 8(2):157, 1977.

46 Vismara, L. A., Foerster, J., Korem, R., et al.: Prospective Identification of Sudden Death Determinants: Specificity of Electrocardiographic Abnormalities and Coronary Risk Factors, *Circulation,* 52(suppl. 2):121, 1975. (Abstract.)

47 Vismara, L. A., Cooper, C., Ikeda, R., et al.: Adverse Effects of Ventricular Hypertrophy on Mortality in Premature Coronary Atherosclerosis: Clinical-Anatomic Correlations in Young Adults, *Am. J. Cardiol.,* 37:179,1976. (Abstract.)

48 Han, J.: Mechanism of Ventricular Arrhythmias Associated with Myocardial Infarction, *Am. J. Cardiol.,* 24:800, 1969.

49. Ecker, R. R., Mullins, C. B., Grammer, J. C., et al.: Control of Intractable Ventricular Tachycardia by Coronary Revascularization, *Circulation,* 44:666, 1971.

50 Vismara, L. A., Miller, R. R., Price, J. E., et al.: Improved Longevity due to Reduction of Sudden Death by Aortocoronary Bypass in Coronary Atherosclerosis, *Am. J. Cardiol.,* 39:919, 1977.

51 Hammermeister, K. E., DeRouen, T. A., and Murray, J. A.: Effect of Aortocoronary Saphenous Vein Bypass Grafting on Death and Sudden Death, *Am. J. Cardiol.,* 39:925, 1977.

Coronary Bypass Surgery: The Total Experience at Baylor College of Medicine[*]

MICHAEL E. DEBAKEY, M.D., and
GERALD M. LAWRIE, M.D.

> In certain cases of angina pectoris, when the mouth of the coronary arteries is calcified, it would be useful to establish a complementary circulation for the lower part of the arteries.
>
> ALEXIS CARREL, 1910[1]

Many surgical techniques have been proposed for the relief of angina pectoris. The senior author's interest in this symptom spans a period when the procedures under consideration ranged from cardiac sympathectomy, thyroidectomy, and stimulation of collateral formation between the heart and thoracic wall[1a] to direct myocardial revascularization, which began in 1964 in the department of surgery at Baylor College of Medicine with successful performance of a left anterior descending coronary bypass graft on a 42-year-old man with left main coronary artery disease. This case was reported briefly in 1970,[2] and a detailed 7-year follow-up was published in 1973.[3]

In 1962, coronary angiography had become available as a result of the pioneering work of Sones[4] and was being used with increasing frequency in the investigation of patients with angina pectoris in our center. The angiographic findings in 313 patients studied at Baylor were reported in 1967.[5]

In the early 1960s, and as a consequence of coronary angiographic visualization of the frequent localizing patterns of occlusive disease of the coronary arteries, increasing efforts were focused on direct surgical methods of restoring circulation, mostly by patch-graft angioplasty with or without endarterectomy, and by excision and vein-graft replacement.[6] The concept of aortocoronary bypass, however, was also being investigated experimentally.[7] From 1964 to 1968, coronary bypass was being cautiously applied, along with coronary endarterectomy, in 32 patients. Of the first eight patients who had endarterectomy and patch-graft angioplasty, three remain well at this writing, about 20 years after operation.

Since 1968, the direct technique of saphenous-vein bypass rapidly replaced all indirect methods of myocardial revascularization. The favorable clinical and angiographic results of this early experience with coronary bypass in a large group of patients were documented in patients followed up to 4 years after operation in a series of reports published between 1970 and 1972.[2,8–10] The largest group analyzed at that time consisted of 1,287 patients followed from 6 months to 4 years after operation.[10] Of these patients, 51 percent were free of angina and about 40 percent were improved after operation. At that time, 77 percent of patients had returned to work. Graft patency was recorded in 325 patients and was 85 percent. During this period of follow-up, 93.6 percent of patients remained alive. The total experience of the senior members of the department of surgery from 1964 until November 1982 now includes 15,812 saphenous vein coronary bypass procedures.

INDICATIONS

A variety of indications have become established for coronary bypass surgery at Baylor College of Medicine.[11] Most have gained general acceptance, but some remain controversial. They are summarized in Table 1.

The most common indication for investigation remains angina pectoris. Mild or absent angina, in itself, has had a decreasing influence on our decision to perform cardiac catheterization and operation. In such mildly symptomatic patients, catheterization is performed if the patient has a strongly positive result of the treadmill exercise test, large perfusion defects on thallium scanning, or a fall in ejection fraction during exercise isotope ventriculography, or if the patient is to have other major operations. These indications are based on the anatomicophysiological concept of the amount of myocardium in danger of ischemic damage.

The beneficial effects of surgical treatment for patients with symptomatic left main and three-vessel coronary disease are well accepted. Both the randomized prospective Veterans Administration Cooperative Study (VA)[12] and the European Coronary Surgery Study Group (ECSSG) trial[13] have examined the survival rates of symptomatic patients in these groups. Surgical treatment for symptomatic patients with left main disease is widely accepted. Although the total experience of

*From the Department of Surgery, Baylor College of Medicine, Houston, Texas.

TABLE 1

Potential indications for cardiac catheterization and coronary bypass

1 Stable angina suddenly increasing in intensity

2 Disabling angina

3 Crescendo (preinfarction) angina and early evolving myocardial infarction

4 Subendocardial infarction

5 Asymptomatic man with positive result of treadmill electrocardiogram or isotope studies

6 Ventricular aneurysms, especially if associated with angina, congestive heart failure, arrhythmias, or embolic phenomena

7 Ventricular septal defect secondary to myocardial infarction

8 Mitral regurgitation secondary to severe papillary muscle dysfunction with congestive heart failure

9 Atypical chest pain

10 Suspected severe left main coronary artery stenosis as indicated by a strongly positive result of treadmill electroencephalogram

11 Associated coronary artery stenosis in patients undergoing investigation for mitral or aortic valvular replacement

12 Patients with aneurysms of the aorta or peripheral vascular disease requiring major surgery who have a history or noninvasive evidence of myocardial ischemia

the VA study on symptomatic patients with three-vessel coronary disease showed a trend toward surgical treatment that was not statistically significant, analyses of the experience of the 10 hospitals in which the aggregate operative mortality rate was 3.3 percent (including 87 percent of the patients) with elimination of the 3 hospitals with an aggregate operative mortality rate of 23 percent showed a significantly improved survival rate with surgical treatment.[12] In the ECSSG study, patients with three-vessel disease treated surgically had a 94 percent 6-year survival rate as contrasted with an 80.4 percent survival rate with medical treatment[13]— a highly significant difference in favor of surgical treatment.

A carefully designed, nonrandomized study from the Seattle Heart Watch used a computer-matched medical control group for comparison with surgical results in three-vessel disease. Significantly better survival rates were reported for the surgical group, at an average follow-up of 5.5 years for patients 48 years old or older with ejection fractions greater than 30 percent and no ventricular arrhythmias in the resting electrocardiogram.[14] Thus, three major studies reported a clear advantage for surgically treated patients with angina pectoris and three-vessel coronary disease with normal or moderately impaired left ventricular function.

The effect of surgical treatment on the survival rate of patients with two-vessel disease is less clear. In the VA study, no difference was reported.[12] In the ECSSG report, the trend was toward better survival rates of

surgical patients, with an 89.4 percent 6-year surgical and an 86.0 percent 6-year medical survival rate.[2] The perioperative mortality rate was, however, unexpectedly high, and an excessive number of surgical patients had proximal left anterior descending (LAD) coronary disease. The 6-year survival rate of the medical group was lower for patients with proximal LAD disease (80.2 percent) than for those without LAD disease (95.0 percent). The 80.2 percent survival rate was almost identical to that of medically treated patients with three-vessel disease. Thus, in this study, proximal LAD disease appeared to be an important factor in the prognosis of patients with two-vessel disease. In the Seattle Heart Watch Study, surgical treatment of symptomatic patients with two-vessel disease yielded significantly higher 4-year survival rates than medical treatment, 98 versus 76 percent.[15]

If symptoms are well-controlled medically, operation usually is not performed for single-vessel disease unless the proximal LAD is affected. Single-vessel proximal LAD disease has been shown to have a deleterious effect on survival.

Medically treated patients with isolated LAD disease have overall annual attrition rates of 3 to 4 percent, compared with rates of about 2 percent for isolated right or circumflex coronary disease[16] and an expected normal attrition rate of about 1 percent. The degree of severity of response to the exercise stress test also increases the mortality rate with, for example, an expected 5-year survival rate of about 75 percent; or an annual attrition rate of about 5 percent, when positive in stage II.[17] The site of the LAD disease influences the magnitude of abnormalities of the left ventricular wall motion observed during exercise and after myocardial infarction. Both are greater with disease just proximal or just distal to the first septal perforator of the LAD.[18] Thus, single-vessel disease of the proximal LAD may be more serious than isolated lesions of other vessels.

Randomized prospective studies have not shown improved overall survival rates for patients with single-vessel disease treated surgically, but multiple factors have not been evaluated in specific subgroups, as for example, results of treadmill testing, the vessel involved, or the amount of myocardium supplied by the LAD that is at risk. These data may therefore be misleading in a patient with specific severe anatomic and pathophysiologic abnormalities.

The role of surgery in the treatment of "asymptomatic" patients is less well established. In these patients the purpose of coronary bypass is to prolong life and preserve myocardial function. It is thus important to determine whether the natural history of "asymptomatic" coronary disease is in fact less serious than "symptomatic" coronary disease of equal angiographic severity and whether surgical treatment favorably influences long-term survival and ventricular function in "asymptomatic" patients.

Absence of symptoms does not ensure a normal prognosis in patients with significant angiographic evidence of coronary disease. Correlation between survival and the presence, absence, or severity of angina has been poor. Although increasing severity of angina pectoris has been shown to be associated with increasingly shorter survival, this is due primarily to the higher prevalence of multivessel disease in patients with more severe symptoms. In one study, joint analysis of 81 clinical and angiographic variables indicated the dominant importance of the angiographic pattern of disease and a variety of clinical and angiographic markers of impaired left ventricular function.[19] Only severe, progressive chest pain and nocturnal chest pain appeared as weak clinical predictors. In another study, the presence, absence, or severity of angina pectoris was not identified as a factor predictive of survival.[20]

In a study from the Duke-Harvard computer bank,[21] asymptomatic patients with three-vessel disease had a 4.7 percent annual attrition rate, which represents at least a fivefold increase over the expected mortality rate of the comparable general population.

Severe myocardial ischemia may occur without angina, as has been shown during treadmill exercise testing[22] as well as by the fact that up to 25 percent of patients complain of no angina during the course of an acute myocardial infarction. About one-half of patients who die from sudden cardiac arrest have had no previous angina. Angiographic studies of asymptomatic survivors of acute myocardial infarction have shown a high incidence of significant multivessel coronary disease.

A common problem is the truly asymptomatic patient who is found to have a positive result of the treadmill exercise test during a routine checkup. Several large studies of apparently healthy asymptomatic men 40 to 60 years of age showed that 3 to 5 percent had significant coronary disease.[23] In from 25 to 33 percent of those who had a positive result of the treadmill test, clinical evidence of coronary atherosclerosis developed.

For these reasons, we advocate early angiography in most asymptomatic patients in whom myocardial ischemia has been shown by treadmill electrocardiography, radionuclide stress ventriculography, or both, and within 6 weeks after hospital discharge in the survivors of myocardial infarction who are younger than 60 years of age.We believe that operation performed only to prolong life is indicated primarily in those younger patients in whom, in our experience, the operation has been very safe.

The best data on surgical treatment for asymptomatic or minimally symptomatic patients come from another study by the Seattle Heart Watch Group,[24] which indicated that only asymptomatic patients with three-vessel disease had improved survival rates after coronary bypass. Three other reports of 125 asymptomatic patients confirm the safety of surgical treatment.[25–27] The operative mortality rate was 0.8 percent (1 of 125 patients), and the late mortality rate (up to 7 years) was 1.6 percent (2 of 125 patients). Of the 113 patients with severe multivessel disease, 99 percent (112 patients) are alive at variable follow-up intervals beyond 19 months—a remarkably low late attrition rate.

We believe that asymptomatic patients with single- or double-vessel disease, in whom no evidence of severe ischemia can be shown by radionuclide stress ventriculography and the proximal LAD is not diseased, have a low sudden-death risk and can be treated medically with reasonable safety. In patients with three-vessel disease or left main stenosis, however, or in those with two-vessel disease and proximal LAD disease or single-vessel proximal and severe LAD disease, we are inclined to operate on the basis of the anatomic situation alone.

We thus offer surgical treatment to most patients with left main or three-vessel disease, regardless of severity of symptoms or response to medical treatment. In patients with two-vessel disease who have high-grade proximal LAD, operation is usually recommended, especially if the other affected vessel is the circumflex coronary artery. If single-vessel disease does not involve the proximal LAD and symptoms are easily controlled, medical treatment is recommended.

The level of preoperative left ventricular function also is a factor in candidates for operation since it influences both the surgical risk and late survival rates. The surgical risk has been shown to be negligible for patients with ejection fractions above 35 percent, whereas below 35 percent the risk, although still low, increases. Surgical treatment, on the other hand, probably produces the greatest improvement in the survival rates of patients with impaired left ventricular function (ejection fractions less than 50 percent) because of their relatively high attrition rates with medical treatment.[12–14,16] Because, however, the ECSSG study showed significantly improved survival rates with surgical treatment for patients with three-vessel and left main disease and ejection fractions over 50 percent,[13] we do not consider normal left ventricular function an indication for medical treatment as suggested by some.[12]

Multivessel coronary artery disease with poor ventricular function (below 35 percent) has the worst prognosis, but surgical treatment is often avoided because relief of symptoms and the perioperative mortality risk have been unpredictable. Over the years, however, selected patients have obtained objective improvement in ejection fraction as well as dramatic relief of symptoms. Now in progress at Baylor is a prospective study of patients with multivessel coronary artery disease and moderate-to-severe ischemic cardiomyopathy—

ejection fraction between 15 and 35 percent (unpublished data). Thus far, left ventricular function has been prospectively evaluated in 36 patients before operation, before hospital discharge, and at late follow-up study by gated cardiac blood pool isotope scanning. In this group, 33 were men and 3 women, with a mean age of 50.0 years and a range from 30 to 73 years. Angina was present in 94 percent of patients and severe symptoms of heart failure in 28 percent. The mean preoperative left ventricular ejection fraction was 26 percent, with a range of 13 to 35 percent. The operative mortality rate (30-day) was 5.5 percent (one death due to myocardial infarction and one to a stroke). No patients required intraaortic balloon pump support. The mean discharge ejection fraction was 35 percent; with a range of 15 to 75 percent, and was significantly higher than before operation. The late ejection fractions (11 months after discharge with a range from 2 to 24 months) in 13 patients was 33 percent (range from 11 to 49 percent) compared with a preoperative value in this subgroup of 28 percent (range from 16 to 35 percent) (Fig. 1). Late improvement of angina occurred in 94 percent of patients, but congestive heart failure improved in only 43 percent of patients. Thus, in some patients improvement in ejection fraction was sustained up to 24 months after operation. Angina, the most common indication for operation, was consistently relieved, but relief of heart failure symptoms was unpredictable. We believe that in patients with severe ischemic myopathy the most predictable favorable results will be obtained in those with severe angina pectoris and a preoperative ejection fraction above 25 percent. In young patients with an even lower ejection fraction, however, we may operate in the hope of prolonging life by preventing recurrent myocardial infarction.

Considerable interest has been shown in early operation for acute myocardial infarction, and excellent results have been reported.[28,29] Although this approach is under active review at our institution, at this writing selected patients in this category are treated by early cardiac catheterization and intracoronary streptokinase therapy rather than immediate operation. "Elective" coronary bypass is performed about 1 week later. Truly emergency operations are reserved for patients in whom intractable angina with or without hypotension develops during or after cardiac catheterization. In our experience, immediate operation has proved safe in these patients and seemed preferable to prolonged attempts at medical stabilization.

In patients with multivessel coronary disease and impaired left ventricular function, intractable ventricular tachyarrhythmias may also develop and require surgical intervention. Coronary bypass alone has proved ineffective for such arrhythmias.[30] We have performed preoperative and intraoperative electrophysiological studies to locate arrhythmogenic foci and have ablated

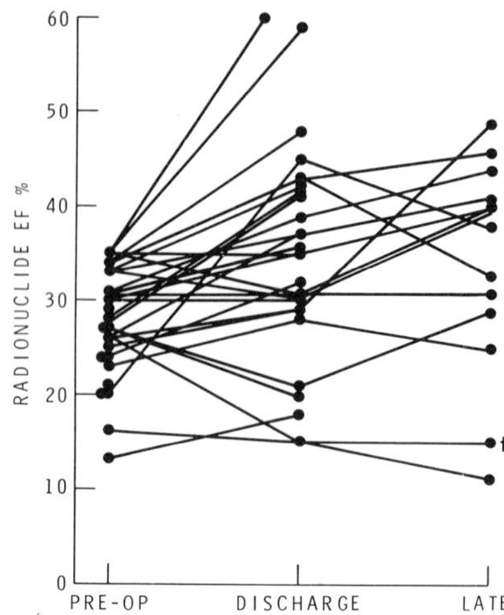

FIGURE 1 Changes in ejection fraction after coronary bypass in patients with preoperative ejection fractions 35 percent or less. Each line represents an individual patient.

them by endocardial resection and cryothermia. Coronary bypass is performed as an adjunct to these procedures. We have treated 14 patients in this manner with a 15 percent hospital mortality rate and 85 percent complete relief of life-threatening ventricular tachycardia.

Another important indication for coronary bypass is coronary as well as some other form of cardiac disease in the same patient. In patients having cardiac operations for noncoronary disease such as valve replacement, we favor correction of coexisting coronary disease by coronary bypass at that time. Although evidence for the benefit of this approach is conflicting, our ability to accomplish this combined procedure without increased risk of perioperative death and the sound physiological basis of the approach have encouraged us to continue using it. The other major indication for coronary bypass is to afford myocardial protection to patients with severe coronary disease who require other major noncardiac operations. Data from our institution suggest that coronary bypass may provide protection against the fatal cardiac complications sometimes encountered during major noncardiac operations in patients with angina pectoris.[31]

In a study[32] of 358 patients operated on for noncoronary conditions who had had previous coronary bypass, the perioperative mortality rate was 1.1 percent. In 70 patients (20 percent), staged operations were planned and subsequent operations performed 6 to 12 weeks after bypass with no cardiac complications and one death. In the remainder, operation was performed from 10 days to 89 months after coronary bypass for urgent reasons or new disease. Three deaths and significant numbers of medical cardiac complications occurred in those patients operated on within 30 days. The subsequent operation was vascular in 232 patients, with three deaths (1.3 percent); thoracic in 43, with no deaths; and general surgical in 113, with one death (0.9 percent). Follow-up study showed 307 patients (87 percent) still alive for periods ranging from 30 days to 7 years. Late death was due to myocardial infarction in only 12 patients (3 percent). This study suggested that the risk of operation was as low in patients who had had successful coronary artery bypass as in those without coronary artery disease and that the risk of subsequent myocardial infarction was slight.

The other study[33] concerned carotid endarterectomy. In 1,546 consecutive carotid endarterectomies performed on 1,238 patients over a period of 10 years, 17 percent of the patients (212 of 1,238) had angina pectoris; an additional 32 percent (396 of 1,238) were asymptomatic but had a history of myocardial infarction. The perioperative mortality rate (30-day) in the 1,306 consecutive endarterectomies in 1,026 patients without symptomatic coronary artery disease was 1.5 percent (15 of 1,026 patients). Of the 212 patients with symptoms, 85 carotid endarterectomies were performed on 77 patients without previous coronary bypass with an operative mortality rate of 18.2 percent (14 of 77). The remaining 135 patients had 155 carotid endarterectomies but were treated by previous coronary artery bypass (84 patients) or simultaneous carotid endarterectomy and coronary artery bypass (51 patients) with an operative mortality rate of 3 percent (4 of 135 patients). The greatly improved survival rate in those patients with symptomatic coronary disease who had coronary artery bypass before, or at the same time as, carotid endarterectomy, and the absence of permanent neurologic deficits in 51 of these 135 patients who had simultaneous carotid endarterectomy and coronary artery bypass suggest that a significantly improved survival rate can be achieved after carotid endarterectomy in these high-risk patients by performance of simultaneous coronary artery bypass.

In light of the results of these studies, we evaluate most patients with angina pectoris who require major noncardiac operations by coronary angiography. Asymptomatic patients with a history or electrocardiographic evidence of myocardial infarction have noninvasive screening, and, if the result is positive, cardiac catheterization is performed. When severe coronary disease is identified, coronary bypass is then performed, either before or simultaneously with the noncardiac operation.

SURGICAL TECHNIQUES AND RESULTS

The standard surgical technique used since 1963 has been the reversed autogenous saphenous vein aorto-coronary bypass operation performed during a period of total cardiopulmonary bypass.[34] The vein is prepared with heparinized saline solution under a pressure less than 300 mmHg. The behavior of these grafts in our patients was examined in detail. The long-term patency of the grafts was studied in 596 vein grafts in 343 patients at a mean follow-up of 15.4 months, with a range from 0 to 84 months.[35] The overall graft patency rate was 84 percent, and after more than 5 years the rate was 89 percent. The patency rate in asymptomatic patients was 91 percent compared with 81 percent in the remainder. The patency of grafts attached distal to total occlusions was 82 percent (78 of 95). The most recent follow-up data (up to 12 years after operation) for 739 vein grafts is shown in Table 2.

The prevalence and clinical significance of intimal proliferation and atherosclerosis of vein grafts in our patients were evaluated in two other studies. In 492 vein grafts from 281 patients, intimal proliferation was examined from 0 to 75 months after operation.[36] The graft patency rates are shown in Table 3.

Vein graft samples were obtained from 41 patients; in 27 patients with 51 grafts (early group), they were obtained from 0 to 30 days (mean 14 days) after operation; in 14 patients with 27 grafts (late group) they were obtained from 7 to 75 months (mean 34 months) after operation. Intimal proliferation was graded from 1 to 4 corresponding to an intima/media thickness ratio of 1, 2, 3, or 4, respectively.

In the early group, all 51 vein grafts showed grades 1 to 2 intimal proliferation; 5 grafts were occluded, all as a result of recent thrombosis. In the late group, 17 of the 27 grafts were studied histologically. All patent vein grafts showed grades 2 to 3 intimal proliferation. Four vein grafts were occluded but only one as a result of grade 4 intimal proliferation. In 14 patients in the late group, angiograms, performed shortly before vein graft samples were obtained, showed 14 patent and 4 occluded grafts. Of the 14 patent grafts 10 showed

TABLE 2

Graft patency of 739 coronary vein grafts studied at a mean follow-up of 47.6 months, range 1 to 136 months

| | | Graft patency | |
Artery	Grafts (no.)	No.	%
Right coronary	263	194	74
Left anterior descending coronary	356	286	80
Left circumflex coronary	120	86	72
Total	739	566	77

SOURCE: Fom G. C. Morris, unpublished data.

TABLE 3
Graft patency rate in 492 vein grafts from 281 patients followed from 0 to 75 months after operation

Duration of follow-up (months)	Graft patency rate	
	No.	%
First	55 of 60	92
1 to 3	49 of 54	91
4 to 6	37 of 44	84
7 to 12	33 of 43	77
13 to 24	113 of 140	81
25 to 36	59 of 72	82
37 to 75	66 of 79	84

grades 2 to 3 intimal proliferation but were of uniformly good caliber angiographically (graft/artery ratio more than 1.5).

This study showed that most grafts had become occluded early, usually because of thrombosis. Late graft occlusion was uncommon and rarely due to intimal proliferation. The angiographic appearance of vein grafts up to 75 months after operation suggested that intimal proliferation was the usual finding in long-term grafts, but that this is compatible with good graft patency. These studies have now been extended beyond 120 months with similar results.

The importance of vein-graft atherosclerosis was evaluated in 99 saphenous vein grafts recovered at necropsy from 55 patients who survived aortocoronary bypass from 0 to 75 months.[37] The severity of vein-graft intimal proliferation and the prevalence of true atherosclerosis were compared in patients with normal and elevated lipid levels. Although intimal proliferation progressed with time in both patient groups, a greater proportion of hyperlipemic patients had high-grade luminal narrowing of vein grafts as the interval after aortocoronary bypass lengthened. True atherosclerosis did not develop before 12 months in any of the 59 vein grafts from the 27 normolipemic and 5 hyperlipemic patients who survived aortocoronary bypass, but it was found in 3 of 26 vein grafts (11.5 percent) from normolipemic and 11 of 14 vein grafts (78.6 percent) from hyperlipemic patients who survived 13 to 75 months after aortocoronary bypass. Because of the generally satisfactory results of these long-term studies, we continue to prefer the saphenous vein unless it is unavailable, when the internal mammary artery or type-specific homograft vein is used.

During the first half of his experience, the senior author preferred the technique of intermittent ischemic arrest for intraoperative myocardial preservation during the period of cardiac arrest required for performing the distal anastomoses. Normothermic total cardiopulmonary bypass was established for venous return by means of bicaval cannulation, ascending aortic arterial return, and a left ventricular sump via the left atrium. Distal anastomoses were performed with use of ischemic arrest accomplished by aortic cross-clamping followed by construction of the corresponding proximal anastomosis. This technique was used for left-sided grafts, whereas for right coronary grafts local clamping of the vessel was used with the heart supported by total cardiopulmonary bypass. During this period, other members of the department had used a single period of normothermic ischemic arrest to perform the distal anastomosis.

After introduction of cold cardioplegic myocardial preservation, it was decided to compare the protection achieved by this technique and intermittent ischemic arrest.[38] A randomized prospective study of 57 patients was done. The comparative effects of normothermic intermittent ischemic arrest and cardioplegia on left ventricular performance were assessed by gated cardiac blood pool imaging in 57 patients undergoing aortocoronary bypass. In 34 patients, intermittent ischemic arrest was used and in 23, cardioplegia. Patients were studied before operation, sequentially in the immediate postoperative period at 30-min intervals, and 1 week after the operation. The two groups did not differ in age, class of angina, number of diseased vessels, previous myocardial infarction, or preoperative ejection fraction (50 $\pm$ 3 percent versus 50 $\pm$ 2 percent [p = ns]).

During the six sequential postoperative studies, transient left ventricular dysfunction (7 percent decrease in absolute ejection fraction) was observed in 10 patients receiving cardioplegia and in 16 receiving intermittent ischemic arrest. By the time of discharge, the preoperative ejection fraction had returned in 24 of 26 patients. The mean ejection fraction at discharge in those having cardioplegia did not differ from the preoperative ejection fraction; in those having ischemic arrest, the ejection fraction increased slightly over the preoperative level. These data suggested that in patients with normal preoperative ventricular performance both cardioplegia and intermittent ischemic arrest afforded satisfactory myocardial preservation. Although the results of this study indicated comparable levels of postoperative left ventricular performance, the improved operating conditions for the surgeon produced by a flaccid, blood-free heart and the ease with which the technique could be applied led to the adoption of cardioplegic protection with a crystalloid-based electrolyte solution as the standard technique since 1977. All distal anastomoses are now performed during a single period of cardioplegic arrest, followed by construction of the proximal anastomoses with the heart beating, during support by total cardiopulmonary bypass.

The surgical techniques for treatment of combined carotid and coronary disease have been detailed elsewhere.[39] In personal experience with 3,182 cases, the mean age was 54.4 years, with a range of 11 to 87 years;

2,669 were male (83.9 percent) and 513 were female patients (16.1 percent). Over the entire period, 1,012 single bypasses were performed, 1,557 double bypasses, 584 triple bypasses, and 29 quadruple bypasses. The number of single bypasses performed has declined sharply since 1976, whereas the number of triple and quadruple bypasses has increased steadily. In 1982, however, the increasing use of coronary angioplasty led to some increase in the number of single-vessel bypasses because of referral for operation after failure of this technique. The use of coronary endarterectomy combined with vein bypass has also steadily declined from a peak in 1973; this procedure is rarely used at this time.

The increase in the number of triple and quadruple bypasses was due to recognition of the importance of revascularization of each of the affected major vessels with avoidance of significant residual disease. Another series of patients was analyzed to determine the effect of site and extent of residual disease on long-term survival rates.

A series of 1,448 consecutive patients operated on between 1968 and 1974 was analyzed to determine the effect of age at operation, number of vessels diseased before operation, preoperative left ventricular function, time period of surgery, and number and site of residual unbypassed coronary lesions after operation.[40] The results showed that residual disease after operation, age at operation, and left ventricular function were the most important variables affecting survival of patients with two-vessel and three-vessel disease at 5 years' follow-up study. Residual disease of the left anterior descending or circumflex coronary arteries was the most important predictor of survival, with residual disease of the right coronary artery exerting a lesser influence. The results suggested that the greatest benefit with regard to improved survival may come from the first two to three grafts performed, and therefore while attempting to place grafts to each major obstructed vessel, we believe, in the absence of evidence to the contrary, that performing more than three to four grafts per patient has no additional benefit.

The perioperative mortality rate (30-day) for the entire experience of the senior author of 3,182 cases, including emergency procedures, left ventricular aneurysmal resection, and associated cerebrovascular procedures, but excluding associated valvular operations, was 4.8 percent. For patients in the sixth decade of life with reasonable left ventricular function, good distal vessels, and no previous cardiac operation, the surgical risk is negligible. Despite steady improvements in surgical techniques and results, however, this overall figure has changed little because of an increasingly older and more severely diseased population of patients, many of whom have had or will require major vascular operations after the coronary bypass procedure. For example, in the personal experience of the senior author, peripheral vascular disease requiring operation was observed in 24.3 percent of a consecutive series of 533 patients who had coronary bypass between 1968 and 1972 and were followed at least 10 years (unpublished data). Vascular procedures were performed before coronary bypass in 64 patients who had 124 operations, and after coronary bypass in 66 patients who had 105 procedures (Table 4).

Interestingly, the 5-year survival rate of patients requiring associated operations was similar to that of those not requiring another operation—about 80 percent. During the next 5 years, however, the survival rates slowly diverged, and at 10 years, the survival rates for the two groups were 46 and 59 percent; these rates reflect the more advanced pathologic condition of the patients who had associated diseases (Fig. 2).

The favorable clinical and angiographic outcome of coronary operations performed by members of our department of surgery has been documented extensively at 5- and 10-year follow-up, along with an analysis of factors influencing the results of operation.[41] The results of operation in 1,144 patients at least 5 years after operation were reported in 1978.[42] Men constituted 1,000 (87.4 percent). The mean age was 50.1 years (range 24 to 75 years). In 1,101 patients (96.2 percent), the indication for operation was angina with reduction of more than 70 percent of the luminal diameter of the coronary arteries. Forty-three patients (3.8 percent) had coronary bypass because of congestive heart failure without angina, and 240 (21 percent) had both conditions. One hundred forty-nine patients (13 percent) had unstable angina, and 675 patients (59 percent) had previous myocardial infarctions. Two hundred twenty-six (19.8 percent) had more than 70 percent stenosis in one vessel, 442 (38.6 percent) in two vessels, and 376 patients (32.9 percent) in three vessels. In 100 patients (8.7 percent), stenosis of the left main coronary artery was greater than 50 percent.

TABLE 4
Incidence of associated vascular procedures in 533 patients followed at least 10 years after coronary bypass

| | Coronary artery bypass | | | |
| | Before (64 pts*) | | After (66 pts) | |
Associated vascular procedures	%	No.	%	No.
Cerebrovascular	32	40	18	19
Aortoiliac occlusive	27	34	29	31
Abdominal aneurysm	15	18	13	14
Femoropopliteal	11	14	24	25
Renovascular	5	6	3	3
Other	10	12	13	13
Total	100	124	100	105

*pts = patients.

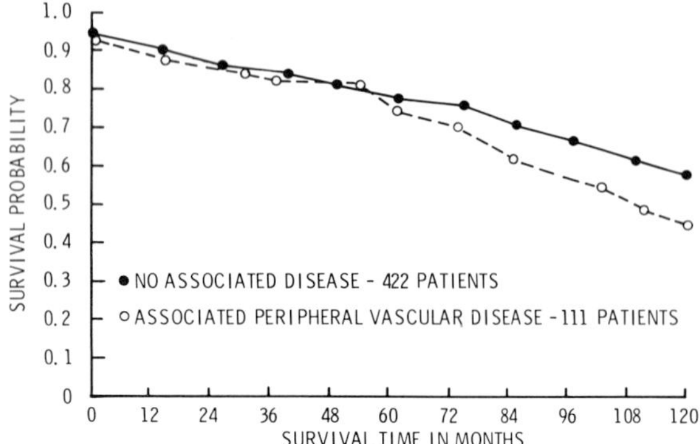

FIGURE 2 Kaplan-Meier curves of survival probability comparing the fate of patients operated on for associated atherosclerotic disease before or after coronary bypass with those who had only coronary bypass during a 10-year follow-up.

The operative mortality rate for the entire series was 4.6 percent (52 patients). For all patients except those with disease of the left main coronary artery it was 3.8 percent (40 of 1,044). The crude 5-year survival rate was 89.1 percent (930 of 1,044).

The survival rates in both sexes were comparable. The survival rates of the men according to the number of vessels operated on were as follows: one vessel, 92.9 percent (169 of 182) overall and 94.9 percent (130 of 137) for patients with good left ventricular function; two vessels, 90.3 percent (352 of 390) overall and 94.3 percent (248 of 263) for those with good left ventricular function; three vessels, 85.7 percent (293 of 342) overall and 90.9 percent (189 of 208) for those with good left ventricular function; and left main coronary, 81.4 percent (70 of 86) overall and 90.6 percent (48 of 53) for those with good left ventricular function. Graft patency in 157 patients was 86.4 percent (247 of 286 grafts), and 94.9 percent (149 patients) had at least one patent graft.

In 1979, a detailed study was published of 134 consecutive patients with more than 50 percent stenosis of the left main coronary artery, all of whom had been followed at least 5 years.[43] Of the 134 patients, 87 percent (117 of 134) were men; the mean age was 57 years (range 37 to 70 years). In addition to left main stenosis, coexistent significant coronary disease was present in other vessels in 128 patients (95.5 percent), with multivessel disease in 109 (81 percent). Ventricular function was good (end-diastolic pressure less than 15 mmHg and no localized contraction abnormality) in 88 patients (66 percent) and poor in 46 patients (34 percent). The perioperative mortality rate was 13 percent (17 patients) in the entire group and 11 percent (10 of 88) among patients with good left ventricular function. Postoperative graft patency in 33 patients was 85 percent (58 of 68). The survival rate was 79 percent (106 of 134) in the entire group, 81 percent (71 of 88) in patients with good ventricular function, and 76 percent (35 of 46) in patients with poor ventricular function. Late annual attrition rates were 1.5 and 2.1 percent in patients with good and poor ventricular function, respectively.

These 5-year survival studies showed that first, men and women had similar late survival rates; second, the annual attrition rate appeared to remain stable despite the passage of considerable time with no acceleration of mortality rate in the later follow-up period; and third, the attrition rates were similar regardless of the number of vessels diseased before operation, a pattern which is different from previously reported medically treated series of patients. Finally, the most common cause of death remained ischemic heart disease, followed by stroke and cancer.

These studies have now been extended to a full 10-year follow-up in more than 1,600 patients operated on between 1968 and 1972. Detailed evaluation of the first 500 patients in this group has been reported.[44] In this group, there were 446 male patients (89.2 percent). Angina pectoris was the major indication for operation. Multivessel coronary disease was present in 81 percent (406 of 500) of patients. Left ventricular function was good (end-diastolic pressure less than 15 mmHg and no evidence of aneurysm or akinesis in the left ventriculogram) in 69.9 percent (348/500) of patients.

At 10-year follow-up, 48 percent of patients were asymptomatic and 41 percent were improved. Propranolol hydrochloride was being used by 36 percent of patients and nitrates by 49 percent. Table 5 shows a comparison of their 5-year and 10-year status. Of the 355 patients under 65 years of age at the time of follow-up examination, 57 percent were employed full-time and 24 percent were working part-time. During the 10-year period, reoperation was performed on 9 percent of patients and was required equally for graft occlusion

TABLE 5

Comparison of symptoms and medication in 500 patients at 5 and 10 years' follow-up

Symptoms and medication	Follow-up	
	5 years (%)	10 years (%)
Symptoms		
Asymptomatic	51	48
Improved	42	41
Unchanged/worse	7	11
Medication		
Propranolol hydrochloride	24	36
Coronary vasodilators	44	49

SOURCE: Lawrie, G.M., et al.: Clinical Results of Coronary Bypass in 500 Patients at Least 10 Years After Operation. *Circulation*, 66 (Suppl. 1): 1, 1982. Reproduced by permission of the American Heart Association.

or appearance of new coronary lesions. This represents an annual reoperation rate of less than 1 percent.

The Cox multivariate analysis technique was used to evaluate the influence of multiple preoperative and intraoperative variables on the 10-year survival rates of this series of 500 patients (Table 6). The most important variables identified were the number of vessels diseased before operation and factors reflecting impairment of left ventricular function: diuretic usage, a history of congestive heart failure, and a history of previous myocardial infarction (Table 7). Because residual disease was not examined, the number of diseased vessels before operation replaced it as a variable.

Kaplan-Meier curves of survival probability were obtained for an overall group of 1,000 consecutive patients followed a full 10 years. The overall 10-year survival rate was influenced most by the quality of preoperative left ventricular function, with a 71.5 percent survival rate for patients with good left ventricular function and 52.8 percent for those with poor left ven-

TABLE 6
Results of the univariate analysis from the Cox model for factors predictive of 10-year survival of 500 patients

Factor	Chi-square	p
Age	5.39	.02
Quality of ventricle	18.35	.00
Number of diseased vessels	25.20	.00
Sex	1.12	.29
Preoperative angina	0.42	.52
History of myocardial infarction	5.39	.02
Preoperative congestive heart failure	22.92	.00
Preoperative stroke	0.45	.50
Preoperative obesity	0.16	.69
Preoperative digoxin	28.81	.0000
Preoperative vasodilator	0.00	.99
Preoperative propranolol hydrochloride	0.71	.40
Preoperative antiarrhythmic drug	1.40	.24
Preoperative diuretic drug	37.34	.0000
Preoperative smoking	0.11	.74
History of diabetes	1.55	.20
Systolic blood pressure	1.89	.17
Diastolic blood pressure	0.01	.93
Preoperative electrocardiogram—myocardial infarction	12.65	.00
Preoperative electrocardiogram—left ventricular hypertension	1.91	.17
Preoperative electrocardiogram—ST changes	8.17	.00
Preoperative electrocardiogram—premature ventricular contractions	5.36	.02
Preoperative electrocardiogram—bundle branch block	0.01	.91
Perioperative electrocardiogram—myocardial infarction	0.93	.34
Left main disease	0.09	.77

TABLE 7
Results of Cox multivariate analysis for factors predictive of 10-year survival in 500 patients

Variable	Beta	Chi-square	p
Preoperative use of diuretic drug	0.76	17.3	.000
Number of diseased vessels	0.59	24.7	.000
Preoperative congestive heart failure	0.53	7.7	.006
Preoperative electrocardiogram—myocardial infarction	0.39	6.3	.012

tricular function (Fig. 3). Unlike many other reports, sex had no significant effect on survival, with overall 10-year rates of 69.4 percent for female patients and 65.1 percent for male patients (Fig. 4).

As the survival curves show, the previously documented[44] lack of an accelerating trend in attrition rate with time is still evident, as is the tendency for the survival curves according to the number of diseased vessels to remain together rather than diverge, and as is the case with medically treated patients (Fig. 5).

The effect of hypertension, diabetes mellitus, hyperlipidemia, and cigarette smoking on 10-year survival rates was analyzed in 332 patients of the senior author (unpublished data). In this preliminary analysis, it was shown that hypertension and hyperlipidemia had a highly significant effect on survival ($p < .05$), whereas diabetes was of borderline significance ($p = .06$), and surprisingly, cigarette smoking had no effect ($p = .31$).

The effect of diabetes mellitus in 1,000 patients followed for 10 years was analyzed in more detail. Of this group, 121 patients had preoperative diabetes, of whom 81 percent (98 of 121) were male patients. Proportion-

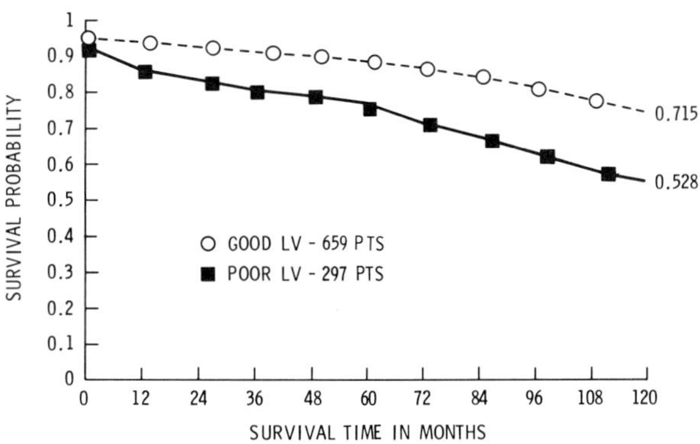

FIGURE 3 Kaplan-Meier curves of survival probability for 956 patients followed 10 years after coronary bypass according to the preoperative state of left ventricular function (LV). (*From G. C. Morris, unpublished data.*)

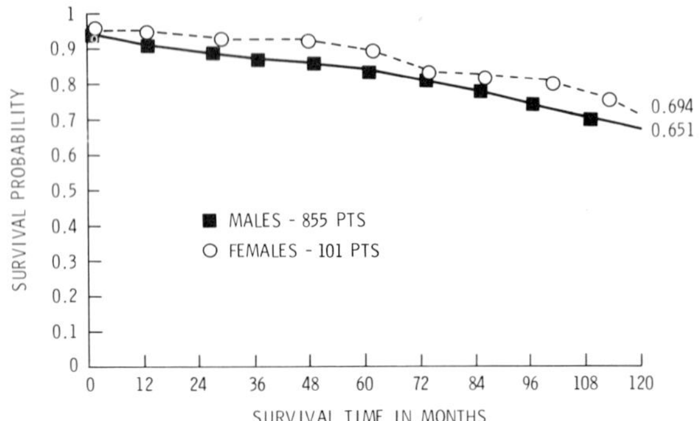

FIGURE 4 Kaplan-Meier curves of survival probability for 956 patients followed 10 years after coronary bypass according to sex. (*From G. C. Morris, unpublished data.*)

ately more of the female patients had diabetes, 23.5 percent compared with 12.2 percent of all male patients. More patients with diabetes were obese, had more multivessel and left main disease, and were taking more antihypertensive medication; but 43 other preoperative variables were similar in diabetic and nondiabetic patients. Diabetes did not affect the perioperative mortality rate, but it adversely influenced the late survival rate. The 10-year survival rate of 63 percent for patients with diabetes was not significantly different from that of the patients without diabetes (68 percent).

The rate of relief of angina of 88 percent in diabetic patients was similar to the 91 percent for nondiabetic patients. More diabetic patients had at least one occluded graft, but initially the diabetic patients had more grafts per patient—1.81 compared with 1.65 grafts per patient in nondiabetic patients and therefore more grafts at risk. Overall patency in diabetic patients was 77.5 percent (62 of 80) compared with 79.5 percent (474 of 596) at a mean follow-up of 48 $\pm$ 36.4 months.

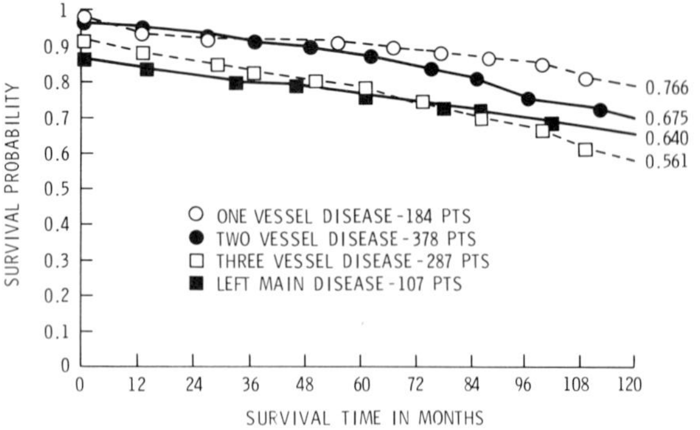

FIGURE 5 Kaplan-Meier curves of survival probability for 956 patients followed 10 years after coronary bypass according to the number of preoperative diseased vessels. (*From G. C. Morris, unpublished data.*)

Thus, although patients with diabetes had less favorable preoperative characteristics than nondiabetic patients, at 10-year follow-up, relief of angina, survival rates, and graft patency were similar. The results of this study suggested that patients with diabetes can expect a long-term prognosis after coronary bypass almost comparable to that of nondiabetic patients.

DISCUSSION

Our experience with coronary bypass has shown unequivocally the remarkable long-term persistence of relief of angina pectoris achieved by this procedure. In many types of multivessel and possibly in single-vessel proximal left anterior descending coronary disease the procedure also enhances survival. The ultimate fate of patients who have had coronary bypass is in large measure dependent on long-term graft patency, the rate of progression of atherosclerotic disease in the native circulation, and sustained preservation of left ventricular function.

Whereas graft patency and ventricular function have remained reasonably stable in our experience over a period of 10 years, progression of atherosclerosis has been documented to occur in the coronary arteries of most patients. In a previous report,[45] however, we documented the rarity of progression of atherosclerosis distal to functioning bypass grafts. Such progression was observed in only 1.8 percent of grafted coronary arteries over a 7-year interval.[4] Bourassa and associates[46] reported high rates of proximal progression of disease but low rates of distal progression (2.4 percent), at 72-month follow-up. Changes in disease of proximal coronary segments accounted for most cases of progression of disease in their study. Bruschke and associates[47] showed that progression in at least one coronary segment had occurred in 92 percent of patients recatheterized after 5 years, but again most progression was proximal. Although this report made the point that lesions distal to previous sites of disease had developed in 29.3 percent of arteries, the distal segments were still operable at the time of latest catheterization.

These observations suggest that the favorable 10-year results of operation obtained despite the frequency of progression of atherosclerosis are indeed due to the fact that progression of atherosclerosis affects mainly the proximal and mid-proximal segments of the coronary arteries and has occurred much less often in the distal segments to which the bypass grafts should have been attached. The distal placement of the grafts combined with a high graft patency rate has reduced considerably the effect of progression of coronary atherosclerosis on the long-term prognosis in these patients.

Subgroups of patients exist who because of metabolic abnormalities have a less favorable long-term prognosis because of abnormally severe progression of atherosclerosis in both native vessel and vein graft. These patients should receive intensive treatment for their risk factors. The results in the diabetic patients, on the other hand, are gratifying and should encourage wider application of operation in this group.

REFERENCES

1 Carrel, A.: On the Experimental Surgery of the Thoracic Aorta and the Heart, *Trans. Am. Surg. Assoc.*, 28:252, 1910.

1a Ochsner, A., and DeBakey, M.: The Surgical Treatment of Coronary Disease, *Surgery*, 2:428, 1937.

2 Morris, G. C., Jr., Howell, J. F., Crawford, E. S., et al.: The Distal Coronary Bypass, *Ann. Surg.*, 172:652, 1970.

3 Garrett, H. E., Dennis, E. W., and DeBakey, M. E.: Aortocoronary Bypass with Saphenous Vein Graft: Seven-Year Follow-Up, *J.A.M.A.*, 223:792, 1973.

4 Sones, F. M., Jr., and Shirey, E. K.: Cine Coronary Arteriography, *Mod. Concepts Cardiovasc. Dis.*, 31:735, 1962.

5 Diethrich, E. B., Liddicoat, J. E., Kinard, S. A., Garrett, H. E., Lewis, J. M., and DeBakey, M. E.: Surgical Significance of Angiographic Patterns in Coronary Arterial Disease, *Circulation* 35,36 (suppl. 1):155, 1967.

6 Garrett, H. E., Diethrich, E. B., and DeBakey, M. E.: Current Surgical Management of Coronary Artery Disease, *Hosp. Med.*, 3:27, 1967.

7 DeBakey, M. E., and Henly, W. S.: Surgical Treatment of Angina Pectoris, *Circulation*, 23:111, 1961.

8 Morris, G. C., Jr., Reul, G. J., Howell, J. F., et al.: Follow-up Results of Distal Coronary Artery Bypass for Ischemic Heart Disease, *Am. J. Cardiol.*, 29:180, 1972.

9 Morris, G. C., Jr., Howell, J. F., Crawford, E. S., Reul, G. J., and Stelter, W.: Operability of End Stage Coronary Artery Disease, *Ann. Surg.*, 175:1024, 1972.

10 Reul, G. J., Morris, G. C., Jr., Howell, J. F., Crawford, E. S., and Stelter, W. J.: Current Concepts in Coronary Artery Surgery: A Critical Analysis of 1,287 Patients, *Ann. Thorac. Surg.*, 14:243, 1972.

11 DeBakey, M. E., and Lawrie, G. M.: Coronary Arterial Bypass: Current Status, in A.R. Billimoria and M.P. Anand (eds.), "Heart and Lung Diseases Update," VI APCDC Education & Award Foundation, Bombay, India, 1982, p. 98.

12 Takaro, T., Hultgren, H. N., Detre, K. M., and Peduzzi, P.: The Veterans Administration Cooperative Study of Stable Angina: Current Status, *Circulation*, 65 (suppl. 2):60, 1982.

13 European Coronary Surgery Study Group: Prospective Randomized Study of Coronary Artery Bypass Surgery in Stable Angina Pectoris: A Progress Report on Survival, *Circulation*, 65 (suppl. 2):67, 1982.

14 Hammermeister, K. E., DeRouen, T. A., and Dodge, H. T.: Comparison of Survival of Medically and Surgically Treated Coronary Disease Patients in Seattle Heart Watch: A Nonrandomized Study, *Circulation*, 65 (suppl. 2):53, 1982.

15 Hammermeister, K. E., DeRouen, T. A., and Dodge, H. T.: Evidence from a Nonrandomized Study That Coronary Surgery Prolongs Survival in Patients with Two-Vessel Coronary Disease, *Circulation*, 59:430, 1979.

16 Webster, J. S., Moberg, C., and Rincon, G.: Natural History of Severe Proximal Coronary Artery Disease as Documented by Coronary Cineangiography, *Am. J. Cardiol.*, 33:195, 1974.

17 Dagenais, G. R., Rouleau, J. R., Christen, A., and Fabia, J.: Survival of Patients with a Strongly Positive Exercise Electrocardiogram, *Circulation*, 65:452, 1982.

18 Kumpuris, A. G., Quinones, M. A., Kanon, D., and Miller, R.R.: Isolated Stenosis of Left Anterior Descending or Right Coronary Artery: Relation between Site of Stenosis and Ventricular Dysfunction and Therapeutic Implications, *Am. J. Cardiol.*, 46:13, 1980.

19 Harris, P. J., Harrell, F. E., Lee, K. L., Behar, V. S., and Rosati, R. A.: Survival in Medically Treated Coronary Artery Disease, *Circulation*, 60:1259, 1979.

20 Hammermeister, K. E., DeRouen, T. A., and Dodge, H. T.: Variables Predictive of Survival in Patients with Coronary Disease: Selection by Univariate and Multivariate Analyses from the Clinical, Electrocardiographic, Exercise, Arteriographic, and Quantitative Angiographic Evaluations, *Circulation*, 59:421, 1979.

21 Cohn, P. F., Harris, P., Barry, W. H., Rosati, R. A., Rosenbaum, P., and Waternaux, C.: Prognostic Importance of Anginal Symptoms in Angiographically Defined Coronary Artery Disease, *Am. J. Cardiol.*, 47:233, 1981.

22 Cumming, G. R., Samm, J., Borysyk, L., and Kich, L.: Electrocardiographic Changes during Exercise in Asymptomatic Men: 3-Year Follow-up, *Can. Med. Assoc. J.*, 112:578, 1975.

23 Morris, S. N., and McHenry, P. L.: Role of Exercise Stress Testing in Healthy Subjects and Patients with Coronary Heart Disease: Controversies in Cardiology—1, *Am. J. Cardiol.*, 42:659, 1978.

24 Hammermeister, K. E., DeRouen, T. A., and Dodge, H. T.: Effect of Coronary Surgery on Survival in Asymptomatic and Minimally Symptomatic Patients, *Circulation*, 62 (suppl. 1):98, 1980.

25 Johnson, W. D., Hoffman, J. F., Jr., and Shore, R. T.: Myocardial Revascularization in the Absence of Cardiac Symptoms, *Am. J. Cardiol.*, 39:268, 1977. (Abstract.)

26 Wynne, J., Cohn, L. H., Collins, J. J., Jr., and Cohn, P. F.: Myocardial Revascularization in Patients with

Multivessel Coronary Artery Disease and Minimal Angina Pectoris, *Circulation,* 58 (suppl. 1):92, 1978.

27 Thurer, R. L., Lytle, B. W., Cosgrove, D. M., and Loop, F. D.: Asymptomatic Coronary Artery Disease Managed by Myocardial Revascularization: Five-Year Results, *Circulation,* 58 (suppl. 2):18, 1978. (Abstract.).

28 DeWood, M. A., Spores, J., Notske, R. N., et al.: Medical and Surgical Management of Myocardial Infarction, *Am. J. Cardiol.,* 44:1356, 1979.

29 Phillips, S. J., Zeff, R. H., Kongtahworn, C., et al.: Surgery for Evolving Myocardial Infarction, *J.A.M.A.,* 248:1325, 1982.

30 Boineau, J. P., and Cox, J. L.: Rationale for a Direct Surgical Approach to Control Ventricular Arrhythmias: Relation of Specific Intraoperative Techniques to Mechanism and Location of Arrhythmic Circuit, *Am. J. Cardiol.,* 49:381, 1982.

31 McCollum, C. H., Garcia-Rinaldi, R., Graham, J. M., and DeBakey, M. E.: Myocardial Revascularization Prior to Subsequent Major Surgery in Patients with Coronary Artery Disease, *Surgery,* 81:302, 1977.

32 Crawford, E. S., Morris, G. C., Jr., Howell, J. F., Flynn, W. F., and Moorhead, D. T.: Operative Risk in Patients with Previous Coronary Artery Bypass, *Ann. Thorac. Surg.,* 26:215, 1978.

33 Ennix, C. L., Lawrie, G. M., Morris, G. C., Jr., et al.: Improved Results of Carotid Endarterectomy in Patients with Symptomatic Coronary Disease: An Analysis of 1,546 Consecutive Carotid Operations, *Stroke,* 10:122, 1979.

34 DeBakey, M. E., and McCollum, C. H., III: Coronary Artery Bypass Procedures, *Compr. Ther.,* 1:14, 1975.

35 Lawrie, G. M., Morris, G. C., Jr., Chapman, D. W., Winters, W. L., and Lie, J. T.: Patterns of Patency of 596 Vein Grafts up to Seven Years after Aorta-Coronary Bypass, *J. Thorac. Cardiovasc. Surg.,* 73:443, 1977.

36 Lawrie, G. M., Lie, J. T., Morris, G. C., Jr., and Beazley, H. L.: Vein Graft Patency and Intimal Proliferation after Aortocoronary Bypass: Early and Long-Term Angiopathologic Correlations, *Am. J. Cardiol.,* 38:856, 1976.

37 Lie, J. T., Lawrie, G. M., and Morris, G. C., Jr.: Aortocoronary Bypass Saphenous Vein Graft Atherosclerosis: Anatomic Study of 99 Vein Grafts from Normal and Hyperlipoproteinemic Patients up to 75 Months Postoperatively, *Am. J. Cardiol.,* 40:906, 1977.

38 Reduto, L. A., Lawrie, G. M., Reid, J. W., et al.: Sequential Postoperative Assessment of Left Ventricular Performance with Gated Cardiac Blood Pool Imaging following Aortocoronary Bypass Surgery, *Am. Heart. J.,* 101:59, 1981.

39 Lawrie, G. M., and Morris, G. C., Jr.: Combined Coronary and Carotid Revascularization, in L. Cohn (ed.), ''Modern Technics in Surgery: Cardiac/Thoracic Surgery,'' Futura Publishing Company, New York, 1980, vol. 4, chap. 33, p. 1.

40 Lawrie, G. M., Morris, G. C., Jr., Silvers, A., Jr., et al.: The Influence of Residual Disease after Coronary Bypass on the 5-Year Survival of 1274 Men with Coronary Artery Disease, *Circulation,* 66:717, 1982.

41 DeBakey, M. E., and Lawrie, G. M.: Factors Influencing the Course of Myocardial Ischemia after Coronary Arterial Bypass, 1983, in press.

42 Lawrie, G. M., Morris, G. C., Jr., Howell, J. F., Tredici, T. D., and Chapman, D. W.: Improved Survival after 5 Years in 1,144 Patients after Coronary Bypass Surgery, *Am. J. Cardiol.,* 42:709, 1978.

43 Lawrie, G. M., Morris, G. C., Jr., Howell, J. F., Hines, M., and Chapman, D. W.: Improved Survival beyond 5 Years after Coronary Bypass in Patients with Left Main Coronary Artery Disease, *Am. J. Cardiol.,* 44:612, 1979.

44 Lawrie, G. M., Morris, G. C., Jr., Calhoon, J. H., et al.: Clinical Results of Coronary Bypass in 500 Patients At least 10 Years after Operation, *Circulation,* 66 (suppl. 1):1, 1982.

45 Lawrie, G. M., Morris, G. C., Jr., Howell, J. F., et al.: Results of Coronary Bypass More than 5 Years after Operation in 434 Patients: Clinical, Treadmill Exercise, and Angiographic Correlations, *Am. J. Cardiol.,* 40:665, 1977.

46 Bourassa, M. G., Lespérance, J., Corbara, F., Saltiel, J., and Campeau, L.: Progression of Obstructive Coronary Artery Disease 5 to 7 Years after Aortocoronary Bypass Surgery, *Circulation,* 58 (suppl. 1):100, 1978.

47 Bruschke, A. V. G., Wijers, T. S., Kolsters, W., and Landmann, J.: The Anatomic Evolution of Coronary Artery Disease Demonstrated by Coronary Arteriography in 256 Nonoperated Patients, *Circulation,* 63:527, 1981.

Coronary Artery Bypass Surgery: The Mayo Clinic Experience[*]

HARTZELL V. SCHAFF, M.D.,
GORDON K. DANIELSON, M.D.,
JAMES R. PLUTH, M.D.,
THOMAS A. ORSZULAK, M.D.,
FRANCISCO J. PUGA, M.D.,
JEFFREY M. PIEHLER, M.D., and
JAMES H. CHESEBRO, M.D.

Through the decade of the seventies myocardial revascularization by direct coronary artery bypass grafting (CAB) has become an established therapy for patients with symptomatic ischemic heart disease. Many surgeons, including Carrel, Beck, and Vineberg, deserve recognition for the pioneering efforts which laid the foundation for coronary artery bypass surgery.[1-3] Although Sabiston in 1962[4] and Garrett in 1964[5] used autogenous saphenous vein for coronary artery bypass, major credit for development of the operation as we know it today is owed to Favaloro[6] and Johnson et al.[7] From its inception, coronary artery bypass surgery has had its champions and its critics. The skepticism of some cardiologists was, perhaps, justified in view of the surgical predecessors, such as internal mammary ligation and pericardial poudrage.[8-11] Initially these operations were enthusiastically endorsed, only later to be proved of little value when subjected to more scientific scrutiny. Cautionary editorials and articles have called for controlled, randomized studies to establish the efficacy of direct coronary artery revascularization in relieving angina and in prolonging patient survival.[12-14] In retrospect, the early pleas for carefully controlled examination of coronary artery bypass surgery have been prophetic, particularly in regard to the widespread application and enormous cost of CAB. It was estimated that in 1980, 110,000 coronary artery bypass operations were performed in the United States at a cost of $15,000 to $20,000 per operation.[15] Surgical treatment of coronary artery disease thus accounts for as much as $2 billion per year in health care costs (or about 1 percent of total health care expenditures).[16] It is true also that coronary artery bypass has become one of the most intensively studied surgical procedures ever. Investigators have compared medical and surgical treatment of coronary artery disease using a variety of techniques including retrospective controls, case-matched controls, and randomized prospective designs.[17-19] The Veterans Administration

Cooperative Study, the European Cooperative Study on Coronary Artery Surgery, the Coronary Artery Surgery Study sponsored by the National Heart, Lung, and Blood Institute are three large multicentered trials directly comparing medical and surgical therapy for patients with angina pectoris.[20-22] These studies have received considerable attention from the medical community as well as the lay press. Although the early results of these trials do not satisfy every clinician, the wealth of information entered prospectively and in a uniform manner has provided an enormous data base for evaluation of coronary artery surgery. In light of these trials we believe that reports from single institutions might best focus on problems in coronary artery surgery which will not be solved by the large randomized trials because of duration of follow-up or, as in the case of graft patency, because these factors have not been incorporated into design of the larger trials. This paper will present an overview of coronary artery surgery at the Mayo Clinic and analyze in detail (1) survival and functional status of patients followed 10 to 12 years after CAB, (2) experience with repeat coronary revascularization, and (3) recent results of a platelet-inhibitor drug trial to improve graft patency after CAB.

From 1969 through 1980, 3,978 patients underwent isolated coronary artery bypass surgery at the Mayo Clinic. Clinical and angiographic features are presented in Table 1. Of our patients 86 percent were men and 50 percent had a myocardial infarction prior to revascularization. Clinical diagnosis of congestive heart failure was made in 25 percent of patients prior to surgery. Almost all patients had significant angina pectoris preoperatively, and 87 percent were New York Heart Association class III or IV. Over half of the patients had three-vessel involvement, and 16 percent of patients had significant (≥ 50 percent) stenosis of the left main coronary artery. During the entire period there were 90 hospital deaths, giving a mortality rate of 2.26 per-

*Mayo Medical School, Rochester, Minnesota.

TABLE 1

Clinical and angiographic characteristics of 3,978 patients undergoing isolated coronary artery bypass at the Mayo Clinic from 1969 through 1980

Clinical characteristics

Mean age (yr)	57
Sex:	
Men	86%
Women	14%
Previous myocardial infarction	50%
Congestive heart failure	25%

Angina classification—NYHA

I	1%
II	12%
III	61%
IV	26%

Coronary artery anatomy

No. of vessels with ≥ 50% stenosis:	
One-vessel disease	12%
Two-vessel disease	36%
Three-vessel disease	52%
Left main coronary artery stenosis ≥ 50%	16%

Left ventricular function

Cardiothoracic ratio ≥ 0.50	13%
Left ventricular ejection fraction (%):	
0–39	10%
40–49	17%
50–59	26%
60–69	26%
≥ 70	21%
Left ventricular end-diastolic pressure (mmHg):	
< 10	13%
10–19	55%
20–29	28%
≥ 30	4%

cent. Causes of hospital death are listed in Table 2. Six additional patients died after discharge but within 30 days of operation (30-day mortality rate 2.41 percent). Some aspects of patient selection for CAB have changed during the years of this review. Assuming patients are otherwise healthy and have significant (≥ 50 percent) stenosis in the proximal coronary arteries with adequate distal vessels for grafting, most symptomatic patients with two- or three-vessel involvement are now offered surgery as an option because of evidence that coronary artery bypass prolongs survival in these subgroups.[21] Management of patients with sin-

TABLE 2

Hospital deaths following isolated coronary artery bypass surgery

Cause	Number of patients
Myocardial failure and/or dysrhythmia	80
Pulmonary embolism	2
Stroke	2
Postoperative hemorrhage	1
Respiratory insufficiency	1
Mesenteric infarction	1
Ascending aortic dissection	1
Wound infection	1
Anesthetic accident	1
Total	90

gle-vessel involvement is individualized according to the amount of disability and estimate of size of the jeopardized myocardial segments. Patients with significant stenosis of the left main coronary artery, particularly those with left dominant circulation or disease in the dominant right coronary artery, are encouraged to undergo coronary artery bypass to improve long-term survival rate.[20] There are few, if any, absolute clinical contraindications for coronary artery revascularization. Poor left ventricular function increases operative risk, but rarely is operation withheld due to left ventricular dysfunction alone in a patient with severe angina pectoris. There is some evidence that mechanical performance of ischemic myocardial segments may be improved after successful revascularization.[24,25] In addition, we have accepted some patients with severe chronic obstructive pulmonary disease, renal failure, or coexisting metabolic disorders. Timing of coronary artery bypass surgery following myocardial infarction remains controversial. We would operate early after myocardial infarction in patients who had evidence of residual myocardial ischemia manifested by unstable angina or strongly positive rehabilitation exercise tests.[23] Mortality rate among 157 patients who underwent coronary revascularization within 60 days of acute myocardial infarction was 4.4 percent. In 76 percent of patients myocardial infarction was subendocardial, and in the remainder there was evidence of transmural injury. Of these patients 72 percent had unstable angina. We favor revascularization on a semiurgent basis for patients with unstable angina not responsive to maximal medical measures. Intraaortic balloon counterpulsation prior to surgery for unstable angina is used infrequently.

Since earlier reports,[26] several trends are noteworthy in anesthetic and operative management of patients undergoing CAB. Generally antianginal medications are maintained preoperatively up to the time of anesthesia. During the period immediately prior to cardiopulmonary bypass maintenance of hemodynamic stability is crucial,[27] and monitoring pulmonary artery pressure in addition to systemic arterial pressure and electrocardiogram is indicated in most patients. Operative technique has become standardized. During cardiopulmonary bypass systemic hypothermia to 20 to 25°C is utilized. All distal anastomoses are completed during a single period of aortic cross-clamping using continuous sutures of no. 7–0 Prolene. Occasionally smaller, more diseased vessels require anastomosis with interrupted no. 7–0 silk sutures, and the interrupted technique is utilized for internal mammary artery grafts. Most proximal anastomoses are made using a partial occlusion clamp on the ascending aorta with the heart in a beating, nonworking state. In recent years the circular sequential vein graft described by Grondin has been used selectively.[28] Myocardial protection using cardioplegia and topical hypothermia is an important feature of the coronary artery bypass operation.[29] Measuring septal temperature we inject cardioplegia solution (4°C) into the proximal aortic root immediately after aortic cross-clamping. Repeat infusions of cardioplegia and repeat application of ice saline are given at 20- to 30-min intervals during the cross-clamp period. There has been a general trend toward bypassing more coronary arteries in patients with multiple-vessel disease; with the use of sequential grafts, we have bypassed as many as eight distal coronary arteries in order to achieve "complete revascularization."

LATE RESULTS

To determine the survival and functional status late after coronary artery bypass grafting we reviewed 500 consecutive patients operated upon between 1969 and 1972.[30] The mean age of the patients was 52 years, and 91 percent were men. Prior to surgery 46 percent of patients had a history of previous myocardial infarction, and 88 percent were New York Heart Association class III or IV with angina. As seen in Table 3, 16 percent of patients had one-vessel disease, 38 percent had two-vessel disease, and 46 percent had three-vessel disease. Fifteen percent of patients had significant stenosis of the left main coronary artery. Sixty-six per-

TABLE 3

Follow-up of 500 patients 10 to 12 years following coronary artery bypass surgery*

	One	Two	Three
Percent by number of vessels diseased (≥ 50% stenosis)	16	38	46
Percent by number of vessels grafted	34	50	16

*Distribution of patients according to the number of diseased coronary arteries and the number of arteries grafted.

cent of patients had two or more saphenous vein bypass grafts. In this early series overall hospital mortality rate was 2.5 percent. Three hundred twenty-six patients had postoperative angiographic assessment of 595 saphenous vein bypass grafts.[31] Overall patency for patients studied during the first month after surgery was 89 percent.

Postoperatively, 484 patients survived more than 1 month, and follow-up was obtained in 483 patients. At the time of last contact 355 patients were living, 88 patients had died due to cardiac-related problems, 20 patients had died due to noncardiac-related diseases, and 7 patients had died of causes possibly related to cardiac disease. In 13 patients the cause of death could not be determined. Figure 1 shows late survival rate stratified according to the number of diseased vessels. Survival rate for patients with one-, two-, and three-vessel disease 5 years after surgery was 96, 93, and 90 percent, respectively. Survival rate 10 years postoperatively was 89, 75, and 62 percent. In Table 4 patient

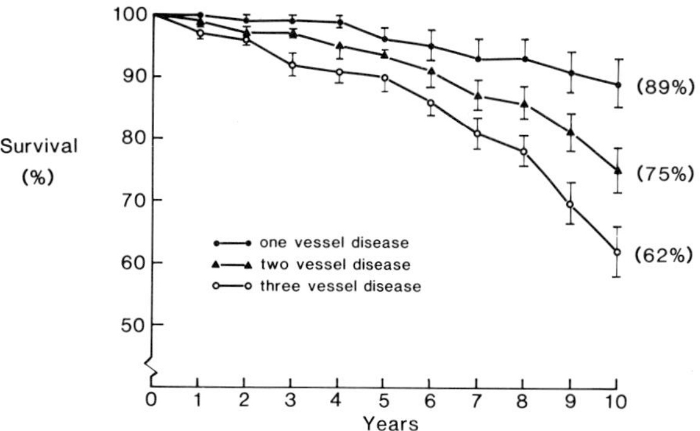

FIGURE 1 Late survival rate following coronary artery bypass surgery in 500 patients stratified according to the number of diseased coronary arteries. This analysis includes only those patients who survived hospitalization. (*From H. V. Schaff, B. J. Gersh, J. R. Pluth, et al., Survival and Functional Status after Coronary Artery Bypass Grafting: Results 10–12 Years Postoperatively in 500 Patients, submitted to Circulation. Used with permission of the American Heart Association, Inc.*)

TABLE 4
Survival of 500 patients following coronary artery bypass expressed as a percentage of that expected from a "normal" age-matched population

	Percent survival				
	Years postoperatively				
Number of vessels diseased	1	3	5	7	10
One vessel	100	102	102	102	102
Two vessels	99	100	99	97	89
Three vessels	99	96	97	91	75

survival rate is expressed as a percentage of that expected for age- and sex-matched population for the same decade. On univariate analysis several variables significantly influenced late survival rate. As seen in Table 5, the extent of coronary artery disease (number of vessels diseased) is the most predictive variable governing late survival rate. In addition, severity of congestive heart failure, presence of previous myocardial infarction, advanced age, presence of diseased ungrafted arteries, and severity of preoperative angina adversely affected 10-year survival rate. Interestingly, variables which were not predictive of late survival rate included sex, presence of left main coronary artery stenosis, and perioperative infarction. When those variables chosen from univariate analysis were analyzed by stepwise linear discriminant analysis (Cox model), the following combination was found to be the best independent predictor of survival: extent of coronary artery disease, severity of congestive heart failure, severity of angina pectoris, and presence of myocardial infarction before coronary artery bypass.

Persistence or recurrence of any angina during the 10- to 12-year follow-up period was reported in 49 per-

TABLE 5
Variables influencing 10-year survival following saphenous vein coronary artery bypass*

	Chi-square	p value
No. of vessels diseased ($\geq$ 50% stenosis)	23.17	.000
Congestive heart failure (NYHA class I–IV)	14.33	.0002
History of preoperative myocardial infarction	13.76	.0002
Age	9.26	.0023
No. of diseased but ungrafted arteries	8.54	.0035
Severity of angina pectoris (NYHA class I–IV)	6.07	.0137

*Variables not predictive were sex, presence of left main stenosis $\geq$ 50%, and perioperative infarction.

SOURCE: From Ref. 52. Used with permission of the American Heart Association, Inc.

cent of patients with one-vessel disease, 51 percent of patients with two-vessel disease, and 55 percent with three-vessel disease. A similar trend was noted for the reported incidence of late postoperative myocardial infarction. For patients with one-vessel disease the incidence of myocardial infarction during the 10-year period was 15 percent, whereas 24 percent of patients with three-vessel disease gave a history of postoperative myocardial infarction ($p = .06$). Eleven percent of patients underwent repeat revascularization during the 10-year follow-up period. There was no difference in frequency of postoperative angina recurrence, myocardial infarction, or need for reoperation when patients were stratified according to the presence or absence of left main coronary artery stenosis ($\geq$ 50 percent). Event-free survival rate was determined using recurrence of angina, repeat coronary artery bypass, myocardial infarction, or cardiac-related death as events. We then used the same variables listed in Table 5 to determine predictors of event-free survival. The single variable which significantly influenced event-free survival was the presence of diseased ungrafted arteries ($p < .0008$). Patients with two- or three-vessel disease were categorized as having complete or incomplete revascularization. As seen in Fig. 2, for patients with complete revascularization (no diseased ungrafted arteries) 5-year survival rate was 94 percent. For patients with incomplete revascularization (one or two

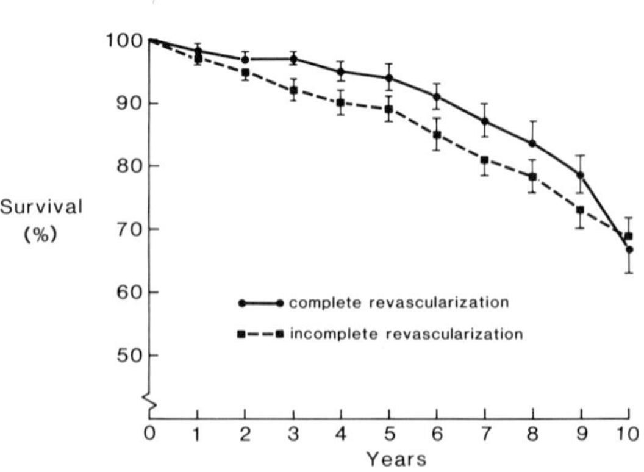

FIGURE 2 Late survival rate following coronary artery bypass surgery among patients with complete and incomplete revascularization. This analysis includes only those patients with two-vessel or three-vessel disease. Patients were considered to have complete revascularization when the number of coronary artery bypass grafts equaled or exceeded the number of diseased coronary arteries. In patients with incomplete revascularization, one or more diseased coronary arteries remained ungrafted postoperatively. (See text for further details.) (*From H. V. Schaff, B. J. Gersh, J. R. Pluth, et al., Survival and Functional Status after Coronary Artery Bypass Grafting: Results 10–12 Years Postoperatively in 500 Patients, submitted to Circulation. Used with permission of the American Heart Association, Inc.*)

diseased ungrafted arteries) 5-year survival rate was 89 percent. This small difference in survival was not maintained over the second 5-year interval, and 10-year survival for both groups was approximately 67 percent. The most common event in the follow-up period was recurrence of angina, and a separate analysis compared the number of diseased ungrafted arteries to the frequency of angina recurrence. As seen in Table 6, when the number of bypass grafts exceeded the number of diseased coronary arteries (using a three-vessel scoring system), the frequency of angina recurrence during the 10-year follow-up period was 33 percent. In these patients the size of secondary branches of the three main coronary arteries permitted individual grafts so that patients with three-vessel disease may have received four grafts, patients with two-vessel disease received three grafts, etc. With one or two diseased but ungrafted arteries, frequency of angina recurrence 10 years postoperatively was 54 and 68 percent. The increased frequency of angina recurrence was significantly associated with the number of diseased ungrafted arteries ($p = .025$).

Of the 355 patients alive at the end of the follow-up period, 69 percent stated they were improved compared to their preoperative angina class, 19 percent were symptomatically unchanged, and 12 percent had more severe angina than preoperatively. Ten years postoperatively 299 patients were under age 65 years. Of these patients 58 percent were working full- or part-time. Thirty-four percent stated that they were unable to work due to their heart condition, and 8 percent of patients were unable to work due to other health problems.

These late results from our earliest series of patients undergoing coronary artery bypass may not be representative of the current practice of coronary artery surgery due to differences in patient selection, anesthetic management, and operative techniques. Several aspects of the follow-up data are, however, pertinent to the present review. First is the remarkable similarity between these results and the other published 10-year survival figures from the Cleveland Clinic and from Baylor University in Houston (Table 7).[32,33] Second,

TABLE 6
Frequency of angina recurrence stratified according to the number of diseased ungrafted coronary arteries

	Number of ungrafted arteries with $> 50\%$ stenosis			
	−1	0	1	2
Incidence of angina recurrence (10 years postoperatively)	33%	52%	54%	68%

SOURCE: From Ref. 52. Used with permission of the American Heart Association, Inc.

TABLE 7
Percent 10-year survival following coronary artery bypass including hospital mortality

No. of vessels diseased	Mayo Clinic (1969–1972)	Cleveland Clinic[32] (1967–1970)	Baylor-Houston[33] (1969–1970)
One	88	81	78
Two	77	76	69
Three	59	62	48

SOURCE: From Ref. 52. Used with permission of the American Heart Association, Inc.

these late follow-up data suggest that coronary artery bypass grafts improve rate of survival compared to medically treated patients. Although there are many pitfalls in comparing nonrandomized groups, natural history studies indicate that annual mortality rate for patients with three-vessel disease may be as high as 11 percent per year.[34] In the present series, annual mortality rate at the 10-year period for patients with three-vessel disease is approximately 4 percent, *including* operative deaths. It has been proposed that current methods of medical therapy, including the use of beta-adrenergic blockers and long-acting nitrates, may improve survival rate in medically treated patients.[35] Nevertheless, it is important to note that in the registry of the Coronary Artery Surgery Study (CASS), the 4-year survival of medically treated patients with three-vessel disease was 68 percent, an annual mortality rate of 8 percent per year.[35] Further evidence of the favorable effect of bypass surgery is seen in follow-up patients with significant stenosis of the left main coronary artery. In such patients treated surgically the effect of left main coronary artery disease on long-term survival was eliminated.

A third important issue raised in this review is the detrimental effects of incomplete revascularization on long-term symptomatic results. This earlier series contains a larger proportion of patients who by current standards would be considered to be incompletely revascularized, that is, having one or more diseased but ungrafted arteries. The presence of diseased but ungrafted arteries was the most important determinant of event-free survival over the 10-year period. Because serial angiographic data were not available in all patients, our definition of complete revascularization applies only to the initial number of grafts inserted compared to the number of diseased coronary arteries. The significant influence of the number of coronary arteries diseased on late survival rate in surgically treated patients may also be related to incomplete revascularization, which occurred most frequently in patients with three-vessel involvement. In our series a poor survival rate in patients with incomplete revascularization was apparent at 5 years, and this might account for the difference in rate of survival of the patients when strat-

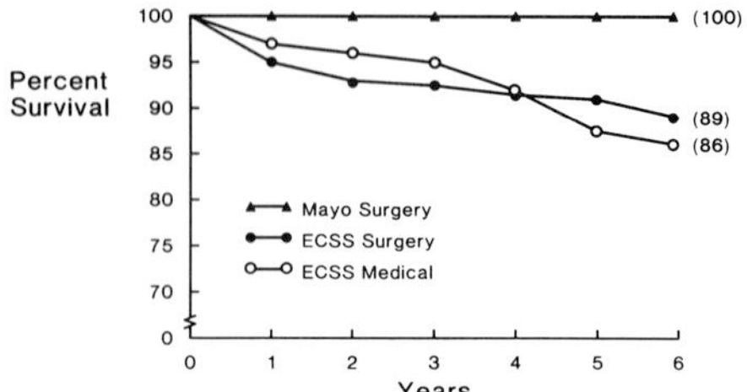

FIGURE 3 Survival rate of patients with two-vessel disease from the European Coronary Surgery Study (ECSS)[21] and from the Mayo Clinic surgical series. The patients included in the Mayo surgical group were those who fit the entrance criteria for the cooperative study during the years of the trial.

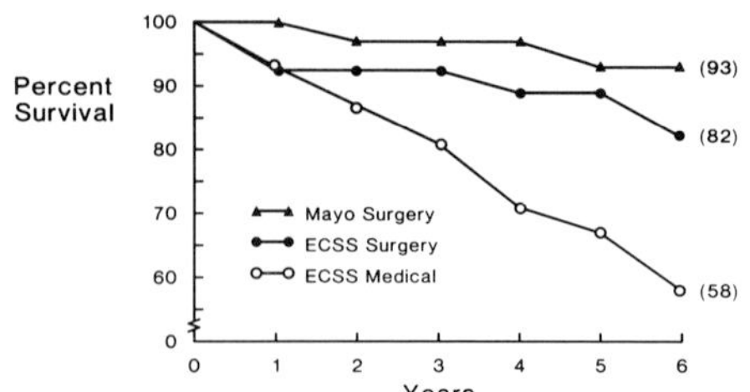

FIGURE 5 Survival rate of patients with left main coronary artery disease from the European Coronary Surgery Study (ECSS)[21] and from the Mayo Clinic surgical series. The patients included in the Mayo surgical group were those who fit the entrance criteria for the cooperative study during the years of the trial.

ified according to the number of diseased arteries. There were even greater differences in survival rate 10 years postoperatively in patients with one-, two-, or three-vessel disease. Yet at this time there is virtually no difference in survival rate among patients with complete or incomplete revascularization. This leads us to conclude that the progression of atherosclerosis in the native coronary arteries and vein-graft attrition are important factors in survival late after coronary artery bypass. With current surgical techniques, the number of patients with diseased ungrafted arteries following operation is low.

It is probable that 10-year results from patients undergoing surgery using current techniques will be even better than those previously described. For example, we have analyzed our results in surgically treated patients eligible for the European Coronary Surgery Study group.[21] Entrance criteria were as follows: (1) men under the age of 65; (2) angina pectoris of at least 3 months' duration; (3) greater than 50 percent obstruction in at least two major coronary arteries; (4) left ventricular ejection fraction greater than 50 percent. Patients with severe angina pain not controlled by medical therapy were excluded.[21] We applied these criteria to our surgical patients undergoing operation

between 1973 and 1976 for purposes of comparison. Six-year survival rates in the Mayo Clinic surgical patients eligible for the European study are shown in Figs. 3, 4, and 5. In each subgroup survival rate in our surgical patients compares favorably with the patients in the European Cooperative Study. The 6-year survival rate in patients with two-vessel disease was 100 percent, and in patients with three-vessel disease was 98 percent. For patients with left main coronary artery stenosis survival rate in the Mayo Clinic surgical group was 93 percent at 6 years.

Reoperation for coronary artery disease As previously discussed, during a 10-year period following initial revascularization as many as 11 percent of patients will become candidates for repeat coronary artery surgery. At the Mayo Clinic the number of reoperations for coronary artery bypass has increased

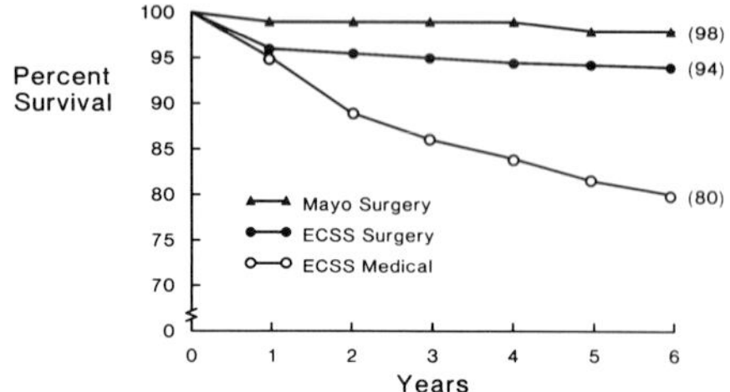

FIGURE 4 Survival rate of patients with three-vessel disease from the European Coronary Surgery Study (ECSS)[21] and from the Mayo Clinic surgical series. The patients included in the Mayo surgical group were those who fit the entrance criteria for the cooperative study during the years of the trial.

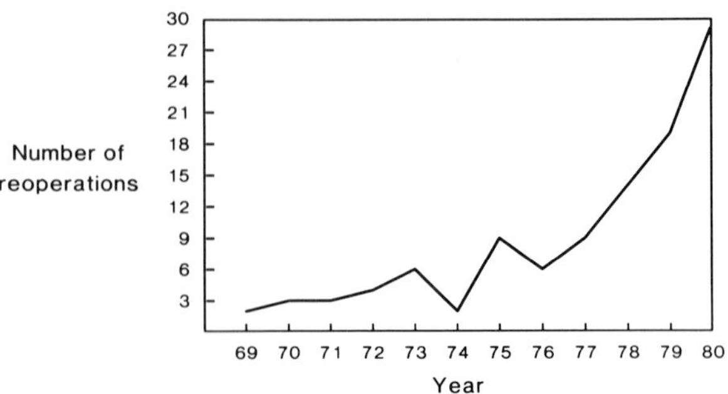

FIGURE 6 The number of second operations for coronary artery disease has increased steadily at our institution. Reoperations accounted for 6.2 percent of all revascularization procedures in 1980. (*From H. V. Schaff, T. A. Orszulak, B. J. Gersh, et al., The Morbidity and Mortality of Reoperation for Coronary Artery Disease and Analysis of Late Results with Use of Actuarial Estimate of Event-Free Interval, J. Thorac. Cardiovasc. Surg., 85:508, 1983. Used with permission.*)

steadily (Fig. 6). In order to define the morbidity and mortality rates of reoperation, the early and late results among the 106 patients who underwent a second revascularization during this 11-year period were reviewed.[36] During this interval, three patients underwent a third operation, and a single patient underwent a fourth operation, but these patients were excluded from the following analysis. There were 96 men and 10 women, mean (± standard deviation) age was 49 ± 8 years (range, 25 to 65 years). Before the first operation all patients had angina pectoris; 8 patients were New York Heart Association (NYHA) class II, 70 patients were in class III, and 28 patients were in class IV (Table 8). Fifty-seven patients (54 percent) had had a documented myocardial infarction before their first revascularization. The distribution of patients according to the number of diseased coronary arteries is shown in Table 9. With the exclusion of patients who had internal mammary artery implants, the average number of coronary arteries bypassed at the first operation was 2.0 per patient. At the time of repeat revascularization, 95 percent of patients were in New York Association class III or IV. Risk factors for coronary atherosclerosis among patients undergoing reoperation are listed in Table 10. The percentages of patients having diabetes mellitus, lipid abnormalities, and hypertension are similar to those from larger groups of patients undergoing primary revascularization.[37] Patients were classified as having recurrent angina due to bypass graft occlusion, progression of atherosclerotic disease in native coronary arteries, diseased but unbypassed arteries at initial operation, or combinations of these factors. As might be expected, more patients had severe three-vessel involvement at the time of reoperation than they did at the time of the first revascularization (Table 9). However, progression of atherosclerotic disease alone was thought to be the cause of recurrent angina in only 9.4 percent of patients (Table 11). The most frequent causes of recurrent angina were bypass graft occlusion alone and in combination with progressive proximal disease (60 patients, 56.6 percent). Marked difference was noted in the interval to the onset of angina as analyzed by the cause

of recurrence. The mean interval to onset of angina in patients who had bypass graft occlusion, diseased but unbypassed arteries at the initial operation, and the combination of unbypassed arteries and bypass graft occlusion was 16 months or less. When recurrent angina was due to progression of atherosclerotic disease, either alone or in combination with other factors, including graft occlusion, the mean interval to onset of angina ranged from 16.4 to 51.6 months. Bypass graft occlusion was noted to be a major cause of recurrent angina in 60 percent of patients.

In our series of repeat coronary artery bypass operations there were three early deaths within 30 days of reoperation for a mortality rate of 2.8 percent. All deaths were due to complications of myocardial infarction. Significant complications included perioperative infarction in eight patients (7.5 percent) and significant low cardiac output in eight patients (7.5 percent). Five patients required reexploration for bleeding. An average of 2.2 coronary arteries were bypassed per patient (Table 12).

At the time of last follow-up (mean, 43 months) 93 patients were living, 5 died of cardiac causes, and 2 died of nonrelated cardiac causes; 2 patients' deaths were judged as possibly due to cardiac causes. Fifty-nine patients had recurrence of angina pectoris, and 23 patients had symptoms of congestive heart failure. The actuarial survival rate of patients dismissed alive

TABLE 8

Results of reoperation for coronary artery disease. Symptomatic status before surgery

New York Heart Association class	Number of patients	
	Before first operation	Before reoperation
I	0	2
II	8	3
III	70	61
IV	28	40

SOURCE: From Ref. 53. Used with permission.

TABLE 9

Extent of coronary artery disease in patients undergoing reoperation for coronary artery disease

Number of diseased coronary arteries	Number of patients	
	Before first operation	Before reoperation
1	20	6
2	33	19
3	53	81

SOURCE: From Ref. 53. Used with permission.

TABLE 10

Risk factors for atherosclerosis among patients undergoing reoperation for coronary artery disease

	Number of patients	Percent
Hypertension	27	25.5
Lipid abnormalities	22	20.8
Diabetes mellitus	4	3.8
Cigarette smoking:		
Continued to smoke	40	37.7
Stopped after first operation	31	29.2
Smoked < 10 pack-years	5	4.7
Never smoked	27	25.5
Unknown	3	2.8

SOURCE: From Ref. 53. Used with permission.

TABLE 11

Cause of recurrence of angina in patients undergoing reoperation for coronary artery disease

	No. of patients	Percent	Mean interval to onset of angina (MOS)
Bypass graft occlusion alone	31	29.2	12.8 ± 19.6
Bypass graft occlusion and progression of disease	29	27.4	51.6 ± 28.3
Unbypassed arteries and progression of disease	19	17.9	16.4 ± 23.7
Progression of disease alone	10	9.4	39.4 ± 28.3
Unbypassed arteries, progression of disease, and bypass graft occlusion	7	6.6	22.1 ± 10.5
Diseased but unbypassed arteries alone	5	4.7	16.0 ± 27.7
Unbypassed arteries and bypass graft occlusion	5	4.7	4.5 ± 3.1

SOURCE: From Ref. 53. Used with permission.

after reoperation for coronary artery disease is 94 percent at 5 years and 89 percent at 7 years. As seen in Fig. 7, all late cardiac-related deaths occurred in patients who had three-vessel disease at reoperation. Event-free survival rate was calculated using end points of cardiac-related death, myocardial infarction, reoperation (a third revascularization), and recurrence of angina. A similar survival curve was constructed in which angina was included as an end point only when patients were New York Heart Association class III or IV; that is, unimproved by reoperation. As illustrated in Fig. 8, the predicted event-free survival rate (freedom from cardiac-related death, myocardial infarction, reoperation, or any angina) is 28 percent at 5 years and 26 percent at 7 years. When mild angina (class II) is not included as a major cardiac event, estimated event-free survival rate was 63 percent at 5 and 7 years.

TABLE 12

Results of reoperation for coronary artery disease

Number of coronary arteries bypassed	Number of patients	
	First operation	Reoperation
0	12*	1
1	30	42
2	35	44
3	24	16
4	5	2
5	0	1

*These 12 patients had an internal mammary artery implant only.
SOURCE: From Ref. 53. Used with permission.

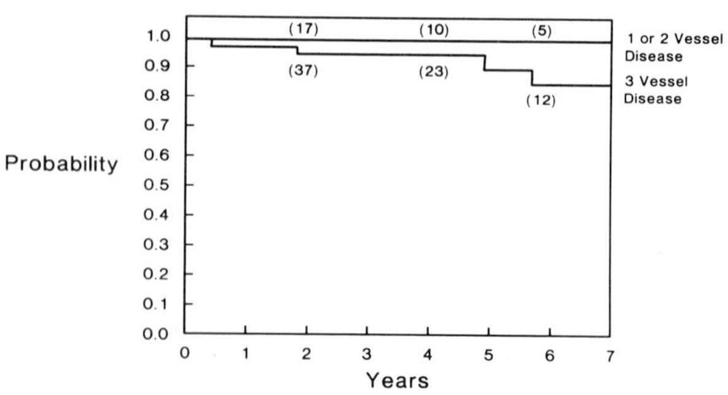

FIGURE 7 Probability of survival rate (cardiac-related deaths) is 94 percent at 5 years and 89 percent at 7 years. All deaths occurred in patients with three-vessel involvement. Numbers in parentheses indicate patients at risk at each interval. (*From H. V. Schaff, T. A. Orszulak, B. J. Gersh, et al., The Morbidity and Mortality of Reoperation for Coronary Artery Disease and Analysis of Late Results with Use of Actuarial Estimate of Event-Free Interval, J. Thorac. Cardiovasc. Surg., 85: 508, 1983. Used with permission.*)

These results suggest that reoperation for second coronary artery bypass is a worthwhile endeavor for many patients. Although operative mortality rate is slightly higher than that of initial operation, it is low enough to justify an aggressive approach in evaluation of recurrent angina. In our series, vein-graft occlusion is a major cause of recurrent angina. We did not, however, observe technical failure because of misidentification of target vessels at the original operation. The

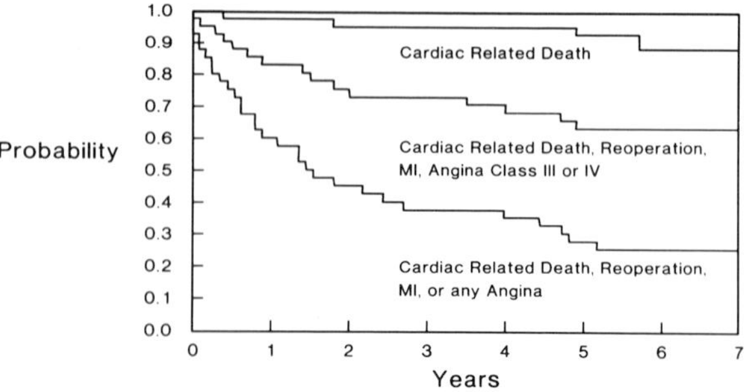

FIGURE 8 Event-free survival rate was computed with cardiac-related death (top curve) as an end point, in addition to reoperation (third revascularization), myocardial infarction (MI), and recurrence of angina. The probability of remaining free of any of these cardiac events is 26 percent at 7 years. However, when mild angina (New York Heart Association class II) is not included as a serious cardiac event, event-free survival is 73 percent 3 years and 63 percent at 5 and 7 years. (*From H. V. Schaff, T. A. Orszulak, B. J. Gersh, et al., The Morbidity and Mortality of Reoperation for Coronary Artery Disease and Analysis of Late Results with Use of Actuarial Estimate of Event-Free Interval, J. Thorac. Cardiovasc. Surg., 85:508, 1983. Used with permission.*)

clinical course of most of our patients who suffered early graft failure was characterized by a variable interval of improvement preceding the recurrence of angina. Early bypass graft occlusion due to improper anastomotic techniques might be expected to result in poor intraoperative flows and little initial reduction of angina. At the time of restudy and reoperation, obvious technical problems leading to graft closure were observed infrequently. In addition, restudy in patients with symptoms often demonstrated vein-graft narrowing but patent distal anastomoses and adequate runoff in the bypassed vessel. This supports the concept that vein-graft failures are primarily due to graft thrombosis, intimal proliferation, or vein-graft atherosclerosis. Even in patients who had progression of disease in native coronary arteries in addition to vein-graft closure, graft failure was seldom caused by new occlusive disease distal to the bypass graft. This impression is consistent with the findings of Guthaner and associates who evaluated patients 5 to 8 years after coronary artery surgery.[38] In their study, vein-graft narrowing occurred in 30 percent of patients during the follow-up period and was not predicted by anastomotic problems in the early postoperative angiograms. In most of their patients who had anastomotic narrowings (which one might expect to lead to vein-graft occlusions), vein grafts remained unchanged and patent. These findings emphasize the need for careful technique during removal of the saphenous vein to minimize intimal injury. In addition, measures such as administration of platelet-inhibiting agents may prevent late vein-graft obstruction and significantly improve long-term relief of angina after saphenous vein bypass grafting.

Platelet-inhibiting drugs for coronary bypass operation Analysis of patients 10 to 12 years following CAB and consideration of etiologies of unsuccessful revascularizations among patients undergoing reoperation for coronary artery disease underscore the importance of bypass graft patency in achieving angina relief and freedom from recurrent myocardial infarction and cardiac-related death. While we recognize that atherosclerosis is a progressive disease, we believe that the majority of coronary artery bypass graft failures are due to inherent problems with the saphenous vein conduit. In this regard the internal mammary artery graft is generally acknowledged to have a high initial patency rate and to be free of late complications such as intimal proliferation or atherosclerosis.[39] This conduit, however, is not useful in all patients and may have inadequate inflow for large coronary arteries.[40] For this reason we reserve the use of the internal mammary artery for bypass of arteries on the anterior surface of the heart with anticipated flows of 50 mL/min or less or for those patients who have inadequate veins. During the first year after surgery the risk of vein-graft

occlusion is 15 to 20 percent but only approximately 2 to 3 percent per year thereafter.[41] Because vein-graft occlusion after operation appears to be the result of platelet deposition, mural thrombus formation, and intimal proliferation, all of which can be suppressed by dipyridamole and aspirin, there has been considerable interest in platelet-inhibitor drugs to enhance early vein-bypass-graft patency. Earlier studies on the efficacy of platelet-inhibitor drugs for coronary artery bypass operations yielded variable results as might be predicted from the widely varying protocols.[42–47] At the Mayo Clinic a large prospective randomized clinical trial of dipyridamole plus aspirin has been performed by Chesebro et al.[48] From September 1977 through March 1981, 407 patients undergoing saphenous vein coronary artery bypass surgery were entered into the drug trial. After giving informed written consent, the patients were randomized to study medication (dipyridamole and aspirin) or placebo in a double-blind fashion. Treated patients received dipyridamole (100 mg) orally four times a day for 2 days before operation. On the day of operation they received dipyridamole (100 mg) orally at 6 A.M., dipyridamole (100 mg) through a nasogastric tube 1 h after operation, and dipyridamole (75 mg) plus aspirin (325 mg) down a nasogastric tube 7 h after the operation. On the day following surgery and daily thereafter patients received dipyridamole (75 mg) and aspirin (325 mg) orally three times a day (Table 13). The preoperative characteristics of the patients are listed in Table 14. The operative procedure was carried out using standard techniques as previously outlined. Saphenous vein grafts were gently irrigated with heparinized saline during preparation. Distal anastomoses were performed during the single period of aortic cross-clamping utilizing systemic hypothermia and multidose cold potassium cardioplegia. Running no. 6–0 or 7–0 Prolene sutures were used for distal anastomoses, and proximal anastomoses were performed using no. 5–0 Prolene. Early postoperative vein angiograms were

TABLE 13

Platelet-inhibitor therapy for aortocoronary vein bypass operations*

Starting 2 days before operation:
  Dipyridamole 100 mg orally qid
Day of operation:
  6 A.M.—dipyridamole 100 mg orally
   1 h after operation—dipyridamole 100 mg, down nasogastric tube (clamp 1½ h)
   7 h after operation—dipyridamole 75 mg and aspirin 325 mg, down nasogastric tube (clamp 1½ h)
Day after operation:
  Dipyridamole 75 mg and aspirin 325 mg orally tid

*No other aspirin or prostaglandin-inhibiting drugs.

TABLE 14
Preoperative characteristics of patients in the platelet-inhibitor drug trial*

	Treatment group	Placebo group
Number of patients	176	184
Mean age (yr) (range)	55 (34–68)	57 (35–68)

	No. of patients (% of group)	
Age > 60 yr	48 (27)	63 (34)
Men	161 (91)	162 (88)
Family history of CAD < 55 yr	63 (35)	73 (40)
Hypertension	56 (32)	61 (33)
Smoking:		
Never	35 (20)	33 (18)
Past	116 (66)	132 (72)
Within 1 wk of surgery	23 (13)	19 (10)
Previous myocardial infarction:		
Transmural	63 (36)	59 (32)
Subendocardial	23 (13)	15 (8)
Peripheral arterial disease	11 (6)	11 (6)
Severity of angina (NYHA functional class):		
I or II	25 (14)	24 (13)
III or IV	148 (84)	155 (84)
Unrelated to exertion	3 (2)	5 (3)

	Median (range)	
Severity of CAD (Gensini score[49])	89 (8–250)	85 (2–224)

*CAD denotes coronary artery disease, and NYHA the New York Heart Association.
SOURCE: From Ref. 54. Used with permission.

performed in 360 of the 407 patients (88 percent) 8 days (median) after operation. The mean number of coronary arteries bypassed per patient was 2.8 in both groups, and an increase in the number of distal anastomoses per patient was observed from the first half of this trial (2.5 per patient) to the second half (3.1 per patient). The number of saphenous vein grafts (individual, sequential, and Y-branch) per patient was 2.1 in the treatment group and 2.0 in the placebo group. Patency rates were calculated for patients, for distal an-

astomoses, and for grafts. Comparisons were made for groups stratified according to sex, risk factors, types of grafts, and interval between operation and angiography.

Treatment with aspirin and dipyridamole resulted in a striking improvement in bypass graft patency. Within 1 month of operation, patency rate per distal anastomosis in the treatment group was 97 percent (341 of 351) versus 90 percent (324 of 362) in the placebo group. The patency rates per distal anastomosis were higher

TABLE 15
Vein bypass patency stratified according to the type of graft

	Number patent of total number (% patent)	
	Treatment group	Placebo group
Type of graft:		
Individual grafts only	224 of 231 (97)	172 of 214 (80)
Sequential grafts only	111 of 115 (97)	126 of 143 (88)
Individual and sequential grafts	118 of 125 (94)	117 of 130 (90)
Y-grafts and individual or sequential grafts	16 of 17 (94)	26 of 33 (79)
Total number of patent distal anastomoses	469 of 488 (96)	421 of 520 (85)

SOURCE: From Ref. 54. Used with permission.

among treatment patients in all subgroups organized by type of grafts (Table 15), number of individual grafts, location of grafts, vein-graft blood flow, or coronary artery diameter (Tables 16 and 17). Considering all patients evaluated within 6 months of operation patency was 96 percent in the treatment group (479 of 488 distal anastomoses) compared to 85 percent in the placebo group (471 of 520 distal anastomoses).

The benefit of aspirin and dipyridamole in patients with individual vein grafts was maintained 1 year postoperatively.[50] There were 101 patients who had individual grafts with early (within 1 month) and late (1 year later) vein-graft angiograms. Patency in the treatment group was 92 percent at the end of 1 year (190 of 207) compared to 78 percent in the control group (123 of 170).[50]

This randomized prospective study documented the effectiveness of perioperative administration of dipyridamole and aspirin in improving patency of saphenous vein bypass grafts. Other investigators have used dipyridamole and aspirin and found no effect on vein-graft patency.[43,44] These previous studies, however, began therapy 1 to 4 days after surgery. In the Mayo Clinic trial, the strategy of platelet-inhibitor therapy was to intervene in the thrombotic process which begins immediately with platelet deposition during the operation.[51] Importantly, there was no difference in postoperative blood loss or transfusion requirements comparing the treatment and control groups. For patients in whom aspirin is contraindicated, dipyridamole is continued, 100 mg qid, postoperatively.

TABLE 16
Patency of all individual vein grafts stratified according to vessel bypassed*

| | Number patent of total number (% patent) | | | |
	Treatment group		Placebo group	
Angiography < 10 days:				
LAD	78 of 78	(100)	53 of 59	(90)
RCA	65 of 69	(96)	48 of 54	(89)
LCX	60 of 62	(97)	40 of 47	(85)
Diagonal	7 of 7	(100)	4 of 5	(80)
Other	1 of 1	(100)	1 of 1	(100)
Total	211 of 217	(97)	146 of 166	(88)
Angiography < 6 months:				
LAD	101 of 104	(97)	78 of 99	(79)
RCA	89 of 94	(95)	78 of 91	(86)
LCX	73 of 76	(96)	59 of 75	(79)
Diagonal	9 of 9	(100)	6 of 7	(86)
Other	1 of 1	(100)	1 of 1	(100)
Total	273 of 284	(96)	222 of 273	(81)

*LAD = left anterior descending coronary artery; RCA = right coronary artery; LCX = left circumflex coronary artery.
SOURCE: From Ref. 54. Used with permission.

TABLE 17
Patency of all individual vein grafts stratified according to blood flow and coronary artery lumen diameter

| | Number patent of total number (% patent) | | | |
	Treatment group		Placebo group	
Blood flow (mL/min):				
≤ 40	45 of 51	(97)	42 of 64	(66)
41–80	129 of 131	(98)	108 of 131	(82)
> 80	91 of 93	(98)	66 of 70	(94)
Total*	264 of 275	(96)	216 of 265	(82)
Lumen diameter (mm):				
≤ 1.0	11 of 13	(85)	10 of 16	(62)
> 1.0–1.5	129 of 135	(94)	102 of 130	(78)
> 1.5–2.0	101 of 102	(99)	79 of 94	(84)
> 2.0	16 of 16	(100)	21 of 21	(100)
Total*	257 of 266	(97)	212 of 261	(81)

*Measurement was not performed in all individual grafts (284 and 273 total grafts in the treatment and placebo groups, respectively).
SOURCE: From Ref. 54. Used with permission.

SUMMARY

Experience from the Mayo Clinic supports the major role for coronary artery bypass surgery in the management of patients with ischemic heart disease. Operative risk is low, and late survival rate and symptomatic improvement are excellent. Refinement in operative and anesthetic techniques have resulted in safer operations and more complete revascularization in patients with multivessel involvement. Perioperative administration of antiplatelet agents dramatically improves patency of individual vein bypass grafts 1 year postoperatively. Late survival rate of patients undergoing operation today may be significantly better than in previous series, thus encouraging the continued and perhaps wider application of coronary revascularization for the management of ischemic heart disease.

REFERENCES

1 Carrel A.: La Technique Opératoire des Anastomoses Vasculaires et de la Transplantation des Vicères, *Lyon Med.*, 98:859, 1902.

2 Beck, C. S.: Revascularization of the Heart, *Ann. Surg.*, 128:854, 1948.

3 Vineberg, A. M., Miller, W. D.: An Experimental Study of the Physiological Role of an Anastomosis between the Left Coronary Circulation and the Left Internal Mammary Artery Implanted in the Left Ventricular Myocardium, *Surg. Forum.*, 1:294, 1950.

4 Sabiston, D. C., Jr.: The Coronary Circulation, *Johns Hopkins Med. J.*, 134:314, 1974.

5 Garrett, H. E., Dennis, E. W., DeBakey, M. E.: Aorto-coronary Bypass with Saphenous Vein Graft: Seven-Year Follow-up, *J.A.M.A.*, 223:792, 1973.

6 Favaloro, R. G.: Saphenous Vein Graft in the Surgical Treatment of Coronary Artery Disease: Operative Technique, *J. Thorac. Cardiovasc. Surg.*, 58:178, 1969.

7 Johnson, W. D., Flemma, R. J., Lepley, D., Jr., et al.: Extended Treatment of Severe Coronary Artery Disease: A Total Surgical Approach, *Ann. Surg.*, 170:460, 1969.

8 Battezzati, M., Tagliaferro, A., Cattaneo, A. D.: Clinical Evaluation of Bilateral Internal Mammary Artery Ligation As Treatment of Coronary Heart Disease, *Am. J. Cardiol.*, 4:180, 1959.

9 Björk, L., Cullhed, I., Hallén, A., et al.: Result of Internal Mammary Artery Implantation in Patients with Angina Pectoris, *Scand. J. Thorac. Cardiovasc. Surg.*, 2:1, 1968.

10 Beecher, H. K.: Surgery As Placebo: A Quantitative Study of Bias, *J.A.M.A.*, 176:1102, 1961.

11 Cobb, L. A., Thomas, G. I., Dillard, D. H., et al.: An Evaluation of Internal-Mammary-Artery Ligation by a Double-blind Technic, *N. Engl. J. Med.*, 260:1115, 1959.

12 Spodick, D. H.: Revascularization of the Heart—Numerators in Search of Denominators, *Am. Heart J.*, 81:149, 1971.

13 Braunwald, E.: Direct Coronary Revascularization. A Plea Not to Let the Genie Escape from the Bottle, *Hosp. Practice*, 6:9, 1971.

14 Braunwald, E.: Coronary-Artery Surgery at the Crossroads, *N. Engl. J. Med.*, 297:661, 1977.

15 Kolata, G. B.: Consensus on Bypass Surgery, *Science*, 211:42, 1981.

16 Weinstein, M. C., Stason, W. B.: Cost-effectiveness of Coronary Artery Bypass Surgery, *Circulation*, 66 (suppl. 3):56, 1982.

17 Loop, F. D., Cosgrove, D. M., Lytle, B. W., et al.: An 11-Year Evolution of Coronary Arterial Surgery 1967–1978, *Ann. Surg.*, 190:444, 1979.

18 DeRouen, T. A., Hammermeister, K. E., and Dodge, H. T.: Comparisons of the Effects on Survival after Coronary Artery Surgery in Subgroups of Patients from the Seattle Heart Watch, *Circulation*, 63:537, 1981.

19 Kloster, F. E., Kremkau, E. L., Ritzmann, L. W., et al.: Coronary Bypass for Stable Angina: A Prospective Randomized Study, *N. Engl. J. Med.*, 300:149, 1979.

20 Read, R. C., Murphy, M. L., Hultgren, H. N., et al.: Survival of Men Treated for Chronic Stable Angina Pectoris: A Cooperative Randomized Study, *J. Thorac. Cardiovasc. Surg.*, 75:1, 1978.

21 European Coronary Surgery Study Group: Prospective Randomised Study of Coronary Artery Bypass Surgery in Stable Angina Pectoris: Second Interim Report, *Lancet*, 2:491, 1980.

22 The Principal Investigators of CASS and their Associates: The National Heart, Lung, and Blood Institute Coronary Artery Surgery Study (CASS), *Circulation*, 63(suppl. 1):81, 1981.

23 Madigan, N. P., Rutherford, B. D., Barnhorst, D. A., et al.: Early Saphenous Vein Grafting after Subendocardial Infarction. Immediate Surgical Results and Late Prognosis, *Circulation*, 56(suppl. 2):1, 1977.

24 Vlietstra, R. E., Chesebro, J. H., Frye, R. L., et al.: Improvement of Left Ventricular Exercise Hemodynamic Function after Aorta-Coronary Bypass Graft, *J. Thorac. Cardiovasc. Surg.*, 81:85, 1981.

25 Chesebro, J. H., Ritman, E. L., Frye, R. L. et al.: Videometric Analysis of Regional Left Ventricular Function before and after Aortocoronary Artery Bypass Surgery: Correlation of Peak Rate of Myocardial Wall Thickening with Late Postoperative Graft Flows, *J. Clin. Invest.*, 58:1,339, 1976.

26 Danielson, G. K., Gau, G. T., Davis, G. D.: Early Results of Vein Bypass Grafts for Coronary Artery Disease, *Mayo Clin. Proc.*, 48:487, 1973.

27 Tarhan, S., Raimundo, H. S.: Coronary Circulation and Anesthesia for Coronary Artery Bypass Graft Surgery, in S. Tarhan (ed.), "Cardiovascular Anesthesia and Postoperative Care," Year Book Medical Publishers, Inc., Chicago, 1982, chap. 8, p. 227.

28 Grondin, C. M., Vouhé, P., Bourassa, M. G., et al.: Optimal Patency Rates Obtained in Coronary Artery Grafting with Circular Vein Grafts, *J. Thorac. Cardiovasc. Surg.*, 75:161, 1978.

29 Berger, R. L., Davis, K. B., Kaiser, G. C., et al.: Preservation of the Myocardium during Coronary Artery Bypass Grafting, *Circulation*, 64(suppl. 2):61, 1981.

30 Schaff, H. V., Gersh, B. J., Pluth, J. R., et al.: Survival and Functional Status after Coronary Artery Bypass Grafting: Results 10–12 Years Postoperatively in 500 Patients, submitted to *Circulation*.

31 Assad-Morell, J. L., Frye, R. L., Connolly, D. C., et al.: Aorta-Coronary Artery Saphenous Vein Bypass Surgery: Clinical and Angiographic Results, *Mayo Clin. Proc.*, 50:379, 1975.

32 Cosgrove, D. M., Loop, F. D., and Sheldon, W. C.: Results of Myocardial Revascularization: A 12-Year Experience, *Circulation*, 65(suppl. 2):37, 1982.

33 Lawrie, G. M., Morris, G. C., Jr., Calhoon, J. H., et al.: Clinical Results of Coronary Bypass in 500 Patients at Least 10 Years after Operation, *Circulation*, 66(suppl. 1):1, 1982.

34 Reeves, T. J., Oberman, A., Jones, W. B., et al.: Natural History of Angina Pectoris, *Am. J. Cardiol.* 33:423, 1974.

35 Mock, M. B., Ringvist, I., Fisher, L. D., et al.: Survival of Medically Treated Patients in the Coronary Artery Surgery Study (CASS) Registry; *Circulation*, 66:562, 1982.

36 Schaff, H. V., Orszulak, T. A., Gersh, B. J., et al.: The Morbidity and Mortality of Reoperation for Coronary Ar-

tery Disease and Analysis of Late Results with Use of Actuarial Estimate of Event-Free Interval, *J. Thorac. Cardiovasc. Surg.*, 85:508, 1983.

37 Kouchoukos, N. T., Oberman, A., Kirklin, J. W., et al.: Coronary Bypass Surgery: Analysis of Factors Affecting Hospital Mortality, *Circulation*, 62(suppl. 1):84, 1980.

38 Guthaner, D. E., Robert, E. W., Alderman, E. L., et al.: Long-term Serial Angiographic Studies after Coronary Artery Bypass Surgery, *Circulation*, 60:250, 1979.

39 Tector, A. J., Schmahl, T. M., Janson, B., et al.: The Internal Mammary Artery Graft. Its Longevity after Coronary Bypass, *J.A.M.A.*, 246:2181, 1981.

40 Flemma, R. J., Singh, H. M., Tector, A. J., et al.: Comparative Hemodynamic Properties of Vein and Mammary Artery in Coronary Bypass Operations, *Ann. Thorac. Surg.*, 20:619, 1975.

41 Hamby, R. I., Aintablian, A., Handler, M., et al.: Aortocoronary Saphenous Vein Bypass Grafts: Long-term Patency, Morphology and Blood Flow in Patients with Patent Grafts Early after Surgery, *Circulation*, 60:901, 1979.

42 Brown, B. G., Cukingnan, R. A., Goede, L., et al.: Improved Graft Patency with Antiplatelet Drugs in Patients for One Year Following Coronary Bypass Surgery, *Am. J. Cardiol.*, 47:494, 1981. (Abstract.)

43 McEnany, M. T., Salzman, E. W., Mundth, E. D., et al.: The Effect of Antithrombotic Therapy on Patency Rates of Saphenous Vein Coronary Artery Bypass Grafts, *J. Thorac. Cardiovasc. Surg.*, 83:81, 1982.

44 Pantely, G. A., Goodnight, S. H., Jr., Rahimtoola, S. H., et al.: Failure of Antiplatelet and Anticoagulant Therapy to Improve Patency of Grafts after Coronary-Artery Bypass. A Controlled, Randomized Study, *N. Engl. J. Med.*, 301:962, 1979.

45 Baur, H. R., VanTassel, R. A., Gobel, F. F. L.: Effect of Sulfinpyrazone on Early Graft Closure Rate after Myocardial Revascularization, *Circulation*, 59,60(suppl. 2):105, 1979. (Abstract.)

46 Mayer, J. E., Jr., Lindsay, W. G., Castaneda, W., et al.: Influence of Aspirin and Dipyridamole on Patency of Coronary Artery Bypass Grafts, *Ann. Thorac. Surg.*, 31:204, 1981.

47 Chesebro, J. H., and Fuster, V.: Drug Trials in Prevention of Occlusion of Aorta-Coronary Artery Vein Grafts, *J. Thorac. Cardiovasc. Surg.*, 83:90, 1982.

48 Chesebro, J. H., Clements, I. P., Fuster, V., et al.: A Platelet-Inhibitor-Drug Trial in Coronary-Artery Bypass Operations: Benefit of Perioperative Dipyridamole and Aspirin Therapy on Early Postoperative Vein-Graft Patency, *N. Engl. J. Med.*, 307:73, 1982.

49 Gensini G. G.: Coronary Arteriography, Futura Publishing Company, Mount Kisco, N.Y., 1975, p. 269.

50 Chesebro, J. H., Fuster, V., Clements, I. P., et al.: Perioperative Dipyridamole Plus Aspirin Therapy Improves Early Aortocoronary Vein Graft Patency with a Continued Late Effect on Individual Grafts, submitted for publication.

51 Josa, M., Lie, J. T., Bianco, R. L., et al.: Reduction of Thrombosis in Canine Coronary Bypass Vein Grafts with Dipyridamole and Aspirin, *Am. J. Cardiol.*, 47:1248, 1981.

52 Schaff, H. V. et al.: Survival and Functional Status after Coronary Artery Bypass Grafting: Results 10-12 Years Postoperatively in 500 Patients, *Circulation* (suppl), September, 1983.

53 Schaff, H. V. et al.: The Morbidity of Reoperation for Coronary Artery Disease and Analysis of Late Results with Use of Actuarial Estimate of Event-Free Interval, *J. Thorac. Cardiovasc. Surg.*, 85:508, 1983.

54 Chesebro, J. H. et al.: A Platelet-Inhibitor-Drug Trial in Coronary-Artery Bypass Operations: Benefit of Perioperative Diphyridamole and Aspirin Therapy on Early Postoperative Vein-Graft Patency, *N. Engl. J. Med.*, 307:73, 1982.

Experience with Coronary Bypass Surgery at the Brigham and Women's Hospital[*]

JOHN J. COLLINS, JR., M.D.,
LAWRENCE H. COHN, M.D., and
RICHARD J. SHEMIN, M.D.

Since July 1970 approximately 3,500 coronary bypass operations have been performed at the Peter Bent Brigham and Brigham and Women's Hospital.[1-6] About 600 coronary bypass operations are presently performed each year for angina pectoris, and an additional number of coronary bypass grafts are performed in patients undergoing surgery primarily for relief of valvular disease or manifestations of coronary artery obstruction other than angina pectoris.

INDICATIONS FOR MYOCARDIAL REVASCULARIZATION SURGERY

Current indications for coronary bypass surgery include the following symptom complexes or angiographic obstruction patterns:

Intractable Angina Pectoris

Angina pectoris is considered intractable when there is failure of medical management to control symptoms or when the side effects of medications necessary for symptom control preclude a satisfactory life-style.

Unstable Angina Pectoris

We consider angina pectoris to be unstable when symptoms have been present for less than 3 months, when there has been worsening of a previously stable angina pattern, when angina occurs at rest or at night, or when anginal pain lasts longer than 20 min, is poorly relieved by nitroglycerin, and is accompanied by reversible ST change (the intermediate coronary syndrome).

Hazardous Coronary Obstruction Pattern

Significant obstruction of the main left coronary artery is considered hazardous regardless of the accompanying symptoms. In addition, obstruction of the left anterior descending coronary artery before the first septal branch or combined obstructions of the proximal anterior descending and proximal dominant posterior coronary circulation are considered hazardous problems independent of the symptom complex. These coronary obstruction patterns, when identified in patients with even minimal symptoms, constitute an indication for myocardial revascularization surgery.

Intermittent Congestive Heart Failure Secondary to Myocardial Ischemia

We have seen a number of patients during the past 10 years with intermittent symptoms of pulmonary venous hypertension sometimes culminating in pulmonary edema due to global myocardial ischemia. This may occur without significant angina pectoris. Often these patients may have normal or near-normal exercise tolerance between episodes of severe congestive heart failure.

Impending or Evolving Acute Myocardial Infarction

Certain patients with symptoms and signs of acute myocardial infarction seen during the first several hours after onset of pain may be candidates for emergency myocardial revascularization; patients with global ischemic change during the first several hours of infarction who have no previous symptom of coronary heart disease should be considered urgent candidates for acute myocardial revascularization. In some instances it may be justifiable to proceed to revascularization surgery without coronary angiography.

Cardiogenic Shock

Patients in cardiogenic shock who are dependent upon intraaortic balloon counterpulsation for maintenance of cardiac output sufficient for peripheral organ per-

[*]From Department of Surgery, Brigham and Women's Hospital. This study was funded by the Brigham Surgical Group Foundation.

fusion may be candidates for emergency revascularization. To be a candidate, a patient should have a recent history of adequate myocardial contractility, adequate distal coronary arteries for grafting, or evidence of motion in at least 60 percent of the peripheral angiographically definable cardiac border area.

Acute Coronary Obstruction

When obstruction of a coronary artery occurs acutely in the cardiac catheterization laboratory and when such an accident is followed by symptoms and electrocardiographic signs of impending myocardial infarction, immediate revascularization is usually indicated.

Revascularization in Anticipation of Extracardiac Surgery

Patients having a stable pattern of angina pectoris who are faced with major extracardiac surgery (most often a peripheral vascular operation) in our institution have been advised to have coronary arteriography. If threatening coronary obstructive lesions are found, myocardial revascularization surgery is recommended before extracardiac surgery is attempted. In some instances, where the extracardiac operation is urgent, such an operation has been performed under the same anesthetic immediately following myocardial revascularization. We have used this approach particularly in operating upon abdominal aortic aneurysms with threatened rupture. Results have been excellent in this group. The most common indication for anticipatory or ancillary myocardial revascularization is seen in patients with valvular heart disease or other noncoronary lesions. It has become our policy to perform revascularization when significant obstructive lesions are seen in proximal coronary arteries in such patients. In our experience, elective cardiac operations combining coronary bypass with other intracardiac surgery do not carry a higher mortality rate. Emergency operations involving myocardial revascularization surgery and noncoronary cardiac surgery carry an extremely high mortality rate (approaching 50 percent). It thus seems advisable that patients known to have coronary heart disease should not be followed too long for other types of cardiac disease which may require operation. When the situation becomes urgent, the risk is higher than a similar degree of urgency would indicate in a patient without accompanying coronary obstruction.

There are perhaps some other instances in which myocardial revascularization surgery may be advised or undertaken. These eight categories, however, include the great majority. During the past several years we have undertaken emergency myocardial revascularization without preliminary angiography in a small group of patients. We feel this is justifiable in patients with immediately life-threatening ischemia when there is no prior history of coronary heart disease or when the prior history includes no significant evidence of heart failure immediately preceding the life-threatening event. Thus, patients with electromechanical dissociation, intractable arrhythmias, or profound shock early in the course of a first myocardial infarction may be candidates. It has become our policy to place a graft to the left anterior descending coronary artery as well as to the dominant posterior coronary arterial vessel. In most persons this will be the right coronary artery, but in some it may be the circumflex, or in some persons, when there are large posterior branches from the right and the circumflex, both vessels should be bypassed.

TECHNIQUE OF MYOCARDIAL REVASCULARIZATION

Our present technique includes general anesthesia (predominantly narcotic and oxygen) with precordial electrocardiographic monitoring. The heart is exposed through a median sternotomy simultaneous with excision of the greater saphenous vein through a series of 10- to 12-cm incisions in the leg. We prefer the vein between the groin and knee for most patients unless this vein exceeds 6 mm in internal diameter. In patients requiring multiple bypass grafts the vein is harvested from the groin to the mid-calf or slightly lower. The vein is irrigated with, and gently distended by, injection of heparinized Ringers lactate solution. Care is taken to be gentle in handling the vein, but we do not use special equipment to measure distending pressure. Venous branches are secured with metal clips rather than ligatures. We have found these clips to be quite satisfactory provided that two clips are placed on any branch 1 mm or greater in diameter. Tiny branches are secured by a single clip. We prefer veins without any evidence of varicosity but on occasion have used veins with small varices without apparent harm. We have not observed late development of an aneurysm in any vein graft.

We do not use direct anastomosis of the left internal mammary artery to the left anterior descending coronary artery as a routine revascularization procedure at the present time. We did several hundred such operations and, our conclusions were as follows:

1 The internal mammary artery is an adequate conduit for revascularization when the internal diameter is 1½ mm or greater or when the free flow from the cut distal end of the internal mammary artery is 40 mL/min or greater.

2 Following mobilization of the internal mammary artery patients have more severe chest pain lasting a longer time after surgery than patients who do not have such mobilization.

3 Some patients will have inadequate flow from the internal mammary artery resulting in the recurrence of angina pectoris despite apparently adequate flow at the time of operation and by subsequent angiography.

All distal anastomoses are performed before proximal aortic anastomoses with the ischemic heart protected by a 500-mL injection of cardioplegic solution into the aortic route. The solution we use is one-half-normal saline at 4°C containing 30 mEq/L potassium chloride buffered to pH 7.4 by addition of sodium bicarbonate. Most patients receive only an initial injection accompanied by topical hypothermia produced by constant drainage of normal saline at 4°C into the pericardial cavity through a sterilized nasogastric tube. When it appears that the ischemic interval may exceed 45 min, a second injection of cardioplegic solution (250 mL) is administered at 30 min following the beginning of ischemia. The usual ischemia interval for performance of three to four distal anastomoses is 30 to 35 min. An ischemic interval of 45 min is unusual, and longer than 60 min is rare.

Distal anastomoses are performed with no. 6-0 Prolene in a continuous fashion. Internal mammary artery anastomoses, when performed, are done either with continuous Prolene or interrupted braided Dacron suture. All obstructed coronary arteries having a diameter greater than 1 mm are considered appropriate for bypass grafts. Those vessels which have been totally obstructed and subsequently recanalized are usually not graftable. Coronary arteries which appear to supply entirely an area of mature scar usually have a very small lumen and are usually not grafted. The average number of distal anastomoses in patients having three-vessel disease presently averages 4.5. This number has gradually increased over the years, but probably will now remain stable.

Intraaortic balloon counterpulsation is only used before operations for patients with cardiogenic shock, or for occasional patients with congestive heart failure or unstable angina with left main coronary artery obstruction. Following myocardial revascularization surgery the intraaortic balloon is used only for those persons having left ventricular power failure.

RISKS OF MYOCARDIAL REVASCULARIZATION

The average probability of death within 30 days of operation for all patients undergoing coronary bypass surgery during the past 10 years is slightly greater than 2 percent. This risk of myocardial revascularization surgery has tended to remain stable over the years. One might believe that it should be gradually reduced, but because the seriousness of illness of the patients has increased proportionately to the improvement of technique, a stable mortality risk has resulted. The risk of significant complications, including neurological, infectious, or hemorrhagic, remains an aggregate of less than 3 percent. The vast majority of these patients eventually pursue a satisfactory course. The probability of perioperative myocardial infarction is approximately 2 percent when judged by the criterion of QRS alteration. About 12 percent of patients have either postoperative ST-segment abnormalities or a significant rise in serum enzymes without QRS change. Transient supraventricular arrhythmias occur in approximately 15 percent of patients and are rarely troublesome.

RESULTS OF MYOCARDIAL REVASCULARIZATION SURGERY

A representative sample of current results in coronary bypass surgery may best be obtained by consideration of all patients who underwent coronary bypass operations at the Peter Brent Brigham Hospital from July 1, 1970 through June 30, 1978. In this series were 1,241 patients, including 202 (16.2 percent) with left main obstruction, 567 (45.8 percent) with three-vessel obstruction, 340 (27.4 percent) with two-vessel obstruction, and 132 (10.6 percent) with single-vessel obstruction. There were 1,051 males and 190 females with an age distribution as shown in Fig. 1. The mean age of males was 52.3 years and of females 55.6 years. There was a tendency toward increased age with wider distribution of coronary obstructive lesions in the men, but this distribution was not definable among women. Distribution of coronary obstruction patterns in the

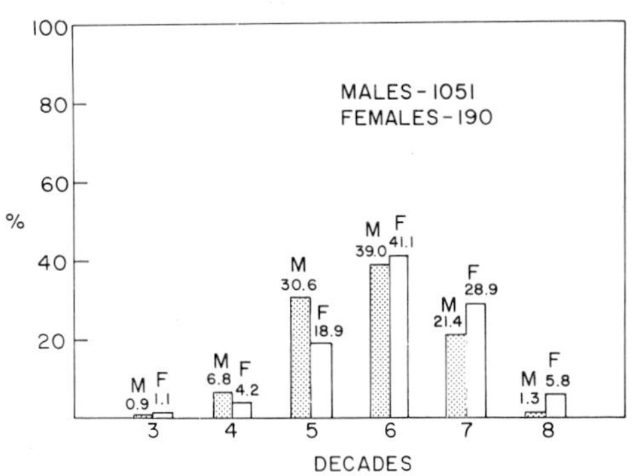

FIGURE 1 Age and sex distribution in 1,241 patients undergoing coronary bypass for angina.

series is shown in Table 1. There were 219 patients with unstable angina pectoris. The incidence of unstable angina pectoris among the various patterns of coronary obstruction is shown in Table 2. Of note is the fact that approximately 40 percent of patients with left main coronary obstruction presented with unstable angina. The probability of unstable angina pectoris for patients with three-vessel and two-vessel disease was about 12 percent. A higher percentage of presentation with unstable angina was observed among patients undergoing surgery for single-vessel disease because the principal indication for surgery in this group was unmanageable angina.

Results of operation were measured in terms of longevity, freedom from myocardial infarction, and freedom from recurrence or persistence of angina pectoris. Actuarial tables showing probability of survival in the total surgical series, patients with three-vessel disease, two-vessel disease, single-vessel disease, and left main coronary obstruction are shown in Figs. 2 to 9.

In Fig. 2, the probability of survival to 7 years after surgery for the entire group is shown. There were 1,241 patients operated upon and the mortality rate within 30 days of operation was 2.1 percent. When this operative mortality rate is included, the survival rate for the surgical group is slightly, but significantly ($p = .001$), less optimistic than for an age- and sex-corrected cohort of the general population. The probability of survival to 7 years following surgery (including operative mortality rate) for this group was approximately 84 percent.

For those persons with three-vessel disease (Fig. 3) the probability of survival to 7 years after surgery, including an operative mortality rate of 2.3 percent, was 83.2 percent. This was significantly lower than the longevity curve for the general population ($p = .01$). Comparison of survival rate in those persons with three-vessel disease who had more complete revascularization, as indicated by the performance of three or more bypass grafts, with those persons who had less complete revascularization is shown in Fig. 4 (see also Figs. 5 and 6). The operative mortality rate was 1.3

percent in those having three or more grafts and 4.1 percent in those having two or fewer grafts in the presence of three-vessel disease. However, the prognosis for survival to 7 years in both groups was not significantly different. Statistical significance was tested by both the Breslow and Mantell-Cox techniques in order to ascertain whether an early significant difference might exist even when the ultimate prognosis for survival was no different. It will be noted, however, that no difference in either early or late survival rate was observed. These data do not support the popular contention that better revascularization portends better survival rate. One possible explanation for this apparent discrepancy from other published reports may relate to the manner of selection of patients for more versus fewer grafts. In this series, every obstructed vessel having a lumen diameter of 1.5 mm or greater was bypassed. Only those vessels having a very small lumen or diffuse obliterative disease were rejected for grafting. It is our opinion that the prognosis for survival is related to the probability of a new myocardial infarction, and the probability of a new myocardial infarction is related to the presence of a significant blood supply subject to loss. It seems probable that those vessels rejected for bypass were either very small, very diffusely diseased, or supplied only areas of scar, so that the blood flow through them did not, even if lost in future, represent

TABLE 2

Incidence of unstable angina among various patterns of coronary obstruction

Classification	Patient distribution		
	Number	Unstable (no.)	Unstable (%)
Left main	202	80	39.6
Three-vessel	567	71	12.5
Two-vessel	340	39	11.5
One-vessel	130	29	22.0

TABLE 1

Distribution of coronary obstruction patterns in patients having CABG* surgery for angina at Peter Bent Brigham Hospital July 1970–June 1978

Classification	No. patients	Percent
Left main	202	16.2
Three-vessel	567	45.8
Two-vessel	340	27.4
One-vessel	132	10.6
Total	1,241	100.0

*CABG = coronary artery bypass grafting.

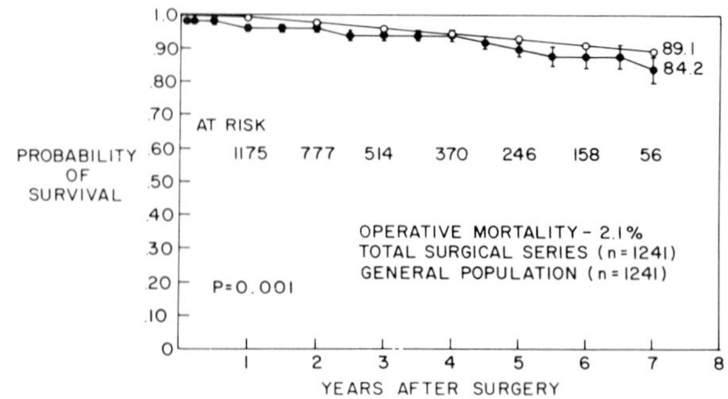

FIGURE 2 Actuarial curves showing comparison of longevity in coronary bypass patients compared to a computer-generated, age- and sex-matched survival probability.

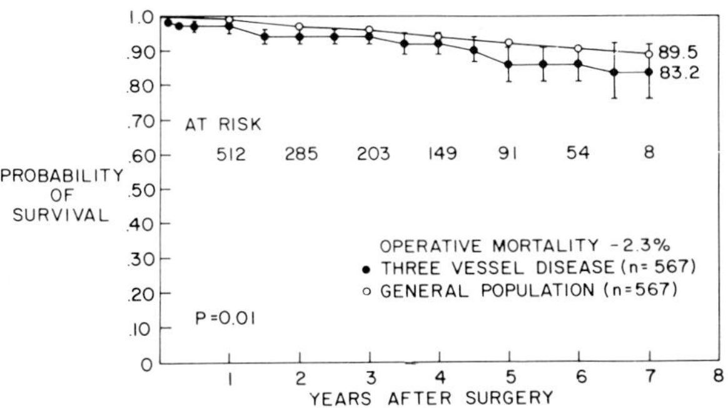

FIGURE 3 Actuarial curves showing comparison of survival probability in coronary bypass patients with three-vessel disease and a computer-generated, age- and sex-matched general population survival probability.

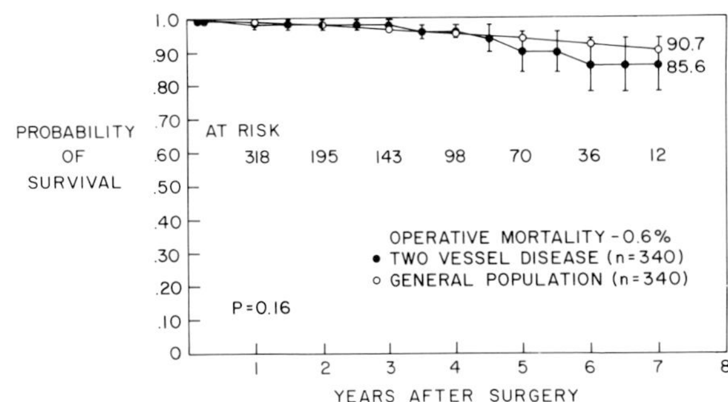

FIGURE 5 Probability of survival in coronary bypass patients with two-vessel obstruction compared to a computer-generated, age- and sex-matched general population curve.

a sufficiently serious deprivation to increase the probability of later myocardial infarction and possible death. If these presumptions are true, it should be unlikely that more complete revascularization would yield a higher short-term survival rate.

Patients having significant obstruction of two major coronary arteries had an operative mortality risk of 0.6 percent and a probability of survival of 85.6 percent. This probability of survival did not significantly differ (including operative risk) from the probability for survival of an age- and sex-matched cohort from the general population ($p = .16$). Comparison of those who had two or more grafts with those who had only one graft in the presence of significant two-vessel coronary obstruction showed no significant difference in rate of survival. The latter portion of these curves does tend to diverge, and a p value of .08 obtained with the Mantell-Cox technique of analysis suggests that further follow-up may show a significant difference in these groups. While the explanation for this observation is not perfectly clear, it may be that patients with two-vessel disease in time will become patients with three-vessel disease. Among those having two or more grafts, the additional perfusion may be a significant advantage in countering progression in previously insignificantly obstructed vessels. Whether this will be proved by further analysis remains to be seen.

Patients with single-vessel disease, as shown in Fig. 7, enjoyed a prognosis for survival which is virtually identical to that for the general population. The operative mortality rate in this group was 0.8 percent.

Patients with left main coronary artery obstruction having a variety of combinations of other lesions were considered as one group. The operative mortality rate was 5.0 percent and was more than twice as high in those with unstable angina as in those with stable symptoms operated upon electively. Even with this relatively high operative risk, the prognosis for survival to 6 years after operation was nearly 90 percent, and the longevity curve for the general population was intercepted at about 5 years after surgery, as shown in Fig. 8. Because of inclusion of the operative risk, it is apparent that the prognosis for survival in patients operated on for left main coronary obstruction must

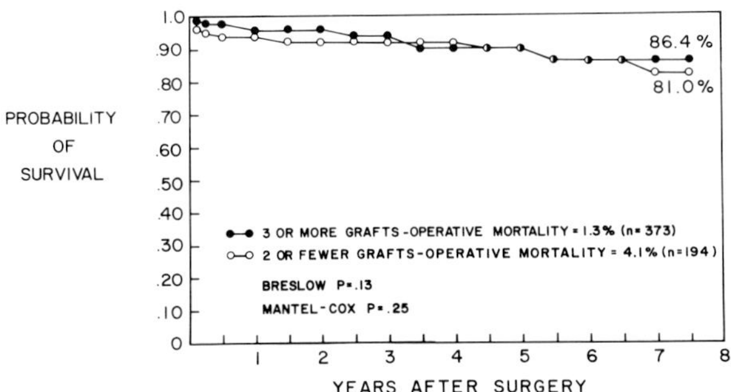

FIGURE 4 Comparison of survival probability in coronary bypass patients with three-vessel disease having more versus fewer grafts.

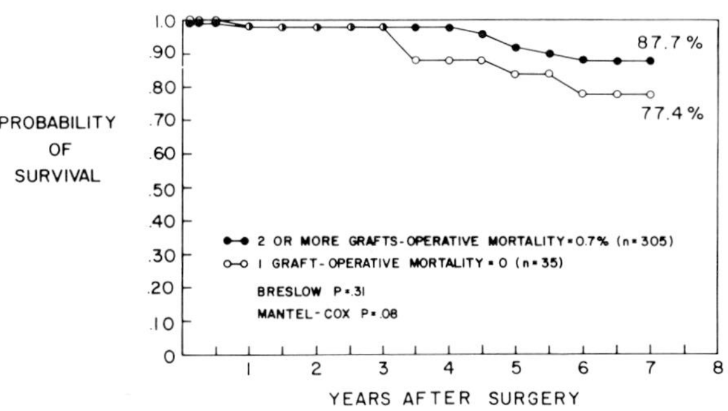

FIGURE 6 Comparison of survival probability in patients with two-vessel obstruction having two or more grafts compared with only one graft.

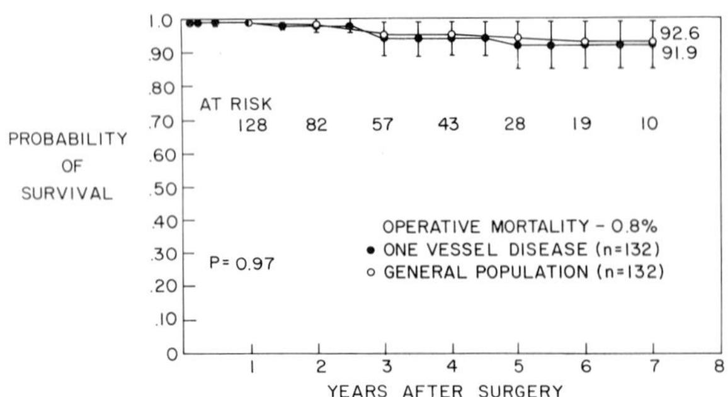

FIGURE 7 Probability of survival in patients with single-vessel disease after coronary revascularization compared with a computer-generated, age- and sex-matched general population sample.

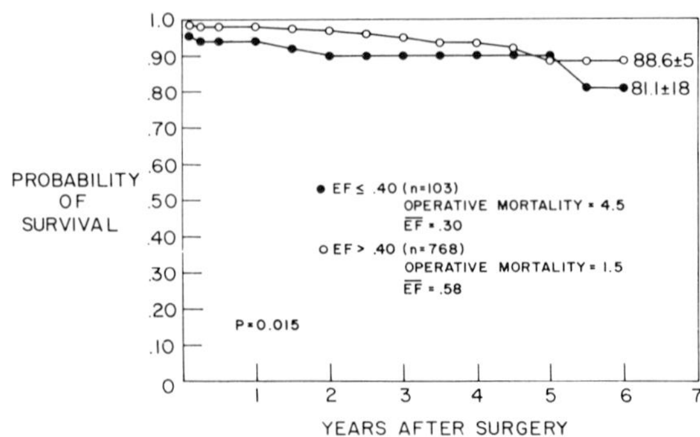

FIGURE 9 Comparison of survival probability in patients with "adequate" and "poor" ejection fractions.

actually be better over the 6 years following operation than the probability of survival for an age- and sex-corrected cohort of the general population. This may seem strange until it is considered that patients undergoing coronary bypass surgery have been carefully screened for elimination of other diseases, particularly malignant tumors, which are the principal short-term mortality risks in patients having similar age characteristics. These data support the concept that revascularization surgery for patients with left main coronary artery obstruction provides a major reversal of a serious risk factor, which is easily demonstrated over a relatively few years following operation.

In Fig. 9 the influence of ejection fraction on probability of survival in patients following coronary bypass surgery is depicted. For patients with an ejection fraction exceeding 0.40, the operative mortality rate was 1.4 percent. For those with an ejection fraction under 0.40 (average 0.30), the operative mortality rate was 4.5 percent. Despite these differences in the risk of operation, the probability of survival at 5 years after surgery was virtually identical. The higher operative mortality rate of patients with impaired left ventricular function accounts for the significant difference in rate of survival over the first several years following surgery. Survivors of operations, however, appear to have a similar prognosis whether the preoperative ejection fraction was high or low. This observation is consistent with the notion that mortality in patients following coronary bypass surgery is related to the occurrence of a new myocardial infarction. It appears that the probability of a new myocardial infarction is more closely related to the adequacy of arterial revascularization than to the impairment of muscular function. There is no specific reason to believe that adequacy of revascularization is impaired by preoperative myocardial damage.

Figures 10 to 17 pertain to the occurrence of myocardial infarction following revascularization surgery. These data were obtained by questionnaire, personal interview, and interview of attending physicians. Any "heart attack" was considered a proven myocardial

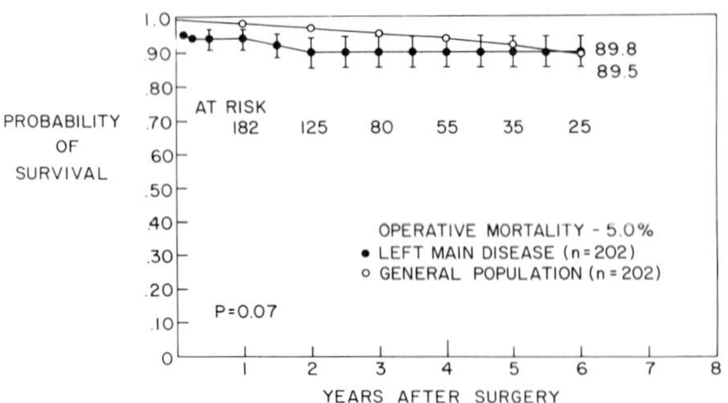

FIGURE 8 Actuarial curves showing survival of patients with left main coronary obstruction compared to a computer-generated age- and sex-matched general population survival probability.

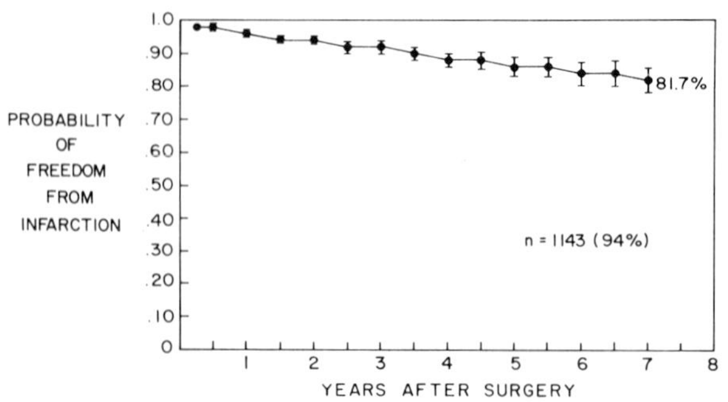

FIGURE 10 Probability of freedom from myocardial infarction after coronary bypass surgery.

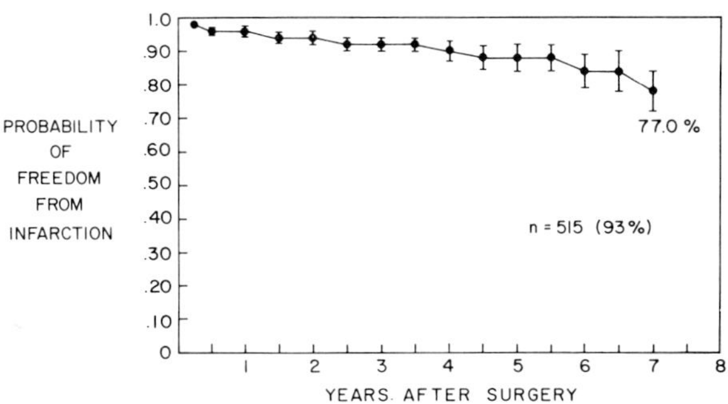

FIGURE 11 Probability of freedom from myocardial infarction in patients with three-vessel disease after coronary bypass surgery.

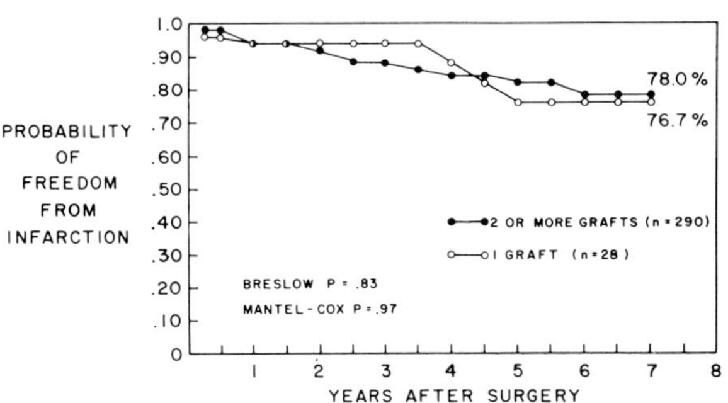

FIGURE 14 Comparison of probability of myocardial infarction in patients with more versus fewer grafts in two-vessel disease.

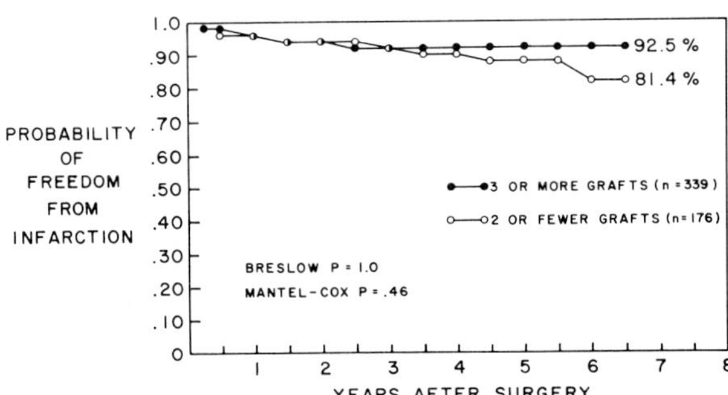

FIGURE 12 Comparison of probability of myocardial infarction in patients with more versus fewer bypass grafts.

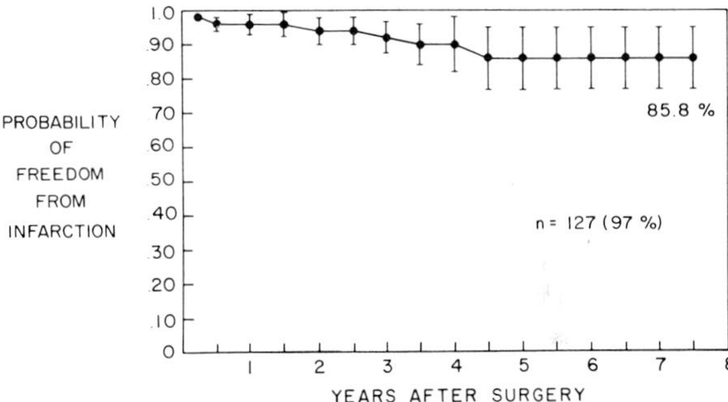

FIGURE 15 Probability of freedom from myocardial infarction following revascularization for single-vessel disease.

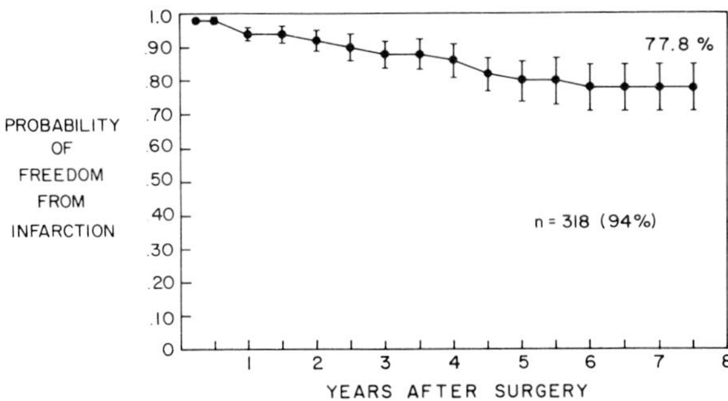

FIGURE 13 Probability of freedom from myocardial infarction in patients with two-vessel coronary obstruction.

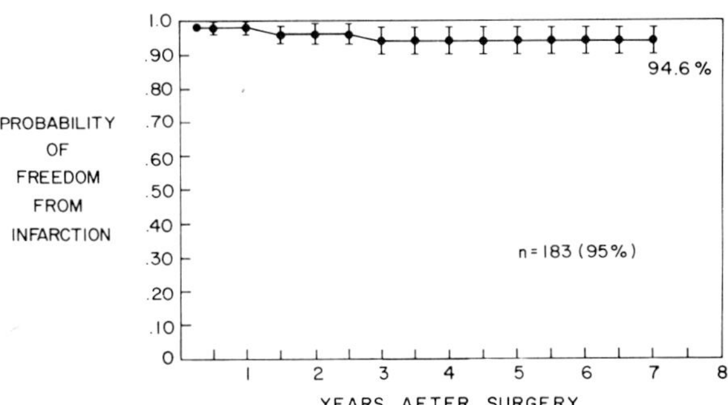

FIGURE 16 Probability of freedom from myocardial infarction following revascularization for left main coronary obstruction.

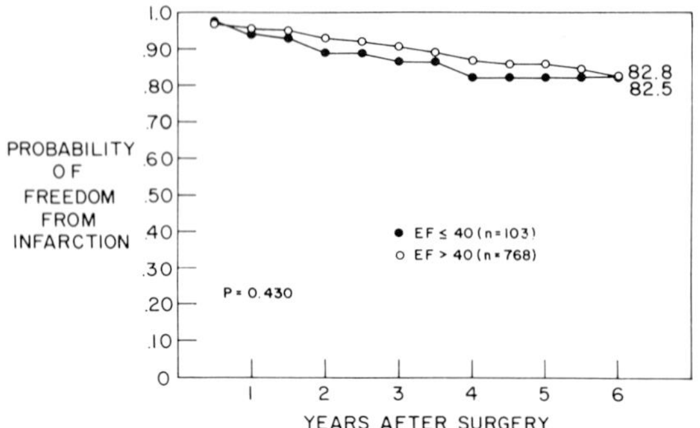

FIGURE 17 Influence of ejection fraction on probability of late myocardial infarction after revascularization surgery.

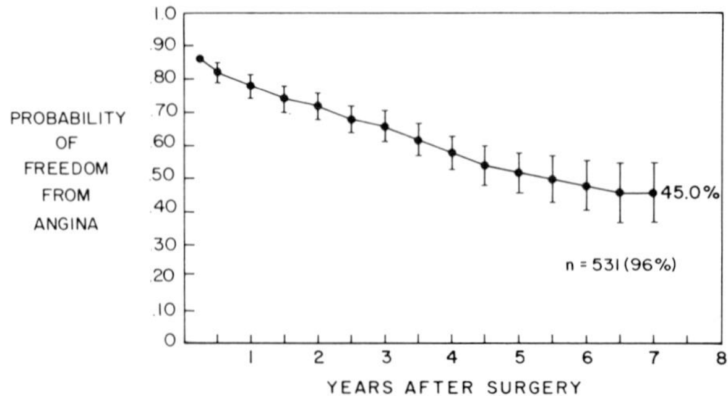

FIGURE 19 Probability of freedom from angina pectoris after revascularization in patients with three-vessel coronary obstruction.

infarction for purposes of this survey. Thus, these data probably represent a somewhat pessimistic view of the probability of occurrence of myocardial infarction.

The probability of freedom from myocardial infarction over 7 years following revascularization surgery for the entire series of patients was approximately 82 percent as shown in Fig. 10. There were 1,143 patients eligible for follow-up, and 94 percent of those were actually interviewed. The probability of remaining free of myocardial infarction for patients with three-vessel disease was 77 percent, with 93 percent of those eligible being interviewed. In Fig. 12 it will be noted that there was no observable significant difference between patients having three or more grafts and those having two or fewer grafts.

Patients with two-vessel disease had an approximately 78 percent chance of being free of myocardial infarction for 7 years following surgery, as shown in Fig. 13. The probability of myocardial infarction following revascularization surgery in patients with two-vessel disease also showed no significant difference when two or more grafts were performed as compared to those patients having only one graft.

Patients with single-vessel disease had an approximately 86 percent chance of being free of myocardial infarction. Patients with left main coronary obstruction had a nearly 95 percent chance of being free of myocardial infarction for 7 years following revascularization surgery. These patients represent the most favorable group, and no doubt this explains the excellent survival rate observed in persons after revascularization for this hazardous condition. In Fig. 17 it is evident that we observed no significant influence of preoperative ejection fraction on probability of myocardial infarction following revascularization surgery in the 871 patients for whom an ejection fraction measurement was available.

The probability of freedom from angina pectoris in the entire surgical series is shown in Fig. 18. The calculation of all data regarding recurrence of angina pectoris was made in a fashion similar to that for occurrence of myocardial infarction in survivors of revascularization surgery. Any patient with a repetitive chest pain syndrome, whether typical of angina pectoris or not, was considered to have recurrent angina. Any patient taking beta blockers or other antianginal

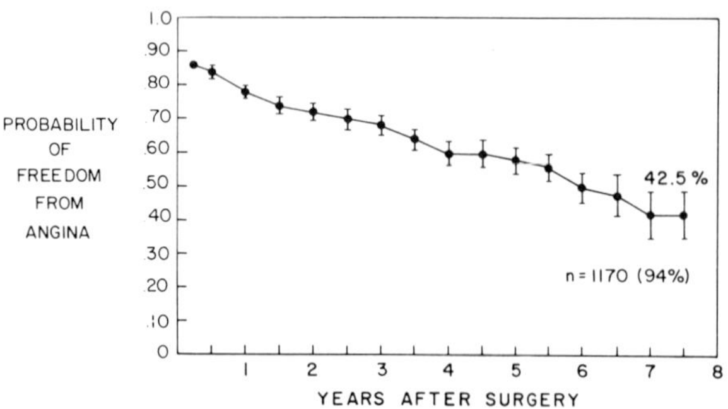

FIGURE 18 Probability of freedom from angina pectoris following revascularization surgery.

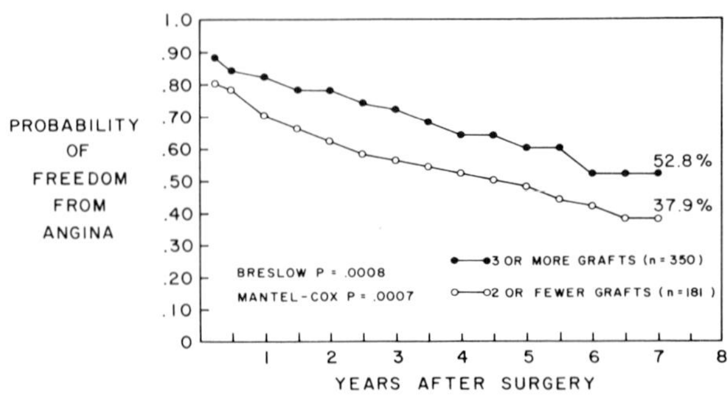

FIGURE 20 Comparison of probability of freedom from angina in patients with three-vessel disease having more versus fewer grafts.

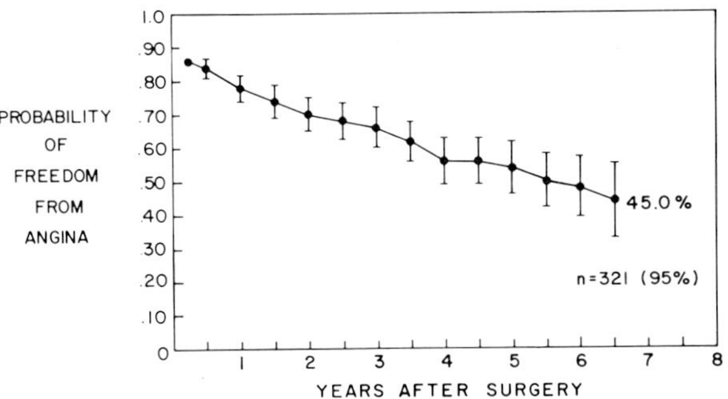

FIGURE 21 Probability of freedom from angina pectoris in patients with two-vessel disease undergoing revascularization surgery.

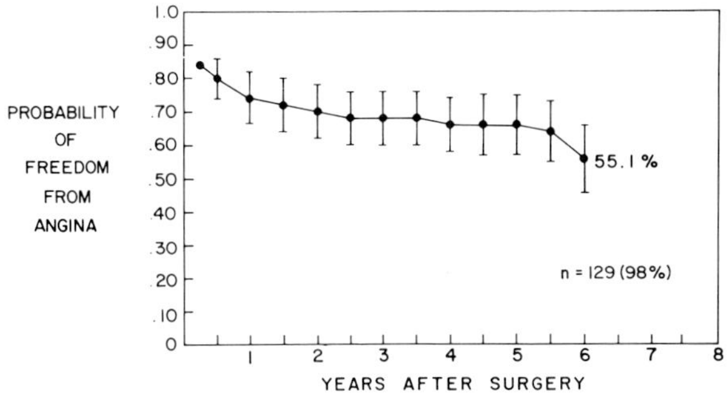

FIGURE 23 Probability of freedom from angina pectoris in patients having revascularization surgery for single-vessel disease.

medication was also considered to have recurrent angina pectoris whether asymptomatic on medication or not. Thus, these data represent a pessimistic, or "worst possible case," analysis.

The entire surgical series showed a probability of being totally free of angina pectoris under all conditions of 42.5 percent. Patients with three-vessel disease showed a probability of freedom from angina of 45 percent at 7 years (Fig. 19). Those patients with three-vessel disease who had three or more grafts had a significantly better probability of remaining free of angina than those who had two or fewer grafts as shown in Fig. 20. It thus appears that small or diffusely diseased vessels not suitable for bypass graft are sufficient to result in a higher proportion of recurrent angina but not enough to produce a higher probability of myocardial infarction or death.

Patients with two-vessel disease had a 45 percent chance of being totally free of angina at 6½ years following surgery (Fig. 21). Similar to the group with three-vessel disease, patients with two-vessel disease who had two or more grafts were significantly less

likely to have recurrent angina at any given interval after surgery than those who had only one graft, as shown in Fig. 22. Patients with single-vessel disease showed a 55 percent chance of total freedom from angina at 6 years following surgery (Fig. 23). The probability of total freedom from angina in those with left main coronary obstruction was 66 percent, as shown in Fig. 24. In Fig. 25 it is demonstrated that there was no significant difference between patients with ejection fraction over 0.40 as compared to those with ejection fraction below 0.40 in the rate of recurrence of angina pectoris following operation.

Analysis of the influence of unstable angina in these various groups of patients with coronary obstructive disease showed a somewhat higher operative mortality rate but no discernible significant difference among survivors in prognosis for longevity, myocardial infarction, or recurrence of angina pectoris.

Based upon these data it has been our policy to pursue a program of complete revascularization, bearing in mind that the principal beneficial effect of multiple grafts to small vessels is probably better reflected

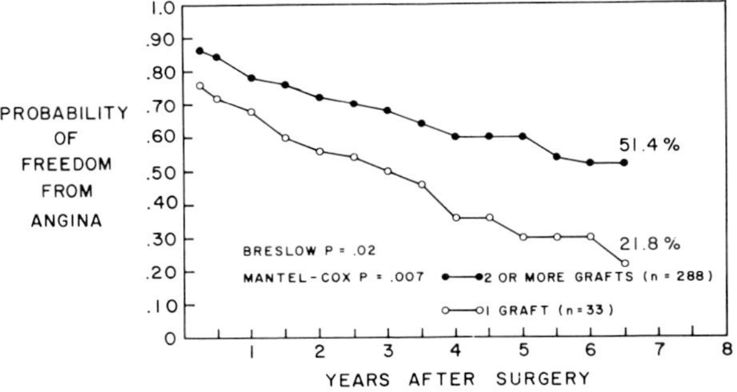

FIGURE 22 Comparison of angina recurrence rate in patients with two-vessel disease having one graft versus two or more grafts.

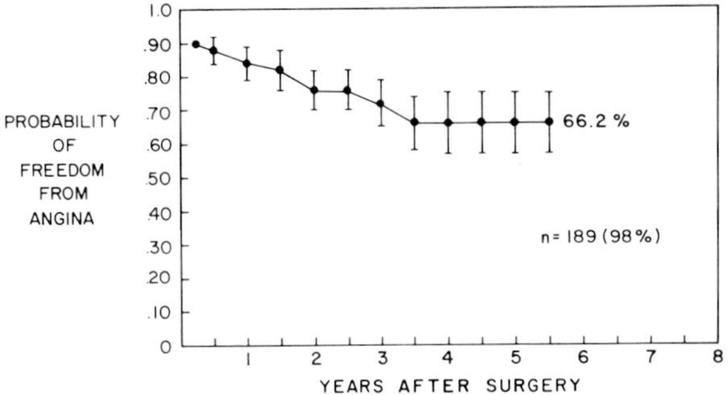

FIGURE 24 Probability of freedom from angina pectoris in patients undergoing revascularization for left main coronary obstruction.

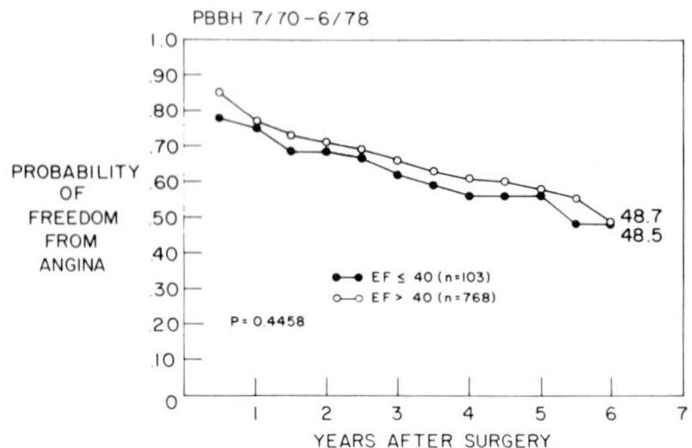

FIGURE 25 Comparison of recurrence rate of angina pectoris in patients with higher versus lower ejection fractions.

in a more optimistic prognosis for angina relief than for advantage in reduction of myocardial infarction or prolongation of life.

REFERENCES

1 "BMOP—Life Tables and Survival Functions," Health Sciences Computing Facility, Regents of University of California, University of California, Los Angeles, 1977.

2 Cohn, L. H., and Collins, J. J., Jr.: The Effect of Coronary Bypass on Longevity. A Nonrandomized Study, in H. Roskamm (ed.), "Coronary Heart Surgery and Rehabilitative Measures," Springer-Verlag, New York, 1979, p. 13.

3 Collins, J. J., Jr., and Cohn, L. H.: Surgical Treatment of Coronary Heart Disease, in P.F. Cohn (ed.), "Diagnosis and Therapy of Coronary Artery Disease: Concepts and Controversies," Little, Brown and Company, Boston, 1979, p. 413.

4 Collins, J. J., Jr., Cohn, L. H., Koster, J. K., Jr., and Mee, R. B. B.: The Influence of Coronary Bypass Surgery on Longevity in Patients with Angina Pectoris, in D.T. Mason (ed.), "Advances in Heart Disease," Grune & Stratton, Inc., New York, 1978, p. 93.

5 Cohn, L. H., Alpert, J., Koster, J. K., Jr., Mee, R. B. B. and Collins, J. J., Jr.: Changing Indications for the Surgical Treatment of Unstable Angina, *Arch. Surg.*, 113:1312, 1978.

6 Collins, J. J., Jr., Koster, J. K., Jr., and Cohn, L. H.: Emergency Coronary Revascularization, in C. E. Rackley (ed.), "Critical Care Cardiology: Cardiovascular Clinics," F.A. Davis Company, Philadelphia, 1981, p. 71.

Coronary Bypass Surgery: A Look from the South[*]

RENÉ G. FAVALORO, M.D.

The attack is very short and like a storm. It usually ends within one hour. I have undergone all bodily infirmities and dangers; but none appears to me more grievous. Why not? Because to have any other malady is only to be sick; to have this is to be dying.

LUCIUS SENECA, 4 B.C.[1]

Direct myocardial revascularization was first performed at the Cleveland Clinic in 1962 using the patch repair technique after coronary endarterotomy (pericardial or vein), mainly on the right coronary artery. The results were acceptable when the operation was performed on patients with localized obstruction. When we decided to use longer patches, total occlusion appeared more frequently in recatheterization studies. As a consequence, longer segmental obstructions were replaced by saphenous vein grafts using end-to-end anastomoses (interposed technique). But very early we realized that this technique also showed limitations, and bypass operation was the next logical step,[1a] thanks to work already done mainly in renal artery reconstruction. At the beginning we went slowly—only 171 operations were performed between May 1967 and December 1968—because we believe patients cannot be a part of our teaching material, agents on whom we practice our favorite treatment.

Full application was undertaken after a good number of patients were restudied several months following the operation demonstrating a high percentage of patent grafts. Nevertheless, already in 1968, the technique was applied in combination with ventricular aneurysmectomy, valvular replacement, and even in a few patients with acute coronary insufficiency (preinfarction angina and acute myocardial infarction).[2] Our work increased steadily in Cleveland, and when I left in 1971 more than 2,000 patients had been operated on. This learning period allowed us to develop a standardized technique[3] with a low mortality rate.[4] In Buenos Aires a total of 8,671 cardiovascular operations were performed up to December 31, 1982; of these 4,438 were revascularization procedures.

PRESENT OPERATIVE TECHNIQUE

Fifteen years have passed since the first utilization of coronary bypass operations at the Cleveland Clinic.

*From the Department of Surgery, El Salvador University School of Medicine, Buenos Aires, Argentina.

Several changes have been made in our operative technique since then. At present I believe only minor variations exist in the different leading centers. Nevertheless, I think it is important to mention the principal landmarks of our routine coronary bypass operation. It is performed under total cardiopulmonary bypass with hypothermia. For uncomplicated cases we keep the temperature around 28°C. If we expect a longer period of extracorporeal circulation (multiple bypasses, combined procedures, reoperation, etc.) the temperature is lowered to 24°C. The aorta is cannulated, and a single cannula is introduced through the right atrium into the inferior vena cava. Once the newly designed cannula is properly placed and the new oxygenators are utilized, there is a minimal blood flow into the right atrium and the right side of the interventricular septum. On the other hand, a left vent is routinely placed in the left ventricle through the right superior pulmonary vein and mitral valve after the aorta is totally clamped and cardioplegia has been initiated. We believe venting of the heart is necessary not only to decompress the left ventricle and prevent subendocardial damage but also to keep the coronary arteries empty, thus allowing the surgeon to perform delicate anastomoses even in very small arteries without difficulty.

We use cardioplegia in all the operations, but I want to make it clear that though I believe it is a significant advantage, nothing replaces a simplified and well-planned operative technique, which is still the most significant factor for good early results. It is difficult to believe the hundreds of papers published related to the proper utilization of cardioplegia, and I do subscribe to McGoon's[5] observation in this regard. I would like to mention only one aspect of this very polemical subject: should we use crystalloid or blood cardioplegia?

It would be wearisome to collect all the papers and we would need several pages to refer to all the literature published on this controversy. In my opinion, it is only of semantic interest if we remember that, even when we do utilize the simplified crystalloid cardioplegia technique at the beginning during the most critical period until the heart stops (energy demands are greater during electromechanical work), the aorta and the heart are full of blood and we are all perfusing the coronary arteries with blood cardioplegia, maybe diluted blood cardioplegia. If we want to be sure that in the brief initial period we induce cardioplegia with blood, we can use a partially occluded clamp, and by leaving the aorta slightly unclamped (1 or 2 mm is enough) we can ensure that oxygen delivery is not impaired until the heart stops. As a consequence, all the sophisticated and expensive equipment designed to deliver blood cardioplegia is not necessary. When heart temperature is kept below 15°C, very little oxygen is utilized to preserve cell viability, and if blood cardioplegia is perfused at low temperature, no oxygen is taken up by the heart cells from the solution.[6] Consequently, we use crystalloid cardioplegia with 15 mg potassium at the first injection, and only 5 mg potassium if more cardioplegia solution is needed. Since we have lowered the potassium level, fewer arrhythmias, mainly atrioventricular block, have been seen and very rarely occur at present.

Cardioplegia solution is given by the root of the aorta. We use the coronary sinus in a retrograde fashion only in a few cases, of course, in severe proximal obstruction of the left main coronary artery disease. The solution is administered slowly, and more solution is given through the graft when the distal anastomosis is completed, starting from the more jeopardized territory (in most patients the anterior descending coronary artery).

Occasionally, in complicated operations, using Buckberg and collaborators' indication,[7] a final dose of 20 mL is given a few minutes after the aorta is unclamped to prevent reperfusion damage. But we would like to stress that operative technique is the most important factor. Cardioplegia is only a help in our present armamentarium, and I tell the young fellows who start on the difficult road of cardiovascular surgery that extracorporeal circulation is an abnormal physiological condition for the patient, and the shorter the period we keep the patient connected to the heart-lung machine, the better our results. As can be seen in Table 1, the amount of cardioplegic solution we utilize is very moderate in comparison to that used by other centers around the world. The heart is bathed, of course, with saline solution using a catheter placed below the heart in the pericardial sac and flushing the left ventricle intermittently, mainly when bypasses are placed in the circumflex coronary artery area.

TABLE 1
Cardioplegia

Dose*	Number of patients
500 mL	456
500–700 mL	156
900 mL	68
900+ mL	54
Total	734

*The maximum dose has been 1,800 mL.

All the distal anastomoses are performed first, with a single running polypropylene suture (no. 7-0 BV-1 needle) and fine needle holders. Sequential grafts are utilized mainly in the circumflex coronary territory, and, though the results are satisfactory, we prefer using two anastomoses per vein in the great majority of patients (22 percent had segmental grafts with two distal anastomoses per vein, and only 1.1 percent had three anastomoses connected to one vein).

Bypasses to the circumflex coronary artery are passed through the transverse sinus in most patients, and the proximal anastomosis is performed on the posterolateral wall of the aorta (Fig. 1). This maneuver prevents kinking of the graft. A correctly implanted graft is an anastomotic technique that increases the number of patent grafts, mainly in the circumflex coronary artery territory that prior to this had the lowest percentage when compared to anterior descending and right coronary artery distribution. Another advantage of this procedure is that shorter venous grafts are necessary to reach the aorta, a significant factor when there are not enough veins available or the quality of the vein is poor in patients who need multiple bypasses.

Retroaortic bypasses are utilized also when the proximal anastomoses are located in the upper third portion of the anterior descending coronary artery, especially in patients with intramuscular location of the vessel or septal branches. With adequate clamps two proximal anastomoses can be performed in the posterolateral wall of the aorta. The transverse sinus provides sufficient room for this. When the ascending aorta is of small caliber and multiple bypasses are needed,

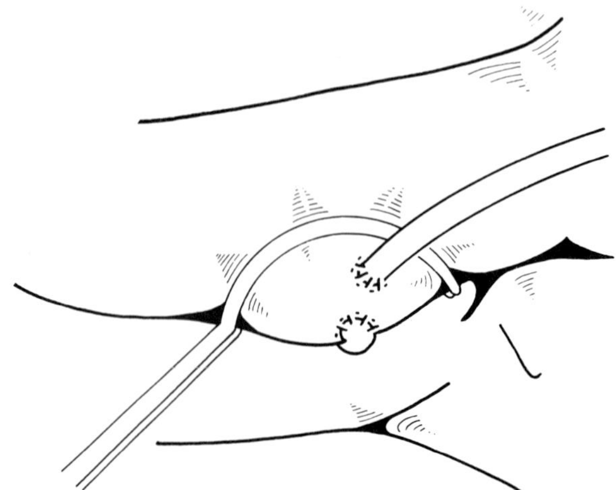

FIGURE 1 Bypasses to the circumflex coronary artery are placed in the posterolateral wall of the ascending aorta. When the anterior wall is severely damaged by atheromatous changes or calcification, bypasses to the right coronary artery may also be placed in the same area.

the proximal anastomosis of the graft to the right coronary artery can also be connected to the posterolateral wall of the aorta.

An increasing number of bypasses are performed, and a satisfactory revascularization is accomplished in the great majority of patients (I think the term *satisfactory* is better than *total revascularization*). In 1982, single bypasses were performed in 15.6 percent of the patients, two bypasses in 34.2 percent, three in 33.7 percent, and four or five in 16.6 percent. Only two patients required six bypasses. Mammary coronary anastomoses were utilized in 5 percent of our patients, most of them to the anterior descending coronary artery. Endarterectomies mainly to the right coronary artery and anterior descending territories were performed in 3.3 percent of the total population. Throughout the operation, cold light and magnifying lenses are used routinely.

CLASSIFICATION OF ISCHEMIC CARDIOMYOPATHY

A proper tabulation is needed to analyze all the data related to coronary arteriosclerosis and draw logical conclusions for proper indications for present medical or surgical treatment and compare the reports from different institutions. In 1978, the World Health Organization and the International Society and Federation of Cardiology[8] prepared a classification in order to unify the different criteria. Even though this classification presents definite landmarks, I think ischemic cardiomyopathy due to coronary arteriosclerosis is a much broader entity. The nomenclature we use in Buenos Aires (Table 2) results from the analysis of our daily work and though it may look complicated, actually it shows the different ways that patients come to us.

Of course, patients with angina may have had episodes of different types of arrhythmias or some degree of heart failure. On the other hand, patients without angina may suffer minor degrees of chest pain. It is also important to note that except for recent-onset angina all the other entities can be divided into two groups: with or without previous myocardial infarction. This is an important factor in the clinical evolution, always depending on the size of myocardial mass destroyed by the acute episode. The definition of the different classes of anginal patients can be found in previous reports from our team.[9–12]

At present, the only change in our classification is that except for stable angina we shorten the period of previous evolution to 1 month. Stable angina is defined as angina pectoris which presents no changes during the last 2 months. Once more we insist on the proper tabulation of patients with unstable angina, which in-

volves entities with significantly different prognoses (percentage of myocardial infarction and death).[9] It is difficult to understand the confusion that still persists in many medical centers. A recent example is from Hultgren et al., who last year defined the following groups of patients as having unstable angina:[13]

(1) Stable angina with an increase in severity or frequency of symptoms over the preceding 2 months; (2) recent onset angina with increasing severity or frequency of symptoms over the preceding 2 months (rest angina was not a requirement of these 2 groups); (3) acute coronary insufficiency with at least 1 episode lasting more than 15 minutes within the preceding 2 weeks. Acute coronary insufficiency was defined as prolonged (more than 15 minutes) anginal pain occurring at rest not promptly relieved by nitrates. Patients with acute myocardial infarction within 3 months of hospital entry were excluded. An additional entry criterion was the presence of transient ST-T wave changes compatible with ischemia. If such changes were not present, a positive electrocardiographic exercise test was required.

Once more patients with different prognoses are put together, and it is difficult to compare medical and surgical treatment. Of course, angina post acute myocardial infarction represents another group of patients with unstable angina even though for practical reasons it is included with the rest of acute myocardial infarction complications.

CLINICAL ANGIOGRAPHIC CORRELATION

Several prospective and one randomized survey on unstable angina were made by our team. It is important to note that the matched populations had similar characteristics: all patients were good candidates for operation and showed similar clinical, electrocardiographic, noninvasive screening, and cineangiographic patterns. Coronary angiography was, of course, the most important study to take into consideration.

We still believe what we have always emphasized in our publications and lectures. Good quality cine coronary angiography with a correct interpretation of the myocardial mass jeopardized by perfusion deficit is the best tool in our armamentarium to predict the future of every single patient. We do not deny that the other factors that determine myocardial perfusion such as spasm, platelet aggregation, and thrombosis are significant, but we think they are overemphasized nowadays in medical literature.

In our cardiac laboratory we were able to detect spasm in any segment of the coronary artery tree, including the left main trunk,[9] and in all the subgroups of our clinical classification with cineangiography per-

TABLE 2
Clinical classification of myocardial ischemia resulting from coronary arteriosclerosis*

I Symptomatic

A With angina

1 Stable angina
- *a* Class I
- *b* Class II
- *c* Class III
- *d* Class IV

2 Recent-onset angina with preserved physical capacity
- *a* Class I
- *b* Class II

3 Unstable angina
- *a* Recent onset angina with loss of physical capacity (class III & IV)
- *b* Progressive angina
- *c* Intermediate syndrome
- *d* Variant angina (Prinzmetal)
- *e* Prolonged myocardial ischemia (acute persistent ischemia)

B Without angina

- *1* Cardiac insufficiency
- *2* Arrhythmias
- *3* Systemic embolization
- *4* Noncharacteristic thoracic pain (atypical pain)
- *5* Dyspnea
- *6* Paroxysmal nocturnal dyspnea
- *7* Acute pulmonary edema
- *8* Fatigue
- *9* Dizziness
- *10* Syncope

C Acute myocardial infarction

1 Uncomplicated
- *a* Transmural
- *b* Nontransmural (*1*) Subendocardial (*2*) Intramural

2 Complicated
- *a* Angina post acute myocardial infarction
- *b* Severe ventricular arrhythmias
- *c* Ventricular septal defect
- *d* Mitral insufficiency
- *e* Left ventricular failure
- *f* Cardiogenic shock

II Asymptomatic

- *A* Following acute myocardial infarction
- *B* Stress test
- *C* Nuclear cardiological test (thallium or technetium)
- *D* Echocardiography
- *E* Arteriosclerosis in other vascular territories
- *F* Valvular diseases
- *G* Family history or risk factors or both
- *H* Abnormal ECG

*Sudden death may appear in any of the different subgroups, including asymptomatic patients.

formed without previous administration of coronary vasodilators. We agree with Freedman et al.[14] that spasm is much more frequent at the sites of the atheromatous lesion, maybe due to increased sensitivity. Consequently, the greater the severity of the mechanical obstruction with concomitant decrease of coronary flow, the greater the danger of other factors aggravating myocardial perfusion deficit.

The new generation of young cardiologists is very much inclined to think of physiological bases without adequate knowledge of the anatomic changes that occur at the coronary level as a result of coronary arteriosclerosis. Twenty-four years have passed since Sones[15] introduced cine coronary angiography, and I am convinced that the confusion that still persists about certain aspects of the disease are due to incorrect interpretation of the cine images; skilled interpretation requires several months' training in a well-organized laboratory.

The clinical angiographic correlation of the population seen at the Guemes Hospital shows the findings discussed below.

Stable Angina

We analyzed 1,618 patients: 563 belonged to classes I and II; of these, 283 had previous myocardial infarction; 1,055 belonged to classes III and IV; of these, 568 had previous myocardial infarction. Patients with stable angina class I and II without previous myocardial infarction showed single-vessel disease, 18 percent, double-vessel disease, 30 percent, triple-vessel disease, 41 percent, left main trunk obstruction, 2 percent, and normal coronary arteries 9 percent. Patients with previous myocardial infarction showed single-vessel disease, 2 percent, double-vessel disease, 30 percent, triple-vessel disease, 64 percent, and left main trunk obstruction, 4 percent. Stable angina class III and IV patients without previous infarction showed single-vessel disease, 22 percent, double-vessel disease, 27 percent, triple-vessel disease, 41 percent, left main trunk obstruction, 4 percent, and normal coronary arteries 6 percent. Patients with previous myocardial infarction showed single-vessel disease, 5.5 percent, double-vessel disease, 27 percent, triple-vessel disease, 62 percent, left main trunk obstruction, 5.5 percent. Certainly, there is a significant increase of triple-vessel disease in patients with previous myocardial infarction.

Recent-Onset Angina

We analyzed 610 patients: 197 (32.3 percent) had preserved physical capacity (class I and II), and 413 had diminished physical capacity (class III and IV). Of the first group, 59.4 percent had one-vessel disease, 33.5 percent, multiple obstructions (24.9 percent two-vessel disease, 8.6 percent three-vessel disease), and 7.1 percent, normal coronary arteries. In the second group, 64.1 percent had one-vessel disease, 31.6 percent, multiple-vessel disease (19.1 percent double-vessel disease, 12.5 percent triple-vessel disease), and 4.7 percent, left main trunk obstruction. In all the groups with one-vessel disease 75 percent corresponded to the anterior descending coronary artery, the great majority of the obstructions were close to the origin, and in 67 percent of class III and IV they were subtotal. The ejection fraction was within normal limits in all patients, but if we studied the first half of the systolic contraction, it showed some decrease in class III and IV patients (between 0.34 and 0.40). Consequently, recent-onset angina shows a specific angiographic pattern. Most patients in classes III and IV were candidates for revascularization.

Progressive Angina, Classes III and IV

The findings of a study of 1,268 patients of whom 768 had previous myocardial infarction have been analyzed; in this group results were very similar to those of patients with stable angina. Of patients without previous myocardial infarction 23 percent had one-vessel disease, 30 percent two-vessel disease, 25 percent, three-vessel disease, 3 percent, left main obstruction, and 19 percent had normal coronary arteries. The incidence of total obstruction (38.7 percent) was greater than in the other clinical groups without previous myocardial infarction. Adequate compromised collateral circulation was present in all of them, which explains the persistent progression of the symptoms.

Intermediate Syndrome

Ninety patients were studied (46.6 percent with previous infarction and 53.4 percent without infarction). Patients with previous myocardial infarction did not differ from the others. In patients without previous myocardial infarction, angiographic patterns depended on the type of angina. If the patients were originally in the group of recent-onset angina, single-vessel disease predominated. On the other hand, if they initially came from the stable angina group, multiple obstructions were found. In our group of 48 patients without previous myocardial infarction there was a predominance of subtotal obstructions (52.3 percent), severe obstructions were found in 38.2 percent and total in 9.5 percent. Of these patients 37.6 percent had one-vessel disease, 24.9 percent, two-vessel disease, 24.9 percent, three-vessel disease, 6.3 percent, left main trunk obstruction, and 6.3 percent, normal coronary arteries. With the new radiological equipment available today, we have the impression that more thrombi are found in this entity, but this requires further corroboration.

Variant Angina (Prinzmetal)

Out of 28 patients studied 10 had severe coronary obstruction, 6 had minor irregularities with mild obstruction, and 12 had normal coronary arteries (in 8 we were able to demonstrate the presence of spasm).

Prolonged Myocardial Ischemia (Acute Persistent Ischemia)

Fifty-five patients were studied, 41 with a previous myocardial infarction: 28 percent had one-vessel disease, 30 percent, two-vessel disease, 26 percent, three-vessel disease, 6 percent, left main trunk obstruction, and 10 percent had normal coronary arteries. There was a predominance of severe obstructions (47 percent) over subtotal (24 percent) and total ones (29 percent). In patients with total obstruction, adequate collateral circulation was present in 30 percent of the patients. I believe this group sustained a minor degree of myocardial necrosis which could not be detected with electrocardiographic and enzyme studies.

Patients without Angina

This group comprises a wide variety of entities. Severe congestive heart failure, severe ventricular arrhythmias, and mitral insufficiency are generally manifestations of far-advanced arteriosclerosis, and they point to multivessel disease in a great number of patients. Occasionally mitral insufficiency is caused by a single lesion in the circumflex coronary territory (only three patients in our entire series).

All the other entities included in this category (dyspnea, paroxysmal nocturnal dyspnea, acute pulmonary edema, fatigue, dizziness, syncope) are equivalent to angina pectoris. We have already pointed out that patients with dyspnea constitute a special group with very poor prognosis. We really do not know why ischemia does not reach the angina threshold even though experimental data, implanting sonomicrometer[16] data (corroborated in our research laboratory) and findings in our catheterization department, show that changes in ventricular contractility and/or electrocardiogram and lactate production occur without clinical manifestations and precede the onset of angina. We have not made enough cineangiographic studies of this type of patient to draw conclusions, but patients range from those with a single obstruction (mainly in the anterior descending coronary artery) to those with multiple obstructions.

Acute Myocardial Infarction

A total of 583 patients have been studied with cine coronary angiography of which 148 were uncomplicated and 435 presented different complications (Table 3). The majority of the uncomplicated cases were transmural acute myocardial infarctions (128 patients). Of the nontransmural, 16 were subendocardial and 4 intramural acute myocardial infarction. The majority (66 percent) were studied during the acute episode (within the first 10 days). The findings are shown in Table 4. In this group of patients, 20 percent had one-vessel disease, 30 percent, two-vessel disease, 43 percent, three-vessel disease, and 7 percent, left main trunk obstruction.

Most of the studies of complicated myocardial infarction come from the group with angina after acute myocardial infarction. The findings are tabulated in Table 5. The angiographic results were previously analyzed[17] and can be summarized as follows: type I, single severe obstruction of a coronary artery that produces a myocardial infarction smaller than the irrigated area; type II, obstruction similar to type I plus further obstruction in other coronary territories; type III, total occlusion of a coronary artery that produces a small infarction because of partial adequate noncompromised collateral circulation; type IV, total occlusion of a coronary artery that produces a small infarction because of the presence of partial adequate compromised collateral circulation; type V, total or

TABLE 3

Cine coronary angiography in patients with acute (within the first 10 days) and subacute (11–30 days) myocardial infarction*

	Number of patients (N = 583)
Uncomplicated AMI	148
Complicated AMI:	
APAMI	340
MI	27
VSD	29
VT and/or VF	29
Severe HF	10

*AMI = acute myocardial infarction; APAMI = angina after acute myocardial infarction; HF = heart failure; MI = mitral insufficiency; VF = ventricular fibrillation; VT = ventricular tachycardia; VSD = ventricular septal defect.

TABLE 4

Uncomplicated myocardial infarction: electrocardiographic classification*

Location of infarction	Number of patients (N = 148)
Transmural myocardial infarction:	
Anteroseptal	33
Anterior	37
Anterolateral	9
Inferior	25
Posterior	9
Inferolateral	6
Lateral	9
Nontransmural myocardial infarction:	
Subendocardial:	
Anterior	13
Inferior	3
Intramural	4

*Twenty-three patients (15 percent) had a previous myocardial infarction, and 104 were studied during the acute phase.

subtotal obstruction that produces a large myocardial infarction with concomitant obstruction in other coronary territories; type VI, total occlusion of a coronary artery that produces an acute ventricular aneurysm with concomitant obstruction in other vascular territories.

In this series, 168 patients were studied during the acute phase and 172 during the subacute phase (between 10 and 30 days); 309 infarctions were transmural, 29 subendocardial, and 2 intramural. Twenty percent of the patients had had a previous myocardial infarction, 8 percent had single-vessel disease, 39 percent, two-vessel disease, 46 percent, three-vessel disease, and 7 percent, left main trunk obstruction.

Twenty-nine patients were studied because of the added complication of a ventricular septal defect. Myocardial infarction was inferior in 19 and anterior in 10. Two patients had previous myocardial infarction, 16 patients were studied within 12 h of the acute episode, 9 between 4 and 7 days, and 4 between 8 and 10 days. Twenty-one patients suffered heart failure, and eight patients were in cardiogenic shock. It is interesting to note that single-vessel disease was present in 10 patients (5 in the right coronary artery); 13 patients had double-vessel disease; and 6 patients had triple-vessel disease. There were no left main trunk obstructions in this series. It must be noted that total occlusion was present in 92 percent of the patients and concomitant ventricular aneurysm in 16 (9 anteroapical and 7 diaphragmatic).

Mitral insufficiency was encountered in 27 patients. Eight patients had a previous myocardial infarction (29 percent), and the site of the acute infarction was inferior in 20 patients; it was posterolateral in 5, and anterior in 2. Nine patients were studied during the first week, 2 during the second, 6 in the third, and 10 within 4 weeks. All had severe mitral insufficiency. The majority—17 patients—had triple-vessel disease; 3 patients had double-vessel disease, 6 patients, single-vessel disease (4 in the right and 2 in the circumflex coronary artery), and one patient, left main trunk obstruction. Total occlusion was present in 98 percent of the patients.

Of the 29 patients studied with iterative episodes of ventricular tachycardia and/or ventricular fibrillation, 7 had anterolateral myocardial infarction, 11, anterior, 3, anteroseptal, 7, inferior, and 1, lateral. Previous infarction was present in only 2 patients. Nine patients had one-vessel disease, 8, two-vessel disease, 11, three-vessel disease, and 1 patient, left main trunk obstruction. Thirty-five percent were studied during the first and second weeks and 65 percent during the third and

TABLE 5

Angina after acute myocardial infarction: clinical groups and their localization

Location	Types						Total
	I	II	III	IV	V	VI	
Anteroseptal	45	30	14	26			115
Anterior					49	3	52
Anterolateral					5	10	15
Inferior	10	8	6	14	43	5	86
Posterior		6	2		9		17
Lateral		6	1	2	14	1	24
Anterior subendocardial	6	9	1	7			23
Anterolateral subendocardial	1	4		1			6
Intramural	2						2
Total	64	63	24	50	120	19	340

fourth weeks. Total occlusion was present in 75 percent of the patients. It is interesting to note that 16 patients had a definite acute ventricular aneurysm.

Ten patients suffered severe left ventricular failure; of these 9 had an anterior infarction and 5 had a previous infarction. Three patients had single-vessel disease, 5 patients, double-vessel disease, and 2 patients had triple-vessel disease. Total obstruction was present in 90 percent of the patients, and 8 had a bona fide acute ventricular aneurysm.

I would like to note that there was no mortality related to the cineangiography performed in the 583 patients studied.

Asymptomatic Patients

The majority were studied because they had previous myocardial infarction. The results can be seen in Table 6. If we divide this group into anterior and posterior infarctions (Fig. 2A and B), approximately 50 percent of the patients with anterior and 60 percent with inferior infarction had multiple-vessel disease. In this group the anterior descending coronary artery was significantly occluded in 72 patients. Left main trunk obstructions were also found though the patients denied any anginal episode in both categories. Theoretically, if a patient had an inferior infarction in the past and is afterwards asymptomatic, he or she should have only one obstruction in the right coronary or circumflex coronary artery. If the infarction was anterior, there should only be one obstruction in the anterior descending coronary territory. But in practice this is far from reality. Many of these patients are indeed candidates for surgery as we will show later on.

The second significant group are those patients who consult us because of arteriosclerotic manifestations in different vascular territories. In our cardiac laboratory we have studied since 1972 all patients with

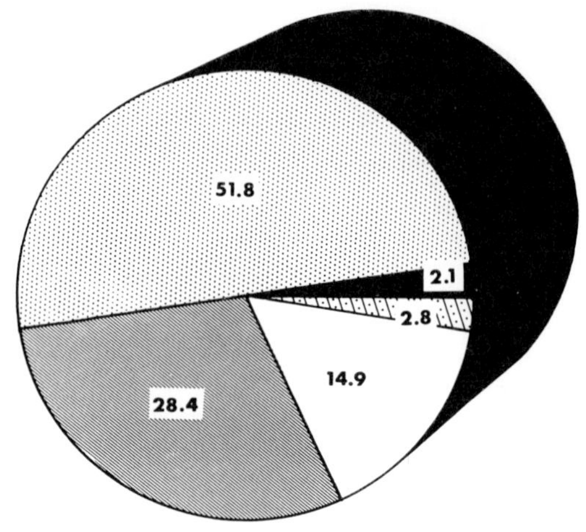

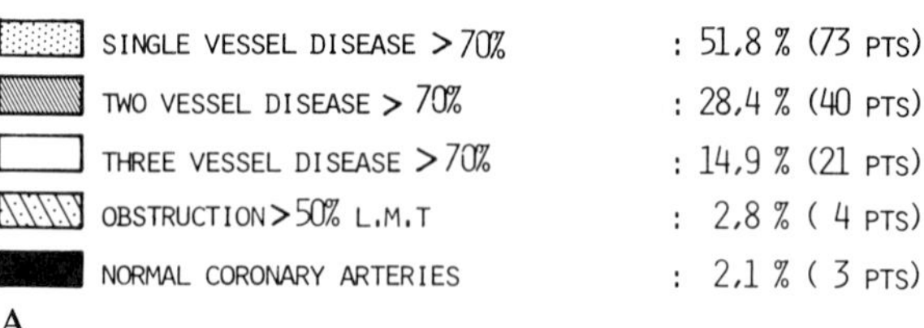

A

FIGURE 2 Angiographic findings. (A) Anterior infarction. (B) Posterior infarction.

vascular disease by cineangiography through the brachial artery with different catheters,[18,19] and concomitant coronary angiography was performed. This has enabled us to collect significant information (Table 7). Two-thirds of these patients had different degrees of angina pectoris. Still, if we analyze the last consecutive 124 patients (78 with peripheral vascular disease and/or abdominal aorta disease, 40 with cerebrovascular

TABLE 6
Chronic asymptomatic infarction: angiographic findings in 344 patients*

ECG	1 v	2 v	3 v	LMO	Normal CA	Total
Anteroseptal	25	18	15	2	3	63
Anterior	19	8	3	1		31
Anterolateral	29	14	3	1		47
Inferior	59	44	25	4		132
Lateral	9	4	1			14
Posterior	3	5	1			9
Posterolateral	2	2	1			5
Inferolateral	1	4	2			7
Inferoposterior	14	8	5	1		28
Inferoposterolateral	2	1	4	1		8

*CA = coronary arteries; ECG = electrocardiogram; LMO = left main obstruction; v = vessel.

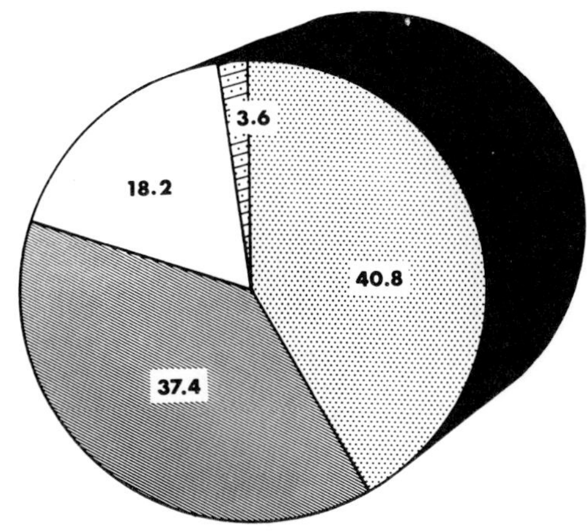

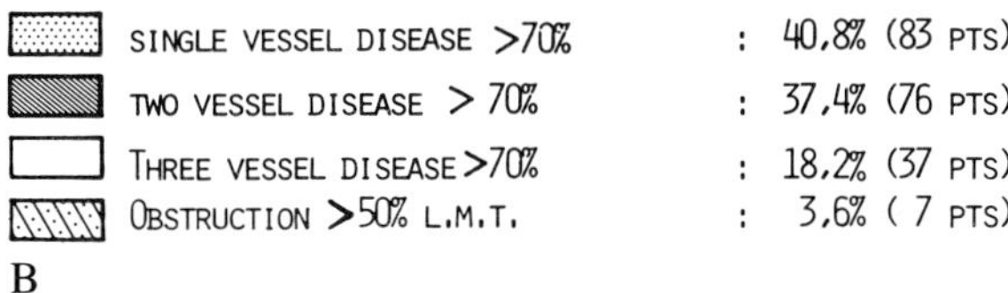

B

insufficiency, and 6 with renal artery obstruction) in whom we studied the coronary arteries even though there was no anginal episode in their clinical history, we find that 38 patients (28.3 percent) had one-vessel disease, 17 patients (14.1 percent) had two-vessel disease, 31 patients (25.8 percent) had three-vessel disease, 7 patients (6 percent) had left main trunk obstruction, and 31 (25.8 percent) had normal coronary arteries.

TABLE 7
Cine coronary angiography associated with cine studies of other vascular territories in 500 consecutive patients and angiographic findings in coronary arteries

Cine coronary angiography associated with cine studies of other vascular territories	Number of patients
Selective arteriography of the limbs	220 (44%)
Selective arteriography of neck vessels	160 (32%)
Abdominal aortogram (with or without selective renal arteriography)	90 (18%)
Selective arteriogram of neck vessels and inferior limbs	30 (6%)
Angiographic findings in coronary vessels	
One-vessel disease	125 (25%)
Two-vessel disease	110 (22%)
Three-vessel disease	150 (30%)
Left main trunk disease	35 (7%)
Normal coronary arteries	80 (16%)

Though all the data about the different clinical entities have been presented following the traditional classification of single-vessel, double-vessel, triple-vessel, and left main trunk obstruction, we are convinced in view of what we know today that this is not sufficient to tabulate the population. Cine coronary angiography is slightly more complicated, as we already mentioned previously, and different types appeared, even in patients with left main trunk obstruction.[9] The length, size, and distribution of each coronary segment vary, and the obstruction site plays an important role. For example, when we examine the anterior descending coronary artery, we should first determine its length, which can extend from the upper portion of the anterior interventricular septum to the beginning of the diaphragmatic distribution. We should determine the number and length of the diagonal branches and the number of septal branches. The site of the obstruction indicates the amount of myocardial mass that is involved in the different coronary patterns. The same approach can be utilized for the circumflex and right coronary artery. This explains, for example, why a single coronary occlusion can produce a widespread bona fide infarction even with concomitant large ventricular aneurysm, ventricular septal defect, mitral insufficiency, or cardiogenic shock, as I already pointed out previously. I recommend that, in the future, patients should be divided into at least five categories: one obstruction, two obstructions, three obstructions, more than three obstructions, and left main trunk obstructions. Otherwise, it will be difficult to explain why we perform more than three bypasses!

Furthermore, I think collateral circulation has not been adequately described. To say that a given number of patients have collateral circulation is meaningless. We should first find the vessel from which it comes and the vessel irrigated (Table 8). In the former, we should carefully examine the artery to see if it is free from obstruction and as a consequence the collateral circulation is not compromised. If there is an obstruction proximal to the site where collateral circulation comes from, it is definitely compromised. The two situations are completely opposed and naturally have different prognoses and therapeutic implications.

TABLE 8
Analysis of collateral circulation

			Anatomic
Compromised or noncompromised	Adequate	Total	
		Partial	Anatomic & functional
	Inadequate		
	Transitory		

Then, we should examine the artery irrigated by the collateral circulation, which, of course, is totally or severely occluded, and the perfused myocardial mass. Collateral circulation is adequate if the myocardium has been preserved. It is totally adequate if the myocardium is within normal limits. It can still be anatomic and functional: the myocardium remains normal even after exercise; or it can be only anatomic: the area perfused deteriorates with exercise. Collateral circulation can still be beneficial if it is partially adequate, i.e., the myocardial mass shows only some impairment in the left cineventriculogram. It is inadequate if all the area has already been replaced by scar tissue. Some examples (Fig. 3A,B,C, and D) will give support to our point of view. Another important issue is that collateral circulation can be transitory, i.e., it can appear and disappear within minutes or even seconds in patients with a severe occlusion who develop spasm during cineangiography. We have seen and documented that if spasm occludes an artery, e.g., the anterior descending coronary artery, collateral circulation appears from the right coronary artery before vasodilators are given. After administration of a sublingual coronary vasodilator spasm disappears and anterograde flow is reestablished. A repeated injection in the right coronary artery will show no collateral circulation.

It is impossible to determine how often this occurs, but it gives us a basis to explain, for example, why a total occlusion of the anterior descending coronary artery at its origin affects the myocardial mass differently, ranging from a normal anterolateral wall to a large ventricular aneurysm.

Finally, if we want to determine the state of the left ventricle, the right anterior oblique projection is not

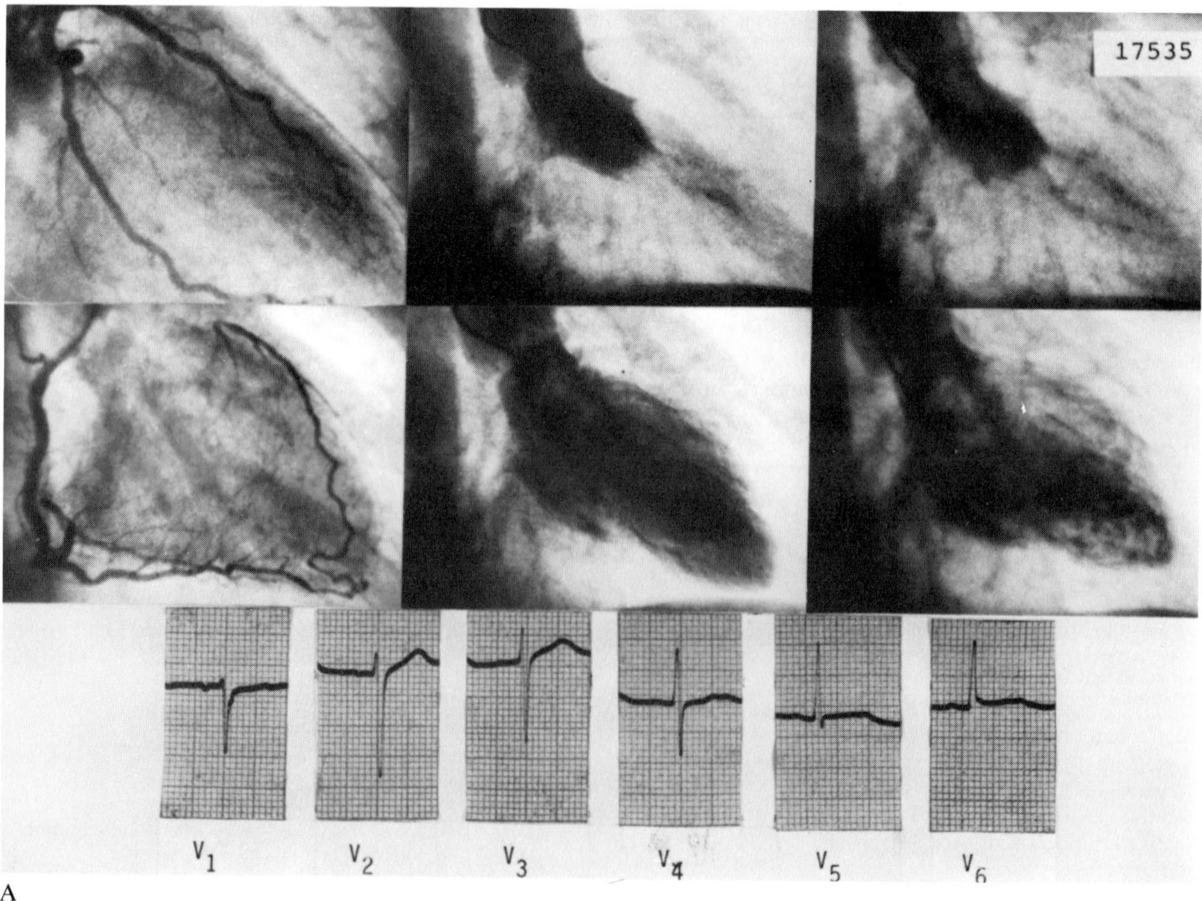

FIGURE 3 Varieties of collateral circulation: (A) Noncompromised adequate, total and functional (in the right normal left ventricular contraction after exercise). (B) Noncompromised partial adequate, ECG: anteroseptal necrosis with anterior ischemia. (C, p. 266) Noncompromised inadequate, ECG: extensive anterior necrosis. (D, p. 267) Compromised, severe obstruction in the right coronary artery (arrow); anatomically adequate, functionally inadequate (in the right, abnormal left ventricular contraction after exercise), ECG: subepicardial anterior ischemia.

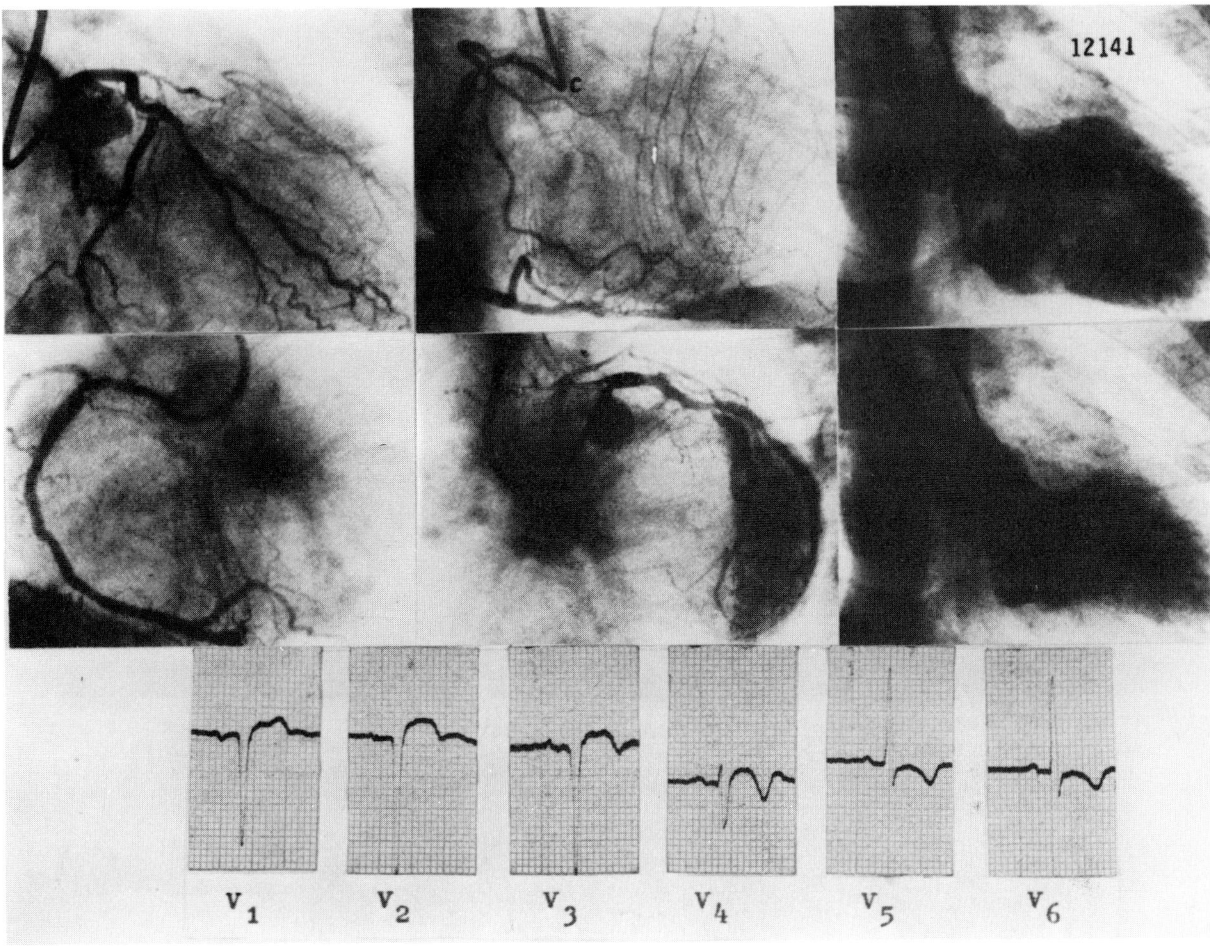

B

enough, because we cannot really see the interventricular septum and the lateral wall of the left ventricle. Following our observations in the operating room, I suggested to Sones that the addition of the left anterior oblique projection should be mandatory mainly in patients with abnormal ventricles if we wanted to obtain proper surgical indications and adequate follow-up. This approach was applied in our routine cine studies at the Cleveland Clinic, and later, since the 1960s, in Buenos Aires.

We are also convinced that the different scoring systems suggested, including our own,[9] are far from making a proper tabulation of the reading of a cine coronary angiogram. They give us an approximation, but on many occasions this is not enough to assess the related risk involved. I would advise all cardiologists who wish to learn about this disease and later on contribute to the proper understanding and implications of coronary arteriosclerosis to spend some time at a cardiac laboratory as a first step in their training. It will be difficult for them to understand what they are doing, for example, in echocardiography or radioisotope techniques, if they do not know the live anatomy with which they will become familiar by looking at hundreds of cine coronary angiograms.

OUR CLINICAL EXPERIENCE IN BUENOS AIRES

We present an analysis of our work in 1982 in order to give an idea of what we are doing at present at the Guemes Hospital in Buenos Aires. A total of 734 patients with coronary arteriosclerosis have been operated upon. Revascularization procedures alone were performed in 687 patients, while 47 had combined concomitant operations (Table 9).

The angiographic findings encountered in the 687 patients with pure revascularization procedures are presented in Table 10. I think it is important to note

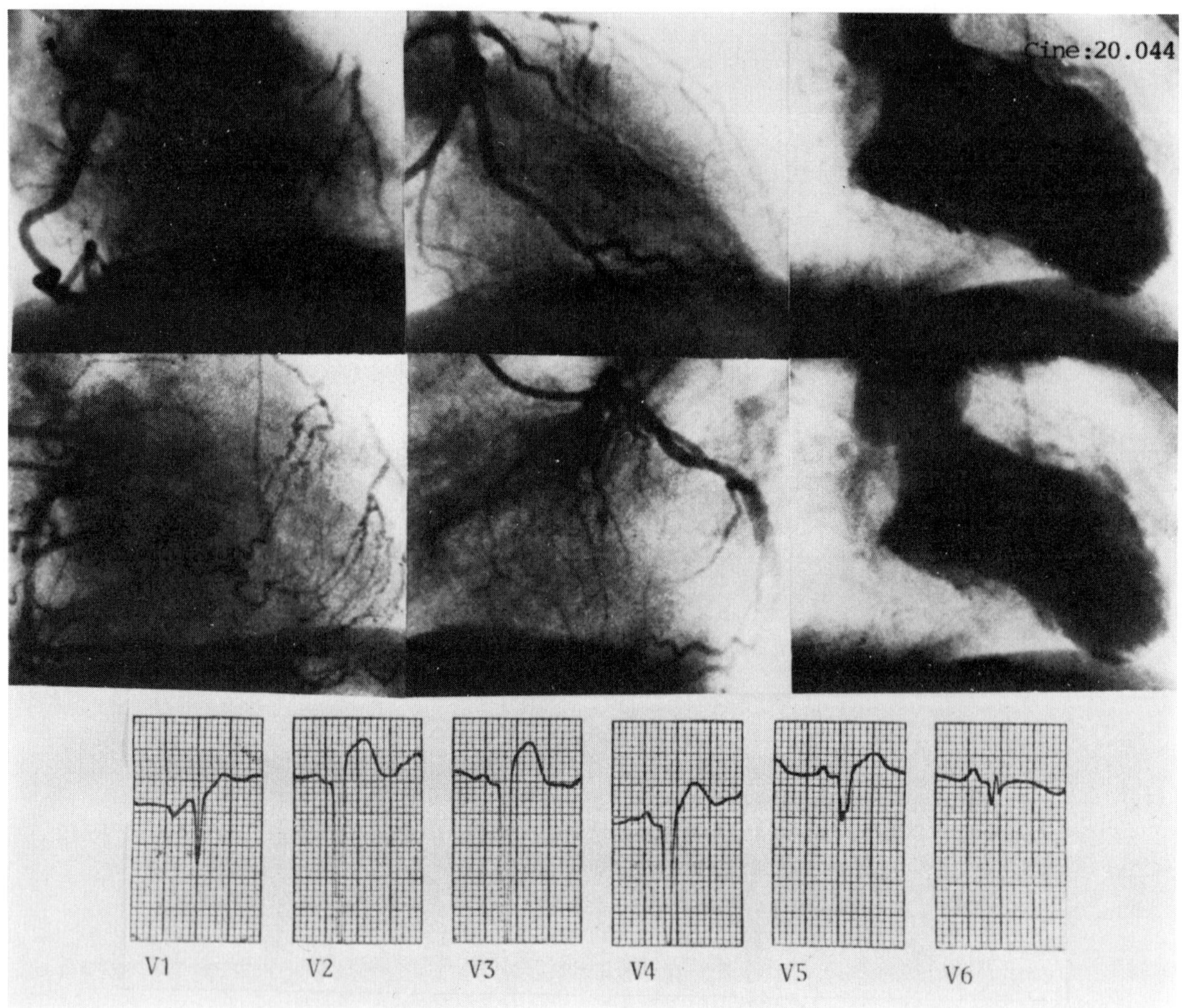

C

that involvement of three or more vessels characterizes 55.4 percent of the population, and 12.6 percent suffered from severe left main coronary artery disease. Three hundred and twenty-seven patients had previous myocardial infarction (47.5 percent) of which 43 percent were diaphragmatic, 36 percent, anterior (anteroseptal or anterolateral), 10.4 percent, anterior and diaphragmatic, and 10.6 percent, at other sites (mainly lateral or posterobasal).

Table 11 shows the state of the left ventricle: 370 patients that were operated on had left ventricular abnormality, an important factor to consider when we compare series from different institutions. Table 12 shows the number of patients in different categories of our clinical classification with the exception of patients who underwent combined procedures. The high incidence of patients with progressive angina is clearly

demonstrated. Most of them belong to class IV, which means that besides having a significant increase of anginal episodes related to stress, they also have anginal episodes at rest. This is certainly very similar to the clinical condition of patients with intermediate syndrome, in which episodes of angina at rest are more frequent and less easily controlled with nitrates. Four patients with dyspnea are separated from the category of "equivalent to angina" because they constitute a poor prognosis group for medical treatment. Our prospective prodromic studies in the coronary care unit showed that 46 percent die during the admission period.

Table 13 shows two distinct clinical groups of patients classified according to surgical risk. As can be seen, the mortality rate is minimal in the low-risk group and increases in the high-risk group. Of the three patients with stable angina who died (class III,1, class

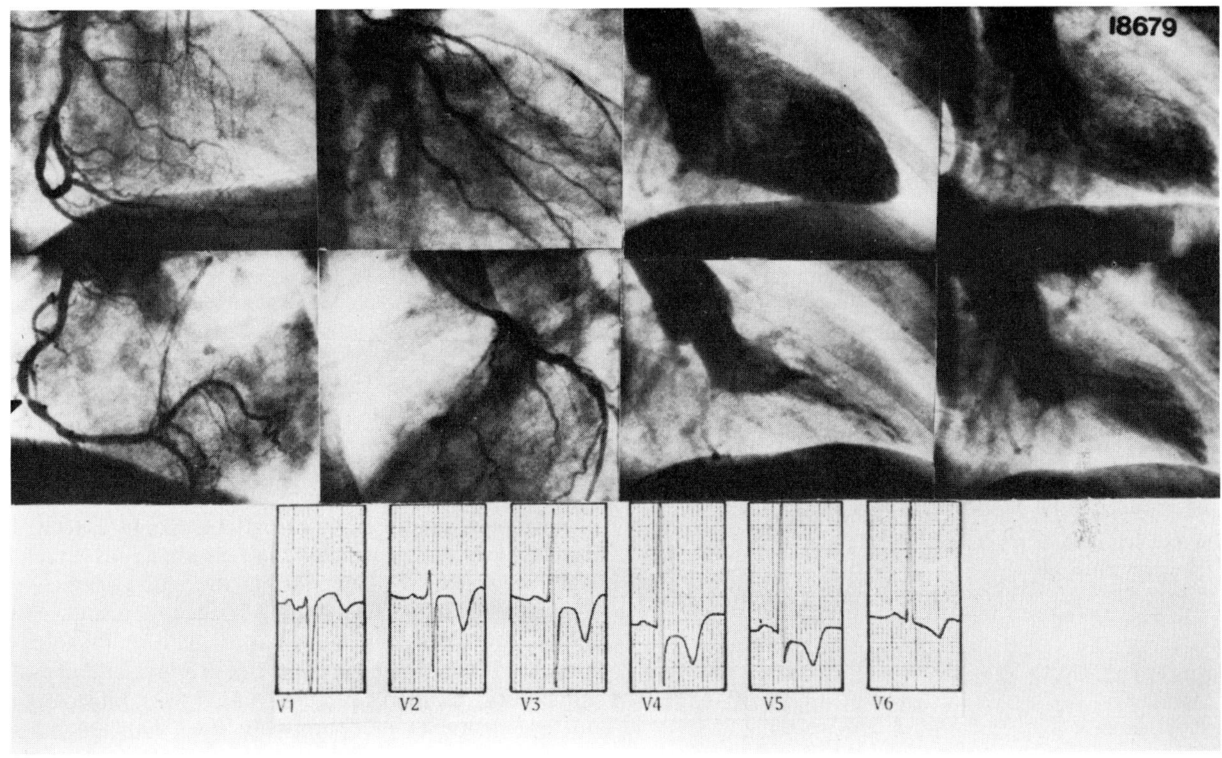

D

IV,2), one had previous myocardial infarction and a severely impaired ventricle with signs of left ventricular failure during the recent clinical evolution.

It is important to note that of the seven patients with progressive angina who died five had previous myocardial infarction of whom two had severely diminished left ventricular contractions and one had a ventricular aneurysm. Of the three deaths in patients with angina post acute myocardial infarction, one had a bona fide acute aneurysm due to a large anterolateral myocardial infarction. Of the two deaths in patients operated on due to an acute infarction, one was a patient who had an anterior aneurysm and a concomitant ventricular septal defect, and the other was a patient in whom we first unsuccessfully tried thrombolytic agents within 4 h of the acute episode, which was due to total occlusion at the beginning of the main anterior descending coronary artery. A single bypass was performed within 12 h. The patient died during the following 24 h even though a balloon pump was inserted through the femoral artery. The operation was indicated because of left ventricular damage, steady fall of the systemic blood pressure, and increased pulmonary wedge pressure.

Table 14 shows the age distribution of the population. The youngest patient was 26 and the eldest 81. Sex did not have a significant incidence on overall mortality rate: 2.7 percent among males and 2.3 percent among females.

Table 15 analyzes risk factors including diabetes, dyslipidemia, hypertension, smoking, obesity, stress, and gout. Even though there was no difference in hospital mortality rate, diabetes alone or with other risk factors increased operative risk: four deaths (4.5 percent in 87 patients). There were also nine deaths (3 percent) in 298 patients with hypertension, but it must be noted that it was difficult to analyze each individual risk factor separately because 62.8 percent of the patients had two or more risk factors present.

Of the entire series 6 patients died in the operating room and 14 between 24 h and 16 days postoperatively (4 due to postoperative myocardial infarction and concomitant left ventricular failure, 3 due to cerebrovascular accidents, 3 due to respiratory insufficiency and superimposed pulmonary infection, 3 due to generalized sepsis, and 1 patient after thrombolytic attempt following revascularization of the main anterior descending coronary artery). Of the patients who died 2 had a single bypass, 5 a double bypass, 7 a triple bypass, 1 four bypasses, 3 aneurysmectomy, and 2 a combined procedure (aortic valve replacement plus two and three bypasses).

The operation nowadays presents very few complications: 19 patients required reoperation for bleed-

TABLE 9
Types of operations performed in 1982*

	Number of patients (N = 734, 20 deaths, or 2.7%)
Single bypass[†]:	
AD	62
Cx	1
RCA	3
Double bypass	199
Triple bypass	216
>3 bypasses	108
Triple bypass plus RCA patch repair	2
Mammary coronary anastomosis:	
Alone	5
Plus 1 bypass	15
Plus 2 bypasses	11
Plus 3 bypasses	2
Endarterectomy plus:	
1 bypass plus IMCA	1
2 bypasses	4
3 bypasses	11
> 3 bypasses	6
Aneurysmectomy:	
Alone	2
Plus 1 bypass	6
Plus 1 bypass plus ligation coronary fistula	1
Plus 2 bypasses	15
Plus 3 bypasses	7
Plus 4 bypasses	2
Plus 4 bypasses plus endarterectomy	1
Plus VSD	2
Ventricular septal defect plus:	
1 bypass	2
1 bypass plus aneurysmectomy	1
2 bypasses plus aneurysmectomy	2
Aortic valve replacement plus:	
1 bypass	13
2 bypasses	9
2 bypasses plus ascending aneurysm	1
3 bypasses	5
3 bypasses plus ascending aneurysm	1
4 bypasses	1
Mitral valve replacement plus:	
1 bypass	2
2 bypasses	8
2 bypasses plus coronary endarterectomy	1
3 bypasses	1
Mitral commissurotomy plus:	
1 bypass plus closure ASD	1
3 bypasses	1
Carotid endarterectomy plus:	
3 bypasses	1
4 bypasses	1
Aorto-bifemoral bypass plus:	
1 bypass	1

*Many combinations occurred in patients with two, three, and more than three bypasses.

†AD = anterior descending; ASD = atrial septal defect; Cx = circumflex; IMCA = internal mammary coronary anastomosis; RCA = right coronary artery.

ing during the first 24 h; wound infection with concomitant mediastinitis occurred in 8 patients; bronchopulmonary complications with prolonged intubation (more than 24 h) in 14 patients—only 2 needed tracheostomy. Gastrointestinal bleeding has practically disappeared (4 patients in the entire medically controlled series). This, I think is due to a decrease in blood utilization, psychological preparation by an expert team when needed, and the prophylactic use of cimetidine. Balloon counterpulsation was utilized only in three patients preoperatively (two with left main trunk obstruction and severe left ventricular dysfunction and one with angina post acute myocardial infarction) and was successfully inserted postoperatively in six patients. Four patients died on the operating table

TABLE 10
Angiographic findings*

Disease	Number of patients (N = 687)	Percent
1 vessel	66	9.6
2 vessels	154	22.4
3 vessels	255	55.4,
>3 vessels	125	combined
Left main:		
<75% stenosis	2	0.29
>75% stenosis	4	0.58
Left main + RCA[†]:		
<75% stenosis	8	1.16
>75% stenosis	11	1.60
100% stenosis	1	0.14
Left main + triple-vessel disease:		
<75% stenosis	34	4.94
>75% stenosis	26	3.78
100% stenosis	1	0.14

(Left main combined = 12.6)

*Sixty-eight percent of the patients had disease of three or more vessels and different varieties of left main trunk obstruction.

†RCA = right coronary artery.

TABLE 11
State of the left ventricle

State of ventricle*		Number of patients (N = 687)	Deaths (N = 18)	% (Total, 2.6%)
Normal or mild				
EF	> 0.58			
MNSER	> 1.56 EDV/s			
Mean VcfB	> 0.81 circ/s			
Mean VcfM	> 0.92 circ/s			
Mean VcfA	> 1.18 circ/s	317	5	1.5
Moderate				
EF	0.57–0.36			
MNSER	1.55–0.57			
Mean VcfB	0.80–0.31			
Mean VcfM	0.91–0.28			
Mean VcfA	1.17–0.60	245	9	3.6
Severe				
EF	≤ 0.35			
MNSER	< 0.56 EDV/s			
Mean VcfB	< 0.30 circ/s			
Mean VcfM	< 0.27 circ/s			
Mean VcFA	< 0.59 circ/s	125	4	3.2

*Circ/s = circumference/s; EDV/s = end-diastolic volume/s; EF = ejection fraction; Mean VcfA = mean circumferential fiber shortening rate, apical segment; Mean VcfB = mean circumferential fiber shortening rate, basal segment; Mean VcfM = mean circumferential fiber shortening rate, equatorial segment; MNSER = mean normalized systolic ejection rate.

TABLE 12
Number of operated patients in relation to the clinical classification

Classification	Class	Number of patients (N = 687, 18 deaths, or 2.6%)
Stable angina	I	6
	II	63
	III	40
	IV	60
Progressive angina	III	66
	IV	191
Intermediate syndrome		7
Angina post acute myocardial infarction		41
Recent-onset angina	I–II	31
	III–IV	66
Prolonged myocardial ischemia (acute persistent ischemia)		10
Equivalent to angina		10 { dyspnea, 4 / others, 6
Atypical angina		26
Asymptomatic		41
Acute myocardial infarction		29

in spite of the addition of this method of assisted circulation.

Since we took the vein from the leg using only one continuous incision, avoiding finger dissection and careful hemostasis of the side branches, very few patients developed local hematomas and thrombophlebitis (eight patients, of whom five developed small-sized pulmonary emboli).

Similarly to the current experience of most cardiovascular centers, we have seen a striking diminution of perioperative myocardial infarction due to improved operative techniques (cold light, magnifying lenses, delicate new sutures, and cardioplegia, as the principal factors).

DISCUSSION

It is very difficult to summarize all the data accumulated in the literature on this subject and compare it to the work we have done since 1967. Approximately 1,300 papers have been published in the short period

TABLE 13

Patients separated according to surgical risk in relation to clinical classification

	Number of patients	Deaths
Low-risk		
Stable angina	169	3
Recent-onset angina, class I & II	31	1
Prolonged myocardial ischemia	10	
Equivalent to angina pectoris	6	
Atypical angina	26	
Asymptomatic	41	
Total	283	4 (1.4%)
High-risk		
Progressive angina:		
Class III	66	7
Class IV	191	
Intermediate syndrome	7	
Angina after acute myocardial infarction	41	3
Recent-onset angina class III & IV	66	2
Dyspnea	4	
Acute myocardial infarction:	29	2
Subendocardial	21	
VSD	5	
MI	2	
Severe arrhythmias	1	
Total	404	14 (3.4%)

between 1977 and 1982. Readers will find an excellent review up to 1980 in "The Heart, Update II," by Hurst et al.[20]

I think there is currently a unanimous recognition of the low hospital mortality rate achieved with this

TABLE 14

Mortality rate in relation to age distribution

Age (years)	Males	Females	Number of deaths*	%
20–30	2	1		
31–40	30	5		
41–50	136	10	1	
51–60	272	36	8	2.6
61–70	182	32	10	4.6
71–75 }	22	3	1	
75+ }	3			3.7
Total	647	87		

*Only two deaths occurred among women.

TABLE 15

Correlation between risk factors and mortality

Factors	Number of patients	%	Deaths	%
Without risk factors	54	7.3	1	1.8
One risk factor	218	29.6	6	2.75
Two risk factors	262	35.7	8	3
Three or more risk factors	200	27.1	5	2.5
Total	734		20	

procedure.[21–27] Obviously this is mainly due to a better selection of surgical candidates, improvement in preoperative preparations and anesthesia, standardized operative techniques, magnifying lenses, cardioplegia, and postoperative care. It is always difficult to compare the results from different institutions, because they depend on the type of patients operated on.

First of all, it is necessary to determine the state of the left ventricle, in my opinion the most important predictor in risk of inhospital and late mortality. For example, it would be difficult to compare our present series (Table 11) with the Coronary Artery Surgery Study[27] because of 6,630 patients operated upon, only 107 had an ejection fraction lower than 30 percent. Even comparison with our preliminary study at the Cleveland Clinic up to 1970, would be hard, because there the majority of our patients had single- and double-vessel disease, and in Buenos Aires in 1982, 55.4 percent had disease of three or more vessels and 12.6 percent, left main trunk obstruction: of these, 8.7 percent had concomitant triple-vessel disease (Table 10).

I feel certain that in most surgical centers the mortality rate has come down due to greater clinical experience, in spite of the fact that the high-risk population is increasing. The clinical state certainly plays a significant role, as shown in Table 13. Nevertheless, it must be noted that 11 patients included in the 20 deaths had a previous myocardial infarction and 4 had an ejection fraction of less than 0.3.

We have not seen any significant increase in mortality rate related to the number of bypasses, but we have seen a significant decrease among patients with left main trunk obstruction since 1977 when mortality rate was 7.2 percent (10 deaths in 139 patients). At present it is very similar to that of the overall population. In 1982 we operated on 87 patients with one death.

Age still is an important factor in our series. As seen in Table 14 there is only one death in the below-50 group; mortality rate increases to 2.6 percent between 51 and 60 years of age, and 4.6 percent between 61 and 70 years. Twenty-eight patients were operated on though they were 70 years of age or more. The eldest was 81 and still is alive at 88. It is always my policy to tell elderly patients that risk increases with age, though a final and adequate biologic evaluation will show if the operation can be performed. The psychological evaluation is also important, and the final decision should finally be made by the patient.

Only two women died. Consequently sex is not as significant a factor in our recent experience as it used to be. This is strictly related to intervention with magnifying lenses, because coronary arteries are much more difficult to handle in women. As previously described, operative mortality rate was not related to risk factors except in the case of diabetes, mainly because of postoperative infection and a slight increase in hypertension.

In our series of 298 patients with hypertension we had nine deaths; however, two had a ventricular aneurysmectomy as well as a revascularization procedure. Hypertension alone was present in only two patients. In the other seven, two were diabetic and five were heavy smokers. Altogether three had two risk factors and four had three or more risk factors. Nowadays, with the use of beta blocking agents, nitroprusside, and intravenous nitroglycerin, hypertension is no longer a contraindication for surgery.

I believe it is important to remark on the significant decrease in mortality rate in combined simultaneous procedures, mainly aortic and mitral valve replacement and direct myocardial revascularization; there were only two deaths in 42 patients in spite of the fact that 2 patients had concomitant ascending aorta graft replacement.

Mortality is also low during ventricular aneurysmectomy and myocardial revascularization. If we exclude the two deaths of patients operated on for an acute aneurysm, there is only one death in the remaining 34 patients. I think this is due to the better protection of the myocardium made possible by the utilization of cardioplegic solution.

Postoperative myocardial infarction, one of the major challenges in our work, has also diminished constantly.[25] In the present series, 23 patients developed new Q waves and concomitant increase of the enzyme level (3 percent). It has been stated that the utilization of radionuclide studies gives greater precision in the determination of myocardial damage.[28–31] It would also appear that the percentage of myocardial infarction may be higher. I would like to point out the need to make a preoperative scan if we want to have accurate studies because some patients without a previous history of myocardial infarction may have positive scintigraphic test.[32]

Cineangiography will undoubtedly give clear evidence as can be seen in nine patients with definite new Q waves and increased enzymes who were restudied in the immediate postoperative recuperation period. In six patients, all the bypasses were patent, and no changes could be detected in the left ventricle in the two oblique projections. In one patient with a single bypass, the graft was occluded; one patient with a triple bypass had two patent grafts and one occluded; and in one patient with five bypasses one was occluded and four were patent, and yet no significant changes were found in the cine studies. It is my belief that the degree of myocardial damage varies significantly, ranging from a small deterioration without clinical manifestations not even detected later by cine coronary angiography to a large necrosis with important clinical manifestations and different degrees of diminished myocardial performance. This conclusion explains the controversies encountered in the literature related to the prognosis of patients with perioperative myocardial infarction.[33–38]

Graft Patency

It would be difficult to judge the present work in Buenos Aires; out of 4,438 coronary operations performed, only 342 patients were restudied because in the majority of cases they became symptomatic (Table 16*A* and *B*). I think one would have to hire some gauchos to catch the Latin American patients with a lasso to be able to catheterize them! Nevertheless, these data confirm that symptomatic patients had a higher proportion of occluded grafts, and this factor is of paramount importance when we compare different statistics. Early occlusions are certainly related to the operative technique used and diminish with clinical experience,[39–44] and late occlusions are mainly caused by atheromatous changes in the vein or progression of the disease in the coronary territory due to arteriosclerotic metabolic disorders. Our findings confirm previous reports that these are much more severe in patients with an abnormal serum lipid level.[45,46]

Though the proportion of patent grafts improves with clinical experience, it reaches a plateau of between 75 and 85 percent in the different coronary territories in the long-term follow-up studies. If we consider that the circumflex coronary artery has the lowest number of patent grafts, utilizing the posterolateral wall of the aorta and placing the graft through the transverse sinus may increase the patency rate. In 32 grafts studied (between 1 month and 2 years), only 3 were occluded. Nevertheless, the number is too small to draw definite conclusions. The best studies on long-term follow-up were made by Bourassa et al. in Montreal, where the average vein graft occlusion rate is 2 percent per year.[43,47]

Opinions vary about the efficacy of anticoagulant and/or antiplatelet therapy in improving the patency rate, ranging from contributions that deny any advantage[48] to a recent paper showing that sulfinpyrazone may reduce the incidence of early closure.[49]

TABLE 16
Repeat cineangiographic studies with selective injection of the grafts

Surgery	Number of patients	Number of bypasses	Open	%	Occluded	%
A **Symptomatic—302 patients***						
1 bypass	76	76	60	78.9	16	21.7
2 bypasses	196	392	316	80.6	1 bypass, 54 2 bypasses, 22	19.4
3 bypasses	24	72	57	79.1	1 bypass, 9 2 bypasses, 6	20.9
3 + bypasses	6	24	15	62.5	1 bypass, 3 2 bypasses, 3	37.5
Total	302	564	448			
B **Asymptomatic—40 patients†**						
1 bypass	6	6	6			
2 bypasses	26	52	50		2	
3 bypasses	6	18	13		5	
3 + bypasses	2	8	7		1	
Total	40	84	76	90.4	8	

*Catheterization was performed because of angina, 171 patients; positive stress test, 60 patients; arrhythmias, 51 patients; myocardial infarction, 24 patients; heart failure, 30 patients. Within 1 month, 30 patients; 1 to 3 months, 35 patients; 3 months to 1 year, 90 patients; 1 to 3 years, 60 patients; > 3 years, 85 patients.

†Within 1 month, 8 patients; 1 to 3 months, 4 patients; 3 months to 1 year, 12 patients; 1 to 3 years, 8 patients; > 3 years, 8 patients.

Nevertheless, we administer antiplatelet therapy to our patients routinely. Very few patients are given anticoagulants, mainly when the coronary arteries or the veins are of poor quality or when we perform coronary endarterectomies.

The mammary artery is an excellent conduit mainly for the anterior descending coronary artery or its diagonal branches and occasionally for lateral branches of the circumflex coronary artery. The results are satisfactory[50,51] with an excellent patency rate, but the previous selection made by the surgeons must be mentioned: only mammary arteries of excellent caliber are used for myocardial revascularization and are connected mainly to the anterior descending coronary artery.

The patency rate of saphenous vein grafts is the highest in the majority of the series reported, on this particlar artery and very close to that obtained with mammary-coronary anastomosis. Since saphenous vein grafts can withstand a greater flow,[52,53] we use the mammary artery mainly for small coronary arteries and in the group of younger patients, knowing from our previous work with the Vineberg procedure that they very seldom present atheromatous plaques and remain free from them for many years.

I am convinced today as I was before[4] that the quality of the saphenous vein and the coronary artery, mainly the distal runoff, and a proper operative technique are the most important factors related to the early patency rate.

Late Evolution

Hundreds of papers have been published on myocardial revascularization with the saphenous vein graft technique. During the last 10 years most of them analyze the data for the purpose of comparing medical versus surgical treatment.

As has been pointed out by Proudfit[54] the results can be analyzed in the following four ways: (1) They can be analyzed only on the clinical basis of angina pectoris and/or myocardial infarction. This is an unsatisfactory method because of the possibility of error in diagnosis. In our hospital, 13,320 cine coronary angiograms were performed up to December 1982. Of these 85 percent were of males and 17 percent of this group had normal coronary arteries; 15 percent were females and in this group 38 percent showed normal coronary arteries.

(2) They can be analyzed on an adequate cine coronary angiogram. The studies can be retrospective or prospective. In the first category, the bias can be that the medically treated patients were chosen over different periods of time from the surgical ones and received different medication, a fact which must be con-

sidered in view of the progress made in recent years. Prospective studies are more logical because they include patients studied over a similar period of time. It is also important to select only patients who had similar indications for surgical treatment when making both the medical and the surgical selection, as was done at the Cleveland Clinic[55,56] and at the Guemes Hospital in all our prospective studies (Fig. 4A,B,C, and D).

(3) They can be analyzed in randomized prospective studies. These have been postulated as the only valid method of therapeutic research.[57] Nevertheless, "good science in randomized clinical trials, as in other investigations, involves simple principles, such as incorporating prior knowledge into the hypotheses and directing analyses toward evaluation of those hypotheses,"[58] but I doubt if some of the centers involved in the most popular randomized study on coronary arteriosclerosis had the proper knowledge of the disease. Furthermore, as mentioned by May et al.,[59] two classes of subjects are often confused—exclusions and withdrawals—and they recommend that reported study results should include outcome data from all subjects randomized in the group to which they were originally assigned.

This is really troublesome if we analyze the data accumulated in the Veterans Administration (VA) randomized study of stable angina[60] and the National Heart, Lung and Blood Institute (NHLBI) study of unstable angina.[61] In the former, a significant selection was made: Patients with acute myocardial infarction in the last 6 months, unstable angina, congestive heart failure 3 weeks prior to catheterization, uncontrolled diabetes, hypertension, ventricular aneurysm, low ejection fraction, elevated end-diastolic pressure (60 percent of this type of patients was operated on and appears in the Cleveland Clinic series[62]) were excluded, only to find in the same VA study in 1981[63] that high-risk patients (ST-segment depression on ECG, previous myocardial infarction, history of hypertension, and angina class III and IV) greatly benefit from surgery even after removal of left main coronary artery disease! These findings were enhanced when patients in the 10 hospitals with the lowest operative mortality (3.3 percent) were compared.

We have already criticized the VA hospital studies.[9] Nevertheless, I think it is important to remember that the majority of patients were from a low-risk population (50 percent coronary obstruction on selection, only 26 percent with triple-vessel disease, exclusion of left main coronary artery), and the operation was done with a low graft patency rate (68 percent), with 18 percent perioperative myocardial infarction, 12 percent of the patients without patent grafts, and 17 percent crossover.

In my opinion, the NHLBI unstable angina study includes patients with different degrees of risk, as we

demonstrated in previous papers.[9,10] Consequently, mortality rate with medical treatment was low.[64,65] Seventeen percent of the patients were excluded because of left main trunk obstruction, and the crossovers were highly significant: 3 percent during initial hospitaliza-

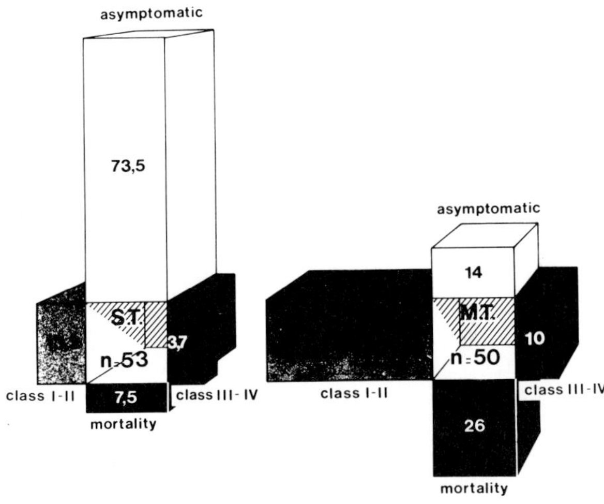

A

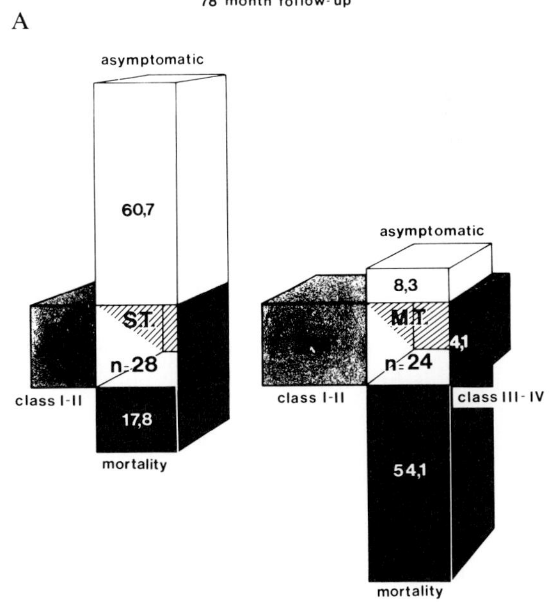

B

FIGURE 4 Prospective study. (A) Stable angina. (B) Intermediate syndrome. (C, p. 274) Angina after acute myocardial infarction. (D, p. 274) Patients with severely deteriorated left ventricle. MT = medical treatment; ST = surgical treatment; n = number of patients. Percentage of mortality and clinical state (classes I, II, III, IV of NYHA classification).

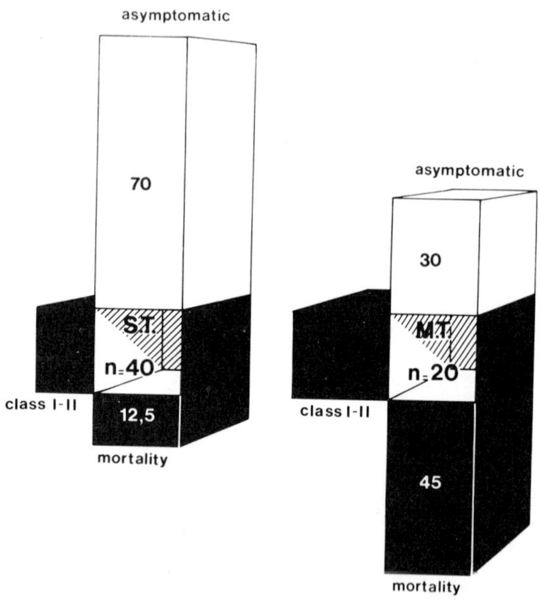

ANGINA AFTER ACUTE MYOCARDIAL INFARCTION
60 month follow-up

C

the medical profession is still confused by these factors: A recent NHLBI article reports on patients with anterior descending coronary artery occlusions with a hospital mortality rate of 9 percent, 23 percent nonfatal perioperative myocardial infarction, and 37 percent crossover, but the final survival curves are plotted following the original randomization of patients![66]

The European Coronary Surgery study of stable angina was designed along the lines of the American VA study. It is so similar that both report six patients who died while they were awaiting surgery as operative deaths! Even though the study showed a low mortality rate in the medically treated group, surgical results were better for the whole series, left main coronary obstruction, triple-vessel disease, and in patients with stenosis in the proximal third of the left anterior descending artery constituting a component of either two- or three-vessel disease. Once more the crossover rate was 27 percent.[67,68]

(4) Results can be analyzed in comparison with the normal population. The original contribution by Green et al.,[69] as well as Lawrie et al.,[70] and the University

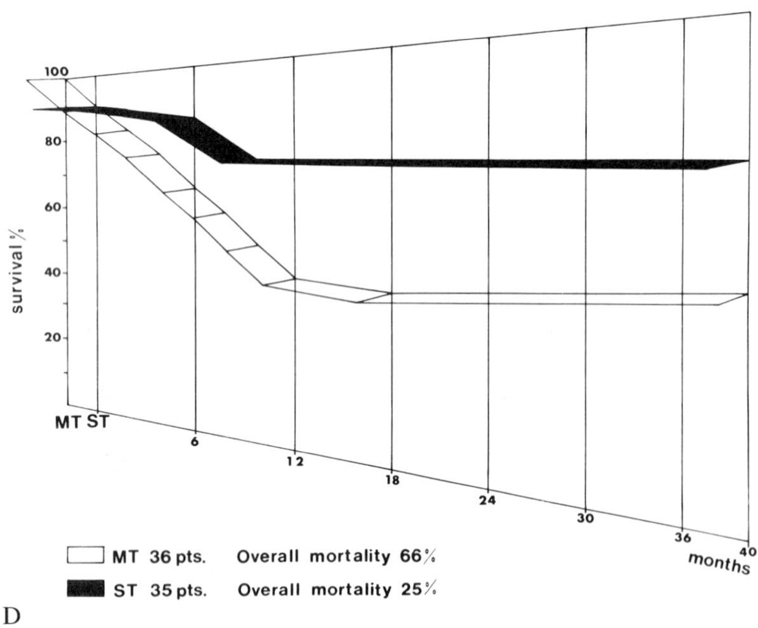

D

tion, 13 percent within 6 months, 19 percent in 1 year, 31 percent in 2 years, and 36 percent in 4 years. Forty-nine percent of patients with triple-vessel disease have been already operated on. We agree with Hultgren et al.[13] that "the high incidence of crossovers and the short follow-up time in the MIRU Study limited the evaluation of comparative survival data." And

of Alabama's Rackley[71] have shown on the basis of U.S. Vital Statistics or insurance actuarial curves that patients with severe coronary artery disease can achieve a mortality rate similar to a matched normal population. The great advantage of this method is that it eliminates the need for randomized studies. However, there are complicating factors, as Proudfit has analyzed.[54] I agree with him nevertheless that this method of comparison may be useful for a limited period of time, perhaps 5 years, even though it has been highly criticized to the point of stating that "patients who undergo cardiac surgery are selected from that patient population because they do not have life-threatening disease and in most instances have not experienced sudden near-death"![72] It is difficult to accept such a criticism, because currently most subjects operated on are high-risk patients, some with acute myocardial infarction and others even resuscitated after a sudden death episode. In conclusion, I certainly agree with Corday,[73] who first endorses the need for randomized series, that these trials "have failed to unfold the true picture because of statistical distortions, small populations, and surgical techniques too poor to provide a true picture." On the other hand, "retrospective and prospective nonrandomized series which incorporate a larger number of patients over a more prolonged period appear to provide more meaningful long-term results and they often demonstrate an improved longevity."

Improvement in Left Ventricular Function

As we have previously pointed out, several observations confirm that oxygen delivery is enhanced by coronary bypass operation.[9] Myocardial contractility improves in consequence. The confusion in the literature is related to the state of the left ventricle prior to surgery: if left ventricular contractions are normal, results can only be compared with exercise, and our experience recently presented at the IX World Congress of Cardiology confirms that even a normal left ventricle with a decrease in ejection fraction during exercise

prior to surgery regains normal limits after myocardial revascularization.[74] Similar results were obtained with contrast ventriculography and radionuclide angiography.[75] Recent studies[76,77] suggest that information may be obtained even from resting studies of ^{201}Tl. If abnormal ventricular function is due to ischemia, the preoperative study with nitroglycerin and postextrasystolic potentiation can demonstrate left ventricular improvement after revascularization.[78–84] Of course, if segments of the ventricle have been replaced by scar tissue, this is irreversible. Nevertheless, even patients with severe left ventricular dysfunction can improve if properly selected.[85]

Prevention of Further Myocardial Infarction

It is difficult to obtain proper data on this question, and we confess that we were not able to reach definite conclusions in our prospective studies. The contribution made by Mason et al.[86] with data compiled from eight referral institutions shows that coronary bypass surgery diminishes the incidence rate of late myocardial infarction when 2,224 surgical patients are compared with 1,118 medically treated ones. It is interesting to note that the incidence of fatal myocardial infarction is also significantly lower among the surgically treated group.

Diminution of Sudden Death

Our findings confirm the report of Vismara et al. as can be seen in Fig. 5.[87] It must be noted that we only include patients with stable and unstable angina with

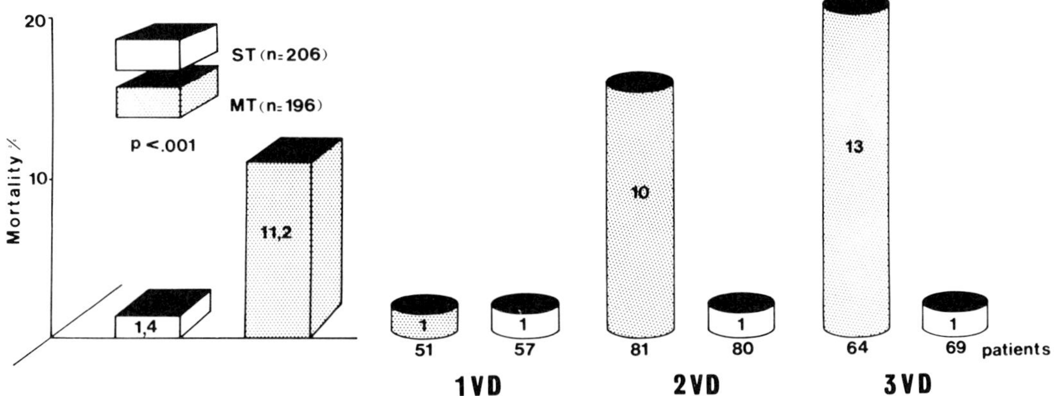

FIGURE 5 Incidence of sudden death in our prospective studies. Most of sudden deaths in the medically treated group occurred in patients with triple-vessel disease. MT = medical treatment; ST = surgical treatment; VD = vessel disease.

similar clinical and angiographic characteristics. Patients from both groups were candidates for the operation.

THE FUTURE

Undoubtedly in the future coronary bypass surgery will concentrate on patients with acute myocardial infarction and patients in the preclinical stage without anginal manifestations.

We have already analyzed cine coronary angiography in patients with acute and subacute myocardial infarction. Our total surgical experience in this field is shown in Table 17. The majority—174—are among patients who had continuing angina of severe degree after an acute infarction and were operated on in the last 10 years (the first operation was performed in July 1972). Most of them were between 40 and 60 years of age (71.8 percent), 20.3 percent were over 60, and the eldest was 71 years old; 44.7 percent were operated on in the acute phase (0 to 10 days), 24.7 percent between 11 and 20 days, and 30.6 percent between 21 and 30 days. Anterior infarctions made up 65 percent, and of the overall population the infarcted area was revascularized in 70.8 percent of the patients. Most grafts (49 percent) were placed in the anterior descending coronary artery. A total of 1.8 grafts per patient were done. The most common were two grafts (42.7 percent) and one graft (32.2 percent). Of the six deaths, four belonged to class IV, one to class V, and one to class II.

Angina after acute myocardial infarction is an entity that plays a secondary role in modern cardiology and is very seldom mentioned in literature. As far as we know, only Chaturvedi et al.[88] remarked in 1974 that 23 patients discharged after an acute myocardial infarction complicated by angina had a poor prognosis: 25 percent died within 3 months and 37 percent within a year, and Hurst also emphasizes the need for possible surgery.[89] Even though the number of patients is too small, our prospective follow-up study (Fig. 4C) shows that these patients can benefit from surgery. There is a striking difference in mortality rate and the percentage of asymptomatic patients. It is interesting to note that 66 percent of the deaths in the medically treated group were sudden. Postoperative cineangiograms were performed in 16 percent of patients of the surgical group in this series. Of the 25 grafts 92 percent were patent, and the analysis of the cineventriculogram showed significant improvement in left ventricular contractility in most patients.[9] We are firmly convinced that angina post acute myocardial infarction should be included in the unstable angina group of patients. The prognosis of this entity is similar to that of patients with intermediate syndrome.[9] We believe that if a patient develops angina after an acute myocardial infarction, he or she should be studied angiographically and revascularized when indicated, regardless of the time elapsed since the acute episode. Patients in class I, II and IV will improve, because the infarction area is small and the area of ischemia is more extensive. The operation is more palliative in patients in class V and VI but can be lifesaving for most of them.

The other complication of acute infarction constitutes the highest risk group of patients in whom medical treatment is obsolete, mainly patients with ventricular septal defect and severe acute mitral insufficiency. Mortality rate may look high, but it is important to emphasize that 8 patients of the ventricular septal defect group were in cardiogenic shock, 18 had a concomitant ventricular aneurysm which was resected or plicated, 10 had concomitant revascularization procedure, and 8 required balloon pump circulatory-assisted device. Two patients with mitral insufficiency were in cardiogenic shock, 18 in severe cardiac insufficiency, and 2 were operated with intractable pulmonary edema. Aneurysmectomy was necessary in 5 patients, and 12 had concomitant revascularization procedure. Balloon pump was needed in 6 patients.

The majority of patients (19) with intractable arrhythmias had a ventricular aneurysm which was resected, and concomitant revascularization procedure was performed in 15 patients. The repetitive episodes of arrhythmias were controlled or diminished significantly in 18 patients. The mortality rate decreased from January 1980. Up to December 1982 there was one death in 15 patients operated on because of a ventricular septal defect, two in 9 patients with severe mitral insufficiency, and one in 11 patients with intractable arrhythmias, mainly due to the improvement in balloon pumping system, operative technique, myocardial protection with cardioplegic solution, and intraoperative mapping.[90–94]

Another type of patient that has definite indications

TABLE 17

Complicated acute myocardial infarction: surgical treatment

Complication*	Number of patients	Deaths	%
APAMI	174	7	4.1
VSD	35	9	25.7
MI	28	12	43.0
IA	26	5	19.0
Total	263	33	

*APAMI = angina after acute myocardial infarction; IA = intractable arrhythmias; MI = mitral insufficiency; VSD = ventricular septal defect.

for cineangiography is the nontransmural myocardial infarction group. A recent publication by Hutter et al.[95] confirms previous observations[96,97] showing that these patients have a poor prognosis after discharge from hospital even though they have a low mortality rate in the coronary care unit. Nontransmural infarction is a more unstable state, because patients with this condition have not suffered a complete infarction of the area perfused by the involved coronary artery, which is not occluded in the majority of the patients studied with cineangiography at our institution. At present, it is our policy to study all the patients with cine coronary angiography before discharging them from hospital, and operations are performed after a careful reading of the cine study. Currently, a total of 32 patients have been operated on using this approach with one hospital death.

The introduction of fibrinolytic agents has opened a new field in acute myocardial infarction.[98–105] They should be used within the first 6 h after onset as demonstrated in our experimental work with monkeys in Buenos Aires.[106] This is the time that the myocardial muscle requires to recover if blood supply is reestablished. Of course, as we already know from the data collected, most patients show severe obstruction after the artery has been cleared by the fibrinolytic agent.[107] Consequently, most patients should be revascularized,[108] not only to prevent rethrombosis and reinfarction but also to treat other obstructions in different coronary territories, knowing in advance that the majority of patients will show obstruction beside that of the artery involved in the infarcted area. In skilled and experienced hands percutaneous transluminal coronary artery reconstruction should be considered mainly for single lesions.[109]

The surgical treatment of uncomplicated myocardial infarction poses significant logistical problems.[110,111] The biggest is how to organize in large cities like Buenos Aires the rapid transfer of patients to a well-equipped center where every measure can be taken fast and efficiently as soon as the diagnosis is made.

Patients without angina need serious consideration in view of all information accumulated in the natural history of coronary arteriosclerosis since 1958. I think cardiologists and cardiovascular surgeons should remember that at least 50 percent of the deaths among patients under medical treatment are sudden (53 percent in our prospective studies) and of this group, in 40 percent sudden death is the first manifestation of the disease. On the other hand, the study of 955 consecutive patients admitted to our coronary care unit with myocardial infarction and analyzed prospectively in search of prodromes shows that in 31 percent of cases, myocardial infarction was the first manifestation of the disease, while another 15 percent did not have angina. Therefore, I firmly believe angina is a late and

luxurious manifestation of coronary arteriosclerosis! It helps us to classify our patients properly only when it is present. As a result of cineangiographic findings analyzed previously in this paper (Tables 6 and 7), 328 patients were operated on even though they were totally asymptomatic or without angina (Table 18). Of course, it is a tremendous responsibility, but I think cardiologists and cardiovascular surgeons should consider it their duty to face it in view of the natural history of the disease.

Even though Norris et al.[112] did not find any difference in a long-term follow-up of patients who were asymptomatic after a previous myocardial infarction, everything depends on the proper interpretation of the cine coronary angiography. Recently, Kent[113] from NHLBI has shown that patients with triple-vessel disease (asymptomatic or mildly asymptomatic) and poor exercise capacity have an extremely grave prognosis, contrary to previous studies by the same institution[114] where they were looking mainly for left main trunk obstruction. In our hospital, 104 totally asymptomatic patients with a previous myocardial infarction have been followed for 40 months with cine coronary angiography as the principal landmark for prognosis. Forty-seven patients (28 with single-vessel and 19 with double-vessel disease) had a good prognosis and were placed on medical treatment. Thirty-nine patients (83 percent) were asymptomatic, and 8 patients (17 percent) developed angina class I or II. Fourteen patients had a bad prognosis (13 had triple-vessel disease and 1 left main trunk occlusion). The follow-up of medical treatment showed 11 deaths (7 sudden and 4 caused by a new infarction). Two patients had angina class I, and one was operated on. Forty-three patients were operated on with three late deaths, only one of cardiac

TABLE 18

Coronary bypass operation in patients without angina pectoris

Patient characteristics	Number of patients	Deaths
Asymptomatic patients after a previous MI*	143	1
Asymptomatic patients with vascular disease in other territories	77	1
Noncharacteristic thoracic pain	54	
Valvular Disease	34	1
Positive stress test	14	
Fatigue	3	
Family history or risk factor	3	
Total	328	3

*MI = myocardial infarction.

origin (sudden death). Thirty-four remained asymptomatic, two had a late myocardial infarction, and the remainder developed angina class I and II. Asymptomatic patients represent, therefore, a group with different prognoses. Noninvasive techniques, mainly radionuclides with exercise and cineangiography, help us to define these entities properly.

The second important group in Table 7 are patients with vascular disease in other territories, mainly abdominal aorta and peripheral and carotid arteries. As described previously, the incidence of silent coronary obstruction is significant, and coronary bypass operation performed as the first step not only diminishes operative risk but also improves long-term survival rate because the main cause of death (early and late) in vascular surgery is myocardial infarction.[115–117]

FINAL COMMENTS

Direct myocardial revascularization using the saphenous vein graft technique and mammary coronary anastomosis introduced in 1967 and 1968 owe their initial development to (1) the pioneer work done at the Cleveland Clinic where the foundations of a new era in the knowledge of coronary arteriosclerosis were laid by Mason Sones with the introduction of cine coronary angiography and by Proudfit and collaborators' with their analysis of the natural history of the disease which gave us, indeed, at the surgical department the basis for the routine and systematic application of coronary bypass surgery since 1967; (2) Johnson et al.[118] in Milwaukee from whom we learned that multiple bypasses can be placed at the distal distribution of the coronary artery tree, and (3) Green[119] in New York, who developed mammary coronary anastomosis.

This period ended in London in 1970 during the VIth World Congress of Cardiology when I had the chance to discuss with Charles Friedberg, an old, respected, and always-remembered friend, all the facets of a controversy that I will never forget, and where, I think, for the first time thousands of colleagues from all over the world had the chance to see important data proving that the myocardial muscle can be oxygenated with a new blood supply. Since then, surgeons have gained confidence with the improvements in the operative technique, significant diminution of operative mortality rate and perioperative myocardial infarction in pure revascularization procedures, combined operations (valvular replacement and ventricular aneurysmectomy), and even in patients at the terminal stage of the disease with ejection fraction of less than 30 percent, though an increasing number of bypasses are being performed, and more and more high-risk patients are being operated on. Maybe the return to endarterec-

tomies will allow us to indicate this procedure even more frequently,[120] particularly in young patients with diffuse disease, poor distal runoff, and preserved heart muscle, if we know in advance that the operative risk and the rate of perioperative myocardial infarction is greater.

With reference to the diagnostic procedures, the noninvasive tests in current use are not 100 percent sensitive or specific.[121–127] Their limitations are related to the prevalence of the disease in the groups studied. The addition of radionuclide studies improves results. Nevertheless, I would like to note that cine coronary angiography will remain the most important tool we have and will have for proper diagnosis of coronary patients. Not even the recent sophisticated method of nuclear magnetic resonance imaging, digital radiography, and new devices from computer tomography can match the accuracy of a good-quality cineangiogram, nowadays performed at a minimal risk. Proper interpretation of cine imaging is, of course, mandatory. If this is not done correctly, results become confusing. For example, if we review the recent papers from the Coronary Artery Surgery Study,[27,128–131] apart from other factors that can be questioned, we will find that patients are generally classified according to a myocardial jeopardized index, using right anterior oblique projection as the only projection for ventricular wall study. This means that the lateral wall and interventricular septum are not included though they play an important role in patients with coronary arteriosclerosis and are even more significant in patients with ventricular aneurysm. I can imagine what confusion the Coronary Artery Surgery Study (CASS) will create from now on. Another example is how poorly collateral circulation is analyzed,[113] and we have already emphasized the need for a proper understanding of its significance.

It must also be pointed out that from now on the crossover factor will make prospective and randomized studies very difficult to perform. For example, we tried to make another study on unstable angina in our hospital, and during the first month alone we had 31, 14, and 17 percent crossovers, respectively, in the group of patients with recent-onset angina class III and IV, intermediate syndrome, and angina post acute myocardial infarction due to a different medical attitude.

I think we have enough evidence in literature to accept that the operation not only improves the quality of life but also prolongs life in (1) left main trunk obstruction; (2) triple-vessel disease; (3) select cases of double-vessel disease;[132,133] (4) possibly select correctly analyzed cases of single-vessel disease (Fig. 6); (5) ventricular aneurysm;[134,135] (6) abnormal ventricle,[136–141] particularly considering the current significant decrease of mortality; (7) unstable angina, if properly tabulated and categorized; (8) angina post acute myocardial infarction; (9) acute myocardial infarction

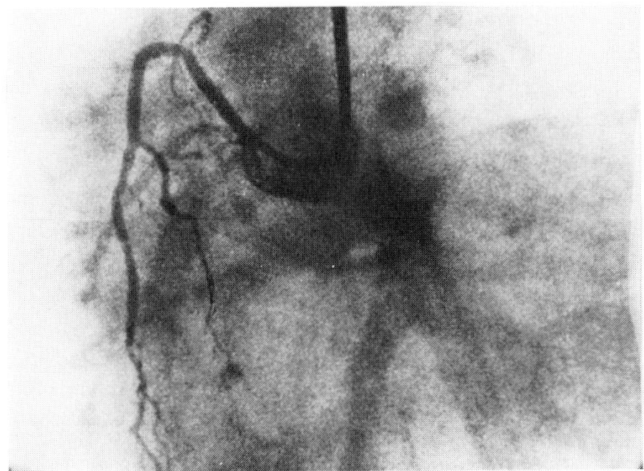

A

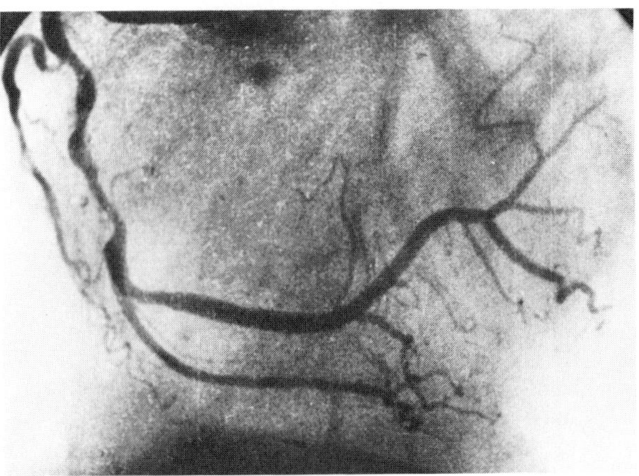

B

FIGURE 6 (*A*) Small right coronary artery. (*B*) Large right coronary artery. The amount of muscle in jeopardy is quite different. Patients with single-vessel disease cannot be placed in only one category.

complicated with ventricular septal defect and mitral insufficiency.

The introduction of percutaneous angioplasty by Gruentzig[142] seems to be beneficial in a limited group of patients,[143] and with more experience we will find its proper place in the treatment of coronary arteriosclerosis. I do not believe that on the basis of the data accumulated to date it can be applied in patients with diffuse disease.[144]

Some social and economic implications recently presented in a symposium held in Washington remain for discussion.[145] I think we have to remember that in the same issue of *The New England Journal of Medicine* in which Braunwald published his controversial editorial[146] discussing the financial implication of the 70,000 or more coronary bypass operations performed in the United States at that time, on page 650 Harris wrote that 75,000 hip replacements were also done in America, I imagine at a similar or even greater financial cost!

It is time to realize that modern medicine, which has increased life-expectancy so much, is very expensive because of present advances in technology which make some equipment obsolete within a year. If this is a problem in the United States, the reader may easily imagine its magnitude in Latin America. We still have to find the most viable way to give the best medical treatment to all the population by means of proper medical system. I speak for all of us who have been involved in this field from the beginning and have had to travel a long and difficult road, full of obstacles, trying to convince our medical colleagues that coronary bypass operation is a good way to treat a select group of coronary patients when I recall having had the courage to write in 1971: "Without being a prophet, I am convinced that the present combined medical and surgical efforts will show that the natural evolution of coronary arteriosclerosis already has been changed."[147] "I am convinced that at present the operation not only improves the quality of life but also prolongs life in properly selected patients."[148] It was gratifying to read the conclusion of the Consensus Development Conference held in Washington by NIH in December 1980:[149]

The symptom of angina pectoris is reported to be relieved in 80 to 90 percent of patients undergoing surgery for chronic stable angina. Bypasses have reduced the subsequent number of cardiac related events, the amount of medication required, and the frequency of hospitalization. The majority of patients have been able to increase their exercise capacity and improve their NYHA functional class after operation . . . The operation has been documented by improvements in functional exercise testing, angina threshold, left ventricular wall motion, left ventricular ejection fraction during exercise, indexes of myocardial oxygen consumption during exercise, and lactate extraction across the myocardium . . . There is the conclusion of the panel that coronary artery bypass represents a major advance in the treatment of patients with coronary artery disease. Evidence has been presented to support the conclusions that an improvement in the quality of life, a decrease in myocardial ischemia, and an increase in survival have been demonstrated after coronary artery bypass in selected subsets of patients.

Here in the south our aim has been mainly directed at organizing well-planned teaching programs. Since July 1971, 51 postgraduate courses have been given at different levels, and 196 residents and fellows have been trained in clinical cardiology, noninvasive techniques, cardiac laboratory, coronary care unit, and cardiovascular surgery. Fifty percent come from Latin American countries. The harvest has been slow because of the conservative cardiology I have found; nevertheless, it has been highly gratifying.

REFERENCES

1 Matthews, M. B.: Historical Background, in D. G. Julian (ed.), "Angina Pectoris," Churchill Livingstone, Edinburgh, 1977, p. 2.

1a Favaloro, R. G.: Saphenous Vein Autograft Replacement of Severe Segmental Coronary Artery Occlusion. Operative Technique. *Ann. Thorac. Surg.*, 5:337, 1968.

2 Favaloro, R. G., Effler, D. B., Cheanvechai, C. H., Quint, R. A., and Sones, F. M., Jr.: Acute Coronary Insufficiency (Impending Myocardial Infarction and Myocardial Infarction). Surgical Treatment by the Saphenous Vein Graft Technique. *Am. J. Cardiol.*, 28:598, 1971.

3 Favaloro, R. G., Effler, D. B., Groves, L. K., Sheldon, W. C., Shirey, E. K., and Sones, F. M., Jr.: Severe Segmental Obstruction of the Left Main Coronary Artery and Its Divisions. Surgical Treatment by the Saphenous Vein Graft Technique, *J. Thorac. Cardiovasc. Surg.*, 60:469, 1970.

4 Favaloro, R. G.: "Surgical Treatment of Coronary Arteriosclerosis," The Williams & Wilkins Company, Baltimore, 1970, p. 66.

5 McGoon, D. W. (ed.): The Quest for Ideal Myocardial Protection, *J. Thorac. Cardiovasc. Surg.*, 79:150, 1980.

6 Magovern, G. J., Jr., Flaherty, J. T., Gott, V. L., Bulkley, B. H., and Gardner, T. J.: Failure of Blood Cardioplegia to Protect Myocardium at Lower Temperatures, *Circulation*, 66 (suppl. 1):60, 1982.

7 Buckberg, G. D.: A Proposed "Solution" to the Cardioplegic Controversy, *J. Thorac. Cardiovasc. Surg.*, 77:803, 1979.

8 Report of the J.I.S. and F. of C./World Health Organization: Nomenclature and Criteria for Diagnosis of Ischemic Heart Disease, *Circulation*, 59:607, 1979.

9 Favaloro, R. G.: Direct Myocardial Revascularization: A Ten Year Journey. Myths and realities, *Am. J. Cardiol.*, 43:109, 1979.

10 Bertolasi, C. A., Trongé, J. E., Carreño, C. A., Jalon, J., and Ruda Vega, M.: Unstable Angina: Prospective and Randomized Study of Its Evolution with and without Surgery. Preliminary Report. *Am. J. Cardiol.*, 33:201, 1974.

11 Bertolasi, C. A., Trongé, J. E., Riccitelli, M. A., Villamayor, R. M., and Zuffardi, E.: Natural History of Unstable Angina with Medical or Surgical Therapy, *Chest*, 70:596, 1976.

12 Bertolasi, C. A., Trongé, J. E., and Mon, G. A.: Clinical Spectrum of Unstable Angina, *Clin. Cardiol.*, 2:113, 1979.

13 Hultgren, H. N., Shettigar, U. R., and Miller, D. C.: Medical Versus Surgical Treatment of Unstable Angina, *Am. J. Cardiol.*, 50:663, 1982.

14 Freedman, B., Richmond, D. R., and Kelly, D. T.: Pathophysiology of Coronary Artery Spasm, *Circulation*, 66:705, 1982.

15 Sones, F. M., Jr., and Shirey, E. K.: Cine Coronary Arteriography. *Mod. Concepts Cardiovasc. Dis.*, 31:735, 1962.

16 Battler, A., Froelicher, V. F., Gallagher, K. P., Kemper, W. S., and Ross, J., Jr.: Dissociation between Regional Myocardial Dysfunction and ECG Changes during Ischemia in the Conscious Dog, *Circulation*, 62:735, 1980.

17 Favaloro, R. G.: Surgical Treatment of Acute Coronary Insufficiency, in J. C. Davila (ed.), "Second Henry Ford Hospital International Symposium on Cardiac Surgery," Appleton-Century-Crofts, New York, 1977, p. 571.

18 Grinfeld, L. R., de la Fuente, L. M., Shinji, K., Zuffardi, E., and Favaloro, R. G.: Total Body Angiography in Patients with Diffuse Atherosclerosis. *Am. J. Cardiol.*, 33:141, 1974. (Abstract.)

19 Londero, H. F., and de la Fuente, L. M.: Transbrachial Selective Arteriography of the Neck Vessels. Our Experience in 258 Cases, *Catheterization Cardiovasc. Diagnosis*, 3:425, 1977.

20 Hurst, J. W.: "The Heart, Update II," McGraw-Hill Book Company, New York, 1980.

21 Sheldon, W. C., Rincon, G., Effler, D. B., Proudfit, W. L., and Sones, F. M., Jr.: Vein Graft Surgery for Coronary Artery Disease. Survival and Angiographic Results in 1000 Patients, *Circulation*, 48 (suppl. 3):184, 1973.

22 Kouchoukos, N. T., Oberman, A., Kirklin, J. W., Russell, R. O., Jr., Karp, R. B., Pacifico, A. D., et al.: Coronary Bypass Surgery: Analysis of Factors Affecting Hospital Mortality, *Circulation*, 60 (suppl. 2):58, 1979. (Abstract.)

23 Campeau, L., Lespérance, J., Crochet, D., Heitz, A., Grondin, C., and Bourassa, M. G.: Clinical and Angiographic Determinants of Early Mortality Related to Aortocoronary Bypass Surgery, *Can. J. Surg.*, 22:221, 1979.

24 Loop, F. D., Cosgrove, D. M., Lytle, B. S., Thurer, R. L., Suripfendorfer, C., Taylor, P. C., and Proudfit, W. L.: An 11 Year Evolution of Coronary Arterial Surgery (1967–1978), *Ann. Surg.*, 190:444, 1979.

25 Kouchoukos, N. T., Oberman, A., Kirklin, J. W., Russell, R. O., Jr., Karp, R. B., Pacifico, A. D., et al.: Coronary Bypass Surgery: Analysis of Factors Affecting Hospital Mortality, *Circulation*, 62 (suppl. 1):84, 1980.

26 Rahimtoola, S. H., Grunkemeier, G., Tepley, J., Lambert, L., Thomas, D. R., Yuen-Fure, S. et al.: Changes in Coronary Bypass Surgery Leading to Improved Survival, *J.A.M.A.*, 246:1912, 1981.

27 Kennedy, J. W., Kaiser, G. C., Fisher, L. D., Fritz, J.

K., Myers, W., Mudd, J. G. et al.: Clinical and Angiographic Predictors of Operative Mortality from the Collaborative Study in Coronary Artery Surgery (CASS), *Circulation*, 63:793, 1981.

28 Platt, M. R., Mills, L. J., Parkey, R. W., Willerson, J. T., Bonte, F. J., Shapiro, W. et al.: Perioperative Myocardial Infarction Diagnosed by Technetium 99m Stannous Pyrophosphate Myocardial Scintigrams, *Circulation*, 54 (suppl. 3):24, 1976.

29 Righetti, A., Crawford, M. H., O'Rourke, R. A., Hardarson, T. H., Schelbert, H., Daily, P. O., et al.: Detection of Perioperative Myocardial Damage after Coronary Artery Bypass Graft Surgery, *Circulation*, 55:173, 1977.

30 Wadhwa, S. K., Schmidt, D. H., and Johnson, W. D.: Myocardial Infarction in Coronary Artery Surgery: Correlation of Scintigram, Enzymes, Electrocardiography and Vectocardiography, *Clin. Res.*, 25:261A, 1977. (Abstract.)

31 Klausner, S. C., Botvinick, E. H., Shames, D., Ullyot, D. J., Fishman, N. H., Roe, B. B., et al.: The Application of Radionuclide Infarct Scintigraphy to Diagnose Perioperative Myocardial Infarction following Revascularization, *Circulation*, 56:173, 1977.

32 Sabom, M. B., Curry, C. H., Curry, S. L., Pepine, C. J., and Conti, C. R.: Technetium Pyrophosphate Myocardial Scintigraphy in Patients with Stable Angina, *Circulation*, 56 (suppl. 3):62, 1977.

33 Codd, J. E., Wiens, R. D., Kaiser, G. C., Barner, H. B., Tyras, D. H., Mudd, J. G., et al.: Late Sequelae of Perioperative Myocardial Infarction. *Ann. Thorac. Surg.*, 26:208, 1978.

34 Ganz, W., Charuzi, Y., Conklin, C., Marcus, E., Wolfstein, R., Matloff, J., et al.: Morbidity and Mortality of Perioperative Myocardial Infarction in Coronary Bypass Surgery: A Two Year Followup, *Circulation*, 58 (suppl. 2):18, 1978. (Abstract.)

35 Oberman, A., Kouchoukos, N. T., Makar, Y. N., Russell, R. O., Jr., Sheffield, L. T., Ray, M., et al.: Perioperative Myocardial Infarction after Coronary Bypass Surgery, *Cleve. Clin. Q.*, 45:172, 1978.

36 Canby, M., McNeer, J. F., Wagner, G., Ross-Duggan, J., Harris, P., and Rosati, R.: Prognostic Significance of Myocardial Infarction Complicating Aortocoronary Bypass, *Circulation*, 58 (suppl. 2):96, 1978. (Abstract.)

37 Fennell, W. H., Chua, K. G., Cohen, L., Morgan, J., Karunaratne, H. B., Resnekov, L., et al.: Detection, Protection, and Significance of Perioperative Myocardial Infarction following Aortocoronary Bypass, *J. Thorac. Cardiovasc. Surg.*, 78:244, 1979.

38 Namay, D. L., Hammermeister, K. E., Zia, M. S., DeRouen, T. A., Dodge, H. T., and Namay, K.: Effect of Perioperative Myocardial Infarction on Late Survival in Patients Undergoing Coronary Artery Bypass Surgery, *Circulation*, 65:1066, 1982.

39 Sheldon, W. C., and Loop, F. D.: Direct Myocardial Revascularization—1976, *Cleve. Clin. Q.*, 43:97, 1976.

40 Walker, J. A., Friedberg, H. D., Flemma, R. J., and Johnson, W. D.: Determinants of Angiographic Patency of Aortocoronary Vein Bypass Grafts, *Circulation*, 45,46 (suppl. 1):86, 1972.

41 Grondin, C. M., Lespérance, J., Bourassa, M. G., Pasternac, A., Campeau, L., and Grondin, P.: Serial Angiographic Evaluation in 60 Consecutive Patients with Aorto-Coronary Artery Vein Grafts 2 Weeks, 1 Year, and 3 Years after Operation, *J. Thorac. Cardiovasc. Surg.*, 67:1, 1974.

42 Lawrie, G. M., Lie, J. T., Morris, G. C., and Beazley, H. L.: Vein Graft Patency and Intimal Proliferation after Aortocoronary Bypass: Early and Long-term Angiopathologic Correlations, *Am. J. Cardiol.*, 38:856, 1976.

43 Bourassa, M. G., Campeau, L., and Lespérance, J.: Effects of Bypass Surgery on the Coronary Circulation: Incidence and Effects of Vein Graft Occlusion, in S. H. Rahimtoola (ed.), ''Coronary Bypass Surgery,'' F. A. Davis Company, Philadelphia, 1977, p. 107.

44 Kouchoukos, N. T., Karp, R. B., Oberman, A., Russell, R. O., Jr., Alison, H. W., and Holt, J. H., Jr.: Long-term Patency of Saphenous Veins for Coronary Bypass Grafting, *Circulation*, 58 (suppl. 1):96, 1978.

45 Lie, J. T., Lawrie, G. M., and Morris, G. C., Jr.: Atherosclerosis of Aortocoronary Bypass Grafts in Normal and Hyperlipoproteinemic Patients, *Am. J. Cardiol.*, 39:285, 1977. (Abstract.)

46 Flemma, R. J., Barboriak, J., Batayias, G. E., et al.: ''Atherosclerosis in Vein Bypass Grafts after Three Years. Implications on Indications and Prognosis in Coronary Surgery,'' (presented at the 57th Annual Meeting of The American Association for Thoracic Surgery, April 1977).

47 Campeau, L., Lespérance, J., Corbara, F., Hermann, J., Grondin, C., and Bourassa, M. G.: Aortocoronary Saphenous Vein Bypass Graft Changes 5–7 Years after Surgery, *Circulation*, 59 (suppl. 1):117, 1978.

48 Pantely, G. A., Goodnigh, S. H., Jr., Rahimtoola, S. H., Harlan, B. J., DeMots, H., Calvin, L., et al.: Failure of Antiplatelet and Anticoagulant Therapy to Improve Patency of Grafts after Coronary Bypass Surgery: A Controlled Randomized Study, *N. Engl. J. Med.*, 301:962, 1979.

49 Baur, H. R., VanTassel, R. A., Pierach, C. A., and Gobel, F. L.: Effects of Sulfinpyrazone on Early Graft Closure after Myocardial Revascularization, *Am. J. Cardiol.*, 49:420, 1982.

50 Green, G. E.: Internal Mammary Artery-to-Coronary Artery Anastomosis. Three-Year Experience with 165 Patients, *Ann. Thorac. Surg.*, 14:260, 1972.

51 Loop, F. D., Lytle, B. W., Cosgrove, D. M., Sheldon, W. C., Irarrazaval, M., and Taylor, P. C.: Atheroscle-

rosis of the Left Main Coronary Artery: 5 Year Results of Surgical Treatment, *Am. J. Cardiol.*, 44:195, 1979.

52 Flemma, R. J., Singh, H. M., Tector, A. J., Lepley, D. Jr., and Frazier, B. L.: Comparative Hemodynamic Properties of Vein and Mammary Artery in Coronary Bypass Operations, *Ann. Thorac. Surg.*, 20:619, 1975.

53 Grondin, C. M., Lespérance, J., Bourassa, M. G., and Campeau, L.: Coronary Artery Grafting with the Saphenous Vein or Internal Mammary Artery: Comparison of Late Results in two Consecutive Series of Patients, *Ann. Thorac. Surg.*, 20:605, 1975.

54 Proudfit, W. L.: Methods Used to Compare the Medical Management of Coronary Atherosclerotic Heart Disease with Coronary Bypass Surgery, in J. W. Hurst (ed.), "The Heart, Update II," New York, McGraw-Hill Book Company, 1980, p. 3.

55 Bruschke, A. V. G., Proudfit, W. L., and Sones, F. M.: Progress Study of 590 Consecutive Surgical Cases of Coronary Disease followed 5–9 Years. Ventriculographic and Other Correlations, *Circulation*, 47:1154, 1973.

56 Proudfit, W. L., Bruschke, A. V. G., and Sones, F. M., Jr.: Natural History of Obstructive Coronary Artery Disease; Supplement to a 10-Year Study, *Cleve. Clin. Q.*, 45:293, 1978.

57 Chalmers, T. C., Smith, H., Ambroz, A., Reitman, D., and Schroeder, B.: In Defense of the VA Randomized Control Trial of Coronary Artery Surgery, *Clin. Res.*, 26:230, 1978.

58 Detre, K. M., Ware, J., and Mantel, N. (eds.): Are Clinical Trials in Coronary Heart Disease Oversold or Undersold?, *Circulation*, 64:667, 1981.

59 May, G. S., DeMets, D. L., Friedman, L. M., Furberg, C., and Passamani, E.: The Randomized Clinical Trial: Bias in Analysis, *Circulation*, 64:669, 1981.

60 Murphy, M. L., Hultgren, H. N., Detre, K., Thomsen, J., Takaro, T., and Participants of the Veterans Administration Cooperative Study: Treatment of Chronic Stable Angina: A Preliminary Report of Survival Data of the Randomized Veterans Administration Cooperative Study, *N. Engl. J. Med.*, 297:621, 1977.

61 Unstable Angina Pectoris Study Group: Unstable Angina Pectoris National Cooperative Study Group to Compare Medical and Surgical Therapy: A Report of Protocol and Patient Population, *Am. J. Cardiol.*, 37:896, 1976.

62 Loop, F. D., Proudfit, W. L., and Sheldon, W. C.: Coronary Bypass Surgery Weighed in the Balance, *Am. J. Cardiol.*, 42:154, 1978. (Editorial.)

63 Detre, K., Peduzzi, P., Murphy, M., Hultgren, H., Thomsen, J., Oberman, A., et al.: Effect of Bypass Surgery on Survival in Patients in Low- and High-Risk Subgroups Delineated by the Use of Simple Clinical Variables, *Circulation*, 63:1329, 1981.

64 Unstable Angina Pectoris Study: Unstable Angina Pectoris National Cooperative Study Group to Compare Surgical and Medical Therapy: II. In-hospital Experience and Initial Follow-up Results in Patients with One, Two and Three Vessel Disease, *Am. J. Cardiol.*, 42:839, 1978.

65 Unstable Angina Pectoris Study Group: Unstable Angina Pectoris National Cooperative Study Group to Compare Surgical and Medical Therapy, III. Results in Patients with S-T Segment Elevation during Pain, *Am. J. Cardiol.*, 45:819, 1980.

66 Unstable Angina Pectoris: National Cooperative Study Group to Compare Medical and Surgical Therapy. IV. Results in Patients with Left Anterior Anterior Descending Coronary Artery Disease, *Am. J. Cardiol.*, 48:517, 1981.

67 European Coronary Surgery Study Group, Varnauskas, E. (ed.): Second Interim Report. Prospective Randomized Study of Coronary Artery Bypass Surgery in Stable Angina Pectoris, *Lancet*, 2:491, 1980.

68 European Coronary Surgery Study Group, Varnauskas, E. (ed.): Long-term Results of Prospective Randomized Study of Coronary Artery Bypass Surgery in Stable Angina Pectoris, *Lancet*, November 27, 1982.

69 Green, D. G., Bunnell, L. L., Arani, D. T., et al.: "Long-term Survival after Coronary Bypass Surgery" (brochure for exhibit at American Heart Association Meeting, Miami, 1977), Buffalo General Hospital, State University of New York, 1977.

70 Lawrie, G. M., Morris, G. C., Howell, J. F., Tredici, T. D., and Chapman, D. W.: Improved Survival after 5 Years in 1,144 Patients after Coronary Bypass Surgery, *Am. J. Cardiol.*, 42:709, 1978.

71 Rackley, C. E.: Prolongation of Life After Coronary Artery Bypass Surgery at the University of Alabama Medical Center, in J. W. Hurst (ed.), "The Heart, Update II," New York, McGraw-Hill Book Company, 1980, p. 151.

72 Conti, C. R.: Influence of Myocardial Revascularization on Survival. Controversies in Cardiology: Part II, *Am. J. Cardiol.*, 42:330, 1978.

73 Corday, E., Swan, H. J. C., and Corday, S. R.: Medical Versus Surgical Treatment of Coronary Artery Disease—1981, *Cardiovasc. Rev. Rep.*, 2:281, 1981.

74 Weinschelbaum, E., Rojo, H., Rodríguez, A., de la Fuente, L., and Favaloro, R.: Pre and Postoperative Left Ventricular Function at Rest and During Ergometric Test in Patients with Previously Normal Left Ventriculogram" (presented at IX World Congress of Cardiology, Moscow, 1982).

75 Kent, K. M., Borer, J. S., Green, M. V., Bacharach, S. L., McIntosh, C. L., Conkle, D. M., et al.: Effects of Coronary Artery Bypass on Global and Regional Left Ventricular Function during Exercise, *N. Engl. J. Med.*, 298:1434, 1978.

76 Beller, G. A., Watson, D. D., Ackell, P., and Pohost, G. M.: Time Course of Thallium-201 Redistribution after Transient Myocardial Ischemia, *Circulation*, 61:791, 1980.

77 Berger, B. C., Watson, D. D., Burwell, L. R., Crosby, I. K., Wellons, H. A., and Teates, C. D.: Redistribution of Thallium at Rest in Patients with Stable and Unstable Angina and the Effect of Coronary Artery Bypass Surgery, *Circulation*, 60:1114, 1979.

78 Chesebro, J. H., Ritman, E. L., Frye, R. L., Smith, H. C., Rutherford, B. D., and Fulton, R. E.: Regional Myocardial Wall Thickening Response to Nitroglycerin. A Predictor of Myocardial Response to Aortocoronary Bypass Surgery, *Circulation*, 57:952, 1978.

79 Stadius, M., McAnulty, J. H., Cutler, J., Rosch, J., and Rahimtoola, S. H.: Specificity, Sensitivity and Accuracy of the Nitroglycerin Ventriculogram as a Predictor of Surgically Reversible Wall Motion Abnormalities, *Am. J. Cardiol.*, 45:399, 1980. (Abstract.)

80 Banka, V. S., Bodenheimer, M. M., Shah, R., and Helfant, R. H.: Intervention Ventriculography: Comparative Value of Nitroglycerin, Post-Extrasystolic Potentiation and Nitroglycerin Plus Post-Extrasystolic Potentiation, *Circulation*, 53:632, 1976.

81 Klausner, S. C., Ratshin, R. A., Tybert, J. V., Lappin, H. A., Chatterjee, K., and Parmley, W. W.: The Similarity of Changes in Segmental Contraction Patterns Induced by Post-Extrasystolic Potentiation and Nitroglycerin, *Circulation*, 54:615, 1976.

82 Helfant, R. H., Pine, R., Meister, S. G., Feldman, M. S., Trout, R. G., and Banka, V. S.: Nitroglycerin to Unmask Reversible Asynergy. Correlation with Post-Coronary Bypass Ventriculography, *Circulation*, 50:108, 1974.

83 Popio, K. A., Gorlin, R., Bechtel, D., and Levine, J. A.: Post-Extrasystolic Potentiation as a Predictor of Potential Myocardial Viability: Preoperative Analysis Compared with Studies after Coronary Bypass Surgery, *Am. J. Cardiol.*, 39:944, 1977.

84 Massie, B., Botvinick, E. H., Brundage, B. H., Greenberg, B., Shames, D., and Gelberg, H.: Relationship of Regional Myocardial Perfusion to Segmental Wall Motion. Physiological Basis for Understanding the Presence and the Reversibility of Asynergy, *Circulation*, 58:1154, 1978.

85 Hellman, C. H., Schmidt, D. H., Kamath, M. L., Anholm, J., Blau, F., and Johnson, W. D.: Bypass Graft Surgery in Severe Left Ventricular Dysfunction, *Circulation*, 62 (suppl. 1):103, 1980.

86 Mason, D. T., Amsterdam, E. A., De Maria, A. N., Smith, J. L., Lee, G., Joye, J., et al.: The Prevention of Myocardial Infarction by Coronary Bypass Surgery, in J. W. Hurst (ed.), "The Heart, Update II," McGraw-Hill Book Company, New York, 1980, p. 103.

87 Vismara, L. A., Miller, R. R., Price, J. E., Karem, R., DeMaria, A. N., and Mason, D. T.: Improved Longevity Due to Reduction of Sudden Death by Aortocoronary Bypass in Coronary Atherosclerosis, *Am. J. Cardiol.*, 39:919, 1977.

88 Chaturvedi, N. C., Walsh, M. J., Evans, A., Munro, P., McC. Boyle, D., and Barber, J. M.: Selection of Patients for Early Discharge after Acute Myocardial Infarction, *Br. Heart J.*, 36:533, 1974.

89 Hurst, J. W. (editor-in-chief): "The Heart," McGraw-Hill Book Company, New York, 1978, p. 1261.

90 Harken, A. H., Horowitz, L. N., and Josephson, M. E.: The Surgical Treatment of Ventricular Tachycardia, *Ann. Thorac. Surg.*, 30:499, 1980.

91 Josephson, M. E., Harken, A. H., and Horowitz, L. N.: Long Term Results of Endocardial Resection for Sustained Ventricular Tachycardia, *Circulation*, 64 (suppl. 4):203, 1981.

92 Guiraudon, G., Fontaine, G., Frank, R., Grosgogeat, Y., and Cabrol, C.: Encircling Endocardial Ventriculotomy. Late Follow-up Results, *Circulation*, 62 (suppl. 3):320, 1980.

93 Gallagher, J. J., Kasell, J., Cox, J. L., Smith, W. M., Ideker, R. E., and Smith, W. M.: Techniques of Intraoperative Electrophysiologic Mapping, *Am. J. Cardiol.*, 49:221, 1982.

94 Ostermeyer, J., Breithardt, G., Kolvenbach, R., Borggrefe, M., Seipel, L., Schulte, H. D., et al.: The Surgical Treatment of Ventricular Tachycardia. Simple Aneurysmectomy Versus Electrophysiologically Guided Procedures, *J. Thorac. Cardiovasc. Surg.*, 84:704, 1982.

95 Hutter, A. M., Jr., DeSanctis, R. W., Flynn, T. H., and Yeatman, L. A.: Nontransmural Myocardial Infarction: A Comparison of Hospital and Late Clinical Course of Patients with that of Matched Patients with Transmural Anterior and Transmural Inferior Myocardial Infarction, *Am. J. Cardiol.*, 48:595, 1981.

96 Cannom, D. S., Levy, W., and Cohen, L. S.: The Short and Long Term Prognosis of Patients with Transmural and Nontransmural Myocardial Infarction, *Am. J. Med.*, 61:452, 1976.

97 Szklo, M., Goldberg, R., Kennedy, H. L., and Tonascia, J. A.: Survival of Patients with Nontransmural Myocardial Infarction: A Population-based Study, *Am. J. Cardiol.*, 42:648, 1978.

98 Rentrop, P., Blanke, H., Wiegand, V., and Karsch, K. R.: Wiedereroffnung verschlossener KranzgefaBe im akuten Infarkt mit Hilfe von Kathetern, *Dtsch. Med. Wochenschr.*, 104:1401, 1979.

99 Rentrop, P., Blanke, H., Karsch, K. R., Rahlf, G., and Leitz, K.: Infarkt-groBenbestimmung durch nich-chirurgische Rekanalisation der Koronararterien. *Dtsch. Med. Wochenschr.*, 106:765, 1981.

100 Reduto, L. A., Smalling, R. W., Freund, G. C., and Gould, K. L.: Intracoronary Infusion of Streptokinase

in Patients with Acute Myocardial Infarction: Effects of Reperfusion on Left Ventricular Performance, *Am. J. Cardiol.*, 48:403, 1981.

101 Ganz, G. W., Buchbinder, N., Marcus, H., Charuzi, Y., Peter, T., Berman, D., et al.: Intracoronary Thrombolysis in Evolving Myocardial Infarction, *Circulation*, 62 (suppl. 3):162, 1980. (Abstract.)

102 Mathey, D. G., Kuck, K. H., Tilsner, V., Krebber, H. J., and Bleifeld, W.: Non-surgical Coronary Artery Recanalization after Acute Transmural Myocardial Infarction, *Circulation*, 63:489, 1981.

103 Effert, S., Merx, W., and Meyer, J.: Revaskularisation des Myokards, Transluminale Koronardilatation—Intrakoronare selektive Thrombolyse, *Dtsch. Arzteblatt*, 78:807, 1982.

104 Meyer, J., Merx, W., Dorr, R., Lambertz, H., Bethge, C. H., and Effert, S.: Successful Treatment of Acute Myocardial Infarction Shock by Combined Percutaneous Transluminal Coronary Recanalization (PTCR) and Percutaneous Transluminal Coronary Angioplasty (PTCA), *Am. Heart J.*, 103:132, 1982.

105 Ganz, W., Buchbinder, N., Marcus, H., Mondkar, A., Maddahi, J., Charuzi, Y., et al.: Intracoronary Thrombolysis in Evolving Myocardial Infarction, *Am. Heart J.*, 101:4, 1981.

106 Favaloro, R. G., Weinschelbaum, E., Laguens, R. P., and de la Fuente, L. M.: ''Experimental Acute Myocardial Infarction in Monkeys. Ultrastructural Study and Effects of Revascularization,'' Rafael Bullrich Award, National Academy of Medicine, Buenos Aires, Argentina, 1975.

107 Merx, W., Dorr, R., Rentrop, P., Blanke, H., Carsh, K. R., Mathey, D. G., et al.: Evaluation of the Effectiveness of Intracoronary Streptokinase Infusion in Acute Myocardial Infarction: Post-Procedure Management and Hospital Course in 204 Patients, *Am. Heart. J.*, 102:1181, 1981.

108 Swan, H. J. C.: Thrombolysis in Acute Myocardial Infarction: Treatment of the Underlying Coronary Artery Disease, *Circulation*, 66:914, 1982. (Editorial.)

109 Meyer, J., Merx, W., Schmitz, H., Erbel, R., Kiesslich, H., Dorr, R., et al.: Percutaneous Transluminal Coronary Angioplasty Immediately after Coronary Streptolysis of Transmural Myocardial Infarction, *Circulation*, 66:905, 1982.

110 Berg, R., Jr., Kendall, R. W., Duvoisin, G. E., Ganji, J. H., Rudy, L. W., and Everhart, F. J.: Acute Myocardial Infarction: A Surgical Emergency, *J. Thorac. Cardiovasc. Surg.*, 70:432, 1975.

111 Duvoisin, G. E., Ganji, J. H., Rudy, L. W., O'Grady, W. P., Grunwald, R. P., and Kendall, R. W.: Surgical Reperfusion for Acute Myocardial Infarction: Ten Year Results in 315 Patients, *Circulation*, 66 (suppl. 2):245, 1982. (Abstract.)

112 Norris, R. M., Agnew, T. M., Brandt, P. W. T., Graham, K. J., Hill, D. G., Kerr, A. L., et al.: Coronary Surgery after Recurrent Myocardial Infarction: Progress of a Trial Comparing Surgical with Nonsurgical Management for Asymptomatic Patients with Advanced Coronary Disease, *Circulation*, 63:785, 1981.

113 Kent, K. M., Rosing, D. R., Ewels, C. J., Lipson, L., Bonow, R., and Epstein, S. E.: Prognosis of Asymptomatic or Mildly Symptomatic Patients with Coronary Artery Disease, *Am. J. Cardiol.*, 49:1823, 1982.

114 Epstein, S. E., Kent, K. M., Goldstein, R. E., Borer, J. S., and Rosing, D. R.: Strategy for Evaluation and Surgical Treatment of the Asymptomatic or Mildly Symptomatic Patient with Coronary Artery Disease, *Am. J. Cardiol.*, 43:1015, 1979.

115 Hertzer, N. R., Young, J. R., Kramer, J. R., deWolfe, V. G., Ruschhaupt, W. F., and Beven, E. G.: Routine Coronary Angiography Prior to Elective Aortic Reconstruction. Results of Selective Myocardial Revascularization in Patients with Peripheral Vascular Disease, *Arch. Surg.*, 114:1336, 1979.

116 Hertzer, N. R.: Fatal Myocardial Infarction following Lower Extremity Revascularization: 276 patients followed 6–11 Postoperative Years, *Ann. Surg.*, 193:492, 1981.

117 Jamieson, W. R. E., Janusz, M. T., Miyagishima, R. T., and Gerein, A. N.: Influence of Ischemic Heart Disease on Early and Late Mortality after Surgery for Peripheral Occlusive Vascular Disease, *Circulation*, 66 (suppl. 1):92, 1982.

118 Johnson, W. D., and Lepley, D.: An Aggressive Surgical Approach to Coronary Disease, *J. Thorac. Cardiovasc. Surg.*, 59:128, 1970.

119 Green, G. E., Stertzer, S. H., and Reppert, E. H.: Coronary Arterial Bypass Grafts, *Ann. Thorac. Surg.*, 5:443, 1968.

120 Halim, M. A., Qureshi, S. A., Towers, M. K., and Yacoub, M. H.: Early and Late Results of Combined Endarterectomy and Coronary Bypass Grafting for Diffuse Coronary Disease, *Am. J. Cardiol.*, 49:1623, 1982.

121 Chaitman, B. R., Waters, D. D., Bourassa, M. G., Tubau, J. F., Wagniart, P., and Ferguson, R. J.: The Importance of Clinical Subsets in Interpreting Maximal Treadmill Exercise Test Results: The Role of Multiple-Lead ECG Systems, *Circulation*, 59:560, 1979.

122 Berger, H. J., Reduto, L. A., Johnstone, D. E., Borkowski, H., Sands, J. M., Cohen, L. S., et al.: Global and Regional Left Ventricular Response to Bicycle Exercise in Coronary Artery Disease, *Am. J. Med.*, 66:13, 1979.

123 Koppes, G., McKiernan, T., Bassan, M., and Froelicher, V.: ''Current Problems in Cardiology,'' Vol. 7, Year Book Medical Publishers, Chicago, 1977, p. 5.

124 Bartel, A. G., Behar, V. S., Peter, R. H., Orgain, E. S., and Kong, Y.: Graded Exercise Stress Tests in An-

giographically Documented Coronary Artery Disease, *Circulation*, 49:348, 1974.

125 Massie, B. M., Botvinick, E. H., and Brundage, B. H.: Correlation of Thallium-201 Scintigrams with Coronary Anatomy: Factors Affecting Region by Region Sensitivity, *Am. J. Cardiol.*, 44:616, 1979.

126 Leppo, J., Yipinstoi, T., Blankstein, R., Bontemps, R., Freeman, L. M., Zohman, L., et al.: Thallium-201 Myocardial Scintigraphy in Patients with Triple-Vessel Disease and Ischemic Exercise Stress Tests, *Circulation*, 59:714, 1979.

127 Conti, C. R., Selby, J. H., Christie, L. G., Pepine, C. J., Curry, R. C., Jr., Nichols, W. W., et al.: Left Main Coronary Artery Stenosis: Clinical Spectrum, Pathophysiology, and Management, *Prog. Cardiovasc. Dis.*, 22:73, 1979.

128 Fisher, L. D., Kennedy, J. W., Chaitman, B. R., Ryan, T. J., McCabe, C., Weiner, D., et al.: Diagnostic Quantification of CASS (Coronary Artery Surgery Study) Clinical and Exercise Test Results in Determining Presence and Extent of Coronary Artery Disease, *Circulation*, 63:987, 1981.

129 Chaitman, B. R., Bourassa, M. G., Davis, K., Rogers, W. J., Tyras, D. H., and Berger, R.: Angiographic Prevalence of High-Risk Coronary Artery Disease in Patient Subsets (CASS), *Circulation*, 64:360, 1981.

130 Faxon, D. P., Ryan, T. H., Davis, K. B., McCabe, C. H., Myers, W., Lesperance, J., et al.: Prognostic Significance of Angiographically Documented Left Ventricular Aneurysm from the Coronary Artery Surgery Study (CASS), *Am. J. Cardiol.*, 50:157, 1982.

131 Mock, M. B., Ringqvist, I., Fisher, L. D., Davis, K. B., Chaitman, B. R., Kouchoukos, N. T., et al.: Survival of Medically Treated Patients in the Coronary Artery Surgery Study (CASS) Registry, *Circulation*, 66:562, 1982.

132 Hammermeister, K. E., DeRouen, T. A., and Dodge, H. T.: Evidence from a Nonrandomized Study that Coronary Surgery Prolongs Survival in Patients with Two-Vessel Coronary Disease, *Circulation*, 59:430, 1979.

133 De Rouen, T. A., Hammermeister, K. E., and Dodge, H. T.: Comparisons of the Effects on Survival after Coronary Artery Surgery in Subgroups of Patients from the Seattle Heart Watch, *Circulation*, 63:537, 1981.

134 Favaloro, R. G., Effler, D. B., Groves, L. K., Westcott, R. N., Suarez, E., and Lozada, J.: Ventricular Aneurysm—Clinical Experience, *Ann. Thorac. Surg.*, 6:227, 1968.

135 Loop, F. D., Effler, D. B., Navia, J. A., Sheldon, W. C., and Groves, L. K.: Aneurysms of the Left Ventricle: Survival and Results of a Ten-Year Surgical Experience, *Ann. Surg.*, 178:399, 1973.

136 Lefemine, A. A., Moon, H. S., Flessas, A., Ryan, T. J., and Ramaswamy, K.: Myocardial Resection and Coronary Artery Bypass for Left Ventricular Failure following Myocardial Infarction. Results in Patients with Ejection Fraction of 40 percent or Less, *Ann. Thorac. Surg.*, 17:1, 1974.

137 Fox, H. E., May, I. A., and Ecker, R. R.: Long-term Functional Results of Surgery for Coronary Artery Disease in Patients with Poor Ventricular Function, *J. Thorac. Cardiovasc. Surg.*, 70:1064, 1975.

138 Isom, O. W., Spencer, F. C., Glassman, E., Dembrow, J. M., and Pasternack, B. S.: Long-term Survival following Coronary Bypass Surgery in Patients with Significant Impairment of Left Ventricular Function, *Circulation*, 52 (suppl. 1):141, 1975.

139 Isom, O. W., Spencer, F. C., and Culliford, A. T.: Coronary Revascularization with Significant Impairment of Left Ventricular Contractility, *Cardiovasc. Clin.*, 8:265, 1977.

140 Zubiate, P., Kay, J. H., and Mendez, A. M.: "Myocardial Revascularization in Patients with Drastic Impairment of Left Ventricular Function—Six Year Follow-up" (presented at Samson Thoracic Surgical Society Meeting, Alberta, Canada, June 1976).

141 Manley, J. C., King, J. F., Zeft, H. J., and Johnson, W. D.: The "Bad" Left Ventricle. Results of Coronary Surgery and Effect on Late Survival, *J. Thorac. Cardiovasc. Surg.*, 72:841, 1976.

142 Gruentzig, A. R., Myler, R. K., Hanna, E. S., and Turina, M. I.: Coronary Transluminal Angioplasty, *Circulation*, 56 (suppl. 3):84, 1977.

143 Kent, K. M., Bentivoglio, L. G., Block, P. C., Cowley, M. J., Dorros, G., and Gosselin, A. J.: NHLBI Percutaneous Transluminal Coronary Angioplasty (PTCA) Registry: Four Years Experience. *Am. J. Cardiol.*, 49:904, 1982. (Abstract.)

144 Stertzer, S., Dorros, G., Myler, R., Cowley, M., Williams, D., Kent, K., et al.: Complex Transluminal Angioplasty in Multivessel Coronary Artery Disease, *Am. J. Cardiol.*, 49:904, 1982. (Abstract.)

145 Technology Assessment Forum on Coronary Artery Bypass Surgery: "Economic, Ethical and Social Issues" (sponsored by the National Center for Health Care Technology in collaboration with the National Heart, Lung, and Blood Institute, April 21–23, 1981, Washington, D.C.), *Circulation*, 66 (suppl. 3): 1982.

146 Braunwald, E.: Coronary-Artery Surgery at the Crossroads, *N. Engl. J. Med.*, 297:661, 1977. (Editorial.)

147 Favaloro, R. G.: Surgical Treatment of Coronary Arteriosclerosis by the Saphenous Vein Graft Technique. Critical Analysis, *Am. J. Cardiol.*, 28:493, 1971.

148 Favaloro, R.: Direct and Indirect Coronary Surgery, *Circulation*, 46:1197, 1972.

149 Consensus Development Conference on Coronary Artery Bypass Surgery: "Medical and Scientific Aspects," National Institutes of Health, Bethesda, Maryland, December 3–5, 1980.

Coronary Artery Revascularization: A Clinical Review of 14 Years' Experience[*]

GIACOMO A. DELARIA, M.D., and
HASSAN NAJAFI, M.D.

> The hope for the damaged myocardium lies in the direction of securing supply of blood through friendly neighboring vessels, so as to restore so far as possible its functional integrity.
>
> JAMES B. HERRICK, 1912
> RUSH MEDICAL COLLEGE

Rush-Presbyterian-St. Luke's Hospital and Medical Center enjoys a midwest location and a tradition of leadership and excellence in the field of cardiovascular surgery. It has a department of cardiovascular and thoracic surgery and a corresponding surgical training program.

Over the past 14 years, 8 surgeons representing two specialty groups have actively participated in the diagnosis and care of nearly 6,000 patients with coronary artery disease. A minimum of rigid institutional guidelines and departmental protocols has allowed each surgeon the opportunity of developing his own approach to these patients. Thus, a large clinical review originating here could provide statistical data more representative of clinical practice than studies obtained from either major clinics or full-time university programs. Accordingly, we have undertaken a review of our entire experience with coronary artery bypass from its inception until December 1981. Only patients who had undergone isolated coronary bypass grafting were selected for this study. Patients who required coronary artery bypass in association with valve replacement, ventricular aneurysmectomy, or repair of ventricular septal rupture were excluded from the review.

DESCRIPTION OF THE PROGRAM OF STUDY

The first direct coronary revascularization at Rush-Presbyterian-St. Luke's Hospital and Medical Center was performed on June 25, 1968. Between that eventful day and December 31, 1981, 4,237 patients who had undergone isolated coronary artery bypass could be identified, and their records were reviewed. Pertinent historical and clinical information was obtained from discharge summaries and hospital charts, many of which had been reduced to microfilm. Data were tabulated and entered into a computer for subsequent recall and correlation. To guarantee accuracy in reporting complications and mortality, the clinical discharge summary data reviews were cross-correlated with existing monthly departmental morbidity and mortality records. Any patient lost from the general review but appearing on morbidity lists was searched out, retrieved, and entered into the general tabulation. Thus, any patient records belonging in the study but lost in the complexities of a 14-year retrospective review would be unlikely to alter morbidity and mortality data and favorably influence overall results.

Follow-up data were obtained on a discrete subset of patients, all operated upon between July 1, 1977 and June 30, 1978. Each was contacted by mail and provided with an information card to fill out. The resulting data were added to the hospital statistics and used in the subsequent evaluation.

Patient Population

For purposes of comparison, three time periods were identified. Each was selected to best represent the three identifiable phases of our coronary bypass experience. The first period began in 1968 and ended in 1971 and included 162 patients, whose cases represented our early experience. During the second period (1972–76), 1,409 patients were added to the study. After 1976, the introduction of better myocardial preservation techniques and cardioplegia defined the final period, 1977–81; 2,666 patients were added to the survey from this group, raising the total number of patients to 4,237.

The sex ratio remained unchanged. Average age did not change significantly over the last two time periods (Table 1). Male patients predominated. Although currently larger numbers of elderly patients are candidates for coronary bypass, their numbers have been balanced by the many patients younger than 40 who require operation. The youngest patient in our series was 23 and the oldest 82.

*Rush Medical College, Chicago, Illinois.

287

TABLE 1
Analysis of risk factors

Factor	1968–1971	1972–1976	1977–1981
Average age	46.7	54.1	54.3
Male patients (%)	81.4	84.6	82.9

Risk Factors

Analysis of risk factors provided a picture typical of most large clinical series of patients with coronary artery disease and is depicted in Fig. 1. With time, the percentage of diabetic patients has slowly increased (11.6 to 14.2 percent). The number of coronary bypass patients who were hypertensive also has increased (17.2 to 34.1 percent). The prevalence of a reported positive family history for coronary disease decreased (34 to 15.6 percent), and there was a gratifying reduction in cigarette smoking (57.4 to 39.2 percent). The presence of either cholesterol elevation or obesity was rarely noted in this series. The increase in the number of patients with elevated cholesterol levels (4.9 to 12.4 percent) probably represents more frequent tests and not a real increase in risk factor. As would be expected, the number of patients who had undergone previous coronary bypass operation increased during each time interval (1.2 to 3.4 percent).

Symptoms

Patient histories were analyzed and compared. Symptoms characteristic of all patients with heart disease were identified and recorded (Fig. 2). There were few differences between the three groups. Angina was the most common complaint and represented the usual indication for coronary revascularization (98.1 to 90.3 percent). Almost 50 percent had experienced a previous myocardial infarction but in fewer than 2 percent was an acute infarct the indication for operation. Cardiogenic shock complicating myocardial infarction was a surgical indication in less than 1 percent of patients. The relative frequency of unstable angina patients increased up to 1971 but thereafter remained stable. Shortness of breath was a remarkably consistent and common complaint, and the relatively high incidence of preoperative congestive heart failure (6.6 percent) helps in characterizing our surgical population and is typical of a medical center referral practice.

The increase in positive treadmill tests (6.7 to 33.5 percent) indicates a more liberal preoperative use of this examination, particularly for patients after myocardial infarction.

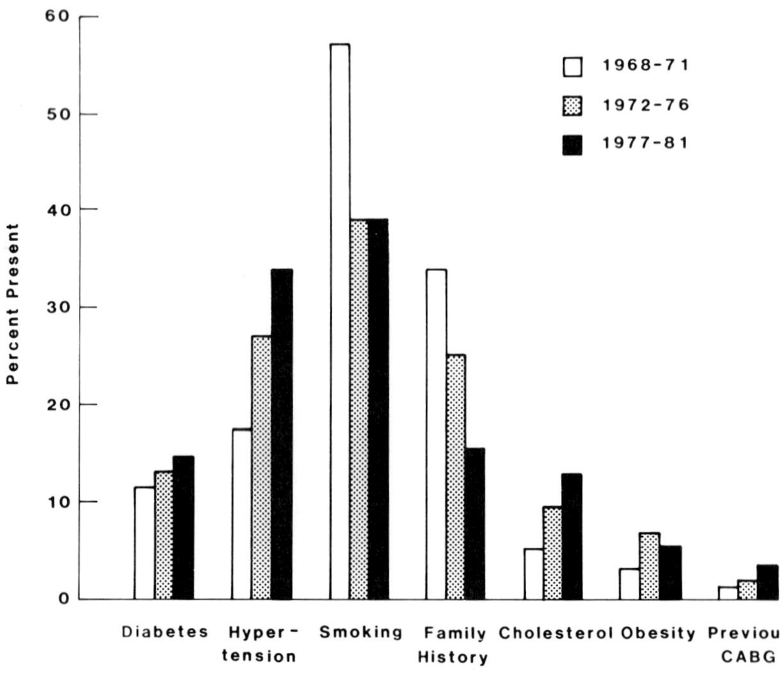

FIGURE 1 Risk factors for coronary artery disease identified in our coronary bypass patients are depicted by time period. The prevalance of a smoking history was the only risk factor which changed dramatically during this 14-year experience.

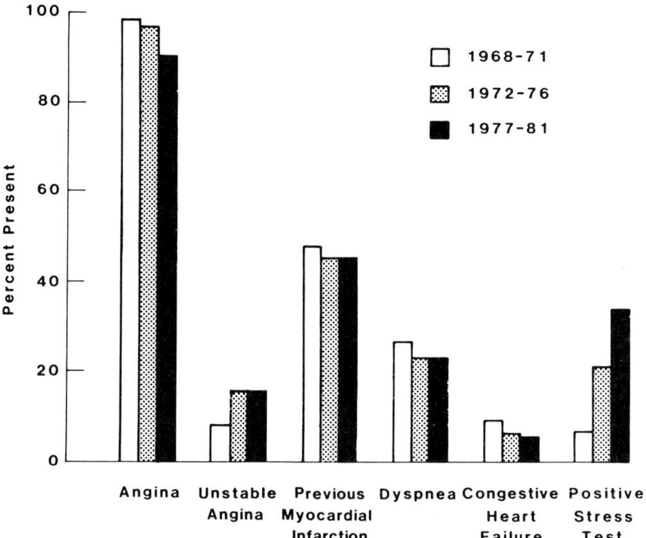

FIGURE 2 Preoperative clinical findings documented in our coronary bypass patients are presented by time period. Angina pectoris was the most common complaint and was reported in 90 percent of patients.

Angiographic Data

All patients underwent coronary angiography and left ventriculography prior to coronary revascularization. Since 1980, complete cardiac catheterization along with coronary angiography has been performed in all patients. Coronary anatomy was divided into five identifiable vessels and included left main (LM), left anterior descending (LAD), diagonal (DIAG), right (RCA), and circumflex (CIRC). Initially, the circumflex anatomy was separated into two categories to distinguish disease in the obtuse marginal branch from that in the posterolateral distribution. However, as too few reports separated these two vessels' domains, they were tabulated together. All vessels were characterized as being without significant disease, stenotic (i.e., narrowed by greater than 70 percent internal diameter), or totally occluded.

The percentage distribution of significant coronary artery stenoses is illustrated by the time period in Fig. 3. Left anterior descending coronary artery stenoses were most frequent in each case (56.1 to 67.3 percent).

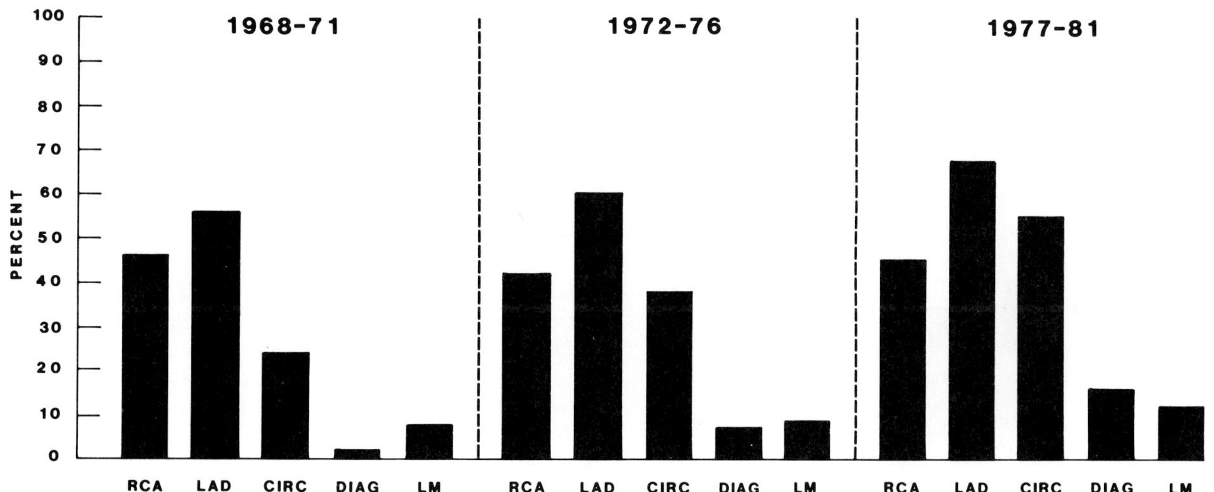

FIGURE 3 Angiographic data from our group of coronary bypass patients are depicted by time period. Only arteries exhibiting > 70 percent intraluminal narrowing were considered to have significant stenosis.

Reports of left main, diagonal, and circumflex stenoses increased with time. On the other hand, the prevalance of stenotic right coronary arteries was stable (45.0 to 42.4 percent). Throughout the observation period, the proportion of stenotic vessels increased and reflected both improvement in diagnosis and a more severely diseased patient population group.

The incidence of total coronary occlusion is depicted in Fig. 4. As there were few differences between time periods, the angiographic data is presented collectively. The right coronary artery was the most commonly occluded vessel (30 percent). The incidence of left anterior descending and circumflex occlusion were respectively 17 and 10 percent. Diagonal occlusions were not usually recorded. Occluded diagonal vessels often represented small diseased arteries, which were unsuitable for bypass and therefore not mentioned in either operative reports or discharge summaries. Six total occlusions of the left main coronary artery were identified in this group of 4,237 patients.

Left ventricular function was not well-characterized for the overall group. Percentage figures for ejection fraction were rarely noted in summaries and, therefore, unavailable for inclusion in the data profile. Enough records had descriptions of ventricular function to develop three classifications: good, fair, and poor. However, in a large percentage of patients, even the requirements for general classifications could not be fulfilled, and this important characteristic remained unknown. The comparison of these results between time periods is shown in Table 2.

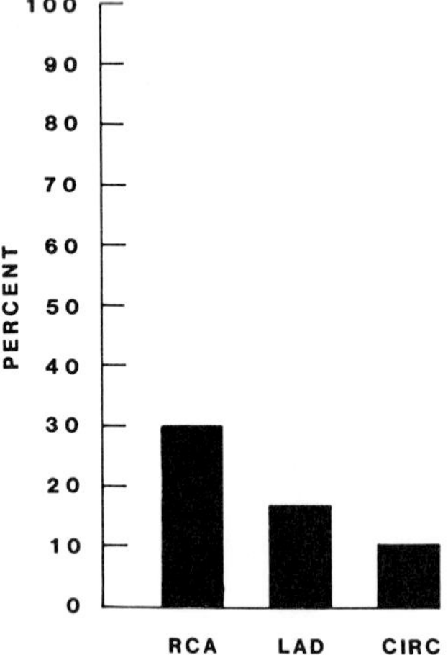

FIGURE 4 The number of coronary arteries found to be totally occluded at angiography remained stable over the 14-year observation period. The right coronary artery was occluded more often, accounting for the increased use of endarterectomy in this vessel.

TABLE 2
Comparison of left ventricular function

Percent	1968–1971	1972–1976	1976–1981
Good	26.5	36.0	35.2
Fair	14.1	27.6	30
Poor	3.0	2.7	8.1
Unknown	56.1	33.5	26.4

It appears that the proportion of patients with poor ventricular function has increased as surgical indications have become more liberal (3.0 to 8.1 percent). However, the large percentage of unclassified ventricular functions, even in the most recent group, made meaningful interpretation difficult.

Surgical Procedure

There have been few changes in the fundamental approach to coronary revascularization in the time period covered by this report. The greatest improvement occurred after the introduction of cold potassium cardioplegic arrest in 1977. Thereafter, all distal bypasses were performed during one uninterrupted period of aortic cross-clamping. Proximal anastomoses were accomplished during the period of myocardial reperfusion and recovery.

Saphenous vein remained the preferred conduit for coronary revascularization. In fact, our entire experience included only 67 internal mammary revascularizations. Most of these (45) were performed between 1972 and 1976. Overall, only 1.5 percent of all bypasses were fashioned with internal mammary arteries.

The average number of bypasses performed per patient was 1.4 by 1971. This figure increased to 1.7 for the period ending in 1976. By 1981, the number of bypassed arteries had increased to 2.2 per patient. These relatively low figures reflect a surgical approach designed to bypass major vessels near to stenoses, thereby minimizing the need for multiple branch bypasses. Also, we share with our colleagues in cardiology an aggressive attitude toward single- and double-vessel disease which helps to reduce our overall average. Nevertheless, as can be appreciated in Fig. 5, the number of bypassed vessels is increasing.

Prior to 1971, the right coronary and left anterior descending arteries were bypassed 67 percent of the time, compared to only 10 percent for circumflex artery bypasses. By 1976, the circumflex artery had become a regular surgical target and was bypassed in almost one-third of cases (31 percent). Diagonal bypass also increased in this time frame. Presently, the left anterior descending is the artery most often bypassed (86 percent). However, the circumflex is now second in frequency (60 percent). The number of diagonal bypasses

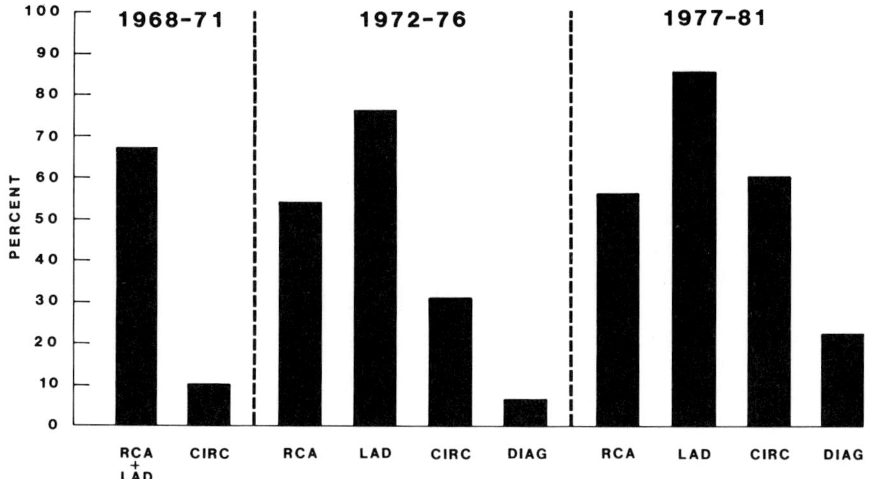

FIGURE 5 Selection of arteries for bypass grafting changed with each time period. As angiographic techniques improved and surgical experience grew, more vessels became suitable for revascularization.

has almost quadrupled (6 to 22 percent). The frequency of right coronary bypasses has remained stable over the past 8 years, dropping slightly from the initial time period (67 to 54 percent).

As demonstrated in Table 3, coronary artery endarterectomy was used with increasing frequency during the observation period. This technical procedure was initially reserved for the right coronary artery. The right coronary artery is totally occluded most often, has fewer branches, and a superficial location which makes it amenable to endarterectomy techniques. However, as experience has grown, endarterectomy has been applied to left-sided vessels, including the LAD and circumflex. Endarterectomy is particularly useful in regions of multiple branch stenoses. Removal of local plaques provides a bypassable artery with a greater domain of study.

decrease in all complications and death rate. Perioperative infarctions were confirmed by diagnostic electrocardiographic changes and appropriate enzyme measurement. Recently, myocardial scans have been used to diagnose this particular postoperative complication. Myocardial enzyme levels were only obtained in those patients with ECG changes indicative of infarction and the presence of unexplained postoperative hemodynamic instability and cardiac arrhythmia.

The overall 30-day mortality rate was 2.1 percent in the last time period. When the patients operated upon as an emergency procedure for acute myocardial infarction, arrhythmia, or cardiogenic shock, or when those with intraaortic balloon counterpulsation were excluded, the mortality rate was reduced to 1.5 percent. The corresponding mortality rate in the excluded emergency group was 14.8 percent.

Complications

The acute 30-day postoperative results were reviewed for the entire series. Perioperative infarction rate, requirement for vasopressors, and mortality rate were tabulated and are illustrated by the time period shown in Fig. 6. Over each period there has been a measurable

TABLE 3
Coronary endarterectomy

Percent	1968–1971	1972–1976	1976–1981
RCA	1.8	9.8	8.2
LAD	————	0.7	1.3
CIRC	————	————	0.2

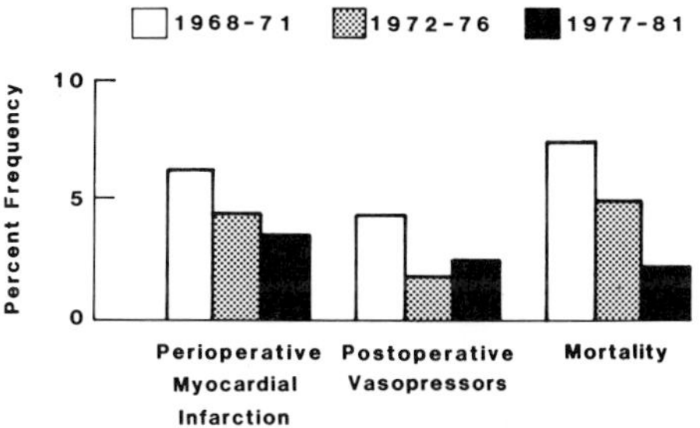

FIGURE 6 The frequency of complications and death rate decreased measurably during successive time periods. The greatest improvement occurred after the introduction of myocardial preservation techniques in 1977.

Late Results

The records of 488 patients who had undergone isolated coronary artery bypass grafting from June 1977 to July 1978 were selected for up-to-date follow-up. Each patient was contacted by mail and asked to fill out a self-addressed inquiry card. Files of patients whose cards were returned as addressee unknown, or not returned at all, were reexamined for clues to possible location. When possible, second and third mailings were sent.

One hundred and eight response cards were never returned. Thus, follow-up was complete on 80 percent of the group. Records of the remaining 20 percent were examined for clinical correlates which could distinguish responders from nonresponders. The average age was 54.4 and not different from the overall study; 82 percent were males. They had undergone an average of 2.4 bypasses per patient. Only 5 percent had experienced a perioperative complication; therefore, a physiological explanation for not responding was unlikely. Probably, a combination of changed addresses, lost employment, retirement moves, and poor motivation provides the best explanation of why none in this group could be contacted. Nevertheless, 80 percent, or 390 patients, did return their cards, and this information can be used to evaluate our long-term results.

Of surviving patients 89 percent were free of angina, and no patients in this group regularly took nitrates or beta blocking agents. However, as 20 percent of patients, including some with angina, experienced mild-to-moderate shortness of breath, along with fatigue and leg swelling, only 69 percent of patients could be classified as symptom-free at 5 years. Four patients, or 1.2 percent of the responders, required repeat coronary bypass surgery.

During the follow-up period, 45 patients died for an overall 5-year mortality rate of 11.2 percent. Twenty patients, or 45 percent, died of heart disease. Three patients, or 7 percent, died of cerebrovascular accidents. Three deaths were noncardiac, and in 19 patients, or 42 percent, the cause of death could not be identified.

SPECIAL TOPICS

Although this present report is the first collective review of our experience, certain areas of our clinical series have been previously examined and give added dimension to this analysis.

Early Results

We first reported a clinical experience with coronary artery bypass in 1973 in a paper presented before the Chicago Surgical Society.[1] The clinical characteristics and course of 400 consecutive patients were reviewed. The age and sex ratio was similar to the first time period in this study. All patients had angina pectoris, and 55 percent gave a history of prior myocardial infarction. The overall mortality rate was 5 percent, but increased to 55 percent in patients operated upon during an acute infarction.

Leg Wound Complications

In 1981, the previous 5 years' operative experience was reviewed to determine the frequency of leg wound complications associated with coronary artery bypass grafting.[2] The series included 2,545 patients, and 27, or 1 percent, experienced a leg wound complication. The complication was serious in 14 patients and resulted in prolonged hospital stay. Additionally, leg wound problems were identified to occur more often in women but not to be influenced by the presence of either diabetes or obesity. Five patients eventually required skin grafting to complete leg closure.

Neurological Complications

Neurological deficits do occur after open heart surgery.[3,4] The frequency of this complication following coronary artery bypass surgery has been variously reported.[5–7] The importance of concomitant carotid artery bypass surgery has received particular emphasis, and combined carotid and coronary surgery is often recommended. Over a 5-year period ending in 1981, our stroke incidence was 1 percent.[8] In 20 patients, or 0.06 percent, the stroke occurred intraoperatively and became manifest in the postanesthesia period. Ten patients remained comatose following operation. Five of these died, two did not regain consciousness, and only three improved. The ten remaining patients exhibited focal neurological deficits. Only one patient died from his neurological complication. The rest improved significantly and were discharged. Most strokes were presumably caused by air or particulate emboli or inadequate cerebral perfusion during cardiopulmonary bypass. No surgically correctable extracranial carotid lesions were identified in patients suffering neurological complications. Accordingly, we select few patients for combined carotid endarterectomy and coronary bypass surgery and limit that operation to patients with symptomatic carotid stenosis in association with unstable angina, left main, or severe triple-coronary disease.

Surgery in Septuagenarians

Elderly patients are often considered as candidates for coronary bypass grafting. The wisdom of this clinical approach and its results were reviewed recently at our institution.[9] Between 1974 and 1980, 105 patients 70 years or older were selected from a group of 2,667 coronary bypass patients. Overall mortality rate for all ages was 3.8 percent. It was 3.5 percent for patients less than 70 and 10.5 percent for patients older than that age ($p = .002$). The operative mortality rate for female patients over 70 was 28.6 percent and four times greater than the 6 percent mortality rate of males reaching a comparable age ($p = .002$). Significant risk factors for subsequent mortality included smoking history and pulmonary hypertension. Coronary bypass is a safe operation in elderly patients. However, only stringent surgical indications are acceptable for elderly female patients with pulmonary hypertension and diffuse small-vessel disease characteristic of their group.

Reoperation

Although a complete analysis of our reoperative statistics is unavailable, a recent report describing a specialized left thoracotomy approach used for reoperation in eight patients has been published.[10] Incorporated in that brief communication is a calculated reoperative rate for our patients of 2.1 percent.

CONCLUSIONS

The past 14 years have been marked by impressive progress in the surgical treatment of coronary artery disease. Morbidity and mortality rates have decreased and results have improved. The population of patients has been stable in age and sex. The incidence of diabetes and hypertension has increased, while smoking has recently become less common. The number of identifiable diseased vessels has risen along with the number of arteries bypassed. More patients with disabled ventricular function are surviving operation and are doing well. The presence of left main disease has had little impact on overall hospital survival, as long as ventricular function was adequate and complete revascularization possible. Emergency operation was associated with increased rate of mortality, particularly in the presence of recent infarction.

Any comparison of our data with other large series is useful and instructive. However, no two series are really equivalent, and, therefore, conclusions cannot be drawn with certainty. The Cleveland Clinic experience, reported in 1982, collected 1,000-patient cohorts from 1971 to 1979 and compared them to their first 740 patients.[11] The patient profiles and surgical indications were similar to ours. Patients operated for either unstable anginal pain or acute infarct were excluded from the operative statistics. Their operative mortality rate was 1.1 percent compared to 1.5 percent

for our last elective time period. The average number of grafts performed in 1979 was 2.7 per patient and higher than our 4-year average of 2.2; however, in 1979 the number of grafts we performed was actually 2.4. Their perioperative myocardial infarction rate decreased from 7.1 to 1.5 percent, much better than our reduction to 3.6 percent from 6.1 percent. On the other hand, their reported incidence of neurological complications was 1.8 percent, higher than the 1 percent rate we identified.

In 1980, Ellis Jones et al. reported their combined coronary statistics:[12] 3,479 patients were collected from a 5-year period ending in 1979. This review, like ours, was retrospective. However, unlike our statistics, theirs had been computerized prospectively and then retrieved for retrospective review. Patient profiles and operative indications differed little from ours. In 1979 the average for number of bypasses was 2.8 combined. Mortality rate was only 0.8 percent. Low mortality rate was attributed to complete revascularization and better myocardial protection. Interestingly, the incidence of perioperative infarction was 4.5 percent and higher than our institutional experience.

The recently published collaborative study in coronary artery surgery (CASS) offers an excellent opportunity for comparison to our data.[13] Many institutions contributed to the data which was reviewed collectively. Operative mortality rate for the CASS report was 2.3 percent, slightly higher than the 2.1 percent noted in our final time period.

Finally, the frequency of coronary artery endarterectomy was surprisingly high in our series. Of all right coronary bypass grafts 8.3 percent were preceded by endarterectomy. These adjunctive procedures were probably associated with a higher perioperative infarction rate as documented by Miller at al. in their comparative study of two patient groups, one with and one without, coronary endarterectomy.[14] These infarcts were rarely transmural and, as described by Burton et al., not associated with long-term disability.[15] A higher infarction rate is acceptable if, as shown by Halim et al., the early patency of endarterectomized arteries is 85 percent and only falls to 77 percent at 1 year.[16]

Coronary artery bypass grafting has established itself as an effective and generally applicable technique for treating patients with symptomatic coronary artery disease. The two requirements for a satisfactory operative result are suitable surgical targets and adequate left ventricular function. Of the two, the quality of the arteries to be bypassed is the more important factor. Angiography is presently unable to identify with certainty those patients whose coronary arteries are irretrievable by standard techniques. Often patients with diffusely diseased and multiple stenotic coronary arteries have poor runoff and low graft flows and do not improve following coronary bypass. Despite adequate

294

myocardial protection, our unexpected mortality rate is always higher in these patients. On the other hand, the patient with disabled ventricular function and severe angina associated with bypassable vessels is easily managed with present anesthetic and myocardial preservation techniques. Here, the patient leaves the operating room improved and correspondingly does well.

Our data is useful only as a review of hospital statistics. Meaningful comparisons with medical series or longevity studies are not possible. However, our retrospective file is now complete, and patients will now be entered into the data bank prospectively. A greater attempt to maintain long-term contact will be made and a program for routine retrieval of follow-up information established. Only by accomplishing this can the population with surgically treatable coronary artery disease be better defined and improved guidelines for operation be developed. Nevertheless, there will always have to be ill-defined qualities which will encourage cardiologists and cardiovascular surgeons to recommend operation in the face of angiographic, hemodynamic, and statistical data which argue differently. These patients will experience a higher rate of morbidity and mortality, but risk-taking will often be rewarded by rehabilitation in otherwise desperate situations.

REFERENCES

1 Najafi, H., Dye, W. S., Javid, H., Hunter, J. A., Goldin, M. D., and Serry, C.: Risk of Aortocoronary Artery Bypass, *Proc. Inst. Med. Chic.*, 29:321, 1973.

2 DeLaria, G. A., Hunter, J. A., Goldin, M. D., Serry, C., Javid, H., and Najafi, H.: Leg Wound Complications Associated with Coronary Revascularization, *J. Thorac. Cardiovasc. Surg.*, 81(3):403, 1981.

3 Gilman, S.: Cerebral Disorders after Open-Heart Operation, *N. Engl. J. Med.*, 272:489, 1965.

4 Javid, H., Turo, H. M., Najafi, H., Dye, W. S., Hunter, J. A., and Julian, O. C.: Neurological Abnormalities following Open Heart Surgery, *J. Thorac, Cardiovasc. Surg.*, 58:502, 1969.

5 Breslau, P. J., Fell, G., Ivey, T. D., Bailey, W. W., Miller, D. W., and Strandness, D. E.: Carotid Arterial Disease in Patients Undergoing Coronary Artery Bypass, *J. Thorac. Cardiovasc. Surg.*, 82:755, 1981.

6 Bernhard, V. M., Johnson, W. D., and Peterson, J. J.: Carotid Artery Stenosis. Association with Surgery for Coronary Artery Disease, *Arch. Surg.*, 105:837, 1972.

7 Breuer, A. C., Hanson, M. R., Furlan, A. S., Lederman, R. J., Loop, F. D., and Cosgrove, D. M.: Central Nervous System Complications of Myocardial Revascularization— A Prospective Analysis of 400 patients, *Stroke*, 11:136, 1980. (Abstract.)

8 Bojar, R. M., Najafi, H., DeLaria, G. A., Serry, C., and Goldin, M. D.: Neurologic Complications of Coronary Revascularization. *Ann. Thorac. Surg.*, in press.

9 Faro, R. S., Goldin, M. D., Najafi, H., et al.: Coronary Revascularization in Septuagenarians, *J. Thorac. Cardiovasc. Surg.*, in press.

10 Faro, R. S., Javid, H., Najafi, H., et al.: Left Thoracotomy for Reoperation for Coronary Revascularization, *J. Thorac. Cardiovasc. Surg.*, 84(3):453, 1982.

11 Cosgrove, D. M., Loop, F. D., and Sheldon, W. C.: Results of Myocardial Revascularization: A 12-Year Experience, *Circulation*, 65 (suppl. 2):37, 1982.

12 Jones, E. L., Craver, J. M., King, S. B., Jr., et al.: Clinical, Anatomic and Functional Descriptors Influencing Morbidity, Survival and Adequacy of Revascularization following Coronary Bypass, *Ann. Surg.*, 192:390, 1980.

13 Kennedy, J. W., Kaiser, G. C., Fisher, L. D., et al.: Multivariate Discriminant Analysis of the Clinical and Angiographic Predictors of Operative Mortality from the Collaborative Study in Coronary Artery Surgery (CASS), *J. Thorac. Cardiovasc. Surg.*, 80:876, 1980.

14 Miller, D. C., Stinson, E. B., Oyer, P. E., et al.: Long-term Clinical Assessment of the Efficacy of Adjunctive Coronary Endarterectomy, *J. Thorac. Cardiovasc. Surg.*, 81:21, 1981.

15 Burton, J. R., FitzGibbon, G. M., Keon, W. J., and Leach, A. J.: Perioperative Myocardial Infarction Complicating Coronary Bypass, *J. Thorac. Cardiovasc. Surg.*, 82:758, 1981.

16 Halim, M. B., Qureshi, M. B., Towers, M. K., and Yacoub, M. H.: Early and Late Results of Combined Endarterectomy and Coronary Bypass Grafting for Diffuse Coronary Disease, *Am. J. Cardiol.*, 49:1623, 1982.

PART III

Coronary Angioplasty in the Treatment of Atherosclerotic Coronary Heart Disease

Percutaneous Transluminal Coronary Angioplasty[*]

JAY HOLLMAN, M.D.,
ANDREAS R. GRUENTZIG, M.D.,
SPENCER B. KING, III, M.D., and
JOHN S. DOUGLAS, JR., M.D.

> Transluminal recanalization appears quite applicable to other arterial systems, particularly those smaller than are usually considered suitable for conventional reconstructive surgery . . . severe proximal narrowing of the coronary artery will be amenable to a manually guided dilator inserted via aortotomy or via the brachial artery by the Sones technique.
>
> C. P. DOTTER and M. P. JUDKINS, 1964[1]

BACKGROUND INFORMATION

The concept of percutaneous angioplasty originated with Charles Dotter and Melvin Judkins. Like so many advances in medicine, the first angioplasty was accomplished by accident. A catheter was passed through an occluded iliac artery in order to perform diagnostic aortography.[2] Following this, and after studies in cadavers, angioplasty was performed on 11 patients.[1]

This technique, largely ignored in the United States, was advanced in Europe under the leadership of Porstmann and Zeitler. The use of a double-lumen catheter, first in the peripheral arteries[3] and later in the coronary arteries,[4,5] by Gruentzig led to the widespread acceptance of this technique for arterial revascularization.

ALTERATION OF PATHOLOGY

The mechanism by which angioplasty alters the obstruction has been investigated in various models. Early investigators advocated a compaction hypothesis, "like footprints on freshly fallen snow."[6,7] This also explained why harder, older, or calcified lesions failed to respond to angioplasty—they were not compactible. As further pathological studies were performed, it became clear that compaction was not the only way the lesions were altered. In fact, compaction may be relatively unimportant compared to splitting, particularly in harder lesions.

Several investigators have described the results of angioplasty in the coronary arteries of fresh cadaver hearts.[8–12] Their work enables us to make the following statements. Dilatation of normal segments results in

*From the Department of Medicine, Division of Cardiology, Emory University School of Medicine, Atlanta, Georgia.

no apparent histological changes, and the tissue adjacent to the atherosclerotic lesion is not damaged by the balloon injury to the lesion.[8] Eccentric stenoses seem to dilate as a result of stretching of the undiseased segment.[11,12] Intimal fractures and tears, as well as plaque rupture, are relatively common.[10,12] Calcified plaques are not likely to respond to 6 atm,[9,12] although it is possible to dilate such areas if the calcium does not extend completely around the artery circumferentially. In such cases the noncalcified segments are compacted and dilated while the calcific areas remain intact.[10] The tunica adventitia is stretched and the muscular media and elastic membrane are disrupted.[10] Overstretching of the atheromatous plaque is the predominant effect with short inflation times. With inflation times of 50 s some degree of compaction is also achieved.[12] Fluid may be expressed from an atherosclerotic lesion during balloon dilatation when lesions are not densely fibrotic.[13]

A variety of live animal models have also been used for the study of the pathological effects of angioplasty. Splitting and tearing of the intima and media occurs in the rabbit model, especially when the balloon's inflated diameter is larger than the diameter of the native artery.[14–16] Although this results in the loss of the endothelium, which is followed by the deposition of platelets enmeshed in fibrin, there is no significant embolization of endothelial cells or plaque fragments.[17] Sequential studies show that reendothelialization of the intima and media is complete by 3 days. Subsequent fibrosis causes retraction of the split areas, which results in a larger lumen at 2 weeks following angioplasty.[18] Scanning electron microscopy of normal canine arteries after dilatation injury shows platelet fibrin deposition on the subendothelial connective tissue. Such deposition could be temporarily inhibited by dextran infusion but not by aspirin or heparin.[19] Experimental studies in miniature pigs confirm the tearing of the intima and media and stretching of elastic fibers. These pathological studies, performed at 10 to 14 days after successful angioplasty, emphasized the destructive changes and dislocation of the atheromatous material between disrupted media.[20] Acute and chronic changes after angioplasty have been studied in two types of induced atherosclerotic lesions in rabbits. Fracture and disruption were important in soft lesions. Intimal fracture did not occur when hard lesions were dilated, but the normal portion of the arterial wall in these lesions appeared to be stretched and damaged. Chronic studies in rabbits showing angiographic evidence of recurrence showed thrombosis with recanalization as well as lipid-laden loose connective tissue. Such studies suggest that recurrence may be an extension of the normal arterial repair process.[18]

Studies from patients dying shortly after angioplasty showed splitting and fracture similar to those seen in animals and cadavers.[21] One patient who died 2 months following angioplasty showed a distinctive intimal proliferation without lipid deposition.[22] Three patients dying from recurrent stenosis at 90, 90, and 180 days after angioplasty showed recurrent lesions indistinguishable from de novo atherosclerosis.[23] A lesion studied 6 months following successful angioplasty showed relatively normal intima for one half of the circumference of the lumen, while the other half of the circumference showed fatty deposition. The endothelial lining was almost absent.[24]

In summary, from animal and human data, it is apparent that intimal fracture and medial splitting and stretching is important for the immediate improvement in luminal diameter in some lesions. In harder, eccentric lesions, stretching of the normal segment may be important. During healing, fibrosis and retraction make the lumen larger.[25] Recurrent lesions develop as a result of excessive intimal proliferation and, when mature, resemble de novo atherosclerotic lesions.

TECHNIQUE

The general technical principles of coronary angioplasty were described in the fifth edition of "The Heart."[26] The technical advances since that communication are the development of balloon catheters that can tolerate up to 12 to 13 atm; the development of lower-profile balloon catheters; the over-the-guide wire system; and the steerable catheter system.

The use of high-pressure balloons has made it possible to dilate hard lesions. In Gruentzig's first 187 patients in whose cases balloon pressures of only 6 atm were possible, there were 12 failures (6 percent) because the obstruction could not be dilated even though the cases were carefully selected.[27] Using less stringent indications, only 3 in 809 (0.3 percent) attempts at Emory University Hospital failed to respond to dilatation after successful crossing.[28] Thus, failure to dilate the obstruction is now a rather unusual reason for failure.

Lower-profile balloons have made passage of more severe stenoses possible. The original Gruentzig balloon (G 20-30) had a body diameter (deflated) of 1.15 mm. This tapered to a tip size of 0.5 mm. Before the development of low-profile balloons, lesions could often be crossed with the tip of the catheter but the deflated balloon would not cross the stenosis. The new catheters, DG 20-20 (USCI) and G-20-20 (Schneider Mediatag, Zürich), have an outer diameter of 1.04 mm and an inflated balloon diameter of 2.0 mm. Twenty-two of 30 lesions were crossed with a lower-profile balloon after the larger balloon failed to cross the stenosis. In 18 of the 22 lesions dilated with the lower-profile balloon, it was possible to recross the vessel with a larger balloon catheter and further dilate the vessel.[29] Similar improvement in primary success was seen after Simpson reduced the outer diameter of the catheter from 1.37 mm to 1.04 mm.[30]

A newer development is the adaptation of a system used in peripheral arteries.[3] The system, developed by Simpson, entails passing a guide wire through the stenosis and following it with a balloon catheter.[30] A guide wire system allows for the confident passage of the catheter through the stenosis once the wire is across the lesion. Also one can withdraw the balloon catheter across the lesion leaving the guide wire, thereby allowing freer flow of blood between dilatations. This is especially advantageous when the patient does not tolerate the procedure well and is having chest pain even during dilatation. When the guide wire is left in place, it ensures safety when the stenosis is passed again. Obviously, a guide wire that can be shaped might pass some lesions when a conventional system might not. The disadvantage of the early Simpson system was the inability to measure distal pressures without withdrawing the guide wire.

The most recent technical advance has been the development of a steerable guide wire (from USCI). In this method a monofilament wire with a spring guide tip is passed through the balloon catheter. Rotation of the proximal end of the wire results in rotation of the distal end of the catheter, thus allowing the distal tip of the wire to be "steered" away from side branches. This 0.018-in. wire when placed through a double-lumen dilatation catheter still allows enough free space for pressure measurements and for the injection of contrast media around the guide wire. Using this system, despite selecting more difficult lesions the primary success rate increased from 89 percent (125 of 134) to 94 percent (120 of 127),[31] and in two patients emergency surgery was avoided by the use of the steerable catheter.[31] The improved primary success rate is most obvious in the right coronary and left circumflex artery, the arteries previously associated with the lowest primary success rates up to now.

Other technical improvements are still being evaluated and tested. Kaltenbach and colleagues have suggested, based on experimental[32] and clinical evidence,[33] that improved primary success might be possible if inflation times are longer at moderate pressure. As indicated earlier, this may not be necessary since the new balloons will tolerate higher pressures.

In summary, while technical advances have expanded the potential applications of this method, there are still enough technical problems remaining to inspire many an innovative catheter engineer.

EVIDENCE THAT ANGIOPLASTY WORKS

A variety of objective methods have been used to prove that angioplasty is of benefit.

Reduction in Diameter Narrowing and Pressure Gradient

The most commonly used descriptors of the effect of coronary angioplasty are a decrease of stenosis as expressed in a reduction of diameter narrowing and reduction in pressure gradient across the stenosis. For instance, in our own experience with more than 1,000 dilatations, the mean reduction in diameter narrowing was from 73 percent to 29 percent (44 percent) and the mean reduction in pressure gradient across the stenosis was from 48 to 13 mmHg. The stenosis is calculated by measuring as many projections of the angiogram as possible and calculating a mean diameter narrowing from these projections. The simultaneous mean blood pressures are measured from the guiding catheter, representing the aortic pressure, and from the main lumen of the dilatation catheter, representing distal arterial pressures. From the mean pressures the gradient across the stenosis before and after dilatation is calculated.

Other Methods Requiring Cardiac Catheterization

Cardiac pacing combined with coronary sinus measurements has been used in the catheterization laboratory to assess coronary angioplasty. After successful angioplasty of the left anterior descending artery there is, at a similar level of atrial pacing, an increase in great cardiac vein flow, a decreased coronary vascular resistance, an increase in myocardial oxygen consumption, and an increase in lactate extraction.[34–37] These data imply that after angioplasty coronary resistance can fall, allowing for increased blood flow and increased oxygen consumption. Aerobic metabolism can thus be preserved as reflected by preservation of lactate extraction.

Using cardiac catheterization techniques six pa-

tients with successful angioplasties of the left anterior descending artery were shown at 6 months to have decreased their exercise end-diastolic pressure from 33.8 to 19.5 mmHg.[38] During comparable exercise, significant improvement of the rate of rise of ventricular pressure (dP/dt maximum) is present in patients after successful percutaneous transluminal coronary angioplasty (PTCA). Following successful angioplasty, normal diastolic relaxation is present even with exercise. Since diastolic relaxation is an active process, requiring energy, its normalization in exercise after PTCA implies improved myocardial metabolism.[38]

The ratio of diastolic to systolic pressure-time index (DPTI/SPTI) during exercise is improved 6 months following successful left anterior descending angioplasty. DPTI/SPTI ratio is a measure of myocardial perfusion, and its normalization with exercise implies improved myocardial perfusion with exercise.[38]

Radionuclide Exercise Tests

A variety of nuclear methods have been used to show the effect on angioplasty on myocardial perfusion and function. Hirzel and colleagues[39] showed improved myocardial perfusion as assessed by thallium stress testing in 28 of 31 patients immediately following coronary angioplasty. All three patients who failed to show an improvement had no thallium defect prior to angioplasty. Moreover, patients on late study showed either a new defect compatible with recurrent stenosis or a more homogeneous image in the exercise study compatible with arterial smoothing and improved perfusion. Thallium exercise testing in follow-up shows a good prediction of recurrence and may identify, in asymptomatic patients, those who will later have recurrent symptoms.[40] It is, however, possible to have an angiographic recurrence with a negative thallium stress test.

Stress radionuclide ventriculography, either by firstpass or gated blood pool scanning, has been used to reveal a salutary effect on ejection fracton during exercise.[38–43] In the normal patient the ejection fraction increases with exercise by at least 5 percent. In the patient with significant coronary artery disease the ejection fraction is usually normal at rest in the absence of previous infarction; however, with exercise the ejection fraction either fails to increase or falls. Restoration of normal ejection fraction responses to exercise after successful angioplasty implies improved myocardial perfusion. In 41 patients stress tested before and after successful angioplasty the mean global ejection fraction fell from 60 percent to 56 percent.[42] After angioplasty the heart rate-matched ejection fraction at rest was unchanged at 61 percent, but with exercise the heart rate-matched ejection fraction rose to 64 percent.

Thus, the ejection fraction at similar exercise load was 56 percent prior to PTCA and 64 percent after PTCA. After successful PTCA 27 patients could be exercised to a higher level; in 9 of these patients the ejection fraction showed a further rise with increased work load, while in 18 the ejection fraction remained the same or fell. Those patients with a further rise in ejection fraction also tended to have a lower residual diameter narrowing and a lower residual gradient across the stenosis after angioplasty.[42] Analysis of exercise-induced regional wall motion abnormalities shows a similar improvement after coronary angioplasty.[41] Thus, radionuclide methods confirm that successful PTCA results in improved myocardial perfusion and improved left ventricular performance with exercise.

The Relief of Angina

While elaborate testing methods are important to confirm the efficacy of the technique, most patients undergo angioplasty for improvement of symptoms. This parameter was assessed by Holmes et al.[44] in an analysis of the National Heart, Lung and Blood Institute (NHLBI) registry data. Of 232 successful angioplasty patients 82 percent were clinically improved, and only 8 percent were still limited by angina. Of 110 patients with unsuccessful angioplasty, 66 percent were clinically improved with further treatment, and 27 percent were limited by their angina. These limitations were present despite the fact that 73 percent of unsuccessful patients underwent coronary bypass surgery. Moreover patients with successful angioplasty returned to work earlier. Follow-up of patients treated in Switzerland between 1977 and 1980 shows similar results.[45] Symptom relief was assessed by performance on a bicycle ergometer. The percentage of patients on medical therapy was similar in the group of successful PTCA patients and in the group of patients in which angioplasty failed and bypass surgery was required.

The Routine Use of Clinical Testing to Assess the Efficacy of PTCA

We continue to use treadmill testing, using the Bruce protocol, for most stable patients before and after angioplasty unless the test is contraindicated. Testing assures the patient that his or her performance is improved. In occasional patients with marginal angiographic and/or marginal hemodynamic results, stress testing may be decisive in assessing the success of the procedure. The discharge stress test also affords the physician a standard that is useful for assessing patients in the follow-up period. For these reasons treadmill or bicycle stress electrocardiography, which is relatively cheap, is effective in the routine assessment of the angioplasty patient.

Summary

Every method used to assess the value of coronary angioplasty on myocardial infarction requires that increased myocardial oxygen demand be created either through exercise or cardiac pacing. Myocardial metabolism, perfusion, and function are usually normal at rest in most stable patients with coronary artery disease. Exercise induces a large number of abnormalities that can be quantitatively or qualitatively measured. Successful PTCA has been shown to reverse or improve all exercise-induced abnormalities of metabolism, perfusion, and function.

PRIMARY SUCCESS

PTCA is an evolving technique. Lesions that are difficult or impossible to reach or dilate early in one's experience may become possible to reach or dilate after more experience and with improved technology. The NHLBI registry data showed a primary success rate of 64 percent in 1,898 patients.[46] However, the success rate was 59 percent in centers performing less than 50 cases (534 of 908), 68 percent in centers performing 50 to 100 cases (536 of 783), and 80 percent in centers performing over 100 cases (161 of 201). In this study younger patients and patients with a short duration of symptoms were more likely to have successful angioplasty. Lack of calcification in the lesion was correlated with improved primary success. Higher inflation pressures and increased number of inflations correlated with a higher primary success rate. Primary success rate was higher in left anterior descending lesions (68 percent) compared to circumflex lesions (44 percent). Success was also higher in single-vessel disease compared to multivessel disease (66 percent versus 54 percent).[47]

In 809 attempts at Emory University Hospital we confirmed the NHLBI registry observation that single-vessel disease is associated with a higher primary success rate. Success was achieved in 87 percent of patients with single-vessel disease; 80 percent of patients with double-vessel disease; and 75 percent of patients with triple-vessel disease. Calcification of the lesion or duration of symptoms was not a marker for primary success in these patients. The access to balloon catheters that will tolerate higher atmospheric pressures has made the hard, calcified lesion more amenable to angioplasty. It should also be remembered that these cases were selected with the anticipation of success despite the presence of calcium. There is agreement in all groups that dilatation of lesions in the left anterior descending coronary artery is associated with a higher primary success rate than is dilatation of lesions in the right coronary or circumflex arteries, but this difference lessened later on in the Emory series when access to the steerable catheter was obtained.[31]

The only predictor of primary success in the Emory patients was lesion eccentricity. Eccentric lesions had an 80 percent primary success rate while concentric stenosis had a 90 percent primary success rate. The principal reason for failure in this series was a failure to cross the stenosis. Raffenbeul et al.[48] also found eccentric stenosis less likely to respond to PTCA, but in this study the difficulty was failure to dilate a successfully crossed stenosis. The NHLBI report did not show a difference between concentric and eccentric stenosis. It is uncertain why this is so, but it might be due to the multicenter nature of the study with variable interobserver interpretation of lesion morphology or because the overall primary success was relatively low.

In our experience, angioplasty for restenosis is associated with a success rate of 95 percent compared to a first-attempt angioplasty success rate of 84 percent.[49] In the Montreal series, the success rate was 91 percent in a group of patients who had repeat angioplasty compared to the 65 percent success rate that was achieved with the first angioplasty.[49a] Centers using either the brachial or femoral artery approach have found that both methods are associated with approximately the same primary success rate.[50] Krajer et al.[51] found the use of a flexible tip guide catheter significantly improved their primary success in right coronary artery lesions. Gruentzig reported an overall improvement in primary success rate from 89 percent to 94 percent after steerable dilating catheters became available.

Primary success statistics can be deceptive since they depend a great deal on patient selection. If only easy stenoses are chosen, the success rate will be higher than if more difficult stenoses are undertaken. As angioplasty technology advances, more and more difficult lesions tend to be attempted.

The optimal primary success rate is 100 percent, but it is unlikely that this figure will be reached. However, even with lesser degress of primary success, substantial financial savings have been shown for angioplasty compared to bypass surgery.[52,53]

INDICATIONS AND CONTRAINDICATIONS FOR CORONARY ANGIOPLASTY

General Indications

As indications change as a result of ongoing developments, the impact of angioplasty on the treatment of patients with coronary artery disease cannot be foreseen at the present time; however, certain indications and relative contraindications have been established.

Using the originally mentioned indication of proximal, discrete, segmental, subtotal, noncalcific stenosis, Hamby and Katz[54] estimated that 8 to 10 percent of patients with significant coronary artery disease might be candidates for coronary angioplasty. Others estimated this incidence as less than 1 percent.[55] Whatever the current indication, the true incidence of angioplasty candidates in a given catheterization practice depends in part on the time in the disease process that the patient undergoes evaluation. Patients with suitable lesions for angioplasty have a shorter duration of symptoms and less myocardial infarctions than other patients with significant disease.[54] Accordingly, a higher percentage of candidates for angioplasty are likely to be found in laboratories where catheterizations are performed soon after the onset of symptoms.

As described under "Technique," technical advances have allowed more and more difficult lesions to be attempted. As complication rates have fallen, one might well ask if the indications for angioplasty should be extended at both ends of the disease spectrum. For example, dilatation of mild stenosis might be attempted in an effort to prevent more advanced disease.

Many hemodynamically insignificant lesions could be dilated by angioplasty. In fact, crossing these lesions is easier, and dilatation is associated with a high primary success rate. Unfortunately, however, mild coronary lesions may reoccur, and the recurrence may be more severe than the original lesion.[56]

There is no evidence that bypass surgery prolongs life in single-vessel coronary artery disease. There is also no current evidence that coronary angioplasty prolongs life. However, with significant proximal left anterior descending coronary artery stenosis, we believe treatment with effective revascularization therapy is justified.[57,58] Thus, with demonstrable ischemia due to an isolated proximal left anterior descending coronary artery lesion coronary angioplasty is recommended even if the patient is asymptomatic.

Apart from this exception, almost all patients receive coronary angioplasty for relief of angina pectoris. It is not possible to give simple rules about the level of symptoms at which revascularization therapy is required. While an elderly patient or a sedentary patient may be content with stable exertional angina, a younger patient with a manual labor job may wish to be free of angina in order to function normally. Nor is the amount of angina always decisive. A single episode of rest pain in a patient with a proximal left anterior descending artery lesion with a large amount of myocardium at risk is much more dangerous than years of pesky, but stable, exertional angina due to a lesion in a small right coronary artery.

Despite early attempts to limit coronary angioplasty

to patients with symptoms sufficiently severe to require bypass surgery, this has not always been possible. The lay public knows that coronary angioplasty is not the same procedure as bypass grafting. Patients as well as physicians are more likely to find angina symptoms unacceptable when a less invasive method for revascularization is available. Ideally for cost-containment purposes, it would be good to wait until a patient's symptoms were so severe that he or she would require bypass surgery to function at an acceptable level of activity, but practically this will not always be possible, particularly as angioplasty becomes a more safe procedure. On the other hand, the presence of a lesion does not constitute an indication for angioplasty. Asymptomatic patients with small amounts of myocardium at risk are not candidates for angioplasty even if their lesions could be dilated with ease. Angioplasty may or may not be of benefit to such patients, it would require a large-scale randomized trial and years of follow-up to prove benefit.

Several subsets of patients have been evaluated for possible benefit of angioplasty. Unstable angina is defined by the National Institutes of Health (NIH) cooperative study as the recent onset of pain or a worsening angina pain pattern sufficient to require hospital admission for stablization.[59] One study showed improvement in symptoms in 13 of 14 patients in whom angioplasty was successful.[35] Another study found the primary success and the complication rate and the reduction in diameter narrowing to be similar between a group of patients with unstable angina pectoris and a group of patients with stable angina pectoris.[60]

Variant angina or angina associated with coronary artery spasm may be associated with underlying severe fixed obstruction or insignificant fixed disease. The indication for angioplasty in such patients is not clearly established.[61–64] While the complication rate and primary success rate are similar to those for angioplasty not associated with variant angina, the recurrence rate appears to be higher in such patients.[61]

Special Subsets

AGE

Elderly patients form a special subgroup of patients. The relief of angina with bypass surgery in the elderly may be similar to the relief obtained in younger patient groups, but the incidence of complications is higher in the elderly.[65,66] Elderly patients (≥70 years), when compared to young patients, have twice the mortality rate[67] and a higher incidence of complications when admitted to a coronary care unit with acute myocardial infarction.[68] The data from the NHLBI registry showed

a mortality rate of 1.4 percent and a myocardial infarction rate of 3.6 percent in 640 older patients (≥60 years old) undergoing angioplasty. The primary success was similar to that of patients less than 60 years of age (61 percent versus 68 percent, respectively).[69] One group reported on 12 patients who were ≥70 years of age. PTCA was successful in 10 patients, and 7 of these were asymptomatic at an average of 5.7 months of follow-up.[70] Although no large series has been reported, preliminary data suggest that PTCA may play a strategic role in the therapy of elderly patients with incapacitating angina.

The patient under the age of 40 years who is suitable for PTCA also deserves special attention. Since atherosclerosis is a progressive disease, one can expect a high percentage of these patients to eventually develop multivessel disease. The average age at *first* coronary bypass operation was 49 years in a series of 500 patients requiring a *second* operation. This was nearly 10 years younger than the average age for all bypass surgery.[71] Perhaps successful PTCA could delay bypass surgery in some patients so that only one operation would be required.

LEFT MAIN DISEASE—A CONTRAINDICATION TO ANGIOPLASTY

Left main stenosis is usually associated with disease in other vessels,[72] and thus it would be an infrequent indication for angioplasty by current indications. Although it may seem to be technically the easiest vessel to dilate, in actuality the stenosis can be difficult to cross. In 11 patients with left main stenosis in the NHLBI registry, 3 died suddenly during the first year following angioplasty.[73] At least one patient dying within a few months following successful PTCA appeared to have spasm of the left main coronary artery. Because bypass surgery has been shown to prolong life in left main coronary artery disease, treatment of this condition seems to belong in the hands of the bypass surgeon.[74]

SPECIAL CONSIDERATIONS

Patients with terminal cancer or other relative contraindications to coronary bypass surgery may benefit from coronary angioplasty.[75]

MULTIVESSEL DISEASE

Gruentzig and Collins debated the issue of multivessel disease with the conclusion by both that any PTCA venture into this disease must be carefully studied and compared with bypass surgery since bypass surgery has been shown to prolong life in these patients.[76] The

NHLBI registry data on angioplasty show that the mortality rate in multivessel disease is 1.9 percent versus 0.7 percent in single-vessel disease.[77] The primary success rate was lower in multivessel-diseased patients (54 percent) compared to that in patients with single-vessel disease (66 percent). In a later study,[78] five experienced centers reviewed their experience in 326 patients with multivessel disease. They found a primary success rate of 72 percent in single-vessel disease and 74 percent in multivessel disease. Mortality rates were not statistically different: 0.4 percent for one-vessel disease and 1.0 percent for multivessel disease. In 102 patients in whom multiple dilatations were attempted (214 total attempts), primary success was achieved in 162 of 214 (76 percent) of lesions. The most significant stenosis was dilated in 100 of 102 patients. The short-term follow-up (2 to 43 months) of the successfully treated patients showed angina relief similar to that achieved with bypass surgery. There was no mortality in the 102 patients. Another experienced center reported 80 patients who underwent multivessel dilatation.[79] They made 168 attempts in 180 lesions with a primary success rate of 91 percent. One death and one transmural myocardial infarction occurred. Follow-up data on 69 patients (mean follow-up 6.9 months) showed that 96 percent of the successfully dilated patients were improved.

A significant barrier to the widespread application of coronary angioplasty to patients with multivessel disease is the large number of patients with diffuse involvement of the coronary arteries. Hamby and Katz,[54] when reviewing 500 patients with clinical symptoms sufficiently severe to justify surgery, found no ideal angioplasty candidates among patients with three-vessel disease and left main coronary artery obstruction. Since the duration of symptoms is shorter in angioplasty candidates than in nonangioplasty candidates, it would be logical to suppose that if one evaluated patients soon after the onset of symptoms of ischemic heart disease, a higher percentage of patients might be found who were candidates for dilatation.

Since some patients develop single-vessel disease and later have double-vessel disease and still later have triple-vessel disease, it is possible that triple-vessel disease might be prevented by the early detection and treatment of single-vessel disease with angioplasty.

What has been shown is that patients with multivessel disease can safely undergo angioplasty. Multiple dilatations can be performed with a high degree of primary success by experienced operators. What remains to be shown is that such therapy gives the same good long-term result as bypass surgery. There is still a very high percentage of multivessel-disease patients who would not be as well revascularized by angioplasty as they would be by bypass surgery because of diffuse disease or total occlusion. In order for angioplasty to have a larger application in the patients going for bypass surgery, either the disease must be diagnosed earlier or the technical problems of diffuse disease and total occlusion must be solved.

At present, 90 percent of the patients undergoing angioplasty at Emory University Hospital have single-vessel disease.

TOTAL OCCLUSION

Although two preliminary reports show that total occlusion can be opened with angioplasty, it is important to understand the special conditions present in these two studies.[80,81] In all patients the underlying lesions were known or the occlusion was relatively recent. Primary success rate was lower than with subtotal stenosis, 67 percent versus 86 percent in one series of 39 patients.[80] The procedure in general is safe, since in almost every case, collateral vessels fill the distal vessel. There were no emergency operations and no myocardial infarctions. In patients with irregular underlying lesions coronary angioplasty is not recommended since this might well result in arterial dissection. There are no data on attempts at crossing total occlusion when the underlying lesion is not known.

EVOLVING OR RECENT MYOCARDIAL INFARCTION

The major problem following successful streptokinase treatment is reocclusion of the artery. In 129 patients with successful streptokinase treatment, 5 cardiac deaths and 20 reinfarctions occurred despite anticoagulation therapy.[82] It is therefore a logical and necessary part of myocardial preservation to treat the underlying stenosis as quickly as possible.[83] Coronary angioplasty performed either immediately following successful streptolysis or during the hospital period results in improved coronary patency and more stable hospital course and follow-up.[84–86] However, Meyer et al.[60] showed that only two of seven patients with cardiogenic shock despite successful opening of the artery were reversed with PTCA of a high-grade underlying stenosis.[60] Although more long-term studies are needed, the preliminary reports of angioplasty after successful streptokinase infusion are encouraging.

In 100 symptomatic patients after acute myocardial infarction, coronary angioplasty was successfully performed on 110 out of 132 lesions (83.3 percent). There were three PTCA deaths, four myocardial infarctions, three emergency bypass operations, and one late death. At an average of 5 months of follow-up, 86 percent of the patients were asymptomatic.[87] Angina symptoms following acute myocardial infarction represent a clear indication for cardiac catheterization and revascularization therapy if appropriate.[88] If these favorable preliminary results can be confirmed (4 percent mortality rate) then the prognosis of the symptomatic patient after acute myocardial infarction will be improved by appropriate angioplasty. Earlier studies showed 25 percent 3-month mortality rate[89] and 57 percent 6-month mortality rate[90] in patients with angina pectoris after acute myocardial infarction.

ANGIOPLASTY AFTER BYPASS SURGERY

The most frequent reason for coronary angioplasty after successful aortocoronary bypass surgery is progression of disease in previously uninvolved coronary arteries or graft failures. Of our patients who had coronary angioplasty 9 percent were status post bypass surgery: 28 patients had bypass graft dilatations, 43 had native vessel dilatations, and 1 patient had both.

One report describes patients who had 16 proximal anastomosis or graft body stenoses and 22 distal bypass anastomosis stenoses. Successful angioplasty was achieved in 15 of 16 proximal or body stenoses, but 7 of these (47 percent) had recurrence in 6 months. Of the 22 distal stenoses primary success was achieved in 95 percent, and only three patients showed restenosis within 6 months.[91] These results are in agreement with the results reported by other centers.[92,93] A high primary success rate can be achieved regardless of the location of the stenosis in a bypass graft; the recurrence rate is high when the obstruction is in the body and proximal anastomosis site. The recurrence rate is low at the distal anastomatic site, and angioplasty would seem to be the treatment of choice in these patients.

ANGIOPLASTY AFTER RECURRENCE OF STENOSIS

One of the principal advantages of PTCA is the ease with which it can be repeated. In one series of patients 26 of 27 repeat attempts were successful, with the one failure not due to technical difficulties but to the requirement of emergency bypass surgery because of acute coronary occlusion.[94] In general terms recurrent lesions tend to be more symmetrical and respond to lower balloon pressures. If technical factors did not prohibit dilatation the first time, a second angioplasty should be technically feasible.

Accordingly, at least one repeat angioplasty appears to be indicated when restenosis occurs. The recurrence rate following a second angioplasty is about 33 percent.[95] After the second recurrence only five of our patients have undergone a third PTCA. We recommend a third PTCA of the same lesion only if the time from PTCA to recurrence is lengthening. If the time interval from the second PTCA to the second recurrence is shorter than the interval from the first PTCA to the first recurrence, then repeat PTCA is not recommended.

INTRAOPERATIVE ANGIOPLASTY

Coronary angioplasty during surgery is done for a variety of indications: distal coronary disease and limited runoff; disease in branch vessels not large enough for grafting; and tandem lesions when separate grafting is not possible.[96] Although done under direct visualization, there is no fluoroscopic control. One study which used 6 atm and two to six inflations per vessel showed improvement in 6 of 18 (33 percent) dilated segments at follow-up angiography. Fifty percent of the lesions showed no change, and two were worse.[97] Another group found that 16 out of 18 (89 percent) dilatations were successful. Success was defined as being able to pass a larger probe through the stenosis. At repeat catheterization in this study seven of eight lesions were improved.[98]

Because the recurrence rate after angioplasty at present is higher than bypass graft closure rate (see below), intraoperative angioplasty should be performed only when further bypass grafting is not possible. Better methods of intraoperative visual assessment need to be developed so that full efforts can be made to dilate the lesion. When this is possible and when the newer methods now used in the percutaneous angioplasty laboratory (i.e., balloons that tolerate higher pressures and steerable systems) are available, results similar to the percutaneous method can be expected. The long-term assessment of intraoperative angioplasty is currently unavailable. Recurrence rates in the small vessels that are dilated at surgery may be different from the recurrence rates in proximal larger vessels that are dilated by the percutaneous method. Until these issues are resolved, intraoperative angioplasty should be done under experimental protocol with careful follow-up. As long as recurrence rate after angioplasty remains higher than the graft occlusion rate, intraoperative coronary angioplasty should be an adjunct rather than a replacement to bypass grafting.

LESION TYPES

Previous studies have considered proximal, discrete, subtotal, and noncalcific lesions as ideal for angioplasty.[5] With the steerable catheter system, lesions as distal as the posterior descending branch of the right coronary artery have been dilated. Distal lesions do not pose major problems as long as they are discrete and the vessel is not tortuous proximal to the lesion. Tortuous vessels absorb the forward force transmitted through the balloon catheter, making it impossible to push the balloon catheter through the lesion. Lesions at a bifurcation of two vessels are not ideal for angioplasty since closure of the nondilated vessel may occur with balloon inflation. However, it is sometimes possible to dilate both vessels simultaneously using Gruentzig's "kissing balloon" technique. The full use of this method of dilating coronary lesions is under investigation.

In one series there was no difference in primary success rate between calcified and noncalcified stenosis.[28] Selection of patients was important, however, since dilatations were attempted with the anticipation of crossing and dilating the stenosis despite the presence of calcium. The low-profile balloon and the ability to dilate at higher pressures have changed the presence of a calcific lesion from an absolute to a relative contraindication.

Lesions just distal to acute bends in the coronary artery form a relative contraindication to angioplasty since these lesions may be more prone to dissection[8] due to errors in crossing or balloon injury during inflation.

COMPLICATIONS

Complications from coronary angioplasty can be classified as major and minor. Major complications are the ones generally reported and include death, the need for emergency bypass surgery, myocardial infarction, and cerebral vascular accident. Less serious complications include groin site hematomas requiring surgical repair and arrhythmias requiring cardioversion.

Early Deaths

In the first 1,000 patients entered into the NHLBI registry there were 13 deaths. Of these 13 deaths, 5 had the onset of chest pain and instability in the catheterization laboratory. Two of these five died despite emergency bypass surgery. Six patients whose chest pain began soon after PTCA died despite elective (three) or emergency (three) bypass surgery. Two patients without chest pain died after elective bypass surgery. The mortality rate was lower in patients with single-vessel disease, occurring in 7 of 780 patients (0.9 percent) compared to patients with multivessel disease, in whom death occurred in 4 of 220 patients (1.8 percent). The death rate was 0.75 percent in patients undergoing angioplasty without prior bypass grafting.[98] In 640 angioplasty patients registered at the NHLBI over the age of 60, the death rate was 1.5 percent for single-vessel

disease and 3.2 percent for multivessel disease.[69] In a combined center study of 852 patients undergoing angioplasty, the mortality rate was higher in patients with multivessel disease (1 percent) compared to the death rate in patients with one-vessel disease; however, this difference was not significant. Multivessel-disease patients with prior bypass surgery had a higher mortality rate of 2.6 percent. There was no death in the 102 patients undergoing multivessel dilatation in this series.[78] In the Zuerich-Emory series of 1,500 attempts at angioplasty, there has been one inhospital death (0.07 percent). This death was due to intracerebral hemorrhage following the use of combined streptokinase and angioplasty. As seen from the NHLBI data, most of the deaths occurred after emergency or elective bypass surgery. Clearly the most important factor in preventing inhospital deaths is the ability of the surgical team and its performance under emergency conditions.[99,100]

Late Deaths

Five late deaths occurred in the Zuerich patients. Three of the five were cardiac: a patient who had dilatation of his left main coronary artery who probably had coronary spasm; an inoperable patient who died of occlusive disease 9 months after dilatation of his left main coronary artery; a patient with double-vessel disease, with a documented good long-term result from dilatation of his left anterior descending coronary artery stenosis, died following occlusion of an anterior marginal artery that was severely stenosed but not dilated at original angioplasty.

At Emory University in Atlanta there have been four late deaths in 1,153 patients who had successful angioplasties. Two of these were cardiac. One died 2 months following angioplasty and 1 day after elective bypass surgery for his recurrent stenosis. Another patient died 1 week following recurrent symptoms and 5 months after successful left anterior descending coronary artery angioplasty.

There have also been two late deaths in our patients who were not successfully dilated. One patient died 10 days after elective single-vessel coronary bypass surgery. Another medically treated patient died suddenly of unknown causes 14 months after attempted angioplasty.

Three late deaths have been reported in the NHLBI registry of 631 patients: one died 3 months following angioplasty of presumed septicemia as a complication of emergency bypass operation. One patient had uncomplicated elective bypass surgery but died 6 months later. Another patient with recurrent stenosis died during anesthetic induction.[101]

The late deaths have indicated that one should endeavor to supply complete revascularization and respond promptly to angina symptoms during the follow-up period.

Emergency Bypass Surgery

Emergency bypass surgery is required when angioplasty precipitates acute coronary occlusion or coronary dissection. In the NHLBI registry of 1,116 angioplasty attempts in 52 centers the emergency bypass surgery rate was 6.6 percent.[102] The reason for the emergency surgery was coronary occlusion (32 percent), dissection (27 percent), prolonged angina (18 percent), coronary spasm (14 percent), coronary embolism (3 percent), and other (7 percent). Although 28 of 74 emergency surgical patients had myocardial infarctions and 6 of 74 (9 percent) died, the indication for surgery, i.e., dissection or occlusion was not predictive of further complication.[102] The emergency surgery risk of patients registered at the NHLBI of patients older than 60 years was 6.0 percent.[69]

Emergency bypass surgery has been required in 3.7 percent of the Emory series of patients. The rate of all complications decline with increasing experience of the operator.[77] We have found a steady decline in the emergency surgery rate such that our current emergency rate is about 2 to 3 percent.[28] Although some of our early dissections were due to crossing errors, i.e., pushing too hard when the tip of the catheter was subintimal, most dissections are intrinsic to the method since intimal tearing occurs in many patients. In an occasional patient it is possible to recross a dissected stenosis and repeat angioplasty and obviate the need for emergency surgery, but this cannot be relied upon.[31] For this reason we doubt that the need for emergency bypass surgery will be completely eliminated.

Early in our experience acute coronary artery occlusion virtually always resulted in emergency bypass surgery,[103] but this is no longer the case. Most acute reocclusions happen less than 2 h after successful PTCA or within 2 to 3 h after discontinuing a heparin infusion. In 13 patients with acute occlusions, 4 resolved spontaneously with nitrates and nifedipine, 4 resolved with repeat emergency PTCA, 5 patients underwent bypass surgery either with (3 patients) or without (2 patients) repeat PTCA attempts.[104] Therefore, in this small series, over one-half of patients who would have ordinarily gone to surgery did not do so because their symptoms resolved with medication or with repeat angioplasty. Others have used streptokinase infusions in this same setting and were successful in three patients in one report and one patient in another.[105,106]

Despite the response to therapy noted, the cause of acute occlusion is frequently uncertain. Patients are premedicated with heparin, nitrates, and nifedipine.

The inconsistent response to intracoronary nitroglycerin makes coronary spasm an unlikely cause of most occlusions. But why should thrombosis occur if the patient is anticoagulated, and if thrombosis has occurred, why is it not apparent angiographically?

Two groups have investigated the possibility that acute occlusion may be related to an imbalance of prostacyclin and thromboxane A_2 metabolism due to arterial injury and platelet activation by the exposed collagen.[107–109] A dramatic rise in thromboxane in the coronary sinus blood is seen,[107] but it is uncertain whether the rise in concentration of this potent arterial constrictor is the cause or the result of acute occlusion.

Regardless of the cause of acute occlusion, we have found that once the artery is reopened, the patient can generally be stabilized with a 24- to 36-h intravenous infusion of heparin and nitroglycerin. If the artery cannot be readily opened within 10 to 15 min of effort while the operating room is being prepared, the patient should go to bypass surgery without delay. In patients manifesting spasm or having a particularly large longitudinal intimal tear after otherwise uncomplicated angioplasty, prophylactic therapy with intravenous heparin and nitroglycerin given for 24 h may prevent acute occlusion.

Myocardial Infarction

The NHLBI angioplasty registry indicates that 38 percent of the patients undergoing emergency bypass surgery following angioplasty have myocardial infarction. In an early report of 631 patients the myocardial infarction rate was 4.4 percent.[101] As stated earlier, the complication rate decreases as experience of the operator increases.[76] Currently the Q wave infarction rate of angioplasty at Emory is about 1 percent.[28]

It is believed that prompt surgical myocardial revascularization after acute decompensation in the angioplasty laboratory will result in limitation of myocardial injury. Seven of the first 25 patients (28 percent) undergoing emergency surgery in the one series had myocardial infarction by Q wave criteria. Of the patients revascularized more than 2 h after the onset of acute occlusion, 4 of 7 (57 percent) had acute infarction, while 3 of 18 patients (17 percent) revascularized less than 2 h after the onset of chest pain had acute infarction.[103] No correlation between the presence or absence of collateral vessels and postoperative infarction has been shown, but the number of patients in both series is small.[100,103]

Margolis[110] and others[100] have advocated the use of intraaortic balloon counterpulsation to stabilize the patient while the transfer to the operating room takes place. In one series of five patients with acute occlusion treated with prompt intraaortic balloon counterpulsation, no evidence of myocardial infarction was present by either electrocardiographic or cardiac enzymatic criteria.[110]

Certain properties of the lesions themselves make them susceptible to complications. When emergency surgery is required after angioplasty in patients with mild coronary stenosis (<60 percent diameter narrowing) a Q wave myocardial infarction is more likely to occur.[56] Eccentric stenoses, particularly long, eccentric stenoses, are more frequently associated with complications after angioplasty.[111]

In summary, to minimize the risk of myocardial infarction prompt bypass surgery is essential. If the total occlusion can be opened during the preparation for surgery, the need for surgery may be aborted. Prompt institution of intraaortic balloon counterpulsation may result in myocardial preservation.

Other Risks

Cerebral vascular accident has not been reported with coronary angioplasty. We have had one fatal intracerebral hemorrhage in nearly 1,500 cases, and this was the only inhospital death. This occurred in a patient who had received streptokinase, heparin, and PTCA. Cardiac tamponade has been reported in two patients; one required surgical decompression and the other responded to percutaneous drainage. Both were due to pacemaker penetration of the right ventricle.[28] Perivascular coronary hemorrhage may be seen in patients requiring bypass surgery,[100] but coronary artery rupture has not yet been reported in living patients. Lee et al. showed that overdistension of the coronary artery of fresh cadavers could result in arterial perforation.[10] Ventricular fibrillation and local arterial complications occur in frequencies similar to that of routine coronary angiography.[28]

Recurrence[41,95,112,113]

Reported recurrence rates vary from 13 to 47 percent. Recurrence rates cannot be determined with accuracy unless all patients undergo routine follow-up angiography. While symptoms are a fairly reliable predictor of recurrence, 11 of 12 patients (92 percent) in one series with recurrent symptoms had recurrent stenosis,[112] the correlation is not perfect. Not all symptomatic patients have recurrent stenosis, and vice versa. At times, repeat catheterization reveals progression of disease at a site other than the site of prior angioplasty. A true recurrence rarely occurs less than 1 month following angioplasty, but patients may have recurrent angina during this time due to coronary spasm superimposed on hemodynamically insignificant disease.[61,62]

About 15 percent of asymptomatic patients will have angiographic evidence of recurrence. By 6 months the artery is usually healed either with a recurrent stenosis or with an open artery.

FACTORS ASSOCIATED WITH RECURRENCE

The analysis of the data in the NHLBI registry indicated that no drug therapy was associated with a decrease in recurrence rates. The data also suggest that patients with improvement in the late follow-up film compared to the initial post-PTCA result were patients with poorer initial results.[113] This is logical since they also were the patients who could improve the most. Others have demonstrated a "cleaning" of the artery on follow-up angiography.[114] This improvement in diameter narrowing may well be due to scarification and retraction of intimal and medial splits, as has been suggested by Cowley and Block.[25] In a study comparing 118 patients with angiographic recurrence and 158 patients with angiographic evidence of nonrecurrence, no statistical differences could be found between patient subgroups when clinical factors such as age, sex, and duration of symptoms prior to PTCA were compared. None of the traditional cardiovascular risk factors (smoking, hypertension, diabetes, history of hyperlipidemia) were shown to correlate with the recurrence of stenosis. Lesion morphology (length, eccentricity, calcification) was not a factor in recurrence, nor was the presence of an intimal tear after angioplasty. Lesions in the left anterior descending coronary artery (47 percent) were more likely to recur than lesions in the right coronary artery or circumflex coronary artery (29 percent, 33 percent).[115]

The Montreal Heart Institute examined the follow-up data from 103 consecutive patients. They concluded that the probability of recurrence was higher in patients with variant angina, class IV effort angina, or with lesions involving branches, in patients older than 60, and when more than nine dilatations per segment were performed.[116] The higher risk of recurrence with variant angina is particularly interesting since it has been suggested that coronary artery spasm may play a role in pathogenesis of recurrence.[22,61] This may be due to the presence of relatively early atherosclerosis in which the muscular media has not been destroyed.[22] Contraction of the muscular media may result in further intimal injury and propagation of the atherosclerotic process.[117] However, there is currently no evidence that the routine treatment of post PTCA patients with antispasm medications is effective in the prevention of recurrent stenosis. In fact, in one nonrandomized study, the recurrence rate was similar in patients on sulfinpyrazone and diltiazem and in patients on sulfinpyrazone alone.[118] Other factors mentioned—older age, class IV symptoms, and lesions involving branches—are not confirmed by other studies. The correlation of an increased number of inflations and higher incidence of recurrence may indicate that an increased number of inflations is harmful or that increased number of inflations are required when the initial results are poor since one monitors the pressure gradient and angiographic result during the performance of coronary angioplasty. A poor initial result (i.e., an increase in diameter of less than 50 percent) in the initial angioplasty has been correlated with a higher incidence of recurrent stenosis.[119]

Data suggesting that an excellent initial result is less likely to be followed by a recurrence are in keeping with bypass surgical data, which suggest that the better the initial flow in a bypass graft, the less likely the graft is to close.[120]

Recurrence is also said to be higher when the stenosis is eccentric rather than concentric,[121] but other studies have not confirmed this.[115]

RECURRENCE IN SPECIAL SUBGROUPS

The recurrence of stenosis following bypass graft angioplasty is variable depending upon the location of the stenosis. Dilatation of the venous graft at the aortic anastomotic site or the graft body has a higher incidence of recurrence (about 50 percent) than dilatation of the vein-graft coronary artery anastomotic site, which has a relatively low recurrence rate (15 percent).[91] Contrary to the experience with peripheral angioplasty, where the recurrence rate of totally occluded vessels is higher than it is with partially occluded arteries, the incidence of recurrent stenosis following angioplasty of totally occluded coronary arteries appears to be no higher than it is of partially occluded arteries.[80]

DRUG THERAPY AFTER CORONARY ANGIOPLASTY

Routine anticoagulation after coronary angioplasty has been recommended. This approach is based on the information that is available on peripheral angioplasty. In one randomized trial the recurrence rate was lower in one group of patients anticoagulated with aspirin (26.2 percent) when compared to a group of patients anticoagulated with coumadin (36.1 percent).[122] Furthermore, the recurrence rate appeared to be even higher in the patients given coumadin but who were poorly compliant. Although these results are not statistically significant ($p < .1$), it is unlikely that coumadin will prove to be more effective than aspirin. Since aspirin is simpler to administer and has fewer serious bleeding complications,[123] one aspirin daily (300 mg) is recommended in an effort to prevent recurrent stenosis. Although aspirin has not been clearly shown to be superior to no treatment, the high recurrence rate in the noncompliant coumadin group and experience from peripheral angioplasty suggest that some form of anticoagulation is useful.

The addition of dipyridamole (Persantin) has theoretical advantages.[124] The combination of dipyridamole and aspirin has been shown to reduce the incidence of bypass graft occlusions following aortocoronary bypass surgery in two studies[125,126] but not in another study.[127] While no definite advantage has been shown for aspirin and dipyridamole over aspirin alone, a trend toward a lower graft occlusion rate was shown for combined therapy.[126] Early institution of therapy may well be important.[125] Insight gained from studies of aortocoronary bypass procedures may well be relevant to angioplasty because of the similarities in the pathology. Stenosis of the distal anastomotic site[128] following bypass grafting and the recurrent stenosis following angioplasty show intimal proliferation.[22] The combined use of aspirin and diypridamole for prevention of recurrent stenosis remains to be investigated.

The use of calcium antagonists in the prevention of recurrence must be carefully studied. The high recurrence rates in patients with variant angina demand that such therapy be investigated.

Intravenous dextran has been a part of the angioplasty protocol of most centers since it was shown to prevent the adherence of platelets to the denuded endothelium in experimental angioplasty in dogs.[19] Although the prevention of platelet adherence may theoretically prevent the development of atherosclerosis by decreasing the release of platelet growth factor, this hypothesis has not been substantiated by clinical studies. There is no evidence that the routine use of dextran prevents the development of recurrence.

In summary, although no drug regimen has been clearly shown to decrease the incidence of recurrence, it is quite probable that some drug combination will eventually be found to decrease the incidence of recurrence.

LIMITATIONS OF STUDIES TO DETERMINE THE RECURRENCE RATE

It is not possible to determine an accurate recurrence rate since all patients will not permit repeated cardiac catheterization. Noninvasive studies are useful but do not show a perfect correlation with angiography.

Several different methods are used in the reporting of recurrence rates. The recurrence of "angina" does not have a perfect correlation with angiographic evidence of recurrence, and the absence of angina does not guarantee that recurrence of stenosis has not occurred. All angiographers do not calculate the recurrence rates the same way. Some divide the total number of angiographic recurrences by the total number of patients; this might result in a falsely low incidence of recurrence since it assumes that all patients without angiography do not have a recurrence. Using the total number of patients in the denominator will further underestimate the percentage of recurrences if patients are included who have not been followed for at least 6 months. Even the angiographic criteria for stenosis are variable. Some use a subjective estimate of lesion severity. Some consider an improvement of 20 percent or more of lumen diameter over preangioplasty diameter to be a continuing success. We personally use a 50 percent loss of the initial gain in diameter narrowing as the definition of recurrence. Obviously, the definition of recurrence is as important as the recurrence rate in comparing the results from various centers.

Summary

The recurrence of stenosis is an unsolved problem following coronary angioplasty. Technical improvements in the method may reduce the recurrence rates in a manner similar to coronary bypass surgery, where improvements in technique were responsible for improved graft patency.[71] But technical advances alone are not likely to prevent recurrence. Drug therapy holds promise, and some form of anticoagulation or platelet inhibition is probably important. At present no therapy has been shown to be superior to aspirin therapy alone. There is no clear correlation between any of the major risk factors and lesion morphology prior to angioplasty.

Dilatation of bypass grafts is possible, but proximal anastomotic and graft body stenoses appear to be subject to a higher incidence of recurrent stenosis. Careful study of recurrence in PTCA patients is justified since any therapy that can prove itself to be effective may also be effective in the prevention of early bypass graft occlusion. Furthermore, since some of these recurrent lesions are indistinguishable from de novo atherosclerosis,[23] prevention of recurrent stenosis may help to elucidate measures or medications that can prevent the development of de novo atherosclerosis.

PERSPECTIVE

Coronary angioplasty is a new and exciting addition to the treatment of coronary artery disease. Since the technique is still evolving, the ultimate role that this method will play in the treatment of coronary disease has yet to be fully realized. Some investigators call for

randomized studies.[129–132] Such trials would be of no value as long as the method continues to rapidly evolve. The Veterans Administration's randomized study of bypass surgery versus medical therapy created much discussion, but by the time the study was completed the surgical mortality and complication rate had changed so much that the data were not comparable to current surgical results. Any randomized study of bypass surgery and coronary angioplasty would be outdated by the time of its publication because improvements in the method of PTCA are continuing.

The evidence for improvement that has been demonstrated for coronary bypass surgery has also been shown for coronary angioplasty. Improved myocardial perfusion during exercise[133,134] and improved left ventricular function with exercise testing[135] has been demonstrated for angioplasty and bypass surgery. Such improvement is expected from both PTCA and coronary bypass since both methods improve myocardial perfusion.

The primary success rate is lower in PTCA when compared to bypass surgery although this comparison is somewhat difficult. It is possible to insert a bypass graft in most vessels attempted; however, by hospital discharge 3 to 12 percent of bypass grafts will be closed. As more experience is gained with angioplasty, the primary success rate will be greater than 90 percent.

The complication rate of angioplasty continues to improve. The Q wave infarction rate for the whole series of Zuerich-Atlanta patients is 2 to 3 percent. The Q wave infarction rate of the most recent 400 patients is about 1 percent. Our inhospital mortality rate in the first 1,500 cases is 1 (0.07 percent). Q wave infarction during single-vessel bypass at Emory Hospital is 4.4 percent (23 of 518). Hospital mortality rate for single-vessel bypass surgery at Emory Hospital between 1973 and 1979 was 0.4 percent.[136] These excellent statistics are now even better because the patients operated on between 1973 and 1976 did not have the benefit of potassium cardioplegia. To prove any statistical difference between the complications of coronary bypass surgery and coronary angioplasty would require an enormous number of patients. One of the main reasons that our PTCA complication is so low is the ability of our surgical team to promptly revascularize the emergency PTCA cases.

The recurrence rate following angioplasty remains a limitation. Although a variety of figures are cited above, the angiographic recurrence rate is probably 25 to 35 percent in patients with initial successful angioplasty treated with aspirin. This rate is higher than the 15 percent 1-year graft closure rate generally accepted for bypass graft surgery.[71] However, in contrast to bypass surgery where repeat surgery is technically more difficult, repeat angioplasty is usually technically easier and associated with fewer complications. Fortunately the late recurrence rate appears to be low, and patients with normal or nearly normal angiograms at 6 months can expect to have a good prognosis.

Extension of angioplasty to new indications requires careful follow-up of patients. Each center performing PTCA should keep careful statistics of the success and complications. If the complications are in gross excess to published reports[137] at a similar point in the learning curve,[138] a reassessment of the angioplasty procedure at that institution is in order.

Coronary angioplasty is a developing technique but currently appears to be the treatment of choice for technically suitable single-vessel disease requiring revascularization therapy. Its future role can be discerned by the careful follow-up of treated patients and by comparing the results with bypass surgery.

REFERENCES

1 Dotter, C. T., and Judkins, M. P.: Transluminal Treatment of Arteriosclerotic Obstruction: Description of a New Technic and a Preliminary Report of its Application, *Circulation*, 30:654, 1964.

2 Dotter, C. T.: Transluminal Angioplasty: A Long View, *Radiology*, 135:561, 1980.

3 Gruentzig, A.: Die Perkutane Rekanalisation chronischer arterieller verschlusse (Dotter-Prinzip) mit einem neuen Doppellumigen Dilatations Katheter, *Fortschr. Rontgenstr.*, 124:80, 1976.

4 Gruentzig, A. R.: Transluminal Dilatation of Coronary-Artery Stenosis, *Lancet*, 1:263, 1978.

5 Gruentzig, A., Senning, A., and Siegenthaler, W. E.: Nonoperative Dilatation of Coronary Artery Stenosis. Percutaneous Transluminal Coronary Angioplasty, *N. Engl. J. Med.*, 301:61, 1979.

6 Dotter, C. T.: Transluminal Angioplasty. Pathologic basis, in E. Zeiter, A. Gruentzig, and W. Schoop (eds.), "Percutaneous Vascular Recanalization," Springer-Verlag, New York, 1978, p. 3.

7 Gruentzig, A.: Percutaneous Transluminal Recanalization (PTR) with the Double Lumen Dilatation Catheter, in E. Zeiter, A. Gruentzig, and W. Schoop (eds.), "Percutaneous Vascular Recanalization," Springer-Verlag, New York, 1978, p. 17.

8 Baughman, K. L., Pasternak, R. C., Fallon, J. T., and Block, P. C.: Transluminal Coronary Angioplasty of Postmortem Human Hearts, *Am. J. Cardiol.*, 48:1044, 1981.

9 Simpson, J. B., Robert, E. W., Billingham, M. E., Myler, R., and Harrison, D. C.: Coronary Transluminal Angioplasty in Human Cadaver Hearts, *Circulation*, 57,58(suppl. 2):80, 1978. (Abstract.)

10 Lee, G., Ikeda, R. M., Joye, J. A., et al.: Evaluation of Transluminal Angioplasty of Chronic Coronary Artery Stenosis, *Circulation*, 63:77, 1980.

11 Freudenberg, H., and Lichtlen, P. R.: The Mechanism of Dilatation in Transluminal Coronary Angioplasty. A Postmortem Study, *Am. J. Cardiol.*, 49:917, 1982. (Abstract.)

12 Freudenberg, H., Wefing, H., and Lichtlen, R.: Risks of Transluminal Coronary Angioplasty. A Postmortem Study, *Circulation*, 57,58(suppl. 2):80, 1978. (Abstract.)

13 Kaltenbach, M., Beyer, J., Klepzig, H., Schmidts, L., and Hubner, K.: Effect of 5 kg/cm^2 Pressure on Atherosclerotic Vessel Wall Segments, in M. Kaltenbach et al. (eds.), "Fourth International Symposium on Coronary Heart Disease, Frankfurt, 1981," Springer-Verlag, Berlin, 1982, p. 190.

14 Block, P. C., Baughman, K. L., Pasternak, R. C., and Fallon, J. T.: Transluminal Angioplasty: Correlation of Morphologic and Angiographic Findings in an Experimental Model, *Circulation*, 61:778, 1980.

15 Block, P. C.: Correlation of the Effect of Transluminal Angioplasty in Experimentally Induced Rabbit Atherosclerosis with Pathological Changes in Human Coronary Artery, in M. Kaltenbach et al. (eds.), "Fourth International Symposium on Coronary Heart Disease, Frankfurt, 1981," Springer-Verlag, Berlin, 1982, p. 183.

16 Castaneda-Zuniga, W. R., Formanek, A., et al.: The Mechanism of Balloon Angioplasty, *Radiology*, 135:565, 1980.

17 Block, P. C., Elmer, D., and Fallon, J. T.: Release of Atherosclerotic Debris after Transluminal Angioplasty, *Circulation*, 65:950, 1982.

18 Ryan, T. J., Faxon, D. P., Weber, V. J., et al.: Acute and Chronic Effects of Transluminal Angioplasty in Three Models of Experimental Atherosclerosis, in M. Kaltenbach et al. (eds.), "Fourth International Symposium on Coronary Artery Disease, Frankfurt, 1981," Springer-Verlag, Berlin, 1982, p. 185.

19 Pasternak, R. C., Baughman, K. L., Fallon, J. T., and Block, P. C.: Scanning Electron Microscopy after Coronary Transluminal Angioplasty of Normal Canine Coronary Arteries, *Am. J. Cardiol.*, 45:591, 1980.

20 Schmidt-Moritz, A. D., Schneider, M., Kunkel, B., and Kaltenbach, M.: Histological Changes following Transluminal Angioplasty of Experimentally Induced Atherosclerosis in Miniature Pigs, in M. Kaltenbach et al. (eds.), "Fourth International Symposium on Coronary Artery Disease, Frankfurt, 1981," Springer-Verlag, Berlin, 1982, p. 176.

21 Block, P. C., Myler, R. K., Stertzer, S., and Fallon, J. T.: Morphology after Transluminal Angioplasty in Human Beings, *N. Engl. J. Med.*, 305:382, 1981.

22 Hollman, J., Austin, G., Gruentzig, A. R., et al.: Recent observations.

23 Waller, B. F., McManus, B. M., Kishel, J. C., et al.: Sudden Death 90 to 180 Days after Percutaneous Transluminal Coronary Angioplasty: Severe Narrowing by Atherosclerotic Plaque at Necropsy at the Site of Previous Angioplasty, *Circulation*, 66(suppl. 2):4, 1982.

24 Lue, H., and Gruentzig, A.: Histopathologic Aspects of Transluminal Recanalization, in E. Zeitler, A. Gruentzig, and W. Schoop (eds.), "Percutaneous Vascular Recanalization," Springer-Verlag, New York, 1978, p. 39.

25 Cowley, M. J., and Block, P. C.: Percutaneous Transluminal Coronary Angioplasty, *Mod. Concepts Cardiovasc. Dis.*, 50:25, 1981.

26 Gruentzig, A. R.: Technique of Percutaneous Transluminal Coronary Angioplasty, in J. W. Hurst (editor-in-chief), "The Heart," 5th ed., McGraw-Hill Book Company, New York, 1982, p. 1904.

27 Gruentzig, A.: Percutaneous Transluminal Coronary Angioplasty, *Semin. Roentgenol.*, 10:152, 1981.

28 Hollman, J., Gruentzig, A., King, S. B., III, et al.: Recent Observations.

29 Palacios, I. F., Block, P. C., Williams, D. O., et al.: Increased Rate of Successful Percutaneous Transluminal Coronary Angioplasty in Patients with High Grade Coronary Artery Stenosis, *Circulation*, 64(suppl. 4):109, 1981. (Abstract.)

30 Simpson, J. B., Baim, D. S., Robert, E. W., and Harrison, D. C.: A New Catheter System for Coronary Angioplasty, *Am. J. Cardiol.*, 49:1217, 1982.

31 Gruentzig, A. R., and Hollman, J.: Improved Primary Success Rate in Transluminal Coronary Angioplasty using a Steerable Guidance System, *Circulation*, 66:11, 1982. (Abstract.)

32 Kaltenbach, M., Beyer, J., Klepzig, H., Schmidts, L., and Hubner, K.: Effect of 5 kg/cm² Pressure on Atherosclerotic Vessel Wall Segments, in M. Kaltenbach et al. (eds.), "Fourth International Symposium on Coronary Heart Disease, Frankfurt, 1981," Springer-Verlag, Berlin, 1982, p. 189.

33 Kaltenbach, M., and Kober, G.: Can Prolonged Application of Pressure Improve the Results of Coronary Angioplasty (PTCA)?, *Circulation*, 66(suppl. 2):123, 1982. (Abstract.)

34 Williams, D. O., Riley, R. S., Singh, A. K., Korr, K. S., and Most, A. S.: Salutory Effect of Percutaneous Transluminal Coronary Angioplasty on Coronary Circulatory Dynamics, in M. Kaltenbach et al. (eds.), "Fourth International Symposium on Coronary Heart Disease, Frankfurt, 1981," Springer-Verlag, Berlin, 1982, p. 81.

35 Williams, D. O., Riley, R. S., Singh, A. K., Gewirtz, H., and Most, A. S.: Evaluation of the Role of Coronary Angioplasty in Patients with Unstable Angina Pectoris, *Am. Heart J.*, 102:1, 1981.

36 Rothman, M., Baim, D., Simpson, S., and Harrison, D.: Improved Hemodynamic and Metabolic Indices after Percutaneous Transluminal Coronary Angioplasty (PTCA), *Circulation*, 64(suppl. 4):253, 1981. (Abstract.)

37 Hartzler, G. O., Smith, H. C., Vlietstra, R. E., Oberle, D. A., and Strelow, D. A.: Coronary Blood Flow Responses during Successful Percutaneous Transluminal Coronary Angioplasty, *Mayo Clin. Proc.*, 55:45, 1980.

38 Sigwart, U., Grbic, M., Essinger, A., et al.: Improvement of Left Ventricular Function after Percutaneous Transluminal Coronary Angioplasty, *Am. J. Cardiol.*, 49:651, 1982.

39 Hirzel, H. O., Nuesch, K., Gruentzig, A. R., and Luetolf, U. M.: Short- and long-term Changes in Myocardial Perfusion after Percutaneous Transluminal Coronary Angioplasty assessed by Thallium-201 Exercise Scintigraphy, *Circulation*, 63:1001, 1981.

40 School, J. M., Chaitman, B. R. and David, P. R.: Evaluation of Percutaneous Transluminal Coronary Angioplasty by Noninvasive Techniques, *Circulation*, 64(suppl. 4):963, 1981. (Abstract.)

41 Kent, K. M., Bonow, R. O., Rosing, D. R., et al.: Improved Myocardial Function During Exercise after Successful Percutaneous Transluminal Coronary Angioplasty, *N. Engl. J. Med.*, 306:441, 1982.

42 Hollman, J., Gruentzig, A., King, S., Douglas, J., and Fajman, W.: The Effect of Percutaneous Transluminal Coronary Angioplasty (PTCA) on Exercise Ejection Fraction (EF), *Circulation*, 64(suppl. 4):253, 1981. (Abstract.)

43 Amor, M., Danchin, N., Godenir, J. P., et al.: Interest of Radionuclide Methods for the Assessment of the Results of Percutaneous Transluminal Coronary Angioplasty, in M. Kaltenbach et al. (eds.), "Fourth International Symposium on Coronary Heart Disease, Frankfurt, 1981," Springer-Verlag, Berlin, 1982, p. 64.

44 Holmes, D. R., Vlietstra, R. E., Mock, M. B., et al.: Follow-up of Patients undergoing Percutaneous Transluminal Coronary Angioplasty (PTCA): A Report from the NHLBI PTCA Registry, *Am. J. Cardiol.*, 49:916, 1982. (Abstract.)

45 Gruentzig, A., Schlumpf, M., and Siegenthaler, N.: Late Functional Results after Success or Failure of Coronary Angioplasty (PTCA), *Circulation*, 64(suppl. 4):193, 1981. (Abstract.)

46 Kent, K. M., Bentivoglio, L. G., Block, P. C., et al.: NHLBI Percutaneous Transluminal Coronary Angioplasty (PTCA) Registry: Four Years Experience, *Am. J. Cardiol.*, 49:904, 1982. (Abstract.)

47 Faxon, D. P., Ryan, T. J., McCabe, C. H., Kelsey, S. F., and Detre, K.: Determinants of a Successful Percutaneous Transluminal Coronary Angioplasty, *Am. J. Cardiol.*, 49:905, 1982. (Abstract.)

48 Rafflenbeul, N., Kaltenbach, M., Engel, H. J., et al.: Morphological and Functional Criteria for a Successful Coronary Angioplasty (PTCA), *Circulation*, 64(suppl. 4):253, 1981. (Abstract.)

49 King, S. B., III, Gruentzig, A. R., Douglas, J. S., Jr., Hollman, J.: Percutaneous Transluminal Coronary Angioplasty for Restenosis following Initial Successful Procedure, *Am. J. Cardiol.*, 49:904, 1982. (Abstract.)

49a Val, P. G., David, P. R., Lespérance, J., et al.: Clinical and Angiographic Follow-up of Successful Percutaneous Transluminal Angioplasty (PTCA), *Circulation*, 66(suppl. 2):330, 1982. (Abstract.)

50 Dorros, G., Stertzer, S., Kaltenbach, M., Myler, R. K., and Spring, D. A.: Percutaneous Transluminal Coronary Angioplasty: Comparison of the Brachial and Femoral Artery Techniques, *Circulation*, 64:162, 1981. (Abstract.)

51 Krajeer, Z., Boskovic, D., Angelini, P., et al.: Transluminal Coronary Angioplasty of the Right Coronary Artery Brachial Cutdown Approach, *Catheterization Cardiovasc. Diagn.*, 8:553, 1982.

52 Jang, G. C., Cowley, M. J., Gruentzig, A. R., et al.: Comparative Cost Analysis of Coronary Angioplasty and Coronary Bypass Surgery: Results from a National Cooperative Study, *Circulation*, 66(suppl. 2):124, 1982. (Abstract.)

53 Jang, G. C., Gruentzig, A. R., Block, P. C., et al.: Delayed Effects of Vessel Restenosis on the Procedure Cost of Coronary Angioplasty, *Circulation*, 66(suppl. 2):330, 1982. (Abstract.)

54 Hamby, R. J., and Katz, S.: Percutaneous Transluminal Coronary Angioplasty: Its Potential Impact on Surgery for Coronary Artery Disease, *Am. J. Cardiol.*, 45:1161, 1980.

55 Berger, S. M., and Gorfinkel, H. J.: Candidates for Transluminal Coronary Angioplasty, *Am. J. Cardiol.*, 48:810, 1981.

56 Ischinger, T., Gruentzig, A. R., Hollman, J., et al.: Should Coronary Arteries with Less than 60% Diameter Stenosis be Treated by Angioplasty?, *Circulation*, 66(suppl. 2):329, 1982. (Abstract.)

57 Hurst, J. W., King, S. B., III, Logue, R. B., et al.: Value of Coronary Bypass Surgery, *Am. J. Cardiol.*, 42:308, 1978.

58 Abedin, Z., and Dack, S.: Isolated Left Anterior Descending Coronary Artery Disease: Choice of Therapy, *Am. J. Cardiol.*, 40:654, 1977.

59 Report of the Unstable Angina Pectoris Study Group: Unstable Angina Pectoris. National Cooperative Group to Compare Medical and Surgical Therapy. I. Report of Protocol and Patient Population, *Am. J. Cardiol.*, 37:896, 1976.

60 Meyer, J., Schmitz, H., Erbel, E., et al.: Transluminal Angioplasty in Patient with Unstable Angina Pectoris, in M. Kaltenbach et al. (eds.), "Fourth International Symposium on Coronary Heart Disease, Frankfurt, 1981," Springer-Verlag, Berlin, 1982, p. 367.

61 David, P. R., Waters, D. D., Scholl, J. M., et al.: Percutaneous Transluminal Coronary Angioplasty in Patients with Variant Angina, *Circulation*, 66:695, 1982.

62 Hollman, J., Gruentzig, A. R., Schlumpf, M., King, S. B., III, and Douglas, J. S., Jr.: Clinical Observations on Coronary Spasm and Percutaneous Coronary Artery Angioplasty, *Am. J. Cardiol.*, 49:965, 1982. (Abstract.)

63 Bentivoglio, L. G., Wolf, M. N., Meister, S. G., and Leo, L. R.: Preliminary Experience with Percutaneous Transluminal Coronary Angioplasty in Patients with Coronary Spasm, in M. Kaltenbach et al. (eds.), "Fourth International Symposium on Coronary Heart Disease, Frankfurt, 1981," Springer-Verlag, Berlin, 1982, p. 347.

64 Kaltenbach, M.: Transluminal Coronary Angioplasty and Coronary Spasm, in M. Kaltenbach (ed.), "Fourth International Symposium on Coronary Heart Disease, Frankfurt, 1981," Springer-Verlag, Berlin, 1982, p. 361.

65 Knapp, W. S., Douglas, J. S., Jr., Craver, J. M., et al.: Efficacy of Coronary Artery Bypass Grafting in Elderly Patients with Coronary Artery Disease, *Am. J. Cardiol.*, 47:923, 1981.

66 Kirklin, J. W., Kouchoukos, N. T., Blackstone, E. H., and Oberman, A.: Research Related to Surgical Treatment of Coronary Artery Disease, *Circulation*, 60:1613, 1979.

67 Williams, B. D., Begg, T. B., Semple, T., and McGuinnes, J.B.: The Elderly in a Coronary Care Unit, *Br. Med. J.*, 2:451, 1976.

68 Noble, R. J., and Rothbaum, D. A.: Heart Disease in the Elderly (Geriatric Cardiology), in J. W. Hurst (ed.), "Update I:The Heart," McGraw-Hill Book Company, New York, 1979, p. 211.

69 Mock, M., Holmes, D., Jr., Vlietstra, R., et al.: Percutaneous Transluminal Coronary Angioplasty (PTCA) in Patients ≥60 Years of Age Registered in the NHLBI Registry, *Circulation*, 66:11, 1982. (Abstract.)

70 McCallister, B. D., Hartzler, G. O., Rutherford, R. D., and McConahay, D. R.: Palliative Percutaneous Transluminal Angioplasty for Unstable Angina in Patients over 70 Years of Age, *Circulation*, 64(suppl. 4):255, 1981. (Abstract.)

71 Loop, F. D., Sheldon, W. C., Lytle, B. W., Cosgrove, D. M., and Proudfit, W. L.: The Efficacy of Coronary Artery Surgery, *Am. Heart J.*, 101:86, 1981.

72 Proudfit, W. L., Shirey, E. K., and Sones, F. M., Jr.: Distribution of Arterial Lesions Demonstrated by Selective Cinecoronary Arteriography, *Circulation*, 36:54, 1967.

73 Levy, R. I., Mock, M. B., Willman, V. L., and Frommer, P. L.: Percutaneous Transluminal Coronary Angioplasty, *N. Engl. J. Med.*, 301:101, 1979. (Editorial.)

74 Takaro, T., Hultgren, H. N., Lipton, M. J., and Detre, K. M.: The VA Cooperative Randomized Study or Surgery for Coronary Arterial Occlusive Disease. II. Subgroup with Significant Left Main Lesions, *Circulation*, 53, 54(suppl. 3):107, 1976.

75 Nuesch, K., Scholer, Y., Pyle, R., and Gruentzig, A.: Percutaneous Transluminal Dilation of Proximal Stenosis of Left Anterior Descending Coronary Artery in Patients with Bronchogenic Carcinoma, *Br. Heart J.*, 46:345, 1981.

76 Gruentzig, A. R., and Collins, J. J. Jr.: Controversies in Cardiology: Proposed Angioplasty Should Be Utilized in Double-Vessel and Triple-Vessel Coronary Disease, *Hospital Prac.*, 17:143, 1982.

77 Kent, K. M., Bentivoglio, L. G., Block, P. C., et al.: NHLBI Percutaneous Transluminal Coronary Angio-

plasty (PTCA) Registry: Four Years' Experience, *Am. J. Cardiol.*, 49(suppl. 2):904, 1982. (Abstract.)

78 Dorros, G., Stertzer, S. H., Cowley, M., Kent, K., and Williams, D.: Complex Transluminal Coronary Angioplasty: Multivessel Disease and Multiple Dilatations, *Circulation*, 66(suppl. 2):329, 1982. (Abstract.)

79 Hartzler, G. O., Rutherford, B. D., McConahay, D. R., and McCallister, S. H.: Simultaneous Multiple Lesion Coronary Angioplasty—A Preferred Therapy for Patients with Multiple Vessel Disease, *Circulation*, 66(suppl. 2):5, 1982. (Abstract.)

80 Savage, R., Hollman, J., and Gruentzig, A. R.: Can Percutaneous Transluminal Coronary Angioplasty Be Performed in Patients with Total Occlusion?, *Circulation*, 66:330, 1982. (Abstract.)

81 Heyndrickx, G.R., Serruys, P. W., Brand, M., Vandormael, M., and Reiber, J. H. C.: Transluminal Angioplasty after Mechanical Recanalization in Patients with Chronic Occlusion of Coronary Artery, *Circulation*, 66(suppl. 2):5, 1982. (Abstract.)

82 Merx, W., Dorr, R., Rentrop, P., et al.: Evaluation of the Effectiveness of Intracoronary Streptokinase Infusion in Acute Myocardial Infarction: Postprocedure Management and Hospital Course in 204 Patients, *Am. Heart J.*, 102:1181, 1981.

83 Swan, H. J. C.: Thrombolysis in Acute Myocardial Infarction: Treatment of the Underlying Coronary Artery Disease, *Circulation*, 66:914, 1982. (Editorial.)

84 Meyer, J., Merx, W., Schmitz, H., et al.: Percutaneous Transluminal Coronary Angioplasty Immediately after Intracoronary Streptolysis of Transluminal Myocardial Infarction, *Circulation*, 66:905, 1982.

85 Hartzler, G. O., Rutherford, B. D., and McConahay, D. R.: Percutaneous Coronary Angioplasty with and without Prior Steptokinase Infusion for Treatment of Acute Myocardial Infarction, *Am. J. Cardiol.*, 49:1033, 1981. (Abstract.)

86 Gold, H. K., Leinbach, R. C., Palacios, I. F., et al.: Effect of Immediate Angioplasty on Coronary Patency following Infarct Therapy with Streptokinase, *Am. J. Cardiol.*, 43:1033, 1982. (Abstract.)

87 McConahay, D., Hartzler, G., and Rutherford, B.: Percutaneous Transluminal Coronary Angioplasty: Use in Management of Symptomatic Patients with Recent Myocardial Infarction, *Circulation*, 66(suppl. 2):329, 1982. (Abstract.)

88 Epstein, S. E., Palmeri, S. T., and Patterson, R. E.: Evaluation of Patients after Acute Myocardial Infarction. Indications for Cardiac Catheterization and Surgical Intervention, *N. Engl. J. Med.*, 307:1487, 1982.

89 Chaturvedi, N. C., Walsh, M. J., Evans, A., et al.: Selection of Patients for Early Discharge after Acute Myocardial Infarction, *Br. Heart J.*, 36:533, 1974.

90 Schuster, E. H., and Bulkley, B. H. Early Post-Infarction Angina: Ischemia at a Distance and Ischemia in the Infarct Zone, *N. Engl. J. Med.*, 305:1101, 1981.

91 Douglas, J. S., Gruentzig, A. R., King, S. B., III, and Hollman, J.: Long-term Results of Percutaneous Transluminal Angioplasty for Aorto-coronary Saphenous Vein Graft Stenosis, *Circulation*, 66(suppl. 2):124, 1982. (Abstract.)

92 Block, P. C., Palacios, I. F., Wholey, M. H., and O'Toole, J.: Percutaneous Transluminal Angioplasty of Stenotic Coronary Artery Bypass Grafts, *Circulation*, 64(suppl. 4):109, 1981.

93 Ford, W. B., Wholey, M. H., Zikria, E. A., et al.: Percutaneous Transluminal Angioplasty in the Management of Occlusive Disease involving the Coronary Arteries and Saphenous Vein Bypass Grafts. Preliminary Results, *J. Thorac. Cardiovasc. Surg.*, 79:1, 1980.

94 King, S. B., III, Gruentzig, A. R., Douglas, J. S., Jr., and Hollman, J.: Percutaneous Transluminal Coronary Angioplasty for Restenosis following Initial Successful Procedure, *Am. J. Cardiol.*, 49:904, 1982. (Abstract.)

95 Gruentzig, A. R.: Results from Coronary Angioplasty and Implications for the Future, *Am. Heart J.*, 103:779, 1982.

96 Mills, N. L., and Doyle, D.: Does Operative Transluminal Angioplasty (OTA) Extend the Limits of Coronary Bypass Procedure?, *Circulation*, 64(suppl. 4):266, 1981. (Abstract.)

97 Roberts, A. J., Feldman, R. L., Pepine, C. J., Knauf, D. G., and Alexander, J. A.: Intraoperative Transluminal Balloon-Catheter Dilatation under Hypothermic Cardioplegic Arrest during Coronary Intraoperative Artery Bypass Surgery, *Am. J. Cardiol.*, 49:957, 1982. (Abstract.)

98 Dorros, G., Bentivoglio, L. G., Block, P. C., et al.: Fatal Complication of Percutaneous Transluminal Coronary Angioplasty (PTCA), *Circulation*, 64:969, 1981. (Abstract.)

99 Turina, M., Gruntzig, A., Krayenbubl, C., and Senning, A.: The Role of the Surgeon in Percutaneous Transluminal Dilation of Coronary Stenosis, *Ann. Thorac. Surg.*, 28:103, 1978.

100 Murphy, D. A., Craver, J. M., Jones, E. L., Gruentzig, A. R., King, S. B., III, and Hatcher, C. R., Jr.: Surgical Revascularization following Unsuccessful Percutaneous Transluminal Coronary Angioplasty, *J. Thorac. Cardiovasc. Surg.*, 84:342, 1982.

101 Kent, K. M., Bentivoglio, L. G., and Block, P. C.: Percutaneous Transluminal Coronary Angioplasty: Report from the Registry of the National, Heart, Lung, and Blood Institute, *Am. J. Cardiol.*, 49:2011, 1982.

102 Cowley, M., Bentivoglio, L., Block, P., et al.: Emergency Coronary Artery Bypass Surgery for complications of Coronary Angioplasty: NHLBI PTCA Registry Experience, *Circulation*, 64(suppl. 4):193, 1981. (Abstract.)

103 Kutcher, M. A., Gruentzig, A. R., Turina, M., et al.: Can Emergency Coronary Bypass Surgery following Acute

Failure of Coronary Angioplasty Prevent Myocardial Infarction?, *Am. J. Cardiol.*, 49:956, 1982. (Abstract.)

104 Hollman, J., Gruentzig, A. R., King, S. B., III, and Douglas, J.: Acute Coronary Occlusion Immediately following Percutaneous Transluminal Coronary Angioplasty, *Circulation*, 66(suppl. 2):4, 1982. (Abstract.)

105 Schofer, J., Krebberer, H. J., Bleifeld, W., and Mathey, D. G.: Acute Occlusion Artery Occlusion during Percutaneous Transluminal Coronary Angioplasty: Reopening by Intracoronary Streptokinase before Emergency Coronary Artery Surgery to Prevent Myocardial Infarction, *Circulation*, 66:1325, 1982.

106 Sigwart, U., Essinger, A., Grbic, M., Gleichmann, U., and Saveghi, H.: Emergency Reopening of Right Coronary Occlusion after Angioplasty using Guide Wire and Thrombolysis, in M. Kaltenbach et al. (eds.), ''Fourth International Symposium on Coronary Heart Disease, 1981, Frankfurt,'' Springer-Verlag, Berlin, 1982, p. 151.

107 Peterson, M., Machaj, V., Watkins, W. D., et al.: Thromboxane Release during Percutaneous Transluminal Angioplasty, *Circulation*, 66(suppl. 2):4, 1982. (Abstract.)

108 Einzig, S., Cragg, A., Rao, G. H. R., et al.: Vasospasm and Angioplasty, *Circulation*, 66(suppl. 2):4, 1982. (Abstract.)

109 Cragg, A., Rysauy, J., Borgwardt, B., et al.: Aspirin Attenuation of Angioplasty-induced Vessel Wall Hyperemia, *Circulation*, 66(suppl. 2):5, 1982. (Abstract.)

110 Margolis, J. R.: The Role of the Percutaneous Intra-Aortic Balloon in Emergency Situations following Percutaneous Transluminal Coronary Angioplasty, in M. Kaltenbach et al. (eds.), ''Fourth International Symposium on Coronary Heart Disease, 1981, Frankfurt,'' Springer-Verlag, Berlin, 1982, p. 145.

111 Meier, B., Gruentzig, A. R., Hollman, J., and Bradford, J. M.: Does Length or Eccentricity of Coronary Stenosis Influence the Outcome of Transluminal Dilatation?, *Circulation*, in press.

112 Jutzy, K. R., Berte, L. E., Alderman, E. L., Ratts, J., and Simpson, J. B.: Coronary Restenosis Rates in Consecutive Patient Series One Year Post-Successful Angioplasty, *Circulation*, 66(suppl. 2):331, 1982. (Abstract.)

113 Holmes, D. R., Vlietstra, R. E., Smith, H. C., et al.: Restenosis following Percutaneous Transluminal Coronary Angioplasty (PTCA): A Report from the NHLBI PTCA Registry, *Am. J. Cardiol.*, 49:905, 1982. (Abstract.)

114 Engel, H. J., Kaltenbach, M., Rafflenbeul, et al.: Changes of Coronary Obstructions in the Months following Transluminal Coronary Angioplasty, in M. Kaltenbach et al. (eds.), ''Fourth International Symposium on Coronary Heart Disease, 1981, Frankfurt,'' Springer-Verlag, Berlin, 1982.

115 Hollman, J., Gruentzig, A., Meier, B., Bradford, J., and Galon, K.: Factors affecting Recurrence after Successful Coronary Angioplasty, *J.A.C.C.*, in press. (Abstract.)

116 Dangoisse, V., Val, P. V., and David, P. R.: Recurrence of Stenosis after Successful Percutaneous Transluminal Coronary Angioplasty (PTCA), *Circulation*, 66:331, 1981. (Abstract.)

117 Gertz, S. D., Uretsky, G., Wajnberg, R. S., Novot, N., and Gotsman, M. S.: Endothelial Cell Damage and Thrombus Formation after Partial Arterial Constriction: Relevance to the Role of Coronary Artery Spasm in the Pathogenesis of Myocardial Infarction, *Circulation*, 63:476, 1981.

118 Val, P. G., David, P. R., Lespaerance, J., et al.: Clinical and Angiographic Follow-up of Successful Percutaneous Transluminal Coronary Angioplasty (PTCA), *Circulation*, 66(suppl. 2):330, 1982. (Abstract.)

119 Schmitz, H. J., Meyer, J., Kiesslich, T., and Effert, S.: Greater Initial Dilatation Gives Better Late Angiographic Results in Percutaneous Coronary Angioplasty (PTCA), *Circulation*, 66:123, 1982. (Abstract.)

120 Mundth, E. D., and Austin, W. G.: Surgical Measures for Coronary Heart Disease, *N. Engl. J. Med.*, 293:13, 1975.

121 Scholl, J. M., David, P. R., Chaitman, B. R., et al.: Recurrence of Stenosis Following Percutaneous Transluminal Coronary Angioplasty, *Circulation*, 64(suppl. 4):193, 1981.

122 Thornton, M. A., Gruentzig, A. R., Hollman, J., King, S. B., III, and Douglas, J.: Coumadin Versus Aspirin in Prevention of Recurrence after Transluminal Coronary Angioplasty—A Randomized Study, *Circulation*, 66(suppl. 2):262, 1982. (Abstract.)

123 EPSIM Research Group: A Controlled Comparison of Aspirin and Oral Anticoagulants in Prevention of Death after Myocardial Infarction, *N. Engl. J. Med.*, 307:701, 1982.

124 Fuster, V., and Chesebro, J. H.: Antithrombotic Therapy: Role of Platelet-inhibitor Drugs. II. Pharmacologic Effects of Platelet-inhibitor Drugs, *Mayo Clin. Proc.*, 56:185, 1981.

125 Chesebro, J. H., Clements, I. P., Fuster, V., et al.: A Platelet-inhibitor-Drug Trial in Coronary Artery Bypass Operations, *N. Engl. J. Med.*, 307:73, 1982.

126 Brown, B. G., Cukingnam, R., Peterson, R. B., et al.: Perianastomotic Arteriosclerosis in Grafted Human Coronary Arteries. Prevention with Platelet-inhibiting Therapy, *Am. J. Cardiol.*, 49:968, 1982. (Abstract.)

127 Sharma, G. V. R. K., Khuri, S. F., Folland, E. D., Josa, M., and Parisi, A. F.: Lack of Benefit from Aspirin-Dipyridamole Therapy in Aorto-Coronary Vein Graft Patency, *Circulation*, 66(suppl. 2):94, 1982. (Abstract.)

128 Bulkley, B. H. and Hutchins, G. M.: Accelerated ''Atherosclerosis''—A Morphologic Study 97 Saphenous Vein Coronary Artery Bypass Grafts, *Circulation*, 55:163, 1977.

129 Spodick, D. H.: Percutaneous Transluminal Coronary Angioplasty, *N. Engl. J. Med.*, 301:1345, 1979. (Letter.)

130 Spodick, D. H.: PTCA, *Circulation,* 61:1061, 1980.

131 Spodick, D. H.: Percutaneous Transluminal Coronary Angioplasty. Opportunity Fleeting, *J.A.M.A.,* 242:1658, 1979. (Editorial.)

132 Spodick, D. H.: Percutaneous Transluminal Coronary Angioplasty *Mayo Clin. Proc.,* 56:526, 1981. (Letter.)

133 Ritchie, J. L., Narahara, K. A., Trobaugh, G. B., William, D. L., and Hamilton, G. N.: Thallium-201 Imaging before and after Coronary Revascularization. Assessment of Regional Myocardial Blood Flow and Graft Patency, *Circulation,* 56:830, 1977.

134 Greenberg, B. H., Hart, R., Botvinick, E. H., et al.: Thallium-201 Myocardial Perfusion Scintigraphy to Evaluate Patients after Coronary Bypass Surgery, *Am. J. Cardiol.,* 42:167, 1978.

135 Kent, K. M., Borer, J. S., Green, M. V., et al.: Effects of Coronary-Artery Bypass on Global and Regional Left Ventricular Function during Exercise, *N. Engl. J. Med.,* 298:1434, 1978.

136 Jones, E. L., Craver, J. M., King, S. B., III, et al.: Clinical, Anatomic and Functional Descriptors influencing Morbidity, Survival and Adequacy of Revascularization following Coronary Bypass, *Ann. Surg.,* 192:390, 1980.

137 Balcon, R., Brooks, N., Layton, C., and Richards, A.: Percutaneous Transluminal Coronary Angioplasty, *Br. Heart J.,* 47:189, 1982.

138 Sowton, E., and Reidy, J.: Complications and Results in Eight Patients undergoing Percutaneous Coronary Angioplasty for Very Severe Lesions, *Br. Heart J.,* 47:190, 1982.

PART IV

Rehabilitation of Patients with Atherosclerotic Coronary Heart Disease

Return to Work or Active Life-Style in Patients with Atherosclerotic Coronary Heart Disease: Rehabilitation of the Coronary Patient[*]

NANETTE K. WENGER, M.D.[†]

You work that you may keep pace with the earth and the
   soul of the earth
For to be idle is to become a stranger unto the seasons,
   and to step out of life's processional that marches in maj-
   esty and proud submission towards the infinite.
When you work you are a flute through whose heart the
   whispering of the hours turns to music.
Which of you would be a reed, dumb and silent, when all
   else sings together in unison?

KAHLIL GIBRAN[1]

MAGNITUDE OF THE PROBLEM

Despite the continuous substantial decline in atherosclerotic coronary heart disease deaths in the United
States in the last decade, almost 1½ million episodes
of myocardial infarction occur each year (Fig. 1). Survivors have a 4 to 5 percent incidence of recurrent
infarction or sudden death annually. About 200,000
persons develop new angina pectoris each year. Coronary disease remains the leading cause of morbidity,
as well as mortality; 20 percent of myocardial infarction survivors have varying degrees of physiological,
psychosocial, and vocational disability.[2]

The economic impact of coronary mortality, morbidity, and disability was over $39 billion in 1977. Of
the almost 500,000 people receiving Social Security
Administration disability allowances in 1975, 33 percent were permanently disabled by coronary heart disease. Atherosclerotic disease is the major cause of permanent disability for both men and women age 40 and
older.

In 1978 there were 18 million days of work lost due
to illness from coronary heart disease as estimated
from a Health Interview Survey (unpublished data);
there were 184 million restricted-activity days (Na-

tional Center for Health Statistics, Ambulatory Medical Care Survey, unpublished data for 1978).

Thus, cardiovascular disease, overwhelmingly due
to arteriosclerosis, ranks first as a cause of limitation
of activity and disabled worker benefits and fourth as
a cause of days lost from work. Of added concern is
that the long-term prognosis after a first myocardial
infarction has not changed from the 1960s to the 1970s,
suggesting that the decline in coronary mortality rate
was probably restricted to the acute phase of the illness.[3]

CURRENT CORONARY REHABILITATION PROGRAM CONCEPTS AND COMPONENTS

The concept that many patients with symptomatic atherosclerotic coronary heart disease can and should return to productive, active, and satisfying lives is the
basis of rehabilitation. During the past decade, the rehabilitative approach to the symptomatic coronary patient has been progressively incorporated into traditional medical care.[4] This approach applies equally to
patients with angina pectoris, myocardial infarction,
and coronary bypass surgery. The ultimate goal of rehabilitation is the patient's rapid return to a normal or
near-normal life-style and role in society. The particular concerns and emphases include the assessment of
the patient's functional status and the application of
measures designed to maintain and enhance function
in a variety of spheres—physiological, psychological,
social, educational, and vocational.[5]

Rehabilitation should begin at the onset of illness
and remain as a continuing feature in the long-term
care of the patient; it should include measures designed
to retard the progression of the disease. The patient's
primary physician thus has a pivotal role in initiating
and coordinating rehabilitative efforts. At each phase
of the illness, the primary physician must formulate a
plan to manage and assess the patient's problems, modifying this plan according to the response to therapy.
The plan of care must include the evaluation of function

*From the Department of Medicine, Division of Cardiology, Emory
University School of Medicine, Atlanta, Georgia.

†With appreciation to Jeanette Zahler for help in preparation of the
manuscript.

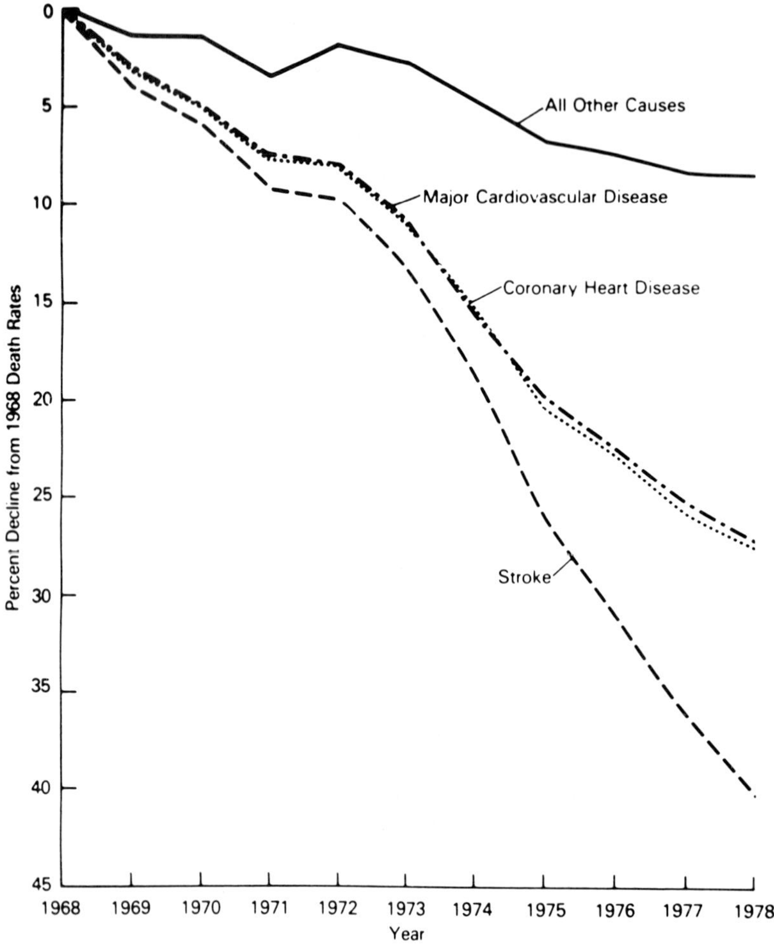

FIGURE 1 Trends in cardiovascular disease and all other causes of mortality: decline by age-adjusted death rates, ages 35–74, 1968–1978, United States. (*From Report of the Working Group on Arteriosclerosis of the National Heart, Lung, and Blood Institute: Summary, Conclusions, and Recommendations, "Arteriosclerosis 1981," vol.1, 1981, p. 2. Used with permission.*)

(such as the severity of the disease, complications, emotional response to illness, etc.), the monitoring of desired and adverse effects of therapeutic maneuvers, and periodic reassessment of function in the several spheres as it is changed by therapy. Ideally, the resources to effect rehabilitation should be available in the local community—in the community hospital, the office of the primary physician, or in public, governmental, and private community agencies and facilities. Although for selected patients with complex diagnostic problems and significant residual cardiac impairment or major psychological, social, or vocational problems referral for consultant assessment and management is necessary, all aspects of the long-term care and rehabilitation of the coronary patient remain the responsibility of the primary physician, ultimately using the personnel, facilities, and services in the local community.[6]

There are two important areas in rehabilitative programming for coronary patients.[7–13] The first involves activity: early ambulation during the hospitalization, and prescriptive exercise training after discharge from the hospital. This incorporates functional evaluation; and reevaluation as function is changed by interventions.

A second component is education of the patient and family; this often begins during the acute hospital stay and continues in the office of the primary physician or in a hospital or community clinic or other community facility. Included is the provision of a variety of counseling services as warranted—psychosocial, educational, vocational—designed to expedite the return of the patient to a satisfying role in the community.

EARLY AMBULATION AFTER MYOCARDIAL INFARCTION AND CORONARY BYPASS SURGERY[6,12]
The Physiological Basis

The deleterious effects of prolonged immobilization at bed rest constitute the physiological basis for recommending early ambulation for most patients after myocardial infarction[14] and coronary bypass surgery.[15]

Important detrimental effects of prolonged bed rest include the following:

1 A 20 to 25 percent decrease in physical work capacity, due to a comparable decrement of cardiac stroke volume. This results from as little as 3 weeks of immobilization. The higher the initial level of fitness, the longer the retraining needed to restore the pre-bed rest status.[14]

2 Orthostatic hypotension and reflex tachycardia when the patient is first mobilized after protracted bed rest. These are manifestations of hypovolemia, as the circulating blood volume may decrease by 700 to 800 mL within a week to 10 days at bed rest.

3 Predisposition to thromboembolism. The hypovolemia is characterized by increased blood viscosity, because plasma volume contracts more than red blood cell mass; circulatory stasis, due to limited use of the leg muscle pump at bed rest, adds to the thromboembolic risk.

4 A modest decrease in pulmonary ventilation (lung volume and vital capacity).

5 A negative nitrogen and protein balance.

6 A decrease in systemic muscle mass and muscular contractile strength. Inefficiently contracting muscle requires more oxygen than trained muscle for comparable work, with this increased demand imposed on an impaired oxygen transport system and potentially ischemic myocardium in the patient with myocardial infarction.

Patient Selection

Early ambulation is appropriate for the patient whose myocardial infarction is characterized by an uncomplicated clinical course. These are patients without significant disturbances of cardiac rhythm, congestive heart failure, persistent or recurrent chest pain, or hypotension or clinical shock. They make up about half of all individuals with infarction admitted to coronary care units,[16,17] and tend to be younger individuals and those with initial infarction; these are also typically patients with the greatest rehabilitation potential. Patients without complications can begin low-level physical activity as early as the first days after infarction. Most patients with an uncomplicated course in the initial days of infarction have little or no inhospital mortality and few significant late complications.[18,19]

Patients whose hospital course is characterized by complications of infarction, dysrhythmia, congestive heart failure, persistent or recurrent chest pain, or clinical shock, require specific measures to control these problems while at bed rest. Gradually progressive ambulation can be begun once stabilization of these problems has been achieved.[20]

Program Components: Coronary Care Unit

The general guidelines for coronary care unit activities are that they be of low-level intensity, 1 to 2 mets (1 met = approximately 3.5 mL O_2 per kilogram of body weight per minute); be gradually progressive in work demand; and be supervised by an individual capable of assessing the patient's response to activity. Self-care activities meet these specifications; patients are permitted to feed themselves, bathe and perform other personal care, use a bedside commode, and sit in bed or in a bedside chair. Activity as low-level as sitting in a chair two or three times a day seems sufficient to limit the hypovolemia resulting from prolonged immobilization and the resultant orthostatic hypotension; it appears that exposure to gravitational stress, rather than the intensity of the activity, may prevent the deterioration of exercise tolerance resulting from protracted bed rest.[21] Selected arm and leg exercises maintain muscle tone and joint mobility, an important aspect for elderly patients.

Guidelines for Activity Surveillance

The electrocardiographic monitor facilitates surveillance of the response to early ambulation in the coronary care unit. Disproportionate responses to low-level activity include the development of chest pain, dyspnea, or palpitations; a heart rate less than 50 beats per minute or greater than 120 beats per minute;* the appearance of dysrhythmias; increased ST-segment displacement suggestive of ischemia on the electrocardiogram or monitor; and a fall of greater than 10 to 15 mmHg in systolic pressure. Systolic pressure normally increases slightly with physical activity; in this clinical setting, a decrease in systolic blood pressure can be equated with inadequacy of the cardiac output to meet the activity demand. An increase in excess of 180 mmHg in systolic blood pressure suggests the need for antihypertensive therapy.

An appropriate response to activity indicates that the patient may be gradually progressed to an activity

---

*An increase in heart rate greater than 20 beats per minute above resting level is an inappropriate response in patients receiving beta-adrenergic blocking drugs.

of greater intensity. An inappropriate response at any stage of activity requires reduction of the level of activity and clinical reassessment of the patient to determine the need for diagnostic and therapeutic interventions.

Program Components: Remainder of the Hospitalization

After transfer out of the coronary care unit, rehabilitative physical activity is designed to enable the patient to attain a functional level permitting the performance of usual personal care and homebound activities at the time of discharge from the hospital. This is currently at 7 to 14 days for patients with an uncomplicated clinical course if the home situation is appropriate. There must be gradual progression from bed rest to the work intensity required to perform household tasks, an energy expenditure of 2 to 3 mets, i.e., two to three times the resting metabolic rate. Additionally, predischarge exercise testing is inappropriate for a patient who has remained at bed rest throughout the hospitalization; progressive ambulation permits an appropriate assessment of exercise capacity to be derived from testing.

Patients continue to perform personal care; sit in a chair for increasing periods of time; and, with supervision, perform selected dynamic exercises involving the arms, legs, and trunk, activities characterized by the rhythmic, repetitive movements of large muscle groups. Subsequent to these "warm-up" exercises, which maintain muscle tone and joint mobility, the major prescriptive component of inhospital activity is walking, with progressive increases in the pace and the distance of walking. More impaired patients are taught energy-conserving techniques for the performance of activities of daily living. Patients who must climb steps at home should practice this before discharge from the hospital, walking down a flight of stairs and returning by elevator, and walking slowly up a flight of steps on the subsequent day. This minimizes the anxiety of the patient and family often associated with initial stair climbing at home.

Inhospital early ambulation physical activities emphasize dynamic (isotonic) activities, with limitation or avoidance of isometric exercise.[22] The latter does not elicit, as does dynamic exercise, a heart rate response proportional to the intensity of the activity. Isometric exercise is associated with little heart rate change, but may evoke a sudden, significant increase in blood pressure, which appears related to the percent of maximum voluntary contraction of the involved muscle group. Isometric activities characterized by less than 20 percent of the maximum voluntary contraction elicit only a minimal blood pressure response, whereas activities involving greater than 20 percent of the maximum voluntary contraction of the muscle group may exert a profound hypertensive effect. This abrupt increase in afterload may be poorly tolerated by a potentially ischemic myocardium and may precipitate chest pain, cardiac dysrhythmias, or both.

The response to physical activity is gauged by criteria comparable to those used in the coronary care unit. Electrocardiographic monitoring during physical activity is required only for selected patients, particularly those with prior serious ventricular ectopy or prior evidence of asymptomatic myocardial ischemia; for these patients, telemetry may be of value.

Ideally, the prescribed daily exercises are associated with a comparable intensity of hospital activities, as well as recreational and educational activities. A wide variety of early ambulation protocols, defining steps or stages in activity progression for the patient, are used in many community hospitals, medical centers, and university complexes. No specific format has major advantage or disadvantage, but there are advantages to a predefined activity format. It is unrealistic to expect a busy clinician to write detailed daily physical activity orders for each patient. Even if feasible, physician-to-physician variations in activity preference would render far less efficient the implementation of early ambulation for a large number of patients by the hospital staff. Also, delineation of hospital activities comparable in intensity to the prescribed exercises facilitates the responses of personnel to questions of permitted and restricted activities; it has the added advantage of ensuring that consistent information about activity is given to the patient and of permitting the hospital staff to describe the predicted progression of activity.

As an example, the early ambulation protocol (with modifications) used at Grady Memorial Hospital under the supervision of the Emory University School of Medicine in Atlanta, Georgia since the early 1960s delineates prescribed exercises, hospital "daily living" activities, and recreational and educational activities of parallel intensity for each of a series of steps. The protocol, incorporated in the patient record, allows the physician to indicate daily approval for progression of the patient from one activity level to the next. The nurse or therapist supervising the physical activity documents each day the patient's clinical response to the level of activity—heart rate, blood pressure, and symptoms if appropriate. The early ambulation protocol format, in addition to structuring and documenting care, facilitates communication among the health professionals caring for the patient. The current revision has seven steps; the initial two steps are designated as coronary care unit activities; the subsequent five, performed on a general medical care area, reflect a simple approach for warm-up exercises and emphasize progressive increases in the pace and distance of walking (Table 1).

TABLE 1

In-patient rehabilitation: Seven-step myocardial infarction program (revised 1980): Grady Memorial Hospital and the Emory University School of Medicine

Step	Date	M.D. initials	Nurse/PT notes	Supervised exercise	CCU/Ward activity	Educational-recreational activity
				CCU		
1	———			Active and passive ROM all extremities, in bed Teach patient ankle plantar and dorsiflexion—repeat hourly when awake	Partial self-care Feed self Dangle legs on side of bed Use bedside commode Sit in chair 15 min 1–2 times/day	Orientation to CCU Personal emergencies, social service aid as needed
2	———			Active ROM all extremities, sitting on side of bed	Sit in chair 15–30 min 2–3 times/day Complete self-care in bed	Orientation to rehabilitation team, program Smoking cessation Educational literature if requested Planning transfer from CCU
				Ward		

3	———			Warm-up exercises, 2 mets:
				  Stretching
				  Calisthenics
				Walk 50 ft and back at slow pace
					Sit in chair ad lib
					To ward class in wheelchair
					Walk in room
						Normal cardiac anatomy and function
						Development of atherosclerosis
						What happens with myocardial infarction
						1–2 mets craft activity

4	———			ROM and calisthenics, 2.5 mets Walk length of hall (75 ft) and back, average pace Teach pulse counting	OOB as tolerated Walk to bathroom Walk to ward class, with supervision	Coronary risk factors and their control
5	———			ROM and calisthenics, 3 mets Check pulse counting Practice walking few stairsteps Walk 300 ft bid	Walk to waiting room or telephone Walk in ward corridor prn	Diet Energy conservation Work simplification techniques (as needed) 2–3 mets craft activity

6	———			Continue above activities
				Walk down flight of steps (return by elevator)
				Walk 500 ft bid
				Instruct on home exercise
					Tepid shower or tub bath, with supervision
					To OT, cardiac clinic teaching room, with supervision
						Heart attack management:
						  Medications
						  Exercise
						  Surgery
						  Response to symptoms
						  Family, community adjustments on return home
						  Craft activity prn

7	———			Continue above activities
				Walk up flight of steps
				Walk 500 ft bid
				Continue home exercise instruction: present information regarding outpatient exercise program
					Continue all previous ward activities	Discharge planning:
						  Medications, diet, activity
						  Return appointments
						  Scheduled tests
						  Return to work
						  Community resources
						  Educational literature
						  Medication cards
						  Craft activity prn

Source: N. K. Wenger: Rehabilitation of the Patient with Symptomatic Atherosclerotic Coronary Heart Disease, in J. W. Hurst (ed.), "The Heart," 5th ed., McGraw-Hill Book Company, New York, 1982, p. 1151. Used with permission.

Safety and Benefits of Early Ambulation

In recent years, in addition to the general acceptability and adoption of early ambulation, there has been unequivocal documentation of its safety for appropriately selected patients.[23–35] Correctly designed and supervised early ambulation has not increased the complications of myocardial infarction: angina, reinfarction, dysrhythmias, congestive heart failure, ventricular aneurysm, cardiac rupture, or sudden cardiac death. Indeed, some studies suggest a more favorable outcome for patients so managed.

The reported benefits of early ambulation include prevention of the deconditioning responses previously described, a decrease in pulmonary atelectasis and thromboembolic complications,[36] and a decrease in anxiety and depression. Emotional complications are common with myocardial infarction, with anxiety reflecting the immediate threat of death, and depression the response to anticipated invalidism and future restrictions of life-style. The reassurance offered by performing progressive physical activity improves the patient's self-confidence and self-image. Additionally, most mood-altering drugs are inadvisable for patients with recent infarction because of their adverse effects on heart rate, blood pressure, and cardiac rhythm; early ambulation therefore assumes greater importance in helping to limit psychological complications.

Early ambulation enables the current shorter hospital stay, with its accompanying saving in medical care costs and the potential improved use of hospital beds.[37] It permits the appropriate performance of predischarge exercise testing. The functional status of the patient is improved at the time of discharge from the hospital, and this has been associated with an earlier and more complete subsequent return to work.[38–40]

EXERCISE TESTING IN REHABILITATION OF THE CORONARY PATIENT

Exercise testing has varied roles in rehabilitation of patients with symptomatic coronary disease.

Predischarge Low-Level Exercise Testing[12]

In recent years formal, low-intensity exercise testing has had increasing application prior to discharge from the hospital after myocardial infarction.[41,42] This is generally performed at 7 days to 3 weeks following infarction. The level of testing typically approximates the physical activity permitted during the last days of hospitalization, i.e., exercise at a work load of 3 to 3.5 mets, or that evoking a heart rate response below 120 to 130 beats per minute.[42] However, in some centers, selected patients are tested to a sign- or symptom-limited end point.[43,44] Predischarge testing requires prior progressive ambulation so that the patient's functional capacity can be reliably ascertained. With appropriate patient selection in experienced exercise testing laboratories, predischarge exercise testing has not been associated with appreciable complications.

This approach offers several potential benefits.[45–48] It may allow more precise definition of safely tolerated activity levels, permitting relatively unimpaired patients to more rapidly resume normal activity. It may permit identification of activity-precipitated, treatable mechanisms of impairment, identifying the incapacitated patient who requires a more prolonged hospitalization, who may need additional diagnostic and therapeutic intervention, or who requires more gradual increases in activity during convalescence. Adverse responses to low-level exercise testing—the precipitation of chest pain and/or ischemic ST-T changes on the exercise electrocardiogram, the appearance of exercise-induced dysrhythmias, and/or the appearance of exercise-induced left ventricular dysfunction (typically evidenced either symptomatically, by hypotension, or by the appearance of a third heart sound or a mitral regurgitant murmur)—may identify the patient requiring additional or more prompt medical or surgical therapy. Poor exercise capacity, often due to left ventricular dysfunction, is commonly associated with the development of angina pectoris and with ST-segment changes and ventricular dysrhythmias on the exercise electrocardiogram.

Finally, the actual performance of a low-level exercise test often decreases the fear, common in patients after myocardial infarction, that physical activity may result in recurrent infarction or sudden death; it thus may exert a positive psychological impact.

Recent data suggest that early exercise testing may be prognostic,[46–53] i.e., that low exercise capacity with electrocardiographic or symptomatic evidence of myocardial ischemia at low levels of exercise may identify the patient with severe and typically multivessel coronary artery obstruction, the patient at high risk who might benefit from earlier medical or surgical intervention. It remains to be defined whether this correlation is better than that offered by traditional exercise testing and whether, indeed, the identification of this feature at the time of hospital discharge is advantageous when compared with the experience with abnormalities identified at the traditional 4- to 8-week sign- or symptom-limited exercise test.

Some physicians, including myself and many of my colleagues at Emory, prefer to have a coronary arteriogram performed on selected patients after myocardial infarction rather than an early exercise test. Some physicians recommend the coronary arteriogram before the patient goes home from the hospital, and others recommend that it be performed a few weeks after infarction. They believe it gives a clearer view of prognosis and the need for bypass surgery than does the exercise test. More follow-up is currently needed to be certain that exercise testing will give answers that duplicate the apparent good results of the present approach using coronary arteriography. This is not the place to debate the issue, but it appears certain that either an exercise test or a coronary arteriogram is indicated in most patients who have recovered from a myocardial infarction.

Traditional Exercise Testing after Recovery from Myocardial Infarction or with Stable Angina Pectoris

Exercise testing for the patient after myocardial infarction is commonly performed at 4 to 8 weeks following the acute event.[54] The performance of a sign- or symptom-limited exercise test in the patient with angina pectoris also has specific guidelines; testing poses no little concern when the anginal pattern is stable, but appears contraindicated in the patient with unstable angina.

Various methods and protocols for exercise testing may be employed, but the test is typically done using a bicycle ergometer or motor-driven treadmill. Leg muscle fatigue may limit performance if patients are unfamiliar with bicycle riding; walking on a treadmill may be a better index of functional capacity. The patient is customarily tested to the limit of tolerance, except that a coronary patient should not exceed the maximum predicted heart rate for age. Exercise testing has documented safety when appropriate guidelines are followed;[55-57] McHenry defines the recent morbidity and mortality rates of exercise testing as 1.8 myocardial infarctions per 10,000 tests and 0.25 cardiac deaths per 10,000 tests.[56] A true "maximal" test is characterized by failure to increase the oxygen consumption with an increase in work load; in practice, the oxygen consumption is rarely measured but the limit of activity tolerance is used. Typically, rather than the test being "maximal," it tends to be a symptom- or sign-limited procedure, i.e., the patient stops because of chest pain, dyspnea, fatigue, claudication, etc., or the physician terminates the test because of an inappropriate response of the heart rate, blood pressure, or electrocardiogram—arrhythmia, conduction abnormality, repolarization abnormality, etc. (Table 2).

TABLE 2
Abnormal responses to exercise

1 Symptoms
Angina pectoris
Inappropriate dyspnea (? L.V. failure)
Fatigue, dizziness, lightheadedness, confusion
Leg pain

2 Signs
Cyanosis, pallor, mottling
Cold sweat, piloerection
Ataxia, glassy stare
Gallop heart sounds
Murmur of valve regurgitation
Abnormal cardiac impulse

3 Heart Rate
Excessive tachycardia
Bradycardia } Chronotropic
Failure to increase } incompetence

4 Blood Pressure
Failure to increase } Inotropic
Progressive decrease } incompetence

5 ECG
ST-segment elevation or depression < Time of onset / Configuration

Arrhythmia—Frequent or multiform PVC
—Ventricular tachycardia
—Atrial tachyarrhythmias
—AV block > first degree

Source: N. K. Wenger: Rehabilitation of the Patient with Symptomatic Coronary Atherosclerotic Heart Disease, Part I, in H. D. McIntosh (ed.), "Cardiology Series," Continuing Education, Baylor College of Medicine, Houston, 1980, p. 18. Used with permission.

Formal exercise testing[58] serves as an extension of the clinical examination at rest, enabling detection of activity-induced chest pain, dysrhythmia, claudication, etc.; and documenting the functional impact of coronary disease. The objective assessment of function may be important in determining prognosis and thus aids in therapeutic decisions; it provides a guideline for assessing the ability of the patient to return to work, for recommendations regarding subsequent exercise training, and for advising occupational and recreational activity levels. Additionally, the performance on an exercise test often affords reassurance of satisfactory functional capability to both the patient and family.

Exercise test data are used to determine the intensity of recommended exercise in writing an individualized exercise prescription in "Individual Prescriptive Exercise in Rehabilitation." Patients should be tested for exercise prescription on their optimal medication regimen, the drugs on which they are to be trained.[59,60] This includes beta-adrenergic blocking agents, digitalis, diuretic drugs, antihypertensive agents, calcium-blocking drugs, etc., and helps ensure that the exercise prescription is appropriate. Major change in medications warrants repeated exercise testing for revision of the exercise prescription, as the changed regimen often reflects an alteration of cardiac status as well.

Each stage of exercise testing is characterized by a defined work load, described in terms of oxygen consumption or mets. This value can be translated into recommendations for occupational and recreational activity. However, most occupational work is intermittent, with brief periods of more strenuous activity and longer low-level interval activity. Since cardiac output, blood pressure response, and oxygen uptake do not approach the steady state until about 2 min after the onset of work, occupational myocardial work demand tends to be lower than for the same level of steady-state exercise. This explains why individuals with modest cardiac impairment can tolerate significant work loads of short duration when adequate rest periods are interspersed. For example, the NYHA class II cardiac patient who can sustain up to 2.5 cal/min of continuous effort can perform intermittent work up to 4 cal/min; comparable values for the class III cardiac patient are 2 and 2.7 cal/min, respectively.[61] When using the results of exercise testing to recommend full-time work, a level of about 30 percent of the physical work capacity is appropriate.[62] Many physicians find tabular or graphic presentations helpful in defining comparable intensity levels of daily living activities, occupational activities, and recreational activities in making recommendations for their patients (Table 3).[63] Once one of these categories has been successfully completed, based on prior exercise test assessment ensuring that this level is appropriate, activities of comparable level in other spheres can also be safely undertaken.

Serial Exercise Testing

Exercise testing after coronary bypass surgery can be used to assess the improvement in physical work capacity; comparable data can determine whether medical therapy has proved effective.

Coronary patients in an exercise program should have serial exercise testing to ascertain whether a training effect has been achieved, i.e., that they can perform more work before the onset of signs or symptoms of myocardial ischemia. This may be done with a "formal" treadmill or bicycle testing protocol or a test monitored by a telemetry lead(s) may be performed in the exercise gymnasium. Alternatively, observation of a patient's symptomatic and heart rate response (with telemetric or directly recorded electrocardiographic

assessment) to a given level of exercise may guide presciption of the next level of activity in a setting where more formal exercise testing is not readily available. This permits revision of the exercise prescription to increase the target heart rate and incorporate training activities of greater intensity. If a training effect is not evident with good adherence to an exercise regimen, careful reevaluation of the patient should be made to assess the need for additional diagnostic and subsequent medical and/or surgical therapy.

Long-term serial exercise testing can define progression of exercise intolerance, which often antedates symptomatic coronary disease. This may identify the need for diagnostic procedures or therapy. Improvement in function and maintenance of that improvement, documented by serial exercise testing, provides motivation for adherence to an exercise regimen.

EXERCISE TRAINING: CARDIAC CONDITIONING PHYSICAL ACTIVITIES AFTER MYOCARDIAL INFARCTION[12,57,64]

Convalescent Physical Activity

To "convalesce" means to grow stronger. During convalescence at home, the initial goal of physical activity is to increase endurance to a level which enables a prompt return to work and/or to usual preinfarction activities. Over 85 percent of individuals with an uncomplicated myocardial infarction employed at the time of infarction currently return to work within 2 to 3 months, typically resuming their former jobs.[16,54,65]

During the first days at home, patients continue the activity level of the last days in the hospital. The amount of rest should also be specified. They perform usual household activities; do predominantly dynamic warm-up exercises; and gradually increase the distance and pace of walking. Patients with limited activity during the hospitalization not uncommonly initially complain of lack of energy on return home; this reflects their perception that increased exertion is necessary to perform a given task, because it entails a greater proportion of their physical work capacity. With continued exercise, their stamina and endurance increase. The "spontaneous" functional improvement[66] described during convalescence may reflect changed community attitudes toward activity for the patient after infarction, enabling nonstructured "training."

Teaching of work simplification techniques may be indicated for more impaired patients. Resumption of sexual activity with the usual partner is recommended when other components of preillness daily life-style are reinstituted. The cardiac work of sexual activity is

TABLE 3
Approximate energy requirements of selected activities

Category	Self-care or home	Occupational	Recreational	Physical conditioning
Very light 3 mets 10 mL/(kg)(min) 4 kcal	Washing, shaving, dressing Desk work, writing Washing dishes Driving auto	Sitting (clerical assembling) Standing (store clerk, bartender) Driving truck* Crane operator*	Shuffleboard Horseshoes Bait casting Billiards Archery* Golf (cart)	Walking (level 2 mph) Stationary bicycle (very low resistance) Very light calisthenics
Light 3–5 mets 11–18 mL/(kg)(min) 4–6 kcal	Cleaning windows Raking leaves Weeding Power lawn mowing Waxing floors (slowly) Painting Carrying objects (15–30 lb)	Stocking shelves (light objects)† Light welding Light carpentry† Machine assembly Auto repair Paper hanging	Dancing (social and square) Golf (walking) Sailing Horseback riding Volleyball (6 man) Tennis (doubles)	Walking (3–4 mph) Level bicycling (6–8 mph) Light calisthenics
Moderate 5–7 mets 18–24 mL/(kg)(min) 6–8 kcal	Easy digging in garden Level hand lawn mowing Climbing stairs (slowly) Carrying objects (30–60 lb)†	Carpentry (exterior home building)† Shoveling dirt† Pneumatic tools†	Badminton (competitive) Tennis (singles) Snow skiing (downhill) Light backpacking Basketball Football Skating (ice and roller) Horseback riding (gallop)	Walking (4.5–5 mph) Bicycling (9–10 mph) Swimming (breast stroke)
Heavy 7–9 mets 25–32 mL/(kg)(min) 8–10 kcal	Sawing wood† Heavy shoveling† Climbing stairs (moderate speed) Carrying objects (60–90 lb)†	Tending furnace† Digging ditches† Pick and shovel†	Canoeing† Mountain climbing† Fencing Paddleball Touch football	Jogging (5 mph) Swimming (crawl stroke) Rowing machine Heavy calisthenics Bicycling (12 mph)
Very heavy >9 mets >32 mL/(kg)(min) >10 kcal	Carrying loads upstairs† Carrying objects (>90 lb)† Climbing stairs (quickly) Shoveling heavy snow† Shoveling 10/min (16 lb)	Lumber jack† Heavy laborer†	Handball Squash Ski touring over hills† Vigorous basketball	Running (≥6 mph) Bicycling (≥13 mph or up steep hill) Rope jumping

*May cause added psychological stress that will increase work load on the heart.

†May produce disproportionate myocardial demands because of use of arms or isometric exercise.

Source: W. L. Haskell: Design and Implementation of Cardiac Conditioning Programs, in N. K. Wenger and H. K. Hellerstein (eds.), "Rehabilitation of the Coronary Patient," John Wiley & Sons, New York, 1978, p. 214. Used with permission.

comparable to the energy expenditure of a brisk walk or of climbing a flight of stairs (peak heart rate of 90 to 145 beats per minute); these data are the basis for recommending resumption of sexual activity.

Walking is a major activity during convalescence. Because patients are taught during the hospitalization to monitor their pulse rate response to exercise, they can ascertain whether walking elicits an appropriate response, in general a heart rate below 120 beats per minute. Alternate recommendations, particularly appropriate for patients taking beta-adrenergic blocking drugs, are that the heart rate increase not exceed 20 beats above resting level. Exercise testing prior to discharge from the hospital can more precisely guide early activity, at times permitting an increased activity level. Although considerable initial emphasis is placed on pulse-monitoring of exercise intensity, patients should be told that this is a temporary feature to teach them the level of exertion required to attain a target heart rate response. Eventually, the rate of perceived exertion, as described by Borg,[67] rather than pulse counting, should guide not only specific exercising, but also the range of activities throughout the day; they should be able to identify an excessive work load, e.g., running to catch a train with a heavy suitcase in hand.

Patients initially walk in and around the home, walking outdoors when they can avoid extremes of temperature and humidity.[68-70] In larger communities, enclosed shopping malls offer temperature- and humidity-controlled sites for walking. Exercise reenforces the promise that the patient can return to a more active life-style. Specific activity recommendations during convalescence help structure the patient's day, which lacks form as compared with the highly routinized hospital stay or preillness occupation. Boredom during convalescence is a major problem among blue-collar workers,[71] who become frustrated with the inactivity imposed by lack of proper advice.

Additional recommendations for convalescence include progressive resocialization and reintegration into community life. Visitors are encouraged (for brief periods of time), and household tasks and low-energy-level hobby activities are identified as appropriate. Social recreational activities are encouraged; patients take car rides, attend church, do simple errands, then resume driving, etc.

Ideally, patients enter a supervised (often hospital-based) progressive activity program within the first month after infarction or coronary bypass surgery. Predischarge exercise testing can be used for the initial exercise prescription; alternatively, the symptomatic, heart rate, and electrocardiographic response to exercise can guide the level of activity. In addition to the safety of using supervised and intermittently monitored exercise to detect potentially dangerous abnormal responses in the early period after infarction, the group setting provides emotional support and facilitates education and counseling.

Patients with a reduced exercise capacity may require more gradual and preferably supervised physical rehabilitation; ventricular ectopy, the development of angina pectoris with low-level exercise, and marked ST-segment depression or exercise-induced hypotension at low levels of activity also identify that when exercise therapy is indicated (as for high-risk patients who are not candidates for coronary bypass surgery), a hospital-based, ECG-monitored cardiac exercise program should be recommended for these patients at increased risk.

The patient's response to early, modest-level convalescent physical activity may help guide the physician's recommendations about return to work, particularly when formal exercise testing is not available. For example, walking at a speed of 3 to 3½ mi/h entails a work intensity of 4 to 5 mets; reassurance can be given to patients who can walk without difficulty at this pace that they can perform most sedentary desk or bench jobs, which entail a 3- or 4-met level.

Patients returning to employment at higher work levels may require more intensive or prolonged exercise training prior to returning to work.

Individualized Prescriptive Exercise in Rehabilitation[72-76]

The prescriptive components of exercise include its "dosage"—the frequency, duration, and intensity of exercise—and the specific type of exercise to be undertaken.[77]

Once the patient has recovered from myocardial infarction or bypass surgery and has often reached a level of endurance sufficient to return to work (commonly within 4 to 8 weeks), more intensive exercise training can be undertaken to enhance cardiovascular function. Conventional exercise testing is necessary to accurately and safely prescribe this exercise. Age-predicted target heart rates cannot be used to prescribe exercise for patients with symptomatic coronary disease; the disease may attenuate the heart rate response to exercise, as may therapy with beta-adrenergic blocking drugs.

The minimum "dosage" of exercise recommended to achieve a training effect requires that the patient exercise at least two or three times weekly, preferably on nonsuccessive days. More than four exercise sessions weekly do not appear to additionally increase maximal oxygen uptake; conversely, unfit individuals or sedentary elderly patients may improve their physical work capacity with as few as one or two exercise sessions each week, although a further increase in $m\dot{V}O_2$ can be attained with more frequent training. Exercise sessions should be 30 to 45 min in duration, including warm-up and cool-down periods; this time is adequate to stimulate aerobic metabolism at the exercise intensity recommended below. During exercise sessions, the intensity (the component requiring prior exercise testing) recommendation is that patients attain a heart rate between 70 and 85 percent of the highest level safely achieved at exercise testing. In general, the 70- to 75-percent target heart rate range is recommended for patients who exercise individually in an unsupervised setting or at home, and the 80- to 85-percent range for supervised group exercise. The 70- to 85-percent heart rate range corresponds to 60 to 78 percent of the peak oxygen uptake, an effective yet safe range within which to stimulate aerobic metabolism and achieve the "training effect."[78] At no time should a coronary patient exercise to a level higher than that documented to maintain an appropriate cardiovascular response during testing. Although an increased duration and/or frequency of exercise can compensate for decreased exercise intensity, this engenders excessive orthopedic complications and poorer adherence to exercise.[79] In the National Exercise and Heart Disease Project, even low-level training (under 70 percent of the heart rate) of patients recovered from myocardial infarction decreased the heart rate and blood pressure response to exercise, particularly in unfit individuals.[80]

Dynamic (isotonic or aerobic) exercise is prescribed, i.e., activities involving the rhythmic repetitive movements of large muscle groups. Recommended activities include walking, running, swimming, bicycling, selected calisthenics, rope-jumping, rowing, skating, aerobic dancing, etc. Although in many structured exercise programs, aerobic games add variety and interest to an exercise session and thus improve adherence, competition and excitement should be limited early in the course of training because they unpredictably increase the heart rate response. Variations in skill also significantly vary the oxygen cost of these activities.

Design of an Exercise Training Program for Patients with Symptomatic Coronary Disease[81]

An individualized exercise prescription varies considerably with the needs and goals of each patient, general health status, age, the initial level of fitness, the level of physical performance, the planned occupational and recreational activities, and the patient's motivation, skills, likes, and dislikes. Accessibility of facilities and equipment must also be considered.

Ideally, patients should initially be encouraged to participate in medically supervised exercise. In addition to enabling proper exercise guidance, medical supervision often increases motivation and reassurance and enables appropriate care for cardiovascular emergencies.[82] Later, as exercise performance and fitness improve, medical supervision can be decreased. The signing of an informed consent document prior to exercise, in addition to its medicolegal implications, affords the physician an additional opportunity to review with the patient the purposes, design, safety features, and potential problems (as well as ways to help avert them) of rehabilitative physical activity. Exercise training should be part of a comprehensive program including education about diet, weight control, smoking cessation, medication taking, etc., and typically is undertaken in the setting of return to gainful employment and reestablishment of normal patterns of social life, recreation, and/or retirement activities. A structured exercise program, particularly in the early weeks after

infarction or bypass surgery, often facilitates this comprehensive approach.

The initial 5- to 10-min warm-up period of stretching and range-of-motion exercises permits musculo-skeletal and circulatory adaptation and readiness for exercise. The 15- to 20-min training or endurance component, designed to stimulate the oxygen transport system, the time during which the target heart rate is to be achieved, typically initially includes either walk-run sequences or exercise on a stationary bicycle or treadmill; these are activities where skill is a minimal component of the intensity of work demand. Since these activities primarily train the legs, they should be supplemented with arm training exercises: selected calisthenics, use of shoulder wheels, rowing machines, etc. The choice of activities varies with the space and equipment available; the availability of routine, continuous ECG monitoring; and the number of patients. Dr. Karl Stoedefalke has defined the characteristics of an ideal program as individual, supervised, therapeutic, dynamic, aerobic, reasonable intensity, educational, recreational, noncompetitive, relaxing, and enjoyable.[83]

Recommendations for unsupervised home exercise vary considerably. Since economic or logistic constraints often limit the availability of supervised exercise for many coronary patients, there is a need to assess the safety and the cost-effectiveness of unsupervised physical activity. Although the cost of supervised exercise is modest when compared with other therapies for coronary patients, sufficient medical and health care resources are not present to provide medical supervision of exercise for all patients with symptomatic coronary artery disease who might benefit from exercise training. Until data are available concerning the safety of unsupervised exercise, interim guidelines[84] define that patients with a low maximal functional capacity, those with severely depressed left ventricular function, with complex ventricular arrhythmias, QT prolongation, exercise-induced hypotension, or the inability to perform effective self-monitoring of exercise heart rate are probably at increased risk for adverse events during exercise and should be trained in a supervised setting; unsupervised exercise may be recommended, on an individual basis, to patients who lack these characteristics, although it is preferable that unsupervised exercise follow a period of observation, instruction, and training in a supervised program.

A review of cardiac arrest occurring during supervised rehabilitative physical activity[85] identified it as more likely to occur among individuals with above-normal exercise capacity, the absence of angina with exertion, poor compliance in maintaining their training heart rate within the recommended range (heart rates often exceeded the recommended level), and a markedly ischemic ST-segment response on the exercise electrocardiogram; the implications are that patients with a markedly abnormal ST-segment response during exercise testing, even at higher levels of exercise, should be considered for arteriography to exclude the possibility of severe coronary obstruction that might place that individual at risk during sustained exercise. Additionally, it identifies the importance of adherence to the exercise prescription. These facts reenforce the recommendation that unsupervised training is unwise for patients with markedly abnormal ST-segment responses at exercise testing. Supervision may not entail an "all-or-none" approach, in that there may be intermittent supervision at periodic exercise sessions in a community facility, or intermittent telephone transmission of the ECG[86] or other physiological data by patients who exercise at home; the technology for tape recording of comparable information is also available, and combinations of these approaches may be used.

Detailed, specific, and quantitative instructions for home exercise should be provided in written form: the type of exercise; intensity, duration, and frequency; target heart rate range and method of checking; recommended clothing; signs and symptoms of excessive exertion; caution regarding exercise relationship to meals, weather conditions, etc. Some initial home exercise regimens involve progressive walking and walk-jog sequences; some progressively increase the intensity and duration of use of a stationary bicycle. As the level of fitness improves, recreational activities where skill is a component of work intensity may add variety to the exercise program: rope jumping, bicycling, skating, swimming, rowing, aerobic dancing, etc. Most coronary patients initially expend about 50 kcal per exercise session, gradually increasing to 200 to 300 kcal (300 kcal is the typical activity expenditure of previously sedentary normal individuals).

Patients in exercise programs without electrocardiographic monitoring should intermittently measure their heart rate response to ensure that it remains in the desired range. Counting of the radial (carotid or temporal) pulse for 10 or 15 s is recommended, multiplying to get the heart rate per minute. Counting for a full minute results in an inappropriately low heart rate because of the gradual postexercise decline during counting. When pulse rhythm irregularities suggest premature beats, patients should have an ECG rhythm strip recorded; this can be readily accomplished using the defibrillator paddles as ECG leads. Intermittent transtelephonic electrocardiographic recording during unsupervised exercise offers a promising alternative for patients in areas remote from exercise centers.[87]

Although continuous training more effectively increases endurance, interval training is more appropriate for coronary patients to avoid an excessive oxygen debt. Interval training may alternate periods of activity and rest or periods of higher and lower intensity activity of 3 to 5 min each. Often activities which primarily produce leg training are alternated with those which selectively involve arm muscles. Interval training also permits a greater total work load to be imposed at each exercise session before the occurrence of activity-limiting symptoms, particularly angina pectoris. Aerobic games—volleyball, basketball, tennis, handball, etc.—add variety and interest to an exercise regimen and encourage adherence; they offer the added advantage of upper body (arm and torso) exercise.[88] However, variations in skill and in the degree of excitement and competitiveness can significantly vary the oxygen cost.

Patients must be taught to identify inappropriate symptomatic responses to exercise—chest pain, palpitations, undue breathlessness or fatigue, etc.—and to report their occurrence to the exercise supervisor. They should be instructed not to exercise during an intercurrent illness, when unusually fatigued or under excessive stress, etc. Patients returning to exercise after a hiatus of days to weeks (because of illness or other reasons) should begin activity at a lesser intensity and gradually progress to higher levels. Overcompetitive individuals may require increased or more prolonged supervision.

The final 5- to 10-min cool-down period involves a gradual decrease in exercise intensity. This allows the heart rate to subside and averts the postexercise hypotension from sudden cessation of activity when maximum peripheral vasodilatation is still present, resulting from pooling of blood in the legs. The exercise heat load can be gradually dissipated. Postexercise showering should be with lukewarm water; extremes of temperature may produce undue peripheral vasoconstriction or vasodilatation.

Standards for exercise programs for cardiac patients define the need for trained personnel and appropriate equipment for emergency cardiac care, including cardiopulmonary resuscitation.[57] Not uncommonly, electrical "death" (i.e., ventricular fibrillation) can be reversed without resultant myocardial infarction. In a 1978 survey of cardiovascular complications of medically supervised exercise for cardiac patients encompassing about 1.6 million exercise hours, one cardiac arrest occurred per 33,000 patient-hours and one myocardial infarction per 233,000 patient-hours of exercise. The fatal complication rate was one death per 116,000 patient-hours in the early years and one death per 212,000 patient-hours in recent years. Although complication rates appear lower in exercise programs with continuous ECG monitoring, it is not known whether the monitoring per se, the closer medical supervision, or the differing intensity of exercise is the determinant.[89] Continuous ECG monitoring is not feasible on a long-term basis and may engender undue dependence of the patient on this type of activity supervision.

The goal of exercise training is the long-term maintenance of fitness; this requires regular physical activity.[64] For physical activity to become a lifetime pattern, it must be enjoyable. Most patients who attain a 7- to 8-met performance level can be progressed to an unsupervised or minimally supervised exercise setting; this not infrequently occurs within 3 to 6 months after infarction or bypass surgery.[90] The initial walk-run-jog sequences can be replaced by bicycle riding, swimming, aerobic dancing, and a number of endurance sport activities. Patients leaving a more formal supervised exercise program require counseling about long-term community exercise activities, particularly individuals with a prior sedentary life-style who have not explored their likes and dislikes in physical activity. This may explain the improved adherence of patients with a prior history of habitual exercise who are familiar with these alternatives.

Patients continuing in supervised exercise[91] and those exercising individually both need serial assessment at 3- to 6-month intervals. Exercise testing can document performance changes, permit revision of the exercise prescription, and/or define the need for a change in medications.

The desire for health maintenance and fear of incapacitation seem equal in motivating adherence to exercise. A positive attitude of the spouse and family toward exercise favorably affects adherence, as do increased severity of the illness, evidence of a prior adequate coping capacity with illness and stress, and higher educational and social class levels. Feedback to the patient regarding functional improvement also helps sustain motivation. Since smoking and blue-collar occupation seem predictive of increased dropout rates from exercise rehabilitation, the subgroup of patients with these characteristics warrants increased attention.[92] The goal of long-term physical activity is reasonable independence in exercising; this mandates a weaning, initially from the monitored setting and subsequently from the ritualization of more formal exercise training, with progressive involvement in exercise that is social, pleasurable, convenient, and appropriate.

The "Training Effect"[93–97]

Training of coronary patients with and without angina pectoris and after myocardial infarction often increases their maximal oxygen uptake as much as 20 percent. In patients with a poor initial level of fitness, further deconditioned after myocardial infarction, the increase in maximal oxygen uptake may be even more dramatic.

The goal of prescriptive physical activity for coronary patients is improvement in cardiovascular function, designated the "training effect." Current data suggest that a peripheral mechanism is primarily responsible for the improved function, related to improved oxygen extraction by trained skeletal muscle. As a result, the heart rate and systolic blood pressure response to submaximal work loads decrease. The training effect is characterized by (1) a lower resting heart rate and systolic blood pressure, and (2) a lesser increase in heart rate and systolic blood pressure for any level of submaximal work. Because these two components, the heart rate and the systolic blood pressure (the rate-pressure product), are major determinants of myocardial oxygen demand, it is understandable that the trained individual will experience less or no angina and demonstrate less or no ischemic electrocardiographic changes at any level of submaximal work. Thus, additional characteristics of the training effect are (3) decreased or absent angina pectoris at work loads which previously induced angina, and (4) decreased or absent ST-electrocardiographic ischemic changes at work loads which previously induced them. Training reduces the myocardial oxygen demand for any body oxygen demand. As the patient exercises at progressive work increments and finally achieves the rate-pressure product at which chest pain and ischemic ECG changes previously occurred, they again appear, but now occur only at a greater work intensity. In the performance of usual daily activities, the trained individual has a lower heart rate and blood pressure response at any submaximal work load, functions farther from the ischemic threshold, and perceives a lesser intensity of exertion for a task because of its lesser percent of the increased physical work capacity; patients describe this as increased "stamina" or "endurance."

Improved peripheral oxygen extraction by working muscle and improved redistribution of cardiac output with exercise result from training and decrease the demand for oxygen transport. Increased oxygen extraction by skeletal muscle, coupled with increased vagal tone, lessened catecholamine release, and a number of other factors may decrease the rate-pressure product and other determinants of myocardial oxygen demand by as much as 18 percent.[98] There is little evidence that short-term, modest-intensity exercise training directly improves intrinsic myocardial performance, especially in older individuals with significant coronary disease, although this aspect remains somewhat controversial.[99] Exercise training of some patients with symptomatic coronary disease increases the resting and exercise end-diastolic volume and stroke volume; at maximum levels of exercise, despite the increase in heart rate, blood pressure, and end-diastolic volume (increased myocardial oxygen demand), the ejection fraction did not fall; the mechanism remains unclear in that no appreciable changes were evident at coronary angiography.[100] Long-term, high-intensity training may improve myocardial contractility, in contrast to the short-term occurrence of peripheral changes.[101,102] Long-term high-intensity training, feasible only in a select subset of patients with coronary disease, may be needed to assess whether exercise improves maximum cardiac output and myocardial oxygenation. The occurrence of angina only at a higher double-product or triple-product than prior to training[94,103] is not well-understood but may reflect an improvement in myocardial oxygen supply or utilization, or changes in myocardial oxygen demand not accounted for by the rate-pressure product.

Both arm and leg exercises must be included in a training program, as their training effects are only modestly interchangeable. In one study,[104] improvement in exercise performance with the untrained limb was only 50 to 75 percent of the change which occurred with the trained limb; this suggests that roughly half of the increase in trained limb performance is due to a generalized training effect, and half is due to changes in the trained skeletal muscle. Most occupational and recreational activities entail arm rather than leg work, mandating arm muscle training for improved performance. The proportion of time spent in arm and leg exercise should be determined by the patient's occupational and recreational goals. The same target heart rate range is used for arm and leg exercise.

Training can be accomplished in the patient receiving concomitant drug therapy,[59,60,105,106] and drug therapy can often improve the ability to exercise. Nitroglycerin and longer-acting nitrate drugs can improve coronary blood flow, alter venous return, improve wall motion, and thereby increase the ejection fraction. An increased exercise capacity of about 1 met is not unusual after the administration of nitrate drugs. The same appears true for calcium-blocking drugs. Despite the decrease in heart rate and blood pressure response with beta-adrenergic blocking drugs, exercise training of patients receiving these agents can increase physical work capacity.[107]

Recent studies suggest that selected patients with severely impaired left ventricular function can safely exercise and achieve a "training effect;"[108] these preliminary data show important peripheral adaptations which may have a beneficial effect on the functional work capacity of these patients. Only a limited number of patients have been so trained in a carefully supervised setting; the safety of this approach without such supervision remains unknown.

Appropriate and Inappropriate Expectations from Exercise Training

The major beneficial effect of exercise is the improvement in functional capacity.[109] This occurs in patients with angina, after myocardial infarction, and after coronary bypass surgery. The hemodynamic determinants of the improved function include an increase in maximal cardiac output and oxygen consumption, a decrease in resting heart rate, a lesser increase in heart rate and systolic blood pressure for any level of submaximal work, and a more rapid return to normal of the exercise heart rate. Myocardial oxygen requirements are less for any level of exercise in the trained individual, enabling an improved intensity and duration of work and a reduction in chest pain symptoms by increasing the exercise threshold for angina.[110]

There is no evidence that exercise alters the angiographic appearance of coronary artery lesions or increases the coronary collateral circulation in human beings.[111–114] Neither have the newer radionuclide techniques shown an increase in myocardial perfusion related to exercise.[115,116] Left ventricular systolic performance, as assessed by ventriculography and the hemodynamic response to exercise, appears unchanged.[113,116] This may reflect the limitations of current methods of evaluation of myocardial perfusion and left ventricular function; and/or the relatively short duration and modest intensity of training of most coronary patients.[117]

Improvement in functional capacity with exercise is primarily a peripheral effect,[118] the decrease in heart rate and blood pressure response, and thus in myocardial oxygen demand, for any level of submaximal work. Whether improvement occurs in myocardial performance remains controversial;[102,119] as does the question of whether exercise alters the incidence of abnormalities of cardiac rhythm.

Neither is there evidence that exercise alters the natural history of coronary disease—the recurrence of myocardial infarction or the incidence of coronary death. The results of a number of randomized clinical trials attempting to define this feature have been inconclusive, primarily due to the small sample size, the high incidence of dropouts among patients randomized to exercise therapy, and the high incidence of patients in the control group exercising regularly although not in a formal exercise program.[80,95,120–126] Exercise training of young or immature animals suggests that long-term physical activity may favorably affect myocardial mitochondrial function and metabolism, increase coronary vascularity even disproportionate to the myocardial hypertrophy, and improve myocardial perfusion and function; whether this occurs in human beings, and particularly in older individuals, remains speculative.[127] A recent multifactorial intervention trial in patients after myocardial infarction showed a reduction in mortality rate, particularly in rate of sudden death and death during the initial 6 months after infarction, associated with an exercise program, excellent medical care, and intensive patient education.[128] A decrease in fatal myocardial reinfarction occurred in the National Exercise and Heart Disease Project.[80]

Serum triglyceride levels decrease with exercise,[129] but the effect on total cholesterol level is not predictable. High-density lipoprotein (HDL) cholesterol is increased in physically active individuals and increases with training.[130-135] The increase in lipoprotein lipase with activity may be the mechanism effecting the lowering of triglyceride levels and the increase in HDL.[136] The effect of exercise on fibrinolysis and platelet function is inconclusive; augmentation of fibrinolysis in response to venous occlusion occurs with moderate physical activity.[137]

Exercise training may exert a beneficial effect on coronary disease by modifying other more powerful coronary risk factors;[138,139] patients who exercise often decrease or discontinue cigarette smoking, weight reduction or weight control is improved, and there is increased health consciousness which may favorably alter diet, encourage blood pressure control when appropriate, etc.

Additional salutary effects of physical activity are psychosocial. Patients who exercise often feel better; have improvement in self-confidence and self-esteem; and show less depression, denial, and dependency on standard psychometric tests; they appear better able to tolerate life crises. The effect of exercise on anxiety is variable. Exercisers tend to participate increasingly in leisure activities and have a better work attendance record; increased return to sexual activity is described.[140] Exercise training has been associated with an improvement in work capacity, income, and job responsibility.[80] Nevertheless, in the National Exercise and Heart Disease Project,[141] no psychosocial differences were noted between the control and exercising groups, despite the increase in work capacity with exercise; possible explanations include the substantial psychological benefit documented during prerandomization which mitigated against a differential outcome in the controlled component of the study; the large dropout rate may have limited the observation of psychosocial change dependent on adherence; the exercise prescription may not have been intense enough, the psychological tests not adequately sensitive or appropriate; or a number of patients may not have obtained psychological benefit from exercise. Emphasis on psychosocial features is appropriate as many patients after myocardial infarction and coronary bypass surgery are more disabled by psychological than by physiological problems.

PATIENT AND FAMILY EDUCATION: MYOCARDIAL INFARCTION[6,12]
Goal and Rationale

Education of the patient and family is designed to provide the necessary knowledge about the coronary disease and its management to enable patients to assume some responsibility for their health care. Education optimally begins during the acute care hospitalization and continues in the physician's office or in a hospital or community clinic or comparable facility. In general, physicians delineate the content of an educational program, and periodically review the material to see that it remains timely, accurate, and appropriate. The actual teaching and the development of teaching materials are often best accomplished by other health professionals—nurses, dietitians, physical or occupational therapists, social workers, etc.—who spend more time with the patient and family, particularly during the hospital stay.

Because myocardial infarction is a life crisis for both the patient and family, it may create motivation for learning. Also, during the hospitalization, a variety of health professionals are available to teach. If benefits of the information presented during the hospital stay are to be maintained—because the content often requires subsequent repetition—the recommendations for care and their implementation must be reenforced after return home to ensure that patients have an adequate understanding of and realistic attitude toward coronary disease. Effort must be made to provide continuity between the education and counseling in the hospital and that done on an ambulatory basis.[142]

Program Components

Fear, pain, anxiety, and fatigue impair the ability to learn while in the coronary care unit; only simple facts should be presented, primarily in response to the patient's questions. Although much of this information may not be remembered, it provides reassurance to both patient and family. There should be a brief explanation of the diagnosis, and presentation of the reasons for the regulations, procedures, and equipment in the coronary care unit. Patients and family aware of this information are less likely to misinterpret staff actions or comments; these explanations help the patient adjust to a life-threatening situation. On occasion, education may provoke anxiety; for the patient coping with the emotional stress of acute infarction by denial, presentation of information about the illness may engender stress, and the teaching may have to be deferred.[143] Emphasis should be on the temporary nature of most restrictions, explaining that as the patient improves and is moved to a general care area, the decrease in surveillance and in the intensity of care reflect progress and recovery. Staff members should transmit their confidence to the patient and family initially that the patient will survive and subsequently of the considerable likelihood of resuming a normal or near-normal life-style.

During the remainder of the hospitalization, once the patient is relatively asymptomatic, has less anxiety about immediate survival, and becomes concerned with planning for return home, more detailed education is appropriate. A teaching program which concentrates on information the patient has to know and which conforms to the patient's perceived needs decreases feelings of helplessness, aids in restoring self-esteem, increases confidence in a successful outcome, and enhances ability to cope with the problems of illness; patients acquire a sense of control and mastery over the threatening illness.

To help patients understand their disease, a brief review must be presented of normal cardiac structure and function and of the atherosclerotic process causing coronary obstruction. Description of the changes should emphasize healing.[71] This information provides a basis for subsequent recommendations for care, including coronary risk modification[143a] and medical or surgical therapy. To decrease unnecessary fear and anxiety, prevalent myths regarding the precipitation of myocardial infarction must be dispelled. Patients often attribute myocardial infarction to excessive work, worry, or stress; a specific preinfarction high-level activity task; excessive pressure by others; excessive alcohol use; straying from religious precepts; etc.[144] Many psychosocial outcomes after an acute coronary episode or coronary bypass surgery appear related to the patient's perception of his or her health status, which may be favorably altered by appropriate information and counseling.

Since management after myocardial infarction entails modification of habit or life-style, the educational curriculum should provide insight into behaviors that may affect the risk of reinfarction and into the value of adopting a healthy life-style.[145] The rationale for dietary changes—calorie, fat, sodium, etc., restriction—should be presented, accompanied by suggestions for implementation. Further adherence is enabled by providing guidelines for food purchasing, food preparation, and restaurant eating; the most important individual to be taught about dietary modifications is the family member responsible for food preparation.

Cessation of cigarette smoking should be recommended both to patients who smoke and to members of their family. Continued smoking following myocardial infarction appears associated with an excessive risk of reinfarction and cardiac death[146–148] and decreases the ability to attain physical fitness. Referral should be made to a hospital or community antismoking program.

Activity plans should identify the reasons for initial activity restriction and provide specific recommendations for progressive activity resumption during recovery and encourage return to work when appropriate.[149] Delineation of exercise programs and facilities in the community help the patient implement physical activity recommendations. Discussion of resumption of sexual activity is important, using the guideline that sexual intercourse is appropriate and safe when other usual daily activities are reinstituted.[150–152] The time to the resumption of sexual activity is typically related to symptoms after recovery from myocardial infarction.[150] Asymptomatic subjects usually resume sexual activity within 8 weeks, while many symptomatic subjects do not resume sexual activity until months later. The physician's advice and instructions can decrease the patient's and spouse's anxiety about resuming sexual relations.[153] Important features in counseling include the age of the patient, the precoronary sexual activity, the general health and level of physical activity, the extent of recovery from myocardial infarction, the associated diseases (diabetes mellitus, diseases of the prostate, etc.), the drugs the patient is taking, etc. In patients with recent infarction, exercise training is associated with increased resumption of sexual activity; a lesser effect is seen with remote infarction.[80] Most patients return to sexual activity several weeks earlier following coronary bypass surgery than after myocardial infarction; patients tend to have a greater decrease in sexual activity prior to surgery than prior to myocardial infarction, and sexual activity tends to increase after surgery; this contrasts with the further decrease in sexual activity which usually follows myocardial infarction.

Education should include advice about control of hypertension, diabetes mellitus, and other coronary risk factors, with specific suggestions for implementation.[154]

Patients must be taught about all medications to be taken—the name, purpose, dosage, desired effects, and potential untoward effects. Many patients have not taken medication prior to infarction, and problems of medication-taking may be unfamiliar to them. Other patients may be discharged home on a large number of complex medication regimens; while the medication schedule should be simplified as much as feasible, the importance of regularly taking medications requires reemphasis. Patients should also be taught the appropriate response to new or recurrent symptoms, emphasizing that immediate medical care is requisite for increased or prolonged chest discomfort. Many hospital centers teach cardiopulmonary resuscitation to families of myocardial infarction survivors.

Community resources should be defined to patients and their families as appropriate, including counseling services, home-care agencies, guidance services, vocational rehabilitation facilities and services for job training and placement, services for financial aid, and postcoronary educational groups or clubs. Prior to discharge from the hospital, discussions should review problems commonly encountered on return home, such as overprotection by the family and possible negative community and job-related attitudes toward coronary patients. Family counseling on life-style adjustments during convalescence should focus on averting unnecessary invalidism of the patient. Travel is usually limited for 2 or 3 months following myocardial infarction or coronary bypass surgery. Patients whose occupation involves travel or who plan a vacation should carry a medical summary, a recent electrocardiogram, and an adequate supply of medications; a leisurely pace of travel is needed, with identification of a physician and medical center at the destination; attention to appropriate cabin pressurization in air travel is necessary.[155]

Major patient and family concerns on returning home relate to tests or procedures planned in the early weeks, specific instructions about activity levels and return to work, and what to anticipate over subsequent months and years; discussions prior to discharge from the hospital should reiterate explanations of these features.

Implementation and Methods

At Grady Memorial Hospital, under supervision of the Emory University School of Medicine, an algorithm for the education of the patient and family after myocardial infarction[156] (Table 4) delineates the information to be presented at each stage of the illness. It includes assessment of the patient's comprehension and learning, and identification of future teaching needs. This format helps ensure that a consistent message is given to the patient and that requisite information is presented, but avoids unnecessary duplication, while allowing repetition where required. Learning may be limited by the complex emotional situations and adjustments, and considerable subsequent repetition may be necessary. However, inhospital teaching is the cornerstone for subsequent education on an ambulatory basis.

An effective educational program is flexible enough to address problems perceived as relevant by a patient at a particular time.[157] Specific patient concerns and problems necessitate some teaching on an individual basis; however, presentation of general information seems best suited to a group format. Only recently has it been appreciated that group education, rather than individual teaching, is often less threatening and anxiety-provoking. It allows the patient to view the group leader as a peer rather than as an authority figure. This group approach is economical of professional time and enables the patient to interact and share experiences with others confronting similar problems. Participation in a group reinforces learning and obviates feelings of uniqueness and deprivation; helping others is supportive of the patient's self-esteem at a time when illness threatens self-image. Involving the patient in planning for recovery and identifying areas of patient decision and responsibility tend to return control to the patient

TABLE 4
Patient education program components*
Problem: myocardial infarction

I Adjustment to coronary care unit
  A Purpose of coronary care unit
  B Regulations of unit (visiting, smoking, flowers)
  C Monitor (sounds and leads)
  D Intravenous infusions and medications
  E Oxygen
  F Activity (leg exercise, etc)
  G ECG, blood tests, x-rays
  H Diet
  I Personal emergencies (e.g., financial, job)
II Adjustment to transfer from unit
  A Constant observation no longer necessary
  B Activity as prescribed
  C Plan for education program (see III)
III Information needed for adaptation to disease
  A Normal anatomy and function of heart
  B Development of coronary atherosclerotic heart disease
  C Heart attack
    1 Risk factors
      a. General discussion
      b. Emphasis on risk factors of individual patient
    2 Warning signs of heart attack
    3 Healing—relation to physical activity
  D Personal response to myocardial infarction
    1 Group discussion
    2 Individual conference with patient, family
IV Plans for care after discharge from hospital
  A Diet
    1 Group discussion
    2 Individual conference with patient, family
  B Discharge medications (each medication, its dosage, is listed for teaching to patient)
  C Activity
    1 General
    2 Sexual
    3 Work simplification
  D Symptoms which should be reported
  E Rehabilitation exercises
  F Clinic or physician appointments
  G Community resources
V Other areas for teaching (e.g., pacemaker, diabetes)
VI Educational materials given to patient (a basic pamphlet list is checked and additional educational materials are recorded)
VII Outpatient (clinic) education
  A Review of IV in class and individual instruction
  B Patient self-learning tapes and slide-tapes

*For each item listed, the date of teaching and instructor's name are recorded, as is the need for further patient education on that topic and the instructor's comments regarding the patient's comprehension.
SOURCE: N. K. Wenger: Rehabilitation of the Patient with Symptomatic Atherosclerotic Coronary Heart Disease, in J. W. Hurst (ed.), "The Heart," 5th ed., McGraw-Hill Book Company, New York, 1982, p. 1155. Used with permission.

and encourage adherence to the medical regimen. Typically, group reenforcement decreases the patient's apprehension about the ability to return to work and/or a near-normal life-style.[158] Teaching should help the patient regain confidence while making realistic plans for resuming or altering the former life-style. The staff must convey their concern for the patient as an individual, and emphasize that in teaching, they confer responsibility on the patient.

Audiovisual materials used in teaching can facilitate learning, ensure coverage of essential information, and provide a varied educational presentation.[159] The information presented during the hospitalization can be reenforced by take-home materials such as books, pamphlets, and instruction sheets. Written directions for care at home provide convenient reference material for the patient and minimize conflicts between patient and family that derive from inadequate or ambiguous instructions.[160] An important reenforcement of learning is the self-test, included as part of an audiovisual or printed presentation; a trained professional should be available to respond to questions or concerns of the patient.

Repetition is needed after the patient returns home. Educational needs not perceived in the hospital become apparent when the patient must make decisions related to health care. Recommended changes must be evaluated before they can be incorporated into the patient's value system; only then can behavioral changes be effected.[161] A patient's attitudes and beliefs about the importance of therapy influence compliance. Health professionals can provide the information, help the patient acquire the skills necessary for life-style change, help the patient set realistic goals, offer continuing encouragement for health-related behavior, and serve as role models, but the patient must effect the changes.

Expectations of Educational Programs

Patients who understand their disease and the rationale for its management have increased incentive and improved ability to cooperate in recommendations for care.[162–164] An educational program creates an atmosphere that encourages patients and their families to ask questions and provides specific information which appears to reduce anxiety. An educational program helps define the patient's responsibility and role, particularly regarding response to symptoms and adherence to therapy. Since many components of care for patients with angina pectoris, after myocardial infarction, or after coronary bypass surgery, involve a lifetime change in habits; intensive serial education appears appropriate.

CORONARY BYPASS SURGERY AS A REHABILITATIVE PROCEDURE
Symptomatic, Functional, and Prognostic Concerns[165–174]

The results of coronary bypass surgery are superior to medical management in the frequency and the extent of relief of angina pectoris. With successful myocardial revascularization the ejection fraction may improve, often with enhancement of function in segments of myocardium with exercise-induced wall motion dysfunction.[166] This improvement is absent in patients with unsuccessful revascularization and those who sustained perioperative myocardial infarction.[175] Reversal of exercise-induced hypotension has also been described postoperatively. The combination of improved ventricular performance and relief of angina pectoris is manifest as improved cardiovascular performance: an improvement in aerobic capacity and physical fitness. In addition to the postoperative improvement in function related to the increase in myocardial oxygen supply, further enhancement of exercise capacity occurred in patients participating in a physical conditioning program; the major reduction in myocardial oxygen demand was evident during the initial few months of exercise training.[176]

Recent data reenforce the improved prognosis, as well as the improvement in symptoms, for appropriately selected patients after coronary bypass surgery. Surgery enhances the rate of survival in patients with critical left main coronary artery obstruction and is requisite in these patients if the remaining arterial anatomy and left ventricular function are appropriate. Improved rate of survival is also evident in patients with triple-vessel and in selected patients with double-vessel disease, but medical and surgical intervention appear associated with comparable outcomes in patients with single-vessel disease. These are, however, relatively crude categorizations, in that the degree of obstruction and the location and number of obstructive lesions in each vessel, as well as the area (mass) of myocardium supplied by the vessel, are major determinants of the significance of the atherosclerotic disease in that vessel.

Vocational and Socioeconomic Concerns

Despite the dramatic symptomatic and functional improvement, rehabilitation, *if* measured by the retention of gainful employment, has been disappointing. Fewer patients return to work after coronary bypass surgery than after uncomplicated acute myocardial infarction.

Among a group of patients undergoing coronary angiography, there was no difference in subsequent full-time employment between patients receiving medical and surgical therapy.[177] Return to work among patients with unstable angina was more likely for those responding to medical management than for those who required either early or late coronary bypass surgery.[178] Increased age at the time of surgery, a lower educational level, the development of angina pectoris postoperatively, prior myocardial infarction, and increased physical requirements of the patient's employment appear related to the decision not to work after surgery.[174,179–182]

A major determinant of employment[174,177,183] in both medically and surgically treated patients appears to be the recent work status. The longer the patient had been unemployed, the less likely the return to work; 6 months or more of unemployment seemed the critical time span. However, in a small series of patients randomized to medical or surgical therapy, surgical intervention with subsequent medical therapy was associated with an increased return to work; the determinant appeared to be improved functional status as evidence of graft patency.[184] In several other reports, a small but significant increase in postoperative return to work occurred in patients not working prior to surgery because of angina pectoris.[185,186] The poor prognostic outlook for return to work after coronary bypass surgery warrants attention because of the combination of medical and nonmedical determinants of this problem. Postoperative clinical results such as the improvement in dyspnea or angina or the improvement of exercise tolerance had a virtually insignificant relationship to return to work in some series[187] (possibly because symptoms were not the reason for discontinuing work), whereas persistent physical disability seemed important in others.[174,188,189] Neither is the severity of the coronary disease or the completeness of myocardial revascularization a constant determinant.[187] This disparity between medical and vocational-social outcomes is evident in many populations.[190] The more routine performance of surgery earlier in the clinical course of the patient; the changing attitudes in the community relative to the surgically treated coronary patient; the increased familiarity of the primary care physician with postoperative patients, etc., did not appear to alter to a major extent the return to work.[180,182,183] This problem warrants attention, as a recent estimate suggests that less than 2 years of resumption of work more than compensates for the costs of surgery, if both taxable income and obviating the need for disability payments are considered.[191]

More recent data[174,191,192] are slightly more optimistic; although most patients not working preoperatively tended to remain unemployed, some patients did seek employment, and 22 percent remained employed 4 years postoperatively. Additionally, surgically treated patients required fewer medications and fewer hospitalizations.[191] In general, the decision not to continue working was more prevalent among older patients and those with prior myocardial infarction. Ninety percent of patients less than 55 years of age employed at the time of surgery were employed 4 years postoperatively, a figure comparable with the 93.5 percent U.S. employment statistics for that age group; 44 percent of patients aged 60 or older at operation were employed 4 years later. For both younger and older individuals reappearance of angina was an important factor in the decision not to work; the physical requirements of employment played a more important role in older patients. A 65 percent return to work, 75 percent to the same job, was defined by 1,602 responses to a mail questionnaire among patients below age 65 who had coronary artery bypass surgery at Emory University Hospital between 1977 and 1980;[174] all patients were either working at the time of surgery or had stopped work because of cardiac symptoms. Absence of chest pain postoperatively and work status prior to surgery best predicted the return to work. Also predictive were younger age, higher education level, completeness of myocardial revascularization, and absence of prior myocardial infarction. The main reasons precluding return to work were physician advice, cardiac symptoms, and an adequate pension.

Rehabilitation after Coronary Bypass Surgery

The initial limited return to work after coronary bypass surgery had been thought to be in part related to the unnecessarily restrictive approach in the early management of these patients. A number of patients had had prolonged preoperative activity restriction because of chest pain, and hence approached surgery in a deconditioned state. Then, in the postoperative period, both patients and the medical team tended to confuse the chest wall pain from the surgical incision and the pain of postoperative pericarditis with ischemic pain. The pain, swelling, numbness, and paresthesias in the leg at the site of saphenous vein removal often restricted activity. The fatigue and activity intolerance, at least in part reflecting the pre- and postoperative deconditioning, were often misinterpreted as cardiac dysfunction.

However, with only occasional exceptions,[185,186] the return to work has not changed in recent years. There is a problem in analysis; patients previously working cannot improve but can only worsen their status by not working; this may be expected with time in older patients. For patients not previously employed, even a small percent return to work is encouraging; patients unemployed preoperatively because of angina pectoris may have increased postoperative employment as symptoms improve.[185,186] If some postoperative patients stay at work, some working preoperatively do not return to work, but some previously unemployed return to work; no net gain is shown despite the satisfactory outcome in the latter group.

Gradually progressive exercise, beginning postoperatively, may reverse the deconditioning related to prior and current immobilization and improve musculoskeletal strength; the long-term caloric expenditure (300 kcal per exercise session) may help control weight. Participation in an exercise program may encourage dietary changes and smoking cessation. Physical activity is associated with increased emotional stability and improved self-image. The psychological benefits may be among the major advantages of exercise, although there is unquestionable additional improvement in exercise tolerance and activity capability in most post-coronary bypass patients after exercise training. Whether exercise alters progression of atherosclerosis after surgery in the native or graft vessels remains unknown; the effect of exercise training and improved physical work capacity on return to work appears overshadowed by more compelling determinants.

Early ambulation and subsequent exercise training[193,194] are comparable to these activities for the patient with myocardial infarction, with some particular concerns. The same therapist can help the postoperative patient with respiratory exercises and early ambulation in the surgical intensive care unit. Low-level, primarily isotonic, exercise can begin as early as the second postoperative day. Patients should initially wear support stockings to prevent edema at the site of saphenous vein removal and to decrease incisional pain. Arm exercise, in addition to bringing about adaptive changes in the arms to decrease myocardial oxygen demand, may increase the strength of the pectoral muscles, improve flexibility, muscle coordination, and joint mobility; and decrease shoulder and chest wall pain. Stretching exercises, with arms raised above the head, are important.

Progressive activity emphasizes walking, with self-monitoring of heart rate. Most patients can readily walk 2 mi in about 30 min by about 4 to 8 weeks after surgery. Subsequent endurance training, guided by exercise test performance either prior to discharge or at 4 to 8 weeks, is as for the postinfarction patient or the patient with stable angina. Typically, all categories of coronary patients participate simultaneously in supervised training.

The problem of how to motivate patients to return to work remains unsolved. Many patients capable of return to work choose not to do so, for a variety of psychosocial and/or monetary reasons, some of which may be appropriate. Cardiac symptoms do not commonly limit employment. As with myocardial infarction patients, return to work is characteristic of individuals who are self-employed, enjoy their jobs, have no satisfactory pension plan, or whose income is needed. Alternatively, the patient whose occupation is associated with stress, who has inadequate financial reward, or who perceives the illness as work-related uses bypass surgery (or myocardial infarction) as a means to retire gracefully.

PSYCHOSOCIAL PROBLEMS AND NEEDS OF CORONARY PATIENTS: PSYCHOLOGICAL FEATURES IN REHABILITATION[195–210a]

Dr. Paul Dudley White emphasized that "it is of importance to realize that the heart may recover more rapidly than the depressed mental state which is so often a complication."[211] The interaction of medical, psychosocial, and behavioral factors at many levels seems important in recovery from myocardial infarction and bypass surgery. Just as infarction impairs the physiological cardiovascular reserve, it encroaches on the emotional reserve, modifying the coping capacity of the patient.

The major psychological reactions in the coronary patient are anxiety, depression, denial, and dependency. Anxiety and depression contribute to the failure to return to work and sexual functioning,[212] to resume social activities, and to make a satisfactory life adjustment; anxiety and depression are typically unrelated to the severity of the physiological disability.[213]

Psychosocial factors also exert a profound impact on care during the acute illness. Prehospital denial is a major factor delaying the access to medical care. Much of the interval between the onset of symptoms and seeking medical care is involved in deciding whether a doctor need be consulted. Knowing the symptoms of infarction and having had a prior infarction does not significantly shorten the delay.[214–216] Once in the hospital, the initial anxiety is realistic, related to fear of dying; but this frequently progresses to depression as patients fear their inability to perform in previous roles. Denial, although associated with an improved prognosis for survival, may become dangerous if excessive; excessive denial may be manifest as a decision to leave the hospital because the patient does not believe a myocardial infarction has occurred. "Appropriate" denial, characterized by confidence in the medical staff and in recovery,[151] is associated with little or no anxiety and depression and correlates with a subsequent rapid return to preinfarction life-style, including return to sexual activity and to work.

Numerous studies identified the supportive nature of the coronary care unit, indicating that ECG and other monitoring are more apt to reassure than to cause distress.[200,217] Anxiety is highest during the first day in the coronary care unit but falls to a more normal level by the second day. Reduction in anxiety is assisted by reassurance from the coronary care unit personnel, who define what is happening and what is to be anticipated. Many patients begin to show signs of depression by the third hospital day, with this response remaining essentially constant until the time of discharge. Depression rarely reaches serious proportions and is characterized primarily by a preoccupation with limitations imposed or anticipated from the myocardial infarction and concern about reduced earning power.[198,199]

The characteristic type A patient,[218] whose life-style involves control and management, adapts poorly to the dependent role in a coronary care unit. There is fear of helplessness, vulnerability, and invalidism, which the patient equates with death. This fear may be expressed as denial, anger, irritability, frustration, anxiety; or a reactive depression may ensue. As a denier, the hospitalized patient will not admit to anxiety, although it is evidenced by autonomic manifestations of rapid heart rate, sighing respirations, and restlessness. Sedation, which diminishes external perception, typically augments the anxiety; the type A patient requires alertness and awareness of self, of body, and of environment. The patient's prior self-image is characteristically one of independence and responsibility for others, devoid of personal problem or illness. Involving the patient in planning for recovery returns control to the patient, and encourages adherence. Denying patients are reluctant to assume the sick role, and are comparably reluctant to discontinue work and be cared for; because of this, they have a high potential for rehabilitation in addition to their increased likelihood of a favorable outcome at least in the early years after infarction.[219]

Depression is the major emotional problem during convalescence and becomes most evident within days after the patient returns home, when the full impact of the illness become apparent. Weakness attendant on relative immobilization during the hospitalization is often misinterpreted as evidence that the heart is more seriously damaged than the patient was told. The patient is frequently overprotected by the family; any tendency toward the self-image of a semi-invalid is encouraged by this behavior. Because most patients are not forewarned about the emotional problems of early convalescence, they see themselves as unique in their depression, and feel that all others recovering from

infarction have made a better adjustment. Many patients who need tranquilizers or sedatives on a temporary basis to reduce anxiety and depression either may have physicians who are loathe to prescribe these drugs or may hesitate to take them because they are seen as an admission of weakness. In most patients, depression resolves within 2 or 3 months, but there are wide variations. Many patients remain anxious about exerting themselves physically or mentally for fear of precipitating pain, recurrent infarction, or sudden death. Nevertheless, high anxiety and depression levels are not characteristic over an extended period of time,[220] and high anxiety and/or depression levels do not appear related to work status.

Fear of activity can cause prolonged and unnecessary abstinence from sexual intercourse; potency disturbances in the male and frigidity in the female are common sequelae of myocardial infarction.[221] The impact of cardiovascular drugs must also be considered in assessing the sexuality of the patient recovering from myocardial infarction; adrenergic-inhibiting drugs, vasodilators, diuretics, antiarrhythmic agents, hypolipidemic drugs, and digitalis may affect the sexual response, with adrenergic-inhibiting drugs having the most serious effects. The result may be interference with the patient's compliance with medication, precipitation of emotional problems, etc.[222] The added restrictions in diet, smoking, and other alterations of life-style engender a discouraged, frustrated, and often angry patient, and this further limits adherence to recommended postcoronary regimens.[150,223,224]

In a small proportion of patients, depression persists and eventuates in prolonged and unwarranted invalidism; in some instances, survival from infarction is viewed by the patient as a disaster. Explanatory features range from the realistic shrinkage of job possibilities to long-standing personality needs which are satisfied when the individual remains in a sick role. The traditional drug therapy of depression carries an increased hazard in symptomatic coronary patients, since most psychotropic drugs alter heart rate, blood pressure, and cardiac rhythm.

The postinfarction change in image profoundly affects life-style. Most patients feel injured and see themselves as individuals whose potential for earning and creativity has been depleted, as less effective as a spouse, parent, and worker. The nonvisible impairment, with an ever-present risk of unexpected death, reenforces the self-perception as a ''cardiac cripple.'' The social and temporal setting of infarction is often that of an individual at or near the peak of employment or professional status, often with people relating to or dependent on his or her function; this role challenges the dependent position required, at least transiently, after myocardial infarction. There is often considerable family responsibility and community visibility. Family and peers may enhance the sense of impairment and potentiate the depression; a spouse who shares the conviction that useful life is at an end adds to the sense of despair. The counterparts at work are colleagues whose attitudes, as well as the patient's, are often shaped by labor and insurance practices and community mores that tend to discriminate against rather than protect the coronary patient. This constellation of situational factors enhances the likelihood of depression, especially in individuals with preillness impairment of personality structure and with little or no job security at the time of illness.

Particularly for these latter patients, the damaged self-image often persists after the restoration of cardiac function. Even after the hospitalization, the patient's self-perception is changed from strength to weakness, from competence to incompetence, and from whole to damaged. There are feelings of resentment, worthlessness, rejection, and abandonment. There is fear of return to the prior life-style: occupation, leisure activity, sexual activity, social pursuits. Fear of recurrence of coronary symptoms or reinfarction may lead to early retirement and withdrawal from an active life-style. Retirement may further damage psychological status, as depression may result from a combination of loss of occupation, income, status, friends and associates, and identity in the community.[219] Reduction or deprivation in smoking, drinking, and physical and sexual activity reenforce the negative self-image. Other factors predictive of the psychological response include the preillness personality structure, the severity of the coronary disease, the patient's relationship with the physician, the meaning of illness to the patient, and financial concerns. Cultural values and attitudes may also influence return to work, compliance with medical management, etc. Unwarranted invalidism also appears related to disparate factors such as sex, ethnic background, socioeconomic status, strength of psychological defenses, family cohesiveness, and the desire to regain the previous life-style patterns. The resultant time lost from work, the personal unhappiness, and the extent of family and social disruption subsequent to myocardial infarction are enormous.

The two interventions which appear to alter the incidence and severity of psychological problems are education and physical activity.[198,201,225] Initial explanation of coronary care unit equipment and procedures; the subsequent specific attention to prepare the patient for transfer out of the coronary care unit;[226] detailed instructions prior to return home and on an ambulatory basis offer reassurance and decrease the anxiety and frustration that results from ambiguous recommendations. Education alleviates the fear and anxiety in part by correcting misinformation or misunderstanding, often based on prevalent community myths about coronary disease. Common myths emphasize the lethal effect of overactivity, excitement, anger, expression of emotion, etc. Educational groups may help reduce psychological morbidity after myocardial infarction.[227,228] Most of these coronary groups or clubs begin while the patient is hospitalized but continue for 3 to 4 months after discharge. They are typically supervised by a physician or nurse who instructs the patients and their families, answers questions, and encourages patients to share their experiences. These groups have not been studied on a large enough scale to objectively assess their value and role.

Progressive physical activity during the hospitalization reenforces the statements that the patient is recovering. The weakness with protracted bed rest often convinces patients of their irreversible and major cardiac damage; it raises concern of their ability to function after leaving the hospital; demonstration that self-care and subsequently that modest levels of physical activity can be engaged in without producing chest pain or danger provides tangible reassurance. Searching for ways to fill the unstructured time of convalescence becomes an arduous task; combination of education and physical activity are appropriate strategies.[213]

Depression[229] after the hospitalization presents a variable constellation of symptoms, many of which may be overlooked or misinterpreted as indicating additional cardiac or other illness. Most common are fatigue, insomnia or fitful sleep, decreased concentration and memory impairment, loss of interest in work or recreation, decreased libido, headache, dizziness, vague chest discomfort, and profound anxiety when confronting new situations. Especially for men and for blue-collar workers, the boredom of convalescence can intensify this presentation. Unanswered concerns about symptoms, medications, planned tests or procedures, allowable activities, long-term prognosis, etc., potentiate depression.[230] Although emphasis is often on problems of men after myocardial infarction, poor rehabilitation outcomes are also frequent among women;[151] anxiety and depression were common in one study, as was the predominance of type A behavior. These women had an increase in hospital readmissions and a high mortality rate; the survivors had limited return to work and to sexual functioning. The problems appeared accentuated among unmarried women. Whether the psychosocial variables were the cause or the effect of the severity of the illness remains unknown; despite their lesser incidence of infarction, women have an increased morbidity and mortality rate after infarction compared with men,[231] and unmarried women have an increased incidence of sudden death.[232] The relationship of these features to the older age at which infarction occurs in women, to the associated diabetes, or to their altered social support systems requires evaluation.[233]

Family relationships assume enormous importance.[234] Family conflicts, anxieties, and guilt are commonly exacerbated by illness and may adversely affect convalescence. Typically, a precarious marriage terminates in divorce after infarction, in part because of the temporary reversal of roles and responsibility and in part related to the emotional support required by the convalescent infarction patient. A wife may deny her dependency by overprotecting her husband or control her aggression by being oversolicitous; both may hinder rehabilitation. Complicating features include feelings of guilt for the patient's disability and fear of sexual involvement causing further harm. Conversely, the family with excessive anxiety and guilt may relegate the patient to an excessively dependent role by their overprotective attitudes, increasing the patient's frustration and depression. If not included in family discussions and decisions, the patient becomes more concerned with self-image; isolation and deprivation of usual family interactions increase depression. The patient with heart disease who loses the ability to resume the preinfarction family role behaves as if reacting to a death in the family, exhibiting a grief and loss reaction.

Comparable emotional responses occur after coronary bypass surgery;[235,236] and comparable intervention strategies seem effective. Psychological problems relate to combinations of initial enjoyment of the excessive attention related to recovery from cardiac surgery; subsequent anxiety about performing in now relatively unfamiliar occupational and family roles; fears of the patient, physician, or employer of cardiac complications; depression related to overprotection by the family; the weakness and fatigue of deconditioning misinterpreted as persistent severe cardiac impairment; unnecessary work restriction because of ambivalent or inappropriate physician recommendations or because of employer or union policies; and frustration and indecision because of financial incentives which encourage invalidism and the disabled role.[237,238] Family members, elated at the patient's safe return home, may not appreciate the patient's ambivalence at having to restrict pleasures or routines while seeing others enjoying the same activities; many related to changes in diet, smoking, etc. Patients commonly become angry at health professionals, family members, and friends who encourage these alterations in life-style, and then feel guilt for their anger at persons trying to help. Anticipating for the patient and family common problems encountered on return home, structuring convalescence with progressive physical activity as an important component, involvement in community heart clubs,[228,239] telephone follow-up or contact systems, etc., appear advantageous. See "Patient and Family Education: Myocardial Infarction." Medications are often not needed, but short-term benzodiazepine therapy early

in convalescence may be helpful; the patient should be cautioned to avoid alcoholic beverages while the medication is used.

Physical activity after the hospitalization, characterized by patients as enabling them to "feel better," has been associated with improvement in the depression, denial, and dependency scores on standardized psychometric tests, although the effect on anxiety is variable.[80] Improvement in physical fitness is associated with psychological improvement in the majority of patients. Patients who exercise have an enhanced self-image and are better able to cope with life stresses; this is often manifest as improved family, occupational, and community relationships.

Participation in physical activity and educational groups during recovery offers emotional and social group support; it obviates feelings of uniqueness and deprivation; provides encouragement by peers more advanced in recovery who have successfully adapted to their illness; and offers the opportunity to express feelings, share frustrations, and exchange solutions.[158] Rehabilitation in great part involves the ability to cope, to attain the behavior and capacities to meet life's demands and goals; coping ability may be enhanced by the acquisition of personal skills, techniques, and knowledge.

The advice and indeed the personality and attitudes of physicians and other health professionals have a major effect on the psychological course of rehabilitation. There is only beginning understanding of the health professional–patient relationship, but what is known of this interaction suggests that it is vital to successful rehabilitation. Attitudes and beliefs, such as resistance to authority, distrust of physicians, low motivation for participating in a health maintenance program, and feelings of alienation, originate in part from the social or cultural background of an individual patient and may lead to behaviors which may interfere with or prevent adequate care. For example, the degree to which patients are able and willing to follow the advice of the physicians may affect rehabilitation. The factors which promote or impede compliance are multifaceted: social, cultural, situational, and physical, as well as psychological.[240] Psychological factors are major barriers to compliance; these may be related to motivation, education, and intelligence.

Osler provided an early description of coronary-prone behavior, characterizing the patient with angina pectoris as one who worked at maximum capacity, incessantly striving for success in commercial, political, or professional life.[241] However, the work environment may also influence the behavior of individuals engaged in the professions and as managers; their jobs are characterized by time pressures, deadlines, competition, and anxieties. Although psychosocial and personality factors appear as risk factors for the development of coronary disease,[218,242–244] data are inadequate to define their role in reinfarction or postinfarction rate of survival. In addition to the effect of psychological factors on the risk and prognosis of coronary disease, it is important to consider the effect of coronary disease on the subsequent psychosocial functioning of the patient. There is insufficient information about the psychology of habit change and the effects of coronary risk intervention; the role of behavior modification (such as group experience including group therapy and patient education) as an adjunct in evoking habit change is unknown.

Much stress is engendered by the patient's perception of a problem and the way it is handled; stress can be characterized as the hidden costs of coping with problems. Stress may derive from diverse situations, reflecting maladaptive coping mechanisms in dealing with family relationships, problems at work, etc. Because the pattern of coping with myocardial infarction or bypass surgery is commonly comparable to responses used with prior illness or other major challenges, patients with habitual unsuccessful adaptation to stress should be anticipated to require support and counseling after infarction or bypass surgery. Patients with prior evidence of ability to cope with problems of adult life appear to have a more favorable outcome; they tend to return to work earlier, and their work efficiency is better.

VOCATIONAL ASPECTS OF REHABILITATION

Vocational concerns impose stress, particularly for younger patients with myocardial infarction who fear for their job security and the family's economic future (see also "Coronary Bypass Surgery as a Rehabilitative Procedure"). Uncomplicated and complicated acute myocardial infarction cannot be directly equated with subsequent less severe and more severe disability, although substantially more patients with a complicated acute illness will be more severely disabled. Conversely, about a third of patients with severe left ventricular dysfunction can attain normal levels of exercise by a variety of compensatory mechanisms.[245] Different rates of return to productive or employed roles have been reported according to the severity of the cardiac disability; these have varied from 65 to 95 percent for less severely disabled cardiac patients to 25 to 33 percent for severely disabled persons.[246]

A longitudinal study of return to work after myocardial infarction identified the lack of correlation between survival and work status.[247] Although the survival rate was 75 to 80 percent at 5 years, employment rates were only 50 percent for salaried workers and 43 percent for wage earners.

In recent years, over 80 percent of previously employed patients with uncomplicated myocardial infarction returned to work within 8 to 12 weeks, typically resuming their former jobs.[16,54] However, long-term studies indicate that despite the high early return to work after uncomplicated infarction, the dropout rate each year is also quite high. Among one group of patients followed during the first year after discharge from the coronary care unit, although 83 percent returned to work by 6 months, only 63 percent were gainfully employed at 1 year.[213] Factors responsible included early retirement, significant depression, worsening health, family illness, and forced retirement by the employer; the latter issue represents a problem in vocational rehabilitation in the United States. Comparable return to work data are not available for patients with complicated infarction and residual impairment, the group more likely to require more extensive rehabilitation services. The return to work rate in this group of patients is estimated at 25 to 33 percent.

Analysis of disability after myocardial infarction delineates that more patients are limited by psychological than physiological problems.[248–250] Only rarely, in patients with marginal cardiac function, does angina pectoris or heart failure preclude or delay return to work, particularly to the low-intensity work load of most jobs in today's mechanized society.[65] In a European study of coal miners and factory workers, patients recovered from myocardial infarction were compared with normal individuals in the same job; postinfarction patients used an increased percent of their maximal oxygen uptake, 42 to 47 percent, compared with 39 percent for normal individuals, but still had an adequate cardiac reserve.[251] Both physical and psychological factors impeding return to work require prompt attention. In 40 percent of over 2,000 patients studied in a Work Classification Clinic,[252] emotional factors were next in importance to the heart disease in affecting the return to work; much of the emotional difficulty was based on fear, anxiety, and tension that developed in previously susceptible individuals; self-perception of health status was a compelling feature.[253] Most patients who return to work do so in the 6 to 10 months after infarction.[254] Therefore, the attitude of the physician in actively encouraging prompt return to work after myocardial infarction or coronary bypass surgery appears important.[255,256] However, return to work without alteration of prior work-related behavior may not constitute optimal rehabilitation; overly ambitious pursuit of work, coupled with high job dissatisfaction, may represent a return to the premorbid, coronary-prone pattern of living.[158] Major psychosocial stress appears associated with jobs characterized by a combination of high work demand (although not necessarily high-level physical work) in association with a low level of control over the working environment, i.e., a limited role in decision-making.

In general, both for patients after infarction and after coronary bypass surgery, recent work status and the type of occupation (the physical effort involved) influence return to work.[257] Features which negatively influence return to work include older age, anxiety or depression, development of symptoms, e.g., pain, dyspnea, palpitations, etc., with effort (i.e., lower functional class), lower social class and less education, a job characterized by higher-level physical activity, patient perception of the illness as job related, and patients who are vocationally disadvantaged.[39,65,174,177,180,182–187,189,190,192,256,258–261] Unfortunately, individuals who do more demanding work, often patients at lower levels of the social class scale, have problems with return to employment. This is magnified because limited educational skills narrow their vocational scope and opportunity for job change.[262] Special training schools, sheltered industrial workshops, and on-the-job evaluation may be required. Additionally, many persons lower on the social class scale appear more likely to smoke, to have a more sedentary lifestyle, less job satisfaction, lesser enjoyment of leisure time pursuits, and fewer social support systems; these may further impede rehabilitation.[219] Federal-state vocational rehabilitation agencies may be valuable in providing employment, counseling, and job retraining.[263]

Although many job-related problems can be counteracted by provision of comprehensive rehabilitative services—functional assessment, counseling, training—some features tend to be counterproductive: inordinate delays in access to services; multiple agencies, differing regulations, and contradictory evaluations of the patient; lack of interagency coordination and inadequate communication between health care and rehabilitative personnel; high personnel turnover limiting the continuity of rehabilitation planning and counseling; and inadequate health education and counseling, particularly for blue-collar workers.

Although patients are physically able to return to prior jobs, they foresee problems: will they be candidates for promotion, salary increases, and more responsible and demanding supervisory positions once identified as an employee with coronary disease? What will be the attitude of coworkers? Will they resent an individual who cannot assume a proportionate share of the work? Will they fear the patient may sustain a recurrent infarction at work? Coronary patients, too, remain aware of the threat of reinfarction or sudden death. These psychosocial-vocational features may not encourage rehabilitation and restored productivity.

Exercise testing permits more precise assessment of function. It may help allay the fears of the patient, physician, and employer regarding the capability and safety of return to work. A number of patients fail to return to work because of lack of professional assurance that they can safely do so. Exercise testing was advocated by a WHO Expert Committee to "estimate probable performance in specific life and occupational situations."[264] However, physical work capacity reflects not only the impact of infarction on cardiovascular function, but the preinfarction fitness and the deconditioning during the hospitalization and convalescence. The physical work capacity of the patient defines the tolerated levels of heart rate and blood pressure under standardized conditions; this correlates moderately well with vocational pursuits when consideration is given to differences in temperature, environment, relationship to meals, intellectual demands, emotional stress, clothing worn when working, etc.[265] Myocardial oxygen demand and cardiac output are greater with arm than leg work of equivalent intensity, although total body oxygen demands are comparable; thus, arm testing is recommended to guide recommendations for arm work.[266–268]

In one series of patients 3 months after myocardial infarction, the average maximum working capacity was 70 percent of normal persons of similar age.[121] Although one-third of patients were limited by angina, and at least one-third experienced cardiac symptoms at a work load so low that they were not considered able to perform some daily life activities, 42 percent of patients limited their physical exertion because of fear rather than physical limitation. The current widespread use of long-acting nitrate drugs, beta-adrenergic blocking agents, and calcium-antagonist drugs provides greater symptomatic relief and may permit increased activity performance. Coronary bypass surgery has even greater implications regarding enhancement of functional status; to date, however, the decrease in symptoms and improvement in function after coronary bypass surgery have not been associated with an increased return to work.[255,256]

Patients in New York Heart Association functional class I[61] can exercise at a work load of at least 7 mets, have little or no cardiac impairment, and remain asymptomatic with usual daily or occupational activities characterized by moderate exertion; their cardiac impairment ranges from 0 to 15 percent. Class II patients, who become symptom-limited with moderate and/or prolonged physical exertion, have a work tolerance of 5 or 6 mets; their degree of cardiac impairment is 20 to 40 percent. Class III patients, typically those with severe angina or heart failure, have a work tolerance in the 3- to 4-met range, and become symptomatic when performing usual daily tasks except at an extremely slow pace; for these individuals, only sedentary work is indicated. Their cardiac impairment is 50 to 70 percent. Class IV patients, symptomatic at rest, may have angina or heart failure, have a work tolerance of 2 mets or less, and are not considered employable (Fig. 2).[269] Their cardiac impairment is 80 to 95 percent. In the National Exercise and Heart Disease Project,[80,270] sign- and symptom-limited patients recovered from myocardial infarction demonstrated 72

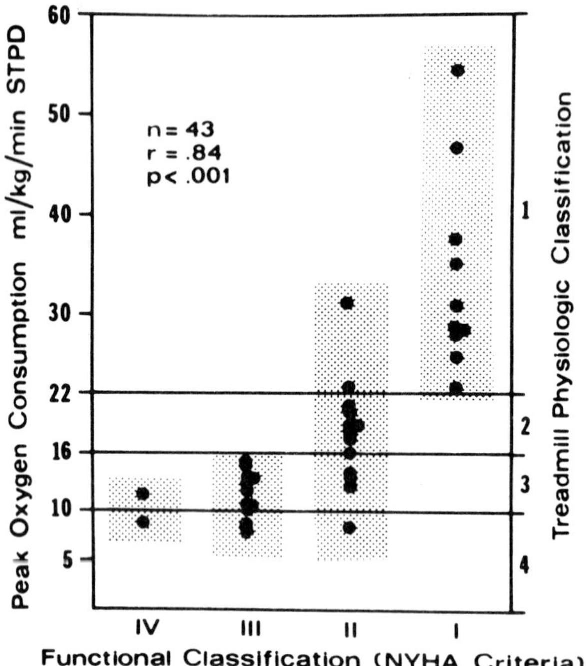

FIGURE 2 Relationship of treadmill physiological classification to clinical functional classification. (*From J. Naughton and R. Haider, Methods of Exercise Testing, in J. P. Naughton, H. K. Hellerstein, and I. C. Mohler (eds.), "Exercise Testing and Exercise Training in Coronary Heart Disease," Academic Press, New York, 1973, p. 79. Used with permission.*)

to 75 percent of the aerobic capacity of heart rate–limited patients.

Other important considerations are the financial, social, disability, and compensation benefits of not returning to work. Industrial, management, and labor and union practices and policies, as well as governmental and private industry disability, pension, and retirement benefits,[124,190] may encourage patients to remain unemployed. Financial incentives of disability or compensation judgments often equal or exceed those possible with employment. Many employers are reluctant to hire patients with coronary disease because of their concerns about extra costs for special physical examinations, decreased employee flexibility and versatility, higher costs associated with paid sick leave within the company, higher cost of employee benefits such as health, disability, and major medical insurance, higher rates of absenteeism, and the possibility of workmen's compensation claims. Many barriers to successful vocational rehabilitation thus lie outside the traditional boundaries of the health care system. In general, the greater the social benefits, the less the incentive to return to work. This major feature of total cost-containment of coronary illness has received inadequate attention.

Factors which favor the return to work of coronary patients include work in industries with a low proportion of heavy labor; management, clerical, or sales occupations; industries with no formal age policies for hiring; experience in the industry or company with the disabled in general; a practice of retaining employees who develop coronary disease; an affirmative action plan for the handicapped by federal contractors; and a low rate of unemployment in the community.[271]

Nevertheless, restrictions limit occupations suitable for coronary patients related to the job, e.g., airline pilot,[272] interstate truck driver, heavy equipment operator, etc., because sudden and unexpected cardiac complications pose excessive hazards to public safety in these occupations, even when the patient's function appears intact.

SOCIOLOGICAL AND SOCIETAL ASPECTS OF REHABILITATION

Other variables related to successful rehabilitation are sociological and societal and occur at many levels: interactions of the patient with spouse, family, and friends; attitudes of physicians, health care, and rehabilitation personnel, employers, unions, and co-workers; and the general social support system in the community. The patient who is viewed as incompetent to perform in prior activities may be relegated to a more dependent position and role in any of these spheres. Family anxieties and fear may result in strife and disruption of family relationships. The factors impeding return to work have been reviewed. Clearly conditions that prevent adjustment to remunerative work may also affect adjustment to life situations such as performing as a housewife, adjusting to retirement, functioning in the community, etc.[273]

The impact of coronary disease thus affects the national economy through reduced worker productivity, loss of taxable revenue, unemployment compensation, death benefits, workmen's compensation, disability benefits, welfare support, and social security benefits. The financial burdens on the family of the patient have even farther-reaching consequences, such as limiting a child's access to higher education, curtailing an improved life-style, limiting the voluntary contributions of the patient and family to the community, etc.; all result in significant subsequent losses to the family and the local and distant community. The effects of coronary disease in costs to the individual, family, community, and nation are staggering. Although it is easy to identify factors which contribute to the dollar cost of illness, equally important "costs," the waste of life and human potential, cannot be measured in these terms.[2,5] To the extent that rehabilitation can be achieved by physiological, psychological, and sociological interventions, the toll in human suffering may be minimized.

KINDS AND AMOUNT OF REHABILITATION MEASURES AND SERVICES CURRENTLY RECEIVED BY CORONARY PATIENTS

A recent survey[54] of U.S. physicians determined changes in the routine care of patients with uncomplicated myocardial infarction between 1970 and 1980. Fifty-three percent of patients with myocardial infarction had their hospital course classified as uncomplicated in 1980. The median length of hospital stay decreased from 21 days in 1970 to 14 days in 1979.

All physicians described a high level (95 to 99 percent) of recommending restriction or cessation of cigarette smoking, and of routine counseling during the hospitalization about diet and about subsequent resumption of sexual activity and return to work. Most counseling was informal rather than in a structured hospital teaching program.

Physicians reported earlier ambulation of patients and earlier return to specific activities such as self-care and walking. Patients were also described as returning to work earlier. Among the guidelines (not mutually exclusive) used to recommend resumption of physical activity, 97 percent of physicians cited clinical judgment, with tolerance to walking cited by 92 percent. Standard exercise tests served as a guideline for 59 percent of family practitioners and internists and for 83 percent of cardiologists; compared with 1970, there was a significant increase in the use of standard exercise tests. Exercise tests, when performed, were done uniformly at about 8 weeks after infarction. There was an increase in the availability and familiarity with standard exercise tests from 1970 to 1980. Among those not using exercise tests, patient safety remained a concern for about 30 percent of family practitioners and internists, unchanged from 1970; there was a significant decrease in concern about patient safety during exercise testing among cardiologists. Significantly fewer 1980 respondents did not consider exercise testing helpful.

Most physicians in both surveys (93 to 95 percent) recommended progressive physical activity on return home. About 45 percent recommended physician-supervised programs, and 45 percent home exercise. Several physicians reported recommending more than one type of program, depending on the patient and the proximity of the program. At least 80 percent of previously employed patients younger than age 65 years returned to work in both survey periods.

The economic impact of the changes is difficult to assess, i.e., the savings related to earlier hospital discharge versus the costs of additional newer diagnostic and therapeutic interventions. Reduction of hospital stay by an average of 7 days and the earlier return to work represent a saving in medical care costs and an increase in taxable income. However, exercise testing, coronary angiography, coronary bypass surgery, etc., are expensive and the cost/benefit ratio is difficult to estimate. The net effect of current practice appears aimed at reducing the physical and vocational invalidism and the morbidity associated with myocardial infarction.

An additional source of data is an American Heart Association survey of cardiac rehabilitation units (Robert M. Levenson, chairman, personal communication). The "Directory of Cardiac Rehabilitation Units" lists over 700 facilities;[274] the survey is based on replies from over 600 of these. Most are housed in hospitals, but some are administered by a hospital but housed in a separate setting, and some are independent or freestanding. Most units offer both inpatient exercise during the acute hospitalization and an outpatient exercise program; half also have patients who exercise without supervision at home but are checked at intervals by the unit, half have a supervised maintenance exercise program, and some units have features in addition to these.

The average duration of inpatient exercise during the acute hospitalization was 2.2 weeks, of outpatient rehabilitative exercise 17.4 weeks, of supervised maintenance exercise 25.0 weeks, and of prescribed home exercise 20.3 weeks. Prior to completion of the program 17.5 percent of participants dropped out. A mean of 45.4 patients were served by each program in a typical month, as well as 23.8 family members; the mean estimated patient capacity was 72.6. Categorized by disease, 17.8 percent of patients had angina pectoris, 62.4 percent myocardial infarction, 25.1 percent coronary bypass surgery, 14.4 percent were coronary prone, and a small percent had other diagnoses. These categories are not mutually exclusive.

Patients with angina pectoris, with or without myocardial infarction, constitute about 20 to 30 percent of the U.S. coronary heart disease population. They do not have as highly structured and developed a system of rehabilitative care as patients with myocardial infarction. Because of their symptoms, these patients may have a greater loss of productivity than patients recovered from uncomplicated myocardial infarction. Because many patients with angina have more physical impairment and limitations and require more medication than many other subsets of coronary patients, their needs for medical and rehabilitative care may exceed those of patients recovered from uncomplicated infarction. Although some programs define that patients with angina pectoris are participants, community facilities will have to expand their coronary rehabilitation programs to meet the needs of this symptom-limited population.

Another unmet need involves the 100,000 or more patients who have coronary bypass surgery in the United States each year. The application of the principles and techniques of coronary rehabilitation used for patients after myocardial infarction to the increasingly large U.S. coronary surgery patient population remains sporadic. The rehabilitative approach, helping in life adjustment after surgery, improves the coping capacity of the individual; important components include physical training, job counseling, coronary risk intervention, and psychosocial counseling. Part of the realistic adaptation to illness includes the patient's acceptance of advice offered by health professionals. Because many of these patients have not sustained myocardial infarction, their rehabilitation potential is great; data about rehabilitation outcomes remain limited.

FRAGMENTATION AND COORDINATION OF REHABILITATION SERVICES AND INSTITUTIONS: PRIMARY CARE DELIVERY, HOSPITALS, SOCIAL SERVICES, OCCUPATIONS, HEALTH CARE

Personnel Involved in the Implementation of Rehabilitation[6]

In the coronary care unit, physicians and nurses with training in acute cardiac care have major responsibility for the patient; the physician in charge may or may not be the patient's primary doctor.

Hospitals admitting patients with myocardial infarction should have the personnel and facilities to assist the physician in providing or implementing rehabilitative services.[145] In a small community hospital, the primary physician and coronary care unit nurse may fulfill all functions of a "rehabilitation team." Larger medical centers with many patients have a more elaborate team including rehabilitation nurses and nurse-educators, dietitians, physical and occupational therapists, social workers, and at times psychologists and rehabilitation counselors. Considerable rehabilitation can be undertaken with minimal additional facilities, equipment, or personnel to those available at most acute care centers and in the community. Rehabilitation requires a realignment of goals and methods, some retraining of personnel, and often a redirection of attitudes and expectations; more optimal use can be made of already trained personnel and available facilities. The responsible physician must institute, direct, and determine the extent of early ambulation, although these activities may be implemented by a nurse, therapist, exercise specialist, or physician assistant; define the content of the educational-informational program; guide the rehabilitation counselor in replying to questions or concerns of the patient's employer; and coordinate these rehabilitative activities with the more traditional aspects of medical care.

During the remainder of the hospital stay, after transfer from the coronary care unit, the roles of the nurse, nurse-educator, nutritionist, social worker, occupational and physical therapists, and vocational counselor increase as the intensity of medical surveillance and therapy diminishes. Progression of physical activity remains under the direction of the responsible physician, as do other prescriptive aspects of therapy. Patients with severe physiological impairment may benefit from learning energy-conserving techniques in self-care and daily activities; the physician must initiate the request for this component of care. Continuity of management must be ensured when different physicians provide acute care in the hospital and subsequent ambulatory care in a distant community.

During convalescence, there is a lessening role for the physician and hospital-based personnel. As the patient leaves the hospital environment, there is progressively greater involvement of supportive family and friends, public health or visiting nurses, social worker, vocational counselor, employer, and other individuals within the community to enhance the function, adjustment, and self-sufficiency of the patient. The patient, too, assumes more responsibility for health care. In smaller communities, and particularly for patients with uncomplicated infarction, the primary physician, at times with a community nurse, may provide the requisite management, guidance, and counseling. As during the hospitalization, with more complex illness, greater functional impairment, and a larger patient population, more elaborate composition and interrelationships of the rehabilitation team are needed. Communication among health professionals is critical to avoid giving conflicting information and advice to the patient and family.

During convalescence, the primary physician (aided by consultants if necessary) must be prepared to assess the patient's physical performance clinically and using exercise test and other data to guide drug, exercise, and/or surgical therapy; and to evaluate the coronary risk factors warranting modification. The physician must also assess the patient's knowledge about coronary disease, its management, and plans for continuing care; and must ascertain the needs of the patient and family for additional counseling and therapy regarding emotional adjustment, return to sexual activity, life-style changes, family relationships, and so forth. Return to work must be evaluated, including the ability to return to the former occupation, the need for job retraining, the need for more intensive physical training prior to return to work, etc. These areas constitute the comprehensive functional capacity of the patient, and their assessment determines the need for additional, specialized services which may be available in the local community or may require referral to a cardiac center. The encouragement and advice of the primary physician has a major impact on the patient's resumption of work and prior life-style.[275]

After recovery, the scope of rehabilitation programming and the personnel involved become more diverse. Although the primary physician continues to coordinate care, emphasis is on decreasing undue dependence on the physician and the medical aspects of care and increasing realistic adaption to illness and return to a normal or near-normal life-style and role in society. The vocational counselor, employer, and industrial physician and nurse may assume significant roles, as do family, friends, coworkers, and so forth. Community endeavors such as exercise programs and educational (including vocational retraining) and recreational programs are important in this phase.

At 4 to 8 weeks after infarction, many patients have improved sufficiently to return to occupational or prior daily living activities. Nearly half of patients who survive a myocardial infarction have an uncomplicated clinical course without significant residual cardiovascular disability. For these patients, the primary physician's long-term medical management involves continued surveillance and therapy and include measures to enhance cardiac function, decrease coronary risk, prevent recurrence or progression of the disease, and encourage return to the former or another occupation. One component of care is prescriptive physical activity. In some instances the primary physician may have the skills, equipment, and facilities for exercise testing and training; alternatively, referral may be made within the community to cardiac consultants, exercise physiologists, physical educators, etc. A gymnasium or large room for exercise training (with trained supervisory personnel and emergency care equipment) may be available in a community hospital, community college, a local school, service club facilities or community centers, in an industrial complex, or in a governmental or privately owned facility. Elaborate and expensive equipment is not required for exercise for coronary patients; simple calesthenics, warm-up exercises, and a walk-run sequence often are the major activity components; however, equipment which permits a variety of activities may provide enjoyment and encourage adherence. Problems include the need to provide transportation services for rehabilitants and the feature that exercise training ideally initially requires at least three activity sessions a week under professional supervision; this represents a dramatic change in the usual pattern of ambulatory care. Accommodations to this difference must be made by the patient and family, the

health care system, and at times the employer. When appropriate, the primary physician must consider surgical intervention (myocardial revascularization) to relieve symptoms and enhance function; and referral must be instituted to appropriate facilities.

Patients with more extensive physiological, psychological, or vocational impairment more frequently require consultative care. An excellent guideline is the report of the Joint Working Party of the Royal College of Physicians of London and the British Cardiac Society on "Cardiac Rehabilitation," which recommends that "any myocardial infarction patient who has not returned to work at 3 months from the onset of his illness should be referred . . . for assessment of his physical and psychosocial state." The timing and scope of this referral are the responsibility of the primary physician.[276]

There is considerable variability in the extent of, attitudes toward, and conduct of rehabilitative practices from one U.S. community to the next. Although these differences have lessened in recent years,[4,54] there remains a lack of transmittal of information about rehabilitation services for coronary patients to the general medical and health care community. Even where community resources are adequate for exercise testing, exercise training, and patient and family education and counseling, including approaches to emotional and family adjustment problems, physicians and other health personnel are not always aware of these services or the means of access to them.

Prevalent Lack of Formal Structured Rehabilitation

Little information is available in the United States about patterns of care from the time of hospital discharge until return to work or prior life-style. There is no structure or organization for the convalescent phase; there is extreme variability in frequency and scope of diagnostic, therapeutic, counseling, and educational care. Even less information is available regarding contact of the physician and other health personnel with the patient's family. This contrasts with formalized approaches to convalescence in some European medical communities, where the patient recovering from myocardial infarction may be sent to a convalescent facility, often in a country resort, with a highly structured physical activity and educational program.[277,278] The physician's office in the United States is geared for crisis intervention in a chronic illness and for the management of sef-limited acute illnesses; physician-patient contact in the average cardiologist's office approximates 6 to 12 min.[279] In the office of a general practitioner, where more than 50 patients are seen daily, the coronary patient is unlikely to have an extended opportunity to discuss problems and receive adequate information and counseling.

Few rehabilitative efforts are currently directed to patients with uncomplicated myocardial infarction, although they appear to have the greatest rehabilitation potential. Most patients after an uncomplicated infarction appear to do well without formal rehabilitation services; they represent successes without formal rehabilitation intervention. These successes appear enhanced by the patient's psychological assets and by family and social support systems; the absence of these features may explain some rehabilitation failures.

Patients in the lower socioeconomic groups appear to receive less relevant advice regarding return to work. Blue-collar patients tend to ask fewer questions about planning for convalescence and rehabilitation, and to receive fewer recommendations for return to specific activities, including sexual activity; they are thus less able to plan their return to work. Additionally, there is a wide discrepancy among hospitals and physicians in dispensing advice to coronary patients; some variables relate to education, social class, intelligence, ethnic group, etc.

The role of the family in rehabilitation of the coronary patient is another neglected area. The interaction between patient and spouse is vital in any illness, but the relationship has unique significance when there is threat to life and when changes in life-style are needed. Subtle changes in role can undermine a patient's self-esteem, reenforce old conflicts, and cause disagreements; this also applies to conflicts of the patient with children and relatives. The family and the support system it furnishes seem important indicators of success or failure in rehabilitation; this support may be maximized by patient-family groups, a system of telephone or other follow-up with families, etc., but the varying means of delivering this care have not been comparatively evaluated.

Communication problems between doctors and other health personnel and patients relate to differences in cultural, sexual, ethnic, religious, philosophical, and socioeconomic factors and background, with varied beliefs regarding health, illness, and work. Difficulties are compounded when communication involves subcultural boundaries; where discrimination, subtle or overt, is present; or where the background of the patient differs significantly from that of the health professionals.[71,279a] The physician must not only explain facts to a patient with a different background, but also do so in terms, concepts, and values that are understandable and acceptable to the patient and family.[280–283]

To summarize, the majority of patients recovered from myocardial infarction have little or no contact with formal government rehabilitation services, but many are apparently rehabilitated. The factors or supportive agents, particularly nongovernment community resources, which influence the success for these patients are not well-defined. The success rate of rehabilitation appears high for patients after uncomplicated infarction, with or without receipt of formal rehabilitation services.[284]

Effectiveness of Rehabilitation Services

Involvement with formal rehabilitative services does not appear to improve recovery when compared with disabled patients who recovered without contact with the traditional rehabilitation service system.[285] The informal supportive social networks constitute a viable community resource and require evaluation and more precise definition.

There are no widely accepted criteria for evaluating rehabilitation services. Most evaluations are based on physical improvement of the coronary patient and return to work. Other important criteria of successful rehabilitation seldom included in the assessment are (1) the patient's evaluation of physical improvement; (2) psychosocial adjustment in family, sexual, and interpersonal roles; (3) the type of vocational rehabilitation and work returned to; (4) the chance for promotion and advancement, level of pay, degree of prestige, and work record; and (5) the extent to which work is commensurate with the patient's knowledge, skills, experience, and ability.[286]

Current Deficits in Social and Psychosocial Rehabilitation of Coronary Patients and Attempts to Overcome These Deficits

Elements within the organizations, facilities, or agencies which provide rehabilitative services may also have negative psychological effects on coronary patients. The organizational arrangements, bureaucratic rules and procedures, administrative policies, professional conflicts and rivalries within agencies, staff motivation and morale, and the quality of performance of workers in an agency may have negative consequences not intended by those responsible for planning and supervision.[286] For example, the transfer of a patient from the coronary care unit to a general care area with fewer nurses may not necessarily be reassuring; it may engender stress if the patient feels vulnerable away from the protection of the coronary care unit. This problem can be obviated by explanations about the decreased need for surveillance reflecting clinical improvement given prior to transfer of the patient. Routine policies restricting visiting in a coronary care unit may create emotional deprivation. Receiving contradictory evaluations, information, and advice from different personnel regarding their illness and its prognosis can have potential serious repercussions.[287,288] The patient who develops rapport with one professional may discover that that individual is no longer available. Although the patient may have progressed in the psychosocial readjustment to illness, there is now necessity to begin once again to explain the circumstances and feelings to new personnel. When this happens repeatedly, the patient bears the added discomforts and delays.[286]

The beliefs and values of the society outside the hospital and rehabilitation agency influence their decisions and performance in many ways.[289,290] Coronary patients may have feelings of helplessness and anger if they believe their experiences with the staff reflect responses to their color, religion, or social class. Feelings of unworthiness, depression, or of being viewed with disdain may emerge, at times with justification, because of ways in which personnel respond to their problems. These feelings influence rehabilitation in a negative way and may cause some patients to discontinue seeking rehabilitative services, even though this may be detrimental to their long-term outcome.

There may be varying need for psychological rehabilitation services among coronary patients. While some patients profit from formal support and intervention, it is advantageous for other patients to deal with emotional adaptations to illness on their own. Additionally, for many coronary patients who might benefit from psychosocial services, lack of access to them may impede rehabilitation.

THE ROLE OF SOCIAL RESOURCES IN CORONARY REHABILITATION[5,273]

The social environment appears to play a role in the development of coronary disease, with predisposing features including social disorganization, rapid social mobility, occupational and geographic mobility, marital status, and so forth. Another common element in increased coronary risk is limited social and community attachments and resources. This observation has accentuated the focus on the role of the social network in enhancing rehabilitation after myocardial infarction.

Interpersonal Relationships: Barriers and Facilitators[5]

RELATIONSHIP OF THE PATIENT WITH HEALTH PROFESSIONALS

Physicians, nurses, and other health professionals interact with the patient in positive and negative ways. Patients cared for in university medical centers and teaching hospitals are also confronted by an array of medical students, student nurses, and resident physicians, with a rapid turnover in attending physicians; these patients are involved in a system-patient relationship rather than the traditional doctor-patient relationship.

While the doctor-patient relationship is often a powerful and constructive force in rehabilitation, potential barriers exist. Iatrogenic illness sometimes occurs because inadequate, misinterpreted, and often forgotten communication between doctor and patient provokes anxiety which interferes with return to normal activity. Communication barriers are more marked when physicians and patients are of widely different social and cultural backgrounds[280,281] and when patients are not encouraged to ask questions and discuss problems.[71]

Another impediment is the lack of provision of sufficient information. This may stem from the physician's giving ambiguous or inadequate information regarding job stress, sexual expectations, or acceptable levels of physical exertion. The physician who is reluctant to permit the recovered patient to return to full activity creates a barrier to rehabilitation.

Frequently the coronary patient's self-perception is of greater impairment than is objectively determined on a medical basis,; these patients consider that the physician has inadequately assessed their extent of disability.

RELATIONSHIP OF THE PATIENT WITH SIGNIFICANT FAMILY, FRIENDS, AND NEIGHBORS[291,292]

The change in family roles due to illness often introduces difficult reorganizations of responsibility, activity, and decision-making powers in the family. When spouse and children must undertake new roles and the patient is placed in a subordinate position, two categories of problems may emerge. If the patient accepts a passive role, the status of a permanent "cardiac cripple" may occur. Alternatively, the patient may fight back, while the spouse and children struggle for dominance, believing this to be in the patient's best interest. Family goals, needs, demands, and life-style may constitute impediments to rehabilitation, particularly when they are associated with status in the community; they may cause the patient to deny the reality of illness to maintain the "normal" family life-style.

Flexibility of both spouses is important in long-term rehabilitation. A high degree of flexibility permits adaptation to changes in relationships, task distribution, decision-making, and responsibilities. A barrier to rehabilitation occurs when a spouse considers the patient to be more dependent and disabled than is the case.[292] For example, a spouse may fear the cardiac risk of sexual intercourse; behaviors which discourage advances may seriously impede the patient's sexual rehabilitation and self-image.

For the coronary patient who is a wife and mother, significant changes may occur in the household; a housekeeper may have to be employed, a nursery found for the children, or other family members may have to assume her former responsibilities. Often these changes engender resentment. The greater the changes the family must make, the poorer the prognosis for rehabilitation of the coronary patient.[292a]

In recovery, inappropriate emphasis tends to be placed on the medical network as the most relevant source of support, often excluding other important sources. Family and friends play a vital role.[293]

INTERPERSONAL RELATIONSHIPS IN THE WORK SPHERE

Some relationships between patients and employers may threaten rehabilitation. Although employers often rehire workers with satisfactory work records, some patients are forced to change jobs and/or to find a new employer after myocardial infarction, especially unskilled and semiskilled workers who perform high levels of physical activity.

Even changing jobs within a firm may impede vocational rehabilitation when seniority rules require the transferred person to start at the bottom of the seniority ladder in terms of pay, pension prospects, and assurance of continued employment.[294]

Because some patients fear losing their jobs for suboptimal physical performance, they may inappropriately overexert, placing themselves at undue risk. Relationships with fellow employees are important. The patient may choose to maintain an image as an effective worker by functioning at an exertional level inappropriately high for physical status. In other instances, a patient may shirk physical work for fear of precipitating symptoms on the job and as a result be resented by fellow workers for inadequate performance. The patient must often make this difficult choice between maintaining status and protecting health.

Legal, Insurance, and Industrial Aspects of Rehabilitation

Many barriers to rehabilitation of the coronary patient stem from laws and regulations, previously intended to protect or compensate the patient, but which are counterproductive to rehabilitation; these require modification and updating. Insurance payments and compensation which discourage rehabilitation must be identified, as well as attitudes in management and labor which have comparable effects; these features also affect the governmental and legislative spheres.

Unions

Unions have an ambivalent role in encouraging impaired workers to return to work. For the coronary patient with a stable work record and good performance, many unions will fight for reinstatement and seniority rights. Within a union-regulated setting, however, seniority rules may become a vocational barrier when a job change is necessary. There is considerable variation in attitudes and practices among unions.

The Role of Social Resources in Recovery

The degree of social integration is a function of social resources and encompasses support derived from a variety of informal and formal social groups.[284,295] The extent to which supportive social resources are effectively utilized[296] appears to favorably affect recovery, both with and without formal rehabilitative intervention.

Since the majority of coronary patients in the United States appear to use informal support services to achieve their rehabilitation outcome, the roles of family members, employers, organizational support systems, churches, community facilities, etc., assume great importance. Since the educated, white-collar, affluent patients typically have greater and more diversified support mechanisms, it is not surprising that discrepancy exists in determinants of ability and disability. Although rehabilitative goals are comparable for all patients, the processes which each patient may require vary considerably, as do the ranges of success.

Productive Roles

A productive role is often defined as return to work; the shortcoming of this definition needs emphasis. Constructive alternatives are available for the survivor of myocardial infarction within the family and community outside of the remunerative, vocational area.

Avocational Rehabilitation

Increasing attention must be devoted to avocational rehabilitation, particularly for patients older than age 65; this aspect is increasingly important as longevity continues to increase. Health professionals often have more difficulty in assessing the work requirements and skills needed for avocational and recreational activities. More physical energy is often expended in recreational than vocational activities. Additionally, more women currently require this aspect of rehabilitation and counseling than vocational counseling after recovery from infarction. The principles used for vocational rehabilitation should be adapted to counsel and recondition patients for recreational tasks as well. A continued active life-style among aging coronary patients may help limit the need for expensive skilled nursing facilities and nursing homes. More rehabilitation services may be required in future years for older patients with coronary disease.

Formal Rehabilitation Organizations, Institutions, and Agencies

Formal rehabilitation services refer to those regularly provided by agencies and individuals; these include hospitals, clinics, physicians, and public agencies such as vocational rehabilitation agencies. Private rehabilitative services and those of voluntary health agencies are also considered.

RESTRICTIVE PATIENT SELECTION

Governmental and other vocational rehabilitation institutions do not accept all working-age patients with work potential. Their financial support, particularly in government agencies, depends on the number of disabled persons successfully returned to work. In effect, eligibility is restricted to coronary patients with a high probability of return to work because they are likely to return to a prior occupation or because they can readily change jobs and/or employers. Thus, coronary patients who are older, have minimal education, have low-grade occupational skills, and/or have severe disability are usually not served by formal rehabilitation programs of state-federal rehabilitation agencies.

Patients with complicated cardiovascular problems, low occupational skill levels, poor work histories, and older patients, i.e., those most in need of rehabilitative services, are often not served by any vocational rehabilitation institution.[297] including governmental agencies. Similarly, women with myocardial infarction are often excluded as poor vocational risks.

AVAILABILITY AND ACCESS

Although there are a large number of rehabilitation institutions and programs in hospitals, clinics, and agencies, they appear sparsely distributed in many areas of the country. Limitation of availability and access in some geographic areas constitutes an inequity in the delivery of rehabilitation services.[196]

Differential access to institutions and services for coronary rehabilitation appears dependent on racial, sexual, ethnic, and socioeconomic categories.[279a,298] Nonreferral is another problem; referral may not occur because physicians are unaware of available services, because they have an uncertain or negative opinion of the value of these services, or because they believe that rehabilitation can occur through the strictly medical care aspect. Thus, some coronary patients may have to make their own contacts with the organizations, institutions, and facilities for needed rehabilitative services.

ALTERNATIVES TO FORMAL REHABILITATION INSTITUTIONS[284]

The majority of disabled coronary patients in the United States do not use formal rehabilitation services and apparently rely on supportive networks in the community.[295,299–302] The informal social network, which includes family, friends, neighbors, unions, employers, fraternal and religious organizations, etc., is an important resource for patients recovering from major medical problems.[293,295,303,304] Only when this support system fails does the individual typically rely on more formal social facilities. The higher the level of social resources, the higher the rate of recovery and rehabilitation as measured by return to work, lack of limitation of activity, source of income, and physician supervision, whether or not formal intervention services are needed or used.

Self-reliance appears to be a key determinant of success. Individuals who need the more structured social services tend to have limited informal and community resources and, perhaps related to this, may not have the necessary self-reliance. Motivation, self-image, and the social support mechanisms determine the outcome almost as much as some clinical considerations.

Societal Factors[305]

Societal factors influence the options open to disabled coronary patients. Some factors are more amenable to change than others; even when societal conditions cannot be altered, it is important to understand how they operate.

Unskilled and many semiskilled workers are frequently underemployed, in part due to continuing technological changes and in part to cyclical economic variations.[306] Many of these individuals have a lifelong record of unemployment and unstable income. Predisability employment problems become forbidding barriers in rehabilitating these individuals; the stable income of workmen's compensation is a desirable alternative to work. High levels of unemployment impede the vocational rehabilitation of coronary patients. Since unemployment is unequally distributed in occupations and is higher in low-skill occupations, persons in these occupations have a lesser chance to return to work after infarction than skilled workers.[286,307] A high level of unemployment is a barrier to the employment of women, blacks, and older patients with coronary disease in the United States.

Some jobs more or less explicitly require overtime work. Lack of part-time and flexible-time work may also limit vocational rehabilitation of moderately disabled coronary patients, especially those who have had a complicated myocardial infarction with residual cardiac dysfunction which mandates limited or part-time work.

Productive roles other than work are acceptable alternatives for disabled coronary patients. Return to remunerative work should not be the sole criterion of rehabilitation success. However, this is an enormously complicated problem because the work ethic can facilitate or impede rehabilitation; it may be a barrier if return to work under any circumstance is overemphasized and other aspects of rehabilitation such as psychological, familial, sexual, and social are neglected.

In many instances, disabled coronary patients are not evaluated on individual merit and ability but are categorized as "heart cases." Discrimination is reenforced when the disabled coronary patient belongs to another societal subgroup in the United States such as women, older individuals, or black patients; multiple subgroup membership may pose a significant barrier to vocational and other aspects of rehabilitation for coronary patients.[308]

People with hidden disabilities, e.g., coronary disease, appear physically nondisabled and thus are expected to be self-sufficient and compete equally in the labor market. An equal problem is that in the disabled community, they are often outcasts because of not being "disabled enough," as they are thought able to compete with active, assertive persons without disabilities.

An additional societal influence on the rehabilitation of coronary patients is the complex of factors constituting the health care system. The level of development, the specific rules and administrative arrangements, the system of financing, and the degree to which provisions are made for coronary patients requiring rehabilitative services and benefits are important components. Molding the complex arrangements in a health care system are societal dimensions, such as political and economic systems, the bureaucracy in government, health care values, the rights of individuals in a society, and the relative importance of rehabilitation to that society. Thus, the way in which an individual coronary patient fares reflects a large number of interrelated complex societal institutions and values.[5]

REFERENCES

1 Gibran, Kahlil: On Work, in "The Prophet," Alfred A. Knopf, Inc., New York, 1923.

2 Report of the Working Group on Arteriosclerosis of the National Heart, Lung, and Blood Institute: Summary, Conclusions, and Recommendations, in "Arteriosclerosis 1981" (NIH Publication No. 81-2034), Vol. 1, U.S. Department of Health and Human Services, Public Health Service, Washington, D.C., 1981.

3 Weinblatt, E., Goldberg, J. D., Ruberman, W., Frank, C. W., Monk, M. A., and Chaudhary, B. S.: Mortality after First Myocardial Infarction. Search for a Secular Trend, *J.A.M.A.*, 247:1576, 1982.

4 Francis, C. K.: Cardiac Rehabilitation: Current Physician Attitudes, in L. S. Cohen, M. B. Mock, and I. Ringqvist (eds.), "Physical Conditioning and Cardiovascular Rehabilitation," John Wiley & Sons, New York, 1981, p. 239.

5 Report of the Task Force on Cardiovascular Rehabilitation, National Heart and Lung Institute: "Needs and Opportunities for Rehabilitating the Coronary Heart Disease Patient" [Department of Health, Education and Welfare Publication No. (NIH) 75-750], Washington, D.C., December 15, 1974.

6 Coronary Heart Disease Study Group: Optimal Resources for the Care of Patients with Acute Myocardial Infarction and Chronic Coronary Heart Disease, *Circulation*, 65:654B, 1982.

7 Zohman, L. R., and Tobis, J. S.: "Cardiac Rehabilitation," Grune & Stratton, Inc., New York, 1970.

8 International Society of Cardiology, Scientific Council on Rehabilitation of Coronary Patients: "Myocardial Infarction: How to Prevent, How to Rehabilitate," Boehringer, Mannheim, West Germany, 1973.

9 Wenger, N. K., and Hellerstein, H. K. (eds.): "Rehabilitation of the Coronary Patient," John Wiley & Sons, Inc., New York, 1978.

10 Pollock, M. L., and Schmidt, D. H. (eds.): "Heart Disease and Rehabilitation," Houghton Mifflin Company, Boston, 1979.

11 Fletcher, G. F., and Cantwell, J. D.: "Exercise and Coronary Heart Disease: Role in Prevention, Diagnosis, Treatment," 2d ed., Charles C Thomas, Publisher, Springfield, Ill., 1979.

12 Council on Scientific Affairs: Physician-supervised Exercise Programs in Rehabilitation of Patients with Coronary Heart Disease, *J.A.M.A.*, 245:1463, 1981.

13 State of the Art, 1983, *J. Cardiac Rehabil.*, 2:429, 1982.

14 Saltin, B., Blomqvist, G., Mitchell, J. H., Johnson, R. L., Wildenthal, K., and Chapman, C. B.: Response to Exercise after Bed Rest and after Training, *Circulation*, 37,38(suppl. 7):1, 1968.

15 Silvidi, G. E., Squires, R. W., Pollock, M. L., and Foster, C.: Hemodynamic Responses and Medical

Problems Associated with Early Exercise and Ambulation in Coronary Artery Bypass Graft Surgery Patients, *J. Cardiac. Rehabil.*, 2:355, 1982.

16 Wenger, N. K., Hellerstein, H. K., Blackburn, H. W., and Castranova, S. J.: Uncomplicated Myocardial Infarction: Current Physician Practice in Patient Management, *J.A.M.A.*, 224:511, 1973.

17 Niemela, K., Takkunen, J. T., Juustila, H., Jounela, A. J., Palatsi, I., and Kaipainen, W. J.: Feasibility of Early Mobilization after Acute Myocardial Infarction, *Ann. Clin. Res.*, 10:328, 1978.

18 Swan, H. J. C., Blackburn, H. W., DeSanctis, R., et al.: Duration of Hospitalization in Uncomplicated Completed Acute Myocardial Infarction, An Ad Hoc Committee Review, *Am. J. Cardiol.*, 37:413, 1976.

19 Lau, Y. K., Smith, J., Morrison, S. L., and Chamberlain, D. A.: Policy for Early Discharge after Acute Myocardial Infarction, *Br. Med. J.*, 280:1489, 1980.

20 Hurst, J. W.: "Ambulation" after Myocardial Infarction, *N. Engl. J. Med.*, 292:746, 1975.

21 Convertino, V., Hung, J., Goldwater, D., and DeBusk, R. F.: Cardiovascular Responses to Exercise in Middle-aged Men after 10 Days of Bedrest, *Circulation*, 65:134, 1982.

22 Mitchell, J. H., and Blomqvist, C. G.: Response of Patients with Heart Disease to Dynamic and Static Exercise, in M. L. Pollock and D. H. Schmidt (eds.), "Heart Disease and Rehabilitation," Houghton Mifflin Company, Boston, 1979, p. 86.

23 Groden, B. M., and Brown, R. I. F.: Differential Psychological Effects of Early and Late Mobilisation after Myocardial Infarction, *Scand. J. Rehabil. Med.*, 2:60, 1970.

24 Groden, B. M.: The Management of Myocardial Infarction. A Controlled Study of the Effects of Early Mobilization, *Cardiac Rehabil.*, 1:13, 1971.

25 Harpur, J. E., Kellett, R. J., Conner, W. T., et al.: Controlled Trial of Early Mobilization and Discharge from Hospital in Uncomplicated Myocardial Infarction, *Lancet*, 2:1331, 1971.

26 Lamers, H. J., Drost, W. S. J., Kroon, B. J. M., van Es, L. A., Meilink-Hoedmaker, L. J., and Birkenhager, W. H.: Early Mobilization after Myocardial Infarction: A Controlled Study, *Br. Med. J.*, 1:257, 1973.

27 Hutter, A. M., Jr., Sidel, V. W., Shine, K. I., and DeSanctis, R. W.: Early Hospital Discharge after Myocardial Infarction, *N. Engl. J. Med.*, 288:1141, 1973.

28 Boyle, J. A., and Lorimer, A. R.: Early Mobilisation after Uncomplicated Myocardial Infarction. Prospective Study of 538 Patients, *Lancet*, 2:346, 1973.

29 Hayes, M. J., Morris, G. K., and Hamptom, J. R.: Comparison of Mobilization after Two and Nine Days in Uncomplicated Myocardial Infarction, *Br. Med. J.*, 3:10, 1974.

30 Bloch, A., Maeder, J.-P., Haissly, J.-C., Felix, J., and Blackburn, H.: Early Mobilization after Myocardial Infarction. A Controlled Study, *Am. J. Cardiol.*, 34:152, 1974.

31 Ahlmark, G., Ahlberg, G., Saetre, H., Haglund, I., and Korsgren, M.: A Controlled Study of Early Discharge after Uncomplicated Myocardial Infarction, *Acta Med. Scand.*, 206:87, 1979.

32 West, R. R., and Henderson, A. H.: Randomised Multicentre Trial of Early Mobilisation after Uncomplicated Myocardial Infarction, *Br. Heart J.*, 42:381, 1979.

33 Sivarajan, E. S., Bruce, R. A., Almes, M. J., et al.: In-hospital Exercise after Myocardial Infarction Does Not Improve Treadmill Performance, *N. Engl. J. Med.*, 305:357, 1981.

34 West, R. R.: Early Mobilization after Uncomplicated Myocardial Infarction, *Am. Heart J.*, 103:311, 1982.

35 Baughman, K. L., Hutter, A. M., Jr., DeSanctis, R. W., and Kallman, C. H.: Early Discharge following Acute Myocardial Infarction. Long-term Follow-up of Randomized Patients, *Arch. Intern. Med.*, 142:875, 1982.

36 Lies, J. L., Carretta, R. F., Amsterdam, E. A., et al.: Lower Extremity Venous Thrombosis in Coronary-Care Unit Patients: Prevention by Early Ambulation and Confirmation by I^{125} Fibrinogen and Venography, *Circulation*, 50(suppl. 3):298, 1974.

37 McNeer, J. F., Wagner, G. S., Ginsburg, P. B., et al.: Hospital Discharge One Week after Acute Myocardial Infarction, *N. Engl. J. Med.*, 298:229, 1978.

38 Thockloth, R. M., Ho, S. C., Wright, H., and Seldon, W. A.: Is Cardiac Rehabilitation Really Necessary?, *Med. J. Aust.*, 2:669, 1973.

39 Schiller, E., and Baker, J.: Return to Work after a Myocardial Infarction, *Med. J. Aust.*, 1:859, 1976.

40 Thornley, P. E., and Turner, R. W. D.: Rapid Mobilisation after Acute Myocardial Infarction: First Step in Rehabilitation and Secondary Prevention, *Br. Heart J.*, 39:471, 1977.

41 Ericsson, M., Granath, A., Ohlsen, P., Sodermark, T., and Volpe, U.: Arrhythmias and Symptoms during Treadmill Testing Three Weeks after Myocardial Infarction in 100 Patients, *Br. Heart J.*, 35:787, 1973.

42 Sivarajan, E. S., Lerman, J., Mansfield, L. W., and Bruce, R. A.: Progressive Ambulation and Treadmill Testing of Patients with Acute Myocardial Infarction during Hospitalization: A Feasibility Study, *Arch. Phys. Med. Rehabil.*, 58:241, 1977.

43 Markiewicz, W., Houston, N., and DeBusk, R. F.: Exercise Testing Soon after Myocardial Infarction, *Circulation*, 56:26, 1977.

44 Wohl, A. J., Lewis, H. R., Campbell, W., et al.: Cardiovascular Function during Early Recovery from Acute Myocardial Infarction, *Circulation*, 56:931, 1977.

45 Jelinek, M. V., Ziffer, R. W., McDonald, J. G., Waser, H., and Hale, G. S.: Early Exercise Testing and Mo-

bilization after Myocardial Infarction, *Med. J. Aust.*, 2:589, 1977.

46 DeBusk, R. F.: Early Exercise Testing after Myocardial Infarction, in N. K. Wenger (ed.), "Exercise and the Heart," F. A. Davis Company, Philadelphia, 1978.

47 Smith, J. W., Dennis, C. A., Gassman, A., et al.: Exercise Testing Three Weeks after Myocardial Infarction, *Chest*, 75:12, 1979.

48 Lindvall, K., Erhardt, L. R., Lundman, T., Rehnqvist, N., and Sjogren, A.: Early Mobilization and Discharge of Patients with Acute Myocardial Infarction. A Prospective Study using Risk Indicators and Early Exercise Tests, *Acta Med. Scand.*, 206:169, 1979.

49 Granath, A., Sodermark, T., Winge, T., Volpe, V., and Zetterquist, S.: Early Work Load Tests for Evaluation of Long-Term Prognosis of Acute Myocardial Infarction, *Br. Heart J.*, 39:758, 1977.

50 Theroux, P., Waters, D. D., Halphen, C., Debaisieux, J. C., and Mizgala, H. F.: Prognostic Value of Exercise Testing Soon after Myocardial Infarction, *N. Engl. J. Med.*, 301:341, 1979.

51 Davidson, D. M., and DeBusk, R. F.: Prognostic Value of a Single Exercise Test Three Weeks after Myocardial Infarction, *Circulation*, 61:236, 1980.

52 Sterling, M. R., Crawford, M. H., Richards, K. L., and O'Rourke, R. A.: Predictive Value of Early Postmyocardial Infarction Modified Treadmill Exercise Testing in Multivessel Coronary Artery Disease Detection, *Am. Heart J.*, 102:169, 1981.

53 Weld, F. M., Chu, K. L., Bigger, J. T., Jr., and Rolnitzky, L. M.: Risk Stratification with Low-Level Exercise Testing 2 Weeks after Acute Myocardial Infarction, *Circulation*, 64:306, 1981.

54 Wenger, N. K., Hellerstein, H. K., Blackburn, H., and Castranova, S. J.: Physician Practice in the Management of Patients with Uncomplicated Myocardial Infarction—Changes in the Past Decade, *Circulation*, 65:421, 1982.

55 Rochmis, P., and Blackburn, H.: Exercise Tests: A Survey of Procedures, Safety and Litigation Experience in Approximately 170,000 Tests, *J.A.M.A.*, 217:1061, 1971.

56 McHenry, P. L., and Morris, S. N.: Exercise Electrocardiography—Current State of the Art, in R. C. Schlant and J. W. Hurst (eds.), "Advances in Electrocardiography," Vol. 2, Grune & Stratton, Inc., New York, 1976, p. 265.

57 "The Exercise Standards Book," American Heart Association, 70-041-A, Dallas, Texas, 1979.

58 Niederberger, M.: Values and Limitations of Exercise Testing after Myocardial Infarction with Special Reference to Quantitative Criteria, *Acta Med. Aust.*, 4(suppl. 9):1, 1977.

59 Jorgensen, C. R., Wang, K., Wang, Y., Gobel, F. L., Nelson, R. R., and Taylor, H.: Effects of Propranolol on Myocardial Oxygen Consumption and Its Hemodynamic Correlates during Upright Exercise, *Circulation*, 48:1173, 1973.

60 Wenger, N. K.: The Coronary Patient: Interactions of Cardiovascular Drugs and Exercise, *Drug Therapy*, 13:59, 1982.

61 Criteria Committee of the New York Heart Association, Inc.: "Diseases of the Heart and Blood Vessels (Nomenclature and Criteria for Diagnosis)," 6th ed., Little, Brown and Company, Boston, 1964.

62 Astrand, P. O., and Rodahl, K.: "Textbook of Work Physiology," McGraw-Hill Book Company, New York, 1970.

63 Gordon, E. E.: The Use of Energy Costs in Regulating Physical Activity in Chronic Disease, *A.M.A. Arch. Indus. Med. Health*, 16:437, 1957.

64 Subcommittee on Exercise/Rehabilitation, Target Activity Group: Standards for Supervised Cardiovascular Exercise Maintenance Programs, *Circulation*, 62:669A, 1980.

65 Kjoller, E.: Resumption of Work after Acute Myocardial Infarction, *Acta Med. Scand.*, 199:379, 1976.

66 Savin, W. M., Haskell, W. L., Houston-Miller, N., and DeBusk, R.: Improvement in Aerobic Capacity Soon after Myocardial Infarction, *J. Cardiac Rehabil.*, 1:337, 1981.

67 Borg, G.: Perceived Exertion as an Indicator of Somatic Stress, *Scand. J. Rehabil. Med.*, 2:92, 1970.

68 Burch, G. E., and Giles, T. D.: The Burden of a Hot and Humid Environment on the Heart, *Mod. Concepts Cardiovasc. Dis.*, 39:115, 1970.

69 Rowell, L. B.: Human Cardiovascular Adjustments to Exercise and Thermal Stress, *Physiol. Rev.*, 54:75, 1974.

70 Raven, P. B.: Heat and Air Pollution: The Cardiac Patient, in M. L. Pollock and D. H. Schmidt, "Heart Disease and Rehabilitation," Houghton Mifflin, Boston, 1979, p. 563.

71 Hackett, T. P., and Cassem, N. H.: White-collar and Blue-collar Responses to Heart Attack, *J. Psychosom. Res.*, 20:85, 1976.

72 Frick, M. H., and Katila, M.: Hemodynamic Consequences of Physical Training after Myocardial Infarction, *Circulation*, 37:192, 1968.

73 Clausen, J. P., Larsen, O. A., and Trap-Jensen, J.: Physical Training in the Management of Coronary Artery Disease, *Circulation*, 40:143, 1969.

74 Committee on Exercise, American Heart Association: "Exercise Testing and Training of Individuals with Heart Disease or at High Risk for Its Development: A Handbook for Physicians," American Heart Association, New York, 70-008-B, 1975.

75 American College of Sports Medicine: "Guidelines for Graded Exercise Testing and Exercise Prescription," Lea & Febiger, Philadelphia, 1975.

76 Mitchell, J. H.: Exercise Training in the Treatment of Coronary Heart Disease, *Adv. Intern. Med.*, 20:249, 1975.

77 Fox, S. M., III, Naughton, J. P., and Gorman, P. A.: Physical Activity and Cardiovascular Health: I. Potential for Prevention of Coronary Heart Disease and Possible Mechanisms; II. The Exercise Prescription: Intensity and Duration; III. The Exercise Prescription: Frequency and Type of Activity, *Mod. Concepts Cardiovasc. Dis.*, 41:17, 1972.

78 Hellerstein, H. K., Hirsch, E. Z., Ader, R., Greenblott, N., and Siegel, M.: Principles of Exercise Prescription for Normal and Cardiac Subjects, in J. P. Naughton, H. K. Hellerstein, and I. C. Mohler (eds.), "Exercise Testing and Exercise Training in Coronary Heart Disease," Academic Press, New York, 1973, p. 129.

79 Pollock, M., Gettman, L., Milesis, C., Bah, M. D., Durstine, L., and Johnson, R. B.: Effects of Frequency and Duration of Training on Attrition and Incidence of Injury, *Med. Sci. Sports*, 9:31, 1977.

80 Shaw, L. W.: Effects of a Prescribed Supervised Exercise Program on Mortality and Cardiovascular Morbidity in Patients after a Myocardial Infarction. The National Exercise and Heart Disease Project, *Am. J. Cardiol.*, 48:39, 1981.

81 Haskell, W. L.: Design and Implementation of Cardiac Conditioning Programs, in N. K. Wenger and H. K. Hellerstein (eds.), "Rehabilitation of the Coronary Patient," John Wiley & Sons, New York, 1978, p. 203.

82 Bruce, R. A., DeRouen, T., Peterson, D. R., et al.: Noninvasive Predictors of Sudden Coronary Death in Men with Coronary Heart Disease, *Am. J. Cardiol.*, 39:833, 1977.

83 Stoedefalke, K. G.: The Principles of Conducting Exercise Programs, in J. P. Naughton, H. K. Hellerstein and I. C. Mohler (eds.), "Exercise Testing and Exercise Training in Coronary Heart Disease," Academic Press, New York, 1973, p. 299.

84 Williams, R. S., Miller, H., Koisch, F. P., Jr., Ribisl, P., and Graden, H.: Guidelines for Unsupervised Exercise in Patients with Ischemic Heart Disease, *J. Cardiac Rehabil.*, 1:214, 1981.

85 Hossack, K. F., and Hartwig, R.: Cardiac Arrest Associated with Supervised Cardiac Rehabilitation, *J. Cardiac Rehabil.*, 2:402, 1982.

86 Capone, R. J., Grodman, R. S., and Most, A. S.: Transtelephonic Surveillance of Cardiac Arrhythmias, *J. Cardiovasc. Med.*, 6:57, 1981.

87 DeBusk, R. F., Houston, N., Haskell, W., Fry, G., and Parker, M.: Exercise Training Soon after Myocardial Infarction, *Am. J. Cardiol.*, 44:1223, 1979.

88 Schwade, J., Blomqvist, C. G., and Shapiro, W.: A Comparison of the Response to Arm and Leg Work in Patients with Ischemic Heart Disease, *Am. Heart J.*, 94:203, 1977.

89 Haskell, W. L.: Cardiovascular Complications during Exercise Training of Cardiac Patients, *Circulation*, 57:920, 1978.

90 Hartung, G. H., and Rangel, R.: Exercise Training in Post-myocardial Infarction Patients: Comparison of Results with High Risk Coronary and Post-Bypass Patients, *Arch. Phys. Med. Rehabil.*, 22:147, 1981.

91 Pyfer, H. R., Mead, W. F., Frederick, R. C., and Doane, B. L.: Exercise Rehabilitation in Coronary Heart Disease: Community Group Programs, *Arch. Phys. Med. Rehabil.*, 57:335, 1976.

92 Oldridge, N. B., Donner, A. P., Buck, C. W., et al.: Predictors of Dropout from Cardiac Exercise Rehabilitation. Ontario Exercise-Heart Collaborative Study, *Am. J. Cardiol.*, 51:70, 1982.

93 Detry, J.-M. R., Rousseau, M., Vandenbroucke, G., Kusumi, F., Brasseur, L. A., and Bruce, R. A.: Increased Arteriovenous Oxygen Difference after Physical Training in Coronary Heart Disease, *Circulation*, 44:109, 1971.

94 Redwood, D. R., Rosing, D. R., and Epstein, S. E.: Circulatory and Symptomatic Effects of Physical Training in Patients with Coronary Artery Disease and Angina Pectoris, *N. Engl. J. Med.*, 286:959, 1972.

95 Kentala, E.: Physical Fitness and Feasibility of Physical Rehabilitation after Myocardial Infarction in Men of Working Age, *Ann. Clin. Res.*, 4(suppl. 91), 1972, p. 1.

96 Rousseau, M. F., Brasseur, L. A., and Detry, J.-M.: Hemodynamic Determinants of Maximal Oxygen Intake in Patients with Healed Myocardial Infarction. Influence of Physical Training, *Circulation*, 48:943, 1973.

97 Detry, J.-M. R., Rousseau, M., and Brasseur, L. A.: Early Hemodynamic Adaptations to Physical Training in Patients with Healed Myocardial Infarction, *Eur. J. Cardiol.*, 2/3:307, 1975.

98 Clausen, J. P.: Circulatory Adjustments to Dynamic Exercise and Effect of Physical Training in Normal Subjects and in Patients with Coronary Artery Disease, *Prog. Cardiovasc. Dis.*, 18:459, 1976.

99 Saltin, B.: The Interplay between Peripheral and Central Factors in the Adaptive Response to Exercise and Training, *Ann. N.Y. Acad. Sci.*, 301:224, 1977.

100 Wallace, A., Rerych, S., Jones, R., and Goodrich, J.: Effects of Exercise Training on Ventricular Function in Coronary Disease, *Circulation*, 57 (suppl. 2):197, 1978.

101 Paterson, D. H., Shephard, R. J., Cunningham, D., Jones, N. L., and Andrew, G.: Effects of Physical Training on Cardiovascular Function following Myocardial Infarction, *J. Appl. Physiol.*, 47:482, 1979.

102 Ehsani, A. A., Martin, W. H., III, Heath, G. W., and Coyle, E. F.: Cardiac Effects of Prolonged and Intense Exercise Training in Patients with Coronary Artery Disease, *Am. J. Cardiol.*, 50:246, 1982.

103 Sim, D. N., and Neill, W. A.: Investigation of the Phys-

iological Basis for Increased Exercise Threshold for Angina Pectoris after Physical Conditioning, *J. Clin. Invest.*, 54:763, 1974.

104 Thompson, P. D., Cullinane, E., Lazarus, B., and Carleton, R. A.: Effect of Exercise Training on the Untrained Limb. Exercise Performance of Men with Angina Pectoris, *Am. J. Cardiol.*, 48:844, 1981.

105 Lester, R. M., and Wallace, A. G.: Cardiovascular Adaptations to Beta-adrenergic Blockade during Physical Training, *Circulation*, 57,58(suppl. 2):140, 1978. (Abstract.)

106 Welton, D. E., Squires, W. G., Hartung, G. H., and Miller, R. R.: Effects of Chronic Beta Adrenergic Blockade Therapy on Exercise Training in Patients with Coronary Heart Disease, *Am. J. Cardiol.*, 43:399, 1979. (Abstract.)

107 Vanhees, L., Fagard, R., and Amery, A.: Influence of Beta Adrenergic Blockade on Effects of Physical Training in Patients with Ischaemic Heart Disease, *Br. Heart J.*, 48:33, 1982.

108 Conn, E. H., Williams, R. S., and Wallace, A. G.: Exercise Responses before and after Physical Conditioning in Patients with Severely Depressed Left Ventricular Function, *Am. J. Cardiol.*, 49:296, 1982.

109 Naughton, J.: Physical Activity for Myocardial Infarction Patients, *Cardiovascular Reviews and Reports*, 3:237, 1982.

110 Ferguson, R. J., Cote, P., Gauthier, P., and Bourassa, M. G.: Changes in Exercise Coronary Sinus Blood Flow with Training in Patients with Angina Pectoris, *Circulation*, 58:41, 1978.

111 Ferguson, R. J., Petitclerc, R., Choquette, G., et al.: Effect of Physical Training on Treadmill Exercise Capacity, Collateral Circulation, and Progression of Coronary Disease, *Am. J. Cardiol.*, 34:764, 1974.

112 Conner, J. F., LaCamera, F., Jr., Swanik, E., Oldham, M. J., Holzaepfel, D. W., and Lyczkowskyj, O.: Effects of Exercise on Coronary Collateralization and Angiographic Studies of Six Patients in a Supervised Exercise Program, *Med. Sci. Sports*, 8:145, 1976.

113 Kennedy, C. C., Spiekerman, R. E., Lindsay, M. I., Jr., Mankin, H. T., Frye, R. L., and McCallister, B. D.: One-Year Graduated Exercise Program for Men with Angina Pectoris. Evaluation by Physiologic Studies and Coronary Arteriography, *Mayo Clin. Proc.*, 51:231, 1976.

114 Cohen, M. V., Yipintsoi, T., Malhotra, A., and Scheuer, J.: Effects of Exercise on Coronary Collateral Function, *Am. J. Cardiol.*, 39:262, 1977.

115 Nolewajka, A. J., Kostuk, W. J., Rechnitzer, P. A., and Cunningham, D. A.: Exercise and Human Collaterization: An Angiographic and Scintigraphic Assessment, *Circulation*, 60:114, 1979.

116 Verani, M. S., Hartung, G. H., Hoepfel-Harris, J., Welton, D. E., Pratt, C. M., and Miller, R. R.: Effects of Exercise Training on Left Ventricular Performance and Myocardial Perfusion in Patients with Coronary Artery Disease, *Am. J. Cardiol.*, 47:797, 1981.

117 Tubau, J., Witztum, K., Froelicher, V., et al.: Noninvasive Assessment of Changes in Myocardial Perfusion and Ventricular Performance following Exercise Training, *Am. Heart J.*, 104:238, 1982.

118 Cobb, F. R., Williams, R. S., McEwan, P., Jones, R. H., Coleman, R. E., and Wallace, A. G.: Effects of Exercise Training on Ventricular Function in Patients with Recent Myocardial Infarction, *Circulation*, 66:100, 1982.

119 Letac, B., Cribier, A., and Desplanches, J. F.: A Study of Left Ventricular Function in Coronary Patients before and after Physical Training, *Circulation*, 56:375, 1977.

120 Rechnitzer, P. A., Pickard, H. A., Paivio, A. V., Yuhasz, M. S., and Cunningham, D.: Long-term Follow-up Study of Survival and Recurrence Rates following Myocardial Infarction in Exercising and Control Subjects, *Circulation*, 45:853, 1972.

121 Sanne, H.: Exercise Tolerance and Physical Training of Non-selected Patients after Myocardial Infarction, *Acta Med. Scand.*, (suppl. 551):1, 1973.

122 Wilhelmsen, L., Sanne, H., Elmfeldt, D., Grimby, G., Tibbins, G., and Wedel, H.: A Controlled Trial of Physical Training after Myocardial Infarction: Effects on Risk Factors, Nonfatal Reinfarction, and Death, *Prev. Med.*, 4:491, 1975.

123 Rechnitzer, P. A., Sangal, S., Cunningham, D. A., et al.: A Controlled Prospective Study of the Effect of Endurance Training on the Recurrence Rate of Myocardial Infarction. A Description of the Experimental Design, *Am. J. Epidemiol.*, 120:358, 1975.

124 Palatsi, I.: Feasibility of Physical Training after Myocardial Infarction and Its Effect on Return to Work, Morbidity, and Mortality, *Acta Med. Scand.*, (suppl. 599–602):1, 1976.

125 Selvester, R., Camp, J., and Sanmarco, M.: Effects of Exercise Training on Progression of Documented Coronary Atherosclerosis, in P. Mulvey (ed.), ''The Marathon: Physiological, Medical, Epidemiological, and Psychological Studies,'' New York Academy of Sciences, 1977, p. 495.

126 Rechnitzer, P. A., Cunningham, D. A., Andrew, G. M., et al.: Relation of Exercise to the Recurrence Rate of Myocardial Infarction in Men. Ontario Exercise-Heart Collaborative Study, *Am. J. Cardiol.*, 51:65, 1983.

127 Scheuer, J.: Effects of Physical Training on Myocardial Vascularity and Perfusion, *Circulation*, 66:491, 1982.

128 Kallio, V., Hamalainen, H., Hakkila, J., and Luurila, O.: Reduction in Sudden Deaths by a Multifactoral Intervention Programme after Acute Myocardial Infarction, *Lancet*, 2:1091, 1979.

129 Oscai, L. B., Patterson, J. A., Bogard, D. L., Beck,

R. J., and Rothermel, B. L.: Normalization of Serum Triglycerides and Lipoprotein Electrophoretic Patterns by Exercise, *Am. J. Cardiol.*, 30:775, 1972.

130 Enger, S. C., Herbjornsen, K., Erikssen, J., and Fretland, A.: High Density Lipoproteins (HDL) and Physical Activity: The Influence of Physical Exercise, Age and Smoking on HDL-Cholesterol and the HDL–Total Cholesterol Ratio, *Scand. J. Clin. Lab. Invest.*, 37:251, 1977.

131 Lampman, R. M., Santinga, J. T., Hodge, M. F., Block, W. D., Flora, J. D., and Bassett, D. R.: Comparative Effects of Physical Training and Diet in Normalizing Serum Lipids in Men with Type IV Hyperlipoproteinemia, *Circulation*, 55:652, 1977.

132 Lehtonen, A., and Viikari, J.: The Effect of Vigorous Physical Activity at Work on Serum Lipids with a Special Reference to Serum High-density Lipoprotein Cholesterol, *Acta Physiol. Scand.*, 104:117, 1978.

133 Williams, P., Robinson, D., and Bailey, A.: High-Density Lipoprotein and Coronary Risk Factors in Normal Men, *Lancet*, 1:72, 1979.

134 Wood, P. D., Haskell, W. L., Stern, M. P., Lewis, S., and Perry, C.: Plasma Lipoprotein Distribution in Male and Female Runners, *Ann. N.Y. Acad. Sci.*, 301:748, 1977.

135 Wood, P. D., and Haskell, W. L.: The Effect of Exercise on Plasma High-Density Lipoprotein, *Lipids*, 14:417, 1979.

136 Nikkila, E. A., Taskinen, M.-R., Rehunen, S., and Harkonen, M.: Lipoprotein Lipase Activity in Adipose Tissue and Skeletal Muscle of Runners: Relation to Serum Lipoproteins, *Metabolism*, 27:1661, 1978.

137 Williams, R. S., Logue, E. E., Lewis, J. L., et al.: Physical Conditioning Augments the Fibrinolytic Response to Venous Occlusion in Healthy Adults, *N. Engl. J. Med.*, 302:987, 1980.

138 Mann, G. V., Garrett, H. L., Farhi, A., Murray, H., and Billings, F. T.: Exercise to Prevent Coronary Heart Disease. An Experimental Study of the Effects of Training on Risk Factors for Coronary Disease in Men, *Am. J. Med.*, 46:12, 1969.

139 Bonanno, J. A., and Lies, J. A.: Effects of Physical Training on Coronary Risk Factors. *Am. J. Cardiol.*, 33:760, 1974.

140 Stein, R. A.: The Effects of Exercise Training on Heart Rate during Coitus in the Post Myocardial Infarction Patient, *Circulation*, 55:738, 1977.

141 Stern, M. J., and Cleary, P.: The National Exercise and Heart Disease Project. Long-term Psychosocial Outcome, *Arch. Intern. Med.*, 142:1093, 1982.

142 Devney, A. M.: Bridging the Gap between Inhospital and Outpatient Care, *Am. J. Nurs.*, 80:446, 1980.

143 Wallace, N., and Wallace, D. C.: Group Education after Myocardial Infarction: Is It Effective?, *Med. J. Aust.*, 2:245, 1977.

143a Zelis, R. F., and Wenger, N. K.: Prevention of Coronary Atherosclerosis, in J. W. Hurst (ed.), "The Heart," 5th ed, McGraw-Hill Book Company, New York, 1982, p. 259.

144 Goble, A.: Folklore and Disability in Heart Disease, *Cardiovasc Dis.*, 5(4): 1969.

145 Schlant, R. C., Forman, S., Stamler, J., and Canner, P.: The Natural History of Coronary Heart Disease: Prognostic Factors after Recovery from Myocardial Infarction in 2789 Men. The 5-Year Findings of the Coronary Drug Project, *Circulation*, 66:401, 1982.

146 Mulcahy, R., Hickey, N., Graham, I., and McKenzie, G.: Factors Influencing Long-term Prognosis in Male Patients Surviving a First Coronary Attack, *Br. Heart J.*, 37:158, 1975.

147 Wilhelmsson, C., Vedin, J. A., Elmfeldt, D., Tibbin, G., and Wilhelmsen, L.: Smoking and Myocardial Infarction, *Lancet*, 1:415, 1975.

148 Salonen, J. T.: Stopping Smoking and Long-term Mortality after Acute Myocardial Infarction, *Br. Heart J.*, 43:463, 1980.

149 Pozen, M. W., Stechmiller, J. A., Harris, W., Smith, S., Fried, D. D., and Voigt, G. C.: A Nurse Rehabilitator's Impact on Patients with Myocardial Infarction, *Med. Care*, 15:830, 1977.

150 Hellerstein, H. K., and Friedman, E. H.: Sexual Activity and the Post-coronary Patient, *Arch. Intern. Med.*, 125:987, 1970.

151 Stern, M. J., Pascale, L., and Ackerman, A.: Life Adjustment Post Myocardial Infarction: Determining Predictive Variables, *Arch. Intern. Med.*, 137:1680, 1977.

152 McLane, M., Krop, H., and Mehta, J.: Psychosexual Adjustment and Counseling after Myocardial Infarction, *Ann. Intern. Med.*, 92:514, 1980.

153 Papadopoulos, C., Larrimore, P., Cardin, S., and Shelley, S. I.: Sexual Concerns and Needs of the Postcoronary Patient's Wife, *Arch. Intern. Med.*, 140:38, 1980.

154 Report of a WHO Expert Committee: Prevention of Coronary Heart Disease, *WHO Tech. Rep. Ser.*, 678, Geneva, 1982.

155 Altman, L. K.: When a Damaged Heart is Part of the Vacation Luggage, "The New York Times," April 23, 1978.

156 Wenger, N. K., and Mount, F.: An Educational Algorithm for Myocardial Infarction, *Cardiovasc. Nurs.*, 10:11, 1974.

157 McWeeney, M. C.: The Patient's Right to Learn or Not to Learn, *Nurs. Admin. Q.*, 4:83, 1980.

158 Rahe, R. H., Ward, H. W., and Hayes, V.: Brief Group Therapy in Myocardial Infarction Rehabilitation: Three- to Four-Year Follow-up of a Controlled Trial, *Psychosom. Med.*, 41:229, 1979.

159 Barbarowicz, P., Nelson, M., DeBusk, R. F., and Has-

kell, W. L.: A Comparison of In-hospital Education Approaches for Coronary Bypass Patients, *Heart Lung*, 9:127, 1980.

160 Scalzi, C. C., Burke, L. E., and Greenland, S.: Evaluation of an Inpatient Education Program for Coronary Patients and Families, *Heart Lung*, 9:846, 1980.

161 Argondizzo, N. T.: Patient and Family Education, in N. K. Wenger and H. K. Hellerstein (eds.), "Rehabilitation of the Coronary Patient," John Wiley & Sons, Inc., New York, 1978, p. 117.

162 Linde, B. J., and Janz, N. M.: Effect of a Teaching Program on Knowledge and Compliance of Cardiac Patients, *Nurs. Res.*, 28:282, 1979.

163 Levine, D. M., Green, L. W., Deeds, S. G., Chwalow, J., Russell, R. P., and Finlay, J.: Health Education for Hypertensive Patients, *J.A.M.A.*, 241:1700, 1979.

164 Hogan, C. A., and Neill, W. A.: Effects of a Teaching Program on Knowledge, Physical Activity, and Socialization in Patients Disabled by Stable Angina Pectoris, *J. Cardiac Rehabil.*, 2:379, 1982.

165 Hurst, J. W., King, S. B., Logue, R. B., et al.: Value of Coronary Bypass Surgery, *Am. J. Cardiol.*, 42:308, 1978.

166 Kent, K. M., Borer, J. S., Green, M. V., et al.: Effects of Coronary-Artery Bypass on Global and Regional Left Ventricular Function during Exercise, *N. Engl. J. Med.*, 298:1434, 1978.

167 Laks, H., Kaiser, G. C., Barner, H. B., Codd, J. E., and Wellman, V. I.: Coronary Revascularization under Age 40 Years, *Am. J. Cardiol.*, 41:584, 1978.

168 Seides, S. F., Borer, J. S., Kent, K. M., Rosing, D. R., McIntosh, C. L., and Epstein, S. E.: Long-term Anatomic Fate of Coronary-Artery Bypass Grafts and Functional Status of Patients Five Years after Operation, *N. Engl. J. Med.*, 298:1213, 1978.

169 Favaloro, R. G.: Direct Myocardial Revascularization: A Ten Year Journey; Myths and Realities, *Am. J. Cardiol.*, 43:109, 1979.

170 Buccino, R. A., and McIntosh, H. D.: Aortocoronary Bypass Grafting in the Management of Patients with Coronary Artery Disease, *Am. J. Med.*, 66:651, 1979.

171 Zir, L. M., Dinsmore, R., Vexerdis, M., Singh, J. B., Harthorne, J. W., and Daggett, W. M.: Effects of Coronary Bypass Grafting on Resting Left Ventricular Contraction in Patients Studied 1 to 2 Years after Operation, *Am. J. Cardiol.*, 44:601, 1979.

172 Li, W., Riggins, R. C. K., and Anderson, R. P.: Reversal of Exertional Hypotension after Coronary Bypass Grafting, *Am. J. Cardiol.*, 44:607, 1979.

173 European Coronary Surgery Study Group: Prospective Randomized Study of Coronary Artery Bypass Surgery in Stable Angina Pectoris. Second Interim Report, *Lancet*, 2:491, 1980.

174 Almeida, D., Bradford, J. M., Wenger, N. K., King, S. B., and Hurst, J. W.: Return to Work after Coronary Bypass Surgery, *Circulation*, in press 1983.

175 Bussman, W.-D., Mayer, V., Kober, G., and Kaltenbach, M.: Regional Ventricular Function at Rest, during Leg Raising and Physical Exercise before and after Aortocoronary Bypass Surgery, in H. Roskamm and M. Schmuziger (eds.), "Coronary Heart Disease," Springer-Verlag, New York, 1979, p. 322.

176 Oldridge, N. B., Nagle, F. J., Balke, B., Corliss, R. J., and Kahn, D. R.: Aortocoronary Bypass Surgery: Effects of Surgery and 32 Months of Physical Conditioning on Treadmill Performance, *Arch. Phys. Med. Rehabil.*, 59:268, 1978.

177 Hammermeister, K. E., DeRouen, T. A., English, M. T., and Dodge, H. T.: Effect of Surgical Versus Medical Therapy on Return to Work in Patients with Coronary Artery Disease, *Am. J. Cardiol.*, 44:105, 1979.

178 Russell, R. O., Wayne, J. B., Kronenfeld, J., et al.: Surgical Versus Medical Therapy for Treatment of Unstable Angina: Changes in Work Status and Family Income, *Am. J. Cardiol.*, 45:134, 1980.

179 Logue, R. B., King, S. B., and Douglas, J. S., Jr.: A Practical Approach to Coronary Artery Disease with Special Reference to Coronary Bypass Surgery, *Curr. Probl. Cardiol.*, 1:1, 1976.

180 Rimm, A. A., Barboriak, J. J., Anderson, A. J., and Simon, J. S.: Changes in Occupation after Aortocoronary Vein-Bypass Operation, *J.A.M.A.*, 236:361, 1976.

181 Lawrie, G. M., Lie, J. T., Morris, G. C., Jr., and Beazley, H. L.: Vein Graft Patency and Intimal Proliferation after Aortocoronary Bypass: Early and Long-term Angiopathologic Correlations, *Am. J. Cardiol.*, 38:856, 1976.

182 Barnes, G. K., Ray, M. J., Oberman, A., and Kouchoukos, N. T.: Changes in Working Status of Patients following Coronary Bypass Surgery, *J.A.M.A.*, 238:1259, 1977.

183 David, P.: Contributing Factors Preventing Return to Work of Cardiac Surgery Patients, in H. Roskamm and M. Schmuziger (eds.), "Coronary Heart Surgery," Springer-Verlag, New York, 1979, p. 370.

184 Frick, M. H., Harjola, P.-T., and Valle, M.: Work Status after Coronary Bypass Surgery. A Prospective Randomized Study with Ergometric and Angiographic Correlations. *Acta Med. Scand.*, 206:61, 1979.

185 Symmes, J. C., Lenkei, S. C. M., and Berman, N. D.: Influence of Aortocoronary Bypass Surgery on Employment, *Can. Med. Assoc. J.*, 118:268, 1978.

186 Wallwork, J., Potter, B., and Caves, P. K.: Return to Work after Coronary Artery Surgery for Angina, *Br. Med. J.*, 2:1680, 1978.

187 Bensch, L., Neuhaus, K. L., Rivas-Martin, J., and Loogen, F.: Clinical Results and Return to Work after Coronary Heart Surgery, in H. Roskamm and M. Schmuziger (eds), "Coronary Heart Surgery," Springer-Verlag, New York, 1979, p. 379.

188 Johnson, W. D., Kayser, K. L., Pedraza, P. M., and Shore, R. T.: Employment Patterns in Males before and after Myocardial Revascularization Surgery. A Study

of 2229 Consecutive Male Patients Followed for as Long as 10 Years, *Circulation,* 65:1086, 1982.

189 Smith, H. C., Hamnes, L., Gupta, S., Vlietstra, R. E., and Elverback, L.: Employment Status after Coronary Artery Bypass Surgery, *Circulation,* 65(suppl. 2):120, 1982.

190 Blumchen, G., Scharp-Bornhofen, E., Brandt, D., van den Bergh, C., and Bierck, G.: Clinical Results and Social Implications in Patients after Coronary Bypass Surgery, in H. Roskamm and M. Schmuziger (eds.), "Coronary Heart Surgery," Springer-Verlag, New York, 1979, p. 375.

191 Crosby, I. K., Wellons, H. A., Jr., Martin, R. P., Schuck, D., and Muller, W. H., Jr.: Employability—A New Indication for Aneurysmectomy and Coronary Revascularization, *Circulation,* 62(suppl. 1):79, 1980.

192 Anderson, A. J., Barboriak, J. J., Hoffmann, R. G., and Mullen, D. C.: Retention or Resumption of Employment after Aortocoronary Bypass Operations, *J.A.M.A.,* 243:543, 1980.

193 Oberman, A. and Kouchoukos, N. T.: Role of Exercise after Coronary Artery Bypass Surgery, in N. K. Wenger (ed.), "Exercise and the Heart," F. A. Davis Company, Philadelphia, 1978, p. 155.

194 Dion, W. F., Grevenow, P., Squires, R. W., et al.: Medical Problems and Physiologic Responses during Supervised Inpatient Cardiac Rehabilitation: The Patient after Coronary Artery Bypass Grafting, *Heart Lung,* 11:248, 1982.

195 Wynn, A.: Unwarranted Emotional Distress in Men with Ischemic Heart Disease, *Med. J. Aust.,* 2:847, 1967.

196 Croog, S. H., Levine, S., and Lurie, Z.: The Heart Patient and the Recovery Process: A Review of the Directions of Research on Social and Psychological Factors, *Soc. Sci. Med.,* 2:111, 1968.

197 Fisher, S.: International Survey on the Psychological Aspects of Cardiac Rehabilitation, *Scand. J. Rehabil. Med.,* 2,3:71, 1970.

198 Cassem, N. H., and Hackett, T. P.: Psychiatric Consultation in a Coronary Care Unit, *Ann. Intern. Med.,* 75:9, 1971.

199 Wishnie, H. A., Hackett, T. P., and Cassem, N. H.: Psychological Hazards of Convalescence following Myocardial Infarction, *J.A.M.A.,* 215:1292, 1971.

200 Cay, E. L., Vetter, N., Philip, A. E., and Dugard, P.: Psychological Status during Recovery from an Acute Heart Attack, *J. Psychosom. Res.,* 16:425, 1972.

201 Hackett, T. P., and Cassem, N. H.: Psychological Adaptation to Convalescence in Myocardial Infarction Patients, in J. P. Naughton, H. K. Hellerstein, and I. C. Mohler (eds.), "Exercise Testing and Exercise Training in Coronary Heart Disease," Academic Press, New York, 1973, p. 253.

202 Ibrahim, M. A., Feldman, J. G., Sultz, H. A., Staiman, M. G., Young, L. J., and Dean, D.: Management after Myocardial Infarction: A Controlled Trial of the Effect of Group Psychotherapy, *Int. J. Psychiatry Med.,* 5:253, 1974.

203 Hackett, T. P., and Cassem, N. H.: "Patient Psychology" (70-029-A), American Heart Association, New York, 1975.

204 Stocksmeier, U.: "Psychological Approach to the Rehabilitation of Coronary Patients," Springer-Verlag, New York, 1976.

205 Cay, E., Philip, A., and Aitken, C.: Psychological Aspects of Cardiac Rehabilitation, in O. W. Hill (ed.), "Modern Trends in Psychosomatic Medicine 3," Butterworth, London, 1976.

206 Doehrman, S. R.: Psycho-social Aspects of Recovery from Coronary Heart Disease: A Review, *Soc. Sci. Med.,* 11:199, 1977.

207 Croog, S. H., and Levine, S.: "The Heart Patient Recovers. Social and Psychological Factors," Human Sciences Press, New York, 1977.

208 Hackett, T. P.: The Use of Groups in the Rehabilitation of the Postcoronary Patient, *Adv. Cardiol.,* 24:127, 1978.

209 Gentry, W. D.: Psychosocial Concerns and Benefits in Cardiac Rehabilitation, in M. L. Pollock and D. H. Schmidt (eds.), "Heart Disease and Rehabilitation," Houghton Mifflin Company, Boston, 1979, p. 690.

210 Naismith, L. D., Robinson, J. F., Shore, G. B., and McIntyre, M. M. J.: Psychological Rehabilitation after Myocardial Infarction, *Br. Med. J.,* 1:439, 1979.

210a Croog, S. H., and Levine, S.: "Life After a Heart Attack. Social and Psychological Factors Eight Years Later," Human Sciences Press, New York, 1982.

211 White, P. D.: "Heart Disease," The Macmillan Company, New York, 1951.

212 Kavanagh, T., and Shephard, R. J.: Sexual Activity after Myocardial Infarction, *Can. Med. Assoc. J.,* 116:1250, 1977.

213 Stern, M. J., Pascale, L., and McLoone, J. B.: Psychosocial Adaptation following an Acute Myocardial Infarction, *J. Chronic Dis.,* 29:513, 1976.

214 Hackett, T. P., and Cassem, N. H.: Factors Contributing to Delay in Responding to the Signs and Symptoms of Acute Myocardial Infarction, *Am. J. Cardiol.,* 24:651, 1969.

215 Moss, A. J., Wynar, B., and Goldstein, S.: Delay in Hospitalization during the Acute Coronary Period, *Am. J. Cardiol.,* 24:659, 1969.

216 Simon, A. B., Feinleib, M., and Thompson, H. K.: Components of Delay in the Pre-Hospital Setting of Acute Myocardial Infarction, *Am. J. Cardiol.,* 30:476, 1972.

217 Hackett, T. P., Cassem, N. H., and Wishnie, H. A.: The Coronary Care Unit: An Appraisal of Its Psychological Hazards, *N. Engl. J. Med.,* 279:1365, 1968.

218 Friedman, M., and Rosenman, R. H.: "Type A Behavior and Your Heart," Alfred A. Knopf, Inc., New York, 1974.

219 Denolin, H. (ed.): Psychological Problems before and after Myocardial Infarction, *Adv. Cardiol.,* vol. 29, S. Karger, Basel, 1982.

220 Stern, M. J., and Cleary, P.: National Exercise and Heart Disease Project: Psychological Changes Observed During a Low Level Exercise Program, *Arch. Intern. Med.,* 141:1463, 1981.

221 Hellerstein, H. K., Hackett, T. P., Kattus, A. A., Stein, R., Witten, C. L., and Zohman, L.: "Sex and the Heart Patient: Truths and Myths," Burroughs Wellcome Company, Research Triangle Park, North Carolina, 1977.

222 Papadopoulos, C.: Cardiovascular Drugs and Sexuality, *Arch. Intern. Med.,* 140:1341, 1980.

223 Marston, M.: Compliance with Medical Regimens: A Review of the Literature, *Nurs. Res.,* 19:312, 1970.

224 Cassem, N. H., and Hackett, T. P.: Psychological Rehabilitation of MI Patients in the Acute Phase, *Heart Lung,* 2:382, 1973.

225 McPherson, B. D., Paivio, A., Yuhasz, M. S., Rechnitzer, P. A., Pickard, H. A., and Lefcoe, N. M.: Psychological Effects of an Exercise Program for Post-Infarct and Normal Adult Men, *J. Sports Med. Phys. Fitness,* 7:95, 1967.

226 Steir, F.: The Effect of Structured Information and Reassurance on the Stress Response of Patients Transferring from the Coronary Care Unit, *Circulation,* 66 (suppl. 2):279, 1982.

227 Adsett, C. A., and Bruhn, J. G.: Short-term Group Psychotherapy in Post-MI Patients and Their Wives, *Can. Med. Assoc. J.,* 99:577, 1968.

228 Bilodeau, C. B., and Hackett, T. P.: Issues Raised in a Group Setting by Patients Recovering from Myocardial Infarction, *Am. J. Psychiatry,* 128:73, 1971.

229 Gulledge, A. D.: Depression after a Heart Attack, *Coronary Club Bull.,* 11:1, 1982.

230 Mayou, R., Foster, A., and Williamson, B.: Medical Care after Myocardial Infarction, *J. Psychosom. Res.,* 23:23, 1979.

231 Moss, A. J., DeCamilla, J., Davis, H., and Bayer, L.: The Early Post-Hospital Phase of Myocardial Infarction: Prognostic Stratification, *Circulation,* 54:58, 1976.

232 Kuller, L., Perper, J., and Cooper, M.: Demographic Characteristics and Trends in Arteriosclerotic Heart Disease Mortality, Sudden Death and Myocardial Infarction, *Circulation,* 52 (suppl. 3):1, 1975.

233 Wenger, N. K.: Coronary Disease in Women: Myth and Fact, *Hosp. Prac.,* 17:114A, 1982.

234 Davidson, D. M.: The Family and Cardiac Rehabilitation. *J. Fam. Prac.,* 8:253, 1979.

235 Heller, S. S., Frank, K. A., Kornfeld, D. S., Malm, J. R., and Bowman, F. D.: Psychosocial Outcome following Open-Heart Surgery, *Arch. Intern. Med.,* 134:908, 1974.

236 Gundle, M. J., Reeves, B. R., Tate, S., Raft, D., and McLaurin, L. P.: Psychosocial Outcome after Coronary Artery Surgery, *Am. J. Psychiatry,* 137:1591, 1980.

237 Hollender, M. H., and Abram, H. S.: Coronary Artery Bypass Operation: Psychological and Medical Problems, *Int. J. Psychiatry Med.,* 5:67, 1974.

238 Rabiner, C. J., Willner, A. E., and Fishman, J.: Psychiatric complications following coronary bypass surgery. *J. Nerv. Ment. Dis.,* 160:342, 1975.

239 Rahe, R. H., Tuffli, C. F., Suchor, R., and Arthur, R. J.: Group Therapy in the Outpatient Management of Post-Myocardial Infarction Patients, *Int. J. Psychiatry Med.,* 4:77, 1973.

240 Davis, M. S.: Physiologic, Psychological and Demographic Factors in Patient Compliance with Doctors' Orders, *Med. Care,* 6:115, 1968.

241 Osler, W.: "Lectures on Angina Pectoris and Allied States," Appleton, New York, 1901.

242 Jenkins, C. D., Zyzanski, S. J., and Rosenman, R. H.: Risk of New Myocardial Infarction in Middle-aged Men with Manifest Coronary Heart Disease, *Circulation,* 53:342, 1976.

243 Rosenman, R. H., and Friedman, M.: Relationship of Type A Behavior Pattern to Prevalence and Incidence of Coronary Heart Disease, *Med. Clin. North Am.,* 58:269, 1974.

244 The Review Panel on Coronary-prone Behavior and Coronary Heart Disease: Coronary-Prone Behavior and Coronary Heart Disease: A Critical Review, *Circulation,* 63:1199, 1981.

245 Litchfield, R. L., Kerper, R. E., Benge, J. W., et al.: Normal Exercise Capacity in Patients with Severe Left Ventricular Dysfunction: Compensatory Mechanisms, *Circulation,* 66:129, 1982.

246 Graham, S., and Reeder, L. G.: Social Epidemiology of Chronic Diseases, in H. E. Freeman, S. Levine, and L. G. Reeder (eds.), "Handbook of Medical Sociology," 3d ed., Prentice-Hall, Inc., Englewood Cliffs, N.J., 1979, p. 71.

247 Pell, S., and D'Alonzo, C.: Immediate Mortality and Five-Year Survival of Employed Men with a First Myocardial Infarction, *N. Engl. J. Med.,* 270:915, 1964.

248 Wigle, R. D., Symington, D. C., Lewis, M., Connell, W. F., and Parker, J. O.: Return to Work after Myocardial Infarction, *Can. Med. Assoc. J.,* 104:210, 1971.

249 Mulcahy, R., and Hickey, N.: The Rehabilitation of Patients with Coronary Heart Disease: A Comparison of the Return to Work Experience of National Health Insurance Patients with Coronary Heart Disease and of a Group of Coronary Patients Subjected to a Specific Rehabilitation Programme, *J. Ir. Med. Assoc.,* 64:541, 1971.

250 Krasemann, E. O., and Jungmann, H.: Return to Work after MI, *Cardiology,* 64:190, 1979.

251 Denolin, H.: Personal communication, 1981.

252 Hellerstein, H. K., and Ford, A. B.: Rehabilitation of the Cardiac Patient, *J.A.M.A.,* 164:225, 1957.

253 Garrity, T. F.: Vocational Adjustment after First Myocardial Infarction: Comparative Assessment of Several Variables Suggested in the Literature, *Soc. Sci. Med.,* 7:705, 1973.

254 Weinblatt, E., Shapiro, S., Frank, C., and Sager, R.: Return to Work and Work Status following First Myocardial Infarction, *Am. J. Public Health,* 56:169, 1966.

255 Wenger, N. K., and Hurst, J. W.: Coronary Bypass Surgery as a Rehabilitative Procedure, *Card. Rehabil.,* 11:1, 1980.

256 National Institutes of Health Consensus-Development Conference Statement: Coronary-Artery Bypass Surgery: Scientific and Clinical Aspects, *N. Engl. J. Med.,* 304:680, 1981.

257 Kushnir, B., Fox, K. M., Portal, R. W., and Aber, C. P.: Factors Influencing the Resumption of Work, Sexual Activity, and Driving Following Acute Myocardial Infarction, *Am. Heart J.,* 93:261, 1977.

258 Danchin, N., David, P., Robert, P., and Bourassa, M. G.: Evolution du statur de travail après pontage aorto-coronarien dans une population Canadienne-française, *Arch. Mal Coeur,* 73:585, 1980.

259 Love, J. W.: Employment Status after Coronary Bypass Operations and Some Cost Considerations, *J. Thorac. Cardiovasc. Surg.,* 80:68, 1980.

260 Niles, N. W., Vander Salm, T. J., and Cutler, B. S.: Return to Work after Coronary Artery Bypass Operation, *J. Thorac. Cardiovasc. Surg.,* 79:916, 1980.

261 Nitter-Hauge, S.: Correlation Studies between Employability, Left Ventricular Hemodynamics and Exercise ECG before and after Aortocoronary Bypass Surgery, *Acta Med. Scand.* (suppl. 645):1, 1981.

262 Gelfand, R., Flanders, B., and Haywood, J.: Return to Work after Myocardial Infarction in a Lower Socioeconomic Population, *J. Natl. Med. Assoc.,* 73:855, 1981.

263 Reedy, C.: The State-Federal Vocational Program in Cardiac Rehabilitation, in J. Naughton and H. K. Hellerstein, and I. C. Mohler (eds.) "Exercise Testing and Exercise Training in Coronary Heart Disease," Academic Press, New York, 1973, p. 17.

264 Report of a WHO Expert Committee: Rehabilitation of Patients with Cardiovascular Disease, *WHO Tech. Rep. Ser.,* no. 270, Geneva, 1964.

265 Astrand, P. O., and Rodahl, K.: "Textbook of Work Physiology," 2d ed., McGraw-Hill Book Company, New York, 1977.

266 DeBusk, R. F., Valdez, R., Houston, N., and Haskell, W.: Cardiovascular Responses to Dynamic and Static Effort Soon after Myocardial Infarction: Application to Occupational Work Assessment, *Circulation,* 58:368, 1978.

267 DeBusk, R., Pitts, W., Haskell, W., and Houston, N.: Comparison of Cardiovascular Responses to Static-Dynamic Effort and Dynamic Effort Alone in Patients with Chronic Ischemic Heart Disease, *Circulation,* 59:977, 1979.

268 Hellerstein, H. K.: Prescription of Vocational and Leisure Activities. Practical Aspects, *Adv. Cardiol.,* 24:105, 1978.

269 Naughton, J., and Haider, R.: Methods of Exercise Testing, in J. P. Naughton, H. K. Hellerstein, and I. C. Mohler (eds.), "Exercise Testing and Exercise Training in Coronary Heart Disease," Academic Press, New York, 1973, p. 79.

270 Naughton, J. (for the Project Staff): The National Exercise and Heart Disease Project: The Pre-Randomization Exercise Program, *Cardiology,* 63:352, 1978.

271 Cardiac Rehabilitation, *Rehab. Brief,* vol. 3, no. 8, June 2, 1980.

272 Sands, M. J., Jr.: Aviator Medical Certification after Coronary-Artery Surgery, *N. Engl. J. Med.,* 307:52, 1982.

273 Monteiro, L. A.: After Heart Attack: Behavioral Expectations for the Cardiac, *Soc. Sci. Med.,* 7:555, 1973.

274 "Directory of Cardiac Rehabilitation Units—1981," American Heart Association, Dallas, 1981.

275 Kushnir, B., Fox, K. M., Tomlinson, I. W., and Aber, C. P.: The Effect of a Pre-Discharge Consultation on the Resumption of Work, Sexual Activity, and Driving following Acute Myocardial Infarction, *Scand. J. Rehabil. Med.,* 8:155, 1976.

276 Joint Working Party of the Royal College of Physicians of London and the British Cardiac Society: Cardiac Rehabilitation, *J.R. Coll. Physicians Lond.,* 9:281, 1975.

277 WHO, 1968: A Programme for the Physical Rehabilitation of Patients with Acute Myocardial Infarction: Report of a WHO Working Group (EURO 5030), Freiburg in Breisgau, March 4–6, 1968.

278 WHO, 1971: Evaluation of Rehabilitation Programmes for Patients with Myocardial Infarction: Report of a WHO Working Group (EURO 8206), Prague, October 4–7, 1971.

279 Adams, F. H., and Mendenhall, R. C. (eds.): Profile of the Cardiologist: Training and Manpower Requirements for the Specialist in Adult Cardiovascular Disease, *Am. J. Cardiol.,* 34:389, 1974.

279a Aday, L. A., and Eichhorn, R.: "The Utilization of Health Services: Indices and Correlates" [DHEW Publication No. (HSM) 73-3003], U.S. Government Printing Office, Washington, D.C., 1972.

280 Mechanic, D.: Inequality, Health Status, and the Delivery of Health Services in the United States, in "Public Expectations and Health Care," Interscience-Wiley, New York, 1972, p. 80.

281 Mechanic, D.: Social Psychological Factors Affecting the Presentation of Bodily Complaints, *N. Engl. J. Med.,* 286:1132, 1972.

282 Twaddle, A.: The Concept of Health Status, *Soc. Sci. Med.,* 8:29, 1974.

283 Waitzkin, H., and Stoeckle, J. D.: The Communication of Information about Illness, in Z. Lipowski (ed.), "Advances in Psychosomatic Medicine," Vol. 8, Karger, Basel, 1972, p. 180.

284 Smith, R. T.: Disability and the Recovery Process. Role of Social Networks, in E. G. Jaco (ed.), "Patients, Physicians, and Illness," 3d ed, Free Press, New York, 1979.

285 Smith, R. T.: Rehabilitation of the Disabled: The role of social network in the recovery process. *Int. Rehabil. Med.,* 1(2):63, 1979. (Table 4.)

286 Safilios-Rothschild, C.: "The Sociology and Social Psychology of Disability and Rehabilitation," Random House, Inc., New York, 1970.

287 Schlesinger, L. E.: Staff Tensions and Needed Skills in Staff-Patient Interaction, *Rehabil. Lit.,* 24:363, 1963.

288 Foster, S., and Andreoli, K. G.: The Postcoronary Patient Behavior following Acute Myocardial Infarction, *Am. J. Nurs.,* 70:2344, 1970.

289 Duff, R. S., and Hollingshead, A. B.: "Sickness and Society," Harper & Row, Publishers, Inc., New York, 1968.

290 Croog, S. H., and Levine, S.: Social Status and Subjective Perceptions of 250 Men after Myocardial Infarction, *Public Health Rep.,* 84:989, 1969.

291 Litman, T. J.: The Family and Physical Rehabilitation, *J. Chronic Dis.,* 19:211, 1966.

292 New, P. K., Ruscio, R. T., Priest, R. P., Petritsi, D., and George, L. A.: The Support Structure of Heart and Stroke Patients: A Study of Significant Others in Patients' Rehabilitation, *Soc. Sci. Med.,* 2:185, 1968.

292a Cobb, A. B.: "Medical and Psychological Aspects of Disability," Charles C Thomas, Publisher, Springfield, Ill., 1973.

293 Kaplan, B. H., Cassel, J. C., and Gore, S.: Social Support and Health, *Med. Care (Suppl),* 15:47, 1977.

294 Warshaw, L. J.: Chronic Disease and Employability: The Physician's Role, *J. Am. Med. Wom. Assoc.,* 20:1120, 1965.

295 Croog, S. H., Lipson, A., and Levine, S.: Help Patterns in Severe Illness: The Roles of Kin Network, Non-Family Resources, and Institutions, *J. Marr & Family,* 34:32, 1972.

296 Anderson, R., and Newman, J.: Societal and Individual Determinants of Medical Care Utilization in the United States, *Milbank Mem. Fund Q.,* 51:95, 1973.

297 Dishart, M.: "A National Study of 84,699 Applicants for Services from State Vocational Rehabilitation Agencies in the United States," National Rehabilitation Association, Washington, D.C., 1964.

298 Andersen, R., and Anderson, O. W.: "A Decade of Health Services," University of Chicago Press, Chicago, 1967.

299 Finlayson, A.: Social Networks as Coping Resources. Lay Help and Consultation Patterns Used by Women in Husbands' Post-Infarction Career, *Soc. Sci. Med.,* 19:97, 1976.

300 Finlayson, A., and McEwen, J.: "Coronary Heart Disease and Patterns of Living," Neale Watson Academic Publications, Inc. Imprints: Prodist, New York, 1977.

301 WHO, 1976: "Disability Prevention and Rehabilitation. 29th World Health Assembly" (A 29/INF Doc/1), 1976.

302 Martin, J. F.: The Active Patient: A Necessary Development, *WHO Chron.,* 32:51, 1978.

303 McKinlay, J. B.: Some Approaches and Problems in the Study of the Use of Services. An Overview, *J. Health Soc. Behav.,* 13:115, 1972.

304 Moos, R. H., and Tsu, V. D.: The Crisis of Physical Illness. An Overview, in R. H. Moos (ed.), "Coping with Physical Illness," Plenum Press, New York, 1977.

305 Smith, R. T.: Role of Social Resources in Cardiac Rehabilitation, in L. S. Cohen, M. B. Mock, and I. Ringqvist, "Physical Conditioning and Cardiovascular Rehabilitation," John Wiley & Sons, Inc., New York, 1981, p. 221.

306 Wolfbein, S.: Employment and Underemployment in the United States, *Sci. Res. Assoc. Chicago,* 194:98, 1964.

307 Strauss, R.: Social Change and the Rehabilitation Concept, in M. B. Sussman (ed.), "Sociology and Rehabilitation," Am. Soc. Assoc., Washington, D.C., 1966.

308 Safilios-Rothschild, C.: The Self-Definitions of the Disabled and Implications for Rehabilitation, in G. Albrecht (ed.), "Socialization in Disability Process," University of Pittsburg Press, Pittsburg, 1974.